CARDIAC
STRESS TESTING & IMAGING

A Clinician's Guide

CARDIAC
STRESS TESTING & IMAGING

A Clinician's Guide

THOMAS H. MARWICK, M.D., Ph.D., F.A.C.C.
Associate Professor of Medicine
Ohio State University College of Medicine
Cleveland Clinic Health Sciences Campus
Director of Cardiac Stress Imaging
Department of Cardiology
The Cleveland Clinic Foundation
Cleveland, Ohio

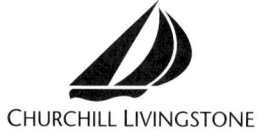

CHURCHILL LIVINGSTONE

New York, Edinburgh, London, Madrid, Melbourne, San Francisco, Tokyo

Library of Congress Cataloging-in-Publication Data
Cardiac stress testing and imaging / a clinician's guide / [edited by]
   Thomas H. Marwick.
       p.   cm.
     Includes index.
     ISBN 0-443-07652-9 (alk. paper)
    1. Stress echocardiography. 2. Heart—Imaging. I. Marwick,
Thomas H.
     [DNLM: 1. Cardiovascular Disease—diagnosis. 2. Exercise Test.
   3. Diagnostic Imaging—methods.   WG 120 C266 1996]
   RC683.5.SS77C37   1996
   616.1'2075—dc20
   DNLM/DLC
     For Library of Congress   96-24943
                                                              CIP

© **Churchill Livingstone Inc. 1996**

All rights reserved. No part of this publication may be reproduced, stored in a retrieval system, or transmitted in any form or by any means, electronic, mechanical, photocopying, recording, or otherwise, without prior permission of the publisher (Churchill Livingstone, 650 Avenue of the Americas, New York, NY 10011).

Distributed in the United Kingdom by Churchill Livingstone, Robert Stevenson House, 1–3 Baxter's Place, Leith Walk, Edinburgh EH1 3AF, and by associated companies, branches, and representatives throughout the world.

Accurate indications, adverse reactions, and dosage schedules for drugs are provided in this book, but it is possible that they may change. The reader is urged to review the package information data of the manufacturers of the medications mentioned.

The Publishers have made every effort to trace the copyright holders for borrowed material. If they have inadvertently overlooked any, they will be pleased to make the necessary arrangements at the first opportunity.

Acquisitions Editor: *Allan Ross*
Assistant Editor: *Jennifer Hardy*
Production Editor: *Robert Carmenini*
Production Supervisor: *Sharon Tuder*
Cover Design: *Jeannette Jacobs*

Printed in the United States of America

First published in 1996   7   6   5   4   3   2   1

THIS BOOK WAS MADE POSSIBLE BY
the personal sacrifice of the contributors and their families,
and it is to them and my family that this book is dedicated.

Contributors

JOZEF BARTUNEK, M.D.
Research Fellow, Cardiovascular Center, Aalst, Onze-Lieve-Vrouw Hospital, Aalst, Belgium

SOREN J. BRENER, M.D.
Interventional Cardiologist, Department of Cardiology, The Cleveland Clinic Foundation, Cleveland, Ohio

DAVID L. BRONSON, M.D.
Clinical Professor, Department of Medicine, Pennsylvania State University College of Medicine, Hershey, Pennsylvania; Chairman, General Internal Medicine, The Cleveland Clinic Foundation, Cleveland, Ohio

RICHARD C. BRUNKEN, M.D.
Staff Physician, Department of Nuclear Medicine, Division of Radiology, The Cleveland Clinic Foundation, Cleveland, Ohio

PAOLO G. CAMICI, M.D.
Professor of Cardiovascular Pathophysiology, Royal Postgraduate Medical School, University of London; Head of Cardiology Cyclotron Unit, MRC Clinical Sciences Centre, Hammersmith Hospital, London, United Kingdom

BERNARD de BRUYNE, M.D., Ph.D.
Co-Director, Cardiovascular Center, Aalst, Onze-Lieve-Vrouw Hospital, Aalst, Germany

ANTHONY C. DE FRANCO, M.D., F.A.C.C.
Assistant Professor, Department of Medicine, Ohio State University College of Medicine, Columbus, Ohio; Co-Director of the Intravascular Ultrasound Laboratory, Department of Cardiology, The Cleveland Clinic Foundation, Cleveland, Ohio

FRANK W. DE GEETER, M.D.
Consultant, Department of Nuclear Medicine, Academic Hospital, Free University Brussels (V.U.B.), Brussels, Belgium

ROBERT DETRANO, M.D.
Professor, Department of Medicine, University of California, Los Angeles, UCLA School of Medicine, Los Angeles, California; Department of Medicine, Harbor–UCLA Medical Center, Torrance, California

MARCELO F. DI CARLI, M.D.
Assistant Professor, Department of Internal Medicine and Radiology, Wayne State University School of Medicine; Director, Department of Cardiac Positron Emission Tomography, Detroit, Michigan

ROBERT L. EISNER, Ph.D.
Associate Professor, Department of Radiology, Emory University School of Medicine; Co-Director, Department of Nuclear Cardiology, Crawford W. Long Memorial Hospital, Atlanta, Georgia

D. FAGRET, M.D., Ph.D.
Professor, Department of Biophysics and Nuclear Medicine, School of Medicine—Grenoble; Professor of Nuclear Medicine, Department of Nuclear Medicine, University Hospital of Grenoble, Grenoble, France

PAOLO M. FIORETTI, M.D., Ph.D.
Cardiologist, Division of Cardiology, Erasmus University; Department of Cardiac Stress Imaging, Academic Hospital, Dijkzigt, Rotterdam, The Netherlands

PHILIPPE R. FRANKEN, M.D., Ph.D.
Clinical Head, Department of Nuclear Medicine, Academic Hospital, Free University Brussels (V.U.B.), Brussels, Belgium

MARCEL L. GELEIJNSE, M.D.
Research Fellow in Cardiology, Department of Cardiac Stress Imaging, Dijkzigt, Rotterdam, The Netherlands

ALAN K. HALPERIN, M.D.
Research Director, Department of General Internal Medicine, The Cleveland Clinic Foundation, Cleveland, Ohio

CHARLES A. HERZOG, M.D.
Assistant Professor, Department of Medicine, University of Minnesota Medical School—Minneapolis; Staff Cardiologist, Division of Cardiology, Department of Medicine, Hennepin County Medical Center, Minneapolis, Minnesota

JAEKYEONG HEO, M.D., F.A.C.C.
Associate Director, Nuclear Cardiology Laboratory, Medical College of Pennsylvania and Hahnemann University School of Medicine, Philadelphia, Pennsylvania

RAINER HOFFMANN, M.D.
Medical Clinic I, Aachen, Germany

AMI E. ISKANDRIAN, M.D.
William Penn Snyder III Professor of Medicine, Department of Medicine, Medical College of Pennsylvania and Hahnemann University School of Medicine; Director, Cardiovascular Research Center; Section Chief, Nuclear Cardiology, Medical College of Pennsylvania and Hahnemann University Hospitals, Philadelphia, Pennsylvania

ISTVAN KOSA, M.D.
Assistant Professor, Second Department of Medicine, Albert Szent-Györgyi Medical School, Szeged, Hungary

JANINE KRIVOKAPICH, M.D.
Professor, Division of Cardiology, Department of Medicine, University of California, Los Angeles, UCLA School of Medicine; Director, Adult Non-Invasive Cardiology Laboratories, Los Angeles, California

MICHAEL S. LAUER, M.D.
Staff Cardiologist, Department of Cardiology, The Cleveland Clinic Foundation, Cleveland, Ohio

J. MACHECOURT, M.D., F.E.S.C.
Professor, Department of Cardiology, School of Medicine—Grenoble; Head of the Intensive Care Unit, Department of Cardiology, University Hospital of Grenoble, Grenoble, France

GEORGES H. MAIRESSE, M.D.
Consultant, Department of Cardiology, Clinique St. Joseph, Arlon, Belgium

THOMAS H. MARWICK, M.D., F.A.C.C., Ph.D.
Associate Professor of Medicine, Ohio State University College of Medicine, Cleveland Clinic Health Sciences Campus; Director of Cardiac Stress Imaging, Department of Cardiology, The Cleveland Clinic Foundation, Cleveland, Ohio

JACQUES A. MELIN, M.D., Ph.D.
Professor, Department of Internal Medicine, University of Louvain, Brussels; Head, Positron Emission Tomography Laboratory, Department of Nuclear Medicine, University Clinic of St. Luc, Brussels, Belgium

NASARAIAH NALLAMOTHU, M.D.
Cardiology Fellow, Department of Nuclear Cardiology, Hahnemann University School of Medicine, Philadelphia, Pennsylvania

STEPHAN NEKOLLA, Ph.D.
Technical University of Munich, Clinic and Policlinic for Nuclear Medicine, Munich, Germany

STEVEN E. NISSEN, M.D.
Professor, Department of Medicine, Ohio State University School of Medicine, Columbus, Ohio; Director of Clinical Cardiology, Vice Chairman, Department of Cardiology, The Cleveland Clinic Foundation, Cleveland, Ohio

OBERDAN PARODI, M.D.
Director of Research, The National Council of Research; Head, Nuclear Medicine Service, CNR Institute of Clinical Physiology, Pisa, Italy

FREDRIC J. PASHKOW, M.D.
Medical Director of Cardiac Health Improvement and Rehabilitation, Department of Cardiology, The Cleveland Clinic Foundation, Cleveland, Ohio

AGNÈS PASQUET, M.D.
Department of Internal Medicine, University of Louvain, Brussels; Fellow, Department of Cardiology, University Clinic of St. Luc, Brussels, Belgium

RANDOLPH E. PATTERSON, M.D.
Professor, Department of Medicine and Radiology, Emory University School of Medicine; Director, Department of Cardiovascular Imaging, Emory Heart Center, Atlanta, Georgia

NICO HJ PIJLS, M.D., Ph.D.
Department of Cardiology, Catharina Hospital, Eindhoven, The Netherlands

DON POLDERMANS, M.D., Ph.D.
Internist, Department of Surgery, Erasmus University, Rotterdam, The Netherlands

ANNIE R. ROBERT, Ph.D.
Associate Professor, Catholic University of Louvain; Head, Division of Biostatistics, Department of Cardiology, University Clinic of St. Luc, Brussels, Belgium

THOMAS RYAN, M.D.
Associate Professor, Department of Medicine, Duke University School of Medicine; Director of Echocardiography, Duke University Medical Center, Durham, North Carolina

MARK SADA, M.D.
Department of Medicine, University of California, Los Angeles, UCLA School of Medicine, Los Angeles, California; Fellow, Harbor–UCLA Medical Center, Torrance, California

GIANMARIO SAMBUCETTI, M.D.
Assistant, Nuclear Medicine Service, CNR Institute of Clinical Physiology, Pisa, Italy

MARKUS SCHWAIGER, M.D.
Professor, University of Munich; Director, Clinic and Policlinic for Nuclear Medicine, Munich, Germany

HENRY G. STRATMANN, M.D.
Associate Professor, Department of Internal Medicine, St. Louis University School of Medicine; Director, Coronary Care Unit, Department of Cardiology, St. Louis Department of Veterans Affairs Medical Center, St. Louis, Missouri

IAN R. THOMSON, M.D.
Professor, Department of Anesthesia, University of Manitoba; Section Head, Cardiovascular Anesthesia, St. Boniface General Hospital, Winnipeg, Canada

ERIC J. TOPOL, M.D.
Chairman and Professor, Department of Cardiology, The Cleveland Clinic Foundation; Director, Joseph J. Jacobs Center for Thrombosis and Vascular Biology, Cleveland, Ohio

E. MURAT TUZCU, M.D.
Associate Professor, Department of Medicine, Ohio State University School of Medicine; Co-Director of the Intravascular Ultrasound Laboratory, Department of Cardiology, The Cleveland Clinic Foundation, Cleveland, Ohio

NEAL G. UREN, M.D., M.R.C.P.
Visiting Scholar, Division of Cardiovascular Medicine, Stanford University School of Medicine, Stanford, Connecticut; Senior Registrar, Department of Cardiology, Glenfield Hospital, Leicester, United Kingdom

JEAN-LOUIS J. VANOVERSCHELDE, M.D., Ph.D.
Assistant Professor, Department of Internal Medicine, University Clinic of St. Luc; Head, Echocardiography Laboratory, Department of Cardiology, University Clinic of St. Luc, Brussels, Belgium

GERALD VANZETTO, M.D.
Assistant Professor, Department of Cardiology, School of Medicine—Grenoble; Department of Cardiology, University Hospital of Grenoble, Grenoble, France

MARIO S. VERANI, M.D., F.A.C.C., F.A.C.P.
Professor, Department of Medicine, Baylor College of Medicine, Baylor University Medical Center; Director, Department of Nuclear Cardiology, The Methodist Hospital, Houston, Texas

DONALD A. WEINER, M.D.
Professor, Department of Cardiology, Boston University Medical Center Hospital; Director, Exercise Laboratory, Section of Cardiology, Boston University Medical Center Hospital, Boston, Massachusetts

WILLIAM WIJNS, M.D., Ph.D.
Cardiologist, Cardiovascular Center, OLV Ziekenhuis, Aalst, Belgium

M. JOHN WILLIAMS, M.B.B.S., F.R.A.C.P.
Senior Imaging Fellow, Department of Cardiology, Echo Laboratory, F-15, The Cleveland Clinic Foundation, Cleveland, Ohio

LIWA T. YOUNIS, M.D., Ph.D.
Assistant Professor, Department of Internal Medicine, St. Louis University School of Medicine; Chief of Cardiology, Department of Internal Medicine, St. Louis Veterans Affairs Medical Center, St. Louis, Missouri

SIBYLLE ZIEGLER, Ph.D.
Technical University of Munich, Clinic and Policlinic for Nuclear Medicine, Munich, Germany

Foreword

For assessment of patients with cardiovascular diseases, our reliance on noninvasive stress testing and imaging has steadily intensified. While exercise treadmill testing ushered in a new era in medicine many years ago, the ongoing revolution of improved echocardiographic and scintigraphic imaging has laid the foundation for a quantum leap in our ability to provide meaningful clinical triage and decision making.

Until now, there has not been a dedicated textbook that comprehensively addresses the field of cardiac stress testing and imaging. Whereas previous texts have concentrated largely on the electrocardiogram, this only accounts for approximately one-third of diagnostic stress testing due to the large number of patients who need pharmacologic stress, or those with uninterpretable electrocardiograms. Furthermore, determination of the actual size of ischemia and viability of cardiac muscle can be critical issues in selected patients.

The topic is exceedingly important. Each year thousands of patients undergo coronary revascularization without any physiologic assessment. For example, in a study we performed in over 2,000 patients in the United States undergoing balloon coronary angioplasty, nearly 70 percent of patients did not have a functional test before the procedure! On the other hand, there are significant difficulties with false-negative treadmill tests, and the confusion of what test to select from an ever-increasing battery of refined stress or pharmacologic imaging studies.

How can we pick from the menu of tests and use the data obtained in an appropriate and meaningful way? To address these questions, Dr. Marwick has been able to recruit over 40 contributing authors from all over the world. These are the recognized authorities in the field, and, importantly, there is remarkable balance achieved. The authors include clinicians, stress-electrocardiography experts, echocardiographers, nuclear medicine specialists, and interventional cardiologists. The merits and disadvantages of particular techniques, as well as the caveats and nuances of interpreting data, are duly emphasized.

The entire approach to *Cardiac Stress Testing and Imaging: A Clinician's Guide* is technical and clinical. While advances in fast computer tomography (CT), magnetic resonance imaging (MRI), and contrast echocardiography are mentioned, the main focus of the book is on the tests which are currently available in clinical practice. The book is highly clinically oriented and does not provide imaging-modality specific data in as much as it poses key clinical questions and situations. There are three sections. The first, addressing diagnostic testing, builds the foundation of the stress imaging testing before delving into key subgroups such as women, patients who cannot exercise, asymptomatic disease, and patients with end-stage renal disease, conduction abnormalities, or left ventricular hypertrophy.

The second section highlights coronary physiologic and anatomic assessment via direct measurement with Doppler and intravascular ultrasound, interrogation of myocardial viability, and critical data to decide whether an intervention is appropriate, or when being performed, has satisfactory or optimal results. The last section is devoted to evaluating prognosis and comprehensively reviews all of the long-term clinical event data for the tests. These findings relate, in particular, to patients with clinically overt ischemic heart disease or those undergoing noncardiac or vascular surgery.

This book will be of immense value for the practicing cardiologist, for whom a decision about whether to test, which test, and how to interpret a particular physiologic assessment represent the crux of day-to-day patient management. In the current era of severe cost-containment, such decisions will be increasingly difficult and determine critical triage paths.

Dr. Marwick directs one of the busiest stress imaging laboratories in the United States, and fully understands the fundamental issues, controversies, and dilemmas. The monograph that he has put together, along with the collective insight of a superb group of contributors, will undoubtedly help advance a burgeoning and important discipline of cardiovascular medicine.

Eric J. Topol, M.D.

Preface

The diagnosis and evaluation of coronary artery disease may be assisted by a substantial number of combinations of stress techniques and imaging and nonimaging methodologies for the diagnosis of ischemia. While exercise electrocardiography maintains a central role in the evaluation of many patients, stress imaging tests have replaced the standard stress test in over 50 percent of patients, who are either unable to exercise maximally (in which case a pharmacologic test is performed) or have a nondiagnostic electrocardiogram. Other books have dealt with either exercise testing or imaging. The purpose of *Cardiac Stress Testing and Imaging: A Clinician's Guide* is to discuss all of these alternatives in relation to specific clinical situations, and to act as a practical guide to assist selection of stress testing approaches by cardiologists and internists. Attention has been directed to techniques in routine clinical use, with reference to less available techniques in special circumstances.

This book is divided into major sections dealing with diagnostic testing, use of testing in the evaluation of patients with known coronary artery disease, and prognostic evaluation. In each section, the author's task was to review the available literature, and to compare the techniques. The book was written by a group of contributors that reflect the consumers and providers of stress testing services—including clinicians, interventionalists, exercise specialists, and experts in imaging, who were selected for their experience in multiple modalities. Unavoidably, some overlap has occurred between chapters, and while attempts have been made to minimize repetition, the merits of allowing different perspectives needs to be recognized. Emphasis has been paid to thorough referencing in the recognition that while many readers may not wish to become experts in the finer nuances of each area, there is a need to gather the literature, much of which originates from specialized journals.

Special thanks and appreciation are due to the editors at Churchill Livingstone for their acceptance of this project, and their practical help and patience.

Thomas H. Marwick, M.D., Ph.D., F.A.C.C.

Contents

DIAGNOSTIC TESTING

1. Role of Routine Exercise Electrocardiographic Testing / **1**
   Fredric J. Pashkow

2. Principles and Methods of Myocardial Perfusion Imaging / **33**
   Istvan Kosa, Sibylle Ziegler, Stephan Nekolla, and Markus Schwaiger

3. Left Ventricular Functional Response to Stress for the Diagnosis of CAD / **67**
   Thomas Ryan

4. Selection of Myocardial Perfusion or Function for the Diagnosis of CAD / **97**
   Marcel L. Geleijnse and Paolo M. Fioretti

5. Cost Analysis of Noninvasive Testing / **113**
   Randolph E. Patterson and Robert L. Eisner

6. Screening for CAD / **125**
   Mark Sada and Robert Detrano

7. Diagnosis of CAD in Women: Multivariate Approaches to Stress Testing / **147**
   Annie R. Robert

8. Stress Echocardiography for the Diagnosis of CAD in Women / **167**
   M. John Williams and Thomas H. Marwick

9. Perfusion Imaging for the Diagnosis and Risk Assessment of CAD in Women / **177**
   Ami E. Iskandrian, Jaekyeong Heo, and Nasaraiah Nallamothu

10. Diagnosis of CAD in the Presence of Left Ventricular Hypertrophy / **189**
    Michael S. Lauer

11. Noninvasive Diagnosis of CAD in Patients with End-Stage Renal Disease / **203**
    Charles A. Herzog

12. Diagnosis of CAD in Patients with Left Bundle Branch Block / **223**
    Georges H. Mairesse

13. Pharmacologic Stress Testing / **233**
    Thomas H. Marwick

KNOWN CORONARY ARTERY DISEASE

14. Can Coronary Angiography Provide Functional Data? / **261**
    Neal G. Uren and Paolo G. Camici

15. Coronary Pressure Measurements in Evaluation of Coronary Stenoses / **281**
    Bernard de Bruyne, Jozef Bartunek, and Nico HJ Pijls

16. Intravascular Ultrasound and Coronary Doppler Flow Measurements / **299**
    E. Murat Tuzcu, Anthony C. De Franco, Sorin J. Brener, and Steven E. Nissen

17. Functional Testing in Patients with Previous Coronary Interventions / **323**
    Anthony C. De Franco and Eric J. Topol

18. Stress Echocardiography Before and After Interventional Therapy / **355**
    Rainer Hoffmann

19. Perfusion Markers after Coronary Interventions / 369
Oberdan Parodi and Gianmario Sambucetti

20. Optimal SPECT Technique for Assessing Myocardial Viability / 385
Philippe R. Franken and Frank W. De Greeter

21. Assessment of Myocardial Viability Using Positron Emission Tomography / 417
Richard C. Brunken

22. Choice of Technique for the Assessment of Myocardial Viability / 463
Jacques A. Melin, Bernard Gerber, William Wijns, and Jean-Louis J. Vanoverschelde

23. Echocardiographic Techniques for the Assessment of Myocardial Viability / 475
Jean–Louis J. Vanovershelde, Angés Pasquet, and Jacques A. Melin

PROGNOSTIC EVALUATION

24. Role of Functional Testing for Prognostic Evaluation / 491
William Wijns and Thomas H. Marwick

25. Routine Exercise Electrocardiographic Testing for Prognostic Evaluation / 499
Donald A. Weiner

26. Implications of Stress-Induced LV Dysfunction on Risk Stratification / 509
Janine Krivokapich

27. Prognostic Evaluation of CAD Patients Using Perfusion Imaging / 525
J. Machecourt, G. Vanzetto, and D. Fagret

28. Prognostic Evaluation of CAD Patients Using Positron Emission Tomography / 559
Marcelo F. Di Carli

29. Clinical Evaluation of Cardiac Risk Before Major Noncardiac Surgery / 571
Alan K. Halperin and David L. Bronson

30. Myocardial Perfusion Imaging in the Preoperative Evaluation of Vascular Patients / 581
Liwa T. Younis and Henry G. Stratmann

31. Pharmacologic Stress Echocardiography for Risk Stratification Prior to Vascular Surgery / 597
Don Poldermans, Paolo M. Fioretti, and Ian R. Thomson

32. Flow Maldistribution Versus Malfunction in Clinical Decision Making / 613
Mario S. Verani

INDEX / 627

Color plates appear following page 48.

Chapter 1

Role of Routine Exercise Electrocardiographic Testing

Fredric J. Pashkow

The evaluation of patients with possible coronary artery disease (CAD) is a challenge to clinicians, who face conflicting pressures in the current practice environment. Sensitivity, accuracy, cost, and access have become considerations in the appropriate selection of various diagnostic studies.[1] The patient's history, however, remains the key to establishing a diagnosis, not just for the more accurate estimation of pretest probability to improve postexercise estimation of disease likelihood, but also for the appropriate selection of test technology and protocol.[2] The exercise electrocardiogram has become a standard diagnostic modality over the last 50 years, but its role is changing.[3]

In this chapter the cardiovascular response to exercise will be discussed mainly in the context of the development of diagnostic exercise testing. A discussion of the evolution of the exercise electrocardiogram (ECG) will be provided with special emphasis on the impact of computerized interpretation and scoring. Chapters 6, 7, and 25 will address pre- and post-test probability, as well as the use of exercise ECG criteria for the determination of prognosis in patients with known CAD. The exercise ECG currently serves as the doorway to special applications of newer imaging technologies such as perfusion or echocardiographic imaging. These developments in the diagnostic application of the technique are the focus of this book.

Current clinical indications for exercise electrocardiographic testing include

    Evaluation of symptoms, especially chest pain.

    Determination of prognosis and staging the severity of disease:

    Pre-event—extent of ischemia.

    Post-event—risk stratification for subsequent myocardial infarction, sudden death or need for revascularization.

    Evaluation of therapy.

    Follow progression of disease.

    Screening for latent coronary disease.

    Evaluation of ventricular function.

    Evaluation of dysrhythmias.

    Assessment of degree of valvular dysfunction.

    Evaluation of functional capacity:

        Exercise prescription.

        Disability determination.

    Evaluation of devices: pacemakers, internal cardioverter defibrillators, left ventricular (LV) assist devices.

The clinical indications for exercise ECG go far beyond diagnosis, but that will be the focus of this chapter.

DEVELOPMENT OF EXERCISE ECG TESTING
ST-Segment Variation as a Marker of Ischemia

Exercise ECG testing has a serendipitous history, but its beginning is attributed[4] to Fiel and Siegel, who reported ST-segment depression in the ECGs of patients with CAD during exercise in 1928.[5] They attributed the alterations observed in the ST segments and T-waves as the result of a decrease in blood flow to the heart. They also demonstrated a return to normal following the administration of nitroglycerine and abatement of the pain. They utilized situps as the exercise stress, and placed manual resistance on the chest to escalate the workload required.

Master described the use of a graded test for measurement of exercise capacity, but did not recognize until later the importance of ECG changes for the demonstration of ischemia.[6] Certainly, he can be credited with the discovery of the importance of functional capacity as a potentially valuable clinical measure. However, it was not until 1941 that he proposed the use of the ECG before and after the exercise tolerance test to detect coronary ischemia.[7]

During the 1930s and 1940s, multiple investigators reported the association of ECG changes during exercise in patients with coronary disease, but the use of the technique, the clinical indications, and the safety of the test were debated.[8,9] The potential significance of silent ischemia was described by Hans Hecht in 1949.[10] The importance of variable work capacity, the value of more strenuous exercise for accuracy of diagnosis, and the reliability of testing at higher work loads were reported by several investigators in the 1940s and 1950s.[4] The establishment of 1.0 mm of ST depression as the threshold for the diagnosis of ischemia is attributed to Yu and Soffer.[11]

Exercise Testing and the Exercise Response

During the next 10 years, pioneering research by Åstrand, Balke, Wasserman, and others defined the physiology of the human exercise response and set the stage for the application of the basic knowledge to the clinical milieu.[12,13] Balke and his associates greatly facilitated this bridging process by performing large studies that consolidated an understanding of the relationship of peripheral muscle function to cardiovascular hemodynamics—a concept that we appreciate today as that of aerobic exercise.[14]

Clausen and others endeavored to characterize the differences in exercise physiology due to CAD.[15-17] In the last decade, the physiology relevant to specific subsets of patients, particularly those with congestive heart failure, has been elucidated.[18-20]

Hellerstein established centers for work assessment and used the treadmill for the measurement of functional capacity and for the determination of occupational fitness.[21] His efforts set the stage for the application of classification schemes such as New York Heart Association (NYHA) functional class designation, that is still in use today. More than 40 years later we still rely upon the plain exercise ECG for the majority of our determinations of occupational and recreational fitness.

Exercise ECG as a Modality of Diagnosis

Modern exercise ECG testing is appropriately credited to Robert Bruce, whose name is attached to the most commonly applied exercise protocol still in use today.[22] Many authorities attribute to Bruce the establishment of guidelines classifying patients by their functional status and the refinement of test protocols based upon his observations of clinical physiology.[4,16]

The power of qualitative and quantitative ST-segment analysis was advanced by the work of Robb and Marks, who presented statistical verification of the predictive value of ST-segment change during exercise stress.[23] They demonstrated that horizontal or down-sloping ST segments after exercise were more reliable in predicting the presence of coronary disease than history, and that deep depression of the ST segment imparted a more severe prognosis. Cardiologists came to the erroneous conclusion, however, that ST-segment depression and anginal chest pain delimit the presence of coronary disease and very many patients were (and still are, unfortunately) submitted to angiography on this basis. The finding of normal coronary arteries in many patients with classical angina and/or abnormal ST segments during exercise has stimulated an effort to clarify the pathophysiology of ischemia and to apply the technique appropriately.

Development of Analytical Techniques

As Ellestad points out, the 10-year period from the early 1970s to the early 1980s should be thought of as the decade of Bayesian analysis.[4] Many investigators addressed the issue of disease prevalence and its influence on test value.[24,25] While the principle really applies to all diagnostic testing in medicine, exercise ECG became the focus of such research, and set the standards by which all newer diagnostic studies would eventually be judged.

If the 1970s should thus be regarded as the era of pretest probability, the following 10 years should be thought of as the decade of post-test probability. Work by Diamond, Detry, and others established the value of the analysis of multiple variables including data measured during the performance of exercise ECG and referred to as multivariate analysis.[26,27] This technique is performed by the selection of a defined subset of patients with known coronary anatomy by angiography, who then have various measured parameters compared in an effort to identify the factors that best discriminate between those with and those without the disease. The performance of multivariate analysis is discussed in more detail in Chapter 7. In summary, this process involves a step wise analysis where the variable that makes the largest contribution to the separation of those with and without the disease (in an initial univariate analysis) is entered first. Finally, all variables are ranked according to their relative discriminatory importance.

The definition of the "defined subset" is quite critical to achieve optimal results. A study population that is assumed to be representative, but that is not, will lead to erroneous conclusions about the merit of a particular variable as a discriminant function. Despite this potential problem with multivariate analysis, Detrano believes that data-based derived descriminant functions are more accurate than literature-based Bayesian derived pretest probabilities.[28]

THE CARDIOVASCULAR RESPONSE TO EXERCISE
Exercise as a Stressor

Exercise is the most common human physiologic stress[29] and provides the most practical available means to test cardiac perfusion and function.[30] Dy-

Table 1-1. Comparison of Cardiovascular Responses to High Intensity Static vs. Dynamic Exercise[a]

Variable	Magnitude of Change from Rest to Exercise	
	Static	Dynamic
Oxygen uptake	↑	↑↑↑
Heart rate	↑	↑↑↑
Stroke volume	±	↑↑
Cardiac output	↑	↑↑↑
Peripheral vascular resistance	±	↓
Systolic blood pressure	↑	↑↑
Diastolic blood pressure	↑↑↑	±
Rate-pressure product	↑↑↑	↑↑↑
Left ventricular Wall stress	Primarily pressure loading	Primarily volume loading

[a] Symbols: ↑, ↑↑, ↑↑↑, relative magnitude of increase; ±, little change. (From Pate et al.,[33] with permission.)

namic (isotonic) exercise puts a volume load on the heart and is preferred for testing since it can be gradually applied and modulated.[31,32] Pure isometric exercise is contraction without movement (such as a hand grip) and because of the diversity in size of peripheral muscle groups, isometric stress can impose a disproportionate LV pressure load[31] (Table 1-1). Most physical activities involve both some isometric and isotonic exercise in varying degrees.[33]

Oxygen Uptake
Maximal Oxygen Uptake

Oxygen is required for cells to metabolize. Oxygen that is taken-up by the body collectively is referred to as ventilatory or total body oxygen uptake,[34] and that which is taken up by heart muscle is referred to as myocardial oxygen uptake. After the second minute of a given level of exercise, the uptake of oxygen is believed to achieve a steady state. During steady state, heart rate (HR), cardiac output, blood pressure, and pulmonary ventilation maintain constant levels. The energy delivered in the beginning of exercise is obtained through anaerobic metabolism and the anaerobic debt is paid during recovery.[13]

Maximal ventilatory oxygen uptake (VO_2max) is the greatest amount of oxygen that a person can extract from inspired air while performing dynamic exercise involving a large part of the peripheral muscle mass.[35] VO_2max can be calculated by measuring expired concentrations of O_2 and CO_2 in exercising subjects.[36–38] Conventionally, oxygen consumption is reported in multiples of basal resting requirements. The "MET" is a unit of basal oxygen consumption or approximately 3.5 ml O_2/kg-min. This value represents the amount of oxygen required to maintain life in the resting state. VO_2max is related to age, gender, predisposing genetic factors, health status, and exercise proclivity. Maximal values of VO_2max peak between 15 and 20 years of age and decline linearly thereafter. In moderately active young men, VO_2max is about 12 METs, while individuals performing aerobic training such as distance running can have maximal oxygen uptakes as high as 60 to 90 ml/kg-min or 18 to 25 METs. By age 60, mean VO_2max in males is about two-thirds of that at the age of 20. VO_2max can be predicted by projection from the HR achieved at submaximal exercise.[12] With sustained bed rest, there is a 25% decrease in VO_2max in normal males over a 3-week period.

Maximal VO_2 is equal to maximal cardiac output (CO) times the maximal arteriovenous oxygen (A-VO_2) difference.[36] Since cardiac output is equal to the product of stroke volume and HR, VO_2 is directly related to HR. The maximal A-VO_2 difference during exercise has a physiologic limit of 15 to 17 volumes percent; hence, if a maximal effort is given, VO_2max correlates nicely with maximal cardiac output.[39]

Myocardial Oxygen Consumption (MVO_2)

Myocardial oxygen consumption (MVO_2) is determined by intramyocardial wall tension (LV pressure times end diastolic volume divided by LV wall thickness), contractility, and HR. Other less important factors include the external work performed by the heart, as well as the energy necessary for electrical activation and basal metabolism of the myocardium.

Accurate measurement of MVO_2 requires cardiac catheterization to assess systolic wall force and myocardial contractility.[34] Noninvasively, MVO_2 may be measured by positron emission tomography (PET)[40–42] or roughly estimated by the product of HR and systolic blood pressure (SBP).[32] This has been called the pressure-rate product[35] or double product.[43] There is a linear relationship between MVO_2 and coronary blood flow.[34] During exercise, coronary blood flow increases up to five times the normal resting value. A patient with obstructive coronary disease cannot increase coronary blood flow enough to supply the metabolic demands of the myocardium during exercise.[32] As a consequence, myocardial ischemia occurs. Angina usually occurs at the same double product rather than at the same workload.[44]

An important basic principle of exercise physiology is that VO_2 and MVO_2 are distinct in their determinants and in the way they are measured or estimated. Though directly related to each other, this relationship can be altered, for example, by exercise training or drugs such as β-blockers.[45]

Peripheral Responses to Dynamic Exercise

The response to dynamic exercise consists of a complex series of cardiovascular adjustments that assure active muscles receive a blood supply appropriate to their metabolic needs, dissipate the heat and byproducts generated by metabolism, and maintain the blood supply to the brain and heart.[46] Since a delivered workload can be accurately calibrated and the physiologic response easily measured, dynamic exercise is appropriate for clinical exercise testing.[31]

As cardiac output increases with dynamic exercise, there is an increase in systemic arterial pressure.[34] Peripheral resistance increases in the tissues that are not functioning in the performance of the ongoing exercise and decreases in active muscles. The net result is a decrease in overall systemic resistance because, while pressure may increase by 25% to 50%, flow can increase by as much as five times during dynamic exercise.[36,46] Since the denominator (flow) increases much more than the numerator (pressure) in the formula for resistance, the result is a decrease in systemic resistance.

Heart Rate Response

An increase in HR is the first measurable response[47] of the cardiovascular system to exercise—as the sympathetic outflow to the heart and systemic blood vessels is increased, the vagal outflow to the heart decreases.[48] The increase in HR is the major mechanism of exercise-induced increases in cardiac output.[49] HR accounts for about 60% to 70% while alteration of preload and afterload (stroke volume) accounts for about 30% to 40% of each L/min pumped.[50] HR during exercise increases linearly with workload and ventilatory oxygen uptake.[34] During low levels of exercise and at a constant work rate, HR will rise and reach a plateau or steady-state within several minutes. At higher workloads, it takes progressively longer to reach a steady-state HR.

There is a decline in mean maximal HR as age increases.[51] This inverse relationship in age appears to be due to intrinsic cardiac changes rather than to neural influences.[52] Individuals who are fit tend to show less rapid declines in maximal HR with age. The HR response to maximal dynamic exercise is dependant upon numerous factors, but particularly age and health. Although a regression line of 220 − age is fairly reproducible, the scatter around this line may be considerable.[31] This makes age-predicted maximal HR relatively useless for clinical purposes. Such predictions are maximal for some individuals and submaximal for others.[53]

HR is also influenced by the type of muscular activity. Dynamic exercise increases HR more so than isometric exercise.[54] Lack of gravitational forces on baroreceptor mechanisms may play a role in the accentuated HR response observed following bed rest.[32] Other factors that influence HR include body position, physical condition, state of health, blood volume, and environment.[55,56] Even in normals, a wide array of regression lines have been reported.[52]

Blood Pressure Response

SBP rises with increasing dynamic work as a result of increasing cardiac output.[57] At each level of work there is a more consistent increase in SBP during the first few minutes, and then a steady state is attained.[46] Systolic blood pressure generally correlates with the maximal exercise level achieved.[32] Normal values of maximal SBP can be defined.[58] In women, the values are alleged to be more variable and not to relate as well as the level of effort.[44] However, the overall LV hemodynamic response to exercise is comparable in both women and men.[59]

After performing maximal exercise, there is a normal decline in SBP, reaching basal levels usually in 6 minutes, and then often remaining lower than pre-exercise levels for several hours.[60] In some patients, higher levels of SBP in recovery phase have been observed exceeding the peak exercise values. Ratios of this rebound phenomenon have been proposed to diagnose coronary disease.[30] Some normals will have precipitous drops in SBP when stopped abruptly due to venous pooling.[60]

During exercise there is an immediate dilation of the arteries in active muscles because of the sudden increase in metabolites. Peripheral resistance increases in the tissues that do not function in the performance of the exercise. The total result is a decrease in overall systemic resistance.[36] While SBP increases simultaneously, diastolic blood pressure usually remains about the same.[60]

INSTRUMENTATION AND METHODS FOR DIAGNOSTIC EXERCISE TESTING

Devices for Exercise Stress

While the treadmill remains the apparatus of choice in most clinical testing laboratories, the cycle ergometer is an important alternative modality. Quality ergometers are available at less cost than comparable quality treadmills. The cycle ergometer allows the application of uniform power increments gradated on the basis of a patient's body mass. It is easier to obtain blood pressure and ECG tracings free of motion artifact with the subject seated and with upper extremities stabilized by the handlebars. This modality of testing may be suitable for patients who may be unsteady when walking or otherwise not capable of exercising on the treadmill. Maximal aerobic capacity is usually lower when measured by the cycle technique, so the treadmill is more sensitive for diagnosis.[61,62]

Treadmills used for exercise testing should have front and side rails for the patients to steady themselves, and some patients may benefit from the helping hand of the person administering the test. Patients should not grasp the front or side rails, as this decreases oxygen uptake and work and increases exercise time and muscle artifact. It is helpful if patients take their hands off the rails, close their fists, and extend one finger touching the side rails to maintain balance while walking after they are accustomed to the treadmill.

Mechanical or electrically braked cycles are calibrated in kiloponds (kpm) or watts. Mechanical cycles must maintain constant revolutions per minute (rpm) but in electrically braked cycles, rpm can range from 40 to 70/min without significant effect on delivered watts. This allows for better workload control since it is common for uncooperative or fatigued patients to decrease their pedalling speed. The highest values of VO_2 and HR are obtained when pedalling speeds of 70 rpm are used. One watt is equivalent to 6 kpm. Since cycle exercise is non-weight-bearing, kiloponds or watts equates directly to calories, which correlates directly to liters of oxygen per minute. METs (in ml O_2/kg) are obtained by dividing the oxygen consumption by the body weight of the individual tested in kilograms.

In addition to its lower cost, the cycle ergometer takes up less space, and makes less noise than a treadmill. Upper body motion is usually reduced, making it easier to obtain blood pressure measurements and to record the ECG. Care must be taken so that isometric exercise is not inadvertently performed by the arms. Maximum VO_2 achieved is lower on a cycle than that achieved on a treadmill.[63]

Numerous other devices have been used to provide the dynamic exercise for exercise testing, including fixed steps and ladder mills. Today, the cycle egometer[64] and treadmill are the most commonly used dynamic exercise devices, the former having greater popularity in Europe, and the latter being clearly more popular in the United States.

ECG Analysis

The revolution that has occurred throughout medicine, related to miniaturization of electronics and the use of large-scale integrated microprocessors, has had a significant impact on instrumentation and the technique of exercise electrocardiographic testing.[30] The influence of computerization on the quality of the tracings and the utility of computer averaged signals is still being debated.[65] The conversion from analog to digital recording systems has allowed for the integration of multiple leads and simultaneous multiple channel recordings with an enormous effect on the convenience and simplification of the performance of the technical procedure.[4] There has also been significant improvement in the signal-to-noise ratio of electrodes and leads.

Patient Preparation

Pretest Instructions

The patient should be instructed not to eat or smoke for 3 hours prior to the test and to come dressed for exercise. No unusual physical efforts should be performed 12 hours prior to testing. The procurement of informed consent is the responsibility of the performing or supervising physician, and has been reviewed in significant detail elsewhere.[33]

Withdrawal of medications should be considered, depending on the indications of the study, as some drugs interfere with exercise responses and complicate the interpretation of the exercise test. In some exercise laboratories, drugs are withdrawn 24 to 48 hours before performing a test. There are no formal guidelines for tapering medications, and life-threatening rebound phenomena may occur with discontinuance of β-blockers.[66] Most testing is done with patients on their usual medication, although it is important to question which drugs have been taken so as to be aware of possible electrolyte abnormalities and other effects.

Pretest Examination

A brief history and physical examination should be accomplished to rule out any contraindications to testing or to detect important clinical signs such as cardiac murmur, gallop sounds, pulmonary bronchospasm, or rales. Patients with a history of increasing or unstable angina should not undergo exercise testing until stabilized. A cardiac physical exam should indicate which patients have concurrent valvular or other heart disease, particularly those with severe aortic stenosis, who should not be exercised.

A standard 12-lead ECG should be obtained. This is essential particularly in patients with known heart disease, since a new abnormality or a change from a previous study may prohibit testing. Recording the ECG after 30 to 60 seconds of hyperventilation prior to starting the exercise has been advocated in an effort to improve analysis of ST-segment changes with stress,[67] but should probably be avoided because of the association of vigorous hyperventilation with syncope,[68] angina in CAD patients[69] and in those with variant angina,[70] and because it can cause false positives.[71] In patients who are felt to have false-positive ST responses, the ECG response to hyperventilation is best observed postexercise or on a day other than the day of the exercise test.[30]

Standing ECG and BP should be recorded to look for vasoregulatory abnormalities, particularly resting ST depression.[60] Orthostatic testing should not be combined with hyperventilation.

Technical Considerations for Optimal ECG Measurement[30,44,61]

Peripheral Electrodes and Cables

There are many available electrodes for performing exercise testing. Silver plate or silver chloride crystal pellets are the best electrode materials with the lowest offset voltage. Electrodes should be constructed with a metal interface that is sunken to create a column to be filled with either an electrolyte solution or a saturated sponge. These fluid column electrodes avoid direct metal-to-skin contact, decreasing motion artifact.

Connecting cables between the electrodes and recorder should be light, flexible, and properly shielded. Most commercial exercise cables are constructed to lessen motion artifact. In general, cables have a life span of a year or so, depending upon use. Eventually they become a source of both noise and electrical discontinuity and must be replaced.

The most critical point of the electrode-amplifier-recording system is the interface between electrode and skin. Removal of the superficial layer of skin significantly lowers its resistance, decreasing the signal-to-noise ratio. The areas for electrode application are first rubbed with an alcohol-saturated gauze. After the skin dries the electrode sites are rubbed with fine sandpaper or rough material. With these procedures, skin resistance should be reduced to 5,000 Ω or less.

ECG Lead Systems

Bipolar lead systems were the first to be used to detect ECG changes during exercise. The relatively short time for placement, freedom from motion artifact, and the ease with which noise problems can be located are the factors that favor their use. The usual positive reference is an electrode with the same placement as the positive reference for V_5 (the fifth intercostal space [ICS] at the midclavicular line). The negative reference for V_5 is Wilson's central terminal, which consists of connecting the limb electrodes—right arm (RA), left arm (LA), and left leg (LL). CM_5 is the most sensitive for ST-segment changes. CC_5 excludes the vertical component included in CM_5 and decreases the influence of the atrial repolarization (Ta), reducing false-positive responses. Electrode placement affects ST-segment slope and amplitude. The various placements do not result in comparable waveforms for analysis.

Since a standard 12-lead ECG with electrodes placed on the limbs cannot be obtained during exercise, other electrode placements have been used. The interpretation of a 12-lead ECG obtained via these recommended exercise electrode sites[72] differs substantially from that of a 12-lead ECG obtained using the standard lead positions.[73] Care must therefore be taken to correctly interpret the baseline tracing and not substitute it for the standard diagnostic ECG. The exercise electrode sites cause the QRS vectors to appear directed inferiorly, posteriorly, and rightward, producing a marked rightward mean frontal axis shift of + 48°. Therefore false lateral and apical infarcts can be seen, while inferior, posterior, and apical infarcts can falsely disappear on the pre-exercise tracings. False-positive or -negative anterior infarctions are not a problem.[73]

Relative Sensitivity of ECG Leads

The precordial leads are capable of detecting 90% of all ST depression observed in multiple lead systems. Other reports relate that using other leads in addition to V_5 will increase the yield of abnormal response by about 10% to 25%. However, the specificity of an abnormal response in other leads is lower.

In subsets with a high prevalence of previous myocardial infarction or symptoms suggesting coronary artery spasm, a more complete lead system is preferable. ST depression in multiple leads (five or more) usually predicts multivessel disease. A three-lead system (V_1, II, and V_5) can be adequate for localizing ischemia due to spasm. In asymptomatic individuals or those with nonspecific chest pain who have a normal resting ECG, recording a single lead such as CC_5 is adequate.

Patients with ECG evidence of myocardial damage or with a history suggestive of coronary spasm may require additional leads. It is advisable to record three leads: a V_5 type lead, an anterior V_2 type lead, and an inferior lead such as aVF. This approach is also helpful for the detection and identification of dysrhythmias. Sometimes abnormalities may not be present or seen as borderline in V_5 while they will be clearly abnormal in V_4, V_6, or other precordial leads.

Exercise Protocols and Testing[30,74]

Exercise Workloads

Exercise ECG is usually performed on a treadmill using a standardized protocol that increases speed and grade in step-wise fashion. Protocol selection is an important consideration. Figure 1-1 illustrates the relationship of workload to stage in several common testing protocols.

The subject should started at low speed (1.5 to 2 mph for 1 minute), to allow for accommodation to the treadmill. The subject is then exercised on a standardized protocol that is likely to result in 9 or more minutes of work. We advocate having the patient exercise to symptom limited level (usually 9 or 10 on the new Borg scale; 17 to 19 on the 6–20 Borg scale, Table 1-2). The subject does a short cool-down walk for 30 to 60 seconds and then may be directed to lie down. Supine recovery increases preload and the diagnostic power of the test.[75] This may not be necessary or desirable in patients with known coronary artery disease,[76] and a more prolonged cool-down walk may be preferable.

Table 1-2. The Borg Scales for Perceived Exertion during Exercise

"New" Borg		"Old" Borg	
0	= Nothing at all	6	= Nothing at all
0.5	= Very, very light	7	= Very, very light
1	= Very light	9	= Very light
2	= Light	11	= Light
3	= Moderate	12	
4	= Somewhat hard	13	= Somewhat hard
5	= Hard	15	= Hard
6		16	
7	= Very hard	17	= Very hard
8		18	
9		19	= Very, very hard
10	= Very, very hard	20	

(From Froelicher,[30] with permission.)

It is important to appreciate the relationship between myocardial and ventilatory oxygen consumption and other exercise test variables.[77] The application of ventilatory oxygen uptake measurements has been increasingly applied. Exercise capacity should not be reported only as total time exercised but also as the VO_2 or MET equivalent of the workload achieved. This permits the comparison of the results of diverse exercise testing protocols and accurate exercise prescription.

The many different protocols for clinical use include an initial low load (warm-up), progressive exercise with an adequate duration at each level and a recovery period. The most commonly used protocols are progressive: they are uninterrupted and the workload is increased in stages. For cycle ergometry, the initial workload is usually 10 to 25 watts (150 kpm/min), and this is usually followed by increases of 25 watts every 2 or 3 minutes until end-points are reached.

Selection of the Appropriate Treadmill Protocol

Numerous treadmill protocols are currently in use; the most widely used is the Bruce protocol. Although the Bruce protocol has advantages such as a final stage that cannot be completed by most individuals and its wide use by investigators in published studies, it also has several disadvantages. Its large increments in work make estimation of VO_2max less accurate, and the fourth stage can either be run or walked, resulting in divergent oxygen costs. Many patients are forced to terminate exercise prematurely because of orthopedic difficulties or inability to tolerate the high workload increments. Some exercise testing laboratories are now trying to use predetermined MET levels for stage advances and to avoid a situation where either walking or running can be performed by the patient. An initial "zero" and "half-stages" (1.7 mph at 0% and then 5% grade) can be used for more limited individuals. Nonetheless, despite these accommodations, the standard Bruce protocol is often too arduous for some elderly or debilitated patients and results in peripheral muscle fatigue before the achievement of true cardiopulmonary limitation. The premature termination of exercise results in too few data points to estimate oxygen consumption accurately.

The Optimal Treadmill Protocol

In an optimally designed protocol there should be a smoother linear relationship between any increase in metabolic reserve and HR reserve.[53] The observed MET increments of the Bruce protocol are large and uneven, and limit the number of submaximal responses that may be observed in relation to the exercise stages. For this reason, modifications of Balke-type protocols, the Naughton protocol or the more recently developed Cornell or chronotropic assessment protocol, that provide four or five stages to achieve maximal exercise, are becoming increasingly prevalent.[30]

The optimal protocol should be adjusted to the individual patient and last 7 to 12 minutes in length—if the test goes longer, then endurance is tested rather than aerobic capacity. It is more important to report workload achieved in METs rather than minutes of total exercise. Shorter durations do not give a patient adequate time to warm-up and longer durations result in peripheral muscle fatigue. Protocols should be tailored according to the type of patient being tested. Three-minute stages are not necessary to achieve steady state at a low workload. Performance can be estimated with the oxygen cost of maximal workload achieved rather than by total treadmill time. In this way, performance in different protocols can be compared. The oxygen costs of the stages of the major exercise protocols are given in Figure 1-1.

Continuous Versus Step-Wise Increase in Speed and Grade

With the availability of computerized, integrated stress testing systems, the use of ramp testing is likely to become more practical in the future. The ramp protocol uses a constant and continuous augmentation in workload by imperceptible changes in speed and grade allowing for a more steady increase in cardiopulmonary responses to exercise. Comparison of the ramp with commonly used clinical protocols shows the ramp to result in a more linear relationship between oxygen uptake for a given increase in work.[63] The ramp rate can be individualized to yield a test duration of approximately 10 minutes.

Systolic Blood Pressure Monitoring[30,74]

Physicians often report that it is difficult to auscultate blood pressure during exercise, but this response is very important to the interpretation of results and deserves significant consideration. We suggest use of the standard sphygmomanometer and stethoscope. A mark with a felt-tip pen over the brachial artery after location by palpation is helpful in locating the point of optimal auscultation during the motion of exercise. The patient's arm should hang relaxed when blood pressure is being taken and, during recording, it is important to be certain that the patient neither tenses the muscles of the arm nor grips the handrails too tightly. Care must be taken to minimize bumping and banging of the tubing. The diastolic blood pressure can drop all the way to zero and still be normal, but a drop in systolic blood pressure below the pre-exercise value is an important marker for cardiac disease.[78]

Test Endpoints

Patient Instructions Concerning Termination

The patient should be instructed to exercise without using any specific pretest estimate of maximal predicted heart rate (MHR), since pretest estimations of MHR are often misleading related to the use of bradycardia-inducing drugs or common intrinsic dysrhythmias such as atrial fibrillation.[79] Perceived exertion responses on the Borg scale are used during the course of the test for this purpose[80] (Table 1-2). The patient is allowed to exercise to a level of maximal effort without adverse signs or symptoms, and is encouraged to achieve a 19 or 20 on the 6–20 Borg scale, or 9 or 10 on the 0–10 Borg scale, after which the exercise is discontinued.

For the submaximal or predischarge exercise study, one of the following should end the test: signs or symptoms of ischemia, achievement of 6 METs, 85% of age predicted maximal heart rate or 110/min if the patient is on β-blockers, and a Borg scale of 17 on the 6–20 Borg scale, or 7 on the 0–10 Borg scale.

Clinical Indications for Termination of an Exercise Test[30]

Absolute Indications

Drop in systolic blood pressure and/or heart rate despite an increase in workload.

Increasing anginal chest pain (more than moderately severe).

Cardiac Stress Testing and Imaging

Functional Class	Clinical Status	O₂ Cost ML/KG/MIN	METS	Bicycle Ergometer (1 Watt = 6 KPDS; For 70 kg body weight) KPDS	Modified Bruce¹ 3 min stages MPH / %GR	BALKE 2 min stages MPH / %GR	Naughton 2 min stages MPH / %GR	Cornell 2 min stages MPH / %GR	CAEP² 2 min stages MPH / %GR	METS
Normal and I (Healthy, dependent on age, activity)		66.5	19		5.5 / 20					19
		63.0	18							18
		59.5	17		5.0 / 18			5.0 / 18.0	7.0 / 15	17
		56.0	16					4.6 / 17.0		16
		52.5	15		4.2 / 16	4.0 / 20.0		4.2 / 16.0	7.0 / 10	15
		49.0	14			3.5 / 20.0		3.8 / 15.0		14
	(Sedentary, Healthy)	45.5	13		3.4 / 14	3.0 / 20.0		3.4 / 14.0	6.0 / 10	13
		42.0	12			3.0 / 17.5	2.0 / 21.0			12
		38.5	11	1500	2.5 / 12	3.0 / 15.0	2.0 / 17.5	3.0 / 13.0	5.0 / 10	11
		35.0	10	1350		3.0 / 12.5	2.0 / 14.0	2.5 / 12.0		10
II (Limited)		31.5	9	1200	1.7 / 10	3.0 / 10.0	2.0 / 10.5	2.1 / 11.0	4.0 / 10	9
		28.0	8	1050		3.0 / 7.5	2.0 / 7.0	1.7 / 10.0	3.5 / 8	8
		24.5	7	900	1.7 / 5	3.0 / 2.5	2.0 / 3.5	1.7 / 5.0	3.0 / 6	7
III (Symptomatic)		21.0	6	750		3.0 / 2.5	2.0 / 0.0	1.7 / 0.0	2.5 / 5	6
		17.5	5	600	1.7 / 0	3.0 / 0.0	2.0 / 0.0		2.0 / 4	5
		14.0	4	450			1.0 / 0.0		1.5 / 3	4
		10.5	3	300					1.0 / 2	3
IV		7.0	2	150						2
		3.5	1							1

Fig. 1-1. Relationship of workload and oxygen costs to stage in several common exercise testing protocols. ¹The Bruce protocol with two additional stages of 1.7/0 and 1.7/5; ²Cleveland Clinic Chronotropic Assessment Exercise Protocol (CAEP).

Central nervous system symptoms.

Signs of poor perfusion (cyanosis, pallor).

Serious arrhythmias (i.e., ventricular tachycardia, sustained).

Technical problems with monitoring the ECG or SBP.

Patient request to stop.

Marked electrocardiograph changes (greater than 0.3 mV of horizontal or downsloping ST-segment depression or more than 0.2 mV of ST-segment elevation).

Discharge of internal cardioverter defibrillator.

Relative Indications

Worrisome ST- or QRS changes as excessive junctional depression or marked axis shift.

Increasing chest pain.

Fatigue, shortness of breath, wheezing, leg cramps, or intermittent claudication.

Worrisome appearance.

Hypertensive response (systolic pressure > 250 mmHg, diastolic pressure > 115 mmHg).

Less serious dysrhythmias including sustained supraventricular tachycardias or ventricular tachycardia, nonsustained.

Development of bundle branch block that cannot be distinguished from ventricular tachycardia.

Second or third degree atrioventricular (AV) block.

Conduction block with pacemaker.

Postexercise Recovery

We usually allow the subject a short cool-down walk or low resistance pedalling on the cycle ergometer for about 30 seconds and then advocate having the patient lie down. Some abnormal responses occur only in recovery or in the postexercise period. According to the law of LaPlace, increased supine heart volume increases wall stress, which then increases myocardial oxygen consumption. If maximal sensitivity is to be achieved with an exercise test, patients should be supine in the postexercise period. Having the patient perform too long a cool-down walk after maximal exercise can delay or eliminate the appearance of ST-segment depression. Investigators have reported that the supine position enhances ST-segment abnormalities and enhances the diagnostic yield of the test.[75]

Monitoring should continue for 6 to 8 minutes after exercise (except in thallium testing) or until changes stabilize.[61] In the supine position, approximately 85% of patients with abnormal responses in a large series were abnormal by 4 to 5 minutes into the recovery period. An abnormal response occurring only in the recovery period is not unusual.[75] It appears to have nearly the same predictive value (84%) of angiographically significant disease as ST-segment depression during exercise (87%), but in subjects without any symptoms or risk factors, these responses seem more likely to be "false positives." Mechanical dysfunction and electrophysiologic abnormalities in the ischemic ventricle after exercise can persist anywhere from minutes to hours.[81-83]

INTERPRETATION OF EXERCISE ECG RESULTS.

Clinical Responses During the Exercise ECG

Symptoms and Signs

The patient's response to physical exercise has value as part of the clinical diagnostic assessment.[30] Cardiac examination made soon after exercise can give some information about ventricular function. Gallop sounds, for example, can be due to LV dysfunction. A mitral regurgitant murmur occurring after exercise suggests papillary muscle dysfunction due to transitory ischemia. Typical exercise-induced angina is a strong marker for CAD.[2] Ischemic chest pain as well as ST-segment depression induced by the exercise test predicts the presence of CAD.[84] When angina and ST-segment changes occur together, they are even more predictive of CAD than either alone.[85] It is, however, important that a careful description of the pain be obtained from the patient to ascertain that it is typical angina rather than nonischemic chest pain. Results from Vassiliadis et al. suggest that the severity of exercise-induced global and regional LV dysfunction is *independent* of the presence of absence of angina during exercise testing.[86]

Perceived Exertion

The use of relative perceived exertion (RPE) scales has helped immeasurably in the clinical monitoring of exercise intensity and duration.[87,88] The original 6–20 or the newer nonlinear 0–10 scale of Borg represents a subjective scaling system that is reliable and valid and correlates closely with objective measures of physical work. Borg's original scale was designed to correlate the subjective work load to the HR of a male of average age and weight; thus the number corresponding to the verbal cue multiplied by the corresponding number for that cue would approximate the subject's HR at that given level of exertion.

The new Borg or 0–10 scale uses a logarithmic progression for perceived work from 0 = "nothing at all" to 10 = "very, very heavy" (almost maximal). In practice, the subject is asked to indicate his or her perceived value while a chart is held up before them during the last 15 seconds of a given stage of exercise. The scale is especially useful in the diagnostic setting, where it provides surprising consistency for the validation of serial results. The Borg scale may be particularly helpful in patients who are on treatment with β-blockers or are taking other bradycardia-inducing medications or have chronotropic incompetence. The scales are useful also in generalizing perceived exertion in the controlled environment of the stress laboratory to the workplace or the recreational realm. Borg has expressed concern, however, that the scale is being applied "linearly" by being misused without the use of the verbal cues and has requested it be withdrawn from common useage.

Exercise Capacity or Functional Capacity

Maximal ventilatory oxygen uptake (VO_2max) is a measure of the functional limits of the cardiovascular system and the best index of exercise capacity. As previously discussed, VO_2max is dependent on many factors and is an indirect estimate of maximal cardiac output. A decline in maximal cardiac output is the major hemodynamic consequence of symptomatic CAD causing a decrease in exercise capacity.

Acute reduction in LV performance, resulting in decreased stroke volume and increasing pulmonary artery pressure, appears to be the mechanism limiting cardiac output. Maximal oxygen uptake is linearly related to maximal cardiac output.

Hemodynamic Responses

Blood Pressure During Exercise

Blood pressure is dependent on cardiac output and peripheral resistance.[89] SBP at maximal exertion, or at immediate cessation of exertion, has been considered a clinically useful first approximation of inotropic capacity of the heart.[60] Since diastolic blood pressure remains generally constant during exercise, the differential blood pressure or systolic pressure gradient should reflect LV function. Cardiac output is the product of HR times stroke volume.[90] An increase in HR alone is not enough to significantly increase the cardiac output sufficiently to perform more than low-level activity.[91]

The normal values for changes in systolic blood pressure during exercise have been defined. The SBP gradient from rest should be 60 ± 25 mmHg in males 40 to 64 years of age. For females of the same age, it should be 40 ± 20 mmHg.[60] Exercise hypertension (defined as > 210 mmHg in men and > 190 mmHg in women at peak exercise) has been found to be associated with less severe coronary disease and a lower mortality rate.[92] This is consistent with earlier findings by Irving and associates that exercise hypertension was associated with a better prognosis.[58] This large study done on the Seattle Heart Watch population did not specifically address the issue of angiographic severity of CAD.

An inadequate SBP rise or fall in SBP during exercise is frequently associated with severe CAD and ischemic dysfunction of the myocardium.[93] An inadequate SBP rise can also be due to aortic outflow obstruction, severe mitral disease, or LV dysfunction. Since changes of blood pressure depend also on peripheral resistance, they reflect more than just the contractile function of the LV. Patients who develop hypotension during exercise also frequently have a poorer prognosis.[94,95]

Heart Rate During Exercise

During dynamic exercise, HR increases linearly with workload and oxygen uptake. During low levels of exercise and at a constant workload, heart rate will rise and gradually reach a plateau or steady state. At higher workloads, it takes progressively longer to reach a steady state.

The issue of chronotropism, or the ability to develop a rate appropriate for a given level of metabolic demand, has been extensively explored.[53] While the presence of absolute chronotropic incompetence is generally considered a primary rhythm anomaly,[96] the documentation of relative chronotropic incompetence is increasingly germane,[97] and may be a manifestation of ischemia.[98] The importance of chronotropic incompetence as a marker of severe coronary disease has been documented as well.[98] The widespread use of β-blockers and other drugs that lower heart rate has complicated the interpretation of HR responses to exercise. Conditions that affect the sinus node, for instance, inferior wall myocardial infarction and intrinsic disease of the sinus node, attenuate the normal response of HR during exercise testing.

In summary, abnormalities of exercise capacity, SBP, and the HR response to exercise can be due to either LV dysfunction or ischemia.

ECG Responses to Exercise Stress[30,99,100]

Normal Responses[99]

For identification of significant ST-segment depression, the PR segment is used as the isoelectric line, since the TP segment disappears during exercise. ST elevation is measured from the isoelectric line—even in the presence of baseline elevation, since early repolarization (ST elevation) is a normal finding and normals shift to the isoelectric line with exercise. If ST depression is present at rest, then the ST depression is measured from the baseline level. ST depression is considered abnormal only if horizontal or downsloping. The ideal ST-level point is the J-junction; criteria that consider upsloping or ST points beyond the J-point increase sensitivity but decrease specificity.

Depression of the J-junction occurs in response to exercise, and is maximal at maximal exercise, gradually returning toward pre-exercise values in recovery. A dramatic increase in ST-segment slope is observed in all leads and is greatest at 1 minute into recovery. These changes return toward pretest values later in recovery. The normal ST-segment vector response to tachycardia and to exercise is a shift rightward and upward. The degree of this shift demonstrates a fair amount of biologic variation.

A gradual decrease in T-wave amplitude is observed in all leads during early exercise. At maximal exercise, the T-wave begins to increase, and at 1-minute recovery the amplitude is equivalent to resting values in the lateral leads.

Abnormal Responses

ST-segment abnormalities have been classically described as the major marker of ischemia (Fig. 1-2).[43] The continuing controversy as to their worth is a consequence of their complexity. The following physiologic constituents influence the surface ECG configuration: oxygen supply versus demand, pressure relationships, contractility and wall motion, preload and afterload, and HR.

On the surface ECG, exercise-induced myocardial ischemia can result in one of the three ST-segment manifestations: depression, elevation, and normalization. ST-segment depression in patients who have had coronary artery bypass surgery[101] or a recent Q-wave myocardial infarction[102] does not appear to have diagnostic value.

ST-Segment Depression

ST-segment depression is the most common manifestation of exercise-induced myocardial ischemia. ST-segment depression occurs due to global subendocardial ischemia, with direction determined largely by the placement of the heart in the chest.[43] The standard criterion for this abnormal response is horizontal or downsloping ST-segment depression of 0.10 mV or more for 80 ms.[99] However, other criteria have been considered. Downsloping ST-segment depression is more serious than horizontal depression.[99] In the presence of baseline abnormalities, exercise-induced ST-segment depression is less specific for ischemia.[103] Other factors have been related to the probability and severity of CAD, including the amount,[104] time of appearance,[105] duration,[106] and number of leads with ST-segment depression. The issue of the significance of magnitude of ST-depression has been questioned by Ellestad[107] and others.[108,109] The severity of coronary disease is also related to the time of appearance of ischemic ST-segment shifts.[110] The lower the workload and double product at which it occurs, the more

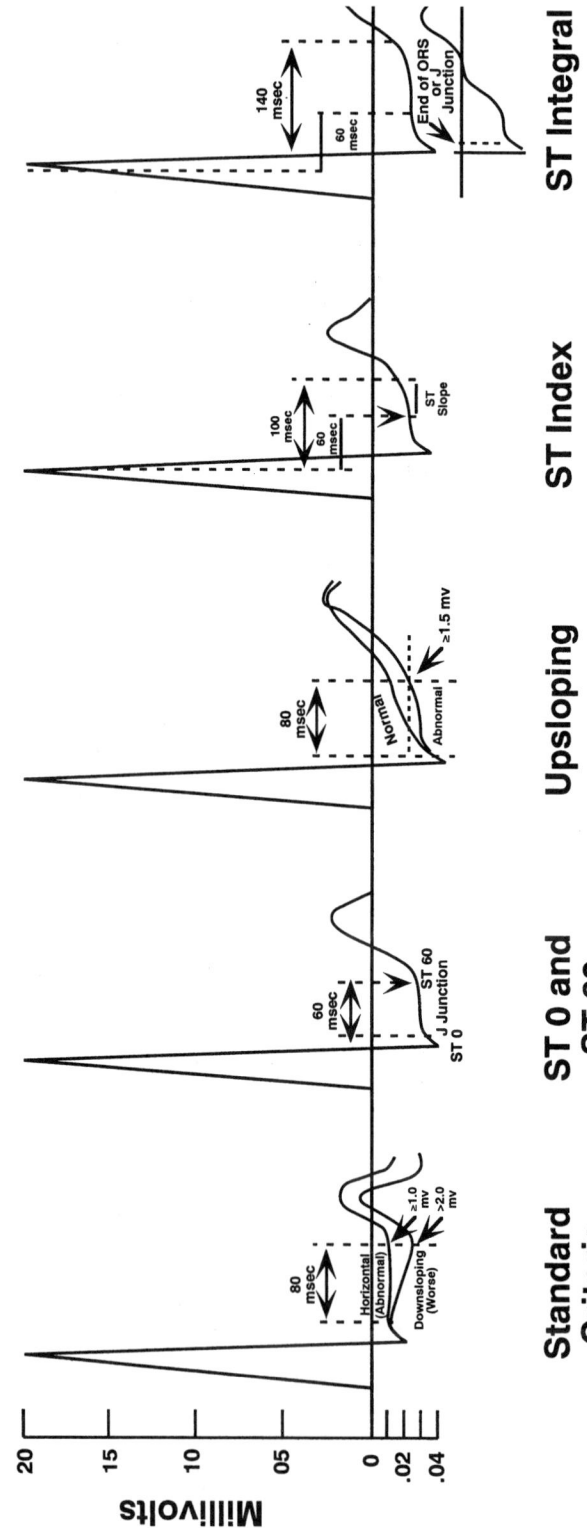

Fig. 1-2. Common approaches for the interpretation of ischemia by ST-segment changes during exercise electrocardiographic testing.

likely the presence of multivessel disease.[111] The persistence of ST depression in the recovery phase in the experience of some investigators is related to the severity of CAD.[99] Figure 1-3 illustrates common ECG patterns observed during exercise.

Siegel and colleagues in a large series from the Cleveland Clinic Foundation reported that up to one-third of patients have ST depression following complete surgical revascularization.[112] The implication is that such baseline ST-segment depressions may interfere with the accuracy of the exercise ECG in those who have undergone bypass surgery.

ST-Segment Elevation

Exercise-induced ST elevation differs in meaning depending upon the status of the myocardium and ECG at baseline.[113] ST elevation is classified by whether it occurs over Q-waves of a myocardial infarction or if it occurs in an ECG area without Q-waves. The mechanisms and implications of these findings are totally different.[102]

ST-Segment Elevation over Q-Waves of Prior MI. Previous myocardial infarction has been considered the most frequent cause of ST-segment elevation during exercise. This appears to be related to the presence of dyskinetic areas or ventricular aneurysms. Approximately 50% of patients with anterior and 15% of patients with inferior infarction exhibit this finding during exercise. Those patients with elevation usually have a lower ejection fraction than those without elevation waves over Q-waves. These changes can result in reciprocal ST depression in other leads simulating ischemia. The underlying extent of the Q-waves for the QRS duration actually determines the amount of ST elevation rather than independently reflecting the amount of dysfunction present. ST-segment elevation has been more frequently observed in anterior leads with Q waves (V_1 through V_2).

ST-Segment Elevation without Q Waves. In patients without previous myocardial infarction (absence of Q waves on the resting ECG), ST-segment elevation during exercise frequently localizes the site of severe transient ischemia due to significant proximal disease or spasm.[114] The mechanism for such ST-segment elevation during exercise is severe transmural ischemia, and the patient should be considered for angiography. An increase in R-wave amplitude has been reported in the lateral leads without Q-waves when ST-segment elevation occurs.

ST-Segment Normalization or Absence of Change

Another manifestation of ischemia can be no change in or normalization of the ST-segment due to cancellation effects. Electrocardiographic abnormalities at rest, including T-wave inversion and ST-segment depression, have been reported to return to normal during attacks of angina and during exercise in some patients with ischemic heart disease. This cancellation effect is a rare occurrence, but it should be kept in mind. Patients with severe coronary disease would be most likely to have cancellation occur, yet they have the highest prevalence of abnormal tests. It has been reported that 20% to 25% of patients with dyskinesia and CAD have normal tests or minimal ST-segment elevation during exercise. When exercise testing fails to produce ST-segment depression or elevation in a patient with known coronary artery disease, this could be due to two or more severely ischemic myocardial segments causing cancellation of ST-segment vectors.

Diagnostic Value of R-Wave Changes

A multitude of factors affect the R-wave amplitude response to exercise, and this response does not appear to have diagnostic significance.[115]

T-Wave and U-Wave Changes

In normal subjects, a gradual decrease in the T-wave amplitude is observed in all leads during early exercise. At maximal exercise, the T-wave begins to increase, and at 1-minute recovery the amplitude is equivalent to resting values in lateral leads.[116] U-wave inversion has been associated with LV hypertrophy, CAD, and aortic and mitral regurgitation. These conditions are associated with abnormal LV distensibility. U-wave inversion induced by exercise in patients with a normal resting ECG appears to be a marker of myocardial ischemia. Several of the newer principles of exercise test interpretation are summarized in Table 1-3.

Factors Effecting Test Sensitivity and Specificity

Definition or Sensitivity and Specificity

Sensitivity is the proportion of those with the disease who are correctly identified with the test. Specificity is the proportion of those without the disease who

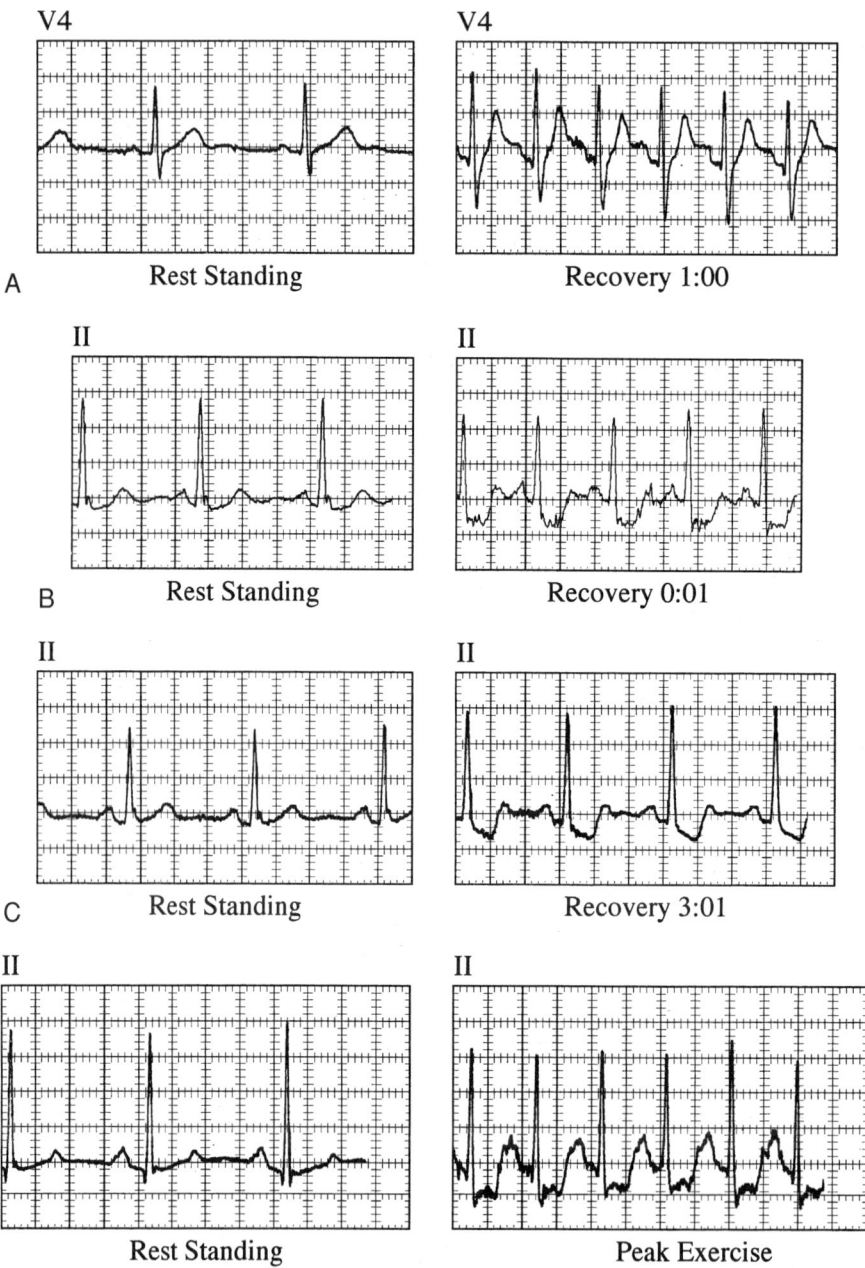

Fig. 1-3. Common electrocardiographic patterns observed during exercise electrocardiogram (ECG) testing. **(A)** Normal. **(B)** Abnormal. Flat and convex ST-segment depression. **(C)** Abnormal. Downsloping ST-segment depression in later recovery. **(D)** False abnormal. Left ventricular hypertrophy (LVH) present only by echocardiogram. *(Figure continues.)*

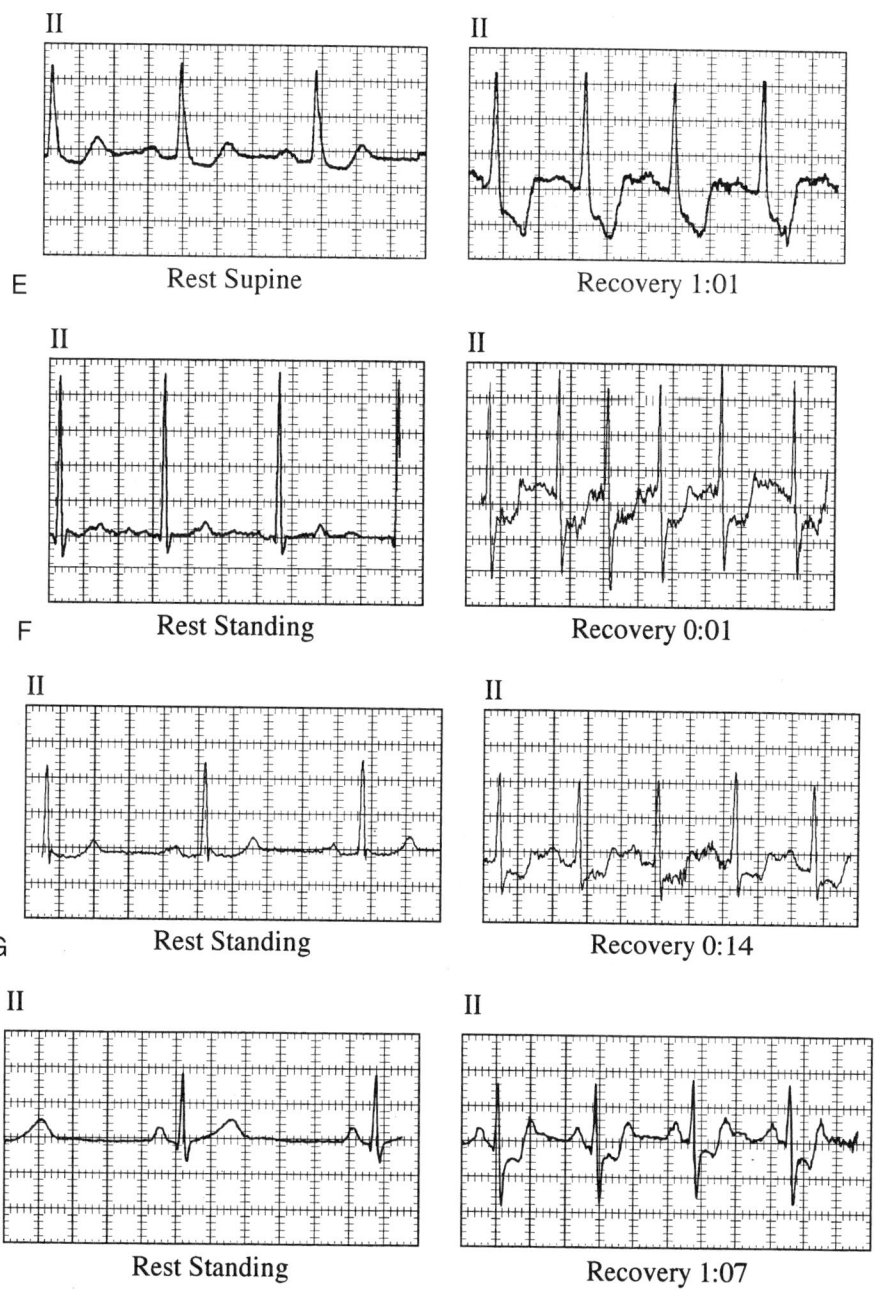

Fig. 1-3 *(Continued).* **(E)** False abnormal. LVH with secondary ST-T's present on resting ECG. **(F)** False abnormal. Subject taking digitalis. **(G)** False abnormal. Subject post-coronary bypass surgery. **(H)** False abnormal. Subject post-coronary angioplasty. *(Figure continues.)*

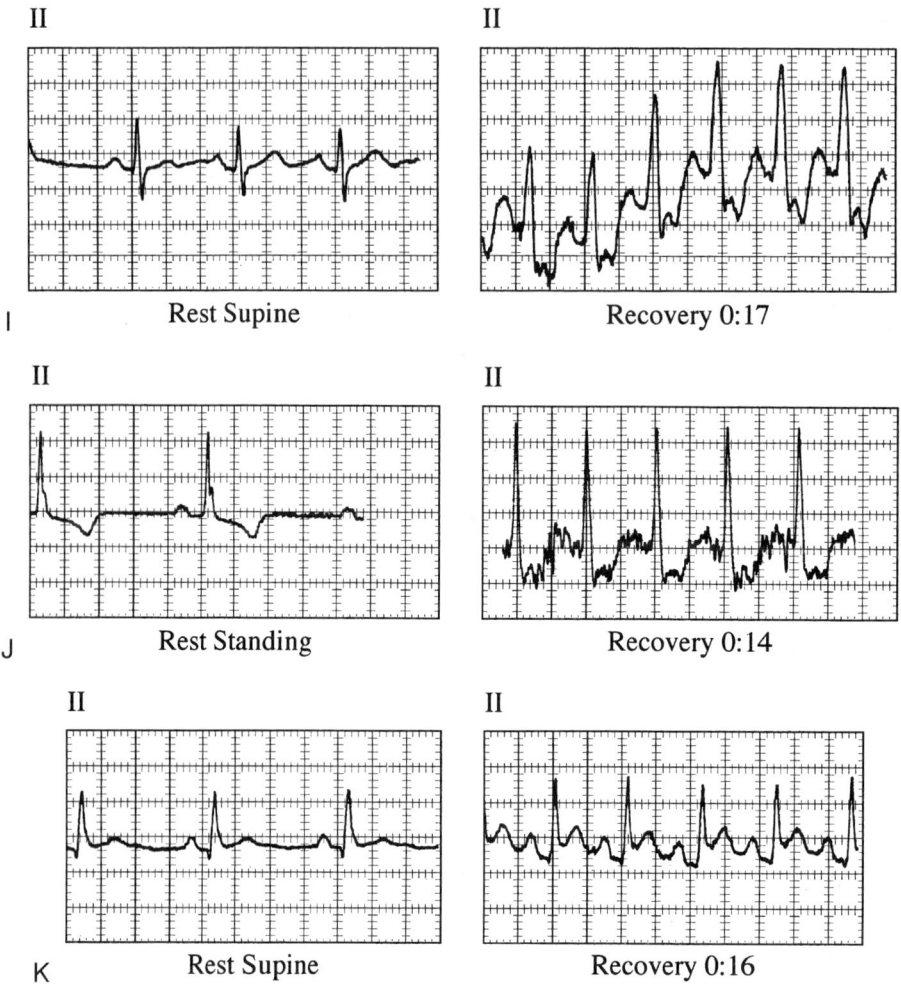

Fig. 1-3 *(Continued).* **(I)** Non-diagnostic. Exercise-induced complete left buncle branch block. **(J)** Abnormal. ST-segment depression with T-wave normalization. **(K)** Abnormal. ST-segment elevation distant from Q-wave infarction. *(Figure continues.)*

are appropriately identified as negative. The sensitivity and specificity of the exercise ECG are also discussed in Chapter 6. The *actual number* of people who will be correctly identified by the test depends on the prevalence (or frequency) of the disease in the group being tested. Several factors have been shown to effect specificity and sensitivity.[103,117]

Sensitivity decreases when equivocal or "nondiagnostic" tests are considered normal.[103] Sensitivity increases when patients with prior myocardial infarction are included or when the test is compared to another method, such as thallium, which identifies physiologically (rather than anatomically) significant coronary disease. Specificity also changes with alteration of interpretative thresholds and decreases, for example, when upsloping ST depression is reported as abnormal, or when pre-exercise hyperventilation is used. Specificity increases when patients with left bundle branch block (LBBB) are excluded.[103]

Provided the baseline ECG does not contain Q-waves, the most reliable and valid lead for analysis during exercise is V_5, or a similarly configured bipolar lead.[118] Exercise ST-segment depression that ap-

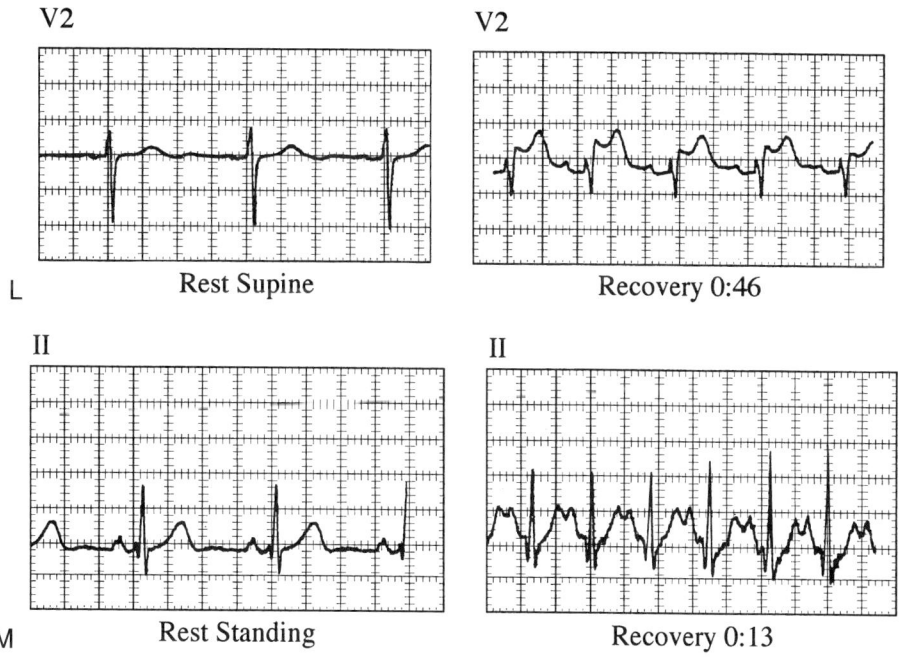

Fig. 1-3 *(Continued).* **(L)** Abnormal. ST-segment elevation at low workload. **(M)** Normal. J-point depression with normal conduction in a subject with pre-excitation (WPW).

pears only in the inferior leads frequently represents a false-positive.[61] We examine the unprocessed analogue strips for the purpose of ST-segment analysis, despite the availability of computerized analysis. Strips should be of 10 seconds or more in duration with minimal baseline deviation ("wander"), and changes are considered as significant if they occur over three beats or more.

The Exercise ECG in Women

For many cardiologists ST-segment depression remains the major focus of interest in exercise ECG testing. With the substantially lower prevalence of coronary disease in premenopausal women, the expectation is that a "positive" test is likely to be a false positive, while a negative test is likely to be a true negative. However, with more young women smoking and the consumption of cigarettes annually smoked by women increasing, the incidence in coronary disease in women may parallel the increasing trend observed with lung cancer.[119] If it does, the lower specificity of the exercise ECG will become increasingly problematic.

The sensitivity and specificity of exercise ECG in women have been variably reported from 50% to 92%.[120,121] Profant was one of the first to report that exercise-induced ST depression was more common in normal women than men.[122] Wu and colleagues further reported a the higher incidence of false-positive results in women under the age of 45 decreased as they aged.[123] Sketch and associates found that 67% of women and 8% of men had false-positive ST changes,[120] whereas Linhart and colleagues reported only 22% false positives following exercise, and only 5% when they excluded those on ST-segment altering drugs or those with abnormal resting ECG.[124] Guiteras found a high false-positive rate in women with probable angina (with ST depression, post-test probability was only 0.5), and in those with nonspecific chest pain, the post-test likelihood was zero.[125] Classical angina associated with ST-segment elevation during exercise was associated with a high likelihood of the presence of disease, but ST depression observed *during exercise only* had a low specificity.[125] Chaitman et al. reported a sensitivity of 79% (vs. 82% in men), with a specificity of 66% using 14 leads after stratification by symptoms.[126] Weiner and his collaborators in the Coronary Artery Surgery

Table 1-3. Newer Principles of Exercise Test Interpretation

1. Ischemic ST depression normally occurs in the lateral leads (I, V_4–V_6)
2. In presence of Q-waves changes may be isolated (II, V_2)
3. Changes in both inferior and lateral leads suggests severe ischemia
4. Isolated inferior or anterior changes are often false positives
5. ST depression does not localize ischemia to an area of myocardium
6. ST depression without angina suggests milder CAD and lower risk
7. ST depression not interpretable in LBBB, previous CABG, Q-wave MI, LVH, digitalis, W-P-W, or ventricular pacemaker
8. ST elevation over Q-wave areas indicates myocardial damage or aneurysm
9. ST elevation over non-Q-wave areas indicates local transmural myocardial ischemia
10. Markers of poor prognosis:
    Exertional hypotension: a drop in SBP below pre-exercise value
    Angina that limits exercise
    Poor exercise capacity (<5 METs)
    Downsloping ST depression especially in recovery
    ST depression starting at a low double product (<15,000)
    ST depression that persists into late recovery

Abbreviations: CAD, coronary artery disease; LBBB, left bundle branch block; CABG, coronary artery bypass grafting; MI, myocardial infarction; LVH, left ventricular hypertrophy; W-P-W, Wolff, Parkinson, White; SBP, systolic blood pressure.
(From Froelicher,[30] with permission.)

Study (CASS), reported on 3153 patients and reported a false-positive rate of 3% in men and 14% in women.[85] The false-negative rate was 38% and 22%, respectively. However, when they matched the subjects for the incidence of prior infarction, by coronary anatomy or age, they found the false-positive and false-negative rates to be nearly the same. Barolsky and associates concluded that the etiology of lower predictive value of the exercise ECG in women is non-Bayesian.[127] In their experience, the prevalence of disease in male and female subjects was similar. The predictive value in males was 77% versus 47% in females. The predictive value of a negative test was similar (81% vs. 78%). Thus, even in women with coronary disease, the exercise ECG is not as accurate as it is in men.

Several explanations have been proposed for this finding. Estrogens have a similar structure to digitalis, a known cause of false-positive ST depression, possibly explaining the differences in specificity related to gender.[128] Androgens have been shown to have a decreasing effect on ST depression.[129] Kusumi and associates studied LV dynamics in women and found higher peripheral vascular resistance and increased oxygen demand in women with abnormal ST-segments than in normals.[130] They speculate that the resultant increase in subendocardial oxygen demand may explain the occurrence of false-positive ECG changes during exercise in females. The range of false-positives in the 1970s and 1980s, before the incorporation of imaging modalities with the exercise ECG, probably reflects in part whether the study originated in a primary or tertiary referral center and the exclusions to interpretation applied.[120,124,131] However, the issue of selection bias remains a significant problem with respect to sensitivity and specificity of the exercise ECG in women in modern office-based practice. A negative exercise ECG in a female is likely to end the work-up at that juncture. The potential affects of various gender-related differences on the exercise ECG are summarized in Table 1-4.

Robert has shown that logistic analysis of exercise variables in women improves the diagnostic value of exercise testing, yielding a significantly better sensitivity (66% to 70%) without a loss of specificity (85%

Table 1-4. Factors That May Affect Exercise ECG Accuracy in Females

Factor	Effect
Higher incidence of SVD	Lowers sensitivity
Lower prevalence of CAD	Lowers specificity
More frequent baseline ST depression	Lowers specificity
Higher prevalence of vasospasm	Lowers specificity
Higher prevalence of MVP	Lowers specificity
Lower average hemoglobin concentration	Lowers specificity
Presence of estrogen, absence of testosterone	Lowers specificity
Hyperventilation, before or during exercise	Lowers specificity

Abbreviations: ECG, electrocardiography; SVD, single-vessel disease; CAD, coronary artery disease; MVP, mitral valve prolapse.

Table 1-5. Some of the Computer-Derived Criteria for Diagnosing CAD

Method	Criteria for Abnormal (Ischemia)
Classic ST-segment depression	Junctional depression of 0.1 mV (1 mm) or more. Exercise-induced ST-segment depression must be flat or downsloping to be abnormal
Upsloping ST80	For upsloping ST-segment with junctional depression of >2 mm from the isoelectric baseline: abnormal if ST segment is depressed 2 mm or more at 0.08 sec (80 ms) after J point (QRS end); normal if less depressed at that point
ST midpoint (ST_4)	Blomqvist divided the ST segment from QS end until the end of the T-wave into eight equal time periods. He found ST_4, or the midpoint, to provide the most discrimination between normal and abnormal. Simoons used a midpoint from QRS end until peak of the T-wave, since peak is easier to identify than T-end
ST index	Abnormal when ST-segment depression is 1.0 mm or greater and the sum of ST-segment depression in mm plus ST slope in mV/sec is equal to or greater than 1.0 (Mean ST-depression measured at 60 to 70 ms after R-wave peak, slope in 40 ms window afterward)
ST/HR slope	As originally described by Elamin and Linden,[144] the maximal rate of progression of ST-segment depression relative to increases in heart rate (maximal ST/HR ratio). The rate of the development of ST-segment depression with respect to increments in heart rate observed in any one lead was represented as the slope of a computed regression line
ST/HR index	Kligfield and Okin[145] divided the change in the ST segment from baseline value to maximum exercise by the change in heart rate over the same period
ST integral	ST integral below isoelectric line greater than 10 μV-sec (1 mm^2 on electrocardiographic paper at standard speed and calibration = 4 μVsec) is considered abnormal. Sheffield originally described measuring the ST integral from the end of the QRS complex to the beginning of the T-wave or where the ST segment crossed the isoelectric line. Others have implemented this by using the peak of the R-wave and measuring the area from 60 to 140 ms after the R-wave
Spatial ST-T magnitudes	Dower and Bruce analyzed magnitudes and slopes at time-normalized areas of $X^2 + Y^2 + Z^2$
ST60 for heart rate	A range of amplitudes at 60 ms after QRS end for exercise heart rate with measurements outside of a normal band and considered abnormal

(From Froelicher,[74] with permission.)

to 93%).[132] This and other implications of multivariate analysis will be discussed in greater detail in Chapter 6. The application of computerized ECG interpretation and analysis has been proposed as a solution to the gender dilemma in the application of exercise ECG by several authors.[133–136] Marwick and colleagues have shown that exercise echocardiography is probably the most accurate and cost-efficient approach for diagnostic exercise ECG testing in women.[137]

COMPUTERIZED ECG INTERPRETATION
Digital Processing of Exercise ECG Data

Computer-derived criteria and scoring systems have been proposed and tested in hopes of improving the diagnostic accuracy of the exercise ECG. Initially, each of the proposed criteria or scores has shown increased accuracy for diagnosis and for the identification of coronary disease severity, but subsequent studies by others, often using populations with more intermediate or low pretest probability, generally have not measured up to the earlier reported experience. Exercise ECG will never be as sensitive or specific as stress studies that incorporate echocardiography or radionuclide imaging, but it is relatively inexpensive and accessible, and thus the search for the "Holy Grail" of accurate and quantitative exercise ECG has continued.

Initial observations suggested that computer signal averaging could distort information and increase the incidence of false-positive studies,[138] but this needs to be reassessed in light of improvements in digital signal processing available during the last

Table 1-6. Summary of Studies Utilizing Computer-Derived Criteria for Identification of CAD

Author	No.	Population	Sensitivity	Specificity	Findings
Quyyumi (1984)	78	Chest Pain	90% (slope)	40% (slope)	ΔST/HR slope does not diagnose the presence or extent of CAD
Kligfield et al. (1986)[145]	17 46	Asymptomatic Angina	57% (standard) 91% (slope) 78% (3VD)	>90% (standard) >90% (slope) 97% (3VD)	ΔST/HR slope improves evaluation of patients with AP
Thwaites et al. (1986)[147]	81	Known CAD	81% (standard) 91% (slope)	64% (standard) 27% (slope)	ST/HR slope performs no better than standard Bruce
Ameisen (1986)	58 55	Angina MI	92% (slope, AP) 38% (slope, MI)	97% (slope, AP) 95% (slope, MI)	Recent MI decreases sensitivity and positive predictive value of ST/HR slope
Detrano et al. (1986)	303	Angiography patients	65% (standard) 68% (slope) 69% (index)	73% (standard, slope, index)	HR-adjusted ST depression is more sensitive than standard
Pruvost (1987)	558	Chest pain	59% (standard) 68% (multivariate analysis)	76% (standard) 83% (multivariate analysis)	Multivariate analysis is more accurate than ST segment alone
Detrano et al. (1987)[139]	271	Consecutive angiography patients	51% (standard) 51% (computer)	87% (standard computer)	Computer assisted interpretation not better than standard
Okin (1988)	606	Asymptomatic	90% (index)	65% (index)	ΔST/HR index and rate-recovery loop improves event prediction
Okin (1988)	128	Angina	50–66% (standard) 93% (slope) 77% (index)	71–73% (standard) 57% (index, slope)	ST/HR slope ≥6 highly sensitive for the identification of 3VD
Sato (1988)	544	Mixed[a]	63% (standard) 70% (slope)	73% (standard) 97% (slope)	ST/HR slope more accurate for diagnosis of CAD and 3VD
Deckers et al. (1989)[64]	123 222	Normals Chest pain	67% (score) 80% (index)	90% (score) 90% (index)	Discriminant analysis and ΔST/HR are accurate and not affected by β-blockers
Kligfield et al. (1989)[148]	100 50 100 50	Normals Chest pain CAD Angina	68% (standard) 95% (slope) 91% (index)	83% (standard) 94% (slope) 98–95% (index-normals vs. chest pain)	ST/HR slope and ΔST/HR index improves sensitivity
Okin and Kligfield (1989)[142]	50	CAD	48% (standard) 96% (slope)	58% (standard) 58% (slope)	Protocol has a significant effect on the accuracy of ST/HR slope
Okin and Kligfield (1989)	117 124	Normals CAD	74% (standard) 93% (loop)	93% (standard) 95% (loop)	ST-segment depression and rate-recovery loop enhances accuracy
Lachterman et al. (1990)[149]	328	Mixed	58% (standard) 54% (index)	73% (standard) 73% (index)	ΔST/HR did not improve diagnostic accuracy for assessing presence or extent of CAD
Okin and Bergman et al. (1991)	50 100	Normals CAD	59% (standard) 90–93% (index, slope)	96% (standard)	ST/HR integral comparable to ΔST/HR index and slope
Okin and Anderson et al. (1991)	3168	Asymptomatic	{2.8% + test (standard) 5.4% + test (index)}	{1.5% − test (standard) 1.7% − test (index)}	ΔST/HR index and rate-recovery loop improves event prediction

Study	N	Population	Results	Additional	Comments
Okin et al. (1991)[150]	50 50 30	Normals Angina CAD	59% (standard at J+60 and J pt); 90–93% (index, slope at J+60); 64–61% (index, slope @ J pt)	96% (standard, index, slope)	J-point measurements significantly degrades performance of HR adjusted indexes of ST depression but less effect on standard criteria
Herbert (1991)	46 154	β-blockers No β-blockers	67% (standard) 63% (index)	58% (standard) 53% (index)	Accuracy unaffected by β-blockers and ΔST/HR index does not improve test
Robert et al. (1991)[132]	135	Mixed	59%–68% (standard) 66%–70% (logistic regression analysis)	85% (standard) 93% (logistic regression analysis)	Logistic regression analysis improves diagnostic accuracy of exercise ECG
Bobbio (1992)	2270	Consecutive angiography patients	75% (standard) 78% (index)	64% (standard) 64% (index)	ΔST/HR index performs better at low HR than standard criteria but overall not significant
Demange et al. (1992)[133]	100	Angina	56% (standard) 73% (index)	71% (standard) 87% (index)	ST 20/HR index improved exercise ECG performance
Morise and Duval (1992)[134]	420	Mixed	48% (standard) 44% (index)	81% (standard) 81% (index)	ΔST/HR index no better than standard criteria
Okin (1992)[141]	100 154	Normals CAD	94% (ST10 index); 88% (ST50 index)	95% (index)	ΔST/HR index more accurate at ST10 than ST50 or ST100
Okin (1992)[135]	150 100 154	Normals Angina CAD	82–93% (index, Female-Male) 93–95% (slope)	97–98% (index, slope)	HR adjustment methods more sensitive, but ΔST/HR index does not identify females as well with CAD
Kligfield (1993)	172	Suspected CAD	73% (standard) 88% (slope) 81% (index)	59% (standard, slope, index)	ST/HR slope superior for detecting 3VD; accuracy is affected by β-blockers
Ribisl et al. (1993)[142]	230	Angiography patients	50% (stan ST0) 57% (standard + exercise capacity)	71% (standard ST0)	Diagnosis enhanced with exercise capacity + ST0; best marker for severity is amount of ST depression
Lehtinen (1994)	161 221	CAD Low likelihood	53% (standard) 51% (slope) 68% (index) 86% (multivariate analysis)	81% (standard) 92% (slope) 84% (index) 72% (multivariate analysis)	ΔST/HR index with multivariate analysis improves diagnostic power of the exercise ECG
Okin (1994)	153 184 212 31	Angina CAD Asymptomatic Negative angiography	82–93% (index, female-male) 93–95% (slope)	97–98% (index, slope)	ΔST/HR index and slope not affected by selection factors; and does not identify females as accurately as males with CAD

Abbreviations: CAD, coronary artery disease; ST/HR, ST-segment heart rate; 3VD, three-vessel disease; MI, myocardial infarction; ppv, positive predictive value; ECG, electrocardiogram.

[a] Mixed represents evaluation of chest pain, screenings, and functional assessment.

several years. Most clinicians are not aware that the sequential beats displayed on some exercise ECG video monitors that are commercially sold today are multiple impressions of a single-averaged beat and that these averaged beats may be influenced by signal noise, respiration, and ectopic beats. Numerical averages can also be misleading: tall T-waves for instance, can cause doubling of the calculated HR.

The computer-derived criteria for diagnosing CAD are summarized in Table 1-5. Hollenberg and associates developed an exercise test score where the area of a curve representing ST-segment amplitude and ST slope in leads V_5 and aVF was divided by the product of exercise duration in minutes and the percent of maximal predicted heart rate achieved during exercise.[139] While improving sensitivity and specificity in cohorts of patients with a high prevalence of CAD, varying experience was reported by other investigators.[140] Detrano and colleagues reported that comparable results could be obtained by consistent visual interpretation of studies in comparison to computer-automated reading.[141] Table 1-6 summarizes the findings of several of the published studies utilizing computerized exercise ECG analysis.

Controversial Issues in Computerized ECG Interpretation

Several areas of controversy have developed over the course of the past 10 years related to computer-generated scores and indexes, and can be summarized as follows:

Does Computerized Interpretation of ST-Segments Improve Diagnostic Accuracy over Standard Interpretive Criteria?

Detrano and others claimed that standard ECG criteria compared favorably overall to computerized interpretation.[141] Nonetheless, other investigators believe that computerized measures are currently quite comparable especially for the determination of disease severity.[142]

What Is the Best Location of ST-Segment Interpretation?

Kligfield, Okin, Detry, and others believe that 50 to 60 ms after the J-junction is the point of measure providing greatest accuracy,[143] whereas Froelicher and associates contend that the J-junction itself (STO) is the optimal point of measurement.[65]

Should Upsloping ST Segments be Considered Abnormal or Should They be Called "Non-Diagnostic" or Borderline Normal?

Specificity is lowered and sensitivity is increased if upsloping ST depression is regarded as abnormal. For clinical purposes, Froelicher and others suggest that upsloping ST depression should be considered normal or borderline.[65]

The ST-Segment/Heart Rate Slope

At about the same time that Hollenberg proposed his treadmill score, Elamin and associates suggested predicting the *severity* of CAD by using the slope of the submaximal ST-segment/heart rate (ST/HR) relationship.[144] This rate-related change in exercise-induced ST-segment depression, most often referred to as the ST/HR slope, attempts to normalize the extent of ST-segment depression for HR, serving as an index of exercise-induced augmentation of myocardial oxygen demand. Initially, the slope had to be manually derived and the analysis was labor intensive. Subsequently, the technique has been incorporated into the software of several stress testing systems. It was reported to significantly improve the accuracy of the exercise ECG for the identification of patients with CAD and for staging the extent of coronary obstruction in patients with known CAD.[145]

Kligfield and associates found an ST/HR slope value of 1.1 μV/beat/min (bpm) as an upper limit of normal improved exercise test sensitivity from 57% to 91% while preserving the specificity of the exercise ECG at greater than 90% in patients with stable angina who were examined using standard Bruce protocols. An ST/HR slope value of 6.0 μV/bpm was found to distinguish patients with and without three-vessel CAD with a sensitivity of 78%, a specificity of 97%, a positive predictive value of 93%, and an overall test accuracy of 90%. They observed that no other criteria based on standard ECG interpretation performed as well as the ST/HR slope for the recognition of three-vessel disease in these patients. Further, patients with high ST/HR slopes who did not have three-vessel coronary disease could be shown to have functionally severe two-vessel disease by radionuclide cineangiography. These data suggested that the ST/HR slope could improve the evaluation and management of patients with possible coronary disease.[145]

Okin observed that the exercise protocol itself could impact the accuracy of the study results[146] and predicted that additional improvement in ST/HR slope accuracy and applicability would likely results from the modification of exercise protocols to reduce heart rate increments between stages, as well as with an increase in the number of monitoring leads from 3 to 12, and with computer analysis of the ST-segment depression. Most published studies found a significant minority of tests where the ST/HR slope was not computable.[147] Whether or not this is important is unclear, but ST/HR slope has not become commonly applied in clinical practice.

ST Segment/HR Index

Kligfield, Okin, and their associates later proposed a simpler approach to HR adjustment than ST/HR slope, by dividing total ST-segment change during exercise by the HR.[148] They derived normal values for the HR-adjusted indexes of ST-segment depression (the ST/HR slope and the delta ST/HR index) during exercise ECG in 150 subjects with a low likelihood of CAD, including 100 normal subjects and 50 subjects with nonanginal chest pain. Sensitivities for detection of myocardial ischemia were calculated from an additional 150 patients with a high likelihood of CAD, including 100 patients with angiographically demonstrated coronary obstruction and 50 patients with stable angina. In contrast to the sensitivity of standard exercise ECG criteria for the detection of disease in this population (68%—102 of 150 subjects), the sensitivity of a delta ST/HR index partition of 1.6 μV/bpm was 91% (137 of 150 subjects, $p < 0.001$). These findings suggested that HR adjustment of ST-segment depression might improve the clinical usefulness of the treadmill exercise ECG.[148]

Lachterman and colleagues attempted to reproduce the findings of Kligfield's group and found the ST/HR index to be of comparable efficacy to standard visual criteria.[149] They evaluated 328 male patients who had undergone both a symptom-limited treadmill test and coronary angiography. The sensitivity of the ST/HR index was 54% at a cut point of 0.021 mm/(beats/min), corresponding to a specificity of 73%. The standard visual ST-segment analysis had a sensitivity of 58% at this same specificity, which corresponded to an ST-segment cut point of 1-mm depression relative to rest (p = NS). Similarly, for the diagnosis of three-vessel or left main coronary disease, no significant difference was found between the sensitivities or the two measurements at cut points of equivalent specificity. The authors concluded that in this consecutive series of patients presenting for routine clinical testing, the ST/HR index did not improve the diagnostic accuracy of the exercise test for identifying the presence or severity of CAD relative to standard visual criteria. Froelicher attributes this finding in part to the exclusion of tests with upsloping ST segments from standard visual analysis, thereby lowering the specificity of the standard group in Kligfield's study,[65] though one would think it would be associated with lowered sensitivity.

The effect of ST-segment measurement position on performance of standard exercise ECG criteria, ST/HR index, and ST/HR slope for the detection of CAD has been studied. Exercise electrocardiograms of 50 clinically normal subjects and 80 patients with known or likely CAD were analyzed using ST depression measured at both the J-junction and 60 msec after the J-junction (ST60). A positive exercise ECG by standard criteria was defined as 0.1 mV or more of additional horizontal or downsloping ST depression at end exercise, and had a specificity of 96% when ST depression was measured at either the J-junction or ST60. There was no difference in sensitivity of standard ECG criteria at ST60 and J-junction (both 59%, p = NS). However, at a matched specificity of 96%, the ST/HR index and ST/HR slope calculated using ST depression at ST60 were significantly more sensitive (90% and 93%) than when calculated using J-junction depression (64% and 61%, both $p < 0.001$). Comparison of areas under the respective receiver operating characteristic curves confirmed the superior performance of ST60 as opposed to J-junction measurements for both the ST/HR index (0.98 vs. 0.89, p = 0.006) and the ST/HR slope (0.96 vs. 0.87, p = 0.007) and also demonstrated modestly improved overall test performance for standard ECG criteria using ST60 measurements (0.88 vs. 0.82, p = 0.001). They concluded that the use of J-junction measurements significantly degrades the performance of heart rate-adjusted indexes of ST depression but has less effect on standard criteria.[150]

The use of normals and patients with known disease to assess test performance has been criticized as unrepresentative of the more common application of studies for the assessment of patients with intermediate probability of disease. Froelicher has questioned the determination of test specificity with a group of normals and sensitivity with a group having a high probability or known CAD. The distinctly different maximal heart rates achieved by the subject groups (highest among the normals, lowest in those with known CAD) would be sufficient in themselves to yield results comparable to the ST-segment analysis.[65]

In conclusion, subset selection will continue to be a problem if the intention is to identify a particular approach that will have universal applicability. Perhaps studies utilizing a sufficiently large database with a huge number of studies from a truly diverse population of subjects will resolve some of the current controversies.

CONCLUSIONS

In an era where stress imaging approaches the standard, the exercise ECG test continues to play an important role. While other markers of ischemia discussed in later chapters are accurate and have become increasingly important, they are universally more expensive than the standard ECG stress test. The stress ECG should still be considered the first investigation for the diagnosis of CAD in most patients who can exercise maximally and in whom the ST segment is interpretable. Recent developments in quantitation may facilitate this process. Important exceptions include those with repolarization abnormalities, those who need to undergo pharmacologic stress testing, and those in whom (for treatment planning) the site or extent of ischemia is important.

REFERENCES

1. Pashkow FJ: Diagnostic evaluation of the patient with coronary artery disease. Cleve Clin J Med 61:43, 1994
2. Ladenheim ML, Kotler TS, Pollock BH et al.: Incremental prognostic power of clinical history, exercise electrocardiography and myocardial perfusion scintigraphy in suspected coronary artery disease. Am J Cardiol 59:270, 1987
3. Chaitman BR: The changing role of the exercise electrocardiogram as a diagnostic and prognostic test for chronic ischemic heart disease. J Am Coll Cardiol 8:1195, 1986
4. Ellestad MH: History of stress testing. p. 1. In Ellestad MH (ed): Stress Testing: Principles and Practice. 3rd Ed. FA Davis, Philadelphia, 1986
5. Feil H, Siegel M: Electrocardiographic changes during attacks of angina pectoris. Am J Med Sci 175:225, 1928
6. Master A, Oppenheimer E: A simple exercise tolerance test for circulatory efficiency with standard tables for normal individuals. Am J Med Sci 177:223, 1929
7. Master A, Jaffe H: The electrocardiographic changes after exercise in angina pectoris. J Mt Sinai Hosp 7:629, 1941
8. Katz L, Landt H: Effect of standardized exercise on the four-lead electrocardiogram: its value in the study of coronary disease. Am J Med Sci 189:346, 1935
9. Riseman J, Waller J, Brown M: The electrocardiogram during attacks of angina pectoris: its characteristics and diagnostic significance. Am Heart J 19:683, 1940
10. Hecht H: Concepts of myocardial ischemia. Arch Int Med 84:711, 1949
11. Yu P, Soffer A: Studies of electrocardiographic changes during exercise. Circulation 6:183, 1952
12. Åstrand P, Rhyming I: Nomogram for calculation of aerobic capacity (physical fitness) from pulse rate during sub maximal work. J Appl Physiol 7:218, 1954
13. Wasserman K, McElroy M: Detecting the threshold of anaerobic metabolism in cardiac patients during exercise. Am J Cardiol 14:844, 1964
14. Balke G, Ware R: An experimental study of physical fitness of Air Force personnel. US Armed Forces Med J 10:675, 1959
15. Clausen J: Circulatory adjustments to dynamic exercise and effect of physical training in normal subjects and in patients with coronary artery disease. Prog Cardiovasc Dis. 28:459, 1976
16. Bruce RA, Kusumi F, Hosmer D: Maximal oxygen intake and homographic assessment of functional aerobic impairment in cardiovascular disease. Am Heart J 85:546, 1973
17. Wasserman K, Whipp BJ: Exercise physiology in health and disease. Am Rev Respir Dis 112:219, 1975
18. Higginbotham MB, Morris KG, Conn EH et al.: Determinants of variable exercise performance among patients with severe left ventricular dysfunction. Am J Cardiol 1:1, 1983
19. Weber KT, Janicki JS: Cardiopulmonary exercise test-

ing for evaluation of chronic cardiac failure. Am J Cardiol 55:22A, 1985
20. Sullivan MJ, Higginbotham MB, Cobb FR: Exercise training in patients with severe left ventricular dysfunction. Hemodynamic and metabolic effects. Circulation 78:506, 1988
21. Hellerstein H: Results of an integrative method of occupational evaluation of persons with heart disease. J Lab Clin Med 38:821, 1951
22. Bruce RA: Evaluation of functional capacity and exercise tolerance of cardiac patients. Mod Concepts Cardiovasc Dis 25:321, 1956
23. Robb G, Marks H: Postexercise electrocardiogram in arteriosclerotic heart disease. JAMA 200:110, 1967
24. Rifkin R, Hood W: Bayesian analysis and electrocardiographic exercise stress testing. N Engl J Med 297:681, 1977
25. Diamond G, Forrester J: Analysis of probability as an aid to the clinical diagnosis of coronary artery disease. N Engl J Med 360:1350, 1979
26. Diamond G: Application of conditional probability analysis to the clinical diagnosis of coronary artery disease. J Clin Invest 65:1210, 1980
27. Detry JM, Robert A, Luwaert RJ et al.: Diagnostic value of computerized exercise testing in men without previous myocardial infarction. A multivariate, compartmental and probabilistic approach. Eur Heart J 6:227, 1985
28. Detrano R, Leatherman J, Salcedo EE et al.: Bayesian analysis versus discriminant function analysis: their relative utility in the diagnosis of coronary disease. Circulation 73:970, 1986
29. Åstrand PO, Rodahl K: Textbook of Work Physiology. 3rd Ed. McGraw-Hill, New York, 1986
30. Froelicher V, Pashkow F: Exercise electrocardiographic testing. p. 49. In Pashkow F, Dafoe W (eds): Clinical Cardiac Rehabilitation: A Cardiologist's Guide. 1st Ed. Williams & Wilkens, Baltimore, 1992
31. Pate R, Blair S, Durstine J et al.: Clinical exercise physiology. p. 19. In Pate R et al. (eds): American College of Sports Medicine: Guidelines for Exercise Testing and Prescription. 4th Ed. Lea & Febiger, Philadelphia, 1991
32. Froelicher V, Myers J, Follansbee W, Labovitz A: Basic exercise physiology. p. 1. In Froelicher V, Myers J, Follansbee W, Labovitz A (eds): Exercise and the Heart. 3rd Ed. Mosby, St Louis, 1993
33. Pate R, Blair S, Durstine J et al.: American College of Sports Medicine: Guidelines for Exercise Testing and Prescription. 4th Ed. Lea & Febiger, Philadelphia, 1991
34. Weber KT: Gas transport and the cardiopulmonary unit. p. 15. In Weber KT, Janicki JS (eds): Cardiopulmonary Exercise Testing: Physiologic Principles and Clinical Applications. WB Saunders, Philadelphia, 1986
35. Weber KT, Janicki JS: Cardiopulmonary Exercise Testing: Physiologic Principles and Clinical Applications. WB Saunders, Philadelphia, 1986
36. Weber KT, Janicki JS, Shroff SG: The mechanics and energetics of ventricular contraction. p. 57. In Weber KT, Janicki JS (eds): Cardiopulmonary Exercise Testing: Physiologic Principles and Clinical Applications. WB Saunders, Philadelphia, 1986
37. Zavala D: Metabolic testing. p. 78 In Pashkow F, Dafoe W (eds): Clinical Cardiac Rehabilitation: A Cardiologist's Guide. 1st Ed. Williams & Wilkins, Baltimore, 1992
38. Froelicher V, Myers J, Follansbee W, Labovitz A: Special methods: Ventilatory gas exchange. p. 32. In Froelicher V, Myers J, Follansbee W, Labovitz A (eds): Exercise and the Heart. 3rd Ed. Mosby, St Louis, 1993
39. Weber KT, Janicki JS, McElroy PA, Reddy HK: Concepts and applications of cardiopulmonary exercise testing. Chest 93:843, 1988
40. Camici P, Ferrannini E, Opie LH: Myocardial metabolism in ischemic heart disease: basic principles and application to imaging by positron emission tomography. Prog Cardiovasc Dis 32:217, 1989
41. Schelbert HR: Positron-emission tomography: assessment of myocardial blood flow and metabolism. Circulation 72:IV122, 1985
42. Sobel BE: Positron tomography and myocardial metabolism: an overview. Circulation 72:IV22, 1985
43. Ellestad MH: Physiology of cardiac ischemia. p. 71. In Ellestad MH (ed): Stress Testing: Principles and Practice. 3rd Ed. FA Davis, Philadelphia, 1986
44. Froelicher VF: Exercise and the Heart: Clinical Concepts. Year Book Medical Publishers, Chicago, Illinois, 1987
45. Ades P, Brammell H, Greenberg J, Horwitz L: Effect of beta blockade and intrinsic sympathomimetic activity on exercise performance. Am J Cardiol 54:1337, 1984
46. Bevegård B, Shepard J: Regulation of the circulation during exercise in man. Physiol Rev 47:178, 1967
47. Petro J, Hollander A, Bouman L: Instantaneous cardiac acceleration in man induced by a voluntary muscle contraction. J Appl Physiol 29:794, 1970
48. Fagraeus L, Linnarsson D: Autonomic origin of heart rate fluctuations at the onset of muscular exercise. J Appl Physiol 40:679, 1976
49. Smith E, Guyton A, Manning D, White R: Integrated mechanisms of cardiovascular response and control

during exercise in the normal human. Prog Cardiovasc Dis 18:421, 1976
50. Eisenhauer AC, McElroy PA, Weber KT: Chonotropic dysfunction and exercise. p. 255. In Weber KT, Janicki JS (eds): Cardiopulmonary Exercise Testing: Physiologic Principles and Clinical Applications. WB Saunders, Philadelphia, 1986
51. Robinson S: Experimental studies of physical fitness. Arbeits-physiologic 10:251, 1930
52. Ellestad MH: Cardiovascular and pulmonary responses to exercise. p. 9. In Ellestad MH (ed): Stress Testing: Principles and Practice. 3rd Ed. FA Davis, Philadelphia, 1986
53. Wilkoff BL, Corey J, Blackburn G: A mathematical model of the chronotropic response to exercise. J Electrophys 3:176, 1989
54. Mitchell J, Blomqvist C, Lind A et al.: Static (isometric) exercise: Cardiovascular responses and neural control mechanisms. Circ Res, suppl. 48:II, 1991
55. Hammond HK, Froelicher VF: Normal and abnormal heart rate responses to exercise. Prog Cardiovasc Dis 27:271, 1985
56. Cotsamire DL, Sullivan MJ, Bashore TM, Leier CV: Position as a variable for cardiovascular responses during exercise. Clin Cardiol 10:137, 1987
57. Guyton A: The relation of cardiac output and arterial pressure control. Circulation 64:1079, 1981
58. Irving J, Bruce R, DeRouen T: Variations in and significance of systolic pressure during maximal exercise (treadmill) testing. Am J Cardiol 39:841, 1977
59. Hakki AH, Iskandrian AS: Effect of gender on left ventricular function during exercise in patients with coronary artery disease. Am Heart J 111:543, 1986
60. Froelicher V, Myers J, Follansbee W, Labovitz A: Interpretation of hemodynamic responses to exercise testing: exercise capacity, heart rate, and blood pressure. p. 71. In Froelicher V, Myers J, Follansbee W, Labovitz A (eds): Exercise and the Heart. 3rd Ed. Mosby, St Louis, 1993
61. Froelicher V, Marcondes G: A Manual of Exercise Testing. Year Book Medical Publishers, Chicago, Illinois, 1989
62. Klein J, Cheo S, Berman DS, Rozanski A: Pathophysiologic factors governing the variability of ischemic responses to treadmill and bicycle exercise. Am Heart J 128:948, 1994
63. Myers J, Buchanan N, Walsh D et al.: Comparison of the ramp versus standard exercise protocols. J Am Coll Cardiol 17:1334, 1991
64. Deckers JW, Rensing BJ, Tijssen JG et al.: A comparison of methods of analysing exercise tests for diagnosis of coronary artery disease. Br Heart J 62:438, 1989
65. Froelicher V, Myers J, Follansbee W, Labovitz A: Special methods: Computerized exercise ECG analysis. p. 48. In Froelicher V, Myers J, Follansbee W, Labovitz A (eds): Exercise and the Heart. 3rd Ed. Mosby, St Louis, 1993
66. Egstrup K: Silent ischemia and beta-blockade. Circulation 84:VI84, 1991
67. Ellestad MH: Hyperventilation and orthostatic changes. p. 270. In Ellestad MH (ed): Stress Testing: Principles and Practice. 3rd Ed. FA Davis, Philadelphia, 1986
68. Buja G, Folino AF, Bittante M et al.: Asystole with syncope secondary to hyperventilation in three young athletes. Pace Pacing Clin Electrophysiol 12:406, 1989
69. Neill WA, Pantley GA, Nakornchai V: Respiratory alkalemia during exercise reduces angina threshold. Chest 80:149, 1981
70. Fujii H, Yasue H, Okumura K et al.: Hyperventilation-induced simultaneous multivessel coronary spasm in patients with variant angina: an echocardiographic and arteriographic study. J Am Coll Cardiol 12:1184, 1988
71. McHenry PL, Richmond HW, Weisenberger BL et al.: Evaluation of abnormal exercise electrocardiogram in apparently healthy subjects: labile repolarization (ST-T) abnormalities as a cause of false positive responses. Am J Cardiol 47:1152, 1981
72. Mason RE, Likar I: A new system of multiple-lead exercise electrocardiography. Am Heart J 71:196, 1966
73. Sevilla DC, Dohrmann ML, Somelofski CA et al.: Invalidation of the resting electrocardiogram obtained via exercise electrode sites as a standard 12-lead recording. Am J Cardiol 63:35, 1989
74. Froelicher V, Myers J, Follansbee W, Labovitz A: Exercise and the Heart. 3rd Ed. Mosby, St Louis, 1993
75. Lachterman B, Lehmann KG, Abrahamson D, Froelicher VF: "Recovery only" ST-segment depression and the predictive accuracy of the exercise test. Ann Intern Med 112:11, 1990
76. Gibbons L, Blair SN, Kohl HW, Cooper K: The safety of maximal exercise testing. Circulation 80:846, 1989
77. Detrano R, Froelicher VF: Exercise testing: uses and limitations considering recent studies. Prog Cardiovasc Dis 31:173, 1988
78. Dubach P, Froelicher VF, Klein J et al.: Exercise-induced hypotension in a male population. Criteria, causes, and prognosis. Circulation 78:1380, 1988
79. Corbelli R, Masterson M, Wilkoff BL: Chronotropic response to exercise in patients with atrial fibrillation. Pace Pacing Clin Electrophysiol 13:179, 1990

80. Borg G, Linderholm H: Perceived exertion and pulse rate during graded exercise in various age groups. Acta Med Scand, suppl. 472:194, 1967
81. Weiner DA, Levine SR, Klein MD, Ryan TJ: Ventricular arrhythmias during exercise testing: mechanism, response to coronary bypass surgery and prognostic significance. Am J Cardiol 53:1553, 1984
82. Detry JM, De Jonghe D: Exercise testing in the evaluation of ventricular arrhythmias in coronary artery disease. Eur Heart J, suppl. 8:55D, 1987
83. Podrid PJ, Venditti FJ, Levine PA, Klein MD: The role of exercise testing in evaluation of arrhythmias. Am J Cardiol 62:24II, 1988
84. Weiner DA, McCabe C, Hueter DC et al.: The predictive value of anginal chest pain as an indicator of coronary disease during exercise testing. Am Heart J 96:458, 1979
85. Weiner DA, Ryan TJ, McCabe CH et al.: Exercise stress testing. Correlations among history of angina, ST-segment response and prevalence of coronary-artery disease in the coronary artery surgery study (CASS). N Engl J Med 301:230, 1979
86. Vassiliadis IV, Machac J, O'Hara M et al.: Exercise-induced myocardial dysfunction in patients with coronary artery disease with and without angina. Am Heart J 121:1403, 1991
87. Borg G, Ottoson D: The Perception of Exertion in Physical Work. Sheridan House Publishers, Dobbs Ferry, NY, 1986
88. Borg G, Hassmen P, Lagerstrom M: Perceived exertion related to heart rate and blood lactate during arm and leg exercise. Eur J Appl Physiol 56:679, 1987
89. Wasserman K, Hansen JE, Sue DY: Principles of Exercise Testing and Interpretation. Lea & Febiger, Philadelphia, 1986
90. Hansen JE, Sue DY, Wasserman K: Predicted values for clinical exercise testing. Am Rev Respir Dis 129:S49, 1984
91. Kristensson BE, Arnman K, Ryden L: The haemodynamic importance of atrioventricular synchrony and rate increase at rest and during exercise. Eur Heart J 6:773, 1985
92. Lauer MS, Pashkow FJ, Harvey S et al.: Angiographic and prognostic implications of an exaggerated exercise systolic blood pressure response and resting systolic blood pressure in adults undergoing evaluation for suspected coronary artery disease. J Am Coll Card 26:1630, 1995
93. Weiner DA, McCabe CH, Cutler SS, Ryan TJ: Decrease in systolic blood pressure during exercise testing: reproducibility, response to coronary bypass surgery and prognostic significance. Am J Cardiol 49:1627, 1982
94. Theroux P, Marpole DG, Bourassa MG: Exercise stress testing in the post-myocardial infarction patient. Am J Cardiol 52:664, 1983
95. Johnston BL: Exercise testing for patients after myocardial infarction and coronary bypass surgery: emphasis on predischarge phase. Heart Lung 13:18, 1984
96. Markewitz A, Fulle P, Wenke K, Weinhold C: Benefit of rate response in patients with sinus node dysfunction. PACE 10:1220, 1987
97. Wilkoff BL, Beck G, Pashkow FJ, Blackburn G: Confidence interval calculation of chronotropic incompetence. PACE 13:1215, 1990
98. Wiens RD, Lafia P, Marder CM et al.: Chronotropic incompetence in clinical exercise testing. Am J Cardiol 54:74, 1984
99. Ellestad MH: ECG patterns and their significance. p. 223. In Ellestad MH (ed): Stress Testing: Principles and Practice. 3rd Ed. FA Davis, Philadelphia, 1986
100. Froelicher V, Myers J, Follansbee W, Labovitz A: Interpretation of ECG responses. p. 99. In Froelicher V, Myers J, Follansbee W, Labovitz A (eds): Exercise and the Heart. 3rd Ed. Mosby, St Louis, 1993
101. Dubach P, Lehmann KG, Froelicher VF: Comparison of exercise test responses before and after either percutaneous transluminal coronary angioplasty or coronary artery bypass grafting. Am J Cardiol 64:1039, 1989
102. Klein J, Froelicher VF, Detrano R et al.: Does the rest electrocardiogram after myocardial infarction determine the predictive value of exercise-induced ST depression? A 2 year follow-up study in a veteran population. J Am Coll Cardiol 14:305, 1989
103. Gianrossi R, Detrano R, Mulvihill D et al.: Exercise-induced ST depression in the diagnosis of coronary artery disease. A meta-analysis. Circulation 80:87, 1989
104. Robb GP, Marks HH, Mattingly TW: The value of the double standard two-step exercise test in the detection of coronary disease: a clinical and statistical follow-up study of military personnel and insurance applicant. Trans Assoc Life Ins Med Dir Am 40:52, 1957
105. Dagenais GR, Rouleau JR, Christen A, Fabia J: Survival of patients with a strongly positive exercise electrocardiogram. Circulation 65:452, 1982
106. Goldschlager H, Selzer Z, Cohn K: Treadmill stress tests as indicators of presence and severity of coronary artery disease. Ann Intern Med 85:277, 1976
107. Ellestad MH, Wan MKC: Predictive implications of stress testing: follow-up of 1700 subjects after maximal treadmill stress testing. Circulation 51:363, 1975

108. Podrid PJ, Graboys TB, Lown B: Prognosis of medically treated patients with coronary-artery disease with profound ST-segment depression during exercise testing. N Engl J Med 305:1111, 1981
109. Colby J, Hakki A-H, Iskandrian AS, Mattleman S: Hemodynamic, angiographic and scintigraphic correlates of positive exercise electrocardiograms: emphasis on strongly positive exercise electrocardiograms. J Am Coll Cardiol 2:21, 1983
110. Ellestad MH: Predictive implications. p. 323. In Ellestad MH (ed): Stress Testing: Principles and Practice. 3rd Ed. FA Davis, Philadelphia, 1986
111. Weiner DA, Ryan TJ, McCabe CH et al.: Prognostic importance of a clinical profile and exercise test in medically treated patients with coronary artery disease. J Am Coll Cardiol. 3:772, 1984
112. Siegel W, Lim JS, Proudfit WL: The spectrum of exercise test and angiographic correlations in myocardial revascularization surgery. Circulation 52:156, 1975
113. Nosratian FJ, Froelicher VF: ST elevation during exercise testing. Am J Cardiol 63:986, 1989
114. Mark DB, Hlatky MA, Lee KL et al.: Localizing coronary artery obstructions with the exercise treadmill test. Ann Intern Med 106:53, 1987
115. Voyles WF, Smith ND, Abrams J: Directional variability in the R wave response during serial exercise testing in patients with coronary artery disease. Am Heart J 108 (4 Pt. 1):983, 1984
116. Surawicz B: ST-segment, T-wave, and U-wave changes during myocardial ischemia and after myocardial infarction: Can J Cardiol, suppl. A:71A, 1986
117. Detrano R, Janosi A, Lyons KP et al.: Factors affecting sensitivity and specificity of a diagnostic test: the exercise thallium scintigram. Am J Med 84:699, 1988
118. Blackburn H, Taylor HL, Vasquez CL et al.: The exercise electrocardiogram during exercise: findings in bipolar chest leads of 1449 middle-aged men, at moderate work levels. Circulation 34:1034, 1966
119. Ellestad MH: Stress testing in women. p. 339. In Ellestad MH (ed): Stress Testing: Principles and Practice. 3rd Ed. FA Davis, Philadelphia, 1986
120. Sketch MH, Muohiuddin SM, Lynch JD et al.: Significant sex differences in the correlation of electrocardiographic exercise testing and coronary arteiograms. Am J Cardiol 36:169, 1975
121. Detry JM, Kapita BM, Cosyns J et al.: Diagnostic value of history and maximal exercise electrocardiography in men and women suspected of coronary heart disease. Circulation 56:756, 1977
122. Profant GR, Early RG, Nilson KL, et al.: Responses to maximum exercise in healthy middle-aged women. J Appl Physiol 33:595, 1972
123. Wu S, Secchi MB, Radice M et al.: Sex differences in the prevalence of ischemic heart disease and in the response to a stress test in a working population. Eur Heart J 2:461, 1981
124. Linhart JW, Laws JG, Satinsky JD: Maximum treadmill exercise electrocardiography in female patients. Circulation 50:1173, 1974
125. Guiteras P, Chaitman BR, Waters DD et al.: Diagnostic accuracy of exercise ECG lead systems in clinical subsets of women. Circulation 65:1465, 1982
126. Chaitman BR: Improved efficiency of treadmill exercise testing using a multiple-lead ECG system and basic hemodynamic exercise response. Circulation 57:71, 1978
127. Barolsky SM, Gilbert CA, Faruqui A et al.: Differences in electrocardiographic response to exercise in women and men: a non-Baysian factor. Circulation 60:1021, 1979
128. Jaffe MD: Effect of oestrogens on postexercise electrocardiogram. Br Heart J 38:1299, 1977
129. Jaffe MD: Effect of testerone cypionate on postexercise ST segment depression. Br Heart J 39:1217, 1977
130. Kusumi F, Buce RA, Ross MA et al.: Elevated arterial pressure and post-exertional ST segment depression in middle-aged women. Am Heart J 92:576, 1976
131. Amsterdam EA, Price JE, Chin R et al.: Exercise stress testing in patients with angiographically normal coronary arteries: similar frequency of false positive ischemic responses in males and females. Am J Cardiol 41:378, 1978
132. Robert AR, Melin JA, Detry JM: Logistic discriminant analysis improves diagnostic accuracy of exercise testing for coronary artery disease in women. Circulation 83:1202, 1991
133. Demange J, Herpin D, Gaudeau B et al.: Improvement of the diagnostic value of exercise test by heart-rate adjusted segment depression. Value of ST 20/HR index. Arch Mal Coeur Vaiss 85:175, 1992
134. Morise AP, Duval RD: Accuracy of ST/heart rate index in the diagnosis of coronary artery disease. Am J Cardiol 69:603, 1992
135. Okin PM, Kligfield P: Identifying coronary artery disease in women by heart rate adjustment of ST-segment depression and improved performance of linear regression over simple averaging method with comparison to standard criteria. Am J Cardiol 69:297, 1992
136. Walling AD, Crawford MH: Exercise testing in women with chest pain: applications and limitations of computer analysis. Coron Artery Dis 4:783, 1993
137. Marwick T, Anderson T, Williams MJ et al.: Exercise echocardiography is an accurate and cost-efficient

137. [no content — continues from previous page] technique for the detection of coronary artery disease in women. J Am Coll Cardiol 26:335, 1995
138. Milliken JA, Abdollah H, Burggraf GW: False-positive treadmill exercise tests due to computer signal averaging. Am J Cardiol 65:946, 1990
139. Hollenberg M, Zoltick JM, Go M et al.: Comparison of a quantitative treadmill exercise score with standard electrocardiographic criteria in screening asymptomatic young men for coronary artery disease. N Engl J Med 313:600, 1985
140. Vergari J, Hakki AH, Heo J, Iskandrian AS: Merits and limitations of quantitative treadmill exercise score. Am Heart J 114:819, 1987
141. Detrano R, Salcedo E, Leatherman J, Day K: Computer-assisted versus unassisted analysis of the exercise electrocardiogram in patients without myocardial infarction. J Am Coll Cardiol 10:794, 1987
142. Ribisl PM, Liu J, Mousa I et al.: Comparison of computer ST criteria for diagnosis of severe coronary artery disease. Am J Cardiol 71:546, 1993
143. Okin PM, Kligfield P: Effect of precision of ST-segment measurement on identification and quantification of coronary artery disease by the ST/HR index. J Electrocardiol 24:62, 1992
144. Elamin M, Mary D, Smith D, Linden R: Prediction of severity of coronary artery disease using slope of submaximal ST segment/heart rate relationship. Cardiovasc Res 14:681, 1980
145. Kligfield P, Okin PM, Ameisen O, Borer JS: Evaluation of coronary artery disease by an improved method of exercise electrocardiography: the ST segment/heart rate slope. Am Heart J 112:589, 1986
146. Okin PM, Kligfield P: Effect of exercise protocol and lead selection on the accuracy of heart rate-adjusted indices of ST-segment depression for detection of three-vessel coronary artery disease. J Electrocardiol 22:187, 1989
147. Thwaites BC, Quyyumi AA, Raphael MJ et al.: Comparison of the ST/heart rate slope with the modified Bruce exercise test in the detection of coronary artery disease. Am J Cardiol 57:554, 1986
148. Kligfield P, Ameisen O, Okin PM: Heart rate adjustment of ST segment depression for improved detection of coronary artery disease. Circulation 79:245, 1989
149. Lachterman B, Lehmann KG, Detrano R et al.: Comparison of ST segment/heart rate index to standard ST criteria for analysis of exercise electrocardiogram. Circulation 82:44, 1990
150. Okin PM, Bergman G, Kligfield P: Effect of ST segment measurement point on performance of standard and heart rate-adjusted ST segment criteria for the identification of coronary artery disease. Circulation 84:57, 1991

Chapter 2

Principals and Methods of Myocardial Perfusion Imaging

Istvan Kosa, Sibylle Ziegler, Stephan Nekolla, and Markus Schwaiger

CORONARY ARTERY DISEASE AND MYOCARDIAL PERFUSION

Atherosclerotic coronary artery disease (CAD) limits coronary flow initially under stress and leads to ischemic symptoms under resting conditions only later in the disease, when normal coronary vasoregulation is exhausted. It is beyond the scope of this chapter to discuss in detail the physiology and pathophysiology of myocardial perfusion, which can be found in several recent reviews.[1-3] However, a brief physiologic framework will be provided to allow for a better understanding of various imaging approaches for the assessment of myocardial perfusion.

Normal Coronary Physiology

The myocardium is almost totally dependent on aerobic metabolism, and therefore oxygen delivery. Thus, the ability of coronary circulation to autoregulate is essential for the heart to respond to changing metabolic demands.[1] The major epicardial coronary vessels contribute little to coronary vascular resistance and act primarily as conductance vessels;[4,5] most of resistance to coronary blood flow arises from the smaller intramural coronary vessels.[6] Certain stimuli, for example hypoxia, relax the smooth muscle of these arterioles, thereby increasing coronary blood flow.[7] The principal mediator of this mechanism is thought to be adenosine, resulting from the metabolism of adenosine triphosphate (ATP),[8] although the role of numerous endothelium-derived vasoactive substances, such as prostacyclin,[9] endothelial-derived relaxing factor-nitric oxide,[10,11] and endothelial-derived hyperpolarizing factor,[12] have recently been discussed.

In healthy young people, maximal vasodilation of these small arterioles provoked by exogenous vasodilators may augment coronary flow to more than three times the resting flow.[13-20] Gould has used the term coronary flow reserve to describe this relative change.[21] This parameter is widely used to characterize the functional extent and severity of CAD. Most perfusion imaging approaches determine the relative coronary reserve, based on comparison of blood flow changes in different myocardial segments. Maximal coronary vasodilation can be achieved with transient coronary occlusion, with intravenous dipyridamole or adenosine administration, or with intracoronary papaverine injection.[16,22] However, not all alterations of flow reserve are due to coronary stenoses; for example, a significant relationship between coronary reserve measurement and age in subjects without CAD has been demonstrated.[23] However, considering hemodynamic parameters such as blood pressure and heart rate, the decreased coronary reserve values in elderly persons may be primarily due to increased resting blood flow, as a consequence of higher heart rate and blood pressure in this patient population.

Clinical Manifestations of CAD

Atherosclerosis is a progressive disease that becomes morphologically manifest only decades after its initiation.[24] According to the most accepted theory of atherogenesis, intimal alteration develops as a response to injuries to the vascular endothelium. The first visible alterations are fatty streaks,[25] which contain foam cells that accumulate large amounts of intracellular lipid and a small number of T lymphocytes.[3] Flow-limiting coronary stenoses are most likely to occur when fatty streaks progress, through platelet adherence and growth factor release, to mature plaques.[26,27] The composition of nonruptured atheromatous plaques is highly variable, reflecting various processes of smooth muscle cell migration and cholesterol accumulation.[28,29]

Early Changes of Blood Flow

In patients with severe CAD in other vascular territories, recent studies have reported a pathological decrease of coronary reserve capacity in regions supplied by angiographically normal epicardial arteries.[30-33] Moreover, patients without clinical evidence of myocardial ischemia, but high risk for the development of CAD based on risk factor profile, have shown an attenuated response to adenosine as assessed by positron emission tomography (PET).[34] The mechanism of this reduction of coronary flow reserve in angiographically normal vessels is not known yet, but may represent the interplay of vascular alterations as well as endothelial dysfunction caused by pharmacologically induced changes in blood flow.[33] If this is so, blood flow measurements may therefore serve as sensitive means to detect CAD before angiographically detectable disease is apparent.

Stable Angina Syndromes

Patients with chronic stable angina usually have critical stenoses of one or more coronary arteries.[24] Because of normal vasoregulation, the enhanced coronary resistance caused by stenosis of major epicardial coronary arteries is compensated by vasodilation of small arteries, maintaining near normal levels of blood flow at rest until a stenosis narrows the lumen by more than 85%.[35] Because this mechanism exploits part of coronary reserve capacity, following administration of vasodilators, the flow reserve in such poststenotic segments is reduced in comparison to normal segments.

According to experimental data derived from a dog model, coronary flow reserve measurements allow for detection of coronary stenosis of about 40 to 50% using a microsphere technique.[35] To noninvasively assess relative flow distribution under rest and stress conditions in humans, imaging methods have become a validated and accepted approach to detect and characterize regional CAD. However, in patients with diffusely decreased coronary reserve due to multivessel disease, absolute flow measurement at stress and rest may be necessary to evaluate regional coronary flow reserve and to functionally define the severity of CAD.

Acute Ischemic Syndromes

Acute ischemic syndromes are caused predominantly by coronary thrombi initiated by the rupture of an atherosclerotic plaque.[36] The clinical presentation of plaque rupture depends on the extent of coronary thrombus formation. Unstable angina, acute myocardial infarction, and sudden cardiac death are possible consequences, which are related to the severity of acute flow reduction in the affected territory.[37]

The timing of plaque rupture is not predictable, although it is known that plaques with high lipid and macrophage content have a greater likelihood of rupture.[28,38,39] While the currently available noninvasive tests are unable to identify such vulnerable plaques, the development of intravascular ultrasound has allowed the assessment of plaque morphology and composition.[40-43] Because plaques causing severe stenosis tend to have a higher fibrous and lower lipid content than those producing less severe lesions,[44-46] a significant part of stenoses considered *insignificant* by diagnostic tests may be prone to later abrupt progression. This hypothesis is supported by the results of Ambrose and Giroud, who studied conservatively treated patients with known coronary morphology, who underwent recatheterization after developing an acute ischemic syndrome. In more than two-thirds of cases, the culprit lesion was in coronary segments that were judged on a previous coronary angiogram to be insignificant.[47,48] These observations may have important consequences for the prognostic evaluation of patients with CAD using stress perfusion studies. Regional myocardial perfusion data may not predict a given patient's risk of suffering acute myocardial infarction.[49] On the other hand, numerous studies (reviewed subsequently by Machecourt and co-authors) have indicated the clinical role of perfusion imaging in the functional assessment of the extent and severity of CAD, and to assess prognostically the consequences of acute myocardial infarction.

Chronically Insufficient Blood Supply at Rest

Severe coronary stenosis may limit the blood supply of the myocardium even under resting conditions, and reduced resting blood flow has been reported in patients with severe CAD using a variety of methods. However, the presence of "chronic ischemia" remains a controversial issue. The term "hibernating myocardium" has been introduced to characterize chronically hypoperfused, dysfunctional myocardium, which recovers function after restoration of perfusion.[50,51] Hibernating myocardium represents a state of reduced blood flow without evidence of ischemia (on the basis of electrocardiographic [ECG] changes, symptoms, or lactate production), but with downregulation of myocardial function. The "sine qua non" of viable cells in dysfunctional myocardium is the presence of residual metabolic activity sufficient to support the integrity of cell membranes.[52] Besides metabolic markers, the relative degree of hypoperfusion as assessed by PET or single photon emission computed tomography (SPECT) may contribute to the clinical differentiation between hibernating and scar tissue.[53,54]

In patients with previous myocardial infarction due to early spontaneous or therapeutic revascularization, a cell injury may not involve the entire vascular territory. The consequence of the acute ischemic injury is often a mixture of viable myocardial cells interlaced with necrotic myocardium (which eventually is replaced by connective tissue). The ratio of viable and necrotic tissue is heterogeneous from region to region, according to the differences of oxygen deficit resulting in a patchy pattern of cell injury.[55,56] Since a transmural gradient of cell damage exists in most patients with previous myocardial infarction, imaging with a high spatial resolution would be required to resolve transmural perfusion heterogeneity. Unfortunately, scintigraphic techniques do not provide sufficient spatial resolution even in combination with gated data acquisition to measure transmural perfusion gradients at the present time. However, scintigraphic data provide an average measurement of flow and metabolism across the myocardial wall, and these data have shown to be useful to predict functional recovery after revascularization and to assess prognosis. The major objective of noninvasive imaging for detection of residual viable tissue is to assist in the improved selection of patients with advanced CAD who benefit most from revascularization. This important clinical issue is discussed in Chapters 20 and 21.

Methods of Measuring Coronary Blood Flow

Although coronary arteriosclerosis is a disease of the coronary artery wall, the consequences are determined by the degree of regional flow restriction by atherosclerotic plaques. The assessment of myocardial blood flow by various techniques plays an important role in the understanding and management of CAD. The invasive and noninvasive methods available for assessment of myocardial blood flow can be classified according to whether they permit absolute or relative measurements of flow. While absolute determinations are necessary for independent characterization of regional blood flow under different conditions, relative measurements allow the comparison of blood flow in different regions in different hemodynamic situations. The latter techniques have proven useful for the clinical application of perfusion imaging.

Invasive Methods of Measuring Coronary Blood Flow

Relative flow distribution may be assessed using quantitative digital subtraction angiography. This measures the changes of absorption, transit times, and myocardial washout after injection of contrast medium.[57] Performance of these measurements at rest and after maximal vasodilation has been shown to provide indices of coronary vascular reserve without the need to compute absolute values of coronary flow at rest and stress.[58]

Absolute coronary flow measurement may be performed invasively, using thermodilution, Doppler, or nuclear methodologies. Historically, timed venous collections from the great cardiac vein, which primarily drains the myocardium supplied by the left anterior descending (LAD) coronary artery, were used to measure coronary flow.[59] Currently, coronary sinus thermodilution[60] and intracoronary Doppler flow measurement[22] are the preferred invasive methods for quantification of coronary flow and flow velocity in humans; discussion of intracoronary Doppler evaluation of coronary disease significance is supplied in Chapter 16. The use of inert gases, such as helium, xenon-133, and krypton-85 with determination of arterial and coronary sinus gas concentrations has only limited applications today because of the necessary intracoronary application and complicated radioactivity measurements[61] The shortcomings of these invasive methods are extensively reviewed elsewhere.[62]

Noninvasive Methods of Measuring Coronary Blood Flow

Tracer approaches for the measurement of relative flow distribution were initially introduced in the early 1970s.[63] Currently, myocardial perfusion scintigraphy with thallium-201 (^{201}Tl)- or technetium-99m (^{99m}Tc)-labeled radiopharmaceuticals is the most widely used imaging method for the clinical evaluation of myocardial blood supply. Modern tomographic imaging approaches, such as SPECT and PET, visualize the relative tracer accumulation in myocardial regions as compared to a reference region with maximal tracer accumulation. Such techniques have been shown to provide high accuracy in detection of CAD, for evaluation of coronary interventions, and allow for prognostic evaluation of patients with known or suspected CAD.

Absolute coronary blood flow measurements may be performed with PET. Data acquisition with attenuation correction allows accurate measurement of myocardial radiotracer distribution. Current systems with dynamic acquisition generate data with high temporal resolution, appropriate for the description of tracer kinetics in myocardial and vascular structures. Such PET measurements can be used to determine noninvasively myocardial blood flow in milliliter per minute per 100 g heart tissue by applying suitable tracer kinetic models.

MYOCARDIAL PERFUSION IMAGING USING CONVENTIONAL NUCLEAR CARDIOLOGY

Flow Tracers

The optimal radionuclide for perfusion imaging by gamma camera should have minimal particulate radiation, a photon energy about 140 keV, and a physical half-life of a few hours necessary for tracer preparation and imaging time. These requirements are currently best met by ^{99m}Tc. However, the appropriate ^{99m}Tc-radiopharmaceuticals for myocardial perfusion scintigraphy became available only in recent years. In its place, ^{201}Tl has been the most widely used radionuclide for myocardial perfusion scintigraphy. This has been used for nearly 2 decades, and represents a clinically accepted and extensively validated flow tracer.

Thallium-201

Physical Characteristics

^{201}Tl is a cyclotron-produced radionuclide that decays by electron capture to mercury-201, and has a half-life of approximately 73.0 hours. On decay, the major emissions are characteristic x-ray of the daughter product, mercury-201, that have an energy range of 69 to 81 keV. ^{201}Tl also emits gamma rays at energies of 167 keV (8%) and 135 keV (2%).

The physical characteristics of ^{201}Tl pose a number of disadvantages for myocardial perfusion imaging. Because ^{201}Tl is not available as a generator product, it requires regular supply every 1 to 2 days to the nuclear medicine laboratory. Its half-life of 73 hours limits the applicable dose to 1 to 3 mCi, with a whole body radiation exposure of 0.21 rads/mCi.[64] Because the majority of emitted radiation has a relatively low energy, a great part of radiation originating from the heart is absorbed by overlying soft tissue. The attenuation coefficient, namely the probability that the emitted photons will be absorbed traveling a certain distance through an absorbent material is 0.18/cm in water[65] (the corresponding value for ^{99m}Tc is 0.15/cm).

Biokinetics

^{201}Tl is a group IIIA metallic element. Since the crystal radii of positive ^{201}Tl and potassium ions are comparable (1.44 and 1.33 Å, respectively), the passive cell membrane transport is similar for these two ions.[66] In cell cultures, approximately 50% of ^{201}Tl influx is blocked by the Na/K-ATPase inhibitor oubain.[67,68] The apparent K_m for Tl$^+$ binding to this protein is approximately 900 times greater than the K_m for K$^+$, explaining the high extraction efficiency of Tl$^+$ by myocardium, despite low blood concentrations.[67] This fraction of Tl$^+$ influx is energy dependent and, hence, requires sufficient cellular ATP concentration. The results of cellular[67] and clinical studies[69–72] support the suitability of Tl$^+$ not only as a flow marker but also as a marker for cell membrane integrity. An additional transport mechanism consistent with the K$^+$ binding site of the Na/K/2Cl transport protein has been identified, which is inhibited with bumetanide.[68] Approximately 30% to 40% of Tl$^+$ influx appears insensitive to transport inhibitors or metabolic blockade.[67,68] This non-energy-dependent association of Tl$^+$ with cellular proteins and membrane elements probably explains nonspecific binding of this tracer to severely injured cells.[73,74] The myocardial extraction fraction of ^{201}Tl determined over physiological flow rates (0.5 to 3.5 ml/min/g) varies between 90% and 68%. It declines with increasing blood flow, due to diffusion limitation at the capillary level during higher flow rates.[75,76] At physiologic flow rates, however, there is a positive linear relationship between the tracer uptake and flow because the increase in flow is proportionally greater than the relatively smaller fall in extraction[77] (Fig. 2-1).

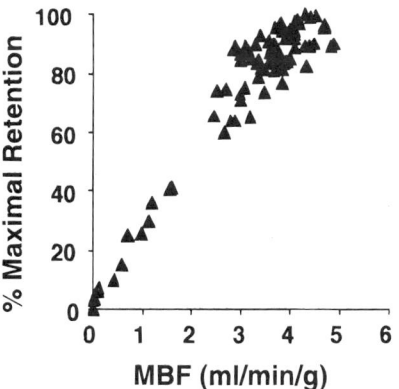

Fig. 2-1. ^{201}Tl absolute retention versus microsphere-determined myocardial blood flow at 5 minutes after tracer injection in open-chested dog model. (From Melon et al.,[77] with permission.)

During resting conditions in a "no recirculation" animal model, the intrinsic washout of ^{201}Tl from myocardial cells shows a $t_{1/2}$ value between 50 and 70 min.[78] A detailed analysis of washout curves describes an early rapid component, with a $t_{1/2}$ of 2.25 minutes, attributed to the ^{201}Tl washout from the interstitial compartment. However, because 93% of injected ^{201}Tl is cleared slowly from myocardial cells, the interstitial washout component is hardly appreciable by slow imaging techniques. The intrinsic washout of ^{201}Tl shows a marked prolongation up to 300 minutes as coronary perfusion pressure is reduced to below 60 mmHg,[78] but net washout accelerates with increasing blood flow.[77] Cellular metabolic dysfunction, independent of blood flow, has little effect on initial capillary–tissue exchange of ^{201}Tl but affects clearance of this tracer.[76] In an animal investigation, Wilson et al. demonstrated that net ^{201}Tl clearance can be accelerated by glucose–insulin–potassium infusion predominantly in postischemic tissue,[79] and by ribose infusion in nonischemic regions.[80] This latter method can be utilized in human investigations to accelerate ^{201}Tl redistribution,[81,82] this being an alternative to 24 hour redistribution imaging with ^{201}Tl.[82]

^{201}Tl Redistribution

The net myocardial ^{201}Tl uptake after intravenous ^{201}Tl administration is considerably influenced by tracer recirculation (Fig. 2-2). However, as consequence of its high extraction, blood ^{201}Tl activity clears rapidly after intravenous (IV) injection of tracer (91.5% of maximal blood activity disappear with a $t_{1/2}$ of about 5 minutes). Because of slow excretion of the isotope from body (only about 4% of total body activity is excreted daily in the urine without significant fecal excretion), a significant blood activity persists for many days (body $t_{1/2}$ of about 40 hours).[64] From this constant ^{201}Tl blood supply the Na/K pump—due to its great affinity for ^{201}Tl—continuously incorporates the isotope into the myocardial cells, which thereafter equilibrates between cellular and vascular space in accordance with its washout rate. The dynamic balance of extraction and washout results in a net myocardial washout having a $t_{1/2}$ value of about 5 to 7 hours in the normal heart.[83] If the distribution of blood flow changes after the initial ^{201}Tl extraction, this dynamic balance shifts in accordance to the new situation. The

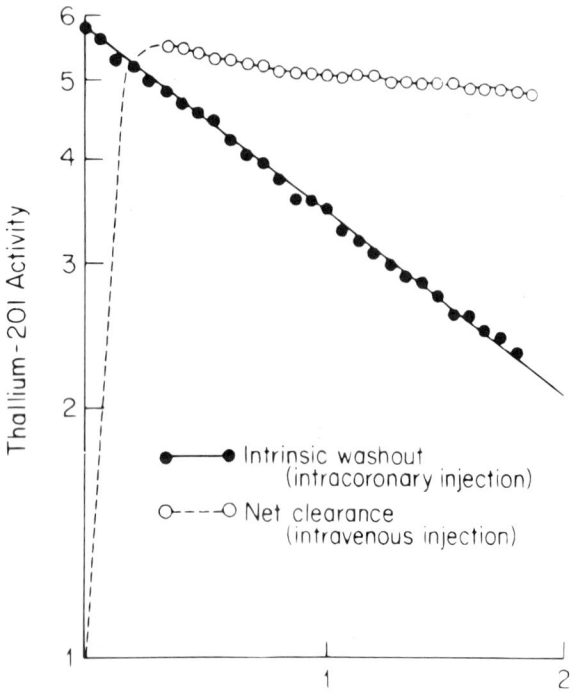

Fig. 2-2. ^{201}Tl net uptake after intracoronary and intravenous tracer injection. (From Grunwald et al.,[78] with permission.)

redistribution process depends on ^{201}Tl blood levels, the regional ^{201}Tl concentration gradient between tissue and vascular space and the regional blood flow. However, redistribution can occur only if the myocardial segment supplied by given stenotic artery contains viable cells.

For the clinical detection of reversible perfusion defects, a 3 to 4 hours redistribution ^{201}Tl imaging protocol has been widely employed.[84] However, in segments with severe perfusion defects and a high degree of coronary stenosis, the process of redistribution is slowed. Prolonged imaging protocols (24 hours) and reinjection imaging protocols have been introduced to enhance the sensitivity of the test to detect reversibility of perfusion defects. Reinjection of 1 mCi ^{201}Tl 3 to 4 hours after stress injection leads to increased ^{201}Tl blood levels supporting the process of redistribution. Reinjection protocols, discussed in more detail in Chapters 20 and 22, are the most commonly used approaches for detection of viable myocardium. Standard redistribution imaging prior to reinjection imaging has been advocated.[85] In recent studies, a minimum delay of 30 to 60 minutes between resting administration or reinjection of ^{201}Tl and imaging has been recommended.[86,87]

^{99m}Tc-Labeled Radiopharmaceuticals

Physical Characteristics

^{99m}Tc-emitted photons have an energy of 143 keV, optimal for camera imaging. This higher energy results in greater penetrability, giving an attenuation coefficient of 0.15/cm, measured in water.[65] Its half-life of 6.03 hours allows the administration of a greater dose of ^{99m}Tc-marked tracer, producing excellent image statistics while keeping the applied radiation dose low. The molybdenum-99/technetium-99m generator (which has a half-life of 67 hours) permits the continuous availability of ^{99m}Tc in nuclear medicine laboratories.

Biokinetics of ^{99m}Tc-MIBI

The first widely used blood flow tracer utilizing the favorable physical characteristics of ^{99m}Tc was hexakis-2-methoxy-2-isobutyl-isonitrile (MIBI).[88] The cellular uptake of ^{99m}Tc-MIBI in myocardium is passively related to the electrochemical gradient generated at the cell membrane level. As a consequence of its lipophilic cationic nature, ^{99m}Tc-MIBI is sufficiently hydrophobic to partition into bilayer cell membranes, but also contains a delocalized charge distributed throughout the molecule, thereby allowing passive translocation across the membrane in proportion to an imposed transmembrane potential.[68] This electrochemical potential concentrates ^{99m}Tc-MIBI in the cytosol relative to extracellular space. Because myocardial cells contain a substantial number of mitochondria that generate a large negative potential across the inner mitochondrial membrane, both potentials contribute a large driving force for its sequestration within the mitochondrial inner matrix. In cultured chick heart, Piwnica-Worms et al. found a intracellular/extracellular concentration gradient as high as 30-fold to 50-fold.[68] At the same time they proved the membrane potential dependency of ^{99m}Tc-MIBI accumulation in these cells. By depolarizing the cell membrane with 130 mM K buffer, the 60 minute net uptake of ^{99m}Tc-MIBI was decrease from 170.7 ± 115.5 to 28.7 ± 13.3 fmol/mg*protein*nM. In addition, the ^{99m}Tc-

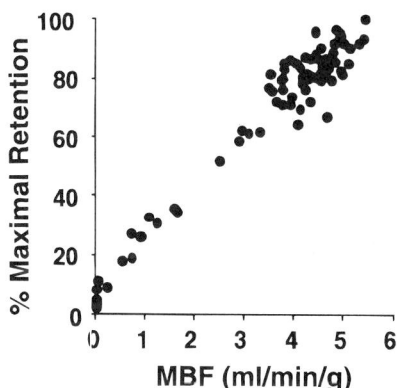

Fig. 2-3. ^{99m}Tc-MIBI absolute retention versus microsphere-determined myocardial blood flow at 5 minutes after tracer injection in open-chested dog model. (From Melon et al.,[77] with permission.)

MIBI initially accumulated in 5.4 mM K buffer was depleted by subsequent exposure to high K buffer.

The uptake of ^{99m}Tc-MIBI in myocardial cells is about 10 times the uptake in fibroblast cell cultures.[89] The factors contributing to this difference are the greater plasma membrane and mitochondrial potential of myocardial cells[89,90] and the greater mitochondrial volume of myocardial cells. The myocardial extraction fraction of ^{99m}Tc-MIBI, like ^{201}Tl, decreases with increasing flow rates, with in an isolated heart model varying between 0.71 and 0.37, depending on flow.[91] Thus, the flow effect on ^{99m}Tc-MIBI tissue uptake is more pronounced than it is with ^{201}Tl. Net tissue retention tends to plateau at flow levels greater than 2.5 ml/min/g, but as with ^{201}Tl, the positive relationship of tracer flux and flow is retained by ^{99m}Tc-MIBI (Fig. 2-3).[77]

The blood clearance of ^{99m}Tc-MIBI in humans is determined by rapid biliary excretion. About 20% of injected dose (ID) accumulates in the liver at 5 minutes after injection, from which it clears quickly into the gallbladder. The gallbladder activity peaks at about 60 minutes. This rapid excretion causes continuous withdrawal of tracer from the vascular space. As a consequence, the blood activity shows after a fast early clearance component (the $t_{1/2}$ is 2.2 minutes) with a moderate, but continuous decrease. The measured blood activity at 10 minutes is still about 2.5% of ID; at 60 minutes it decreases to 1%, and at 24 hours to 0.3% of ID.[88] Because the myocardial membrane potential does not support a concentration gradient greater than 30-fold to 50-fold[68] myocardial net tracer extraction ceases several minutes after injection.

In isolated rat hearts, ^{99m}Tc-MIBI shows an intrinsic washout rate of 0.0071 min^{-1} under normal conditions equivalent to a washout $t_{1/2}$ of 98 minutes).[92] In human investigations using imaging approaches, the net washout seems to be much slower, as discussed in Chapter 20. Franceschi et al. observed a 27% reduction in myocardial activity after ^{99m}Tc-MIBI stress injection during a 6-hour period in normal myocardium. These investigators noted different washout rates of normal and ischemic segments (27 ± 18% and 16 ± 16%, respectively) leading to reduced activity differences between normal and hypoperfused segments as a function of time. These results are in agreement with animal data of Melon et al., which demonstrated an acceleration of washout with increasing flow. However, during the 20-minute observation period of this investigation, the positive correlation of net myocardial tracer uptake and blood flow was retained in spite of increasing washout. The relatively stable tissue retention of MIBI provides unique advantages of this tracer, since imaging can be delayed several hours after injection. The distribution of regional tracer retention reflects even at a later time point the relative blood flow values at the time of injection.[88]

Biokinetics of ^{99m}Tc-Tetrofosmin

Tetrofosmin is the first of ^{99m}Tc- marked diphosphines to become commercially available for perfusion imaging. Like MIBI it is a cationic ^{99m}Tc- complex, with similar heart uptake and retention and blood clearance kinetics but significantly faster clearance from both lung and liver.[93] In a dog model involving left anterior descending occlusion, Sinusas et al. demonstrated the effect of diffusion limitation at flow values exceeding 2.0 ml/min/g using pharmacological stress.[94] After normalization to values in a nonischemic region they found a correlation coefficient of 0.87 between myocardial ^{99m}Tc-tetrofosmin activity and microsphere flow (Fig. 2-4). The blood clearance of ^{99m}Tc-tetrofosmin is rapid, showing less than 5% of the injected activity in the whole blood volume by 10 minutes.[93] After stress injection, the blood clearance of ^{99m}Tc-tetrofosmin is further ac-

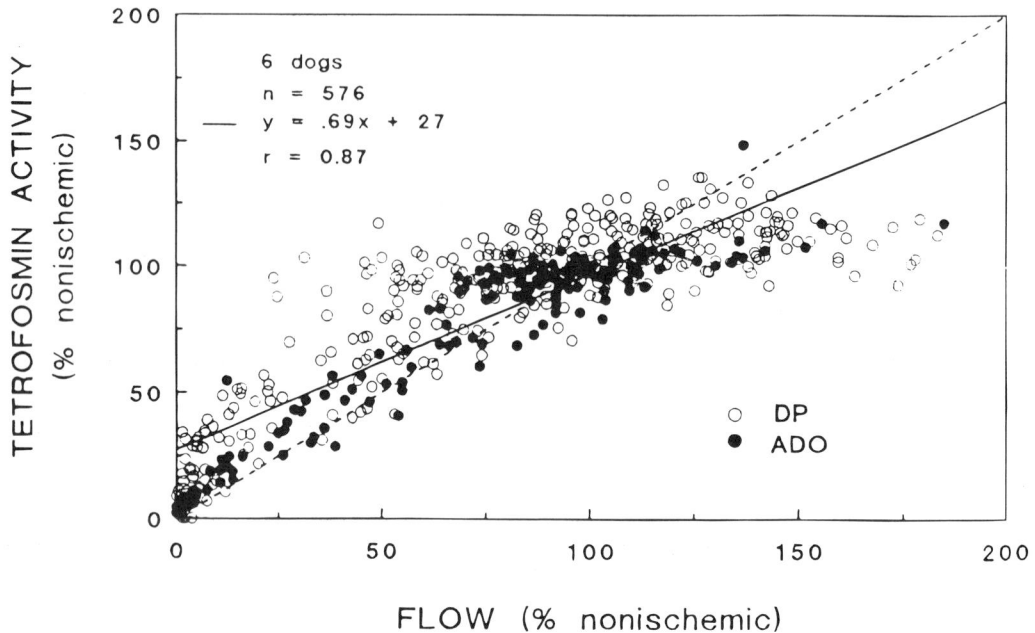

Fig. 2-4. ^{99m}Tc-tetrofosmin activity and microsphere flow normalized to nonischemic values. A total of 576 segments in six experiments. (From Sinusas et al.,[94] with permission.)

celerated, due to the affinity of the complex for skeletal muscle, which consumes a greater proportion of the cardiac output during stress.

^{99m}Tc-tetrofosmin has a notable urinary excretion accounting for 13% and 9% of injected dose at 2 hours after stress and rest injection, respectively. Fecal clearance is of roughly similar importance, resulting in a whole-body clearance at 48 hours of 72 ± 6% at rest and 67 ± 6% after exercise.[93] Due to the moderate liver activity observed after tracer injection, Jain et al. proposed starting the acquisition 5 to 10 minutes after stress and 30 to 45 minutes after rest injection of the tracer.[95] On the other hand, Schroter et al. found the heart-to-liver organ ratio very similar during the first 20 minutes after stress injection of ^{99m}Tc-MIBI and ^{99m}Tc-tetrofosmin in a clinical study (Fig. 2-5).[96]

Biokinetics of ^{99m}Tc-Teboroxime

^{99m}Tc-teboroxime is a highly lipophilic, neutral boron tris oxime compound. Its proposed mode of myocardial uptake is based solely on the ability to partition into a nonaqueous environment,[97,98] behaving purely as flow tracer. The depletion of cellular ATP stores with carbonylcyanide m-chlorophenyl hydrazone (CCCP) does not significantly influence its accumulation in cultured chick heart cells.[99] As a consequence of its nonspecific binding, in contrast to ^{201}Tl and ^{99m}Tc-MIBI, it also accumulates in relation to flow in necrotic tissue.[97]

^{99m}Tc-teboroxime shows greater myocardial extraction fraction than ^{201}Tl and the effect of diffusion limitation appears only at high flow values (> 4.0 ml/min/g). The measured extraction values at flows between 0.5 and 3.5 ml/min/g are between 0.75 and 0.94.[100] The blood clearance of ^{99m}Tc-teboroxime is rapid and biexponential, with a first $t_{1/2}$ of 0.8 minutes (88%) and a second of 2.5 hours (12%).[101] The small quantity of teboroxime remaining in the blood is altered into a form that does not undergo reuptake by the heart.[102,103] The process responsible for this decreasing uptake may be substitution of the chloro with the hydroxyl group on the technetium atom of teboroxime. Another explanation for this change is the time-dependent increase in the affinity of teboroxime for blood cells and plasma proteins.[103]

The biexponential myocardial clearance of ^{99m}Tc-teboroxime in patient studies is dominated by its first

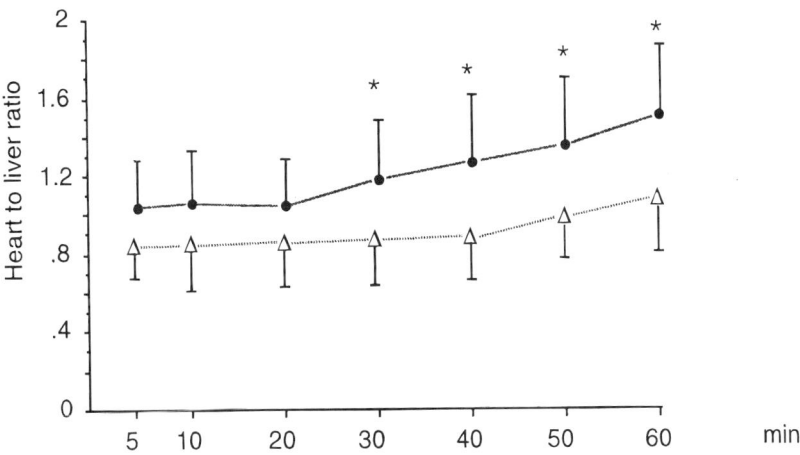

Fig. 2-5. Heart-to-liver activity ratio in dynamic planar images of 12 patients after stress injection of ^{99m}Tc-tetrofosmin and ^{99m}-MIBI, respectively (* $p < 0.05$).

phase, showing a half-life between 10 and 15 minutes. At 60 minutes postinjection, little activity remains in the heart.[104] Furthermore, ^{99m}Tc-teboroxime washout is more rapid in "high flow" than in "low flow" regions (Fig. 2-6).[105,106] The initial pattern of myocardial ^{99m}Tc-teboroxime uptake changes rapidly due to early redistribution.[107] The rapid kinetics of ^{99m}Tc-teboroxime posed a challenge to the temporal resolution of imaging protocols—SPECT requires a multihead data acquisition with short frame durations. On the other hand, animal,[108,109] and preliminary human studies[110,111] demonstrate that this differential washout can be utilized in detecting significant coronary stenosis. In a dog model, Stewart et al. observed a prolongation of myocardial clearance during adenosine infusion in regions supplied by stenosed arteries in comparison to normal myocardial regions (11.2 ± 3.7 versus 6.3 ± 1.5 min; $p < 0.05$).[108] This differential washout can be used to detect poststenotic perfusion abnormalities in dogs with a sensitivity, specificity and diagnostic accuracy of 62%, 100%, and 81%, respectively. Chiao et al.[110] used a two-compartment model for fitting of dynamic teboroxime SPECT data to characterize the kinetics of ^{99m}Tc-teboroxime from the blood to the myocardium (k^1) and from the myocardium to the blood (k_2). Using this method, they demonstrated a significant increase of teboroxime uptake and clearance (stress/rest values 2.7 ± 1.1 and 1.5 ± 0.3, respectively) in humans during adenosine-induced coronary vasodilation. Nonetheless, although ^{99m}Tc-teboroxime displays excellent physiologic properties, its rapid tissue clearance limits widespread clinical application using standard SPECT imaging approaches. High temporal resolution imaging is needed to take advantage of the high initial extraction of this tracer, and rapidly changing activity levels in normal and ischemic myocardium following tracer injection limit the application of standard tomographic imaging protocols for detection of CAD.

Other ^{99m}Tc-Labeled Pharmaceuticals

Numerous new ^{99m}Tc flow tracers are currently under investigation. The clinical value of these tracers is not yet defined. Furifosmin,[112] Q12,[113,114] and Q3[114] belong to the group of phosphins, like tetrofosmin. NOET[115–117] is a neutral lipophilic nitrido complex that displays redistribution kinetics like ^{201}Tl. The clinical place of each of these agents remains to be defined.

Imaging Protocols

Various imaging protocols have been proposed depending on tracer selection and clinical objective (Fig. 2-7). The prime goal of these protocols is to delineate accurately the location, extent, and severity of stress-induced perfusion defects as well as to define their reversibility. Many of the protocols are also used to define the extent of viable tissue, and

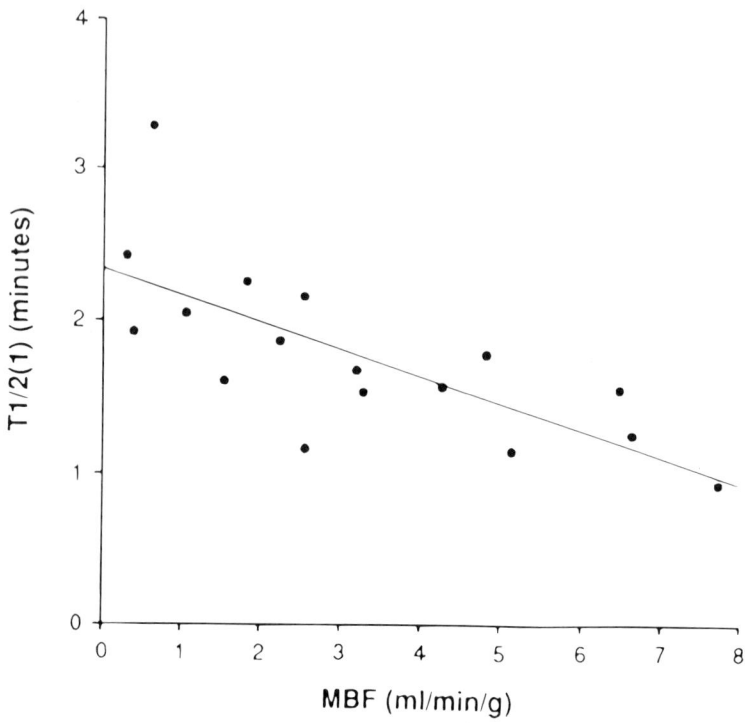

Fig. 2-6. Clearance half-time of the ^{99m}Tc-teboroxime versus mean myocardial tissue blood flow in open-chested dogs. $r = 0.72$, $P = 0.001$. (From Stewart et al.,[106] with permission.)

are discussed further in a subsequent chapter. Cost and throughput considerations favor imaging protocols that can be completed within a few hours.

^{201}Tl Protocols

Stress Redistribution

The classical ^{201}Tl protocol consists of a stress injection of 2 to 3 mCi ^{201}Tl with immediate stress acquisition and a redistribution imaging performed 3 to 4 hours later (Fig. 2-7a). Because of the phenomenon of redistribution, commencement of imaging within 20 minutes of tracer injection at peak stress is crucial in this protocol.[84,118] However, initiation of SPECT imaging too early after stress may increase the incidence of motion artifacts due to hyperventilation ("upward creep").[119] Completion of a standard stress-redistribution study takes about 5 to 6 hours. Recent studies have shown that this redistribution protocol leads to significant underestimation of viable tissue.[120,121]

Stress 4 Hour and Late Redistribution

To increase the diagnostic accuracy of ^{201}Tl to detect viable tissue in regions with fixed 4-hour redistribution defects, late imaging was proposed 24 to 72 hours after stress tracer injection (Fig. 2-7b).[122-124] However, this time delay is inconvenient for patients and affects image quality.

Stress Redistribution–Reinjection

As an alternative to delayed imaging, Dilsizian proposed to perform a third data acquisition 10 to 15 min after resting reinjection of 1 mCi ^{201}Tl, administered immediately after the completion of the 4-hour redistribution imaging (Fig. 2-7c).[54] The need for three acquisitions and the timing of the reinjection are a subject of some controversy. Dilsizian et al. demonstrated that early (10 to 15 minutes) imaging after the ^{201}Tl reinjection cannot be used as a substitute for redistribution imaging.[85] Early images delineate resting perfusion defects in regions supplied

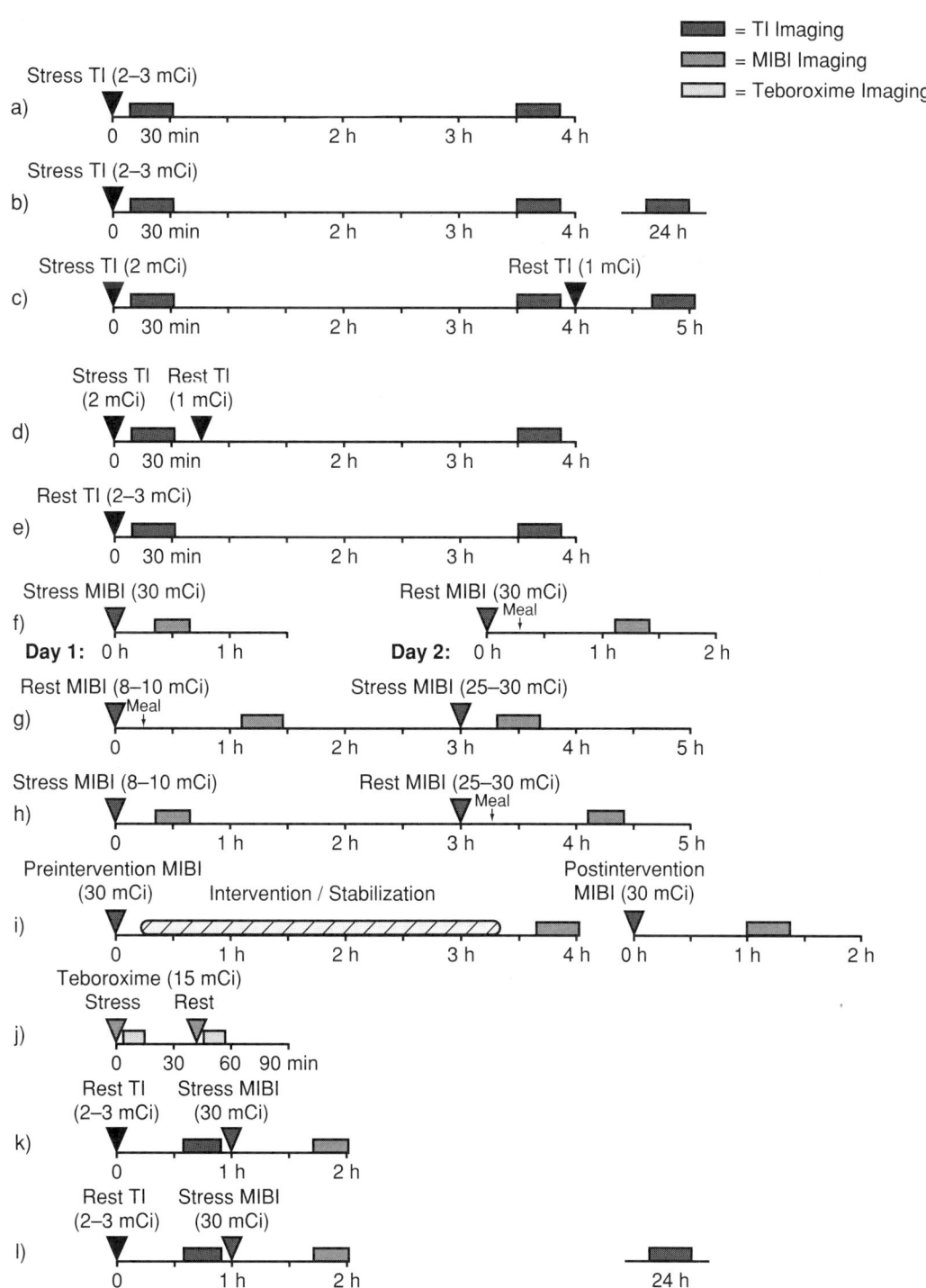

Fig. 2-7. (a–l) Imaging protocols with ^{201}Tl- and ^{99m}Tc-labeled pharmaceuticals in the evaluation of patients with suspected or known CAD.

by severely stenosed or occluded arteries, which can normalize at later imaging.

Stress Reinjection

Galli et al. proposed the reinjection of ^{201}Tl immediately after stress imaging, with repeat imaging 4 hours later (Fig. 2-7d).[125] They found clinically negligible differences between images acquired 4 and 24 hours after resting injection of ^{201}Tl (in only 3% of 94 patients). The reinjection of ^{201}Tl immediately after the completion of stress acquisition and repeated acquisition 60 minutes after this resting injection was proposed by van Eck-Smit et al. to further reduce imaging time.[87] In patients with anterior wall myocardial infarction, the results of such 60-minute resting and imaging 4 hours after resting injection of ^{201}Tl showed high concordance (0.97). The stress/reinjection protocols combine the identification of stress-induced perfusion defects and hibernating myocardium. The advantage of these methods is to delineate all regions that can benefit from a revascularization procedure (ischemic burden).

Rest Redistribution

The preferred protocol with ^{201}Tl for assessment of hibernating myocardium is rest/redistribution imaging (Fig. 2-7e). With this protocol, hibernating myocardium is characterized by reduced ^{201}Tl uptake on initial images (because of reduced regional myocardial resting blood flow) with redistribution on late images due to net accumulation of ^{201}Tl in viable segments.[126,127] However, clinically important, reversible resting wall motion abnormalities in severe CAD may not only represent myocardial hibernation, but also repeated periods of myocardial stunning, a condition that is coupled with normal resting blood flow. Accordingly, the demonstration of myocardial uptake of ^{201}Tl in regions of wall motion abnormality defines viability independent of a reversibility criteria. For this purpose, delayed imaging after resting ^{201}Tl injection seems to be clinically sufficient if the relative regional ^{201}Tl uptake is considered. A threshold of greater than 50% of maximal ^{201}Tl activity has been proposed as a marker of tissue viability.[72]

^{99m}Tc-Labeled Pharmaceuticals without Significant Washout

^{99m}Tc-MIBI and ^{99m}Tc-tetrofosmin allow delayed imaging protocols without the risk of losing information regarding blood flow distribution at the time of injection. On the other hand, these tracers require separate injections under rest and stress conditions. If the primary indication of stress perfusion scintigraphy is the diagnosis of CAD, it appears to be more practical to begin with stress imaging, as a negative result may not require a second resting control. If both injections are needed, they can be performed according to the "separate-day" or "1-day" protocol.

Separate-Day Protocols

Because of the 6-hour physical half-life of technetium, less than 6% of initial activity can be detected after 24 hours. As the myocardial activity is further decreased by a slow washout of tracers, a 2-day protocol is optimal for avoiding residual tracer activity from previous injection. Recommended doses range between 25 and 30 mCi for both rest and stress imaging, exploiting the potential of good count statistics for both image sets (Fig. 2-7f). Stress image acquisition may be started as early as 15 minutes after the exercise injection, minimizing hepatobiliary or gastrointestinal interference and avoiding the need to give milk or a fatty meal prior to imaging (Fig. 2-7f).[128] Due to the different organ–blood distribution at rest, imaging after the resting injection requires a 60 to 90-minute waiting period and administration of milk 15 minutes before imaging to clear gallbladder activity. Although in cases of normal first day stress results, no second day study is necessary, the initial uncertainty as to when the diagnostic procedure will be completed, and the possible image acquisition on the second day are still inconveniences for both the patient and the referring physician.

One-Day Protocols

The 1 day protocol requires a dose increment for the second tracer injection of four to five times the initial dose. This overcomes the background activity of the first injection. The recommended doses vary between 8 and 10 mCi for the early injection and 25 to 30 mCi for the late injection. The low dose, early imaging usually requires a longer imaging time per stop (25 to 40 seconds) to produce appropriate imaging quality. A time delay of 3 to 4 hours can further reduce background count before the second investigation, however, this unfavorably influences the convenience of the study.

For the 1-day protocol, the rest/stress imaging sequence is more widely used than the stress/rest sequence (Fig. 2-7g). With the rest/stress method, the high activity and good image quality of the second images are utilized to identify perfusion defects at stress, which reflect the most important clinical information for disease detection and prognosis. Theoretically, background activity from the rest study in the regions of stress perfusion defects could reduce the sensitivity for CAD detection, however, such effect has not been reported to date.

The stress/rest protocol, with a timing sequence similar to the classical ^{201}Tl stress/redistribution protocol, offers the simplest conversion from ^{201}Tl to ^{99m}Tc-MIBI, and allows for a morning stress procedure, which is preferred by many cardiologists (Fig. 2-7h). However, this approach has been shown to be less effective than the rest/stress sequence in assessing defect reversibility.[129]

Preintervention and Postintervention Tracer Injection

The characteristic of ^{99m}Tc-MIBI and ^{99m}Tc-tetrofosmin to "save" the information about blood flow distribution at the time of injection can be used to extend image acquisition 5 to 6 hours after tracer injection. Even when giving the tracer before reperfusion therapy of acute myocardial infarct patients, imaging can be performed after therapy.[130] The acquired "frozen images" depict the pretreatment status. Later repetition of the study, with comparison of these results to the initial results, poses a unique method for evaluating the efficacy of revascularisation procedures (Fig. 2-7i).

^{99m}Tc-Labeled Pharmaceuticals with Significant Washout

The fast clearance of teboroxime requires rapid commencement and completion of imaging after stress injection of the tracer. The proposed imaging interval is between 2 and 8 minutes (Fig. 2-7j).[102] On images acquired 5 minutes after stress injection, significant redistribution is already detectable in regions of stress-induced perfusion defects.[131] As rapid positioning of the patient after an exercise test is difficult to execute, pharmacological stresses are preferred for teboroxime studies. If SPECT imaging is chosen, the use of triple-head camera is recommended to obtain rapid accumulation of data and appropriate image quality.[132,133] With such a system, the completion of stress-rest studies is possible within 60 to 90 minutes.

Dual Isotope Protocols

Performance of resting imaging with ^{201}Tl and stress imaging with ^{99m}Tc-MIBI[128] or ^{99m}Tc-tetrofosmin[134] combine the advantages of these two tracers (Figure 2-7k). Injection of ^{99m}Tc-labelled pharmaceuticals at peak stress produces excellent tomographic image quality. The detection of viable myocardium may be enhanced by delayed imaging (greater than 30 minutes) after resting injection of ^{201}Tl. Due to the shorter half-life of ^{99m}Tc, late ^{201}Tl imaging after 24 to 72 hours can be performed (Fig. 2-7l). In patients who have perfusion defects on the initial rest ^{201}Tl stress ^{99m}Tc-MIBI study, a 10% to 15% increase in reversibility of the resting defects during the dual-isotope study has been reported when imaging was repeated 24 hours after ^{201}Tl injection.[135] Another benefit is the logistic advantage of such stress procedures and delayed imaging; minimizing the waiting period between imaging decreases the investigation time to about 2 hours. However, due to different radiation characteristics of ^{201}Tl and ^{99m}Tc there are differences in the apparent cavity size, and the extent of attenuation artifacts. Clinical experience, however, has shown that the dual-isotope approach provides accurate diagnostic information.[128]

Imaging Techniques

Planar Techniques

Beside the introduction of new radiopharmaceuticals, the development of improved imaging equipment has played an important role in the clinical acceptance of nuclear cardiological procedures. The Anger gamma camera was initially introduced in the 1960s, and became the first technique to obtain images of regional radiotracer distribution in humans.[136] Using planar imaging techniques in combination with ^{201}Tl the gamma camera became the most important cardiac nuclear medicine imaging technology in the 1970s and early 1980s.

SPECT

Three-dimensional representation of myocardial tracer distribution became possible with the introduction of tomographic data reconstruction using single photon emission tomography.[137] Several tomographic imaging approaches are currently in use. Single camera data acquisition using a 180° acquisition presents the most commonly used technique.[138–140] Modern multihead camera systems increase the sensitivity and may reduce the time required for data acquisition. Reduced data acquisition time is not important only for the throughput in a cardiovascular laboratory, but also for the avoidance of motion artefacts occurring during data acquisition. The recent introduction of triple-head cameras allows myocardial data acquisition with high temporal resolution in tomographic mode. Tracer kinetics can be characterized by dynamic data acquisition using frame durations as short as 10 to 30 s/frame.[111] The most important recent advance for cardiac SPECT imaging has been the introduction of attenuation correction. Using an external radiation source, simultaneous transmission and emission scanning can be performed using different energy windows.[141,142] From these results, the regional attenuation factors can be calculated with either filtered backprojection or iterative reconstruction algorithm and applied to correct the attenuation artifacts produced by soft tissue attenuation. Initial clinical results indicate that such an approach allows successful correction of soft tissue attenuation in the inferior wall of the left ventricle, as demonstrated in Plate 2-1.

Gated SPECT

The advent of ^{99m}Tc-labeled radiopharmaceuticals has led to an improvement of the counting statistics for myocardial perfusion imaging. This advantage can be exploited by gated data acquisition to produce end-diastolic and end-systolic images. Gated SPECT may provide several attractive features: (1) regional wall motion may permit the separation of attenuation artefacts and true perfusion defects,[143] (2) spatial resolution can be increased by avoiding blurring of images by cardiac motion,[144] and (3) indices of cardiac function may be derived by measuring changes in count density occurring during the cardiac cycle. These count changes indirectly reflect wall thickening (partial volume effect) and can be used as indices of regional function. Volumetric sampling approaches allow the calculation of global parameters such as end-diastolic and -systolic volumes and ejection fraction. The use of gated SPECT together with three-dimensional visualization of perfusion and function may provide unique functional and morphological information.

A full discussion of technical details of gamma camera or PET camera design is beyond of the scope of this chapter. Several recent reviews are recommended for a more detailed discussion of the technical principles of scintigraphic equipment.[145–151]

Assessment of Relative Cardiac Perfusion

Semiquantitative Approaches

Most clinical perfusion studies are interpreted visually, and the accuracy and reproducibility of such visual analysis have been established in the literature. However, most of the published literature reflects the careful visual data analysis of "expert readers" in sophisticated academic centers. A recent article by Wackers et al. suggests considerable intraobserver variability even between different academic centers.[152] As shown in this article, the introduction of semiquantitative data analysis reduces variability and increases reproducibility of test results. In addition, analysis software provided by the manufacturers supports standardization not only of data interpretation, but also data acquisition. It is expected that semiquantitative and truly quantitative analysis will further improve by the more widespread availability of powerful workstations and sophisticated software packages. However, despite these advances, visual evaluation of scintigraphic studies will remain the most widely used method of interpretation. At this time point, semiquantitative analysis provides only supportive data, which may increase the standardization of interpretation.

Quantitative Approaches

Numerous approaches have been reported in the literature for quantitation regional tracer distribution on SPECT and PET images. The analysis of static studies has employed various normalization strategies to obtain semiquantitative indices of tracer distribution. Dynamically acquired data sets require appropriate tracer kinetic models to extract quantitatively parameters of perfusion.

Static images, which represent relative perfusion based on regional activity concentration, are most often acquired. The analysis of these data sets assumes that the uptake of tracer is a direct measure of blood flow in the myocardium. Tracer uptake is expected to be homogeneous in the normal heart, which allows simple normalization schemes for the detection of hypoperfused tissue.

Derivation of Semiquantitative Information from Myocardial Perfusion Images

The types of analysis of static data sets differ mostly in their degree of computational sophistication. The methods can be separated in three categories: (1) manual procedures require the user to draw representative regions of interest (ROI) in transaxial images or, more efficiently, reoriented short-, horizontal-, and long-axis views; (2) automated routines use short-axis slices or the data volumes to calculate circumferential profiles of activity maxima or their analogues in a volume; and (3) algorithms where the endocardial and epicardial border is defined either manually or automatically and the average activity within these borders is calculated.

Manually positioned ROIs introduce operator depending variabilities and offer limited spatial resolution, but the circumferential profile-based techniques have proven to be more reliable. Developed for the analysis of planar views,[153-155] this circumferential profile approach requires definition of a central point in the image (e.g., a short axis slice). Radial profiles are extracted from the center of the left ventricular passing perpendicularly to the cardiac wall (Fig. 2-8) for typically 30 to 60 angles sampling the entire myocardium (Fig. 2-9). Along each radial profile the area of maximal counts is determined and used to generate the circumferential profile. This scheme is performed for all slices from base to apex. Long-axis slices can be used to optimize apical sampling to avoid apical undersampling.[156] Alternatively, using a more volume-oriented approach, the long axis of the heart may be defined interactively and oblique rays sampling the myocardium in a perpendicular fashion can be used to extract activity profiles from the data volumes.[157-160] All these approaches use a combination of a half-spherical sampling scheme in the apex and a cylindrical scheme in the remaining heart. Thus, inherently, the problems of apical sampling are minimized.

The development of fully three-dimensional

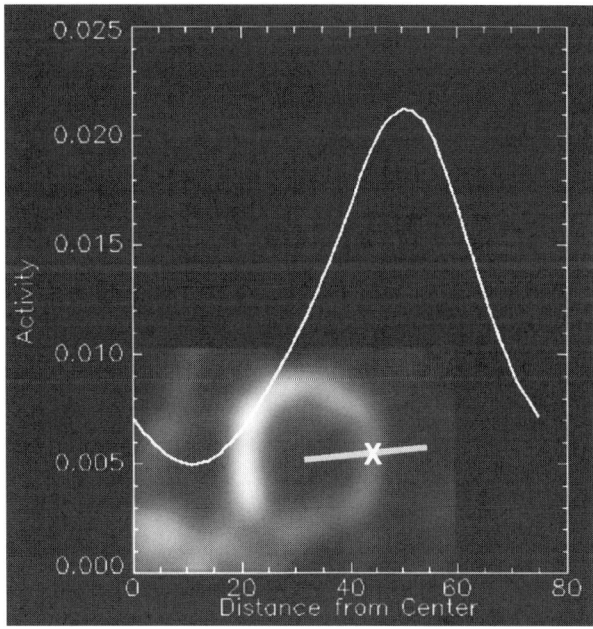

Fig. 2-8. Determination of maximal activity in a profile curve through the myocardial wall in a short axis slice.

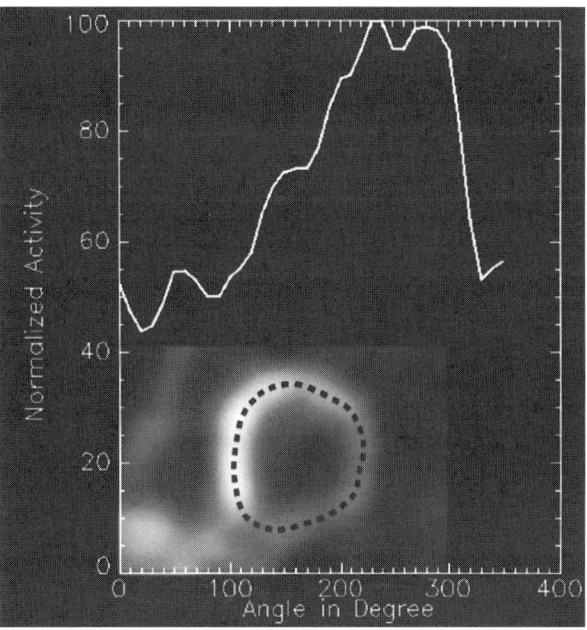

Fig. 2-9. Creation of circumferential profile curve along the myocardial wall.

methods has been accelerated by the reduced cost of computer memory together with increased processing speed. This third approach makes optimal use of the available scintigraphic information. The use of template shapes such as ellipses decreases the time required for manual analysis, although this may not reflect accurately the individual shape of the left ventricle. For automated routines the accurate detection of myocardial activity is challenging, as a spatially varying point-spread function is inherent to SPECT imaging. Furthermore, these approaches may benefit from a gated acquisition, as this approach minimizes "motional blur" and regional quantification is improved.

Depiction and Analysis of Semiquantitative Data

The activity maxima derived from the above approaches are further processed using filtering and continuity criteria to avoid sampling artifacts in segments with reduced tracer uptake. For visualization and analysis purposes, the sampled values are displayed in a spreadsheet style for the ROI-based methods or in "bullseye" or polarmap projection.[156]

The polar map can be described as a two-dimensional representation of a three-dimensional tracer distribution (Plate 2-2). As the sampled values reflect relative count density but no truly quantitative information, they are scaled to provide relative uptake values. Several strategies have been described, normalizing either each circumferential profile individually ("Cedars-Sinai") or the entire heart ("Emory").[161] For the latter, the individual polar map may be scaled to the sector with the highest counts or the mean of several connected sectors having the highest mean counts in the total polar map. This technique assumes that each polar map contains myocardium exhibiting normal tracer accumulation. Finally, these normalized values of regional tracer distribution can be processed, for example, using a 50% threshold, to identify abnormally perfused tissue.

More advanced techniques compare the normalized maps with so called "normal databases," generated from the maps of healthy individuals without evidence of cardiovascular disease, to perform an additional calibration. These normal maps can correct to some extent limitations of the imaging equipment and the physics of the imaging process (finite resolution, scatter, attenuation, etc.). From the gender-matched set of normal maps (gender matching is necessary in nonattenuated corrected SPECT imaging), a regional mean and a standard deviation map is calculated. The processing of individual patient maps is realized by the defining differences of this map from the normal map, by units of standard deviations. However, as the size of the human heart is not constant, the sampling procedure requires a homogeneous sampling of the individual hearts, using for example a threshold of greater than 2.5 standard deviations below normal as the criterion of abnormal perfusion. To facilitate the interpretation of polar maps, sectors can be statistically combined into standard regions (e.g., left anterior descending [LAD], right coronary artery [RCA], right circumflex [RCX]), permitting measurement of means, standard deviations, and the percentage of underperfused sectors. Thus, a comprehensive report page may combine selected short, horizontal, and vertical long axis rest and stress images together with the corresponding polar maps and semiquantitative information (severity, extent) extracted from the maps.

The three-dimensional nature of SPECT imaging may be utilized to limit the spatial distortions introduced through the polar map approach.[157,160] With suitable graphics hardware, this information can be used to display the polar map (i.e., the three-dimensional maximum count surface) and allow the interactive manipulation of the virtual heart (Plate 2-3).

POSITRON EMISSION TOMOGRAPHY

The radionuclides used for PET imaging emit a β particle with positive charge (i.e., a positron). The energy of this positron varies from 1 to 3.5 MeV, depending on the isotope, and, consequently, these particles travel several millimeters in tissue before colliding with an electron. This annihilation event releases two photons of 511-keV energy in nearly opposite directions. PET imaging is based on the detection of these high-energy photons, which experience only little attenuation in tissue (attenuation coefficient is 0.096/cm).[65] The distance between the decaying isotope and the detectable annihilation (i.e., the positron travel) is a limiting factor for the resolution in the image. This factor, however, be-

Color Plates

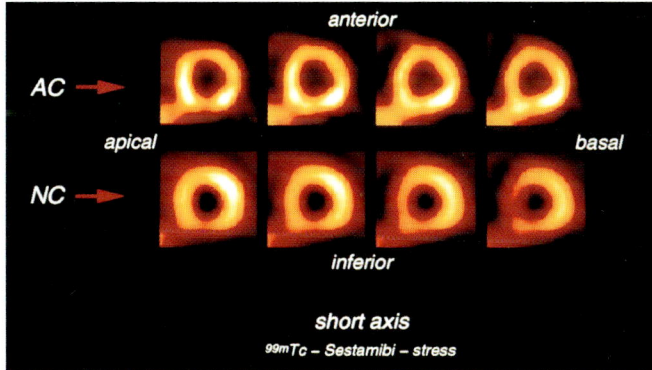

Plate 2-1

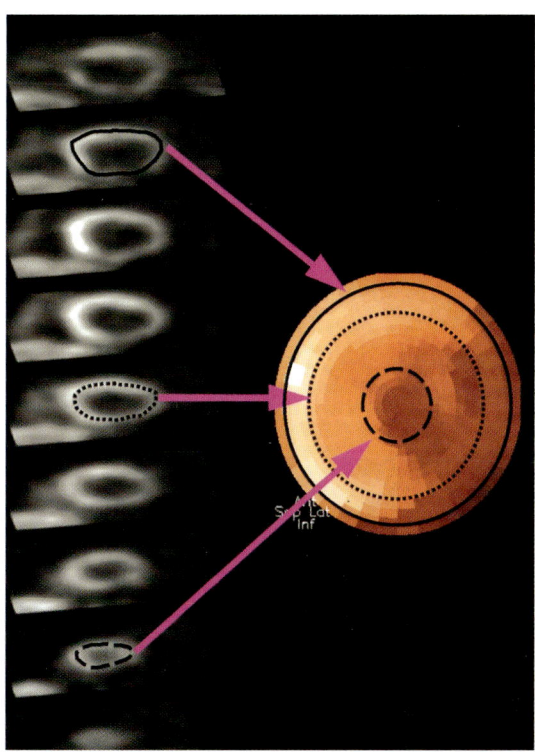

Plate 2-2

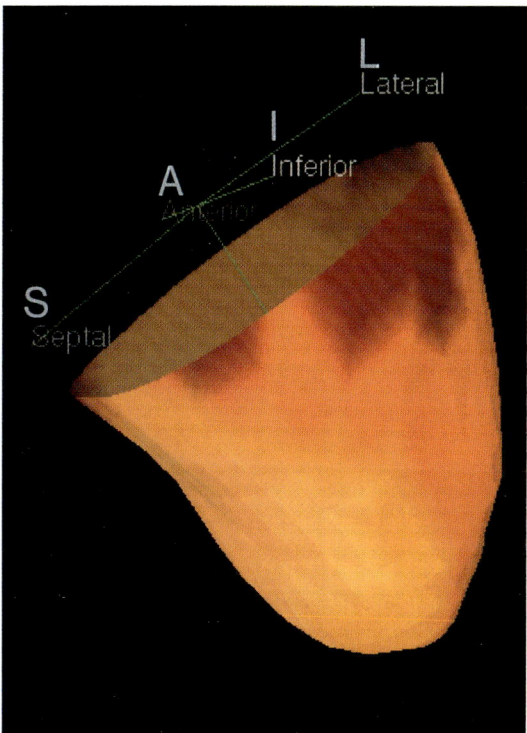

Plate 2-3

Plate 2-1. ^{99m}Tc-MIBI single photon emission tomography (SPECT) images without (NC) and with (AC) attenuation correction in a 67 kg male 72 years of age.

Plate 2-2. Generation of polar map from circumferential profile curves.

Plate 2-3. Three-dimensional display of myocardial activity distribution. L, lateral; I, inferior; A, anterior; S, septal.

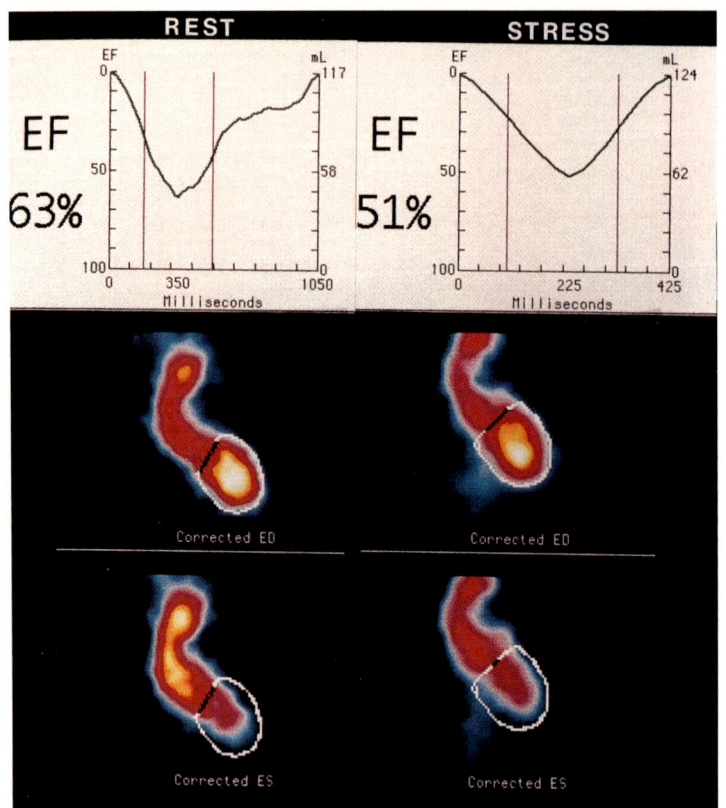

Plate 3-1

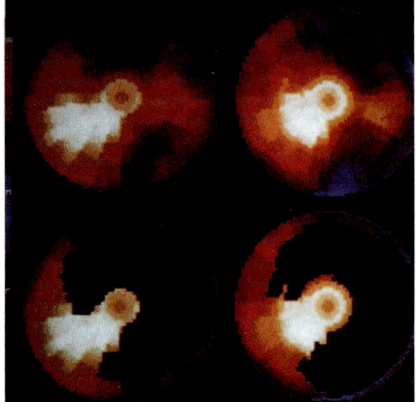

Plate 10-1

Plate 3-1. First pass radionuclide angiograms from a 48 year old male patient with hyperlipidemia are shown. The rest study (left) demonstrates normal wall motion and preserved overall left ventricular (LV) systolic function with a LV ejection fraction (EF) of 63%. The ventricular volume curve is shown at the top, from which ejection fraction is calculated. Corresponding stress images (right) demonstrate an exercise-induced decrease in LVEF to 51%. Wall motion reveals hypokinesis of the basal and apical anterolateral wall and apex. The study demonstrates exercise-induced ischemia probably involving the left anterior descending coronary artery. ED, end-diastole; ES, end-systole. (Courtesy of Michael Hanson, M.D., Duke University School of Medicine.)

Plate 10-1. Thallium-201 SPECT bullseye circumferential profile in a patient with hypertension and end-stage renal disease (immediate poststress images right and delayed images left) showing a false-positive fixed lateral defect mimicking an extensive lateral wall myocardial infarction. The lower left and right images reflect comparisons with gender-specific normal files and the black areas correspond to count density 32 standard deviations below normal. (Modified from DePuey EG, Guertler-Krawczynska E, Perkin JV et al: Alterations in myocardial thallium-201 distribution in patients with chronic systemic hypertension undergoing single-photon emission computed tomography. Am J Cardiol 62:234, 1988.)

Plate 18-1. Two-chamber transesophageal dobutamine echocardiography in a patient with left anterior descending artery disease. **(A)** Diastolic (left) and systolic images at rest. **(B)** Diastolic (left) and systolic images at peak dobutamine dose, with an inducible wall motion abnormality of the anterior wall (arrows).

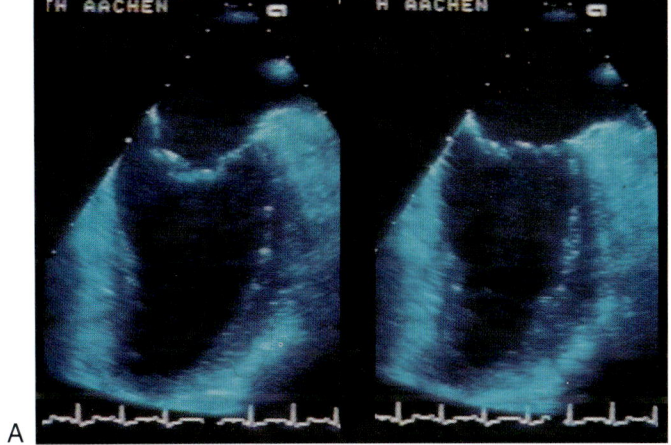
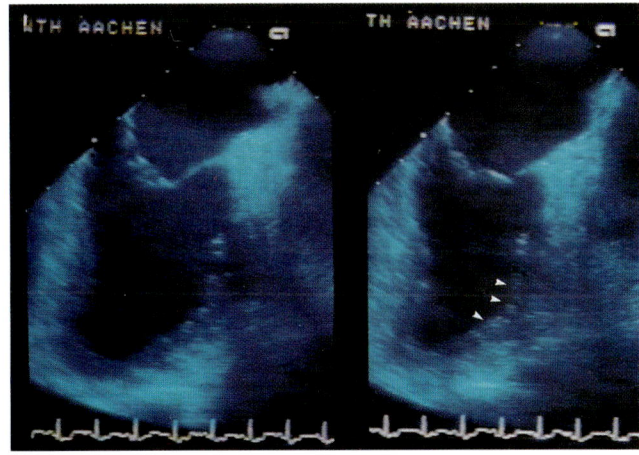

Plate 19-1. Positron emission tomographic images of myocardial blood flow distribution **(A & B)** before and **(C & D)** after coronary angioplasty of a severe stenosis of the proximal left anterior descending (LAD) coronary artery in a patient who also had a mild stenosis of the left circumflex branch. Before angioplasty, a perfusion defect was evident in the anterior regions after dipyridamole **(B)**. Following revascularization, the left circumflex stenosis became evident, causing a reduction in vasodilator reserve in the posterolateral wall after dipyridamole **(C & D)**. PTCA, percutaneous transluminal angioplasty.

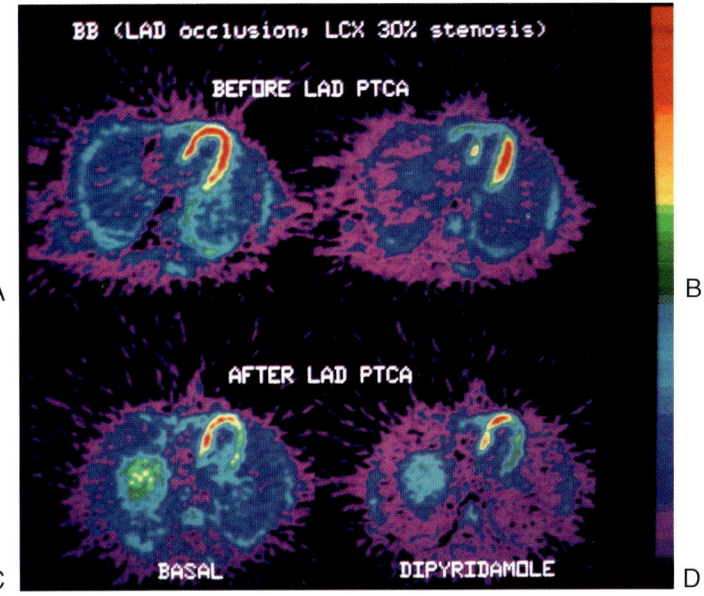

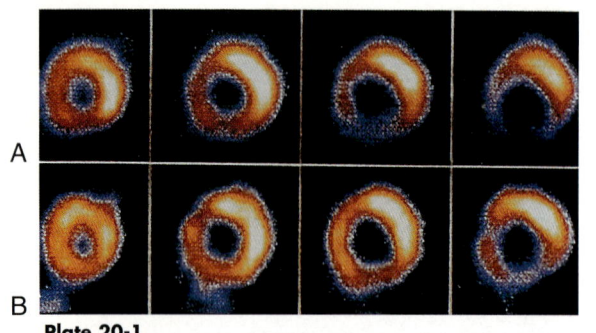

Plate 20-1.

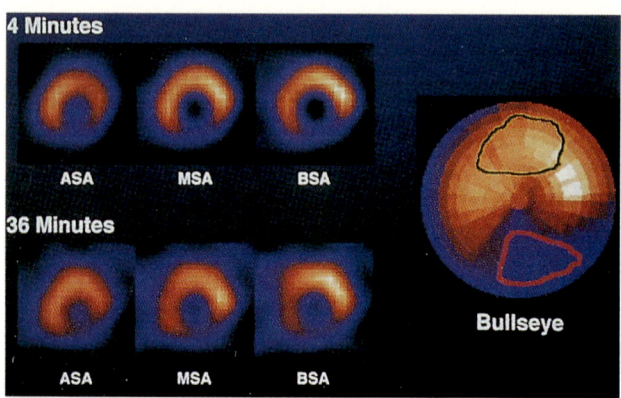

Plate 20-2.

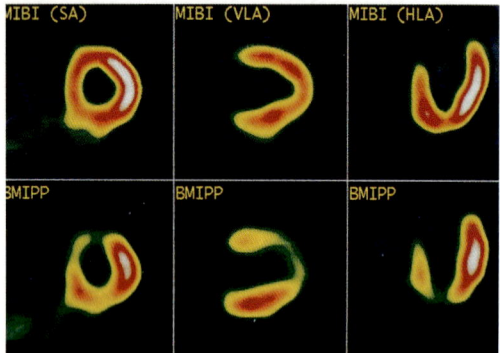

Plate 20-3.

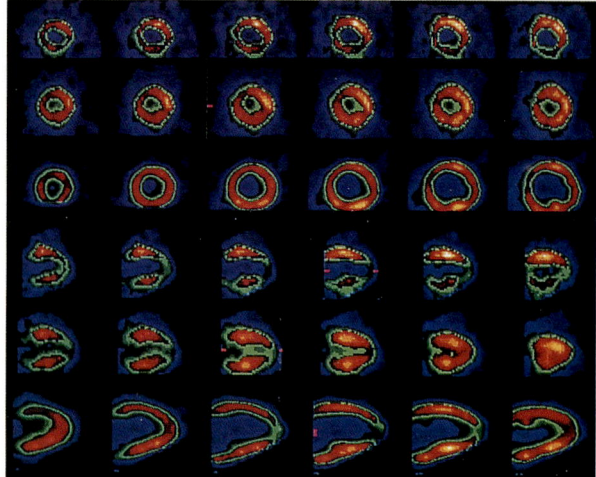

Plate 20-4.

Plate 20-1. Rest **(A)** -redistribution **(B)** thallium SPECT imaging in a patient with inferior wall and septal abnormalities. Left ventricular short-axis slices are shown from apical to basal level (from left to right) are shown. (From Iskandrian et al. J Nucl Cardiol 2:101, 1995.)

Plate 20-2. Representative short axis slices from a man with unstable angina and three-vessel coronary artery disease. There is a moderately decreased activity in the inferolateral wall that shows relative improvement over time (see Fig. 20-13).

Plate 20-3. Example of BMIPP and sestamibi mismatched defects. Short axis (SA), vertical long axis (VLA), and horizontal long axis (HLA) slices obtained with sestamibi (MIBI) and with BMIPP in a patient studied 1 week after acute anterior myocardial infarction. The study shows reduced BMIPP but normal sestamibi uptake in the infarct-related coronary artery territory, indicating the presence of viable, but jeopardized myocardium. (From Knapp et al., J Nucl Med 36:1022, 1995.)

Plate 20-4. Rest thallium (rows 1 and 4), FDG-SPECT (rows 2 and 5), and FDG-PET (rows 3 and 6) short axis and vertical long axis slices in a patient with a fixed apical thallium defect and inferior wall abnormalities. FDG-SPECT and FDG-PET show some increased uptake in these areas but with essentially little uptake in the apex. There is a near equality between the FDG-PET and FDG-SPECT images. (From Burt RW, Perkins OW, Oppenheim BE et al: Direct comparison of fluorine-18-FDG SPECT, fluorine-18-FDG PET and rest thallium-201 SPECT for detection of myocardial viability. J Nucl Med 36:176, 1995.)

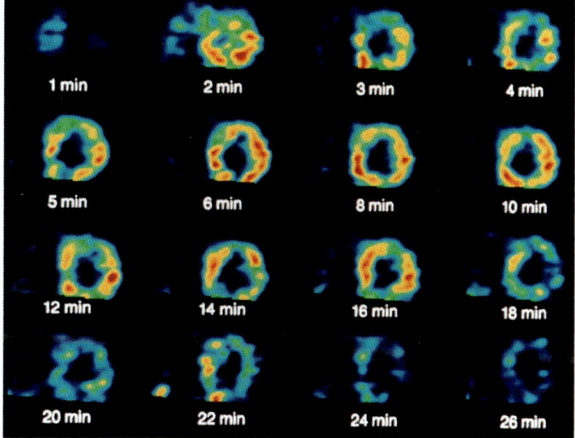

Plate 21-1

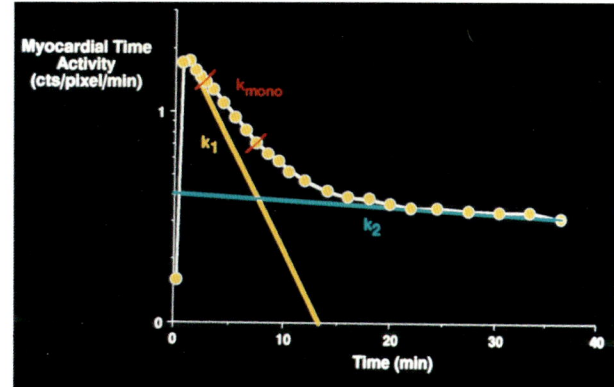

Plate 21-2

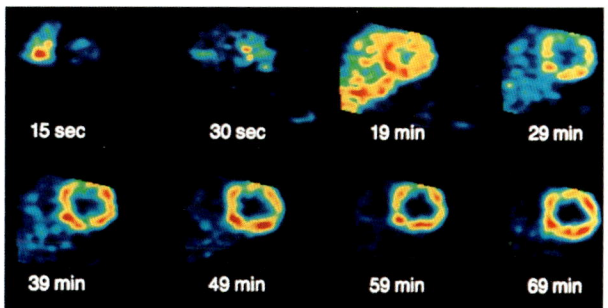

Plate 21-3

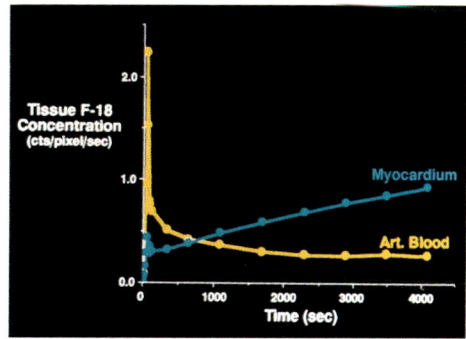

Plate 21-4

Plate 21-1. Sequential short axis carbon-11 acetate images. The images obtained one and two minutes following intravenous tracer administration demonstrate activity within the blood pool. Subsequent images demonstrate progressive uptake and then clearance of the carbon-11 label from the myocardium.

Plate 21-2. Analysis of myocardial time-activity curves obtained from dynamic carbon-11 acetate positron emission tomography (PET) images. Biexponential curve fitting yields two parameters, k_1 and k_2. The first parameter, k_1, is linearly related to myocardial oxygen consumption while k_2 is believed to reflect the conversion of labeled glutamate to labeled glutamine. K_{mono}, derived from monoexponential fitting of the initial portion of the curve, can also used to quantitatively assess myocardial oxygen consumption. As indicated on the graph, K_{mono} slightly underestimates k_1.

Plate 21-3. Sequential myocardial short axis fluorine-18 deoxyglucose positron emission tomography (FDG-PET) images. Early images at 15 and 30 seconds depict blood pool activity, while subsequent images demonstrate progressive myocardial accumulation of the glucose metabolic tracer. In contrast to carbon-11 acetate images, the myocardial to background activity progressively improves over the period of imaging.

Plate 21-4. Myocardial and vascular time activity curves from an fluorine-18 deoxyglucose (FDG) imaging study. As activity clears from the vascular space there is an on-going accumulation of activity within the myocardium, reflecting tissue trapping of radioactive tracer

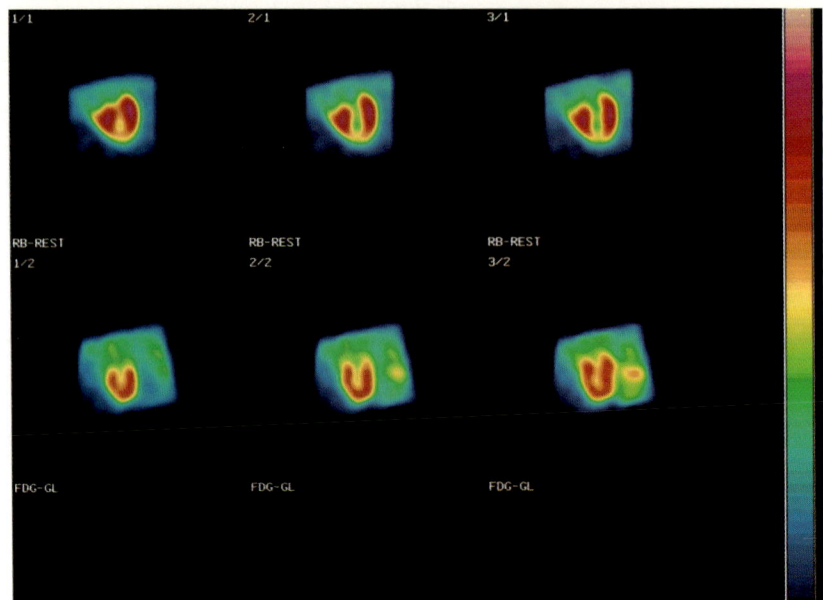

Plate 21-5.

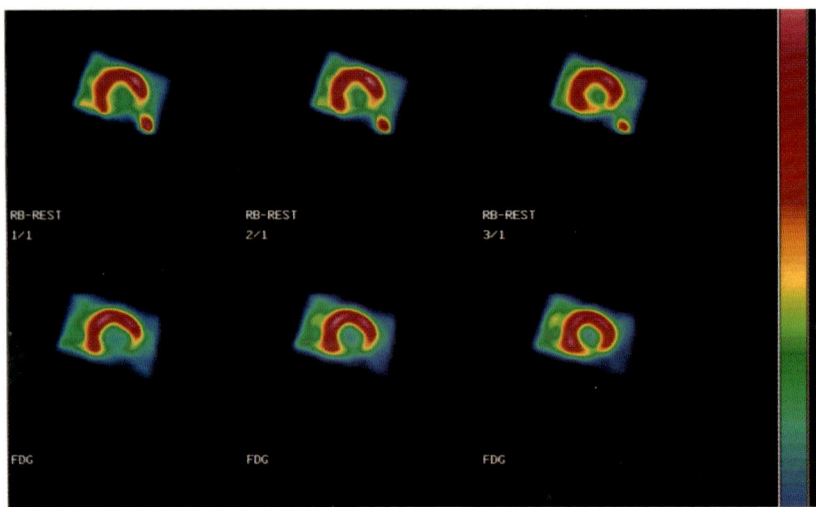

Plate 21-6.

Plate 21-5. Horizontal long axis rubidium-82 perfusion and fluorine-18 deoxyglucose (FDG) metabolic positron emission tomography (PET) images in a patient with a history of anterior infarction. An extensive defect is present in the anterior and apical ventricular regions on the resting rubidium-82 perfusion images. In contrast, FDG activity is well preserved in the hypoperfused ventricular areas ("perfusion-metabolism mismatch") denoting residual tissue viability.

Plate 21-6. Representative rubidium-82 perfusion and fluorine-18 deoxyglucose (FDG) metabolic short axis positron emission tomography (PET) images obtained at the midventricular level in a patient with a history of previous inferior wall infarction. Concordant perfusion and metabolic defects are present in the inferior region of the ventricle, indicating completed infarction.

Plate 24-1. Transverse histological sections of coronary plaque stained with Sirius red dye. **(A)** The unstable plaque seen under polarized light shows that the large lipid core is devoid of connective tissue. The cap between the lumen (L) and the lipid core is thin. **(B)** The stable plaque has no lipid core but contains a considerable quantity of connective tissue. **(C)** The luminal edge of the plaque shows an area of young collagen (yellow) contrasting with the collagen that is remnant from the original cap (blue). The appearance indicates healing of a previous disruption. **(D)** In the area of young collagen, staining for smooth muscle actin shows abundant smooth muscle cells. (Adapted from Davies MJ: Acute coronary thrombosis—the role of plaque disruption and its initiation and prevention. Eur Heart J 16:L-3, 1995, with permission.)

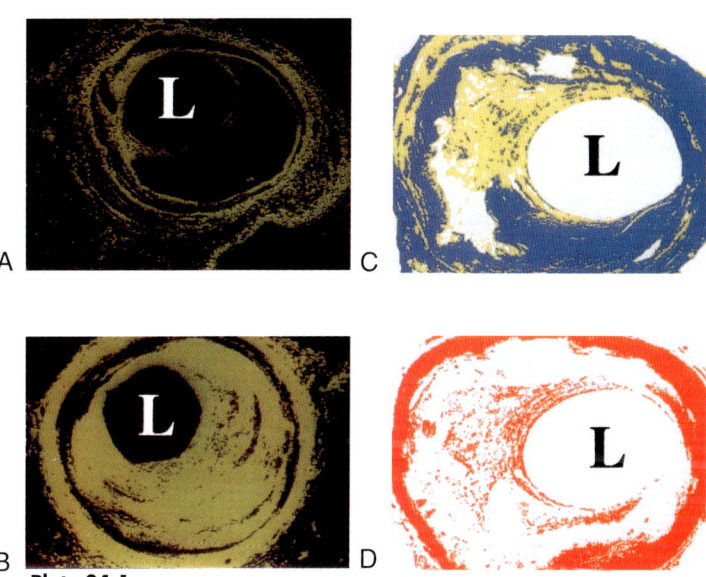

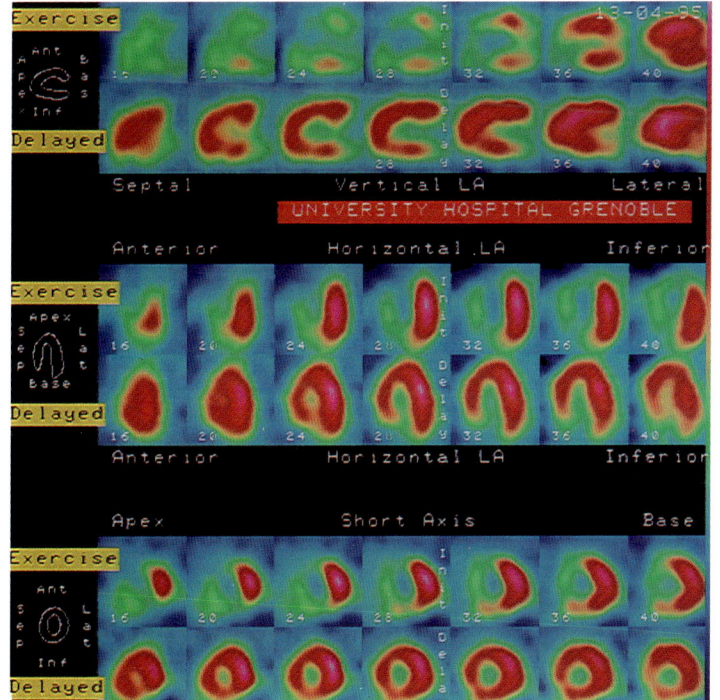

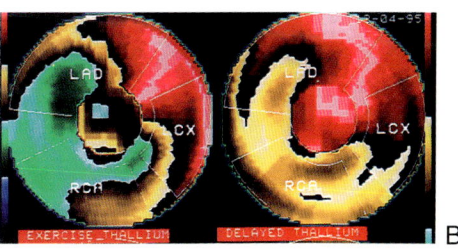

Plate 27-1. SPECT-thallium imaging in a 50-year-old patient with chronic stable angina. Tomographic images **(A)** show a largely reversible perfusion defect in the anterior, septal, apical, and inferior zones. The extent of this is more readily quantified using a polar map display **(B)**, which shows initial uptake in these segments to be less than 50% of normal (green), and residual mild defects (50% to 74% of reference zone, yellow) on the redistribution scan. This extensive ischemia is associated with high risk and provoked interventional therapy.

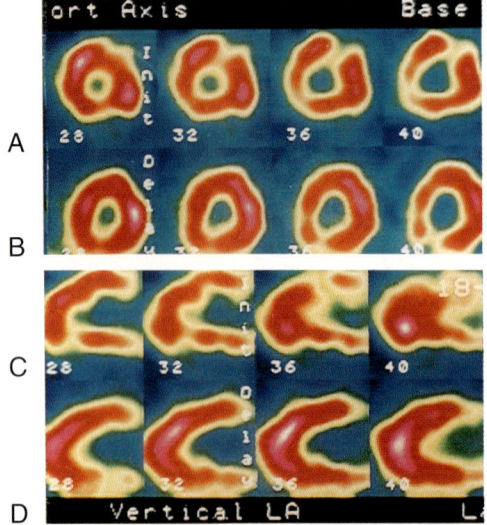

Plate 27-2. (A –D) SPECT thallium short axis (A & B) and vertical long axis (C) small anterior perfusion defect induced by stress (A & C) and absent on the redistribution scan. SPECT, single photon emission computed tomography.

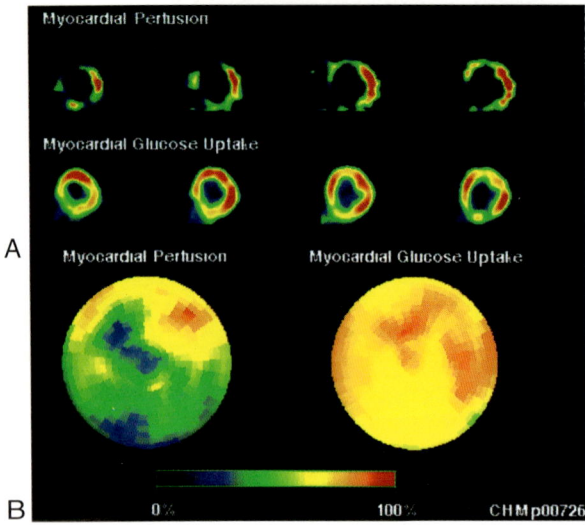

Plate 28-1. Positron emission tomography images of a 65-year-old man with severe three-vessel coronary artery disease and poor left ventricular function (LVF) admitted to the hospital with pulmonary edema. (A) Images of regional perfusion ([^{13}N]ammonia, top row) and glucose utilization ([^{18}F]deoxyglucose, bottom row) in corresponding midventricular short-axis views from apex (left) to base (right). Anterior wall is on top, the inferior wall is on the bottom, the interventricular septum is on the left, and the lateral wall is on the right. Resting perfusion images demonstrate large and severe blood flow defects in the anterior, septal, apical, and inferior ventricular walls. Glucose metabolism is preserved in all hypoperfused regions (perfusion–metabolism mismatch). (B) Normalized polar map displays of the extent, magnitude, and location of regional perfusion abnormalities (left) and glucose utilization (right) confirm the visual findings.

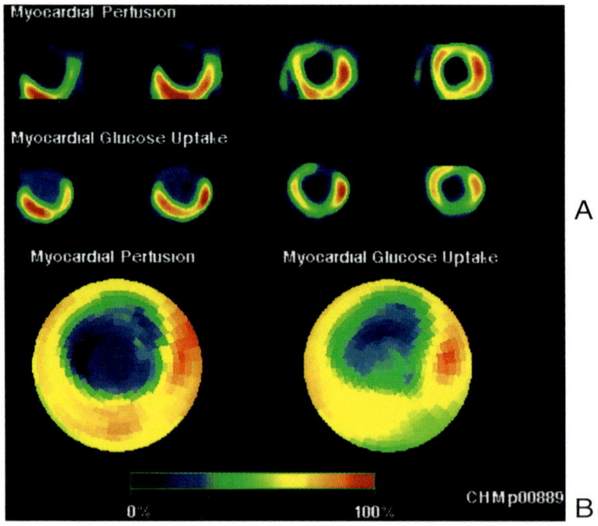

Plate 28-2. Positron emission tomography images of a 70-year-old woman with a history of an anterior wall infarct admitted to the hospital with congestive heart failure and mild angina. (A) Images of regional perfusion ([^{13}N]ammonia, top row) and glucose utilization ([^{18}F]deoxyglucose, bottom row) in corresponding midventricular short-axis views from apex (left) to base (right), with the same orientation as in Plate 28-1. There is a large and severe resting blood flow defect involving the anterior, anteroseptal, and apical ventricular walls with aneurysmal dilatation of the left ventricular cavity. Glucose metabolism is concordantly decreased in all hypoperfused regions (perfusion–metabolism match). (B) Normalized polar map displays of the extent, magnitude, and location of regional perfusion abnormalities (left) and glucose utilization (right) confirm the visual findings.

comes important only if high-resolution PET instrumentation as well as cardiac gating is employed.

PET Flow Tracers

The positron emitting isotopes are generally short lived (several minutes) and, thereby, permit rapid sequential measurements. On the other hand, their short half-life requires the local production of the isotope. Several blood flow tracers are available for the evaluation of myocardial perfusion using PET (Table 2-1). Based on the mode of production, these radiopharmaceuticals are divided into two groups. Rubidium-82 (^{82}Rb) and copper-62-pyruvaldehyde-bis(N-4-methylthiosemicarbazone) (^{62}Cu-PTSM) are generator produced radiopharmaceuticals. Nitrogen-13-ammonia (^{13}NH$_3$) and oxygen-15-water (H$_2$^{15}O) require an on-site cyclotron for their production.

Direct Cyclotron Products

Nitrogen-13-Ammonia

At the present time ^{13}NH$_3$ is the most frequently used cyclotron-produced blood flow tracer. It is produced in ^{16}O(p)^{13}N reaction by reduction of ^{13}N-nitrate with a purity greater than 99%.[162] The 10 minute half-life of this isotope is optimal for most PET systems, but it has the disadvantage of requiring a 30- to 40- minute waiting period for ^{13}N decay between repeated images. Nevertheless a stress-rest protocol can be completed within 1.5 to 2.0 hours.[163] Because of low positron energy (1.2 MeV), this radiotracer offers excellent image quality.

In blood, more than 95% of total ^{13}NH$_3$ circulates as nitrogen-13-ammonium (^{13}NH$_4^+$).[164] As ammonium leaves the vascular space, it is rapidly converted to ammonia[165] to permit almost complete extraction of activity.[166] Because this initial extraction is followed by competing flow-dependent back diffusion and metabolic trapping, the single pass extraction fraction determined by extrapolation from residue function is about 80% at normal flow values, falling to around 60% at flow values of 3 ml/min/g.[166] The metabolic fixation of ammonia within myocardium may occur in several ways,[167] but the glutamic acid–glutamine pathway appears to be the predominant.[167–170] Although metabolic factors might be expected to interfere with metabolic trapping, this process demonstrates relative constancy over a wide range of physiological hemodynamic and metabolic conditions, making this pharmaceutic suitable for myocardial flow imaging.[166] The blood activity of ^{13}NH$_3$ clears rapidly; 5 minutes after administration, less than 2% of the maximum activity remains in the blood.[166] The significantly slower clearance half-time from the myocardium yields a high contrast between myocardial and blood activity, optimal for visual analysis (Fig. 2-10).

The kinetics of ^{13}NH$_3$ for quantification of myo-

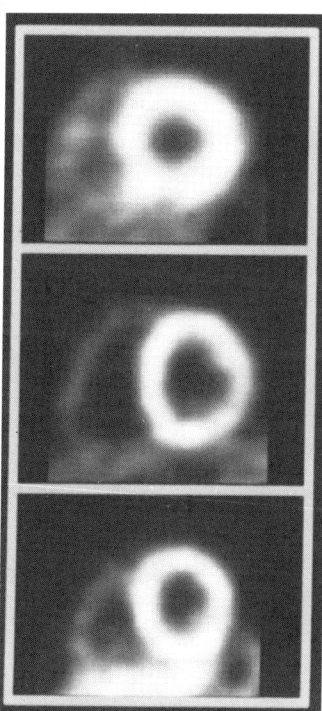

Fig. 2-10. Comparison of positron emission tomography (PET) flow tracers. Cross-sectional images obtained in normal volunteers after the injection of various blood flow tracers. **(A)** ^{82}Rb, **(B)** ^{13}NH$_3$, and **(C)** ^{62}Cu-PTSM.

Table 2-1. PET Tracers for the Measurement of Myocardial Perfusion

	Physical Half-Life (min)	Energy
^{13}NH$_3$	10.0	1.0
H$_2$^{15}O	2.0	1.7
$_{82}$Rb	1.3	3.3
$_{62}$Cu-PTSM	9.8	1.2

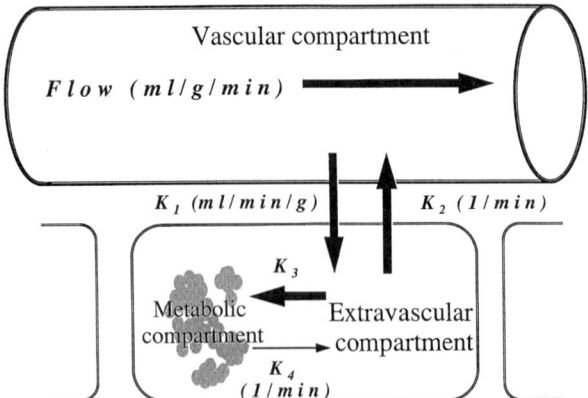

Fig. 2-11. Three-compartmental tracer kinetic model employed for determination of blood flow using $^{13}NH_3$ positron emission tomography (PET) data.

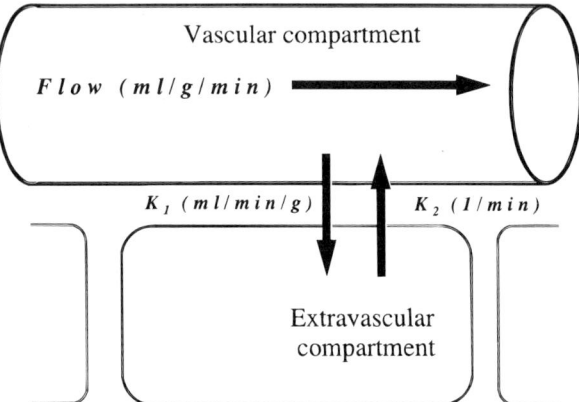

Fig. 2-12. Two-compartmental tracer kinetic model employed for determination of blood flow using $H_2{}^{15}O$ positron emission tomography (PET) data.

cardial blood flow can be described by a three-compartmental model, first proposed by Hutchins et al. (Fig. 2-11).[18] The first compartment of this model, the intravascular space, is anatomically separated from the two extravascular compartments (2 and 3), which represent different chemical states of the tracer but do not distinguish between anatomically separable spaces. Because $^{13}NH_3$ is almost totally extracted to the extravascular space, the rate constant (k_1) is determined by blood flow. Within the extravascular compartment, the tracer competes for back diffusion into the vascular space (k_2) and transfer into metabolic compartment (k_3). These parameters k_1, k_2, and k_3 can be determined with an appropriate nonlinear fitting routine of the myocardial time-activity curve. Detailed descriptions of the tracer kinetic models for $^{13}NH_3$ are provided by Hutchins et al.[18] and Krivokapich et al.[171]

Oxygen-15-Water

$H_2{}^{15}O$ is a radiopharmaceutical with excellent physiologic properties for quantitative blood flow determination and a short physical half-life (120 seconds). ^{15}O is produced in cyclotron, usually with the ^{15}N-(p,n)^{15}O- reaction. $H_2{}^{15}O$ can be utilized either by direct intravenous injection of tracer, or as it is formed in vivo after inhalation of ^{15}O-labeled CO_2.[17,19,172]

$H_2{}^{15}O$ represents a metabolically inert flow tracer, which diffuses freely across membranes and is highly extracted by myocardial tissue. Animal studies have shown its stable single first-pass extraction over a wide range of flow.[173] However, extracted $H_2{}^{15}O$ diffuses rapidly back into the vascular space, yielding a blood-to-myocardium ratio near 1 within 60 to 90 seconds after injection. Thus, the separation of myocardial and vascular ^{15}O activity for quantitative analysis requires the delineation of vascular space using ^{15}O-labeled red blood cells after separate administration of $_{15}O$-labeled carbon monoxide.[17]

Because, unlike $^{13}NH_3$, $H_2{}^{15}O$ does not show any metabolic trapping, its kinetics can be depicted by a two-compartment model of vascular and extravascular space for quantitative flow determination (Fig. 2-12). The tracer delivered into the vascular space diffuses immediately and almost totally to the extravascular space (k_1); k_2 represents the clearance of activity from tissue. In cases of such freely diffusable tracers, values for blood flow are usually derived from the estimation of k_2.[174] Although there is little doubt about the suitability of $H_2{}^{15}O$ dynamic PET for clinical research, further advances in data processing are necessary for routine application in the clinical environment.

Generator Products

Rubidium-82

Rubidium was the first radiotracer used for coronary flow studies in the late 1950s.[175] The positron emitting isotope of rubidium (^{82}Rb) was introduced into nuclear medicine laboratories in the early 1980s as the first generator produced PET-radiopharmaceutical. The 25 day half-life of strontium-82, the parent of the generator system, makes the ultrashort-lived ^{82}Rb (half-life 75 seconds) a simple-to-use radionuclide source. Because of this ultrashort half-life, an automatic elution and an on-line injection system are required for human imaging.

The emitted positron of ^{82}Rb has a 3.3-MeV energy, the highest value of all available PET flow tracers. Because this high-energy positron travels up to 1 cm before colliding with an electron to produce two gamma rays, ^{82}Rb PET images have the lowest intrinsic resolution (Fig. 2-10).

The kinetic characteristics of the positive rubidium ion is determined by the similarity of its crystal radius to that of the potassium ion (1.48 and 1.33 Å, respectively). The myocardial extraction fraction is lower than that of ^{201}Tl, around 65%, and it decreases considerably with increasing blood flow.[176] This nonlinear relationship limits the ability to quantitate myocardial perfusion based on tissue tracer concentration alone. However, correction factors or mathematical models can be employed to compensate for known decreases of tracer extraction at higher flow states.[176]

Copper-62-PTSM

An alternative generator-produced flow agent, copper-62-pyruvaldehyde bis(N-methylthiosemicarbazone) copper(II) (^{62}Cu-PTSM) has recently been evaluated.[177] The ^{62}Cu isotope has 100% positron decay with a physical half-life of 9.7 minutes, making it ideal for most PET instrumentation. However, the relatively short (9.13 hour) half-life of parent isotope ^{62}Zn ^{62}Cu requires a generator to be delivered to the PET laboratory every 1 to 2 days.[178,179] ^{62}Cu has a lower positron energy compared to ^{82}Rb (2.7 and 3.3 MeV, respectively), which offers a theoretical advantage for better image resolution. ^{62}Cu-PTSM can be produced in about 30 minutes[180] using a rapid and simple method to label H$_2$(PTSM) with ^{62}Cu.[181-183] The resulting lipophilic compound produces high-quality cardiac images.

Kinetic studies in animals have shown that ^{62}Cu-PTSM has a single pass extraction similar to ^{13}NH$_3$,[184] and rapid blood-pool clearance.[177] In contrast to ^{13}NH$_3$, the maximal extraction fraction is lower than 60%, and decreases further at flow rates greater than 2.5 ml/min/g.[177] Data from tumor cell studies show that ^{62}Cu-PTSM appears to be reduced within the cell by sulfhydryl groups, liberating ionic copper. Tissue retention occurs because of subsequent binding of the liberated copper ion to intracellular macromolecules.[185-187] Liver activity exceeds myocardial activity by 5 minutes post-injection, and this difference tends to increase with time.[180] Because of the close proximity of the liver to the inferior wall, excessive liver activity may lead to scatter contribution to inferior wall activity, which may reduce the sensitivity for disease in this region. Another undesirable characteristic after intravenous administration is the binding of ^{62}Cu-PTSM to red blood cells, making it unavailable for myocardial reuptake and possible influencing quantitative flow calculations. However, after correction of the input function to this activity, Herrero et al. found good correlation between data gained by ^{62}Cu-PTSM and H$_2$^{15}O dynamic PET with a two-compartment model.[188]

Imaging Techniques

The PET detector system has to perform linearly over a wide range of count rates and be sensitive to allow for short scan time intervals to monitor the rapid uptake and release of tracers. Most of the current commercial tomographs employ block detectors made of scintillation crystals (bismuth germanate) that are divided into up to 24 detector rings.[189-191] Although cost effective, this design limits the count rate performance of these scanners. Systems built with fast scintillation materials (barium fluoride) permit inclusion of information on the time-of-flight of the annihilation quanta and generally show a better signal-to-noise ratio and excellent high count rate performance.[192-194] Unfortunately, their lower sensitivity and the requirement for increased data handling prohibit the widespread use of these systems in cardiac applications. Correction of photon attenuation is a prerequisite for tracer distribution measurements in the heart. The attenuation factors are measured with external sources in a transmission scan. Ring or rotating pin sources made of positron emitters are used for this purpose.

Table 2-2. Coronary Flow Values Determined at Rest and Stress by Positron Emission Tomography

Study	Tracer	Rest Flow ml/min/100 g	Stress Flow ml/min/100 g	Coronary Flow Reserve	Type of Stress
Araujo et al. (1991)[19]	$H_2^{15}O$	88 + 8	352 + 113	4.0 + 1.6	Dipyridamole
Bergmann et al. (1989)[17]	$H_2^{15}O$	90 + 22	355 + 112	3.9 + 2.2	Dipyridamole
Camici et al. (1989)[232]	$H_2^{15}O$	92 + 13	367 + 94	4.0 + 1.6	Dipyridamole
Chan et al. (1992)[233]	$^{13}NH_3$	110 + 20	430 + 13	3.9 + 0.8	Dipyridamole
		110 + 20	440 + 90	4.0 + 1.5	Adenosine
Czernin et al. (1993)[23]	$^{13}NH_3$	76 + 17	300 + 80	3.9 + 1.9	Dipyridamole
Geltman et al. (1990)[234]	$H_2^{15}O$	125 + 28	462 + 158	3.7 + 2.1	Dipyridamole
Hutchins et al. (1990)[18]	$^{13}NH_3$	88 + 17	417 + 112	4.7 + 2.2	Dipyridamole
Krivokapich et al. (1989)[171]	$^{13}NH_3$	70 + 17	135 + 22	1.9 + 0.8	Bicycle
Krivokapich et al. (1993)[235]	$^{13}NH_3$	77 + 14	225 + 25	2.9 + 0.8	Dobutamine
Sambuceti et al. (1993)[236]	$^{13}NH_3$	103 + 25	366 + 92	3.5 + 1.7	Dipyridamole

Several methods have been tested to reduce transmission scan time without loss in data quality. Smoothing of the transmission data increases the accuracy of the correction without any resolution loss in the emission images.[195] Other approaches include segmentation of transmission images for classifying different regions as specific tissue types.[196] Recent attempts to measure the transmission scans in single data acquisition mode overcome the deadtime problems of coincidence counting with high activity rotating sources and show promising results. Scanning time would be greatly reduced if transmission and emission data can be measured simultaneously. This is possible if adequate masking in the sinograms is implemented,[197,198] a method already in use for brain studies and being tested for whole body applications.

Quantitative Assessment of Myocardial Blood Flow
Measurement of Absolute Myocardial Blood Flow

The potential of PET for the quantitative assessment of myocardial blood flow represents a major advantage over SPECT imaging. Such measurements provide flow estimates in milliliters per minute per 100 g tissue, which can be used to assess myocardial blood flow under resting and stress conditions as well as before and after pharmacological interventions. Regional coronary reserve can be quantitated based on absolute flow values.

PET blood flow measurements obtained with $^{13}NH_3$ and $H_2^{15}O$ in normal volunteers as well as in patients with CAD are summarized in Table 2-2. There is good reproducibility of blood flow measurements under resting as well as stress conditions among various imaging laboratories, as shown by the consistent measurements of coronary reserve values. The variation of individual resting and maximal flow values suggest that some of the methods may lead to systematic underestimation or overestimation of "true" myocardial blood flow. In most studies, coronary flow reserve over 2.5 times resting flow can be considered "normal", based on the standard deviation of the measurements in control groups with a low likelihood of CAD.[32,199]

For flow measurements, dynamic data acquisition is important to describe arterial input function as well as tissue response. Current PET instrumentation allows the acquisition of such scintigraphic data with high temporal resolution. In contrast to other organs, the large blood chambers of right and left ventricle allow simultaneous measurements of radioactivity in blood and tissue. Several studies have validated the accuracy of this approach for the noninvasive determination of the arterial input function without the need of arterial blood sampling.[200–202] By combining temporal sequences of activity changes in blood and myocardium, tracer tissue uptake rates as well as clearance of activity from tissue can be quantitated. Depending on the radiopharmaceutical used, tracer kinetic models (involving two or three compartments) can be applied to derive estimates of myocardial blood flow, metabolic rate, and tissue tracer retention. While physiologic processes are undoubtedly more complicated than can be described by such simple models, limitation in counting statistics and duration of data acquisition require a simplification of the physiologic process.[203] It is important to remember that the quantitation of physiologic processes using tracer approaches requires steady-state conditions, and only under steady-state conditions can the flux of substrates be quantitated using simplified tracer kinetic models. Moreover, PET measurements under various physiologic and pathophysiologic states assume a similar distribution volume of the tracer within the different compartments of the model.

Quality control of data acquisition is necessary to optimize the accuracy and reproducibility of quantitative measurements.[204] Tracer administration should be standardized according to the technical performance of the PET instrument used.[202] Data processing requires three-dimensional correction for possible displacement of the heart during the dynamic acquisition as well as automated region assignment for efficient analysis of large data sets.[204] The tracer kinetic model approach employed by most institutions also includes a term correcting for the geometric distortion due to limited image resolution provided by PET (partial volume effect, activity cross-contamination).[17,53,173,205]

Limitations of Cardiac PET Measurements

Scatter, dead time, counting statistics, and spatial resolution limit quantitative measurements in cardiac PET scanning.[189] The effect of scattered radiation is small as long as the myocardial activity is high and lung activity is low. At very high count rates, mispositioning of counts and loss of count rate due to dead time of block detector tomographs are noticeable. In current whole body scanners, correction methods are implemented that compensate for deadtime loss associated with activities of 10 to 20 mCi in the field of view. Since such activity levels are typically encountered in cardiac images, prolonged tracer injection schemes are preferred to avoid high bolus activity during the first pass of the tracer.

The spatial resolution (6 to 7 mm) of a whole body scanner results in spillover and partial volume effect that has to be addressed in quantitative cardiac measurements. Myocardial activity contaminates the neighboring blood pool activity in the left ventricle and vice versa. Since the activity concentration in the blood decreases and the myocardial count rate increases over time, the amount of spillover is not a constant. The use of small regions of interest placed in the tissue minimize this spillover effect. As a consequence of finite resolution, real activity concentration is recovered only in structures that extend over more than twice the full width at half maximum (FWHM) of the tomograph (partial volume effect). If the actual width of the myocardial wall is known (either estimated by edge detection methods or by morphological imaging modalities such as ultrasound or magnetic resonance imaging [MRI]), correction methods can be applied using the information on resolution distortion from phantom measurements. Another approach determines the extravascular space by subtraction of a blood volume scan from the transmission data and uses this as myocardial tissue fraction in a given region of interest.[53] No further reference measurements are needed if the unknown fraction of blood pool contamination is included in the tracer kinetic model that is used to describe the measured tissue curve.[206] In the last frames of the dynamic scan, the tissue ROIs are defined so that they contain some blood pool activity. The input function is generated by placing a very small ROI in the left ventricle, assuming that this region contains pure blood activity. The model parameters are determined by fitting the model equation including a fourth parameter of tissue/blood fraction to the measured tissue curves. With this method, spillover and partial volume effect are corrected at the same time resulting in less biased rate constants.[53]

Some of the current limitations in quantitative measurements will be solved when three-dimensional data acquisition is routinely available.[207-209] Data are usually acquired in two-dimensional transaxial slices. New scanner developments that work without interplane septa are aimed to facilitate the three-dimensional acquisition of coincident events. The count rate will increase drastically, allowing lower radiation doses while the count rate limitations of the detector system have to be kept in mind. Although the contribution of scattered events increases in these setups, an improvement by a factor of 3 to 4 is expected in sensitivity, leading to a factor of 2 in noise equivalent count rates for cardiac studies.[210] New problems might arise from the increased amount of scattered radiation originating in the liver and appropriate correction methods have to be developed.

DIAGNOSTIC PERFORMANCE OF STRESS PERFUSION INVESTIGATIONS

Evaluation and reevaluation of a diagnostic test is challenging when that test is already widely used as a part of the diagnostic work-up. Referral of patients to angiography based upon the results of the diagnostic test generates posttest referral bias, which may lead to a decreased specificity as discussed by Rozanski et al.[211] For example, if only patients with abnormal perfusion scintigrams are referred for coronary angiography, an accurate determination of specificity becomes impossible.

A second important aspect of studies validating the diagnostic performance of perfusion scintigraphy is the disease prevalence in the patient population under study, as well as that of previous myocardial infarction. The sensitivity of the diagnostic test is augmented in patients with previous myocardial infarction, but inclusion of such patients does not reflect the typical group undergoing this test, for diagnosis of suspected CAD.

The use of different diagnostic criteria often complicates the comparison of different studies. Values for sensitivity and specificity depend on such criteria, which may therefore vary from study to study. The use of receiver operating characteristic (ROC) analysis approaches allows a more appropriate statistical comparison of different diagnostic modalities,[212] and allows the direct comparison of various diagnostic procedures over a wide range of criteria used to define abnormal results.

Finally, the most objective evaluation of diagnostic procedures requires the performance of multicenter studies with defined patients selection criteria and standardized reference techniques. The test results should be evaluated without knowledge of the clinical data using a core-laboratory facility. However, such evaluation is almost impossible at the current time, due to financial and logistic restrictions, but may be required in the future to satisfy the requirements of insurance carriers and policymakers to reimburse a new diagnostic test.

Planar Imaging

Using pooled data of exercise ^{201}Tl planar studies (Table 2-3), Okada reported a sensitivity of 82% and a specificity of 91% for detection of CAD.[213] However, using this method, the recognition of individual stenoses of the major coronary vessels was relatively poor, with reported sensitivities varying from 63 to 78% in the LAD, 21 to 45% in the left circumflex (LCx), and 50 to 85% in the RCA (Table 2-4).[214–217] Previous myocardial infarctions in the vascular territories of LAD and RCA were detectable by planar techniques with a high sensitivity (95% and 85%, respectively) while the recognition of persistent defects in the region of LCx was relatively low (48%).[214]

SPECT Imaging

After the adaptation of SPECT for cardiac imaging, comparative studies at the late 1980s reported an approximately 10% increase of accuracy in the global detection of CAD, by use of SPECT rather than planar techniques.[217–220] Using receiver operating characteristic curves, Fintel et al. demonstrated that SPECT is more accurate than planar imaging over the wide range of criteria for the overall detection and exclusion of CAD and the identification of LAD and LCx involvement. SPECT did not provide improved diagnosis in patients with previous myocardial infarction.[217] Studies analyzing the sensitivity of SPECT in the detection of individual stenosis reported sensitivity values from 70% to 88% in the LAD, from 50% to 79% in the LCx, and from 75% to 96% in the RCA. In spite of a global increase in vessel sensitivity, the detection of stenoses in LCx region appears limited.

The adaptation of semiquantitative evaluation for relative myocardial tracer distribution using a normal database has shown a similar diagnostic effectiveness as experienced specialists in the detection of CAD, but the intraobserver and interobserver variability of the interpretation was reduced.[221,222] Consequently, we recommend the use of semiquantitative evaluation for studies depicting small changes of myocardial perfusion (e.g., follow-up of therapeutic procedures). The sensitivity and specificity of this method in various patient subpopulations have been studied by pooling semiquantitatively evaluated SPECT data.[223] This study demonstrated the in-

Table 2-3. Global Detection of Coronary Artery Disease with Various Nuclear Perfusion Imaging Techniques

Study	Patient Number	Stenosis Threshold (%)	Tracer	Stress	Imaging	Planar Sensitivity (%)	Planar Specificity (%)	SPECT Sensitivity (%)	SPECT Specificity (%)	PET Sensitivity (%)	PET Specificity (%)
Massie et al. (1979)[214]	78	70	Tl	Exercise	Planar	89	93				
Rigo et al. (1980)[215]	133	50	Tl	Exercise	Planar	89	81				
Okada et al. (1980)[213]	1817	No data	Tl	Exercise	Planar	82	91				
Tamaki et al. (1984)[237]	104	50	Tl	Exercise	Qu-SPECT			95	93		
DePasquale et al. (1988)[238]	210	50	Tl	Exercise	Qu-SPECT			95	74		
Iskandrian et al. (1989)[239]	461	50	Tl	Exercise	Qu-SPECT			82	60		
Fintel et al. (1989)[217]	135	50	Tl	Exercise	Planar/SPECT	84	90	91	90		
Maddahi et al. (1990)[240]	138	50	Tl	Exercise	Qu-SPECT			95	56		
Mahmarian et al. (1990)[241]	360	50	Tl	Exercise	Qu-SPECT			87	87		
Van Train et al. (1990)[242]	318	50	Tl	Exercise	Qu-SPECT			94	43		
Schelbert et al. (1982)[225]	45	50	NH₃	Dipyridamole	PET					97	100
Yonekura et al. (1987)[226]	58	75	NH₃	Exercise	PET					97	100
Demer et al. (1989)[243]	193	50	NH₃; Rb	Dipyridamole	PET					82	95
Go et al. (1990)[229]	135	70	Rb	Dipyridamole	SPECT/PET			79	76	95	82
Stewart et al. (1991)[228]	81	50	Rb	Dipyridamole	SPECT/PET			84	53	84	88
Grover-McKay et al. (1992)[227]	31	50	Rb	Dipyridamole	PET					91	86
Simone et al. (1992)[230]	225	67	Rb	Dipyridamole	PET					83	91
Laubenbacher et al. (1993)[159]	52	75	NH₃	Dipyridamole	PET					93	80
Williams et al. (1994)[231]	287	67	Rb	Dipyridamole	PET					87	88
Van Train et al. (1994)[138]	161	50	Tc — MIBI	Exercise	SPECT			87	36[a]		
Heo et al. (1994)[140]	148	50	Tl + Tc — MIBI	Exercise	SPECT			77	65[b]		
Matzer et al. (1994)[244]	109	50	Tl + Tc — MIBI	Adenosine/Dipyridamole	SPECT			92	85		
Pennel et al. (1995)[245]	407	50	Tl	Adenosine (+ Exercise)	SPECT			96	78		

Abbreviations: Qu-SPECT, quantitative evaluated single photon emission computed tomography; PET, positron emission tomography.
[a] Normalcy rate = 81%.
[b] Normalcy rate = 97%.

Table 2-4. Sensitivity (%) of the Detection of the Individual Coronary Stenosis in Various Vascular Territories

Study	Patient Number	Stenosis Threshold (%)	Tracer	Imaging	Planar LAD	Planar LCx	Planar RCA	SPECT LAD	SPECT LCx	SPECT RCA	PET LAD	PET LCx	PET RCA
Massie et al. (1979)[214]	78	70	Tl	Planar	78	45	73						
Rigo et al. (1980)[215]	33	50	Tl	Planar	63	21	50						
Nohara et al. (1984)[216]	58	75	Tl	Planar/SPECT	73	39	85	88	78	96			
Fintel et al. (1989)[217]	135	50	Tl	Planar/SPECT	69	30	83	76	50	88			
Tamaki et al. (1984)[224]	75	50	Tl	SPECT				88	70	89			
DePasquale et al. (1988)[238]	210	50	Tl	SPECT				70	50	88			
	210	50	Tl	Qu-SPECT				78	65	89			
Tamaki et al. (1984)[237]	104	50	Tl	Qu-SPECT				87	78	92			
Maddahi et al. (1990)[240]	138	50	Tl	Qu-SPECT				78	79	82			
Mahmarian et al. (1990)[241]	360	50	Tl	Qu-SPECT				81	77	75			
Van Train et al. (1990)[242]	318	50	Tl	Qu-SPECT				78	68	84			
Allman et al. (1992)[222]	76	50	Tl	SPECT				57	49	81			
Yonekura et al. (1987)[226]	60	75	NH_3	PET							95	78	89
Grover-McKay et al. (1992)[227]	31	50	Rb	PET							91	75	75
Laubenbacher et al. (1993)[159]	52	75	NH_3	PET							86	80	83

Abbreviations: LAD, left anterior descending; LCx, left circumflex; RCA, right coronary artery; PET, positron emission tomography; Qu-SPECT, quantitative single photon emission computes tomography.

creasing sensitivity in the detection of CAD in relation with severity of disease (83%, 93%, and 95% for single-vessel, two-vessel, and three-vessel disease, respectively). Similarly, an increase of sensitivity was demonstrated in patients with previous myocardial infarction (85% and 99% for patients without and with previous myocardial infarction, respectively). On the other hand, Tamaki et al. demonstrated decreasing sensitivity for the detection of individual artery stenosis in the presence of an increasing number of stenosed arteries (92%, 50%, and 44% for single-vessel, two-vessel, and three-vessel disease, respectively).[224] Similarly, in a study of patients without previous myocardial infarction and less advanced CAD reported by Allman et al., accurate characterization of the extent of CAD could not be provided either with visual or with computer analysis of pharmacological stress ^{201}Tl SPECT. In the population of 76 patients, they demonstrated a sensitivity, specificity, and accuracy in detection of multivessel disease of 48%, 68%, and 58%, respectively.[222]

PET Imaging

The initial PET studies, similar to earlier methods, have shown excellent accuracy for myocardial perfusion PET in the global detection of CAD.[225,226] More recent reports indicate sensitivity, specificity, and accuracy values ranging from 83% to 95%, from 80% to 91%, and from 85% to 92%, respectively.[159,227–231] The two published studies that have compared the diagnostic effectiveness of SPECT and PET in the same patient populations show an approximate 10% increase in accuracy.[228,229] In the identification of individual coronary stenoses, PET also shows the highest sensitivity in the regions of LAD and RCA; however, sensitivity values for the identification of LCx lesions (from 75% to 80%) appear higher than with SPECT. Laubenbacher et al. reported accuracy in detection of LCx lesion of 79%, similar as to that in the LAD and RCA (85% and 82%, respectively) with ^{13}NH$_3$-PET, using semiquantitative analysis.

The accuracy for the detection of CAD has increased with the evolution from planar to PET imaging, but this has been paralleled by increasing cost, largely due to the expense of imaging equipment. Although SPECT is well accepted in the routine diagnosis of CAD, there are still not sufficient data available to define the diagnostic differences and cost-effectiveness between SPECT and PET in a large patient populations. These investigations are necessary to calculate the cost-to-benefit ratios of various clinical situations where PET should replace SPECT for myocardial perfusion studies in patients with suspected CAD.

CONCLUSIONS

The improvements of imaging equipment and the introduction of ^{99m}Tc radiopharmaceuticals have extended the successful clinical implementation of perfusion scintigraphy in the work-up of patients with coronary artery disease. As outlined in this chapter, a variety of radiopharmaceuticals allow a number of imaging protocols for specific clinical indications. The most widely used approach remains ^{201}Tl SPECT scintigraphy due to the extensive clinical experience and cost considerations. However, the ^{99m}Tc-labeled radiopharmaceuticals produce improved image quality, which together with attenuation correction and gated data acquisition provide not only assessment of myocardial perfusion but also evaluation of left ventricular function with one radiopharmaceutical. Combination of ^{99m}Tc-labeled radiopharmaceuticals for flow and functional imaging together with ^{201}Tl scintigraphy for tissue viability may exploit the full potential of modern tomographic cardiovascular scintigraphy. PET technology is necessary to quantitatively assess regional perfusion. Such noninvasive measurements are especially attractive for clinical research, but still await a defined clinical indication. However, if early detection of CAD or monitoring of regression or progression of disease become important clinical questions, PET measurements of perfusion may become more widely employed. The means of visualization and quantitative analysis provided by modern workstations yield important and objective information of relative and absolute myocardial perfusion to the referring cardiologist, not only for diagnostic but also prognostic purposes as outlined in Chapters 27 and 28 of this book.

REFERENCES

1. Bradley JA, Alpert JS, Mass W: Coronary flow reserve. Am Heart J 122:1116, 1991
2. Clark LT: Atherogenesis and thrombosis: mecha-

nism, pathogenesis, and therapeutic implications. Am Heart J 113:1106, 1992
3. MacIsaac AI, Thomas JD, Topol EJ: Toward the quiescent coronary plaque. J Am Coll Cardiol 22:1228, 1993
4. Nellis SH, Liedtke AJ, Whitesell L: Small coronary vessel pressure and diameter in an intact beating rabbit heart using fixed-position and free-motion techniques. Circ Res 49:342, 1981
5. Chilian WM, Bohling BA, Marcus ML: Capacitance function of epicardial coronary arteries. Fed Proc 40:603, 1981
6. Tillmanns H, Steinhausen M, Leinberger H et al: Pressure measurements in the terminal vascular bed of the epimyocardium of rats and cats. Circ Res 49:1202, 1981
7. Provenza DV, Scherlis S: Demonstration of muscle sphincters as a capillary component in the human heart. Circulation 20:35, 1959
8. Berne RM: The role of adenosine in the regulation of coronary blood flow. Circ Res 47:807, 1980
9. Moncada S, Vane JR: Pharmacology and endogenous roles of prostaglandin endoperoxides, thromboxane A2, and prostacyclin. Pharmacol Rev 30:293, 1978
10. Palmer RM, Ferrige AG, Moncada S: Nitric oxide release accounts for the biological activity of endothelium-derived relaxing factor. Nature (London) 327:524, 1987
11. Moncada S, Palmer RM, Higgs EA: The discovery of nitric oxide as the endogenous nitrovasodilator. Hypertension 12:365, 1988
12. Feletou M, Vanhoutte PM: Endothelium-dependent hyperpolarization of canine coronary smooth muscle. Br J Pharmacol 93:515, 1988
13. Merlet P, Mazoyer B, Hittinger L et al: Assessment of coronary reserve in man: comparison between positron emission tomography with oxygen-15-labeled water and intracoronary Doppler technique. J Nucl Med 34:1899, 1993
14. Hoffman JIE: Maximal coronary flow and the concept of coronary flow reserve. Circulation 70:82, 1984
15. McGinn AL, White CW, Wilson RF: Interstudy variability of coronary flow reserve. Circulation 81:1319, 1990
16. Wilson RF, White CW: Intracoronary papaverin: an ideal coronary vasodilatator for studies of the coronary circulation in conscious humans. Circulation 73:444, 1986
17. Bergmann S, Herrero P, Markham J et al: Noninvasive quantitation of myocardial blood flow in human subjects with oxygen-15-labeled water and positron emission tomography. J Am Coll Cardiol 14:639, 1989
18. Hutchins GD, Schwaiger M, Rosenspire K et al: Noninvasive quantification of regional myocardial blood flow in the human heart using N-13 ammonia and dynamic positron emission tomographic imaging. J Am Coll Cardiol 15:1032, 1990
19. Araujo LI, Lammertsma AA, Rhodes CG et al: Noninvasive quantification of regional myocardial blood flow in coronary artery disease with oxygen-15-labeled carbon dioxide inhalation and positron emission tomography. Circulation 83:875, 1991
20. Uren NG, Melin JA, De-Bruyne B et al: Relation between myocardial blood flow and the severity of coronary-artery stenosis. N Engl J Med 330:1782, 1994
21. Gould KL, Lipscomb K, Calvert C: Compensatory changes of the distal coronary vascular bed during progressive coronary constriction. Circulation 51:1085, 1975
22. Wilson RF, Laughlin DE, Ackell PH et al: Transluminal, subselective measurement of coronary artery blood flow velocity and vasodilator reserve in man. Circulation 72:82, 1985
23. Czernin J, Muller P, Chan S et al: Influence of age and hemodynamics on myocardial blood flow and flow reserve. Circulation 88:62, 1993
24. Luther TC: Atherogenesis and thrombosis: mechanisms, pathogenesis, and therapeutic implications. Am Heart J 123:1106, 1992
25. Stary HC: Evolution and progression of atherosclerotic lesions in children and young adults. Arteriosclerosis 99:119, 1989
26. Collins P, Fox P: The pathogenesis of atheroma and the rationale for its treatment. Eur Heart J 13:560, 1992
27. Ross R, Raines EW, Bowen-Pope DF: The biology of platelet-derived growth factors. Cell 46:155, 1986
28. Davies MJ, Woolf N, Katz DR: The role of endothelial denudation injury, plaque fissuring, and thrombosis in the progression of human atherosclerosis. p. 105. In Weber PC, Leaf A (eds): Atherosclerosis: Its Pathogenesis and the Role of Cholesterol. Raven Press, New York, 1991
29. Davies MJ, Woolf N, Rowles PM et al: Morphology of the endothelium over atherosclerotic plaques in human coronary arteries. Br Heart J 60:459, 1988
30. Uren NG, Marraccini P, Gistri R et al: Altered coronary vasodilator reserve and metabolism in myocardium subtended by normal arteries in patients with coronary artery disease. J Am Coll Cardiol 22:650, 1993
31. Sambuceti G, Parodi O, L'Abbate AL: Evidence for a

global impairment of coronary artery disease. Circulation 84:II-652, 1991
32. Beanlands R, Muzik O, Melon P et al: Non-invasive quantification of regional myocardial flow reserve in patients with coronary atherosclerosis using nitrogen-13 ammonia positron emission tomography: Determination of extent of altered vascular reactivity. J Am Coll Cardiol 26:1465, 1995
33. Maseri A, Crea F, Cianflone D: Myocardial ischemia caused by distal coronary vasoconstriction. Am J Cardiol 70:1602, 1992
34. Dayanikli F, Grambow D, Muzik O et al: Evaluation of coronary flow reserve in asymptomatic males with hyperlipidaemia and family history of coronary artery disease (CAD) (abstract). J Nucl Med 34:155P, 1993
35. Gould KL: Quantification of coronary artery stenosis in vivo. Circ Res 57:341, 1985
36. Davies MJ, Thomas A: Thrombosis and acute coronary-artery lesion in sudden cardiac ischemic death. N Engl J Med 310:1137, 1984
37. Kolibasch AJ, Bush CA, Wepsic RA: Coronary collateral vessels: spectrum of physiological capabilities with respect to providing rest and stress myocardial perfusion, maintainance of left ventricular function and protection against infarction. Am J Cardiol 117:296, 1989
38. Ridolfi RF, Hutchins GM: The relationship between coronary artery lesion and myocardial infarcts: ulceration of atherosclerotic plaques precipitating coronary thrombus. Am Heart J 93:468, 1977
39. Gertz SD, Kragel AH, Kalan JM et al: Comparison of coronary and myocardial morphologic findings in patients with and without thrombolytic therapy during fatal first acute myocardial infarction. The TIMI Investigators. Am J Cardiol 66:904, 1990
40. Liebenson PR, Klein LW: Intravascular ultrasound in coronary atherosclerosis: a new approach to clinical assessment. Am Heart 123:1643, 1992
41. Werner GS, Sold G, Buchwald A et al: Intravascular ultrasound imaging of human coronary arteries after percutaneous transluminal angioplasty: morphologic and quantitative assessment. Am Heart J 122:212, 1991
42. Honye J, Mahon DJ, Jain A et al: Morphological effects of coronary balloon angioplasty in vivo assessed by intravascular ultrasound imaging. Circulation 85:1012, 1992
43. Bartorelli AL, Neville RF, Keren G et al: In vitro and in vivo intravascular ultrasound imaging. Eur Heart J 13:102, 1992
44. Hangartner JR, Charleston AJ, Davies MJ et al: Morphological characteristics of clinically significant coronary artery stenosis in stable angina. Br Heart J 56:501, 1986
45. Kragel AH, Reddy SG, Wittes JT et al: Morphometric analysis of the composition of coronary arterial plaques in isolated unstable angina pectoris with pain at rest. Am J Cardiol 66:562, 1990
46. Kragel AH, Reddy SG, Wittes JT et al: Morphometric analysis of the composition of atherosclerotic plaques in the four major epicardial coronary arteries in acute myocardial infarction and in sudden coronary death. Circulation 80:1747, 1989
47. Ambrose JA, Tannenbaum MA, Alexopoulos D et al: Angiographic progression of coronary artery disease and the development of myocardial infarction. J Am Coll Cardiol 12:56, 1988
48. Giroud D, Li JM, Urban P et al: Relation of the site of acute myocardial infarction to the most severe coronary arterial stenosis at prior angiography. Am J Cardiol 69:729, 1992
49. Wackers FJ: Planar, SPECT, PET: the quest to predict the unpredictable? (editorial). J Nucl Med 31:1906, 1990
50. Braunwald E, Rutherford JD: Reversible ischemic left ventricular dysfunction: evidence for the hibernating myocardium. J Am Coll Cardiol 8:1467, 1986
51. Rahimtoola SH: The hibernating myocardium. Am Heart J 117:211, 1989
52. vom-Dahl J, Eitzman DT, al-Aouar ZR et al: Relation of regional function, perfusion and metabolism in patients with advanced coronary artery disease undergoing surgical revascularization. Circulation 90:2356, 1994
53. Iida H, Rhodes CG, de-Silva R et al: Myocardial tissue fraction-- correction for partial volume effects and measure of tissue viability. J Nucl Med 32:2169, 1991
54. Dilsizian V, Rocco TP, Freedman NM et al: Enhanced detection of ischemic but viable myocardium by the reinjection of thallium after stress- redistribution imaging. N Engl J Med 323:141, 1990
55. Hutchins GM, Bulkley BH: Correlation of myocardial contraction band necrosis and vascular patency. A study of coronary artery bypass graft anastomoses at branch points. Lab Invest 36:642, 1977
56. Kloner RA, Ellis SG, Lange R et al: Studies of experimental coronary artery reperfusion. Effects on infarct size, myocardial function, biochemistry, ultrastructure and microvascular damage. Circulation 68:18, 1983
57. Vogel R, Le-Free M, Bates E et al: Application of digital techniques to selective coronary arteriography. Am Heart J 107:153, 1982
58. Mancini GB, Williamson PR, DeBoe SF: Effect of cor-

onary stenosis severity on variability of quantitative arteriography, and implications for interventional trials. Am J Cardiol 69:806, 1992
59. Rayford CR, Khouri EM, Lewis FB et al: Evaluation of use of left coronary inflow and O2 content of coronary sinus blood as a measure of left ventricular metabolism. J Appl Physiol 14:817, 1959
60. Ganz W, Tamura K, Marcus HS et al: Measurement of coronary sinus blood flow by continuous thermodilution in man. Circulation 44:181, 1971
61. Cannon PJ, Weiss MB, Sciacca RR: Myocardial blood flow in coronary artery disease: studies at rest and during stress with inert gas washout techniques. Prog Cardiovasc Dis 20:95, 1977
62. Marcus ML: Methods of measuring coronary blood flow. In The Coronary Circulation in Health and Disease. McGraw-Hill, New York, 1983
63. Strauss HW, Zaret BL, Martin ND et al: Noninvasive evaluation of regional myocardial perfusion with potassium-43. Radiology 108:85, 1973
64. Atkins HL, Budinger TF, Lebowitz E et al: Thallium-201 for medical use. Part 3: Human distribution and physical imaging properties. J Nucl Med 18:133, 1977
65. Bacharach SL: Quantitation in cardiac PET: a few remaining challenges. p. 89. In Zaret BL, Beller GA (eds): Nuclear Cardiology: State of the Art and Future Directions. Mosby, St. Louis, Missouri, 1992
66. Mullins LJ, Moore RD: The movement of thallium ions in muscle. J Gen Physiol 43:759, 1960
67. McCall D, Zimmer LJ, Katz AM: Kinetics of thallium exchange in cultured rat myocardial cells. Circ Res 56:370, 1985
68. Piwnica-Worms D, Kronauge JF, Marsh JD et al: Effect of metabolic inhibition on technetium-99m-MIBI kinetics in cultured chick myocardial cells. J Nucl Med 31:464, 1990
69. Dilsizian V, Arrighi JA, Diodati JG et al: Myocardial viability in patients with chronic coronary artery disease. Comparison of 99mTc-sestamibi with thallium reinjection and 18F fluorodeoxyglucose. Circulation 89:578, 1994
70. Tamaki N, Ohtani H, Yonekura Y et al: Viable myocardium identified by reinjection thallium-201 imaging: comparison with regional wall motion and metabolic activity on FDG-PET. J Cardiol 22:283, 1992
71. Ohtani H, Tamaki N, Mohiuddin IH et al: Minimal redistribution of thallium-201 representing reversible ischemia after coronary bypass surgery: value of quantitative analysis of exercise thallium-201 SPECT. J Cardiol 21:835, 1991
72. Bonow RO, Dilsizian V, Cuocolo A et al: Identification of viable myocardium in patients with chronic coronary artery disease and left ventricular dysfunction. Comparison of thallium scintigraphy with reinjection and PET imaging with 18F-fluorodeoxyglucose. Circulation 83:26, 1991
73. McCall D, Zimmer LJ, Katz AM: Effect of ischemia-related metabolic factors on thallium exchange in cultured rat myocardial cells. Can J Cardiol 2:176, 1986
74. Piwnica-Worms D, Chiu ML, Kronauge JF: Divergent kinetics of 201Tl and 99mTc-sestamibi in cultured chick ventricular myocytes during ATP depletion. Circulation 85:1531, 1992
75. Leppo JA, Meerdink DJ: Comparison of the myocardial uptake of a technetium-labeled isonitrile analogue and thallium. Circ Res 65:632, 1989
76. Meerdink DJ, Leppo JA: Myocardial transport of hexakis (2-methoxyisobutylisonitrile) and thallium before and after coronary reperfusion. Circ Res 66:1738, 1990
77. Melon PG, Beanlands RS, DeGrado TR et al: Comparison of technetium-99m-sestamibi and thallium-201 retention characteristics in canine myocardium. J Am Coll Cardiol 20:1277, 1992
78. Grunwald AM, Watson DD, Holzgrefe HH et al: Myocardial thallium-201 kinetics in normal and ischemic myocardium. Circulation 64:610, 1981
79. Wilson RA, Okada RD, Strauss HW et al: Effect of glucose-insulin-potassium infusion on thallium myocardial clearance. Circulation 68:203, 1983
80. Angello DA, Wilson RA, Gee D: Effect of ribose on thallium-201 myocardial redistribution. J Nucl Med 29:1943, 1988
81. Perlmutter NS, Wilson RA, Angello DA et al: Ribose facilitates thallium-201 redistribution in patients with coronary artery disease. J Nucl Med 32:193, 1991
82. Hegewald MG, Palac RT, Angello DA et al: Ribose infusion accelerates thallium redistribution with early imaging compared with late 24-hour imaging without ribose. J Am Coll Cardiol 18:1671, 1991
83. Strauss HW, Pitt B: 201-thallium as a myocardial imaging agent. Semin Nucl Med 7:49, 1977
84. Pohost GM, Zir LM, Moore RH et al: Differentiation of transiently ischemic from infarcted myocardium by serial imaging after a single dose of thallium-201. Circulation 55:294, 1977
85. Dilsizian V, Bonow RO: Differential uptake and apparent 201Tl washout after thallium reinjection. Options regarding early redistribution imaging before reinjection or late redistribution imaging after reinjection. Circulation 85:1032, 1992
86. Inglese E, Brambilla M, Dondi M et al: Assessment of myocardial viability after thallium-201 reinjection

or rest-redistribution imaging: a multicenter study. J Nucl Med 36:555, 1995
87. van-Eck-Smit BL, van-der-Wall EE, Baur LHB et al: Concordance between thallium-201 stress-immediate reinjection imaging and rest-redistribution imaging for the identification of viable myocardium (abstract). J Nucl Cardiol X2:S21, 1995
88. Wackers FJ, Berman DS, Maddahi J et al: Technetium-99m hexakis 2-methoxyisobutyl isonitrile: human biodistribution, dosimetry, safety, and preliminary comparison to thallium-201 for myocardial perfusion imaging (phase I and II studies). J Nucl Med 30:301, 1989
89. Chiu ML, Kronauge JF, Piwnica-Worms D: Effect of mitochondrial and plasma membrane potentials on accumulation of hexakis (2-methoxyisobutylisonitrile) technetium(I) in cultured mouse fibroblasts. J Nucl Med 31:1646, 1990
90. Davis S, Weiss MJ, Wong JR et al: Mitochondrial and plasma membrane potentials cause unusual accumulation and retention of rhodamine 123 by human breast adenocarcinoma-derived MCF-7 cells. J Biol Chem 260:13844, 1985
91. Marshall RC, Leidholdt EMJ, Zhang DY et al: Technetium-99m hexakis 2-methoxy-2-isobutyl isonitrile and thallium-201 extraction, washout, and retention at varying coronary flow rates in rabbit heart. Circulation 82:998, 1990
92. Beanlands RSB, Dawood F, Wen WH et al: Are the kinetics of technetium-99m methoxyisobutyl isonitrile affected by cell metabolism and viability? Circulation 82:1802, 1990
93. Higley B, Smith FW, Smith T et al: Technetium-99m, 2-bi bis (2-ethoxyethyl) phosphino ethane: human biodistribution, dosimetry and safety of a new myocardial perfusion imaging agent. J Nucl Med 34:30, 1993
94. Sinusas AJ, Shi Q, Saltzberg MT et al: Technetium-99m-tetrofosmin to assess myocardial blood flow: experimental validation in an intact canine model of ischemia. J Nucl Med 35:664, 1994
95. Jain D, Wackers FJ, Mattera J et al: Biokinetics of technetium-99m-tetrofosmin: myocardial perfusion imaging agent: Implication for a one-day imaging protocol. J Nucl Med 34:1254, 1993
96. Schroeter G, Schneider-Eicke J, Leitner G et al: Tracer kinetics of ^{99m}Tc tetrofosmin and ^{99m}Tc MIBI (abstract). Nuklearmedizin 34:A115, 1995
97. Kronauge JF, Chiu ML, Cone JS et al: Comparison of neutral and cationic myocardial perfusion agents: characteristics of accumulation in cultured cells. Int J Rad Appl Instrum B 19:141, 1992
98. Linder KE et al: Neutral tris oxime complexes of technetium (III): chemistry and biodistribution of TcX(oxime)3. J Nucl Med 29:800, 1988
99. Piwnica-Worms D, Kronauge JF: Transport mechanisms of SPECT perfusion tracers in cultured cells, p. 25. In Zaret BL, Beller GA (eds): Nuclear Cardiology: State of the Art and Future Directions. Mosby, St. Louis, Missouri, 1992
100. Leppo JA: Cardiac transport of single photon myocardial perfusion agents. p. 35. In Zaret BL, Beller GA (eds): Nuclear Cardiology: State of the Art and Future Directions. Mosby, St. Louis, Missouri, 1992
101. Bisson G, Hendel RC, Taillefer R: Newer technetium-99m-labeled myocardial perfusion imaging agents: clinical indications. Am J Cardiac Imaging 8:213, 1994
102. Johnson LL: Clinical experience with technetium 99m teboroxime. Semin Nucl Med 21:182, 1991
103. Rumsey WL, Rosenspire KC, Nunn AD: Myocardial extraction of teboroxime: effects of teboroxime interaction with blood. J Nucl Med 33:94, 1991
104. Hendel RC, McSherry B, Karimeddini M et al: Diagnostic value of a new myocardial perfusion agent, teboroxime (SQ 30,217), utilizing a rapid planar imaging protocol: preliminary results. J Am Coll Cardiol 16: 855, 1990
105. Gray WA, Gewirtz H: Comparison of 99mTc-teboroxime with thallium for myocardial imaging in the presence of coronary artery stenosis. Circulation 84: 1796, 1991
106. Stewart RE, Schwaiger M, Hutchins GD et al: Myocardial clearance kinetics of technetium-99m-SQ30217: A marker of regional myocardial blood flow. J Nucl Med 31:1183, 1990
107. Beanlands R, Muzik O, Nguyen N et al: The relationship between myocardial retention of technetium-99m-teboroxime and myocardial blood flow. J Am Coll Cardiol 20:712, 1992
108. Stewart RE, Heyl B, O-Rourke RA et al: Demonstration of differential post-stenotic myocardial technetium-99m-teboroxime clearance kinetics after experimental ischemia and hyperemic stress. J Nucl Med 32:2000, 1991
109. Johnson G, Glover DK, Hebert CB et al: Myocardial clearance kinetics of technetium-99m-teboroxime following dipyridamole: differentiation of stenosis severity in canine myocardium. J Nucl Med 36:111, 1995
110. Chiao PC, Ficaro EP, Dayanikli F et al: Compartmental analysis of technetium-99m-teboroxime kinetics employing fast dynamic SPECT at rest and stress. J Nucl Med 35:1265, 1994
111. Carretta RF, Weiland FW, Vande-Streek PR et al: Technetium-99m-teboroxime resting washout imag-

112. Daher E, Sinusas A, Natale D et al: Tc99m-furofosmin organ clearance and heart/organ ratio: Implication for timing of imaging (abstract). J Nucl Med 36:24P, 1995
113. Gerson M, Lukes J, Deutsch E et al: Comparison of ^{99m}Tc Q12 and Tl-201 imaging for detection of angiographically documented coronary artery disease in humans. J Nucl Cardiol 1:499, 1994
114. Gerson MC, Lukes J, Deutsch E et al: Comparison of imaging properties of technetium 99m Q12 and technetium 99m Q13 in humans. J Nucl Cardiol 2:224, 1995
115. Giganti M, Duatti A, Uccelli L et al: Biodistribution and preliminary clinical evaluation of 99mTc-NOET as myocardial perfusion tracer (abstract). J Nucl Cardiol 2:S44, 1995
116. Fagret D, Marie PY, Brunotte F et al: Myocardial perfusion imaging with technetium-99m-Tc NOET: Comparison with thallium-201 and coronary angiography. J Nucl Med 36:936, 1995
117. Ghezzi G, Fagret D, Arvieux CC et al: Myocardial kinetic of TcN-NOET: A neutral lipophilic complex tracer if regional myocardial blood flow. J Nucl Med 36:1069, 1995
118. Pohost GM, Alpert NM, Ingwall JS et al: Thallium-redistribution: mechanisms and clinical utility. Semin Nucl Med 10:70, 1980
119. Friedman J, Van-Train K, Maddahi J et al: "Upward creep" of the heart: a frequent source of false-positive reversible defects during thallium-201 stress-redistribution SPECT. J Nucl Med 35:1718, 1989
120. Gibson RS, Watson DD, Taylor GJ et al: Prospective assessment of regional myocardial perfusion before and after coronary revascularization surgery by quantitative thallium-201 scintigraphy. J Am Coll Cardiol 1:804, 1983
121. Liu P, Kiess MC, Okada RD et al: The persistent defect on exercise thallium imaging and its fate after myocardial revascularization: does it represent scar or ischemia? Am Heart J 110:996, 1985
122. Gutman J, Berman DS, Freeman M et al: Time to completed redistribution of thallium-201 in exercise myocardial scintigraphy: relationship to the degree of coronary artery stenosis. Am Heart J 106:989, 1983
123. Cloninger KG, DePuey EG, Garcia EV et al: Incomplete redistribution in delayed thallium-201 single photon emission computed tomographic images: an overestimation of myocardial scarring. J Am Coll Cardiol 12:955, 1988
124. Kiat H, Berman DS, Maddahi J et al: Late reversibility of tomographic myocardial thallium-201 defects: an accurate marker of myocardial viability. J Am Coll Cardiol 12:1456, 1988
125. Galli M, Marcassa C: Thallium-201 redistribution after early reinjection in patients with severe stress perfusion defects and ventricular dysfunction. Am Heart J 128:41, 1994
126. Gewirtz H, Beller GA, Strauss HW et al: Transient defects of resting thallium scans in patients with coronary artery disease. Circulation 59:707, 1979
127. Iskandrian AS, Hakki A, Kane SA et al: Rest and redistribution thallium-201 myocardial scintigraphy to predict improvement in left ventricular function after coronary artery bypass grafting. Am J Cardiol 51:1312, 1983
128. Berman DS, Kiat H, Friedman JD et al: Separate acquisition rest thallium-201/stress technetium-99m-sestamibi dual-isotope myocardial perfusion single-photon emission computed tomography: A clinical validation study. J Am Coll Cardiol 22:1455, 1993
129. Heo J, Kegel J, Iskandrian AS et al: Comparison of same-day protocols using technetium-99m-sestamibi myocardial imaging. J Nucl Med 33:186, 1992
130. Wackers FJ: Thrombolytic therapy for myocardial infarction: assessment of efficacy by myocardial perfusion imaging with technetium-99m-sestamibi. Am J Cardiol 66:36E, 1990
131. Weinstein H, Dahlberg ST, McSherry BA et al: Rapid redistribution of teboroxime. Am J Cardiol 71:848, 1993
132. Iskandrian AS, Heo J, Nguyen T et al: Tomographic myocardial perfusion imaging with technetium-99m-teboroxime during adenosine-induced coronary hyperemia: correlation with thallium-201 imaging. J Am Coll Cardiol 19:307, 1992
133. Sasaki M, Ichiya Y, Kuwabara Y et al: Rapid myocardial perfusion imaging with 99Tcm-teboroxime and a three-headed SPECT system: a comparative study with 201Tl. Nucl Med Commun 13:790, 1992
134. Mahmood S, Gunning M, Bomanji JB et al: Combined rest thallium/stress technetium-99m-tetrofosmin SPECT: Feasibility and diagnostic accuracy of a 90-minute protocol. J Nucl Med 36:932, 1995
135. Kiat H, Biasio Y, Wong FP: Frequency of reversible resting hypoperfusion in patients undergoing rest Tl-201/stress Tc-sestamibi separate acquisition dual isotope myocardial perfusion SPECT. J Am Coll Cardiol 21:222A (abstract), 1993
136. Anger HO: Scintillation camera. Rev Scientific Instrument 29:27, 1958
137. Kuhl DE, Edwards RQ: Reorganizing data from trans-

verse section scans using digital processing. Radiology 91:975, 1968
138. Van-Train KF, Garcia EV, Maddahi J et al: Multicenter trial validation for quantitative analysis of same-day rest-stress technetium-99m-sestamibi myocardial tomograms. J Nucl Med 35:609, 1994
139. Kiat H, Germano G, Friedman J et al: Comparative feasibility of separate or simultaneous rest thallium-201/stress technetium-99m-sestamibi dual-isotope myocardial perfusion SPECT. J Nucl Med 35:542, 1994
140. Heo J, Wolmer I, Kegel J et al: Sequential dual-isotope SPECT imaging with thallium-201 and technetium-99m-sestamibi. J Nucl Med 35:549, 1994
141. Chang LT: A method for attenuation correction in radionuclide computed tomography. IEEE Trans Nucl Sci 25:638, 1978
142. Ficaro EP, Fessler JA, Rogers WL et al: Comparison of americium-241 and technetium-99m as transmission sources for attenuation correction of thallium-201 SPECT imaging of the heart. J Nucl Med 35:652, 1994
143. DePuey EG: How to detect and avoid myocardial perfusion SPECT artifacts. J Nucl Med 35:699, 1994
144. Faber TL, Akers MS, Peshock RM et al: Three-dimensional motion and perfusion quantification in gated single-photon emission computed tomograms. J Nucl Med 32:2311, 1991
145. Galt JR: New instrumentation for cardiovascular nuclear medicine news. J Nucl Med 35:20N, 1994
146. Rogers WL, Ackermann RJ: SPECT instrumentation. Am J Physiol Imaging 7:105, 1992
147. Watson DD, Smith WH: SPECT: current and future developments. J Nucl Biol Med 36:108, 1992
148. DePuey EG, Salensky H, Melancon S et al: Simultaneous biplane first-pass radionuclide angiocardiography using a scintillation camera with two perpendicular detectors. J Nucl Med 35:1593, 1994
149. Tan P, Bailey DL, Meikle SR et al: A scanning line source for simultaneous emission and transmission measurements in SPECT. J Nucl Med 34:1752, 1993
150. Fahey FH, Harkness BA, Keyes JWJ et al: Sensitivity, resolution and image quality with a multi-head SPECT camera. J Nucl Med 33:1859, 1992
151. Tsui BM, Zhao X, Frey EC et al: Quantitative single-photon emission computed tomography: basics and clinical considerations. Semin Nucl Med 24:38, 1994
152. Wackers FJT: Science, art, and artifacts: How important is quantification for the practicing physician interpreting myocardial perfusion studies? J Nucl Cardiol 1:S109, 1994
153. Meade RC, Bamrah VS, Horgam JD et al: Quantitative methods in the evaluation of thallium-201 myocardial perfusion images. J Nucl Med 19:1175, 1978
154. Burow RD, Pond M, Schafer AW et al: "Circumferential profiles": a new method for computer analysis of thallium-201 myocardial perfusion images. J Nucl Med 20:771, 1979
155. Caldwell JH, Williams DL, Hamilton GW et al: Regional distribution of myocardial blood flow measured by single-photon emission tomography: comparison with in vitro counting. J Nucl Med 23:490, 1982
156. Garcia EV, Van-Train K, Maddahi J et al: Quantification of rotational thallium-201 myocardial tomography. J Nucl Med 26:17, 1985
157. Miller TR, Starren JB, Grothe RA: Three-dimensional display of positron emission tomography of the heart. J Nucl Med 29:530, 1988
158. Faber TL, Akers MS, Peshock RM et al: Three-dimensional motion and perfusion quantification in gated SPECT. J Nucl Med 32:2311, 1991
159. Laubenbacher C, Rothley J, Sitomer J et al: An automated analysis program for the evaluation of cardiac PET studies: initial results in the detection and localization of coronary artery disease using nitrogen-13-ammonia. J Nucl Med 34:968, 1993
160. Faber TL, Cooke CD, Peifer JW et al: Three-dimensional displays of left ventricular epicardial surface from standard cardiac SPECT perfusion quantification techniques. J Nucl Med 36:697, 1995
161. Garvin AA, Cullom SJ, Garcia EV: Myocardial perfusion imaging using single-photon emission computed tomography. Am J Cardiac Imaging 8:189, 1994
162. Krizek H, Lembares N, Dinwoodie R et al: Production of radiochemically pure 13-NH3 for biomedical studies using the 16-O(p, = E0)13-N reaction. J Nucl Med 14:629, 1973
163. Schwaiger M, Muzik O: Assessment of myocardial perfusion by positron emission tomography. Am J Cardiol 67:35D, 1991
164. Warren KS: Ammonia toxicity and pH. Nature (London) 195:47, 1962
165. Phelps ME, Hoffman EJ, Raybaud C: Factors which affect cerebral uptake and retention of 13NH3. Stroke 8:694, 1977
166. Schelbert HR, Phelps ME, Huang SC et al: N-13 ammonia as an indicator of myocardial blood flow. Circulation 63:1259, 1981
167. White A, Handler P, Smith EL et al: p. 651. Principles of Biochemistry. McGraw-Hill, New York, 1978
168. Kobayashi T: Myocardial amide-nitrogen metabolism with special reference to ammonia metabolism. Stud-

ies by the use of the coronary sinus catheterization technique. Jpn Circ J 31:33, 1967
169. Davidson S, Sonnenblick EH: Glutamine production by the isolated perfused rat heart during ammonium chloride perfusion. Cardiovasc Res 9:295, 1975
170. Watanabe T: Significance of ammonia in myocardial metabolism. Jpn Circ J, suppl. 32:1811, 1968
171. Krivokapich J, Smith GT, Huang SC et al: 13N ammonia myocardial imaging at rest and with exercise in normal volunteers. Quantification of absolute myocardial perfusion with dynamic positron emission tomography. Circulation 80:1328, 1989
172. Iida H, Takahashi A, Ono Y et al: Quantitative and noninvasive measurement of myocardial blood flow using H2-15-O and dynamic positron emission tomography. J Nucl Med 27:976, 1986
173. Bergmann S, Fox K, Rand A et al: Quantification of regional myocardial blood flow in vivo with H2-15-O. Circulation 70:724, 1984
174. Kety S: Measurement of local blood flow by the exchange of an inert, diffusable substance. Methods Med Res 8:228, 1960
175. Love WD, Burch GE: A study in dogs of methods suitable for estimating the rate of myocardial uptake of Rb-86 in man, and the effect of norepinephrine and pitression on Rb-86 uptake. J Clin Invest 36:468, 1957
176. Mullani NA, Goldstein RA, Gould KL et al: Myocardial perfusion with rubidium-82: I. Measurement of extraction fraction and flow with external detectors. J Nucl Med 24:898, 1983
177. Shelton ME, Green MA, Mathias CJ et al: Assessment of regional myocardial and renal blood flow with copper-PTSM and positron emission tomography. Circulation 82:990, 1990
178. Robinson GD, Zielinski FW, Lee AW: The zinc-62/copper-62 generator: a convenient source of copper-62 radiopharmaceuticals. Int J Appl Radiat Isotopes 31:111, 1980
179. Mathias CJ, Welch MJ, Raichle ME, et al: Evaluation of a potential generator-produced PET tracer for cerebral perfusion imaging: single-pass cerebral extraction measurements and imaging with radiolabeled Cu-PTSM. J Nucl Med 31:351, 1990
180. Beanlands RS, Muzik O, Mintun M et al: The kinetics of copper-62-PTSM in the normal human heart. J Nucl Med 33:684, 1992
181. Green MA: A potential copper radiopharmaceutical for imaging the heart and brain: copper-labeled pyruvaldehyde bis(N4-methylthiosemicarbazone). Nucl Med Biol 15:59, 1987
182. Green MA, Klippenstein DL, Tennison JR: Copper(II) bis(thiosemicarbazone) complexes as potential tracers for evaluation of cerebral and myocardial blood flow with PET. J Nucl Med 29:1549, 1988
183. Green MA, Mathias CJ, Welch MJ et al: Copper-62-labeled pyruvaldehyde bis(N4-methylthiosemicarbazonato)copper(II): synthesis and evaluation as a positron emission tomography tracer for cerebral and myocardial perfusion. J Nucl Med 31:1989, 1990
184. Shelton ME, Green MA, Mathias CJ et al: Kinetics of copper-PTSM in isolated hearts: a novel tracer for measuring blood flow with positron emission tomography. J Nucl Med 30:1843, 1989
185. Petering DH: The reaction of 3-methoxy-2-oxobutyraldehyde bis(thiosemicarbazonato)copper(II) with thiols. Bioinorg Chem 1:273, 1972
186. Winkelmann DA, Bermke Y, Petering DH: Comparative properties of the antineoplastic agent 3-ethoxy-2-oxobutyraldehyde bis(thiosemicarbazone)-copper(II) and related chelates. Bioinorg Chem 3:261, 1974
187. Minkel DT, Saryan LA, Petering DH: Structure-function correlations in the reaction of bis(thiosemicarbazone)copper(II) complexes with Ehrlich ascites tumor cells. Cancer Res 38:124, 1978
188. Herrero P, Markham J, Weinheimer CJ et al: Quantification of regional myocardial perfusion with generator-produced 62Cu-PTSM and positron emission tomography. Circulation 87:173, 1993
189. Spinks T, Araujo L, Rhodes C et al: Physical aspects of cardiac scanning with a block detector positron tomograph. J Comput Assist Tomogr 15:893, 1991
190. Wienhard K, Eriksson L, Grootoonk S et al: Performance evaluation of the positron scanner ECAT EXACT. J Comput Assist Tomogr 16:804, 1992
191. Wienhard K, Dahlbom M, Eriksson L et al: The ECAT EXACT HR: performance of a new high resolution positron scanner. J Comput Assist Tomogr 18:110, 1994
192. Ter-Pogossian M, Mullani N, Ficke D et al: Photon time-of-flight-assisted positron emission tomography. J Comput Assist Tomogr 5:227, 1981
193. Mazoyer B, Trebossen R, Schoukroun C et al: Physical evaluation of TTV03, a new high spatial resolution time-of-flight positron tomograph. IEEE Trans Nucl Sci 37:778, 1990
194. Lewellen T, Bice A, Harrisson R et al: Performance measurements of the SP3000/UW time-of-flight positron emission tomograph. IEEE Trans Nucl Sci NS-35:665, 1988
195. Meikle S, Dahlbom M, Cherry S: Attenuation correction using count-limited transmission data in positron emission tomography. J Nucl Med 34:143, 1993
196. Xu E, Mullani N, Gould K et al: A segmented attenuation correction for PET. J Nucl Med 32:161, 1991

197. Thompson C, Ranger N, Evans A: Simultaneous transmission and emission scans in positron emission tomography. IEEE Trans Nucl Sci 36:1011, 1989
198. Thompson C, Ranger N, Evans A et al: Validation of simultaneous PET emission and transmission scans. J Nucl Med 32:154, 1991
199. Muzik O, Beanlands R, Dayanikli F et al: Quantification of myocardial blood flow reserve using PET and N-13 ammonia in patients with angiographically documented CAD. J Nucl Med 34:35P (abstract), 1993
200. Weinberg I, Huang S, Hoffman E et al: Validation of PET acquired input functions for cardiac studies. J Nucl Med 29:241, 1988
201. Gambhir S, Schwaiger M, Huang S et al: Simple noninvasive quantification method for measuring myocardial glucose utilization in humans employing positron emission tomography and fluorine-18 deoxyglucose. J Nucl Med 30:359, 1989
202. Raylman R, Caraher J, Hutchins G: Sampling requirements for dynamic cardiac PET studies using image derived input functions. J Nucl Med 34:440, 1993
203. Huang S, Phelps M: Principles of tracer kinetic modeling in positron emission tomography and autoradiography. p. 287. In Phelps M, Mazziotta J, Schelbert H (eds): Positron Emission Tomography and Autoradiography: Principles and Applications for the Brain and Heart. Raven Press, New York, 1986
204. Muzik O, Beanlands R, Wolfe E et al: Automated region definition for cardiac nitrogen-13-ammonia PET imaging. J Nucl Med 34:336, 1993
205. Iida H, Kanno I, Takahashi A et al: Measurement of absolute myocardial blood flow with H2150 and dynamic positron-emission tomography. Strategy for quantification in relation to the partial-volume effect. Circulation 78:104, 1988
206. Hutchins G, Caraher J, Raylman R: A region of interest strategy for minimizing resolution distortions in quantitative myocardial PET studies. J Nucl Med 33:1243, 1992
207. Cherry S, Dahlbom M, Hoffman E: Three-dimensional PET using a conventional multi-slice tomograph without septa. J Comp Assist Tomogr 15:655, 1991
208. Colsher JG: Fully three-dimensional positron emission tomography. Phys Med Biol 25:103, 1980
209. Townsend D, Spinks T, Jones T et al: Three-dimensional reconstruction of PET data from a multi-ring camera. IEEE Trans Nucl Sci 36:1056, 1989
210. Bailey D, Lee K, Stocks G et al: Clinical 3D PET for improved patient throughput (abstract). J Nucl Med 34:P184, 1993
211. Rozanski A: Referral bias and the efficacy of radionuclide stress tests: Problems and solutions. J Nucl Med 33:2074, 1992
212. Metz CE: Basic principles of ROC analysis. Semin Nucl Med 8:283, 1978
213. Okada RD, Boucher CA, Strauss HW, Pohost GM: Exercise radionuclide imaging approaches to coronary artery disease. Am J Cardiol 46:1188, 1980
214. Massie BM, Botvinick EH, Brundage BH: Correlation of thallium-201 scintigrams with coronary anatomy: factors affecting region by region sensitivity. Am J Cardiol 44:616, 1979
215. Rigo P, Bailey IK, Griffith LSC, Pitt B, Burow RD, Wagner HN, Becker LC: Value and limitation of segmental analysis of stress thallium myocardial imaging for localization of coronary artery disease. Circulation 61:973, 1980
216. Nohara R, Kambara H, Suzuki Y, Tamaki S, Kadota K, Kawai C, Tamaki N, Torizuka K: Stress scintigraphy using single-photon emission computed tomography in the evaluation of coronary artery disease. Am J Cardiol 53:1250, 1984
217. Fintel DJ, Links JM, Brinker JA et al: Improved diagnostic performance of exercise thallium-201 single photon emission computed tomography over planar imaging in the diagnosis of coronary artery disease: a reciever operating characteristic analysis. J Am Coll Cardiol 13:600, 1989
218. Go RT, Cook SA, MacIntyre WJ et al: Comparative accuracy of stress and redistribution thallium 201 cardiac single photon emission transaxial tomography and planar imaging in the diagnosis of myocardial ischemia (abstract). J Nucl Med 23:P25, 1982
219. Links JM, Fintel DF, Becker KC, Wagner HN: Comparison of planar and SPECT thallium imaging in men and women (abstract). J Nucl Med 26:P49, 1985
220. Taylor DM, Choraria SK, Maugham J et al: Diagnosis of coronary artery disease using thallium imaging: tomographic versus planar imaging. Nucl Med Comm 10:401, 1989
221. Nishimura S, Mahmarian JJ, Boyce TM, Verani MS: Quantitative thallium-201 single photon emission computed tomography during maximal coronary vasodilatation with adenosine for assessing coronary artery disease. J Am Coll Cardiol 18:736, 1991
222. Allman KC, Berry J, Sucharsky LA et al: Determination of extent and location of coronary artery disease in patients without prior myocardial infarction by thallium-201 tomography with pharmacologic stress. J Nucl Med 33:2067, 1992
223. Mahmarian JJ, Verani MS: Exercise thallium-201 perfusion scintigraphy in the assessment of coronary artery disease. Am J Cardiol 67:2D, 1991

224. Tamaki N, Yonekure Y, Mukai T et al: Segmental analysis of stress thallium myocardial emission tomography for localization of coronary artery disease. Eur J Nucl Med 9:99, 1984
225. Schelbert HR, Wisenberg G, Phelps ME et al: Noninvasive assessment of coronary stenoses by myocardial imaging during pharmacological coronary vasodilatation VI.: Detection of coronary artery disease in human beings with intravenous N-13 ammonia and positron computed tomography. Am J Cardiol 49:1197, 1982
226. Yonekura Y, Tamaki N, Senda M et al: Detection of coronary artery disease with 13N-ammonia and high-resolution positron-emission computed tomography. Am Heart J 113:645, 1987
227. Grover-McKay M, Ratib O, Schwaiger M et al: Detection of coronary artery disease with positron emission tomography and rubidium 82. Am Heart J 123:646, 1992
228. Stewart RE, Schwaiger M, Molina E et al: Comparison of rubidium-82 positron emission tomography and thallium-201 SPECT imaging for detection of coronary artery disease. Am J Cardiol 67:1303, 1991
229. Go RT, Marwick TH, MacIntyre WJ et al: A prospective comparison of rubidium-82 PET and thallium-201 SPECT myocardial perfusion imaging utilizing a single dipyridamole stress in the diagnosis of coronary artery disease. J Nucl Med 31:1899, 1990
230. Simone GL, Mullani NA, Page DA, Anderson BAS: Utilization statistics and diagnostic accuracy of a non-hospital-based positron emission tomography center for the detection of coronary artery disease using rubidium-82. Am J Physiol Imaging 7:203, 1992
231. Williams BR, Mullani NA, Jansen DE, Anderson BA: A retrospective study of the diagnostic accuracy of a community hospital-based PET center for the detection of coronary artery disease using rubidium-82. J Nucl Med 35:1586, 1994
232. Camici P, Marracini P, Marzilli M et al: Coronary hemodynamics and myocardial metabolism during and after pacing stress in normal humans. Am J Physiol 257:E309, 1989
233. Chan S, Brunken R, Czernin J et al: Comparison of maximal myocardial blood flow during adenosine infusion with that of intravenous dipyridamole in normal men. J Am Coll Cardiol 20:979, 1992
234. Geltman E, Henes C, Senneff M et al: Increased myocardial perfusion at rest and diminished perfusion reserve in patients with angina and angiographically normal coronary arteries. J Am Coll Cardiol 16:586, 1990
235. Krivokapich J, Huang S, Schelbert H: Assessment of the effects of dobutamine on myocardial blood flow and oxidative metabolism in normal human subjects using nitrogen-13 ammonia and carbon-11 acetate. Am J Cardiol 71:1351, 1993
236. Sambuceti G, Parodi O, Marcassa C et al: Alteration in regulation of myocardial blood flow in one-vessel coronary artery disease determined by positron emission tomography. Am J Cardiol 72:538, 1993
237. Tamaki N, Yonekura Y, Mukai T et al: Stress thallium-201 transaxial emission computed tomography: quantitative versus qualitative analysis for evaluation of coronary artery disease. J Am Coll Cardiol 4:1213, 1984
238. DePasquale EE, Nody AC, DePuey EG et al: Quantitative rotational thallium-201 tomography for identifying and localizing coronary artery disease. Circulation 77:316, 1988
239. Iskandrian AS, Heo J, Kong B, Lyons E: Effect of exercise level on the ability of thallium-201 tomographic imaging in detecting coronary artery disease: analysis of 461 patients. J Am Coll Cardiol 14:1477, 1989
240. Maddahi J, Van-Train K, Prigent F et al: Quantitative single photon emission computed thallium-201 tomography for detection and localization of coronary artery disease: optimization and prospective validation of new technique. J Am Coll Cardiol 14:1689, 1989
241. Mahmarian JJ, Boyce TM, Goldberg RK et al: Quantitative exercise thallium-201 single-photon emission computed tomography for the enhance diagnosis of ischemic heart disease. J Am Coll Cardiol 15:318, 1990
242. Van-Train KF, Maddahi J, Berman DS et al: Quantitative analysis of tomographic stress thallium-201 myocardial scintigrams: a multicenter trial. J Nucl Med 3:1168, 1990
243. Demer L, Gould KL, Goldstein RA et al: Assessment of coronary artery disease severity by positron emission tomography: comparison with quantitative arteriography in 193 patients. Circulation 79:825, 1989
244. Matzer L, Kiat H, Wang FP et al: Pharmacologic stress dual-isotope myocardial perfusion single-photon emission computed tomography. Am Heart J 128:1067, 1994
245. Pennell DJ, Mavrogeni SI, Forbat SM et al: Adenosine combined with dynamic exercise for myocardial perfusion imaging. J Am Coll Cardiol 25:1300, 1995

Chapter 3

Left Ventricular Functional Response to Stress for the Diagnosis of CAD

Thomas Ryan

The detection of myocardial ischemia is one of the most important and fundamental goals of stress testing. To do this successfully, a test must be capable of first *inducing* ischemia and then *detecting* some aspect of the ischemic event. The induction of ischemia is generally accomplished either through exercise or pharmacologic means. If a progressive increase in myocardial oxygen demand occurs in the presence of a coronary artery lesion, the delivery of oxygen will be inadequate to meet the rising demand and ischemia will develop.

Several techniques are available to detect the various manifestations of ischemia, each one focusing on a different component of the ischemic process. In its most basic form, cardiac stress testing relies on the development of ST-segment depression (as well as symptoms, such as angina) as markers of ischemia. The advantages of this approach are cost and simplicity. Unfortunately, it is now well established that the stress electrocardiogram provides only modest accuracy and is limited in its ability to yield information regarding the location and extent of disease. In certain subsets, such as women or patients with left bundle branch block (LBBB), nonimaging stress tests are of little value.

To overcome these shortcomings, the addition of some form of cardiac imaging to the stress electrocardiogram (ECG) has been widely implemented. Such approaches focus on either myocardial perfusion or left ventricular (LV) function as the end point of ischemia. More complex and costly than the "nonimaging" stress test, it is implicit that these techniques provide greater accuracy as well as more detail about the ischemic process. In doing so, both the diagnostic and prognostic value of the test are enhanced.

This chapter will focus on the principles, techniques, and clinical applications of those stress testing modalities that measure LV function as the marker of ischemia. The various imaging methods used to evaluate regional and global LV function will be described and their relative advantages and disadvantages will be compared. Finally, guidelines for the optimal use of each technique and their role in clinical decision making will be covered.

LV FUNCTIONAL INDICES AS MARKERS OF ISCHEMIA

Normal Physiology of the LV Response to Exercise

The heart's response to exercise involves an interaction between the various determinants of cardiac performance—heart rate, contractility, and loading conditions. The normal response to exercise is a global increase in LV contractility, the development of hyperdynamic wall motion, and a gradual rise in heart rate. The magnitude of these changes depends on the intensity and duration of the effort and the amount of muscle mass involved. The changes are also posture dependent. In the supine position, end-diastolic volume is near maximal at rest and changes little during exercise.[1] The hyperdynamic response is less pronounced and most of the increase in cardiac output is heart rate mediated.[2,3] The upright posture is associated with a lower resting LV end-diastolic volume. During exercise, however, a greater increase in stroke volume and end-diastolic volume occur making the hyperdynamic response more apparent.[1,4] Following exercise, the hyperdynamic state may persist for 2 to 4 minutes before returning to baseline.[5]

In the normal subject, when cardiac performance is monitored during exercise, the most striking physiologic changes are the increase in LV contractility and the decrease in LV end-systolic volume. These physiologic alterations can be detected in a variety of ways including wall motion analysis (which evaluates *regional* LV systolic function) and ejection fraction response (which assesses *global* function). Failure of these changes to occur in response to exercise is abnormal. Possible causes include cardiomyopathy, a marked increase in blood pressure, reduced exercise capacity, medications (such as β-blockers), and ischemia.

Ischemia and the LV Response to Exercise

The process of ischemia can be thought of as a sequence of interrelated events (the *ischemic cascade*), each of which has been used as a marker of disease. In most cases, regional myocardial dysfunction occurs *after* the development of a perfusion defect, but *before* some of the more common manifestations of ischemia such as ST-segment depression or angina pectoris. In the experimental setting, myocardial dyssynergy develops very soon after the interruption of coronary blood flow. This predictable phenomenon, initially described in the 1930s by Tennant and Wiggers,[6] can be demonstrated using echocardiography or radionuclide angiography. The reduction in systolic function is manifest as both a decrease in endocardial excursion and wall thickening. By comparing regional function at baseline and during stress, resting abnormalities (due to either infarction or hibernating myocardium) can be distinguished from transient dyssynergy (an indicator of induced ischemia). When stress is terminated, the time course of functional recovery is variable.[7,8] Most induced abnormalities will persist for several minutes permitting their detection by methods that rely on postexercise imaging. Although regional wall motion abnormalities have occasionally been demonstrated up to 30 minutes after cessation of exercise,[9] rapid resolution of regional dyssynergy also occurs, an observation with important implications for postexercise imaging.[7,10]

It must be emphasized that regional and global LV function, though inherently linked, may behave differently during stress. For example, a patient with single-vessel coronary artery disease (CAD) may develop an isolated wall motion abnormality due to limited ischemia. If the remainder of the LV wall motion becomes hyperdynamic, ejection fraction will rise appropriately during stress. Thus, a *regional* abnormality will be present without evidence of *global* dysfunction. Conversely, a patient who develops severe hypertension in the absence of a significant coronary stenosis may demonstrate a blunted exercise ejection fraction response without an associated regional wall motion abnormality. Recognition of the inherent differences between regional and global manifestations of induced ischemia is essential to understand and compare test results.

Clinical Application of LV Function Response to Exercise

There are several advantages of these functional indices as markers of ischemia. LV dysfunction is a *fundamental* aspect of the ischemic process. As such, a regional wall motion abnormality requires clinically important ischemia in order to develop. Regional dyssynergy is a *specific* marker of ischemia and is rarely seen in other situations. Its assessment permits a direct evaluation of the extent and location of ischemia and allows both global and regional LV function to be assessed.

The major disadvantage of functional indices of ischemia is that they are inherently load dependent. This is particularly true of global parameters such as ejection fraction, which is highly dependent on changes in both preload and afterload as well as alterations in contractility. A theoretical disadvantage of the LV functional indices relates to the sequence of events that comprises the ischemic cascade. Because the development of regional dyssynergy occurs *after* a perfusion defect, functional abnormalities may be less sensitive than perfusion imaging for the detection of ischemia. It is conceivable that a stress test would be terminated *after* the development of hypoperfusion but *before* a wall motion abnormality appears, thereby yielding discordant results and a false-negative functional study.

STRESS METHODOLOGIES

Exercise Echocardiography

Exercise echocardiography relies on a comparison of two-dimensional echocardiographic images obtained before, during, and after exercise (Table 3-1). The test is versatile and can be performed using either treadmill or bicycle protocols. Although a variety of views can be obtained, the most common approach utilizes the long and short axis and the apical four- and two-chamber views. Alternatively, the apical long axis or subcostal views may be used. If treadmill exercise is performed, imaging during exercise is rarely possible[11] and immediate postexercise imaging is necessary.[12] Using this protocol, it is essential that the patient move from the treadmill to the imaging (left lateral decubitus) position as quickly as possible so that postexercise imaging is completed within 1 to 2 minutes. The primary limitation of treadmill exercise echocardiography is the dependence on postexercise imaging. If wall motion abnormalities recover before imaging is completed, false-negative results occur.[7,10,13]

Bicycle exercise echocardiography can be done in either an upright or recumbent position. The patient pedals against a gradually escalating workload while imaging is performed. The patient must be sufficiently coordinated and cooperative to undergo this form of stress testing. The primary advantage of bicycle exercise is the opportunity to obtain images during exercise. In theory, imaging throughout exercise allows determination of the onset of regional dyssynergy. In practice, images are obtained at baseline and peak exercise and the interpretation is based on a comparison of these two stages.

Fundamental differences exist between supine and upright ergometry. During supine exercise, all the standard views (including subcostal images) can be obtained. Image acquisition has recently been improved by the implementation of ergometers that allow left lateral decubitus positioning.[14] Imaging is more challenging in the upright position and is usually limited to the apical and subcostal windows.[15] In most cases, the apical views are most easily recorded with the patient leaning slightly forward, arms extended.[16] A lordotic position is generally necessary to obtain subcostal views. Although this has the advantage of minimal lung interference, apical foreshortening may occur and must be carefully avoided.

In most patients, upright exercise allows a greater level of exertion to be obtained. Fatigue occurs at an earlier stage during supine exercise, especially when proper leg support is not provided. These limitations of supine exercise are overcome in part by the occurrence of ischemia at a lower workload.[17] During exercise, both arterial blood pressure and LV volume are greater in the supine position.[1] These differences contribute to a higher myocardial oxygen demand and the potential for the earlier development of myocardial ischemia. Despite these differences, both techniques are effective means to induce myocardial ischemia and have been widely utilized in clinical practice. Although patients generally will prefer an upright form of exercise, the ease of image acquisition favors the supine position.

Exercise Radionuclide Angiography

There are two basic forms of radionuclide angiography. *First pass angiography* involves analysis of the radionuclide bolus (usually containing technetium-99m) as it initially traverses the central circulation.

Table 3-1. Stress Echocardiographic Methods

Stress Techniques	Imaging Options
Exercise	Two-dimensional echocardiography
Treadmill	Transthoracic
Bicycle (upright, supine)	Transesophageal
Hand grip	Contrast-enhanced
Pharmacologic	Doppler
Dobutamine	Pulsed
Arbutamine	Continuous wave
Dipyridamole	Color flow imaging
Adenosine	
Atrial pacing	

Once the tracer has mixed with the blood, changes in counts correlate with changes in volume. As the tracer-containing blood passes through the cardiac chambers, sufficient spatial and temporal resolution are achieved to permit quantitative analysis of left and right heart function. *Equilibrium radionuclide angiography*, or gated blood pool imaging, permits repetitive imaging over time after injection of radiolabeled red blood cells.[18] Once the labeled material is uniformly distributed, imaging is performed by sampling counts over several minutes. Temporal resolution is accomplished by ECG gating. Spatial resolution depends on summation of data derived from several hundred cardiac cycles to provide optimal definition of blood pool boundaries.

The advantages of the equilibrium technique include the opportunity to perform several studies over time. This allows acquisition of multiple cardiac views so that regional function can be more thoroughly assessed. In addition, because sampling is performed over several minutes, statistical reliability is improved and the study is less prone to errors introduced by arrhythmias. The effectiveness of blood pool labeling, acquisition of adequate counts, and avoidance of chamber overlap are important factors that affect data quality.

Both techniques have been utilized in conjunction with stress testing for assessment of cardiac function. For many applications, the two techniques provide similar results. Global LV function (i.e., ejection fraction) can be measured with either modality. Right ventricular function is better evaluated using the first pass technique.[19] Regional wall motion analysis is more accurately assessed with the equilibrium method.

Radionuclide angiography is generally performed in the upright posture. Although both treadmill and bicycle exercise can be utilized, the relatively greater stability of the thorax while seated on an ergometer favors this modality and helps to minimize motion artifact during data acquisition. This is especially important with the equilibrium technique when excessive patient motion during the sampling period can introduce significant artifact. Using the equilibrium method, images can be obtained for several hours once the blood is labeled. Each acquisition requires several minutes after which the data are summed and presented as a representative cardiac cycle.

Therefore, it is essential that a steady state be maintained during each sampling period to ensure accuracy.[20] After baseline imaging is completed, exercise is undertaken and sampling is repeated at peak. Again, it is important that the patient maintain a steady and near maximal level of exertion while data are collected.

Nonexercise Stress

Pharmacologic stress testing can be performed using either positive inotropic agents (which increase myocardial oxygen demand) or vasodilator agents (which create perfusion abnormalities by preferentially shunting blood away from regions supplied by stenotic coronary arteries). The following segments are meant to summarize the salient features of pharmacologic and pacing stress. These subjects are dealt with in more detail in Chapter 13 on pharmacologic stress testing.

Dobutamine Stress

Of the positive inotropic agents, dobutamine is the drug with which there has been the greatest experience. Dobutamine stress testing involves step-wise administration of the drug,[21] which in the presence of CAD causes myocardial ischemia and subsequently regional dyssynergy (Fig. 3-1). Longer stage duration may provide a greater level of stress at a lower maximal dose.[22] If heart rate fails to increase appropriately, some investigators have utilized atropine (0.25 to 2.0 mg intravenously), which is safe and has been shown to enhance the sensitivity of the dobutamine stress test for the detection of coronary artery disease.[23] The normal response to dobutamine involves the development of hyperdynamic wall motion, with little change of end-diastolic LV volume, reduction of end-systolic volume, and a significant increase in ejection fraction. Failure to develop a hyperdynamic response is abnormal and is most likely the result of induced myocardial ischemia. Dobutamine is generally considered safe and well tolerated as a stress agent,[24] with the commonest side-effects being due to arrhythmias.[24] Up to 20% of patients may experience hypotension during dobutamine infusion,[25] but in contrast to exercise testing, a decrease in blood pressure during dobutamine infusion is not necessarily a marker of severe ischemia.[26-28] There are several potential causes for

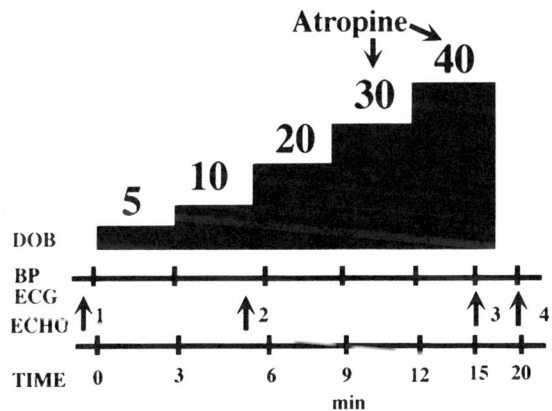

Fig. 3-1. A dobutamine stress echocardiography (DSE) protocol. Following acquisition of baseline data, dobutamine (DOB) is administered at a starting dose of 5 μg/kg/min then increasing, every 3 minutes, to a peak dose of 40 μg/kg/min. The electrocardiogram (ECG) and blood pressure (BP) are obtained at each stage. Echocardiograms are obtained prior to infusion (No. 1) at low dose (No. 2) at maximum dose (No. 3), and 5 minutes after termination of the infusion (No. 4). When heart rate response is suboptimal, atropine is administered to augment the heart rate response. min, minutes (From Ryan,[125] with permission.)

this phenomenon, including vagal reflexes,[28] intracavitary obstruction due to hyperdynamic wall motion, inadequate preload due to hypovolemia, and baseline hypertension.

Vasodilator Stress

Dipyridamole is the agent most often employed for vasodilator stress testing. This drug causes maximal coronary hyperemia by potentiation of the effects of endogenous adenosine. The usual protocol employs a dose of 0.56 mg/kg infused over 4 minutes, with an additional 0.28 mg/kg is administered over 2 minutes if the test remains negative. Common side effects include headache, nausea, hypotension, and flushing. There has now been extensive experience with dipyridamole echocardiography, especially in Europe, where the safety and efficacy of the test have been demonstrated.[29] Dobutamine and dipyridamole can be used sequentially in a single protocol,[30] which appears feasible and sensitive for the detection of CAD.

Adenosine is a potent vasodilator with a very rapid onset and a brief duration of action, and may itself be used in conjunction with echocardiography as a stress agent. This drug is administered intravenously at a dose of 0.14 mg/kg/min over 6 minutes for a total dose of 0.84 mg/kg.[31] Adverse effects, while common, are transient. However, identification of ischemia during adenosine infusion is challenging because the brief duration of action is associated with short-lived and often subtle wall motion abnormalities.

Cardiac Pacing Echocardiography

Cardiac pacing has also been used to increase heart rate during echocardiographic monitoring, most commonly using transesophageal atrial pacing, often in conjunction with transesophageal imaging.[32–34] The pacing rate is typically initiated at 100 beats/min and then increased every 2 to 3 minutes. Potential limitations include an inability to capture the atria, the development of atrioventricular (AV) block at higher heart rates, and poor patient tolerance. Echocardiographic imaging may be either transthoracic or transesophageal. Although the test has limited application, studies have demonstrated that it is feasible in the majority of patients.[35]

IMAGING TECHNIQUES

Two-Dimensional Echocardiography

Transthoracic

Transthoracic two-dimensional echocardiography provides most of the relevant information in patients with CAD. The tomographic nature of echocardiography allows multiple imaging planes to be recorded, thereby providing the opportunity to assess the LV completely. Using this method, both endocardial excursion and wall thickening can be evaluated. This in turn provides diagnostic information on regional and global systolic function. In conjunction with stress testing, two-dimensional echocardiography is ideally suited to detect and localize wall motion abnormalities and to distinguish ischemia from prior myocardial infarction (Fig. 3-2). The administration of intravenously injected left heart contrast agents may enhance the accuracy of wall motion analysis by improving endocardial border definition.[36]

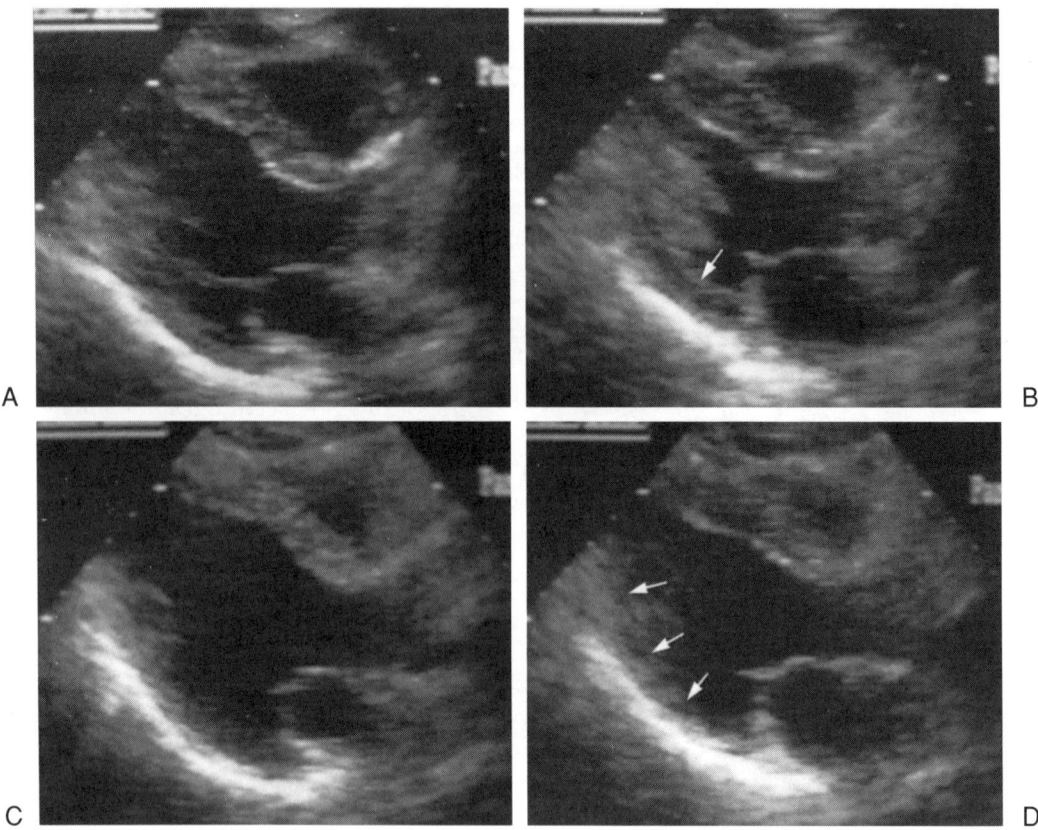

Fig. 3-2. A quad screen display of a stress echocardiogram. (**A** & **C**) End-diastolic frames and (**B** & **D**) end-systolic frames. (**A** & **B**) The resting study and (**C** & **D**) the stress study. At baseline, a small area of posterobasal akinesis is noted by the single white arrow. With stress, the posterior wall motion abnormality becomes more extensive (white arrows) and the end-systolic cavity size increases.

Transesophageal

Transesophageal echocardiographic imaging may be necessary, particularly when transthoracic image quality is poor. This is usually performed during either pharmacologic or pacing stress.[33,37–39] This approach is clearly more invasive than transthoracic imaging, but generally provides excellent image quality. If single-plane imaging technology is utilized, transesophageal stress echocardiography is limited with respect to the number of views that are obtained. This limitation is avoided through the use of biplane or multiplane transducers which allow a more complete assessment of the LV. In most cases, the transducer is positioned in the mid esophagus from which long-axis views are recorded. The endoscope is then advanced to the stomach to provide short-axis imaging, yielding a more complete evaluation of LV wall motion.

Doppler

The Doppler technique can be used to yield quantitative information on global ventricular function. By recording flow through the aortic or mitral valve, the flow velocity integral can be calculated from which stroke volume and cardiac output are derived.[40–43] During treadmill exercise, a small nonimaging probe can be positioned in the suprasternal notch permitting changes in aortic flow to be monitored throughout the protocol. If aortic cross-sectional area is assumed to be constant, changes in the flow velocity integral correlate directly with alterations in systolic function. In addition to LV stroke volume, flow acceleration can be measured as an additional marker of LV function. These parameters have been used to predict the presence and severity of coronary disease and LV dysfunction.[42] The addition of Doppler information may enhance the sensitivity of wall motion analysis for the detection of coronary disease.[41,44] Other potential applications of exercise Doppler echocardiography include the ability to assess the effect of drugs on ventricular function[43] and the evaluation of ischemic mitral regurgitation through the use of color flow imaging.[45]

However, the role of Doppler in the field of stress echocardiography has been limited by a variety of factors. First, the limited time frame during which imaging is performed makes the acquisition of ancillary data impractical. Second, factors other than LV function may influence flow parameters—for example, diastolic function changes due to ischemia may be blunted by increased left atrial pressure caused by ischemic LV dysfunction.

Digital Echocardiography

The development of digital imaging techniques has contributed greatly to the growth of stress echocardiography.[46,47] Digitization is the process of converting the analog video image into discrete bits of information recorded in binary code. The data are stored and then reassembled into a series of digital images. Digital acquisition of ultrasound images begins with identification of the R-wave of the ECG. Beginning at this point in time, the computer then captures a series of frames of video images. Eight or more frames are typically recorded and displayed in a cine loop (Fig. 3-3). The digital recording may be as short as a single cardiac cycle (as little as 8 frames of video images covering 350 ms) or as long as several minutes, the equivalent of a digital videotape. A major advantage of the digital processing technique is the ability to display the echocardiogram in a variety of ways. Displaying rest and stress views in a side-by-side format is commonly employed for most stress echocardiographic protocols.

There are several advantages to digital stress echocardiography. The opportunity to display images in a side-by-side format is perhaps the most important. When a stress echocardiogram is recorded on videotape, detection of stress-induced wall motion abnormalities is dependent on *remembering* the resting study while viewing the stress study. With digital technology, the display of rest and stress images simultaneously permits subtle abnormalities to be detected and provides a more efficient and convenient approach to analysis. Digital processing also allows the operator to select the cardiac cycles that are used

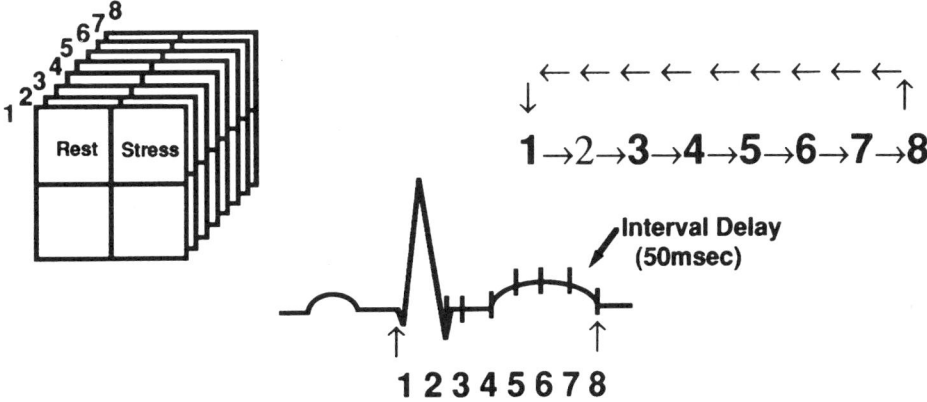

Fig. 3-3. The concept of digital cine loop recording, as applied to stress echocardiography, is illustrated. Eight equally spaced frames of echocardiographic information are captured and digitized, beginning with the R-wave and extending throughout systole. The interval delay between frames (50 ms in the example) may be adjusted depending on heart rate. The eight frames are played in an endless loop recording. Images at rest and during stress are displayed in a side-by-side fashion as shown on the left side of the figure. This permits wall motion at different stages of stress to be compared.

in the final display. Those cycles that are degraded by respiratory interference can be eliminated and the highest quality and most representative cycles can be used. Finally, digital techniques permit post-exercise imaging to be completed quickly, because only a single cycle from each view is needed to create the cine loop. This reduces the likelihood that an induced wall motion abnormality will resolve before it can be recorded.

Radionuclide Angiography

Radionuclide angiography involves the detection and localization of scintillation events using a gamma camera. Utilizing a lead collimator, a large sodium iodide thallium crystal (or multiple crystals) and an array of photomultipliers, gamma-rays emitted by the circulating radionuclide are detected. These events are defined in space and counted through the use of sophisticated electronic processing. Localization is accomplished by simultaneous analysis of an event by three adjacent phototubes. Spatial resolution is primarily determined by the physical characteristics of the gamma camera, including the speed of electronic signal processing. Temporal resolution is a function of the radioactive counts available to the camera, the counting rate, and the rate of signal processing.

First Pass Radionuclide Angiography

For the assessment of cardiac function, the radioactivity of the tracer within the heart and circulation must be mapped in time and space. With first-pass imaging, a discrete bolus of the radiopharmaceutical is injected while imaging is performed. For purposes of stress testing, individual injections are done at baseline and during exercise. Using the newer technetium-based agents, such as sestamibi or teboroxime, it is possible to simultaneously assess both LV function and myocardial perfusion in a single test.[48] Either supine or upright exercise can be used. The camera is usually positioned firmly against the anterior chest wall providing an anterior projection. A left anterior oblique view may be used to provide better separation between the left and right ventricles. Resolution is maximized by locating the camera as close as possible to the heart. Excess patient motion during data collection will adversely affect the quality of results.

If data are acquired at 25 ms intervals for 20 seconds, 800 frames of information are collected. This will generally contain the entire initial transit of the bolus. Counts are gathered over time as the tracer circulates through a given chamber. The curve generated by the passage of the radionuclide represents the total quantity of the tracer at a given point in time. Information about chamber volume, flow, valvular regurgitation, and shunting is available. In contrast to echocardiography, the information is usually planar. The primary limitation of this technique relates to chamber overlap and the difficulty in separating counts collected from different locations within the heart. Background correction and attention to beat selection are additional factors affecting data quality.

Equilibrium Radionuclide Angiography

This technique differs from the first-pass technique in several ways. Once equilibrium is attained following tracer injection, image construction requires data acquisition over several cardiac cycles. Each cardiac cycle is divided into intervals, defined by R-wave gating. Images for each time point within the R–R interval are obtained by summing counts from multiple cycles. The counts from multiple cardiac cycles are combined into a composite cine loop, displayed as a "single" representative beat.

Exercise protocols are similar to those employed in first-pass angiography. An advantage of equilibrium radionuclide angiography is the opportunity to acquire images at several stages throughout exercise (without the need for multiple injections of the tracer). Because data from many cardiac cycles are summed, arrhythmias will affect the final composite image. A limitation of equilibrium radionuclide angiography is the duration of acquisition of each image, generally 2 to 3 minutes. For representative data to be obtained, steady-state hemodynamics must be maintained throughout the acquisition.[20]

Magnetic Resonance Imaging

Magnetic resonance imaging (MRI), like echocardiography, produces high-resolution, tomographic images of cardiac structures. The patient is positioned within a strong magnetic field generated by a superconducting magnet, a radiofrequency pulse is applied, and the nuclear magnetic resonance signal from hydrogen nuclei are detected and utilized to construct the image. There are two basic forms of MRI: *spin-echo* and *gradient-echo* imaging. To assess LV function, gradient-echocardiographic, or cine, MRI is most often utilized. To create a cine MR image, ECG gating is required. Images are recorded in a predefined tomographic plane at fixed intervals throughout the cardiac cycle. The still images are then displayed in a *cine loop*, from which cardiac function can be assessed.

Thus, to construct an MRI cine loop, the patient must remain stationary within the magnet while imaging is performed. To image the LV in multiple slices, several minutes of data collection are necessary. Slice thickness is usually 8 to 10 mm, similar to echocardiography. Temporal resolution is in the range of 30 to 50 ms, yielding up to 30 frames per cardiac cycle at a heart rate of 60 per minute.

The advantages of MRI include the high resolution of the individual images, permitting both wall thickness and endocardial excursion to be analyzed. The technique allows unlimited options for segmenting the LV. Currently, however, time constraints limit the number of slices that can be collected and this is particularly critical during the performance of a stress test. In the future, the potential use of MRI for tissue characterization and to directly visualize coronary arteries and vein grafts will enhance the application of the technique to ischemic heart disease.

The major limitation is that MRI can be used only in conjunction with pharmacologic stress. Because of the need for the patient to remain motionless within the magnet during data collection, exercise is currently not feasible. Finally, the method has been performed in relatively few patients at a limited number of centers. Greater experience is necessary to demonstrate the accuracy and clinical utility of this technique. In the future, it is likely that additional improvements in technology will further shorten imaging time, thereby increasing the number of slices that can be recorded at various stages throughout the pharmacologic stress protocol.

INTERPRETATION OF TESTS OF LV FUNCTION
Stress Echocardiography

The interpretation of stress echocardiograms relies on assessment of both wall thickening and endocardial excursion. The entire LV can be interrogated using multiple views. Wall motion is subjectively graded as either normal, hypokinetic, akinetic, or dyskinetic. In the normal heart, stress will result in an increase in regional and global function, that is, ventricular function and wall motion will become hyperdynamic. Lack of a hyperdynamic response is generally considered abnormal and is most often the result of induced myocardial ischemia. In some cases, however, *absence* of a hyperdynamic response (i.e., wall motion is normal, but unchanged) may be normal. For example, the development of hyperkinesis may not occur in the presence of a low level of stress, severe hypertension, or drug therapy such as β-adrenergic blocking agents. *Postexercise* wall motion may not be hyperkinetic, particularly if there is a lengthy delay in image acquisition.

Both wall thickening and endocardial excursion should be analyzed. Of the two, reduced wall thickening is a more specific marker of ischemia, but wall motion changes are more easily identified (Fig. 3-4). Several schemes are currently available to assess LV regional wall motion. The 16-segment model advocated by the American Society of Echocardiography is used most often and should be encouraged (Fig. 3-5).[49,50]

To distinguish between infarction and ischemia, rest and stress images are compared. A segment that is akinetic at baseline is most likely infarcted. A segment that is normal at rest and deteriorates during stress is ischemic. *Worsening* of wall motion in an area *abnormal* at rest may be the result of ischemia developing in an area of partial infarction.[51] Other possibilities, such as a change in local loading conditions, may also occur and the finding of deterioration of an akinetic segment at stress echocardiography is not specific for ischemia. Improvement in mild resting hypokinesis with stress is probably a normal phenomenon.[52] Stress-induced improvement in akinetic or dyskinetic segments is uncommon and is most likely the result of a tethering effect of normal adjacent segments. A summary of the possible wall motion responses that occur during stress echocardiography is provided in Table 3-2.

Stress echocardiography is often used to predict coronary anatomy. This process involves an assessment of the location and extent of wall motion ab-

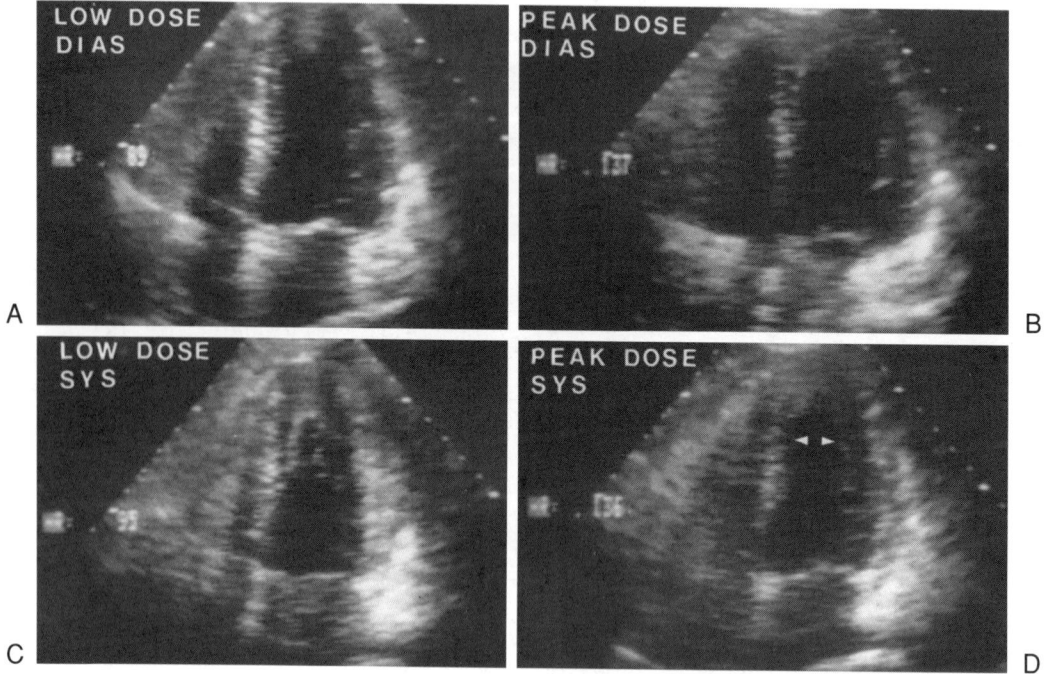

Fig. 3-4. An abnormal dobutamine stress echocardiogram is shown. (**A** & **C**) Low-dose images left and (**B** & **D**) peak-dose images. (**A** & **B**) End-diastolic (DIAS) frames and (**C** & **D**) end-systolic (SYS). At low-dose dobutamine, wall motion is normal, the end-systolic left ventricle (LV) cavity is small, and wall thickening of the septum and apex are well preserved. At peak-dose dobutamine, there is an abnormality involving the LV apex (**D**). The end-systolic cavity is increased, wall thickening is reduced, and the apex is relatively dilated compared to the low-dose stage. This is indicative of myocardial ischemia involving the septum and apex, probably due to disease in the left anterior descending coronary artery.

normalities. One scheme that can be utilized to predict coronary anatomy is shown in Figure 3-6. It must be emphasized that individual variability in coronary artery distribution limits the precision of such predictions. This is especially true in the posterior circulation. The approach described in Figure 3-6 employs four echocardiographic views and divides the LV into 16 segments. Some of these segments are referred to as "overlap" regions. Dyssynergy in these regions should be interpreted in context, based on the presence or absence of abnormalities in adjoining segments. Using such an approach, predicting coronary artery anatomy is possible in the majority of patients. Accuracy is generally greater for identifying lesions in the left anterior descending and right coronary arteries[53,54] and somewhat lower for detecting obstruction within the left circumflex artery.[14]

Radionuclide Ventriculography

Interpretation of a radionuclide angiogram includes both a subjective and a quantitative component. Quantitation of LV function and the changes that occur during stress are optimally performed using a left anterior oblique view. The degree of obliquity is varied to obtain the maximum separation between the right and left ventricles, often called the "best septal view." When the radionuclide is in equilibrium within the circulation, radioactive counts are proportional to volume (Plate 3-1). To quantify volume changes, a region of interest is defined and counts are calculated throughout the cardiac cycle; the change between diastole and systole is proportionate to ejection fraction (Fig. 3-7). An advantage of this approach is that it is relatively operator independent. Once the optimal viewing angle is determined and the region of interest is defined, obtain-

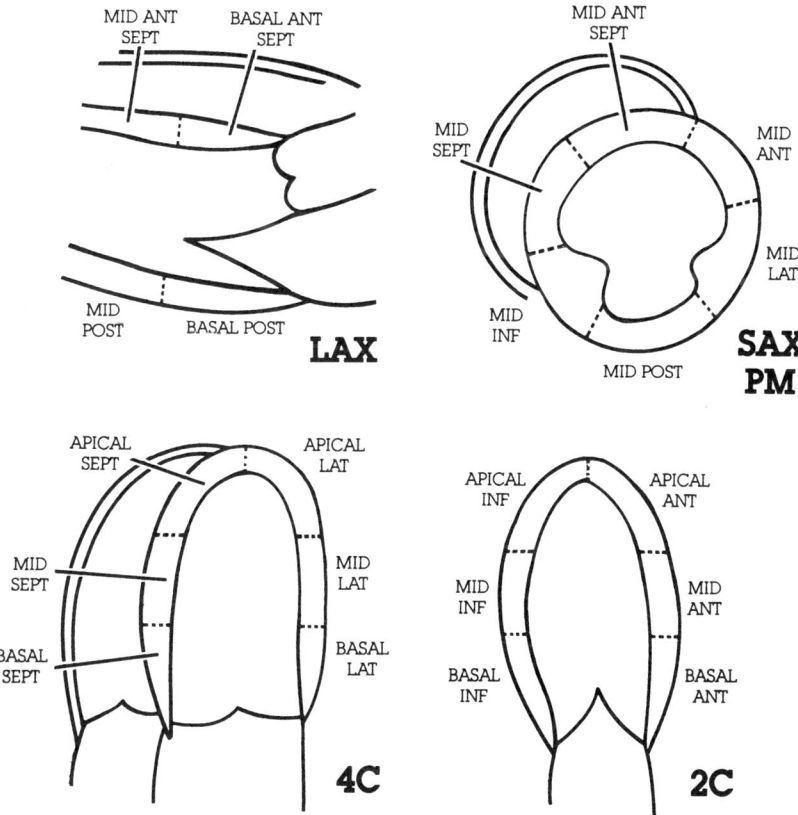

Fig. 3-5. The four echocardiographic views used in most stress echocardiographic protocols are shown. The long-axis (LAX) and short-axis (SAX) at the papillary muscle (PM) level are obtained from the parasternal window. The four-chamber (4C) and two-chamber (2C) views are recorded from the apex. The left ventricle can be divided into 16 segments as illustrated. Wall motion is graded in each segment at different levels of stress. Abnormal wall motion in the different regions can be correlated with coronary anatomy, as described in the text. (From Feigenbaum,[126] with permission.)

ing the quantitative information is straightforward. Because the calculations are count based, the results are independent of ventricular geometry and assumptions about LV shape are avoided. The main source of error involves attenuation measurements reflecting the variability of distance between the camera and targets.

Information on regional wall motion can also be obtained from equilibrium radionuclide angiography.[55] Cine loops of a composite cardiac cycle are generated from multiple views. The left anterior oblique projection permits septal, inferior, and lateral wall motion to be evaluated. The apex and anterior wall are best visualized in an anterior projection and the inferior wall and inferobasal segments are recorded in a lateral projection. Wall motion is graded from visual analysis of the cine loops. Alternatively, regional ejection fraction can be calculated by planimetry of borders at end-diastole and end-systole.[56] Although the feasibility of this quantitative technique has been demonstrated, most analyses rely on subjective wall motion interpretation. Correlation between radionuclide angiography and contrast ventriculography is good[57] and interobserver variability is acceptable.[58,59] Unlike echocardiography, which is a tomographic technique, most radionuclide angiographic methods are planar. This important difference must be taken into account when wall motion is analyzed and when the two techniques are compared.

Table 3-2. Interpretation of Regional Wall Motion with Stress Echocardiography

Wall Motion		
Baseline	Stress	Interpretation
Normal	Hyperkinetic	Normal
Normal	Unchanged	Variable
Normal	Deteriorates	Ischemia
Hypokinetic	Hyperkinetic	Normal (viable)[a]
Hypokinetic	Unchanged	Infarction
Hypokinetic	Akinetic	Infarction ± Ischemia
Akinetic	Improves	Stunned or hibernating[a]
Akinetic	Unchanged	Infarction
Akinetic	Worsens	Infarction

[a] With dobutamine only.

CLINICAL APPLICATIONS

Stress Echocardiography

Detection of CAD

Using angiography as the standard, the sensitivity of exercise echocardiography to detect CAD has ranged from 71%[60] to 97%.[61] The results of several of these studies are summarized in Table 3-3. The accuracy of dobutamine stress echocardiography is discussed in more detail in Chapter 13, but in summary, the sensitivity has ranged from 70%[23] to 96%.[62] In part, these differences are explained by patient selection criteria used in the various studies. For example, if a high percentage of patients with prior myocardial infarction are included, the presence of a resting wall motion abnormality suggests disease whether or not ischemia is induced. In patients without prior myocardial infarction, i.e., those with normal wall motion at rest, sensitivity has ranged from 66%[63] to 91%.[14] In this setting, detection of disease requires the induction and detection of a transient wall motion abnormality.[10,63,64]

The ability of stress echocardiography to detect disease is affected by several other factors (Table 3-4). Sensitivity is lower in patients with less severe coronary stenosis, poor exercise tolerance, and less extensive coronary artery disease (i.e., single-vessel disease).[65] Sensitivity will be increased in the presence of severe coronary stenoses, adequate exercise capacity and multivessel disease. Lesion morphology may also affect sensitivity, being greater in those patients with complex morphology.[66] Finally, sensitivity has been correlated with location of disease, generally being greatest for the left anterior descending artery and lowest for the left circumflex coronary artery.

Among patients with prior myocardial infarction, the detection of CAD per se is not an issue. Instead, the goal of stress testing usually involves risk stratification, and the detection of multivessel disease and myocardial ischemia. Both exercise and dobutamine stress echocardiography have been shown to be useful in patients with resting wall motion abnormalities.[10,63,64,67] The extent of coronary disease, with the presence or absence of multivessel involvement, and the degree LV dysfunction can be identified.

When stress echocardiography is compared to coronary angiography, it is essential to recognize that stenosis severity as well as angiographic criteria will influence the accuracy of the functional test. Investigators have traditionally used a 50% reduction in coronary artery diameter to define significant disease. It is well recognized that coronary lesions of intermediate severity may or may not be flow limiting. In such cases, stress echocardiography can be used to determine the functional significance of intermediate lesions.[14,68] The relationship between lesion severity and the sensitivity of exercise echocardiography is well established. Salustri et al.[69] studied 44 patients with single-vessel CAD using bicycle exercise echocardiography. Lesion severity was stratified on the basis of angiographic findings. The likelihood of a wall motion abnormality was directly related to the severity of narrowing and there was a moderate correlation between the ischemic wall motion score index and the percent diameter stenosis ($r = 0.62$).

No study has yet demonstrated the superiority of one form of exercise echocardiography over another. However, inherent differences exist between treadmill and bicycle stress testing, which may impact on accuracy. For example, the possibility that an induced wall motion abnormality could normalize prior to postexercise imaging suggests that bicycle stress echocardiography (which allows imaging during stress) may be more sensitive than treadmill testing (which relies solely on post-exercise imaging).

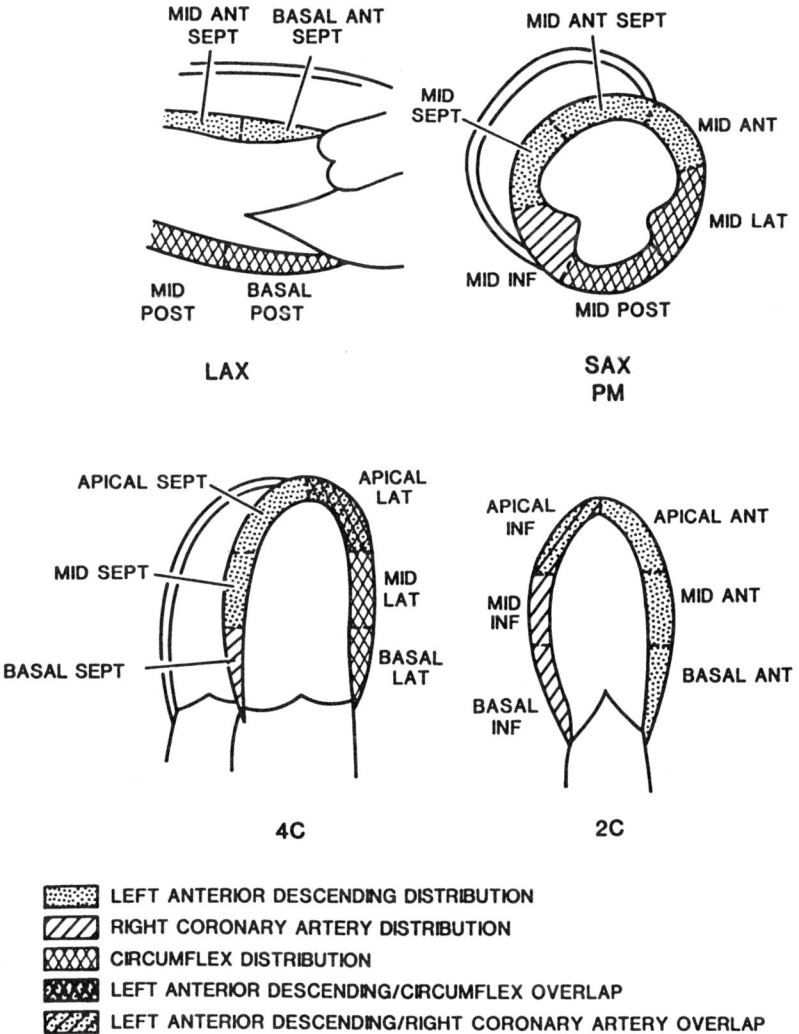

Fig. 3-6. The relationship between coronary artery distribution and the 16 left ventricular segments is demonstrated. Using the four standard views, predictions about coronary anatomy are possible. Potential regions of coronary artery overlap include the apical lateral and apical inferior segments. See text for details. (From Segar,[53] with permission.)

The persistence of an induced wall motion abnormality following cessation of exercise is variable and is affected by a variety of factors including the severity of hypoperfusion, the duration of ischemia, and the extent of coronary collateral flow.[8,9,70,71] It is well established that most induced abnormalities persist for at least 1 to 2 minutes after exercise, permitting their detection using postexercise protocols.

The importance of rapid recovery of wall motion and its impact on sensitivity have been examined in several studies (Fig. 3-8). Presti et al.[7] were the first to demonstrate rapid resolution of regional dyssynergy following bicycle ergometry. They studied 104 consecutive patients and identified rapid recovery in 10 of the 29 with an inducible wall motion abnormality. Among these 10 patients, 6 had completely normal wall motion on post-exercise imaging causing a decrease in sensitivity from 100% at peak to 70% at

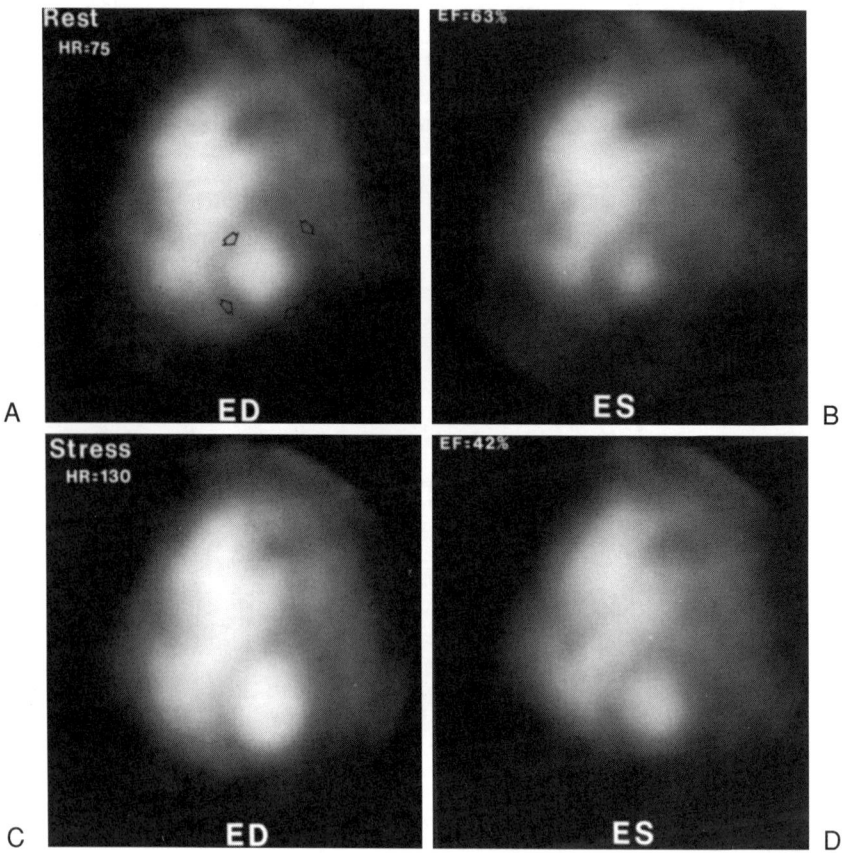

Fig. 3-7. Equilibrium radionuclide angiograms from a 56-year-old male; 5 years S/P coronary artery bypass surgery are shown. The rest (**A** & **B**) and stress (**C** & **D**) images at end-diastole (**A** & **C**) and end-systole (**B** & **D**) demonstrate significant exercise-induced abnormalities. The best septal projection (approximately 45° LAO) was utilized and the left ventricle is outlined (**A**) by the arrows. The heart rate (HR) at baseline was 75 bpm. The patient exercised 9 minutes to a maximum heart rate of 130 bpm and a peak blood pressure of 190/86 mmHg. At rest, wall motion and systolic function are normal with a left ventricular ejection fraction (EF) of 63%. At peak exercise, at end-systole, severe hypokinesis of the low posterolateral and inferoapical walls develop. The ejection fraction decreases to 42%. The results are consistent with multivessel inducible myocardial ischemia. (Courtesy of Michael Hanson, M.D.)

postexercise. Similar results were reported by Ryan et al.[10] in a series of 309 patients. These investigators reported a sensitivity of 83% at post-exercise and 91% at peak exercise.

The specificity of exercise echocardiography in published series ranges from 64%[61] to 100%.[72] Similar values have been reported for dobutamine stress echocardiography.[62,73] False-positive results may occur in patients with other forms of cardiac disease, such as nonischemic cardiomyopathy (Table 3-4). Stress-induced wall motion abnormalities have occasionally been reported in patients without CAD.[74,75] Wall motion abnormalities in the absence of coronary disease are often small and frequently involve the posterobasal segments.[76] When the presence or absence of coronary disease is based on angiographic findings, some false-positive echocardiograms may actually represent cases of ischemia in patients in whom the severity of disease is underestimated by angiography.

Because of the small number of patients without CAD included in many series, the issue of specificity

Table 3-3. Accuracy of Exercise Echocardiography: Comparison with Coronary Angiography

Reference	Method	n	Sensitivity (%) Overall	SVD	MVD	No MI	Specificity (%)
Armstrong et al. (1986)[64]	Treadmill	95	88			80	87
Armstrong et al. (1987)[78]	Treadmill	123	87	81	93	78	86
Crouse et al. (1991)[61]	Treadmill	228	97	93	100		64
Quinones et al. (1992)[99]	Treadmill	289	74	58	89		88
Marwick et al. (1992)[63]	Treadmill	150	84	79	96	87	86
Ryan et al. (1988)[72]	Treadmill	64	78	76	80	78	100
Galanti et al. (1991)[101]	Bicycle	53	93	93	92		96
Pozzoli et al. (1991)[60]	Bicycle	75	71	60	94		96
Sawada et al. (1989)[80]	Treadmill or bicycle	57[a]	86	88	82		86
Hecht et al. (1993)[14]	Bicycle	180	93	78	90	91	86
Hecht et al. (1993)[13]	Bicycle	136	94	84	100	92	88
Ryan et al (1993)[10]	Bicycle	309	93	84	100	91	78
Marwick et al. (1995)[119]	Treadmill or bicycle	161[a]	80	75	85		81

Abbreviations: MI, myocardial infarction; MVD, multivessel coronary artery disease; n, number of patients; SVD, single-vessel coronary artery disease.
[a] Women only; all studies except Galanti et al.[101] used ≥50% luminal narrowing as the angiographic criterion for disease.

is often difficult to address. The pretest likelihood of disease may influence the reader making it more likely that a study be interpreted as abnormal. For these reasons, *normalcy rate* is often used as an alternative to specificity. Normalcy refers to the likelihood of a normal result when the test is applied to a population of patients with a very low pretest probability of disease. The normalcy rate reported in the literature has ranged from 93% to 100%.[14,63,77]

Table 3-4. Factors That Reduce Sensitivity and Specificity

Causes of False-Negative Results	Causes of False-Positive Results
Single-vessel disease (especially in the left circumflex artery)	Nonischemic cardiomyopathy Left bundle branch block
Mild coronary stenosis (~50% luminal narrowing)	Postoperative septal motion
Inadequate stress	Excessive afterload response
Rapid recovery	Interpreter bias (e.g., basal inferior wall)
Poor image quality	Poor image quality

Localization of Coronary Artery Lesions

The ability of functional stress testing to localize ischemia and make predictions regarding coronary anatomy is important in several circumstances. This capability may be especially useful in patients with known coronary anatomy, to demonstrate the functional significance of a stenosis or to identify the "culprit" lesion. Several factors will influence the accuracy with which coronary anatomy can be predicted (Table 3-5). The known variability of coronary distribution in different individuals must be taken into account. This is especially true of the posterior circulation where either the right coronary artery or left circumflex coronary artery may be dominant. The ability of stress echocardiography to identify individual lesions in patients with multivessel disease is further affected by the relative severity of each stenosis. For example, if ischemia in one area leads to test termination, only the most severely diseased vessel will be identified and other more moderate lesions will be missed.

These same factors affect the ability of stress echocardiography to distinguish multivessel from single-vessel disease. As expected, the technique is more sensitive in patients with more extensive disease, such as those with multivessel involvement. How-

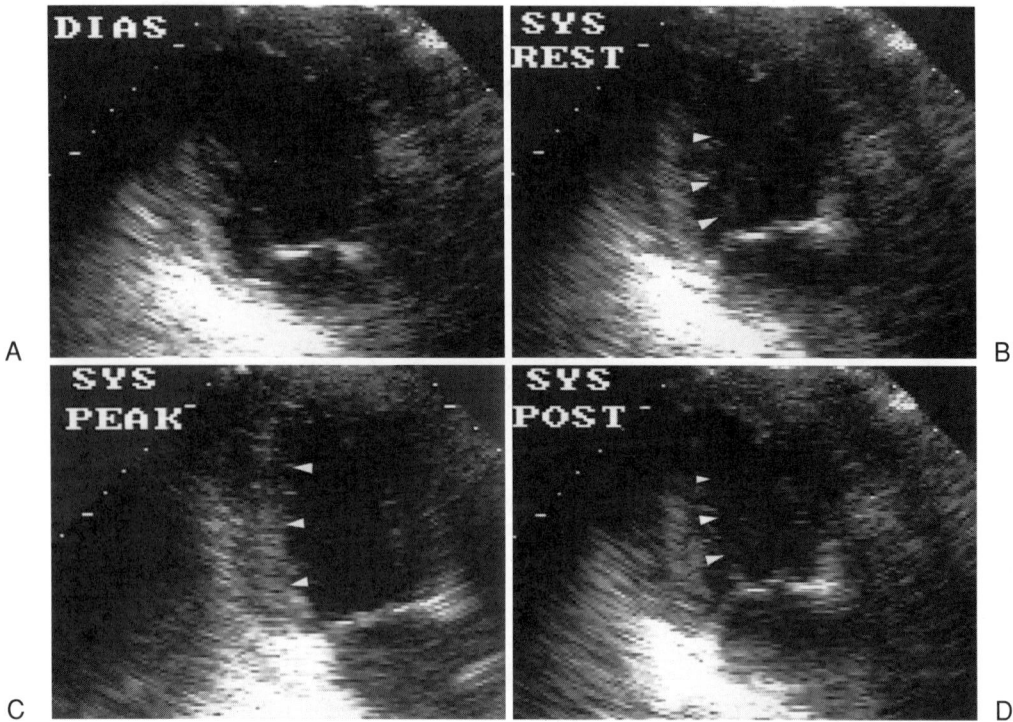

Fig. 3-8. A quad screen echocardiogram obtained using upright bicycle stress testing. The phenomenon of "rapid recovery" is demonstrated. **(A)** The end diastolic (DIAS) two-chamber view. Wall motion is normal at baseline **(B)** (SYS REST). At peak exercise, akinesis develops in the inferobasal wall (SYS PEAK, **C**). **(D)** Obtained during early recovery (SYS POST), recovery of endocardial excursion and systolic wall thickening is demonstrated. (From Ryan,[125] with permission.)

Table 3-5. Localization of Coronary Artery Lesions Using Stress Echocardiography

Reference	Method	Sensitivity (%)		
		LAD	LCx	RCA
Armstrong et al. (1987)[78]	Treadmill	71[a]	13[a]	85[a]
Pozzoli et al. (1991)[60]	Bicycle	69	45	65
Hoffman et al. (1993)[54]	Bicycle	85[a]	60[a]	82[a]
	Dobutamine	83[a]	50[a]	82[a]
Marwick et al. (1992)[63]	Treadmill	77	67	70
Hecht et al. (1993)[14]	Bicycle	95	78	81
Ryan et al. (1993)[10]	Bicycle	79	36	79
		80[a]	17[a]	83[a]
Segar et al. (1992)[53]	Dobutamine	79	70	77

Abbreviations: LAD, left anterior descending coronary artery; LCx, left circumflex coronary artery; RCA, right coronary artery.
[a] Patients with single-vessel disease only.

ever, the specific demonstration of multivessel disease requires detection of wall motion abnormalities in more than one vascular territory. For example, an early study from Indiana University[78] using treadmill exercise echocardiography demonstrated a sensitivity of 97% for detecting CAD in patients with multivessel involvement. However, for the *specific identification* of multivessel disease, sensitivity was only 54%. Hecht et al.[13] on the other hand, used supine bicycle exercise to correctly identify the presence of multivessel disease in 93% of patients. It is possible that the use of peak exercise imaging may account for this difference. In a more recent study from Indiana University, also using a bicycle protocol,[10] the number of stenotic major coronary arteries was correctly predicted in 186 of 309 patients (60%). The extent of disease was underestimated in 26% and overestimated in 14% (Fig. 3-9).

Left Ventricular Functional Response to Stress for the Diagnosis of CAD

	Angio			
	0	1	2	3
Echo 0	**76**	12	4	2
1	17	**57**	25	14
2	5	14	**37**	23
3	0	2	5	**16**

Fig. 3-9. Correlation between echocardiography (Echo) and angiography (Angio) for predicting extent of coronary artery disease, without regard to localization. Overall, 186 patients were correctly classified (76 without coronary artery disease, 57 with single-vessel, and 53 with multivessel disease). Understimation of extent of disease occurred in 80 (26%) patients and overestimation in 43 (14%) patients. (From Ryan et al.,[10] with permission.)

Similar findings have been reported using dobutamine stress echocardiography. Cohen et al.[73] studied 70 men with dobutamine stress echocardiography prior to coronary angiography. Sensitivity for the detection of three-, two-, and one-vessel disease was 100%, 89%, and 69%, respectively. For *specifically* identifying multivessel disease, the presence of *multiple* wall motion abnormalities had an accuracy of 71%. However, the induction of a wall motion abnormality at low dose (≤ 15 µg/kg/min) had an accuracy of 84%. Olson et al.[79] have also demonstrated that an abnormal LV volume response to dobutamine stimulation may further enhance the ability of the test to detect more extensive and severe coronary disease.

Comparison with Stress Testing Results

The incremental value of stress echocardiography to ECG monitoring has been extensively evaluated. In each of these studies, echocardiography has been demonstrated to be more sensitive and specific for detecting disease. Part of the enhanced accuracy provided by echocardiography depends on the prevalence of ambiguous or nondiagnostic stress ECG results.[80] However, even when such patients are excluded, the higher sensitivity of echocardiography is maintained.[63] The superiority of the exercise echocardiogram is greatest in patients with single-vessel CAD. In such patients, the predictive value of the stress ECG is quite low. Among patients with a nondiagnostic stress ECG, wall motion analysis has been shown to be useful for the diagnosis of coronary disease. In a series of 309 patients studied at Indiana University,[10] a nondiagnostic stress ECG occurred in 104 patients (Fig. 3-10). In this subset, the negative and positive predictive values of echocardiography were 82% and 93%, respectively. This superior diagnostic accuracy was maintained even when patients with resting wall motion abnormalities were excluded.

Comparison of Stress Echocardiographic Techniques

Several clinical series, mostly from Europe, have demonstrated the utility of vasodilator stress echocardiography.[81,82] Severi and colleagues[83] examined 429 consecutive patients who were hospitalized for evaluation of chest pain. Sensitivity and specificity for the detection of angiographic CAD (defined as a $\geq 75\%$ reduction in luminal diameter) were 75% and 90%, respectively. In some series, however, accuracy has been less. Mazeika et al.[84] studied 58 patients, 69% of whom had CAD. In this series, sensitiv-

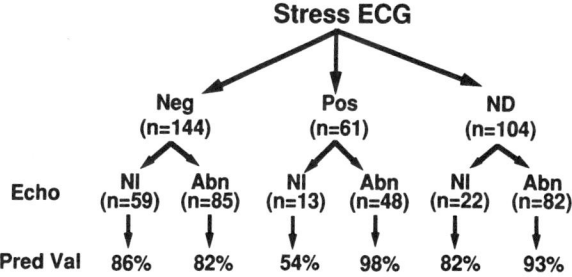

Fig. 3-10. The accuracy of exercise echocardiography when combined with stress electrocardiographic (ECG) results is presented. The positive and negative predictive value (PRED VAL) within each subgroup is shown on the bottom line. The accuracy of echocardiography is high in all groups except those with a positive stress ECG and a normal echocardiogram. In this subset, echocardiography had a negative predictive value of only 54%. Neg, negative stress ECG; Pos, positive stress ECG; ND, nondiagnostic stress ECG; NI, normal stress echo; Abn, abnormal stress echo. (From Ryan et al.,[10] with permission.)

ity was only 40% and inducible wall motion abnormalities developed only in patients with multivessel disease. By combination of dipyridamole with dobutamine in patients without evidence of ischemia at the conclusion of a high-dose dipyridamole study, Ostojic et al.[30] reported a sensitivity and specificity of 92% and 89%, respectively. The test appeared capable of detecting more mild forms of coronary disease that were missed by dipyridamole alone, and was safe and well tolerated with a feasibility of 96%.

One advantage of dipyridamole echocardiography is the ability to stratify a positive result by carefully determining the time of onset of the wall motion abnormality following completion of the infusion. Picano et al.[85] correlated this parameter with coronary flow reserve (determined using positron emission tomography [PET] scanning) in a group of 11 patients with single-vessel coronary disease. The investigators demonstrated a significant relationship ($r = 0.87$) between the dipyridamole time and the functional severity of the coronary lesion.

Atrial pacing is an alternative to pharmacologic stress in patients who are unable to exercise. Overall sensitivity has been reported as high as 93% and specificity has ranged from 76% to 100%.[32,34,35,86] Among patients with single-vessel coronary disease, the test may be more sensitive than other forms of stress echocardiography.[32,34,86] The accuracy of this technique has also been compared to other forms of stress echocardiography. Iliceto et al.[86] examined 78 consecutive patients with transesophageal atrial pacing and postexercise echocardiography. Atrial pacing echocardiography was slightly more sensitive (90% vs. 82%), but less specific (84% vs. 95%) than postexercise imaging. A limitation of this approach is the invasive nature of the technique, which reduces patient tolerance somewhat. In general, image quality is excellent, an important factor in overall accuracy. The test may be optimally applied in patients who are unable to exercise and have poor transthoracic image quality.

The various stress echocardiographic techniques have been compared in several clinical studies (Table 3-6). When choosing among these various modalities, it is important to consider the patient population and the goal of testing in addition to the accuracy of each test. The different pharmacologic stress methodologies have been compared in several series. In most studies, dobutamine echocardiography has been found to be more sensitive and less

Table 3-6. Comparing the Accuracy of Various Stress Echocardiographic Methods

Reference	n	Method	Sensitivity (%)	Specificity (%)	Accuracy (%)
Marwick et al. (1993)[89]	97	Dobutamine	85	82	84
		Adenosine	58	87	69
Hoffman et al. (1993)[54]	66	Bicycle	80	87	82
		Dobutamine	79	81	80
Cohen et al. (1993)[97]	52	Bicycle	78	87	81
		Dobutamine	86	87	87
Marangelli et al. (1994)[35]	104	Treadmill	89	88	88
		TAP	83	76	80
		Dipyridamole	43	92	63
Beleslin et al. (1994)[90]	136	Treadmill	88	82	87
		Dobutamine	82	77	82
		Dipyridamole	74	94	77
Iliceto et al. (1986)[86]	58	Bicycle	82	95	—
		TAP	90	84	—
Marwick et al. (1994)[98]	86	Dobutamine	54	83	64
		Bicycle	88	80	85
Sochowski et al. (1995)[91]	46	Dipyridamole	67	86	76
		Dobutamine	71	82	76

Abbreviations: TAP, transesophageal atrial pacing.

specific than dipyridamole or adenosine echocardiography.[87-90] However, in one study,[91] the accuracy and feasibility of dobutamine and dipyridamole were equivalent. In theory, vasodilating agents may redistribute coronary blood flow without inducing myocardial ischemia. In such a situation, an abnormality may be detected using a perfusion imaging agent (such as thallium-201) without resulting in an associated wall motion abnormality.[92-94] This possibility suggests that dipyridamole stress testing with perfusion scintigraphy would be more sensitive than with echocardiography.[95] The severity of regional dysfunction induced by the two agents may also differ. In an animal study, dobutamine was associated with a consistently greater degree of dyssyngery than dipyridamole.[96]

Exercise and pharmacologic stress echocardiographic methods have also been compared.[54,90,97] When evaluating these studies, patient selection criteria should be carefully considered. Any comparison between exercise and pharmacologic stress should address two issues: (1) the *accuracy* of the various modalities in a group of patients able to successfully complete each protocol, and (2) the *feasibility* of the test in an unselected population. Marwick et al.[98] recently compared dobutamine and bicycle exercise echocardiography in 86 active patients. Both methods resulted in submaximal stress in a similar number of patients, dobutamine because of inadequate heart rate response or the development of side effects, and bicycle ergometry because of reduced exercise capacity. Among patients in whom maximal stress was achieved, sensitivities were not significantly different (73% for dobutamine and 77% for exercise echocardiography).

Other investigators have reported similar findings suggesting that exercise and pharmacologic stress echocardiography yield equivalent results in patients able to successfully complete the various protocols. Cohen et al.[97] studied 52 patients with dobutamine stress echocardiography and supine bicycle exercise. Overall sensitivity and specificity of the two tests, as well as the ability to specifically identify extent of disease, were similar. During dobutamine infusion, however, ischemia consistently developed at a lower heart rate and blood pressure compared to exercise. The investigators suggested that, while the two modalities have equivalent accuracy, they may produce ischemia by different physiologic mechanisms.

Marangelli et al.[35] examined the feasibility of different stress echocardiographic techniques in a series of 104 consecutive patients with suspected CAD. A successful treadmill exercise test was possible in only 77% of patients. Of 82 patients subjected to nonexercise stress testing, dipyridamole echocardiography was successfully completed in 96% and transesophageal atrial pacing in 77%. However, due to a significantly higher accuracy of exercise echocardiography for the detection of CAD, the authors suggested that exercise testing is superior if patients are able to adequately perform the test. Among patients in whom exercise is inadequate, either pharmacologic or pacing stress echocardiography could be performed in the majority of patients and should be utilized.

Comparison between Stress Echocardiography and Perfusion Imaging

When echocardiographic and perfusion imaging modalities are compared, it must be recognized that there are inherent differences between these two approaches to the detection of myocardial ischemia. Because hypoperfusion must precede regional dyssynergy, it can be argued that a perfusion defect will occur before the development of abnormal wall motion. As a result, perfusion scintigraphy may be more sensitive than stress echocardiography in cases in which stress is terminated *after* the development of hypoperfusion, but *before* a change in wall motion occurs. Alternatively, echocardiography may be more specific than perfusion scintigraphy since it relies on the development of a wall motion abnormality to define ischemia.

Stress echocardiography and perfusion scintigraphy have now been compared in several clinical series, and these comparisons are discussed in detail in Chapter 4. Despite the theoretical differences described above, it is reasonable to expect the two modalities to provide concordant information concerning the presence, extent, and location of CAD. A summary of the studies comparing the various methods is presented in Table 3-7. In most, the overall accuracies of the different modalities are equivalent. Quinones et al.[99] studied a series of 289 patients with treadmill exercise echocardiography and tomo-

Table 3-7. Concordance and Relative Accuracy of Stress Echocardiography and Radionuclide Imaging

Reference	n	Echocardiography			Perfusion Imaging			Agreement
		Method	Sensitivity (%)	Specificity (%)	Method	Sensitivity (%)	Specificity (%)	
Pozzoli et al. (1991)[60]	75	Bicycle	71	96	MIBI	84	88	88
Hecht et al. (1993)[100]	71	Bicycle	90	80	SPECT	92	65	79
Quinones et al. (1992)[99]	289	Treadmill	74	88	SPECT	76	81	88
Hoffman et al. (1993)[54]	66	Bicycle	80	87	Treadmill-SPECT	89	71	
Galanti et al. (1991)[101]	53	Bicycle	93	96	Planar thallium-201	100	92	
Marwick et al. (1993)[104]	217	Dobutamine	72	83	MIBI	76	67	
Marwick et al. (1993)[89]	97	Dobutamine	85	82	Adenosine-MIBI	86	71	
Forster et al. (1993)[102]	105	Dobutamine	75	89	MIBI	83	89	74
Takeuchi et al. (1993)[105]	120	Dobutamine	85	93	SPECT	89	85	81
Mairesse et al. (1994)[103]	129	Dobutamine	76	89	MIBI	76	65	65

Abbreviations: MIBI, ^{99m}Tc-methoxyisobutyl isonitrile; SPECT, single-photon emission computed tomography (using thallium-201).

graphic thallium-201 scintigraphy. Among 112 patients who also underwent coronary angiography, the sensitivity of the two tests was similar regardless of the extent of coronary disease. Specificity was slightly higher for echocardiography (88%) compared to thallium imaging (81%). Hecht et al.[100] compared treadmill tomographic thallium-201 imaging and supine bicycle echocardiography in 71 patients. Accuracy, overall sensitivity, and specificity were similar for both tests.

Several studies have also evaluated the concordance of echocardiography and perfusion imaging.[63,99–101] In the series of 289 patients described above from Baylor University,[99] echocardiography and tomographic thallium imaging were in agreement regarding the presence or absence of coronary artery disease in 88% of patients. Agreement regarding the type of abnormality (i.e., distinguishing between baseline and induced abnormalities) was 82%. Within the abnormal regions, thallium detected more reversible segments while echocardiography detected a greater number of resting abnormalities.

Thus, most discordant results involved segments that exhibited partial reversibility with scintigraphy but a resting wall motion abnormality by echocardiography.

In comparisons using pharmacologic stress, a variety of different protocols and stress agents have been studied. In most series, similar degrees of accuracy have been reported.[54,102–105] Marwick and colleagues[89] compared echocardiography and single-photon emission computed tomography (SPECT) imaging (with ^{99m}Tc-methoxyisobutyl isonitrile [MIBI]) during both dobutamine and adenosine stress in 97 consecutive patients. The four different stress tests were then compared to coronary angiography. With the exception of adenosine echocardiography, the tests were similar with respect to overall accuracy and sensitivity. Adenosine echocardiography, however, was less sensitive (58%) and less accurate (69%) compared to the other three modalities.

When these comparative data are analyzed, several additional issues must be considered. When the different modalities are performed under optimal circumstances, concordance is quite high and the various techniques appear similar with respect to diagnostic yield. In specific clinical situations, certain advantages must be recognized. For example, for the detection of ischemia within an area of prior myocardial infarction, perfusion scintigraphy may be preferable. Because wall motion will be abnormal at baseline in these segments, exercise echocardiography will be limited in its ability to detect superimposed ischemia. Echocardiography has higher specificity than perfusion scintigraphy and this may be especially important in certain clinical situations. Additional advantages of echocardiography include lower cost, lack of radiation exposure, and immediate availability of diagnostic information. The additional diagnostic information provided by echocardiography, regarding LV function and valvular heart disease, for example, is an additional advantage. Finally, it is important to consider local expertise when choosing among the different stress test modalities. All forms of stress imaging are operator dependent and technically challenging. This important issue must be considered when attempting to extrapolate the published literature to individual laboratories.

Radionuclide Angiography

Criteria for Positivity

When ischemia is induced during stress testing, regional dyssynergy develops, leading to a decrease in LV function and, in some cases, an increase in LV volume. Using exercise radionuclide angiography, evidence of ischemia may be detected as an induced wall motion abnormality, an abnormal volume response to stress, or a decrease in LV ejection fraction. In most clinical series, some aspects of baseline LV ejection fraction and/or an abnormal ejection fraction response are utilized for the diagnosis of CAD. Although the "normal" response to exercise is an increase of 5% or greater in LV ejection fraction, the factors that determine this response in an individual patient are complex.[106] Resting ejection fraction, gender, medications, age, and exercise protocols are factors known to affect the LV ejection fraction response during exercise. Due to the number of factors that influence this parameter, it is not surprising that the change in ejection fraction is quite variable[107-109] and may be affected by parameters unrelated to the extent and severity of CAD.

Accuracy for Diagnosis of CAD

For the detection of angiographic CAD, exercise radionuclide angiography has sensitivity and specificity of approximately 90% and 58%, respectively.[110-112] Of the criteria that can be measured, the resting ejection fraction is most useful to identify patients with evidence of prior myocardial infarction.[106] When baseline LV function is normal, the ejection fraction response to exercise is a sensitive, but not specific, marker of disease.[106] In comparison, an inducible wall motion abnormality is more specific, but less sensitive. Given the limited accuracy of any one parameter, a combination of variables is most helpful to distinguish normal from abnormal results (Table 3-8).[110]

These findings have important implications for the application of exercise radionuclide angiography in different patient cohorts. When applied to patients with a low or intermediate pretest likelihood of disease, achieving a definitive diagnosis may not be possible and further diagnostic testing is often necessary.[113] The accuracy of exercise radionuclide angiography is further affected by the severity of the underlying disease. In patients with left main or three-vessel disease, exercise ejection fraction is a useful parameter.[114] Among patients with single-vessel coronary disease, radionuclide angiography has limited sensitivity and may be inferior to other techniques such as thallium perfusion imaging.[112]

Magnetic Resonance Imaging

Cine MRI is an alternative form of noninvasive cardiac imaging that can be used in conjunction with stress testing. Like echocardiography, MRI is a tomographic technique that permits evaluation of both endocardial excursion and ventricular wall thickening. Gradient echocardiographic, or cine, sequence protocols allow the creation of cine loops for the evaluation of systolic function. Technical improvements in the past few years now permit high-resolution imaging in the majority of patients. Using current methodology, cine MRI is currently the most accurate imaging technique for the assessment of myocardial thickening.

Several reports have demonstrated the utility of combining MRI with dobutamine stress for the detection of myocardial ischemia. The first such report,[115] published in 1992, utilized a gradient-refo-

Table 3-8. Accuracy of Radionuclide Angiography for the Detection of CAD

Reference	n	Criteria	Sensitivity (%)	Specificity (%)	Normalcy[a] (%)
Berger et al. (1979)[120]	73	Abnormal EF	73		100
		RWM	47		
Johnstone et al. (1980)[121]	48	Abnormal EF	85	100	
Jengo et al. (1980)[122]	58	Abnormal EF	86		100
		RWM	67		
Bodenheimer et al. (1979)[123]	75	Regional EF	82		
Borer et al. (1979)[124]	84	Abnormal EF	89	100	
		RWM	94		
Osbakken et al. (1984)[111]	120	Abnormal EF	80	62	
Jones et al. (1981)[106]	496	Abnormal EF	82	73	
		RWM	56		
Port et al. (1985)[112]	46[b]	Abnormal EF	56		

Abbreviations: n, total number of patients and normal subjects; abnormal EF, abnormal exercise response of LVEF; regional EF, abnormal exercise response of regional LVEF; RWM, exercise-induced regional wall motion abnormality; LVEF, left ventricular ejection fraction.
[a] Percentage of normal subjects with a negative test result; all studies utilized either supine or upright bicycle exercise.
[b] Patients with single-vessel disease only.

cused, velocity-compensated echo protocol to create cine MRI images during dobutamine infusion in 25 patients with exertional chest pain. Both long-axis and short-axis views of the LV were obtained and wall motion was analyzed qualitatively (Fig. 3-11). Of 22 patients with angiographic CAD, reversible wall motion abnormalities were detected in 20 patients (91%). This compared favorably to dobutamine thallium scintigraphy which identified 21 patients. Agreement between thallium and MRI occurred in 96% of patients at baseline and 90% of patients during stress.

A potential advantage of stress MRI is the high resolution of the technique, which permits the endocardium and epicardium to be clearly visualized in the majority of patients. This, in turn, allows various quantitative approaches to regional LV function to be utilized. Van Rugge and colleagues[116] applied a modified centerline technique to quantify changes in wall thickening during dobutamine infusion in a series of 39 patients with CAD and 10 normal volunteers. Although the tracing of endocardial and epicardial contours was performed manually, this quantitative approach permitted detection of ischemic changes in 91% of patients with CAD. As with other forms of pharmacologic stress imaging, sensitivity was greatest in patients with three-vessel disease and lowest in patients with one-vessel disease or lesions involving the left circumflex coronary artery.

The ability to accurately record wall thickening may be particularly valuable in the assessment of myocardial viability. Baer and colleagues[117] compared low-dose dobutamine MRI and PET scanning in 35 patients with a history of myocardial infarction and regional LV dysfunction. The authors identified two MRI criteria that correlated with PET evidence of viability. Using metabolic integrity on PET scanning as the standard, preserved end-diastolic wall thickness and dobutamine-induced wall thickening were 72% and 81% sensitive, respectively. If both MRI parameters were combined in an effort to predict viability, sensitivity increased to 88% and specificity was 87%.

There are several limitations to pharmacologic stress testing using MRI. The technique remains a research tool and is practiced in only a few specialized centers. An important limitation is the time required to perform imaging. The total duration of imaging is dependent on the number of tomographic slices that are recorded and the heart rate of the patient. Acquisition time is inversely related to heart rate. In one clinical study, in which six views were recorded, mean acquisition time for the baseline study was 42 ± 4 minutes.[118] During dobutamine infusion, due to the increased heart rate, acquisition time decreased to 24 ± 6 minutes. In a later study by the same group of investigators,[116] only four

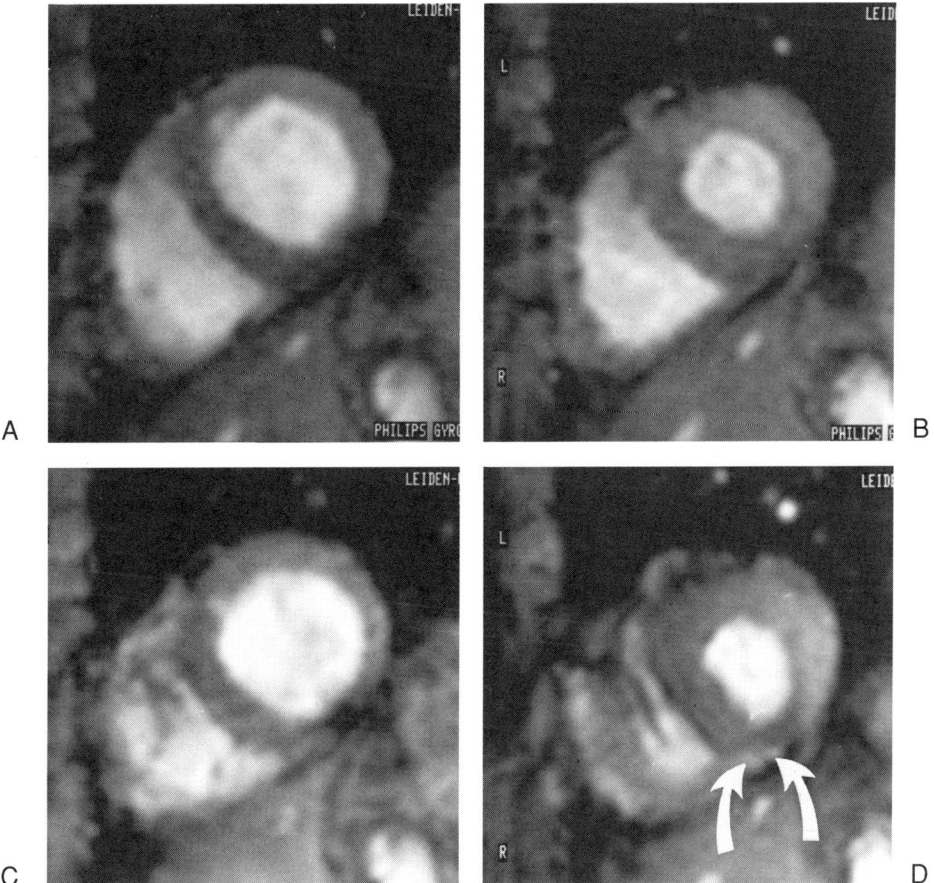

Fig. 3-11. Baseline (**A** & **B**) and dobutamine stress (**C** & **D**) cine magnetic resonance imaging tomograms at end-diastole (**A** & **C**) and end-systole (**B** & **D**) in a patient with right coronary artery stenosis. The baseline contraction pattern is normal with homogeneous systolic wall thickening (**B**). At peak dobutamine stress, the posterior wall fails to demonstrate systolic wall thickening, an indication of regional ischemia (**D**, white arrows). (From van Rugge et al.,[168] with permission.)

tomographic slices were utilized. Mean acquisition time decreased to 26 ± 3 minutes at rest and 12 ± 6 minutes at peak dobutamine infusion. In the future, the development of "ultrafast" MRI will likely lead to a significant shortening of acquisition time, and this will enhance the utility of the technique.

CONCLUSIONS

The currently available techniques for examining the LV function response to exercise are stress echocardiography, nuclear ventriculography, and MRI. Nuclear ventriculography provides global functional data, but is less useful for detection of regional wall motion abnormalities. The accuracy of nuclear ventriculography varies, depending upon the criteria used for positivity and the population studied; of the three, it is currently the least attractive. Magnetic resonance imaging offers excellent endocardial definition and promises to provide a truly quantitative approach. If pharmacologic stress MRI can be combined with MRI angiography, this method will likely play an increasingly important role in the evaluation of coronary artery disease. However, it is expensive, not widely available, and requires the use of pharmacologic stress. Stress echocardiography is accurate and may be performed with exercise and pharmacologic approaches, but limited by image quality, and its subjective interpretation requires a well-trained observer. In view of its availability and low cost, it is the most attractive of the alternatives for examining the global LV response to stress, and may be enhanced by technical advances such as contrast echocardiography, tissue Doppler imaging, and the use of transesophageal imaging in selected patients.

REFERENCES

1. Poliner LR, Dehmer GJ, Lewis SE et al.: Left ventricular performance in normal subjects: A comparison to the responses to exercise in the upright and supine positions. Circulation 62:528, 1980
2. Steingart RM, Wexler J, Slagle S, Scheuer J: Radionuclide ventriculographic responses to graded supine and upright exercise: critical role of the Frank-Starling mechanism at submaximal exercise. Am J Cardiol 53:1671, 1984
3. Thadani U, West RO, Mathew TM, Parker JO: Hemodynamics at rest and during supine and sitting bicycle exercise in patients with coronary artery disease. Am J Cardiol 39:776, 1977
4. Iskandrian AS, Hakki AH, DePace NL: Evaluation of left ventricular function by radionuclide angiography in normal subjects and in patients with chronic coronary heart disease. J Am Coll Cardiol 1:1518, 1983
5. Koike A, Itoh H, Doi M et al.: Beat-to-beat evaluation of cardiac function during recovery from upright bicycle exercise in patients with coronary artery disease. Am Heart J 120:316, 1990
6. Tennant R, Wiggers CJ: The effect of coronary artery occlusion on myocardial contraction. Am J Physiol 112:351, 1935
7. Presti CF, Armstrong WF, Feigenbaum H: Comparison of echocardiography at peak exercise and after bicycle exercise in the evaluation of patients with known or suspected coronary artery disease. J Am Soc Echo 1:119, 1988
8. Athanasopoulos G, Marsonis A, Joshi J et al.: Significance of delayed recovery after digital exercise echocardiography. Br Heart J 66:104, 1991
9. Robertson WS, Feigenbaum H, Armstrong WF et al.: Exercise echocardiography: a clinically practical addition in the evaluation of coronary artery disease. J Am Coll Cardiol 2:1085, 1983
10. Ryan T, Segar DS, Sawada SG et al.: Detection of coronary artery disease using upright bicycle exercise echocardiography. J Am Soc Echo 6:186, 1993
11. Heng MK, Simard M, Lake R, Udhoji VH: Exercise two-dimensional echocardiography for diagnosis of coronary artery disease. Am J Cardiol 54:502, 1984
12. Berberich SN, Zager JRS, Plotnick GD, Fischer ML: A practical approach to exercise echocardiography: Immediate post exercise echocardiography. J Am Coll Cardiol 3:284, 1984
13. Hecht HS, DeBord L, Sotomayor N et al.: Supine bicycle stress echocardiography: peak exercise imaging is superior to postexercise imaging. J Am Soc Echo 6:265, 1993
14. Hecht HS, DeBord L, Shaw R et al.: Digital supine bicycle stress echocardiography: a new technique for evaluating coronary artery disease. J Am Coll Cardiol 21:950, 1993
15. Ginzton LE, Conant R, Brizendine M et al.: Exercise subcostal two-dimensional echocardiography: a new method of segmental wall motion analysis. Am J Cardiol 53:805, 1984
16. Feigenbaum H: Stress echocardiography: an overview. Herz 16:347, 1991
17. Currie PJ, Kelly MJ, Pitt A: Comparison of supine and erect bicycle exercise electrocardiography in coronary heart disease: accentuation of exercise-induced ischemic ST depression by supine posture. Am J Cardiol 52:1167, 1983
18. Thrall TJ, Freitas JE, Swanson D et al.: Clinical comparison of cardiac blood pool visualization with technetium-99m red blood cells labeled in vivo and with technetium-99m human serum albumin. J Nucl Med 19:796, 1995
19. Morrison DA, Turgeon J, Ovitt T: Right ventricular ejection fraction measurement: contrast ventriculography versus gated blood pool and gated first-pass radionuclide methods. Am J Cardiol 54:651, 1984
20. Seaworth JF, Higginbotham MB, Coleman RE, Cobb FR: Effect of partial decreases in exercise workload on radionuclide indices of ischemia. J Am Coll Cardiol 2:522, 1983
21. Ryan T: Dobutamine stress echocardiography. Coronary Artery Dis 2:552, 1991
22. Weissman NJ, Nidorf SM, Guerrero JL et al.: Optimal stage duration in dobutamine stress echocardiography. J Am Coll Cardiol 25:605, 1995
23. McNeill AJ, Fioretti PM, El-Said ME et al.: Enhanced sensitivity for detection of coronary artery disease by addition of atropine to dobutamine stress echocardiography. Am J Cardiol 70:41, 1992
24. Mertes H, Sawada SG, Ryan T et al.: Symptoms, ad-

verse events, and complications associated with dobutamine stress echocardiography: experience in 1118 patients. Circulation 88:15, 1993
25. Marcovitz PA, Bach DS, Mathias W et al.: Paradoxic hypotension during dobutamine stress echocardiography: clinical and diagnostic implications. J Am Coll Cardiol 21:1080, 1993
26. Rosamond TL, Vacek JL, Hurwitz A et al.: Hypotension during dobutamine stress echocardiography: initial description and clinical relevance. Am Heart J 123:403, 1992
27. Pellikka PA, Oh JK, Bailey KR et al.: Dynamic intraventricular obstruction during dobutamine stress echocardiography. A new observation. Circulation 86:1429, 1992
28. Mazeika PK, Nadazdin A, Oakley CM: Clinical significance of abrupt vasodepression during dobutamine stress echocardiography. Am J Cardiol 69:1484, 1992
29. Picano E, Marini C, Pirelli S et al.: Safety of intravenous high-dose dipyridamole echocardiography. Am J Cardiol 70:252, 1992
30. Ostojic M, Picano E, Beleslin B et al.: Dipyridamole-dobutamine echocardiography: A novel test for the detection of milder forms of coronary artery disease. J Am Coll Cardiol 23:1115, 1994
31. Zoghbi WA, Cheirif J, Kleiman NS et al.: Diagnosis of ischemic heart disease with adenosine echocardiography. J Am Coll Cardiol 18:1271, 1991
32. Lambertz H, Kreis A, Trumper H, Hanrath P: Simultaneous transesophageal atrial pacing and transesophageal two-dimensional echocardiography. A new method of stress echocardiography. J Am Coll Cardiol 16:1143, 1990
33. Zabalgiotia M, Gandhi DK, Abi-Mansour P, Rosenblum J: Feasibility and safety of transesophageal stress echocardiography. Am J Med 303:90, 1992
34. Iliceto S, Sorino M, D'Ambrosio G et al.: Detection of coronary artery disease by two-dimensional echocardiography and transesophageal atrial pacing. J Am Coll Cardiol 5:1188, 1985
35. Marangelli V, Iliceto S, Piccinni G et al.: Detection of coronary artery disease by digital stress echocardiography: Comparison of exercise, transesophageal atrial pacing and dipyridamole echocardiography. J Am Coll Cardiol 24:117, 1994
36. Porter TR, Xie F, Kricsfeld A et al.: Improved endocardial border resolution during dobutamine stress echocardiography with intravenous sonicated dextrose albumin. J Am Coll Cardiol 23:1440, 1994
37. Panza JA, Laurienzo JM, Curiel RV et al.: Transesophageal dobutamine stress echocardiography for evaluation of patients with coronary artery disease. J Am Coll Cardiol 24:1260, 1994
38. Stoddard MF, Prince CR, Morris GL: Coronary flow reserve assessment by dobutamine transesophageal Doppler echocardiography. J Am Coll Cardiol 25:325, 1995
39. Frohwein S, Klein JL, Lane A, Taylor WR: Transesophageal dobutamine stress echocardiography in the evaluation of coronary artery disease. J Am Coll Cardiol 25:823, 1995
40. Mitchell GD, Brunken RC, Schwaiger M et al.: Assessment of mitral flow velocity with exercise by an index of stress-induced left ventricular ischemia in coronary artery disease. Am J Cardiol 61:536, 1988
41. Labovitz AJ, Pearson AC, Chaitman BR: Doppler and two-dimensional echocardiographic assessment of left ventricular function before and after intravenous dipyridamole stress testing for detection of coronary artery disease. Am J Cardiol 62:1180, 1988
42. Bryg RJ, Labovitz AJ, Mehdirad AA et al.: Effect of coronary artery disease on Doppler-derived parameters of aortic flow during upright exercise. Am J Cardiol 58:14, 1986
43. Harrison MR, Smith MD, Nissen SE et al.: Use of Doppler echocardiography to evaluate cardiac drugs: effects of propranolol and verapamil on aortic blood flow velocity and acceleration. J Am Coll Cardiol 11:1002, 1988
44. El-Said EM, Roelandt JRTC, Fioretti PM et al.: Abnormal left ventricular early diastolic filling during dobutamine stress Doppler echocardiography is a sensitive indicator of significant coronary artery disease. J Am Coll Cardiol 24:1618, 1994
45. Heinle SK, Tice FD, Kisslo J: Effect of dobutamine stress echocardiography on mitral regurgitation. J Am Coll Cardiol 25:122, 1995
46. Feigenbaum H: Exercise echocardiography. J Am Soc Echo 1:161, 1988
47. Feigenbaum H: Digital recording, display, and storage of echocardiograms. J Am Soc Echo 1:378, 1988
48. Borges-Neto S, Coleman RE, Potts JM, Jones RH: Combined exercise radionuclide angiocardiography and single photon emission computed tomography perfusion studies for assessment of coronary artery disease. Semin Nucl Med 21:223, 1991
49. Ewy GA, Ronan JA, Jr, Appleton CP et al.: ACC/AHA guidelines for the clinical application of echocardiography. A report of the American College of Cardiology/American Heart Association Task Force on assessment of diagnostic and therapeutic cardiovascular procedures. (Subcommittee to develop

50. Schiller NB, Shah PM, Crawford M: Recommendations for quantitation of the left ventricle by two dimensional echocardiography. J Am Soc Echo 2:358, 1989
51. Takeuchi M, Araki M, Nakashima Y, Kuroiwa A: The detection of residual ischemia and stenosis in patients with acute myocardial infarction with dobutamine stress echocardiography. J Am Soc Echo 7:242, 1994
52. Ginzton LE, Conant R, Brizendine M et al.: Quantitative analysis of segmental wall motion during maximal upright exercise: variability in normal adults. Circulation 73:268, 1986
53. Segar DS, Brown SE, Sawada SG et al.: Dobutamine stress echocardiography: Correlation with coronary lesion severity as determined by quantitative angiography. J Am Coll Cardiol 19:197, 1992
54. Hoffman R, Lethen H, Kleinhaus E et al.: Comparative evaluation of bicycle and dobutamine stress echocardiography with perfusion scintigraphy and bicycle electrocardiogram for identification coronary artery disease. Am J Cardiol 72:555, 1993
55. Okada RD, Pohost GM, Nichols AB et al.: Left ventricular regional wall motion assessment by multigated and end-diastolic, end-systolic gated radionuclide left ventriculography. Am J Cardiol 45:1211, 1980
56. Wackers FJ, Terrin ML, Kayden DS et al.: Quantitative radionuclide assessment of regional ventricular function after thrombolytic therapy for acute myocardial infarction: results of phase I thrombolysis in myocardial infarction (TIMI) trial. J Am Coll Cardiol 13:998, 1989
57. Pfisterer ME, Ricci DR, Schuler G et al.: Validity of left-ventricular ejection fractions measured at rest and peak exercise by equilibrium radionuclide angiography using short acquisition times. J Nucl Med 20:484, 1979
58. Wackers FJT, Berger HJ, Johnstone DE et al.: Multiple gated cardiac blood pool imaging for left ventricular ejection fraction: validation of the technique and assessment of variability. Am J Cardiol 43:1159, 1979
59. Okada RD, Kirshenbaum HD, Kushner FG et al.: Observer variance in the qualitative evaluation of left ventricular wall motion and the quantitation of left ventricular ejection fraction using rest and exercise multigated blood pool imaging. Circulation 61:128, 1980
60. Pozzoli MMA, Fioretti PM, Salustri A et al.: Exercise echocardiography and technetium-99m MIBI single-photon emission computed tomography in the detection of coronary artery disease. Am J Cardiol 67:350, 1991
61. Crouse LJ, Harbrecht JJ, Vacek JL et al.: Exercise echocardiography as a screening test for coronary artery disease and correlation with coronary arteriography. Am J Cardiol 67:1213, 1991
62. Marcovitz PA, Armstrong WF: Accuracy of dobutamine stress echocardiography in detecting coronary artery disease. Am J Cardiol 69:1269, 1992
63. Marwick TH, Nemec JJ, Pashkow FJ et al.: Accuracy and limitations of exercise echocardiography in a routine clinical setting. J Am Coll Cardiol 19:74, 1992
64. Armstrong WF, O'Donnell J, Dillon JC et al.: Complementary value of two-dimensional exercise echocardiography to routine treadmill exercise testing. Ann Internal Med 105:829, 1986
65. Mazeika PK, Nadazdin A, Oakley CM: Dobutamine stress echocardiography for detection and assessment of coronary artery disease. J Am Coll Cardiol 19:1203, 1992
66. Lu C, Picano E, Pingitore A et al.: Complex coronary artery lesion morphology influences results of stress echocardiography. Circulation 91:1669, 1995
67. Sawada SG, Segar DS, Ryan T et al.: Echocardiographic detection of coronary artery disease during dobutamine infusion. Circulation 83:1605, 1991
68. Sheikh KH, Bengtson JR, Helmy S et al.: Relation of quantitative coronary lesion measurements to the development of exercise-induced ischemia assessed by exercise echocardiography. J Am Coll Cardiol 15:1043, 1990
69. Salustri A, Pozzoli MMA, Hermans W et al.: Relationship between exercise echocardiography and perfusion single-photon emission computed tomography in patients with single-vessel coronary artery disease. Am Heart J 124:75, 1992
70. Homans DC, Sublett E, Dai XZ, Bache RJ: Persistence of regional left ventricular dysfunction after exercise-induced myocardial ischemia. J Clin Invest 77:66, 1986
71. Gavrielides S, Kaski JC, Tousoulis D et al.: Duration of ST segment depression after exercise-induced myocardial ischemia is influenced by body position during recovery but not by type of exercise. Am Heart J 121:1665, 1991
72. Ryan T, Vasey CG, Presti CF et al.: Exercise echocardiography: detection of coronary artery disease in patients with normal left ventricular wall motion at rest. J Am Coll Cardiol 11:993, 1988
73. Cohen JL, Greene TO, Ottenweller J et al.: Dobutamine digital echocardiography for detecting coronary artery disease. Am J Cardiol 67:1311, 1991

74. Douglas PS, O'Toole ML, Woolard J: Regional wall motion abnormalities after prolonged exercise in the normal left ventricle. Circulation 82:2108, 1990
75. Fisman EZ, Pines A, Ben-Ari E et al.: Left ventricular exercise echocardiographic abnormalities in apparently healthy men with exertional hypotension. Am J Cardiol 63:81, 1989
76. Bach DS, Muller DWM, Gros BJ, Armstrong WF: False positive dobutamine stress echocardiograms: characterization of clinical, echocardiographic and angiographic findings. J Am Coll Cardiol 24:928, 1994
77. Bach DS, Hepner A, Marcovitz PA, Armstrong WF: Dobutamine stress echocardiography: Prevalence of a nonischemic response in a low-risk population. Am Heart J 125:1257, 1993
78. Armstrong WF, O'Donnell J, Ryan T, Feigenbaum H: Effect of prior myocardial infarction and extent and location of coronary artery disease on accuracy of exercise echocardiography. J Am Coll Cardiol 10:531, 1987
79. Olson CE, Porter TR, Deligonul U et al.: Left ventricular volume changes during dobutamine stress echocardiography identify patients with more extensive coronary artery disease. J Am Coll Cardiol 24:1268, 1994
80. Sawada SG, Ryan T, Fineberg NS et al.: Exercise echocardiographic detection of coronary artery disease in women. J Am Coll Cardiol 14:1440, 1989
81. Picano E, Lattanzi F, Masini M et al.: High dose dipyridamole echocardiography test in effort angina pectoris. J Am Coll Cardiol 8:848, 1986
82. Picano E, Distante A, Masini M et al.: Dipyridamole-echocardiography test in effort angina pectoris. Am J Cardiol 56:452, 1985
83. Severi S, Picano E, Michelassi C et al.: Diagnostic and prognostic value of dipyridamole echocardiography in patients with suspected coronary artery disease: comparison with exercise electrocardiography. Circulation 89:1160, 1994
84. Mazeika P, Nihoyannopoulos P, Joshi J, Oakley CM: Uses and limitations of high dose dipyridamole stress echocardiography for evaluation of coronary artery disease. Br Heart J 67:144, 1992
85. Picano E, Parodi O, Lattanzi F et al.: Assessment of anatomic and physiologic severity of single-vessel coronary artery lesions by dipyridamole echocardiography: comparison with positron emission tomography and quantitative angiography. Circulation 89:753, 1994
86. Iliceto S, D'Ambrosio G, Sorino M et al.: Comparison of postexercise and transesophageal atrial pacing two-dimensional echocardiography for detection of coronary artery disease. Am J Cardiol 57:547, 1986
87. Martin TW, Seaworth JF, Johns JP et al.: Comparison of adenosine, dipyridamole, and dobutamine in stress echocardiography. Ann Intern Med 116:190, 1992
88. Previtali M, Lanzarini L, Ferario M et al.: Dobutamine versus dipyridamole echocardiography in coronary artery disease. Circulation 83:27, 1991
89. Marwick TH, Willemart B, D'Hondt A et al.: Selection of the optimal nonexercise stress for the evaluation of ischemic regional myocardial dysfunction and malperfusion. Circulation 87:345, 1993
90. Beleslin BD, Ostojic M, Stepanovic J et al.: Stress echocardiography in the detection of myocardial ischemia: head-to-head comparison of exercise, dobutamine, and dipyridamole tests. Circulation 90:1168, 1994
91. Sochowski RA, Yvorchuk KJ, Yang Y et al.: Dobutamine and dipyridamole stress echocardiography in patients with a low incidence of severe coronary artery disease. J Am Soc Echocardiog 8:482, 1995
92. Fung AY, Gallagher KP, Buda AJ: The physiologic basis of dobutamine as compared with dipyridamole stress interventions in the assessment of critical coronary stenosis. Circulation 76:943, 1987
93. Jain A, Suarez J, Mahmarian JJ et al.: Functional significance of myocardial perfusion defects induced by dipyridamole using thallium-201 single-photon emission computed tomography and two-dimensional echocardiography. Am J Cardiol 66:802, 1990
94. Whitfield S, Aurigemma G, Pape L et al.: Two-dimensional Doppler echocardiographic correlation of dipyridamole-thallium stress testing with isometric handgrip. Am Heart J 121:1367, 1991
95. Simonetti I, Rezai K, Rossen JD et al.: Physiological assessment of sensitivity of noninvasive testing for coronary artery disease. Circulation, suppl. III, 83:43, 1991
96. Segar DS, Ryan T, Sawada SG et al.: Pharmacologically induced myocardial ischemia: a comparison of dobutamine and dipyridamole. J Am Soc Echocardiog 8:9, 1995
97. Cohen JL, Ottenweller JE, George AK, Duvvuri S: Comparison of dobutamine and exercise echocardiography for detecting coronary artery disease. Am J Cardiol 72:1226, 1993
98. Marwick TH, D'Hondt AM, Mairesse GH et al.: Comparative ability of dobutamine and exercise stress in inducing myocardial ischaemia in active patients. Br Heart J 72:31, 1994
99. Quiñones MA, Verani MS, Haichin RM et al.: Exercise echocardiography versus thallium-201 single-photon

emission computed tomography in evaluation of coronary artery disease: analysis of 292 patients. Circulation 85:1026, 1992
100. Hecht HS, DeBord L, Shaw R et al.: Supine bicycle stress echocardiography versus tomographic thallium-201 exercise imaging for the detection of coronary artery disease. J Am Soc Echo 6:177, 1993
101. Galanti G, Sciagrà R, Comeglio M et al.: Diagnostic accuracy of peak exercise echocardiography in coronary artery disease: comparison with thallium-201 myocardial scintigraphy. Am Heart J 122:1609, 1991
102. Forster T, McNeill AJ, Salustri A et al.: Simultaneous dobutamine stress echocardiography and technetium-99m isonitrile single-photon emission computed tomography in patients with suspected coronary artery disease. J Am Coll Cardiol 21:1591, 1993
103. Mairesse GH, Marwick TH, Vanoverschelde JLJ et al.: How accurate is dobutamine stress electrocardiography for detection of coronary artery disease? Comparison with two-dimensional echocardiography and technetium-99m methoxyl isobutyl isonitrile (Mibi) perfusion scintigraphy. J Am Coll Cardiol 24:920, 1994
104. Marwick T, D'Hondt AM, Baudhuin T et al.: Optimal use of dobutamine stress for the detection and evaluation of coronary artery disease: combination with echocardiography or scintigraphy, or both? J Am Coll Cardiol 22:159, 1993
105. Takeuchi M, Araki M, Nakashima Y, Kuroiwa A: Comparison of dobutamine stress echocardiography and stress thallium-201 single-photon emission computed tomography for detecting coronary artery disease. J Am Soc Echo 6:593, 1993
106. Jones RH, McEwan P, Newman GE et al.: Accuracy of diagnosis of coronary artery disease by radionuclide measurement of left ventricular function during rest and exercise. Circulation 64:586, 1981
107. Gibbons RJ, Lee KL, Cobb FR et al.: Ejection fraction response to exercise in patients with chest pain, coronary artery disease and normal resting ventricular function. Circulation 66:643, 1982
108. Port S, McEwan P, Cobb FR, Jones RH: Influence of resting left ventricular function on the left ventricular response to exercise in patients with coronary artery disease. Circulation 63:856, 1981
109. Hanley PC, Zinsmeister AR, Clements IP et al.: Gender-related differences in cardiac response to supine exercise assessed by radionuclide angiography. J Am Coll Cardiol 13:624, 1989
110. Austin EH, Cobb FR, Coleman RE, Jones RH: Prospective evaluation of radionuclide angiocardiography for the diagnosis of coronary artery disease. Am J Cardiol 50:1212, 1982
111. Osbakken MD, Okada RD, Boucher CA et al.: Comparison of exercise perfusion and ventricular function imaging: an analysis of factors affecting the diagnostic accuracy of each technique. J Am Coll Cardiol 3:272, 1984
112. Port SC, Oshima M, Ray G et al.: Assessment of single vessel coronary artery disease: results of exercise electrocardiography, thallium-201 myocardial perfusion imaging and radionuclide angiography. J Am Coll Cardiol 6:75, 1985
113. Gibbons RJ, Lee KL, Pryor D et al.: The use of radionuclide angiography in the diagnosis of coronary artery disease—a logistic regression analysis. Circulation 68:740, 1983
114. Gibbons RJ, Fyke FE, III, Clements IP et al.: Noninvasive identification of severe coronary artery disease using exercise radionuclide angiography. J Am Coll Cardiol 11:28, 1988
115. Pennell DJ, Underwood RS, Manzara CC et al.: Magnetic resonance imaging during dobutamine stress in coronary artery disease. Am J Cardiol 70:34, 1992
116. Van Rugge FP, Van der Wall EE, Spanjersberg SJ et al.: Magnetic resonance imaging during dobutamine stress for detection and localization of coronary artery disease. Quantitative wall motion analysis using a modification of the centerline method. Circulation 90:127, 1994
117. Baer FM, Voth E, Schneider CA et al.: Comparison of low-dose dobutamine-gradient-echo magnetic resonance imaging and positron emission tomography with [^{18}F]fluorodeoxyglucose in patients with chronic coronary artery disease. Circulation 91:1006, 1995
118. Van Rugge FP, Van der Wall EE, de Roos A, Bruschke AVG: Dobutamine stress magnetic resonance imaging for detection of coronary artery disease. J Am Coll Cardiol 22:431, 1993
119. Marwick TH, Anderson T, Williams MJ et al.: Exercise echocardiography is an accurate and cost-efficient technique for detection of coronary artery disease in women. J Am Coll Cardiol 26:335, 1995
120. Berger HJ, Reduto LA, Johnstone DE et al.: Global and regional left ventricular response to bicycle exercise in coronary artery disease. Am J Med 66:13, 1979
121. Johnstone DE, Sands MJ, Berger HJ et al.: Comparison of exercise radionuclide angiocardiography and thallium-201 myocardial perfusion imaging in coronary artery disease. Am J Cardiol 45:1113, 1980
122. Jengo JA, Freeman R, Brizendin M, Mena IS: Detection of coronary artery disease: Comparison of exercise stress radionuclide angiocardiography and thal-

lium stress perfusion scanning. Am J Cardiol 45:535, 1980
123. Bodenheimer MM, Banka VS, Fooshee CM, Helfant RH: Comparative sensitivity of the exercise electrocardiogram, thallium imaging and stress radionuclide angiography to detect the presence and severity of coronary heart disease. Circulation 60:1270, 1979
124. Borer JS, Kent KM, Bacharach SL et al.: Sensitivity, specificity and predictive accuracy of radionuclide cineangiography during exercise in patients with coronary artery disease. Circulation 60:572, 1979
125. Ryan T: Stress echocardiography. In Marcus' Cardiac Imaging: A companion to Braunwald's Heart Disease. 2nd Ed. W.B. Saunders, Philadelphia, 1996
126. Feigenbaum H: Echocardiography. 5th Ed. Lea & Febiger, Philadelphia, 1994

Chapter 4

Selection of Myocardial Perfusion or Function for the Diagnosis of CAD

Marcel L. Geleijnse and Paolo M. Fioretti

Stress echocardiography and stress myocardial perfusion scintigraphy have gained wide acceptance as accurate techniques for the detection and localization of coronary artery disease (CAD). In addition to their use in combination with exercise, their clinical availability has been broadened by the use of pharmacologic stress agents. This chapter attempts to define the place of stress echocardiography in the context of perfusion scintigraphic techniques for the detection of CAD.

A number of variables (referral bias, extent and severity of coronary disease, the definition of significant coronary disease, different stress protocols, medications) may potentially influence the results of either test, so that comparisons will focus on studies involving performance of both echocardiographic and nuclear imaging in the same patients for each of the most widely used stress techniques: exercise, dobutamine, and vasodilators (adenosine and dipyridamole). For these comparisons to be valid, we are assuming that the investigators in these studies are equally expert in either technique. Likewise, we assume that practitioners making choices between echocardiography and scintigraphy have equivalent expertise available in each. Indeed, the availability of expert performance and interpretation promises to be a paramount issue in the relative clinical diffusion of these approaches.

BASIC PRINCIPLES OF FUNCTION VERSUS PERFUSION FOR DIAGNOSIS OF CAD

A sequence of functional events follows increasing myocardial oxygen demand due to exercise or pharmacological stress, in the presence of a flow limiting coronary artery stenosis. According to the "ischemic cascade" theory,[1] perfusion abnormalities due to limited coronary flow reserve are followed by diminished left ventricular compliance (diastolic dysfunction), decreased myocardial contractility (systolic dysfunction), and increased left ventricular end-diastolic pressure. These changes are evidenced at perfusion scintigraphy by relatively reduced tracer uptake and at echocardiography by alterations of transmitral flow patterns, abnormal regional systolic function, and eventually left ventricular cavity enlargement and reduction of overall left ventricular systolic function.

The development of myocardial perfusion defects with either exercise or pharmacologic stressors depends on the induction of regional heterogeneity of myocardial blood flow. As discussed in Chapter 2, coronary blood flow to the vascular bed of a normal artery dramatically increases during stress, whereas perfusion through a stenosed artery may change minimally. Because the initial uptake of radiopharmaceuticals is flow-dependent within physiologic ranges,[2] the relative myocardial radionuclide concentration will be greater in vascular beds supplied by a normal artery relative to that in beds perfused by an artery with significant obstruction. Classically, a twofold difference in relative count activity is required to detect a perfusion abnormality scintigraphically.[3]

Regional malperfusion severe enough to cause metabolic consequences of ischemia can be identified by echocardiography, based upon the response of the left ventricle. The normal response of the left ventricle to exercise or pharmacologic stress is to increase endocardial excursion, the speed of contraction, and the degree of myocardial thickening. Indices pointing to the presence of myocardial ischemia include stress-induced deterioration of regional endocardial excursion, delayed excursion ("tardokinesis"), and a reduction of myocardial thickening. Classically flow must be reduced to 50% in at least 5% of the myocardium to detect new wall motion abnormalities.[4]

STRENGTHS AND LIMITATIONS OF STRESS ECHOCARDIOGRAPHY

Before reporting the diagnostic accuracies, the strengths and limitations of the two competing imaging modalities, echocardiography (function) and nuclear imaging (perfusion), will be discussed (see Table 4-1).

Benefits of Stress Echocardiography Compared with Perfusion Imaging

Clinical Considerations

Several aspects of stress echocardiography are attractive from the standpoint of clinical feasibility. In comparison with single-photon emission computed tomography (SPECT) cameras, echocardiography machines are smaller in size and more easy portable, allowing studies in the coronary care unit and emergency room, for example. The shorter time for performance and interpretation of a stress echocardiogram is attractive in the outpatient setting, although the superseding of the conventional 4-hour thallium protocol by more "patient friendly" dual isotope techniques discussed in Chapter 2 may reduce the importance of this benefit of echocardiography. The absence of ionizing radiation may be attractive to the public, for whom nuclear tests have a bad image, at least in The Netherlands. In contrast, demonstration of echocardiographic images may assist with patient education.

Two-dimensional echocardiography has the abil-

Table 4-1. Comparison of Advantages and Disadvantages of Stress Echocardiography and Myocardial Perfusion Scintigraphy for the Diagnosis of Coronary Artery Disease

	Stress Echocardiography	Stress Perfusion Scintigraphy
Equipment	Low cost Portable	Relatively expensive Laboratory-based
Personnel	"Learning curve" for acquisition and reading	Relatively automated
Imaging	No radiation Rapid, instant results On-line, real-time imaging Function Tomographic	Radiation exposure Time consuming Off-line, "snapshot" at peak stress Perfusion Planar vs. SPECT
Reporting	Regional function/thickening Usually qualitative Global function (EF, ESV)	Regional flow heterogeneity Quantitation well accepted Global function (lung-heart ratio, gated SPECT)

Benefits	Identifies other sources of chest pain
	Ischemic threshold
	   Safety
	   Therapy assessment
		Widespread experience
		Less vulnerable to submaximal stress

Problems	Variable echo window Endocardial border definition Treadmill exercise	Artifacts due to breast tissue, left bundle branch block or left ventricular hypertrophy

Abbreviations: SPECT, single-photon emission computed tomography; EF, ejection fraction; ESV, end-systolic volume.

ity to visualize the heart using a noninvasive, real-time approach. As ischemia may be observed "on-line," appropriate action can be taken if imaging is performed during the test. Especially in patients in whom safety is a major concern (patients with suspected unstable angina or severe coronary disease), this "cinematographic" aspect of echocardiographic monitoring is very attractive. Documentation of the "ischemic threshold" (during pharmacologic or bicycle stress) can give important information about the severity and extent of underlying coronary disease, and can assess the adequacy of therapy, by measuring the ischemia-free stress time. In contrast, SPECT offers a "snapshot" of perfusion at the time of peak stress, without the ability to examine function "on-line."

Echocardiography has excellent spatial resolution and, combined with Doppler techniques, is capable of accurately defining systolic and diastolic function, chamber dimensions, volumes, and wall thickness. Nonischemic explanations for the patient's symptoms (such as mitral valve prolapse or pericardial disease) may be apparent from visualization of valve anatomy and gradients and pericardial effusion. These aspects are unique among the noninvasive techniques in common usage for the detection of coronary disease.

The interpretation of stress echocardiography is performed by cardiologists, who often feel that they have a better grasp of the clinical questions that need to be answered in cardiac patients than radiologists or nuclear medicine physicians. While any stress imaging study should be interpreted apart from the clinical and exercise data to obtain independent information, these data should then be applied to the clinical situation of the patient. In this respect, the nuclear physician may be put at a disadvantage in being unaware of the patient's clinical data, and the final synthesis of the results is less clinically oriented. For example, the response to the finding of minor inferior perfusion defects or minor hypokinesia of the inferior wall may be modulated by accurate knowledge of the patient's clinical data.

Finally, artifacts that are problematic with SPECT (breast and diaphragmatic attenuation) are not problematic with echocardiography. The benefits of this on the relative specificity of the technique will be discussed subsequently.

Availability and Cost

Additional strengths of echocardiography are its widespread availability and relatively low cost. In contrast to gamma cameras, most cardiologists have access to an echocardiography machine, and their clinical use is not regulated or constrained by any regulatory agencies. The average prices for these machines are lower than those of the average SPECT gamma camera systems, and additionally the need for technical support is less. As a consequence of lower purchasing and maintenance costs, the total cost of an echocardiographic study is less compared with a scintigraphic study; in The Netherlands, dipyridamole thallium scintigraphy costs about $531 (US dollars) compared to about $185 for dobutamine stress echocardiography.[5]

Benefits of Stress Perfusion Imaging Compared with Echocardiography

Imaging Considerations

In a large number of laboratories, especially in the United States, cardiac stress is routinely performed using the treadmill. In contrast to bicycle stress, echocardiographic imaging cannot be performed during treadmill exercise because of excessive patient motion. Consequently, the first images are taken immediately after cessation of exercise, putting the patient on a bed in the left lateral decubitus position. Unfortunately, wall motion abnormalities present at peak stress may revert rapidly to normal after the discontinuation of exercise, and may be missed using post-exercise imaging. While thallium may undergo redistribution between exercise and imaging, this is minimal if the delay between stress and imaging is brief, and if ^{99m}Tc sestamibi is used, the image corresponds to the perfusion status at the time of injection.

Despite the well-established standardization of the routine echocardiographic examinations, the availability of standard echocardiographic windows is variable from patient to patient, and, in some cases, especially in patients with chronic obstructive pulmonary disease, poor "echogenicity" results in suboptimal images that may make a correct interpretation difficult or impossible. In our experience, noninterpretable studies constitute a small minority of the patients (about 5%), although referral bias obviously influences these results. Importantly, it is sometimes difficult to predict which patients have poor echocardiographic images during the test, since paradoxically, the images may improve during stress. In contrast, although soft tissue attenuation may pose problems for SPECT (more with thallium than ^{99m}Tc), chronic lung disease does not pose a problem for image quality.

Even if the echocardiogram is of interpretable quality, technical problems may remain. In contrast to the relatively automated acquisition of nuclear images, with their relatively easy interpretation and computer quantitation, echocardiography is characterized by manual, technician-dependent image acquisition, problems with endocardial border definition, and visual, subjective interpretation. Inexpert use of the electrocardiographic (ECG) gating, comparison of nonidentical cross sections, and failure or delayed visualization of abnormal segments are all avoidable, operator-dependent problems. However, images suffer from poor endocardial border definition even in the hands of the best sonographer.

Interpretation

The interpretation of stress echocardiograms requires an important "learning curve" even for experienced echocardiographers. As discussed previously, there is an important difference in the accuracy of echocardiographers who are and are not trained in stress echocardiography.

Subjective analysis is further hampered by the absence of clear consensus about the definition of the "ischemic response." Whereas segments deteriorating from normal contraction to akinesis or dyskinesis are universally called ischemic segments, controversy exists about the interpretation of basal segments, segments showing minimal hypokinesis at peak stress (in particular, basal inferoposterior segments), and segments with absence of physiologic hyperkinesis during stress. Even for experts, the interpretation of studies in patients with abnormal resting contraction or left bundle branch block is sometimes very difficult. Moreover, at present, few data are available about the intra- and interobserver variability, especially between observers working in different centers. While training is also important for scintigraphic interpretation, this may be facilitated by quantitation, as discussed in Chapter 2.

Influence of Drug Therapy

As a positive stress echocardiogram requires the induction of wall motion abnormalities (and hence, "true" ischemia), the use of anti-ischemic drugs may decrease the sensitivity of the test. As a submaximal heart-rate response may compromise the development of maximal vasodilation, the same is true for exercise or dobutamine perfusion imaging, but this problem may be avoided by pharmacologic vasodilation. Performance of stress echocardiography in patients with ongoing anti-ischemic therapy is appropriate if the clinical question pertains to the efficacy of treatment for the control of angina, but is inappropriate if the test is performed for diagnostic purposes.

COMPARISONS OF STRESS ECHOCARDIOGRAPHY AND PERFUSION SCINTIGRAPHY

Exercise or Dobutamine Stress Echocardiography versus Perfusion Scintigraphy

Exercise results in a marked increase in heart rate and blood pressure. As discussed in Chapter 13, dobutamine can simulate exercise by activating β_1-, β_2-, and α_1-receptors.[6] Its main initial effect is a positive inotropic effect and, at higher doses (≥ 20 μg/kg/min), heart rate and to a lesser extent systolic blood pressure increase. This augmentation of myocardial contractility, heart rate, left ventricular pressure, and wall stress increases oxygen requirements. However, in the presence of a critical coronary stenosis, the enhanced myocardial oxygen demand is not matched by a concomitant increase in blood flow. This creates a condition of regional supply–demand imbalance that results in regional myocardial dysfunction. When dobutamine is used, its strong inotropic effect facilitates the echocardiographic detection of ischemic segments with abnormal function, as normal segments become hyperkinetic in response to the drug.

Either exercise or dobutamine can also be used in conjunction with myocardial perfusion scintigraphy, since both alter relative regional myocardial blood flow reserve. Normally, a dose-related increase in subepicardial and subendocardial blood flow occurs within myocardium supplied by normal coronary arteries. However, blood flow increases minimally within vascular beds supplied by significantly stenosed arteries, with most of the increase occurring within the subepicardium rather than the subendocardium.[7] This heterogeneity in myocardial blood flow can be visualized by perfusion scintigraphy.

Table 4-2 reports the sensitivity and specificity for the detection of CAD in 7 studies, directly comparing *exercise* echocardiography and perfusion scintigraphy in the same 390 patients.[8-14] In these patients, both tests were done simultaneously and coronary angiography was used as the reference standard. The sensitivities of both tests for the identification of CAD were comparable (80% vs. 84%, respectively), although there was a higher sensitivity for perfusion imaging in the setting of single vessel disease (80% vs. 69%, respectively, $p < 0.05$). There was a trend toward a better specificity for echocardiography (91% vs. 83%, $p < 0.10$).

The sensitivity and specificity values reported in 4 studies, comprising 318 patients who underwent simultaneous *dobutamine* stress echocardiography and perfusion scintigraphy, are summarized in Table 4-3.[15-18] The sensitivities of both tests for the identification of CAD were comparable (76% vs. 81%, respectively), although again there was a trend toward a higher sensitivity for perfusion imaging in the setting of single vessel disease (68% vs. 76%, respectively). The overall results for specificity showed that dobutamine echocardiography was a more specific test (85% vs. 71%, $p < 0.01$). These data are consistent with previous data that indicate that the high sensitivity of myocardial perfusion imaging with SPECT may be at the cost of a sacrifice in specificity.[19]

The results of direct comparisons of exercise and exercise simulating (dobutamine) stress echocardiography and perfusion scintigraphy presented in this chapter suggest that the two imaging techniques offer comparable levels of accuracy in the diagnosis of coronary artery disease (82% and 81%, respectively, Fig. 4-1). The finding that echocardiography is more specific, but may be less sensitive (particularly in the detection of single vessel disease), is in line with the "ischemic cascade" model. As the development of a perfusion disturbance is expected to precede the development of true ischemia, perfusion imaging might be expected to be more sensitive than wall motion imaging for the detection of mild stenosis. Indeed, the difference in sensitivity is less than might be expected. This might be explained by two major factors: suboptimal inducement of flow heterogeneity by exercise or dobutamine[7] or inherent compensating strengths of echocardiography over perfusion scintigraphy, including improved spatial resolution, and the ability to categorize wall motion independently in each segment (contrasting with the relative flow comparisons used in myocardial perfusion imaging). Some ischemic regions may even be identified by echocardiography rather than scintigraphy, for example, abnormal wall motion due to subendocardial ischemia may be evident before malperfusion is extensive enough to be apparent at perfusion scintigraphy.

Vasodilator Stress Echocardiography versus Perfusion Scintigraphy

The performance of adenosine and dipyridamole stress testing is discussed in more detail in Chapter 13. In brief, adenosine is a naturally occurring molecule that regulates blood flow in various vascular beds including the myocardium, by activation of specific cell surface receptors.[20] In particular, α_2-receptor activation in vascular smooth muscle cells ultimately leads to smooth muscle relaxation and dilatation. Dipyridamole is an indirect coronary vasodilator that increases the extracellular concentration of adenosine by blocking its intracellular transport, metabolism, and inactivation.[21]

In normal arteries, these vasodilators cause an increase in coronary flow—both subendocardial and subepicardial—of threefold to fivefold.[22] However, in stenosed arteries this augmentation is limited (dependent on stenosis severity), creating flow heterogeneity, which can be detected by perfusion scintigraphy. Echocardiographically detected functional evidence of ischemia is not caused by marked changes in blood pressure or heart rate (which change only minimally) but by coronary steal—either "vertical"[7,23] (subepicardium from subendocardium) or "horizontal" (nonstenotic from stenotic vessel territory).[24]

As seen in Table 4-4, pooling data from five studies[25-29] directly comparing vasodilator (dipyridamole or adenosine) echocardiography and perfusion scintigraphy in the same 222 patients showed that the sensitivity of vasodilator perfusion scintigraphy was superior to that of vasodilator echocardiography

Table 4-2. Direct Diagnostic Comparisons between Exercise Echocardiography and Perfusion Scintigraphy

Author	Number of Patients	Stress	Imaging Modality	CAD %DS	Sensitivity	Specificity	Sensitivity SVD	Sensitivity MVD	Exclusions
Maurer and Nanda (1981)[8]	36	Treadmill	Echo	≥50	19/23 (83%)	12/13 (92%)	3/6 (50%)	16/17 (94%)	MI
			^{201}Tl Planar		17/23 (74%)	12/13 (92%)	—	—	
Quiñones et al. (1992)[9]	112	Treadmill	Echo	≥50	64/86 (74%)	23/26 (88%)	24/41 (58%)	40/45 (89%)	—
			^{201}Tl SPECT		65/86 (76%)	21/26 (81%)	25/41 (61%)	40/45 (89%)	
Wann et al. (1979)[10]	6	Supine bike	Echo	≥50	1/3 (33%)	3/3 (100%)	0/1 (0%)	1/2 (50%)	MI, rest WMA
			^{201}Tl Planar		2/3 (67%)	3/3 (100%)	0/1 (0%)	2/2 (100%)	
Hecht et al. (1993)[11]	71	Supine bike	Echo	≥50	46/51 (90%)	16/20 (80%)	17/22 (77%)	29/29 (100%)	—
			^{201}Tl SPECT		47/51 (92%)	13/20 (65%)	21/22 (95%)	26/29 (90%)	
Pozzoli et al. (1991)[12]	75	Upright bike	Echo	≥50	35/49 (71%)	25/26 (96%)	20/33 (61%)	15/16 (94%)	—
			MIBI SPECT		41/49 (84%)	23/26 (88%)	27/33 (82%)	14/16 (88%)	
Galanti et al. (1991)[13]	53	Upright bike	Echo	≥70	25/27 (93%)	25/26 (96%)	13/14 (93%)	12/13 (92%)	MI, rest WMA
			^{201}Tl Planar		27/27 (100%)	24/26 (92%)	14/14 (100%)	13/13 (88%)	
Salustri et al. (1992)[14]	37	Upright bike	Echo	≥50	19/23 (83%)	12/14 (86%)	19/23 (83%)	—	MI, rest WMA
			MIBI/^{201}Tl SPECT		20/23 (87%)	10/14 (71%)	20/23 (87%)	—	
Total	390		Function		209/262 (80%)	116/128 (91%)	93/134 (69%)[a]	97/105 (92%)	
			Perfusion		219/262 (84%)	106/128 (83%)	107/134 (80%)	95/105 (90%)	

Abbreviations: CAD %DS, percent diameter stenosis value for significant coronary artery disease; Echo, echocardiography; MI, myocardial infarction; MIBI, technetium-99m sestamibi; MVD, multivessel disease; SVD, single vessel disease; SPECT, single-photon emission computed tomography; ^{201}Tl, thallium-201; WMA, wall motion abnormalities.
[a] $P < 0.05$.

Table 4-3. Direct Diagnostic Comparisons between Dobutamine Echocardiography and Perfusion Scintigraphy

Author	Number of Patients	Dobu Dose	Imaging Modality	CAD %DS	Sensitivity	Specificity	Sensitivity SVD	Sensitivity MVD	Exclusions
Günalp et al. (1993)[15]	19	Dobu 30	Echo MIBI SPECT	≥50	7/10 (70%) 9/10 (90%)	8/9 (89%) 8/9 (89%)	5/7 (71%) 6/7 (86%)	2/3 (67%) 3/3 (100%)	MI, rest WMA
Marwick et al. (1993)[16]	217	Dobu 40	Echo MIBI SPECT	≥50	102/142 (72%) 108/142 (76%)	62/75 (83%) 50/75 (67%)	45/68 (66%) 50/68 (74%)	57/74 (77%) 58/74 (78%)	MI
Forster et al. (1993)[17]	21	Dobu 40 + A	Echo MIBI SPECT	≥50	9/12 (75%) 10/12 (83%)	8/9 (89%) 8/9 (89%)	1/4 (25%) 3/4 (75%)	8/8 (100%) 7/8 (88%)	MI, rest WMA
Senior et al. (1994)[18]	61	Dobu 40	Echo MIBI SPECT	≥50	41/44 (93%) 42/44 (95%)	16/17 (94%) 12/17 (71%)	12/14 (86%) 12/14 (86%)	29/30 (97%) 30/30 (100%)	—
Total	318		Function Perfusion		159/208 (76%) 169/208 (81%)	94/110 (85%)[a] 78/110 (71%)	63/93 (68%) 71/93 (76%)	96/115 (83%) 98/115 (85%)	

Abbreviations: A, atropine; CAD %DS, percent diameter stenosis value for significant coronary artery disease; Dobu dose, dobutamine dose in $\mu g/kg/min$; Echo, echocardiography; MI, myocardial infarction; MIBI, technetium-99m sestamibi; MVD, multivessel disease; SVD, single vessel disease; SPECT, single-photon emission computed tomography; WMA, wall motion abnormalities.

[a] $P < 0.01$.

Table 4-4. Direct Diagnostic Comparisons between Vasodilator Echocardiography and Perfusion Scintigraphy

Author	Number of Patients	Stress Dose	Imaging Modality	CAD %DS	Sensitivity	Specificity	Sensitivity SVD	Sensitivity MVD	Exclusions
Marwick et al. (1993)[25]	97	Adeno 0.18	Echo MIBI SPECT	≥50	34/59 (58%) 51/59 (86%)	33/38 (87%) 27/38 (71%)	16/31 (52%) 25/31 (81%)	18/28 (64%) 26/28 (93%)	MI
Nguyen et al. (1990)[26]	25	Adeno 0.14	Echo ^{201}Tl SPECT	≥50	12/20 (60%) 18/20 (90%)	5/5 (100%) 5/5 (100%)	— —	— —	—
Amanullah et al. (1993)[27]	40	Adeno 0.14	Echo MIBI SPECT	≥50	25/34 (74%) 32/34 (94%)	6/6 (100%) 6/6 (100%)	— —	— —	—
Perin et al. (1991)[28]	25	Dipy 0.56	Echo ^{201}Tl Planar	≥50	11/19 (58%) 18/19 (95%)	6/6 (100%) 3/6 (50%)	— —	— —	—
Simonetti et al. (1991)[29]	35	Dipy 0.84	Echo ^{201}Tl Planar	≥75	19/22 (86%) 20/22 (91%)	12/13 (92%) 13/13 (100%)	— —	— —	MI
Total	222		Function Perfusion		101/154 (66%)[a] 139/154 (90%)	62/68 (91%)[b] 54/68 (79%)	16/31 (52%)[c] 25/31 (81%)	18/28 (64%)[d] 26/28 (93%)	

Abbreviations: Adeno, adenosine (dose in mg/kg/min); CAD %DS, percent diameter stenosis value for significant coronary artery disease; Dipy, dipyridamole (dose in mg/kg); Echo, echocardiography; MI, myocardial infarction; MIBI, technetium-99m sestamibi; MVD, multivessel disease; SVD, single vessel disease; SPECT, single-photon emission computed tomography; ^{201}Tl, thallium-201.

[a] $P < 0.0001$.
[b] $P < 0.05$.
[c] $P < 0.02$.
[d] $P < 0.01$.

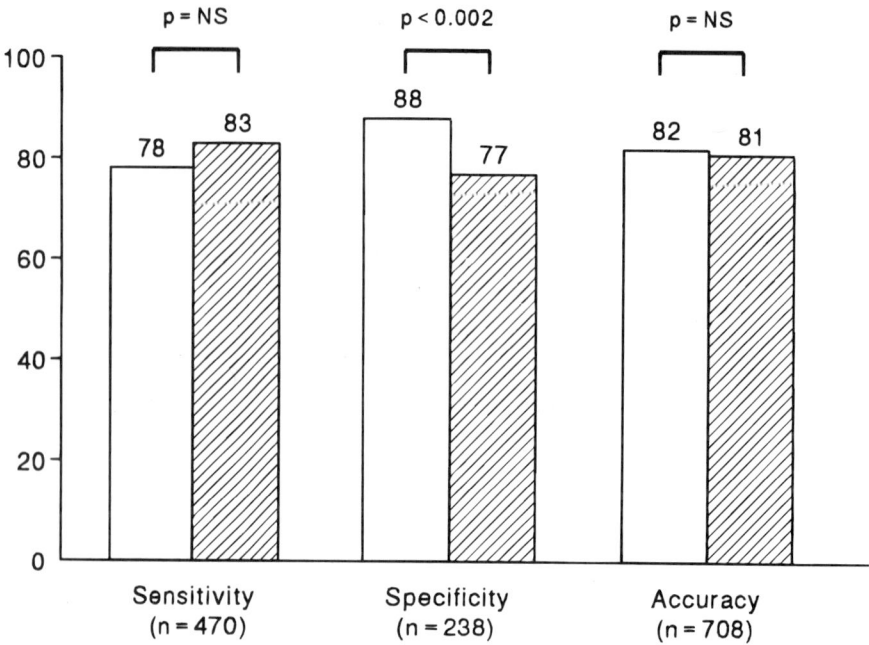

Fig. 4-1. Sensitivity, specificity, and accuracy of exercise or exercise-simulating (dobutamine) stress echocardiography and perfusion imaging for the detection of coronary artery disease. White bars, function; striped bar, perfusion.

(90% vs. 66%, $p < 0.0001$). Only Marwick et al.[25] reported sensitivities according to the extent of disease. In this study, the sensitivity of vasodilator perfusion scintigraphy was superior to echocardiography, both for single (81% vs. 52%, $p < 0.02$) and multivessel disease (93% vs. 64%, $p < 0.01$). These results are not surprising, since vasodilators create primarily blood flow heterogeneity (detected by perfusion scintigraphy and not echocardiography) and "true" ischemia in only in a limited number of patients.

Dobutamine Stress Echocardiography versus Vasodilator Perfusion Imaging

In the many patients who are unable to exercise, the optimal pharmacologic techniques for echocardiography and scintigraphy are fundamentally different. On the basis of the underlying principles of the tests, the necessity of ischemia for the development of abnormal wall motion would suggest that dobutamine would be more effective than a vasodilator for stress echocardiography. Indeed, a comparison performed in an animal model[7] suggested that dobutamine was the most appropriate stress to demonstrate abnormal wall motion due to ischemia. Pooled data from seven published studies[30] directly comparing dobutamine versus vasodilator for stress echocardiography in the same 517 patients showed that dobutamine was more sensitive, compared to both dipyridamole (78% vs. 67%, $p < 0.002$) and adenosine (82% vs. 52%, $p < 0.001$) and equally specific. Of note, up to this moment there are no direct comparisons available using the new promising dipyridamole–atropine stress echocardiography protocol.[31]

In the same animal model,[7] dipyridamole caused the greatest flow heterogeneity, making it particularly suited for myocardial perfusion studies. Published clinical data, however, are conflicting about the superiority of vasodilators to dobutamine for perfusion scintigraphy. Kumar et al.[32] found that dipyridamole thallium scintigraphy correlated better with coronary score. However, these results were based on a very small group of patients; the authors did not report test accuracy, used an insufficient dobutamine dose (20 µg/kg/min) and included patients with previous myocardial infarction. Marwick et al.[25] found in a larger series of 97 patients—without previous myocardial infarction and using high-dose dobutamine—that the accuracy of dobutamine MIBI SPECT was comparable with adenosine MIBI SPECT (accuracies of 77% and 80%, respectively).

The most appropriate means of comparing pharmacologic stress echocardiography and scintigraphy seems, therefore, to use dobutamine with the former and a vasodilator stress with the latter. Unfortunately, reports directly comparing dobutamine stress echocardiography with vasodilator perfusion scintigraphy are scarce. The only two published reports with available angiographic data in 97 and 120 patients[25,33] showed that the tests were equally sensitive (85% vs. 86% and 85% vs. 89%, respectively). However, there was a trend toward a higher specificity of dobutamine stress echocardiography (82% vs. 71% and 93% vs. 85%, respectively). Based on these results, and considering the advantages of echocardiography over perfusion scintigraphy (Table 4-1) it can be anticipated that the use of dobutamine stress echocardiography in patients who are unable to exercise will grow further in the future.

Assessment of Disease Localization

The detection of disease in the circumflex coronary artery is a major problem for both perfusion scintigraphy and echocardiography. In addition to the variation in coronary anatomy (with a small circumflex territory in some patients), perfusion scintigraphy suffers from a less reliable assessment of the posterior regions of the heart, due to problems of photon attenuation. Echocardiography suffers from problems with resolution of the lateral wall endocardium because of the parallel orientation of the wall and the ultrasound beam, and problems of lateral resolution. These circumflex disease detection problems are reflected in Figure 4-2, showing the sensitivities (Fig. 2A) and specificities (Fig. 2B) of exercise or exercise-simulating (dobutamine) stress echocardiography and perfusion scintigraphy for the individual vessels as reported in three studies.[11,12,18] Comparison of regional function versus perfusion studies showed the respective sensitivities to be 83% vs. 73% (p = NS) for the left anterior descending artery, 60% vs. 60% (p = NS) for the left circumflex artery, and 80% vs. 84% (p = NS) for right coronary disease. Specificities were 90% vs. 89% (p = NS), 94% vs. 95% (p = NS), and 89% vs. 80% ($p < 0.05$), respectively. The sensitivity for the detection of left circumflex coronary artery (LCx) versus left anterior descending/right coronary artery (LAD/RCA) disease was lower for both imaging techniques (60% vs. 82% for function, $p < 0.002$ and 60% vs. 78% for perfusion, $p < 0.01$, respectively). To compensate for the variation in blood supply of the posterior wall (by either the right or circumflex artery, depending on their relative size) Marwick et al.[16] divided the blood supply of the heart into two systems: an anterior (LAD) system and a posterior (RCA or LCx) system. Neither imaging modality was found to be superior on a regional basis; in 34 patients with only LAD territory disease, the sensitivity of echocardiography was 62%, compared with 76% by scintigraphy (p = NS) and in 34 with only LCx or RCA disease both modalities had a sensitivity of 71%.

Assessment of Disease Extent

The relative ability of echocardiography and perfusion scintigraphy to predict coronary disease extent has been investigated at two centers. In a study by Senior et al.[18] dobutamine stress echocardiography identified 70% of the 30 patients with multivessel coronary disease as having functional abnormalities in more than 1 coronary territory, compared with scintigrams showing a multivessel pattern in 77% (p = NS). Specificities were 90% and 94%, respectively. In 74 patients with multivessel coronary disease *but without prior infarction*, Marwick et al.[16] reported the recognition of multivessel disease by echocardiography to be only 18%, compared with scintigrams showing a multivessel pattern in 34% (p = NS). On the other hand, echocardiography was more specific for multivessel disease, which it predicted incorrectly in 9% of patients having single vessel disease, compared with 19% falsely predicted as being multivessel by perfusion imaging. The ability of each test to recognize multivessel disease was also analyzed by correlating the echocardiographic or perfusion extent score (calculated from the number of segments demonstrating abnormal regional function or perfusion, expressed as a percentage of the visible segments), with an angiographic score of disease extent (modified from the Gensini score). The echocardiographic and scintigraphic correlation with the angiographic score corresponded to a similar degree, with respective R values of 0.45 and 0.35. These data indicate that functional and perfusion indices of coronary

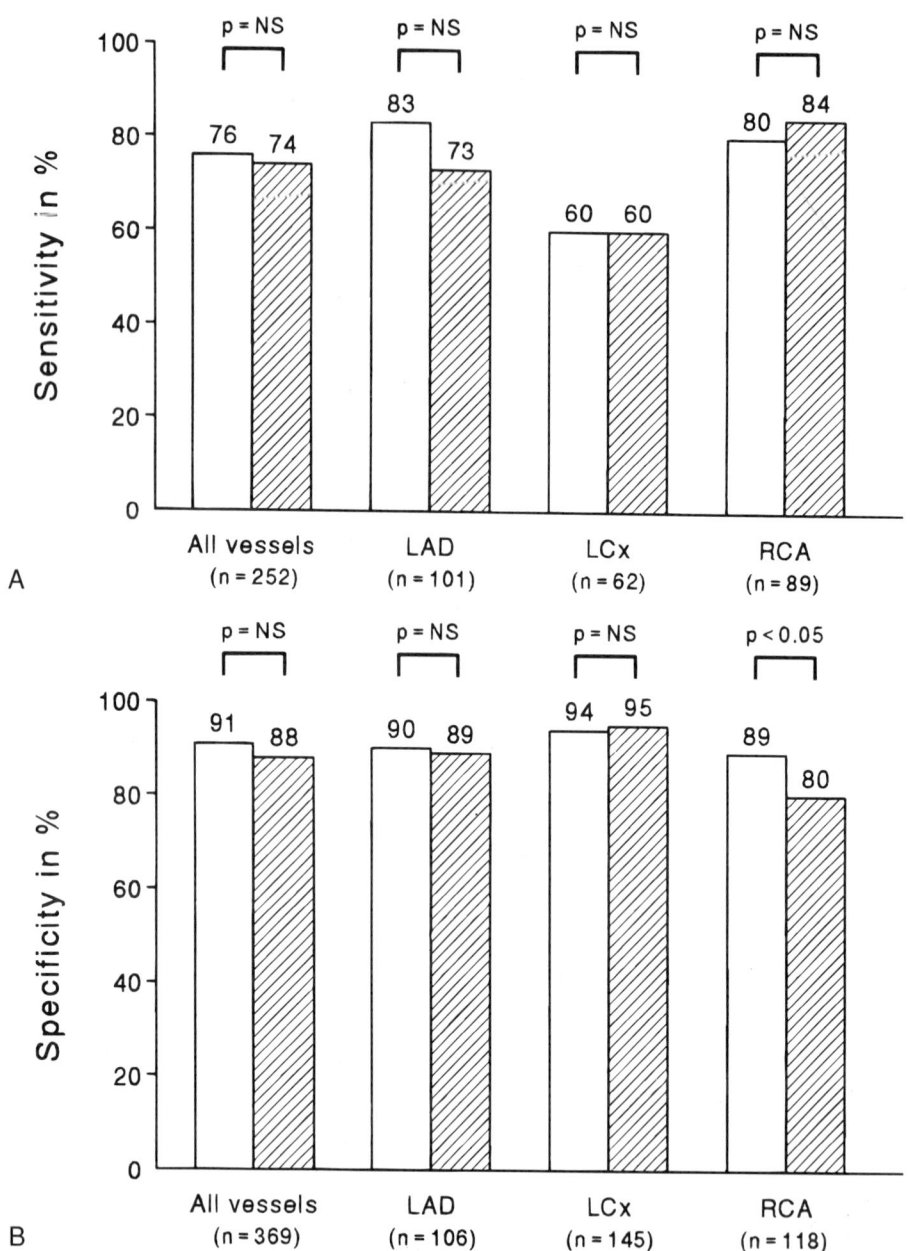

Fig. 4-2. **(A)** Sensitivity and **(B)** specificity of exercise or exercise-simulating (dobutamine) stress echocardiography and perfusion imaging for identification of disease in individual coronary arteries. LAD, left anterior descending coronary artery; LCx, left circumflex coronary artery; RCA, right coronary artery; white bars, function; striped bars, perfusion.

disease extent are comparable, and have similar overall accuracy for the detection of multivessel disease, although both probably underestimate this problem.

The recognition of multivessel disease is more difficult in patients with normal resting function than those with prior myocardial infarction. The underestimation of multivessel disease can be explained by the premature cessation of stress because of the development of limiting ischemia in one region, imperfect assignment of myocardial regions to coronary arteries, collateral circulation, anatomically significant but functionally nonsignificant lesions, and (for perfusion imaging) diffuse hypoperfusion.

COMBINATION OF STRESS ECHOCARDIOGRAPHY AND PERFUSION SCINTIGRAPHY

The roles of functional and perfusion imaging might potentially be complementary in the diagnosis of CAD. In particular, a strategy starting with echocardiography (because of the lower cost) and addition of perfusion in subgroups of patients seems attractive. Two studies have analyzed the usefulness of the addition of perfusion to echocardiography. Both Marwick et al.[16] and Senior et al.[18] found that addition of perfusion to all echocardiography studies negative for ischemia maximized sensitivity (from 72% to 89% and from 93% to 98%, respectively), but compromised the specificity markedly (from 83% to 52% and from 94% to 71%) by combining the false positives of each methodology. In these two studies, additional perfusion studies were required in 47% and 31% of the patients, respectively. Clearly, this option is, therefore, not feasible on grounds of cost or results.

A more attractive alternative is to add perfusion to those echocardiographic tests in which the yield is most likely to be the highest, for example, in patients with submaximal dobutamine stress, since perfusion scintigraphy is known to be less compromised by submaximal stress.[34,35] Only Marwick et al.[16] looked to this option and found that with the addition of perfusion only to negative, submaximal echocardiography studies (14% of the patients) sensitivity increased from 72% to 80% and specificity decreased from 83% to 77%. Their definition of submaximal stress was the presence of β-blocking drugs or failure to attain the maximal dobutamine dose. The option of addition of perfusion to function in studies simply not reaching target heart rate or a target rate-pressure product was not examined. Such a strategy may, perhaps, improve the results of combining the two techniques.

STRESS ECHOCARDIOGRAPHY VERSUS PERFUSION SCINTIGRAPHY: A PROBABILISTIC APPROACH

While values for sensitivity and specificity have a useful role in comparing tests, the use of these investigations in diagnostic practice is to assist in the clinical recognition of coronary disease. In this sense, tests are used to reclassify the initial clinical impression of the probability of coronary disease into high-, low-, and intermediate-risk subgroups. According to Bayes' theorem, the likelihood of a positive test result is determined by the probability of disease in the patient studied, as well as the accuracy of the test. A comparison of tests using probability analysis permits examination of their performance in groups with various pretest likelihoods of disease.

We performed this analysis in 223 patients (without a previous myocardial infarction, bundle branch block, or ventricular hypertrophy), studied with dobutamine echocardiography and ^{99m}Tc sestamibi perfusion imaging.[30] The pretest disease probability, and the posttest probability (derived from the pretest probability and the likelihood ratios calculated from values for sensitivity and specificity) were estimated in all patients. The population was grouped into those at high- (> 80%), intermediate- (10% to 80%), and low-probability (< 10%) of disease, before and after the performance of each test, and the ability of each test to restratify patients was analyzed (Fig. 4-3A & B). According to the pretest likelihood of disease, 68 patients (30%) were regarded as having a low- or high-probability of disease. By application of Bayes' theorem, echocardiography defined 121 patients (54%) as being in the high or low posttest probability groups, compared with 97 (43%) using scintigraphy ($p < 0.05$), thus leaving more patients in the intermediate-probability group after scintigraphy. Importantly, the accuracy of predicting coronary disease in the high-probability group and the absence of disease in the low-

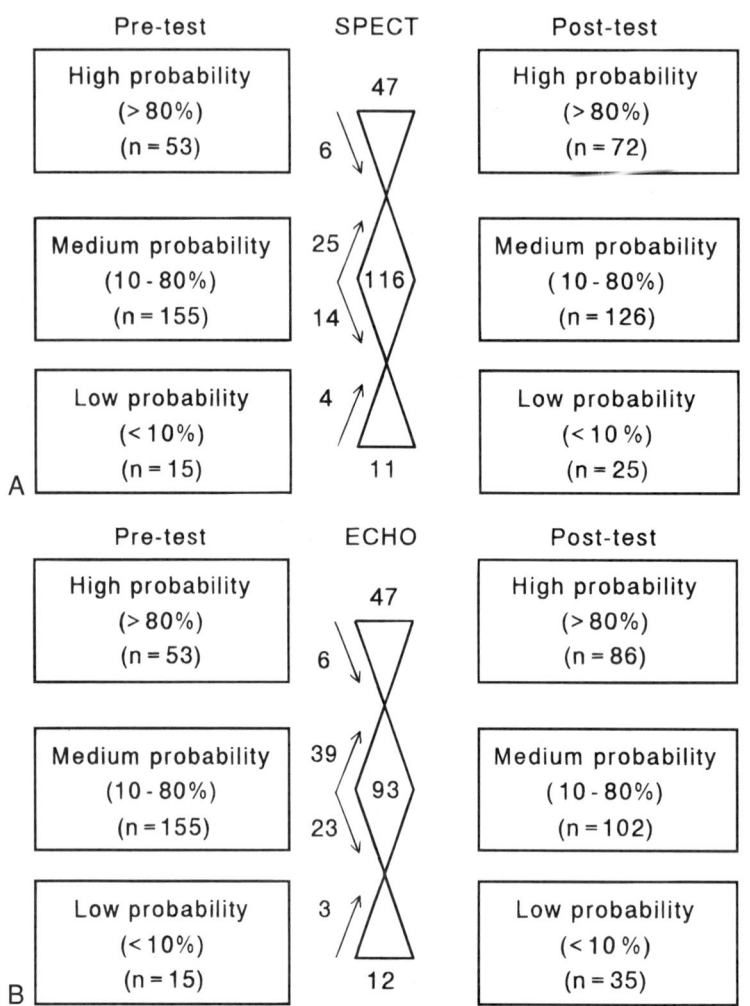

Fig. 4-3. Bayesian approach to the comparison of dobutamine perfusion scintigraphy (SPECT, **A**) and echocardiography (ECHO, **B**). Patients are classified before and after the test into low-, intermediate-, and high-probability of coronary artery disease, and the ability of each test to accurately reclassify them is compared. (From Geleijnse et al.,[30] with permission.)

probability group were similar for echocardiography (105/121, 87%) and scintigraphy (88/97, 91%).

CONCLUSIONS

This chapter has concentrated on the direct comparisons of stress myocardial perfusion imaging and echocardiography for diagnostic purposes; comparisons related to other aspects will be discussed in other chapters.

Some features of stress testing with echocardiography and perfusion scintigraphy are comparable, for example, their accuracy for the diagnosis of coronary disease and their ability to identify the site (and to a lesser degree, the extent) of disease. Both techniques also have their strong and weak points. Echocardiography requires less equipment (and costs less) than scintigraphy. However, at the present state of development, stress echocardiography is highly operator dependent. Irrespective of other considerations, if there is limited local expertise in stress echocardiography, its use in preference to the nuclear techniques is highly inappropriate. However, once the condition of adequate training is fulfilled, we believe that the selection of one or the other test should be tailored to clinical circumstances rather than as a uniform decision. To this end, we propose the following guidelines.

Perfusion imaging is more useful in
1. Patients with poor echocardiographic windows.
2. Patients requiring vasodilator stress (those unable to exercise and also unable to undergo dobutamine testing, e.g., because of history of arrhythmias). Only perfusion imaging is recommended for diagnostic purposes, as vasodilator echocardiography is insensitive, particularly for single vessel disease.

Echocardiography is more useful in
1. Patients requiring dobutamine stress (those unable to exercise and also unable to undergo vasodilator testing, because of obstructive pulmonary disease).
2. Patients in whom safety is a major concern (potentially unstable or severely ischemic). Using echocardiography, ischemia may be observed "on-line" and the appropriate action taken.
3. Studies being performed to assess the adequacy of therapy—as echocardiography visualizes ischemia rather than perfusion heterogeneity, and provides an additional index of disease severity by measuring the ischemia-free stress time.
4. Patients with a suspicion of significant valvular, myocardial, or pericardial components to their presentation.
5. Patients with left ventricular hypertrophy and left bundle branch block. Stress echocardiography seems to be more specific than perfusion scintigraphy in these situations (although these data await confirmation).

The combination of echocardiography and perfusion scintigraphy cannot be recommended because of cost constraints. However, as particular features of stress testing have been identified in which echocardiography is inaccurate (submaximal stress), it may be useful to perform stress echocardiography as the procedure of choice, with the ability to inject MIBI in such circumstances. This option has become feasible only with the availability of MIBI, which does not undergo redistribution, and is a potentially cost-efficient strategy.

FUTURE DEVELOPMENTS

Important technical improvements are expected in the near future (some of which are already available) in both echocardiography and perfusion imaging that will probably require the reassessment of the relative role of the two modalities.

The assessment of stress echocardiography has been mainly visual (semiquantitative), leading to the potential of a low reproducibility, especially if the studies are read by investigators of different institutions.[36] Edge detection based on backscatter analysis and acoustic quantification[37] with color coding for the assessment of the time course of endocardial motion, tissue Doppler imaging,[38,39] and the use of contrast agents will hopefully enhance the ability to characterize and quantify wall motion in the near future, and may provide a new and more reproducible approach to stress echocardiography. Contrast echocardiography may eventually offer a means of evaluating both myocardial perfusion and function using the same technique, at both rest and stress. Finally, the role of three-dimensional echocardiography has to be explored.

Perfusion scintigraphy also has great potential for improvement due to some new technical developments. The use of multiple headed gamma cameras will reduce the acquisition time and improve spatial resolution. Likewise, the examination of left ventricular function (with first-pass studies) and perfusion after the same injection of technetium-labeled radiotracers, and the use of new algorithms for the attenuation correction using transmission scans[40] are factors that will strengthen the information obtainable from scintigraphic studies.

It is very difficult to forsee the "winner" among the different available methods, in this era of very rapid developments. New techniques (e.g., coronary magnetic resonance angiography[41] and electron beam tomography[42]) that are not yet in routine practice (and hence are not discussed in this book) permit noninvasive imaging of the coronary artery. It is unlikely that these new methods will replace stress imaging, but they will hopefully assist the evaluation of patients among whom the interpretation of stress imaging is more problematic.

REFERENCES

1. Nesto RW, Kowalchuck GJ. The ischemic cascade: temporal sequence of hemodynamic, electrocardiographic and symptomatic expressions of ischemia. Am J Cardiol 57:23C, 1987
2. Leppo JA, Meerdink DA: Comparison of the myocardial uptake of a technetium-labeled isonitrile analogue and thallium. Circ Res 64:632, 1989
3. Gould KL: Noninvasive assessment of coronary stenoses by myocardial perfusion imaging during pharmacologic coronary vasodilation. I. Physiologic basis and experimental validation. Am J Cardiol 41:267, 1978
4. Armstrong WF: Echocardiography in coronary artery disease. Progr Cardiovasc Dis 30:267, 1988
5. Poldermans D, Fioretti PM, Forster T et al.: Dobutamine stress echocardiography for assessment of perioperative cardiac risk in patients undergoing major vascular surgery. Circulation 87:1506, 1993
6. Ruffolo RR Jr: The pharmacology of dobutamine. Am J Med Sci. 294:244, 1987
7. Fung AY, Gallagher KP, Buda AJ: The physiologic basis of dobutamine as compared with dipyridamole stress interventions in the assessment of critical coronary stenosis. Circulation 76:943, 1987
8. Maurer G, Nanda NC: Two dimensional echocardiographic evaluation of exercise-induced left and right ventricular asynergy: correlation with thallium scanning. Am J Cardiol 48:720, 1981
9. Quiñones MA, Verani MS, Haichin RM et al.: Exercise echocardiography versus thallium-201 single-photon emission computed tomography in evaluation of coronary artery disease. Analysis of 292 patients. Circulation 85:1026, 1992
10. Wann LS, Faris JV, Childress RH et al.: Exercise cross-sectional echocardiography in ischemic heart disease. Circulation 60:1300, 1979
11. Hecht HS, Debord L, Shaw R et al.: Supine bicycle stress echocardiography versus tomographic thallium-201 exercise imaging for the detection of coronary artery disease. J Am Soc Echocardiogr 6:177, 1993
12. Pozzoli MMA, Fioretti PM, Salustri A et al.: Exercise echocardiography and technetium-99m MIBI single-photon emission computed tomography in the detection of coronary artery disease. Am J Cardiol 67:350, 1991
13. Galanti G, Sciagrà R, Comeglio M et al.: Diagnostic accuracy of peak exercise echocardiography in coronary artery disease: comparison with thallium-201 myocardial scintigraphy. Am Heart J 122:1609, 1991
14. Salustri A, Pozzoli MMA, Hermans W et al.: Relation between exercise echocardiography and perfusion single-photon emission computed tomography in patients with single-vessel coronary artery disease. Am Heart J 124:75, 1992
15. Günalp B, Dokumaci B, Uyan C et al.: Value of dobutamine technetium-99m-sestamibi SPECT and echocardiography in the detection of coronary artery disease compared with coronary angiography. J Nucl Med 34:889, 1993
16. Marwick T, D'Hondt A, Baudhuin T et al.: Optimal use of dobutamine stress for the detection and evaluation of coronary artery disease: combination with echocardiography or scintigraphy, or both? J Am Coll Cardiol 22:159, 1993
17. Forster T, McNeill AJ, Salustri A et al.: Simultaneous dobutamine stress echocardiography and 99m-technetium isonitrile single photon emission computed tomography in patients with suspected coronary artery disease. J Am Coll Cardiol 21:1591, 1993
18. Senior R, Sridhara BS, Anagnostou E et al.: Synergistic value of simultaneous stress dobutamine sestamibi single-photon emission computerized tomography and echocardiography in the detection of coronary artery disease. Am Heart J 128:713, 1994
19. Van Train KF, Maddahi J, Berman DS et al.: Quantitative analysis of tomographic stress thallium-201 myocardial scintigrams: A multicenter trial. J Nucl Med 31:1168, 1990
20. Berne RM: The role of adenosine in the regulation of coronary blood flow. Circ Res 47:807, 1980
21. Fitzgerald GA: Dipyridamole. N Engl J Med 316:1247, 1987
22. Wilson RF, Wyche K, Christensen BV et al.: Effects of adenosine on human coronary arterial circulation. Circulation 82:1595, 1990
23. Flameng W, Wunsten B, Schaper W: On the distribution of myocardial blood flow: II. Effects of arterial stenosis and vasodilation. Basic Res Cardiol 69:435, 1974
24. Demer L, Gould KL, Kirkeeide R: Assessing stenosis severity: coronary flow reserve, collateral function, quantitative coronary arteriography, positron imaging, and digital subtraction angiography: a review and analysis. Prog Cardiovasc Dis 30: 307, 1988
25. Marwick T, Willemart B, D'Hondt AM et al: Seletion of the optimal nonexercise stress for the evaluation of ischemic regional myocardial dysfunction and malperfusion. Comparison of dobutamine and adenosine using echocardiography and 99m Tc-MIBI single pro-

ton emission computed tomograpy. Circulation 87: 345, 1993
26. Nguyen T, Heo J, Ogilby JD et al: Single photon emission computed tomography with thallium-201 during adenosine-induced coronary hypermie: correlation with coronary arteriography, exercise thallium imaging and two-dimensional echocardiography. J Am Coll Cardiol 16:1375, 1990
27. Amanullah AM, Bevegard S, Lindvall K et al: Assessment of left ventricular wall motion in angina pectoris by two-dimensional echocardiography and myocardial perfusion by technetium-99m sestamibi tomography during adenosine-induced coronary vasodilation and comparison with coronary angiography. Am J Cardiol 72:983, 1993
28. Perin EC, Moore W, Blume et al: Comparison of dipyridamole echocardiography with dipyridamole thallium scintigraphy for the diagnosis of myocardial ischemia. Clin Nucl Med 16:417, 1991
29. Simonetti I, Rezai K, Rossen JD et al: Physiological assessment of sensitivity of noninvasive testing for coronary artery disease. Circulation, suppl III, 83:III-43, 1991
30. Geleijnse ML, Marwick TH, Boersma E et al.: Optimal pharmacological stress testing for the diagnosis of coronary artery disease: a probabilistic approach. Eur Heart J, suppl. M:3, 1995
31. Picano E, Pingitore A, Conti U et al.: Enhanced sensitivity for detection of coronary artery disease by addition of atropine to dipyridamole echocardiography. Eur Heart J 14:1216, 1993
32. Kumar EB, Steel SA, Howey S et al. Dipyridamole is superior to dobutamine for thallium stress imaging: a randomised crossover study. Br Heart J 71:129, 1994
33. Takeuchi M, Araki M, Nakashima Y et al.: Comparison of dobutamine stress echocardiography and stress thallium-201 single-photon emission computed tomography for detecting coronary artery disease. J Am Soc Echocardiogr 6:593, 1993
34. Marwick TH, D'Hondt AM, Mairesse GH et al.: Comparative ability of dobutamine and exercise stress in inducing myocardial ischemia in active patients. Br Heart J 72:31, 1994
35. Elhendy A, Geleijnse ML, Roelandt JRTC et al.: Dobutamine-induced hypoperfusion without transient wall motion abnormalities: Less severe ischemia or less severe stress? J Am Coll Cardiol 27:323, 1996
36. Hoffmann R, Lethen H, Marwick T et al.: Analysis of interinstitutional observer agreement in the interpretation of dobutamine stress echocardiogram. J Am Coll Cardiol 27:330, 1996
37. Yvorchuk KJ, Davies RA, Chang KL: Measurement of left ventricular ejection fraction by acoustic quantification and comparison with radionuclide angiography. Am J Cardiol 74:1052, 1994
38. Sutherland GR, Stewart MJ, Groundstroem KWE et al.: Color Doppler myocardial imaging: a new technique for the assessment of myocardial function. J Am Soc Echocardiogr 7:441, 1994
39. Uematsu M, Miyatake K, Tanake N et al.: Myocardial velocity gradient as a new indicator of regional left ventricular contraction: detection by a two-dimensional tissue Doppler imaging technique. J Am Coll Cardiol 26:217, 1995
40. Jaszczak RJ, Gilland DR, Hanson MW, et al.: Fast transmission CT for determining attenuation maps using a collimated line source, rotable air-copper-lead attenuators and fan-beam collimation. J Nucl Med 34:1577, 1993
41. Manning WJ, Li W, Edelman RR: A preliminary report comparing magnetic resonance coronary angiography with conventional angiography. N Engl J Med 328: 828, 1993
42. Simons BD, Schwartz RS, Edwards WD et al.: Noninvasive definition of anatomic coronary artery disease by ultrafast computed tomographic scanning: A quantitative pathologic comparison study. J Am Coll Cardiol 20:1118, 1992

Chapter 5

Cost Analysis of Noninvasive Testing

Randolph E. Patterson and Robert L. Eisner

THE BALANCE OF ACCURACY AND COST

Technology has improved the quality of cardiovascular diagnostic procedures dramatically in recent years, but these technologic improvements are costly.[1] Primarily because of economic concerns, many have questioned whether or not these technological improvements are worth their cost.[1-3] To some, technology has come to be considered the chief villain in the rising cost of health care. The purpose of this chapter is to focus on a narrow topic that is of direct concern to physicians who perform or order diagnostic tests for coronary artery disease (CAD). Specifically, we will compare the cost-effectiveness of different diagnostic tests for CAD. Since CAD is the leading cause of death and heart failure in the Western world,[3] it is especially important to optimize its diagnostic assessment.

In 1996 several modalities are being used to diagnose CAD,[4] and many criteria can be used to compare their cost-effectiveness: risk of complications, sensitivity, specificity, rate of nondiagnostic tests, and costs.[5,6] The best criteria would consider quality of care or patient outcomes (which depend importantly on complications and accuracy of the test) as well as total costs. Total costs start with the initial cost of the test but also depend on the cost of subsequent medical care related to the patient's outcome.[7-9] Unfortunately, it is very difficult to obtain accurate data for patient costs and outcomes in enough patients to draw reliable conclusions.

This chapter reviews a model that uses literature data to estimate patient outcomes and costs.[5,6] Specifically, we tried to estimate the differential costs of diagnosis of CAD using different modalities.[5,6] We compared five modalities for diagnosis of CAD: exercise electrocardiography (ECG), stress echocardiography, stress single photon emission computed tomography (SPECT) myocardial perfusion imaging (MPI), stress positron emission tomographic (PET) MPI, and cardiac catheterization with coronary arteriography.[4,5] We focus on how the different costs and accuracies of various tests affect total costs, patient outcomes, and cost effectiveness.

METHODOLOGY FOR EVALUATION OF COST-EFFECTIVENESS

Effectiveness of Cardiac Care

As discussed above, to compare the relative value of these procedures, one must consider effectiveness as well as cost of each procedure.[4,5] Effectiveness of health care is more difficult to calculate than cost because one must consider not only the accuracy of a diagnostic test but also the quality of the patient's outcome with or without an accurate initial diagnosis.[7-11] For instance, some patients will suffer complications such as acute myocardial infarction because CAD was missed by a false negative test result. Calculating the effectiveness or quality of medical care is difficult[8,11-13] but has become more important than ever in medicine. Not only health care providers but also health care payers and consumers are very interested in this question. Factors that must be considered in calculating effectiveness include (1) whether the patient lives or dies (mortality rate); (2) the presence and severity of the patient's symptoms (morbidity rate); (3) whether the patient can carry on his or her usual life-style (e.g., activities of daily living, social interactions, and employment), and (4) how much time and effort the patient must devote to health maintenance.[5,11] These factors are often combined in the expression of a patient's own perception of his or her quality of life. One can then combine quantity of life (survival), with the other factors (quality) as quality-adjusted life-years (QALY). Calculation of QALY allows one to express the patient's outcome[11] in quantitative terms but does not require placing a dollar value on human life. Such estimates involve the patient's subjective response to his or her situation, and these responses are very important to understanding the total impact of illness on a person. Some distinction has been made between an objective measurement of illness such as mortality rate (effectiveness) and the other four factors that relate to quality of life. Utility includes both survival and quality of life. Thus, in the present analysis, we selected variables for effectiveness (or utility) that include quantity and quality of life (QALY), estimated from data available for the accuracy and complication rates of tests, the mortality and morbidity rates of CAD with different treatment approaches, and estimates of quality of life based on the above. Most values of variables were from published empirical studies.[5,6,14-46] Specifically, we compared the improvement (Δ) in QALY resulting from accurate initial diagnosis of CAD and institution of treatment with initially missing the diagnosis of CAD.

Cost of Cardiac Care

The difficult task of calculating costs deserves further consideration. Costs are very difficult to calculate accurately because they must include not only the initial or direct cost of each test but also the costs of subsequent procedures induced by the results of the first test (e.g., coronary arteriography[4,5] to determine whether a positive exercise ECG is true or false as an indicator that a patient has CAD). Costs must also consider complications (e.g., the cost of an occasional surgical repair of a femoral artery after angiography).[4-8]

A central issue is to decide whether to use charges (fees) or reimbursement rates for medical care or the true cost required to provide the care. It is much easier to obtain a list of charges or reimbursements for health care procedures than it is to determine the true cost of providing the care.

Some of the difficult questions involved in determining actual costs include

What is fair reimbursement for physicians in different specialties, nurses, technologists, administrators, and all the other people necessary to make a health care organization work properly?

What is a fair price for medical equipment and supplies? Vendors of supplies must hire people to design, manufacture, sell, deliver, and service the medical equipment and supplies. How should the vendors' employees and owners be reimbursed?

How should one calculate the cost of the physical space in which health care is provided?

The complexity of these questions is obvious and has led most studies to use other more easily obtained data for cost variables. As capitated health care plans become more prevalent, it will be increasingly important for health care providers to determine their true costs in order to offer coverage at a price that is high enough to maintain quality but is also low enough to compete with other providers.

Cost-Effectiveness Model and Sensitivity Analysis

Having defined cost and effectiveness or utility, the next task is to determine a means of comparing these parameters. One way is to review a large clinical data base that includes all test results, clinical outcomes, and costs. Unfortunately, such data are not currently available in an accurate, complete form, and when

Table 5-1. How Changes in the Rates of False (+),[a] Nondiagnostic, and False (−)[b] Results Influence Overall Costs of Health Care

Diagnostic Test Has	Outcomes that Decrease Costs	Outcomes that Increase Costs	Net Effect On Costs
Fewer false (+) results	Fewer arteriographies Fewer complications of arteriographies Fewer PTCA or CABG after test for physiologic significance of anatomic lesions	Physicians more likely to refer patients for arteriography for (+) test, thus more arteriographies and complications (small effect)	Decrease
Fewer nondiagnostic results	Fewer arteriographies Fewer complications of arteriographies	None	Decrease
Fewer false (−) results	Fewer complications of CAD in patients with missed diagnosis Fewer malpractice cases for CAD missed Fewer arteriographies for patients with (−) tests when physician was not confident that result was correct Fewer arteriography complications, because fewer arteriographies performed	More arteriographies for patients with (+) tests and CAD More arteriography complications More PTCA or CABG after (+) test for physiologic significance of anatomic lesions (small effect)	Decrease

Abbreviations: CABG, coronary artery bypass graft; CAD, coronary artery disease; PTCA, percutaneous transluminal coronary angioplasty.
[a] Positive
[b] Negative

such data become available, they will likely be proprietary because of their value in the current health care market. An alternative approach is to calculate effectiveness and costs based on available data. Such calculations require use of an approach or model[5,6,47] to organize the data, and they require some assumptions. Computing cost effectiveness from a model requires consideration of why one possible value of any variable is selected over alternatives. To help validate the model and its assumptions and variables, one can vary systematically the values of one or more variables to test the impact of changes in these variables on cost effectiveness. This procedure is called sensitivity analysis of a model[5,6,48] (i.e., analyzing the sensitivity of the conclusions [output data] to systematic changes in variables or assumptions [input data]) (Table 5-1).

Effects of Pretest Probability of CAD on Cost-Effectiveness

Clearly, the spectrum of patients undergoing noninvasive diagnostic testing must be considered. These heterogeneous groups demonstrate variations in the accuracy of tests, complications, outcomes, and costs.[29,49] It is very difficult to obtain accurate data for any one population and even harder for individual subgroups of that population. One would need to study a very large number of populations or a group just like the one in which one is interested. The use of pooled data inevitably uses results from different populations collected in different ways and may have so many hidden differences that any conclusions from one population cannot be generalized.

While detailed characterization of patient populations is very complex, one of the most important characteristics that can be estimated reliably is the pretest clinical probability of disease in the population being tested.[29,49] Thus an alternate and more feasible approach to determine the impact on cost-effectiveness of different types of patients is to study outcomes and costs in populations with different prevalences of CAD. We used data from published studies with known prevalences of disease, and calculated the effectiveness of changing prevalence of CAD, based on Bayes' theorem.[5,6,50,51]

The focus of our analysis was on differences result-

Table 5-2. Accuracies of Different Diagnostic Approaches for CAD

	ECG	Echo	SPECT	PET	Angio
Sensitivity	0.68	0.75	0.84	0.95	0.99
Specificity	0.77	0.90	0.87	0.95	0.99
Nondiagnostic	0.18	0.10	0.09	0.01	0.01

Abbreviations: Angio, arteriography; CAD, coronary artery disease; Echo, echocardiography; ECG, exercise electrocardiography; PET, positron emission tomography; SPECT, single photon emission computed tomography.

ing from variations in diagnostic testing approaches, related to their variable accuracies, complication rates, and costs. We were less interested in the absolute outcome or cost than in the relative changes in the cost required to achieve a particular outcome. On the basis of these general considerations, we can determine how cost effectiveness (cost per ΔQALY) changes for patients being evaluated for possible CAD, when the diagnostic approach utilizes different diagnostic tests.[5,6]

Assumptions of This Model

We used ΔQALY (improved QALY owing to diagnosis and treatment minus QALY without diagnosis or treatment of CAD) over a 10-year follow-up period to indicate utility of care for CAD.[5,6] We assumed that accurate diagnosis and appropriate treatment of CAD led to an improvement (Δ) of 3.0 years of life at full quality, over a 10-year follow-up period, compared with not making the diagnosis or instituting any specific treatment for CAD. This figure was derived from literature values of mortality and morbidity rates and impact of treatment on quality of life.[14–46]

Our data regarding the assumed accuracy, complications, and the rate of nondiagnostic tests and costs are summarized in Tables 5-2 and 5-3.

In these diagnostic strategies, if the noninvasive test used initially was positive or nondiagnostic, then the patient was referred for angiography (Fig. 5-1B). The detailed methods and assumptions of the above analysis are explained more fully elsewhere.[5,6]

COST-EFFECTIVENESS OF NONINVASIVE TESTING

Patients at Low to Intermediate Probability of CAD

Comparison of different modalities is easiest to understand by comparing each modality to one standard approach, such as the exercise ECG, for one particular type of patient. We will make these comparisons for one patient example, a 50-year-old woman with atypical chest discomfort (0.30 probability of CAD).[50] Figure 5-2 illustrates the total costs per patient tested expressed as a percentage of the cost per patient tested for exercise ECG ($3821). The costs per patient tested were somewhat lower for echocardiography (-4.7%) and PET (-0.6%). The costs per patient tested are slightly higher for SPECT ($+2.3\%$), but much higher for arteriography ($+48.8\%$).

These results suggest that the higher specificity and lower nondiagnostic rate of stress echocardiography (Table 5-2) avoided use of arteriography for false positive tests in enough patients to reduce the total cost of care (by 4.7%) for patients with pCAD $= 0.30$, despite its higher initial cost (Table 5-3 and Fig. 5-2). Stress SPECT generated slightly more (by 2.3%) cost per patient tested because of its greater initial cost (Table 5-3) and its greater sensitivity to detect CAD (Table 5-2 and Fig. 5-2). More true positive tests generated more arteriography than did exercise ECG, despite its greater specificity and lower nondiagnostic rate (Table 5-2). PET showed essen-

Table 5-3. Costs, Complications, and Mortality Rates of Different Approaches for CAD

	ECG	Echo	SPECT	PET	Angio
Cost/test	$330	$900	$1,200	$1,800	$4,800
Complications/test	0.0005	0.0005	0.0005	0.0005	0.02
Mortality/test	0.00005	0.00005	0.00005	0.00005	0.0015
Complications of CAD missed/year	0.025	0.025	0.025	0.025	0.025
Mortality of CAD missed/year	0.02	0.02	0.02	0.02	0.02

Abbreviations: Angio, arteriography; CAD, coronary artery disease; Echo, echocardiography; ECG, exercise electrocardiography; PET, position emission tomography; SPECT, single photon emission computed tomography.

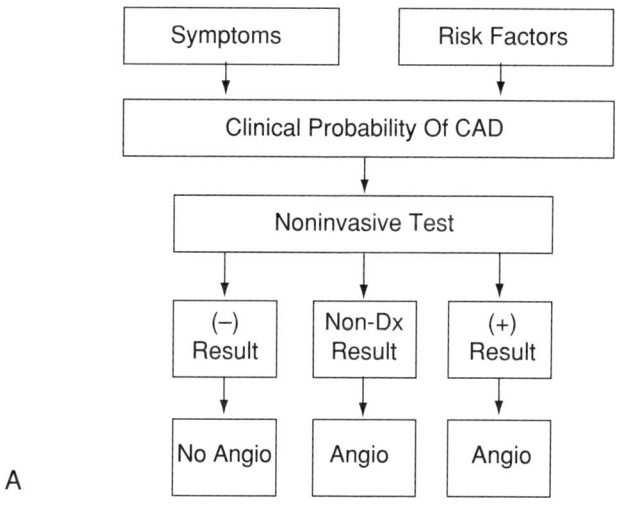

Fig. 5-1. (A) Diagnostic algorithms for coronary artery disease. (B) Results of analysis.

tially no differences in total cost per patient tested (Fig. 5-2), compared with exercise ECG. This is a remarkable result in that the greater accuracy of PET (by 18% to 27%) (Table 5-2) was sufficient to offset its 5.5-fold greater initial cost (Table 5-3 and Fig. 5-2). Arteriography generated a (48.8%) higher total cost because its 14.5-fold higher initial cost offset its almost perfect accuracy (Table 5-2 and Fig. 5-2).

The improvement in QALY over 10 years for patients like this would be 0.548 with ECG, but higher for all other modalities (expressed as % change from exercise ECG), related to sensitivity of the test: Echocardiography (+9.4%) is less than SPECT (+27.7%), which is less than PET (+50.5%), which is less than arteriography (+55.6%); each % figure represents the difference compared with exercise ECG (Fig. 5-1B and Fig. 5-3). Thus, any test that misses more people with CAD allows more deaths

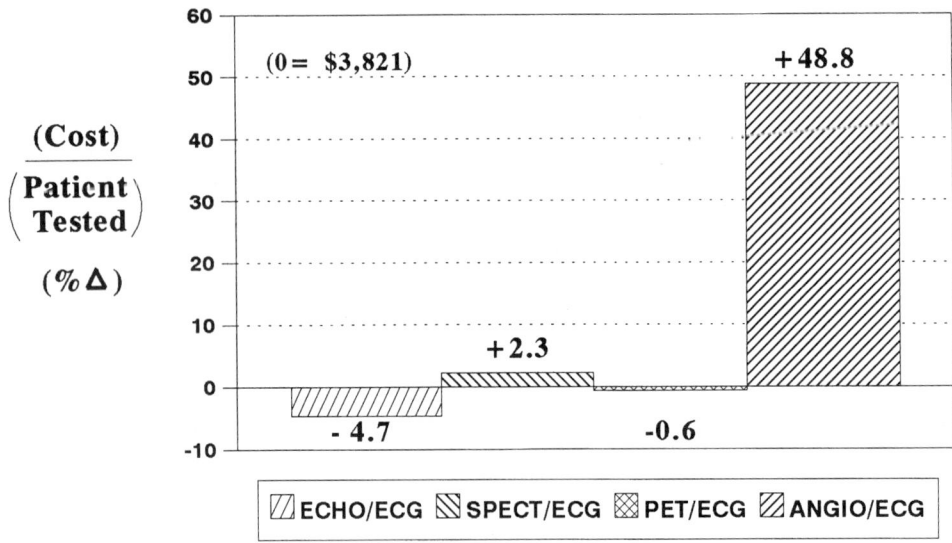

Fig. 5-2. These bar graphs show cost per patient tested. Each result is expressed as the % difference from exercise electrocardiography (ECG), using diagnostic approaches that start with stress echocardiography (ECHO), stress single photon emission computed tomography myocardial perfusion imaging (SPECT) MPI stress positron emission tomography (PET) MPI and arteriography (ANGIO). Data are for a population with a probability of coronary artery disease (CAD) of 0.3 (e.g., 50-year-old women with atypical chest discomfort). Note that cost/patient tested changes little among noninvasive modalities but increases dramatically with ANGIO.

and other complications of the disease. The more sensitive the test, the better the outcomes because of more appropriate treatment of the disease.

Cost-effectiveness is easiest to express as its inverse, cost per change (Δ) in QALY. This value was highest (least favorable) for exercise ECG ($6,977/$\Delta$QALY), compared with the other tests, because of its limited accuracy. Compared with exercise ECG, stress echocardiography was 13% more cost-effective because it was more specific and reduced the number of nondiagnostic results (to avoid unnecessary arteriography), and it was slightly more sensitive than exercise ECG (Table 5-2 and Fig. 5-4). Thus greater accuracy (0.07 to 0.17) offset the 2.7-fold greater initial cost of stress echocardiography compared with exercise ECG (Table 5-3 and Figure 5-4). Stress SPECT MPI was 20% more cost-effective than exercise ECG because its greater sensitivity (by 0.16) and specificity (by 0.10) and lower nondiagnostic rate (by 0.09) (Table 5-2 and Figure 5-4) offset its 3.6-fold higher initial cost (Table 5-3). The results were even more dramatic for PET (34% more cost-effective), for which a much higher sensitivity (by

0.27) and specificity (by 0.18) and lower nondiagnostic rate (by 0.09) (Table 5-2) offset a 5.5-fold higher initial cost (Table 5-3 and Figure 5-4). The almost perfect accuracy of arteriography (Table 5-2) failed to offset its 14.5-fold greater initial cost and higher complication rate (Table 5-3) in this population, so that arteriography was slightly more cost-effective (4.4%) than exercise ECG in patients with a 0.30 clinical probability of CAD (Figure 5-4).

Intermediate Pretest Probability of Disease

When considering populations of patients with different clinical pCAD (e.g., between 0.3 and 0.8) there were major increases in cost per patient tested for exercise ECG (84%), stress echocardiography (76%), SPECT (65%), and PET (72%), but no real change for arteriography (1%) where the % represents the increase in cost for each diagnostic approach in patients with pCAD of 0.8 versus 0.3 (Table 5-4). Costs increase because of the greater need for arteriography in patients whose CAD creates positive test results.[5,6,47]

The improvement (Δ) in QALY over 10 years also

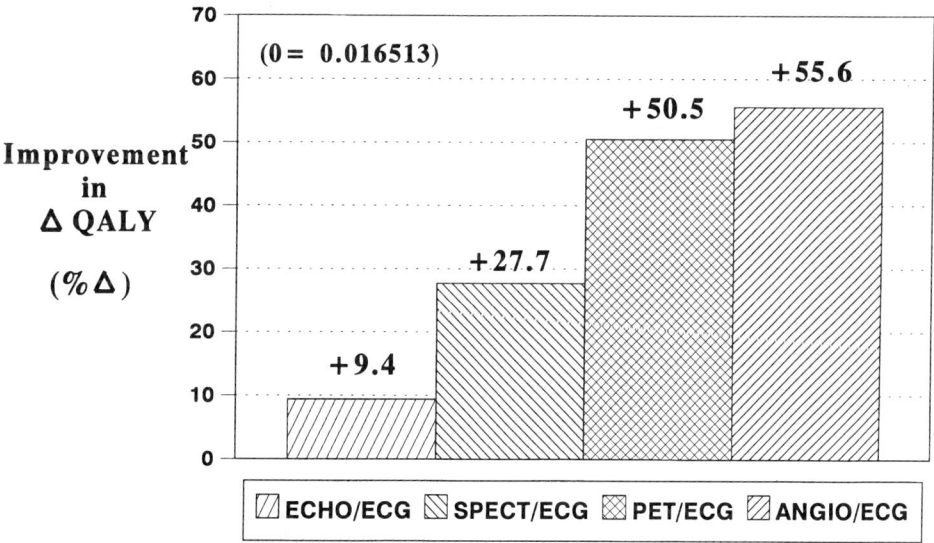

Fig. 5-3. These bar graphs show improvement in the net change in quality-adjusted life years (ΔQALY) over 10 years. Each result is expressed as the % difference from exercise electrocardiography (ECG), using diagnostic approaches that start with stress echocardiography (ECHO), stress single photon emission computed tomography myocardial perfusion imaging (SPECT) MPI, stress positron emission tomography (PET) MPI, and arteriography (ANGIO). Data are for a population with a probability of coronary artery disease (CAD) of 0.3 (e.g., 50 year-old women with atypical chest discomfort). Note that ΔQALY increases steadily as sensitivity of the test increases.

increased as expected, as pCAD increased (e.g., between 0.3 and 0.8) for exercise ECG (171%), echocardiography (169%), SPECT (169%), PET (167%), and arteriography (174% increase) (Table 5-5). The 166% greater prevalence of CAD increased ΔQALY comparably for all diagnostic procedures.

In contrast, cost-effectiveness improved as pCAD increased (i.e., cost per effect [ΔQALY] decreased as pCAD increased between 0.3 and 0.8) with exercise ECG (-55%), echocardiography (-34%), SPECT (-39%), PET (-36%), and arteriography (-63% decrease) (Table 5-6). Higher prevalence of CAD in the population tested makes any diagnostic testing more cost-effective because there are more patients to benefit from making the diagnosis and treating CAD.[5,6]

The most remarkable change between pCAD of 0.3 and 0.8 was that arteriography changed from being the second least cost-effective test (to ECG) at the low pCAD (0.3) to being the most cost-effective approach at the high pCAD (0.8) population (e.g., 60-year-old women with typical angina pectoris)

Table 5-4. Cost/Patient Tested

pCAD	ECG	Echo	SPECT	PET	Angio
0.2	3352	3089	3401	3250	5676
0.3	3821	3642	3909	3799	5686
0.4	4290	4194	4416	4347	5696
0.6	5228	5300	5431	5444	5715
0.8	6166	6405	6446	6541	5735

Abbreviations: Angio, arteriography; ECG, electrocardiography; Echo, echocardiography; pCAD, probability of coronary artery disease; PET, positron emission tomography; SPECT, single photon emission computed tomography.

Table 5-5. ΔQALY

pCAD	ECG	Echo	SPECT	PET	Angio
0.2	0.36048	0.39701	0.46343	0.54861	0.55659
0.3	0.54766	0.59933	0.69929	0.82445	0.85238
0.4	0.73485	0.80166	0.93514	1.10029	1.14817
0.6	1.10923	1.20632	1.40686	1.65198	1.73976
0.8	1.48361	1.61097	1.87858	2.20367	2.33134

Abbreviations: Angio, arteriography; ECG, electrocardiography; Echo, echocardiography; pCAD, probability of coronary artery disease; PET, positron emission tomography; SPECT, single photon emission computed tomography.

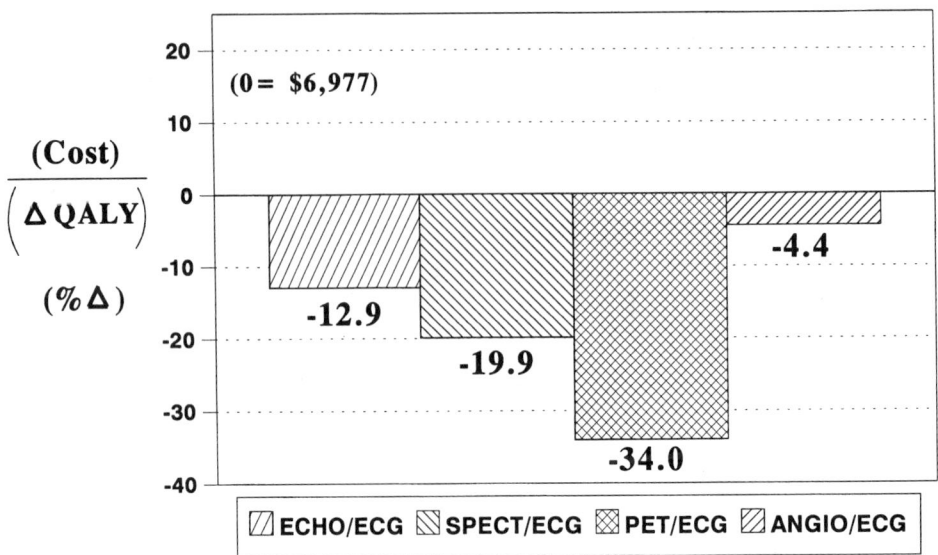

Fig. 5-4. These bar graphs show cost/net change in quality-adjusted life years (ΔQALY). Each result is expressed as the % difference from exercise electrocardiography (ECG), using diagnostic approaches that start with stress echocardiography (ECHO), stress single photon emission computed tomography myocardial perfusion imaging (SPECT) MPI, stress positron emission tomography (PET) MPI, and arteriography (ANGIO). Data are for a population with a probability of coronary artery disease (CAD) of 0.3 (e.g., 50-year-old women with atypical chest discomfort). Decreases in cost/ΔQALY means increased cost-effectiveness, and cost/ΔQALY decreases among noninvasive tests as their accuracy increases, despite the higher initial cost of more accurate tests.

(Table 5-6). Compared with ECG, arteriography was 4.4% more cost-effective at the low pCAD (0.3) but was 40.8% more cost-effective at the high pCAD (0.8) (Table 5-6). This finding of the model is consistent with the clinical practice pattern of most physicians (i.e., arteriography is usually recommended as the first test in a person with a high (0.8) pCAD because of typical angina at an appropriate age). Most noninvasive tests would be positive and lead to arteriography anyway, but only after more delay and expense in patients with high pretest probability of CAD.

Table 5-6. Cost/ΔQALY

pCAD	ECG	Echo	SPECT	PET	Angio
0.2	9299	7781	7339	5924	10198
0.3	6977	6076	5590	4607	6670
0.4	5838	5232	4722	3951	4961
0.6	4714	4393	3860	3295	3285
0.8	4156	3976	3431	2968	2460

Abbreviations: Angio, arteriography; ECG, electrocardiography; Echo, echocardiography; pCAD, probability of coronary artery disease; PET, positron emission tomography; SPECT, single photon emission computed tomography.

As emphasized by McKean,[48] the ratio of cost to effect can sometimes present a different picture of the relationship between cost and effect than is apparent by simply describing the relationship (Figure 5-5). The relatively large differences in QALY and smaller differences in cost are much easier to see for the five different diagnostic approaches in Figure 5-5.

Sensitivity Analysis of Model

Large changes in several variables, individually or in groups, produced some changes in total costs, clinical outcomes, and cost-effectiveness, but there was no real change in the rank order of the different diagnostic testing approaches.[5,6] Thus the conclusions about the value of each diagnostic modality relative to the others were not significantly influenced by moderate changes in initial costs, test accuracies, or clinical outcomes.[5,6] (See Appendix for further analysis.)

CONCLUSION

This chapter has discussed a model to test the relative costs, outcomes, and cost-effectiveness of different clinical approaches to diagnose CAD. The model

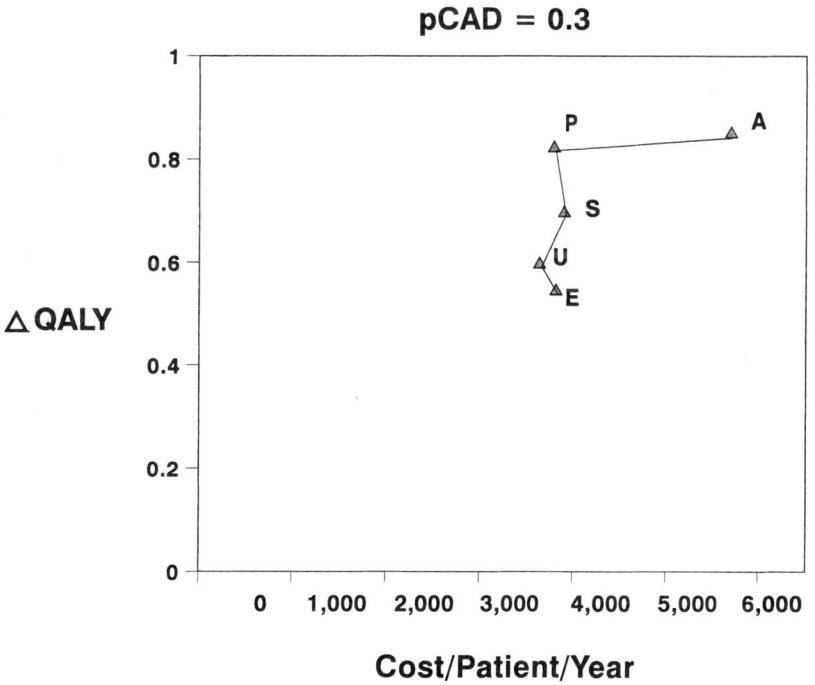

Fig. 5-5. Relationships between cost/patient tested/year in dollars (x-axis) and the net change in quality-adjusted life years (ΔQALY) (y-axis). The data are for a patient with a probability of coronary artery disease (CAD) of 0.3. Arteriography (ANGIO) (A) shows largest increase in ΔQALY, but cost is also much greater. Positron emission tomography (PET) (P) shows the largest increase in ΔQALY of all noninvasive approaches—close to ΔQALY for ANGIO, but at a much reduced cost. Single photon emission computed tomography (S) shows slightly lower ΔQALY than PET at a slightly greater cost than PET. Echocardiography (U) shows a very low cost but a much lower ΔQALY. Exercise electrocardiography (E) shows the lowest cost but also the lowest ΔQALY.

is useful because it allows testing many hypotheses, and real data are almost impossible to obtain. The model indicates that the cost-effectiveness of a noninvasive test is greater when the test is more accurate. More accurate (sensitive) noninvasive tests detect more CAD so that treatment can prevent many complications. More accurate (specific) noninvasive tests create fewer false positive results that lead to arteriography for correct diagnosis. Pretest or clinical probability (p) of CAD exerts a powerful effect on cost-effectiveness, because patients with CAD benefit more from testing than do patients without CAD. For example, arteriography is second to ECG the least cost-effective test at low (0.3) pCAD but becomes the most cost-effective test at high (0.8) pCAD. Among noninvasive tests, the rank order of cost-effectiveness for patients at all pCAD is listed from best to worst as follows: stress PET-MPI, stress SPECT-MPI, stress echocardiography, exercise ECG. The greater accuracy seemed to offset the higher initial cost of the more accurate tests. The key issue seems to be that the initial cost of any test is only a small part of the total cost, which includes the cost of subsequent care and procedures performed because of the initial test result.

SUMMARY

Although accurate accounting of all costs of health care for patients with CAD is difficult, measurement of the effectiveness of health care for CAD is even more difficult. The limited feasibility of collecting these data in patient populations led us to develop a clinical-econometrics model. We used this model to calculate the relative cost-effectiveness (cost per effect) of different diagnostic approaches to diagnose CAD. We compared four noninvasive tests and arteriography, and we assumed that patients with positive or nondiagnostic noninvasive tests would be referred for arteriography. We used literature values for the costs, accuracies, and complication rates of each test: exercise ECG, stress echocardiography, stress SPECT MPI, stress PET MPI, and arteriography. Analysis of the model indicated that total cost per patient tested was higher for arteriography (followed by SPECT, exercise ECG, and PET, respectively) in patients with low clinical probability (p) of CAD (e.g., 0.30) and lowest for echocardiography. In patients with high clinical pCAD e.g., 0.8. arteriography had the lowest cost per patient tested (followed by exercise ECG, ECHO, SPECT, and PET).

Improvement in quality-adjusted life years (ΔQALY) was highest in proportion to sensitivity to detect CAD: arteriography was better than PET, followed by SPECT, echocardiography, and exercise ECG. Cost-effectiveness was greatest (lowest cost/ΔQALY) at low pCAD (e.g., 0.3 for PET) followed by SPECT, echocardiography, arteriography, and exercise ECG. At high pCAD e.g., 0.8 cost-effectiveness was greatest for arteriography (followed by PET, SPECT, echocardiography, and exercise ECG). The critical point that emerges from this analysis is that the cost of a test must account for its outcomes (e.g., arteriography to determine whether a positive test is true or false) and the complications of CAD missed by false negative test results.

ACKNOWLEDGMENTS

The authors are most grateful to Susan L. Schmarkey, B.S., C.N.M.T., for editorial assistance, to T.S. Chu, B.S., M.S.B.M.E., for assistance with computer programming, and to Gail Nechtman for expert preparation of the manuscript.

APPENDIX

Thomas H. Marwick

The unique work of Patterson and Eisner is based upon assumptions that are very clearly defined by the authors. The two that are most subject to variation are test accuracy and cost. In the following tables, Medicare reimbursement (ETT $117, echocardiography $281, SPECT $617, PET $727, arteriography $2510) has been substituted for the cost quoted by the authors, and the sensitivity/specificity data have been adjusted to follow the levels quoted elsewhere in this book (ECG sensitivity 0.7, specificity 0.7; echocardiography 0.8, 0.85; SPECT 0.9, 0.70; PET 0.95, 0.9; arteriography 0.99, 0.99). Echocardiography is the least expensive approach in low probability patients (Table A5-1).

However, as discussed by the authors, analysis of cost alone ignores efficacy, but this is more difficult to measure. The following tables evaluate efficacy according to the assumptions proposed by the authors. The reader needs to remember, however, that the consequence of missing disease at a stress test may be less onerous than the authors assume (and hence the gain in QALY may be less than assumed). This would tend to reduce the effectiveness (and hence cost-effectiveness) of the more accurate tests (Appendix Tables A5-2 & A5-3).

Table A5-1. Cost/Patient Tested

pCAD	ECG	ECHO	SPECT	PET	ANGIO
0.2	2256	1826	2382	1764	3363
0.3	2611	2200	2654	2092	3373
0.4	2965	2573	2925	2420	3383
0.6	3674	3321	3469	3076	3403
0.8	4384	4068	4012	3732	3422

Table A5-2. ΔQALY

pCAD	ECG	ECHO	SPECT	PET	ANGIO
0.2	0.37269	0.43368	0.50512	0.54722	0.55659
0.3	0.56700	0.65513	0.76454	0.82324	0.85238
0.4	0.76130	0.87659	1.02395	1.09925	1.14817
0.6	1.14990	1.31949	1.54278	1.65129	1.73976
0.8	1.53851	1.76240	2.06161	2.20332	2.33134

Table A5-3. Cost/ΔQALY

pCAD	ECG	ECHO	SPECT	PET	ANGIO
0.2	6054	4211	4716	3223	6042
0.3	4605	3358	3471	2541	3957
0.4	3895	2936	2857	2201	2946
0.6	3195	2517	2248	1863	1956
0.8	2849	2308	1946	1694	1468

REFERENCES

1. Eckholm E: The Technology Imperative. Solving America's Health Care Crisis. p. 69. New York Times, New York, 1993
2. D'Agincourt L: Health reform collides with nuclear medicine. Diagn Imag 51, 1994
3. National Heart, Lung, and Blood Institute: Morbidity from Coronary Heart Disease in the United States. National Heart, Lung, and Blood Institute Data Fact Sheet, Bethesda, MD, 1990
4. Patterson RE, Horowitz SF, Eisner RL: Comparison of modalities to diagnose coronary artery diseases. Sem Nucl Med 24:286, 1994
5. Patterson RE, Eng C, Horowitz SF et al: Bayesian comparison of cost-effectiveness of different clinical approaches to diagnose coronary artery disease. J Am Coll Cardiol 4:278, 1984
6. Patterson RE, Eisner RL, Horowitz SF: Comparison of cost-effectiveness and utility of exercise ECG, SPECT, PET and coronary angiography for diagnosis of coronary artery disease. Circulation 91:54, 1995
7. McNeil BJ, Varady PD, Burrows BA, Adelstein SJ: Measures of clinical efficacy: cost-effectiveness calculations in the diagnosis and treatment of hypertensive renovascular disease. N Engl J Med 293:216, 1975
8. Bell RS: Efficacy...what's that? Semin Nucl Med 8:316, 1978
9. Roper WL, Winkenwerder W, Hackbarth GM, Krakauer H: Effectiveness in health care: an initiation to evaluate and improve medical practice. N Engl J Med 319:1197, 1988
10. Enthoven AC: Shattuck lecture: cutting costs without cutting the quality of care. N Engl J Med 298:1229, 1978
11. Ellwood P: Special report—Shattuck guest lecture: outcome management, a technology of patient experience. N Engl J Med 18:1549, 1988
12. Weinstein MC, Fineberg HV, Elstein AS et al: Clinical decisions and limited resources. p 228. In: Clinical Decision Analysis. WB Saunders, Philadelphia, 1980
13. Sox HC Jr, Blatt MA, Higgins MC, Martin KI: Medical Decision Making. Butterworths, Boston, 1988, pp. 147, 317
14. Proudfit WL, Bruschke AVG, Sones FM Jr: Natural history of obstructive coronary artery disease: ten-year study of 601 nonsurgical cases. Prog Cardiovasc Dis 21:53, 1978
15. Kent KM, Bentvoglio LG, Block PS et al: Long term efficacy of percutaneous transluminal angioplasty (PTCA): Report from the NHLBI registry. Am J Cardiol, Suppl. C, 53:27C, 1984
16. Talley JD, Hurst JW, King SB III et al: Clinical outcome five years after attempted percutaneous coronary angioplasty in 427 patients. Circulation 77:820, 1988
17. Frye RL, Frommer PL, McCallum BD: Consensus development conference on coronary artery bypass: introduction. Circulation, Suppl. II, 65:1, 1982
18. Hurst JW, King SB III: The prolongation of life by coronary bypass surgery—the Emory University Hospital experience. p. 141. In Hurst JW (ed): The Heart: Bypass Surgery for Obstructive Coronary Disease. Update II. McGraw-Hill, New York, 1980
19. Cosgrove DM, Loop FD, Sheldon WC: Results of myocardial revascularization: a 12-year experience. Circulation 65 (Suppl II):37, 1982
20. Hammermeister KE, DeRouen TA, Dodge HT: Comparison of survival of medically and surgically treated coronary disease patients in Seattle Heart Watch: a non-randomized study. Circulation, Suppl. II, 65:53, 1982
21. Hall RJ, Elayda MA, Gray A et al: Coronary artery bypass: long-term follow-up of 22,284 consecutive patients. Circulation, Suppl. II, 68:20, 1983
22. The Veterans Administration Coronary Artery Bypass Surgery Cooperative Study Group: Eleven-year survival in the Veterans Administration randomized trial of coronary bypass surgery for stable angina. N Engl J Med 311:1333, 1984
23. Peduzzi P, Hultgren H, Thomsen J, Detre K: Ten-year effect of medical and surgical therapy on quality of life: Veterans Administration Cooperative Study of Coronary Artery Surgery. Am J Cardiol 59:1017, 1987
24. Varnauskas E. European Coronary Surgery Study Group: survival, myocardial infarction, and employment status in a prospective randomized study of coronary bypass surgery. Circulation, Suppl. V, 72:90, 1985
25. Killip T, Passamani E, Davis K, the CASS Principal Investigators, and their associates: The Coronary Artery Surgery Study (CASS): a randomized trial of coronary bypass surgery. Eight year follow-up and survival in patients with reduced ejection fraction. Circulation, Suppl. V, 72:102, 1985
26. Califf RM, Pryor DB, Greenfield JC Jr: Beyond randomized clinical trials: applying clinical experience in the treatment of patients with coronary artery disease. Circulation 74:1191, 1986
27. McNeer JR, Margolis JR, Lee KL et al: The role of the exercise test in the evaluation of patients for ischemic heart disease. Circulation 57:64, 1978
28. Weiner DA, Ryan TJ, McCabe CH et al: The role of exercise testing in identifying patients with improved survival after coronary artery bypass surgery. J Am Coll Cardiol 8:741, 1986

29. Diamond GA, Forrester JS: Analysis of probability as an aid in the clinical diagnosis of coronary artery disease. N Engl J Med 30:1350, 1979
30. Gianrossi R, Detrano R, Mulvihill D et al: Exercise-induced ST depression in the diagnosis of coronary artery disease: a meta-analysis. Circulation 80:87, 1989
31. Beller GA: Diagnostic accuracy of thallium-201 myocardial perfusion imaging. Circulation, Suppl. I, 84:1, 1991
32. Patterson RE, Horowitz SF, Eng C et al: Can exercise electrocardiography and thallium-201 myocardial imaging exclude the diagnosis of coronary artery disease? Am J Cardiol 49:1127, 1982
33. Bungo MW, Leland OS: Discordance of exercise thallium testing with coronary arteriography in patients with atypical presentations. Chest 83(1):112, 1983
34. DePasquale EE, Nody AC, DePuey EG et al: Quantitative rotational thallium-201 tomography for identifying and localizing coronary artery disease. Circulation 77:316, 1988
35. Iskandrian AS, Heo J, Kong B, Lyons E: Effectiveness of exercise level on the ability of thallium-201 tomographic imaging in detecting coronary artery disease: analysis of 461 patients. J Am Coll Cardiol 14:1477, 1989
36. Van Train KF, Maddahi J, Berman DS et al: Quantitative analysis of tomographic stress thallium-201 myocardial scintigrams: A multicenter trial. J Nucl Med 31:1168, 1990
37. Mahmarian JJ, Boyce TM, Goldberg RK et al: Quantitative exercise thallium-201 single photon emission computed tomography for the enhanced diagnosis of ischemic heart disease. J Am Coll Cardiol 15:318, 1990
38. Schwartz RS, Jackson WG, Celio PV, Richardson LA, Hichman JR Jr: Accuracy of exercise Tl^{201} myocardial scintigraphy in asymptomatic young men. Circulation 87:165, 1993
39. Tamaki N, Yonekura Y, Senda M et al: Value and limitation of stress thallium-201 single photon emission computed tomography: Comparison with nitrogen-13 ammonia positron tomography. J Nucl Med 20:1181, 1988
40. Demer LL, Gould KL, Goldstein RA et al: Assessment of coronary artery disease severity by positron emission tomography: comparison with quantitative arteriography in 193 patients. Circulation 79:825, 1989
41. Williams BR, Jansen DE, Wong LF et al: Positron emission tomography for the diagnosis of coronary artery disease: A non-university experience and correlation with coronary angiography, abstracted. J Nucl Med 30:845, 1989
42. Go RT, Marwick TH, MacIntyre WJ et al: A prospective comparison of rubidium-82 PET and thallium-201 SPECT myocardial perfusion imaging utilizing a single dipyridamole stress in the diagnosis of coronary artery disease. J Nucl Med 31:1899, 1990
43. Stewart RE, Schwaiger M, Molina E et al: Comparison of rubidium-82 positron emission tomography and thallium-201 SPECT imaging for detection of coronary artery disease. Am J Cardiol 67:1303, 1991
44. Garcia EV, Eisner RL, Patterson RE: What should we expect from cardiac PET? J Nucl Med 34:978, 1993
45. Bruce RA, Irving JB: Exercise electrocardiography. p. 336. In Hurst JW, Logue RB, Schlant RC, Wenger NK (eds): The Heart, Arteries and Veins. 4th Ed. McGraw-Hill, New York, 1978
46. Adams DF, Abrams HL: Complications of coronary arteriography: a follow-up report. Cardiovasc Radiol 2:89, 1979
47. Gould KL, Goldstein RA, Mullani NA: Economic analysis of clinical positron emission tomography of the heart with rubidium-82. J Nucl Med 30:707, 1989
48. McKean R: Efficiency in Government Through Systems Analysis. John Wiley & Son, New York, 1958, pp 21–96
49. Diamond GA, Forrester JS: Analysis of probability as an aid in the clinical diagnosis of coronary artery disease. N Engl J Med 30:1350, 1979
50. Patterson RE, Horowitz SF: Importance of epidemiology and biostatistics in deciding clinical strategies for using diagnostic tests: A simplified approach using examples from coronary artery disease. J Am Coll Cardiol 13:1653, 1989
51. Lusted LB: Introduction to Medical Decision-Making. Charles C Thomas, Springfield, IL 1968, pp 1–46

Chapter 6

Screening for CAD

Mark Sada and Robert Detrano

PRECLINICAL ATHEROSCLEROTIC HEART DISEASE
The Prevalence of Atherosclerosis

In 1953, Enos and colleagues, intending to study wound ballistics in Korean war combat victims, eventually turned their attention instead to the coronary arteries.[1] After postmortem coronary artery dissections and angiography, they concluded that 77% of subjects had "gross evidence of atherosclerosis" with 3% of subjects showing complete occlusions and approximately 12% with greater than 50% stenosis of at least one major epicardial artery. The high prevalence of atherosclerosis in these young men had profound implications regarding the prevalence in the population at large.

Almost two decades later, McNamara and colleagues performed an autopsy series on Vietnam War casualties and concluded that 45% of subjects (young, asymptomatic males) had some evidence of atherosclerosis.[2] Although they noted less severe lesions than those found in the Korean war casualties, atherosclerosis was quite prevalent. Subsequent work has confirmed the findings from these two landmark studies.[3-7]

These results were concordant with findings in civilian life. Hollman and colleagues, in an autopsy series from the New Orleans area, showed that aortic fatty streaking was present in all subjects older than 3 years.[3] Extending their study to the coronary arteries, Strong and McGill reported on the prevalence and extent of coronary atherosclerosis from 548 autopsied subjects, ranging in age from 1 to 69 years.[4] The levels of atherosclerosis paralleled the respective coronary heart disease (CHD) mortality rates for age, gender, and race. Lesions were present early in life, on average 20 years before the onset of disease. In an extension of this work, they showed that by the third decade, 90% of subjects, regardless of gender or race, had fatty streaking of the coronary arteries.[8] By the end of the fourth decade, "fibrous plaques and more advanced lesions were present in a majority of subjects, black and white, men and women."[9] The International Atherosclerosis Project, a 14 country study, showed large geographic and ethnic differences in the extent of coronary atherosclerosis, which corresponded to coronary heart disease death rates.[7]

More recently, the Primary Determinants of Atherosclerosis in Youth (PDAY) study has shown a correlation between degree of atherosclerosis and conventional risk factors, including serum lipoproteins.[10] This ongoing study is a multicenter collaborative project investigating atherosclerosis in 15- to 34-year-old victims of violent death. Careful collection of clinical and pathologic data has confirmed the high prevalence of atherosclerosis in young, asymptomatic adults.

The results of the above studies confirm the frequency of fatty streaking of the intima—an early stage of atherosclerosis—in our society. As lesions progress, raised plaques can be seen within the arterial wall.[11] These lesions may progress slowly over time. Acute plaque rupture, often accompanied by hemorrhage and thrombosis, can lead to rapid progression of luminal stenosis.[12] If significant luminal compromise occurs in this fashion, sudden death, acute myocardial infarction, or unstable angina can result. Coronary artery disease (CAD) at this point is labeled as symptomatic. Thus, a continuum exists between the earliest atherosclerotic lesions and symptomatic coronary heart disease. On the day before a myocardial infarction, a patient has just as much atherosclerosis as on the day after; however, his symptom status has clearly changed.

Clinical and Economic Implications

Coronary heart disease is responsible for 535,000 deaths each year in the United States, with nearly 1.5 million hospitalizations for myocardial infarction.[13] The economic costs are staggering—over $117 billion per year for the treatment of cardiovascular disease.[14] Historically, the medical community has focused on the treatment of patients once coronary heart disease has been established. Less attention has been given to the management of asymptomatic individuals with occult disease, who represent the majority of those with coronary atherosclerosis. Should asymptomatic subjects be screened for occult coronary atherosclerosis? If so, what are the options for management if it is detected?

Identification and Significance of Occult Lesions

Coronary angiography is often regarded as the "gold standard" to identify coronary atherosclerosis. The degree of luminal stenosis is visually estimated, using an adjacent arterial segment for comparison. This then serves as a measure of the "severity of disease" and is often equated with the chance that the patient may sustain a subsequent myocardial infarction: the "tighter" the stenosis, it is argued, the greater the chance of infarct or death.

The angiographic gold standard has been criticized based on a number of grounds. Technical concerns include the subjectivity of visual assessment. When visual estimates of lesional severity are compared to quantitative assessments, significant interobserver variability is found.[15] Moreover, the lack of a normal adjacent arterial segment for reference may lead to underestimation of lesional severity.[16] Recent work using intracoronary ultrasound, which demonstrates significant atherosclerosis in many angiographically normal segments, supports this concept.[17]

A number of recent observations challenge the concept that angiographically important stenosis causes cardiac events. Angiographic studies before and after myocardial infarction have demonstrated that most lesions resulting in cardiac events are not severely stenotic.[18] Additionally, lipid-lowering trials demonstrate a reduction in cardiac events out of proportion to the reduction in angiographic disease.[19,20] This has been attributed to favorable changes in the lipid composition of atherosclerotic plaques[21] and improvement in endothelial vasomotor function.[22,23]

Given these recent observations, does the presence of flow limiting disease, and hence myocardial ischemia, have any prognostic importance? The fact is that patients with severe stenoses *do* have a worse prognosis than those with mild disease.[24,25] Even though clinical events may not be attributable to occlusion of the most severe stenosis, they are more likely to occur in those individuals with more extensive angiographic disease. Similarly, the presence and severity of myocardial ischemia have proven prognostic significance in both the symptomatic[26–29] and asymptomatic[30–40] patient. In this context, the exercise test can be viewed as a marker for extent of disease. Thus, although we cannot predict the behavior of any *individual* lesion, we can make the probabilistic argument that the more extensive the disease, the more likely the patient is to develop a cardiac event.

EXERCISE TESTING AS A SCREENING TOOL

Stress testing is one strategy to identify patients with occult coronary atherosclerosis. Physiologic stress, in the form of exercise, is employed to induce myocardial ischemia, identified as electrocardiographic (ECG) changes. Hence, coronary stenoses severe enough to induce ischemia, dubbed "flow limiting lesions," should be identified through this technique. Historically, it was argued that lesions less than 50% do not produce flow limitations. However, recent work using positron emission tomography has shown that ischemia can sometimes occur with less severe lesions.[41] On the other hand, lesions of greater than 50% may *not* produce ischemia. Recall that myocardial ischemia develops if myocardial oxygen demand outstrips supply. Oxygen demand for a given segment of myocardium is determined by the level of exercise attained. Supply is determined by many factors, including the extent of luminal compromise, the oxygen-carrying capacity of blood, and the presence or absence of collateral vessels. Thus, the severity of lumenal compromise is only one of *several* factors that affect the supply–demand balance.

Accuracy for the Diagnosis of Coronary Artery Disease

The "accuracy" of the exercise ECG can be defined as its ability to discriminate between those with and without flow limiting stenosis. As discussed by Pashkow and Robert, wide variations in sensitivity, specificity, and positive and negative predictive values have been reported for exercise ECG testing.[42–44] Variations in predictive value are expected since this is dependent on disease prevalence. However, sensitivity and specificity, which define the accuracy of a test, should not vary from population to population, that is, they should be independent of the prevalence of disease.

What Contributes to the Wide Range of Reported Accuracy?

Ransohoff and Feinstein identified problems of "spectrum" and "bias" as potential sources of such inconsistencies. If too narrow a spectrum of diseased and nondiseased patients is included in a study, the test accuracy may be falsely elevated (problem of spectrum).[45] If the interpretation of the test and the establishment of the true diagnosis are not done independently (problem of bias), again the test efficacy is falsely elevated. Additionally, technical factors such as the type of exercise protocol, the definition of a positive test, and the definition of angiographic disease could also contribute to these differences.[42] Philbrick and colleagues analyzed 33 studies comprising 7,501 patients undergoing both exercise testing and angiography.[43] They found the spectrum of patients was adequate, with a variety of anatomic lesions seen. However, problems of bias were quite frequent. Detrano and colleagues, using meta-analysis, showed that work-up bias and publication year affected sensitivity, and inclusion of men and patients with prior history of infarction influenced specificity of the exercise thallium test.[46] Technical factors, such as type of exercise used and use of tomographic imaging, did not influence accuracy. A similar analysis applied to exercise-induced ST depression revealed methodologic factors, such as exclusion of patients taking digitalis and those with right bundle branch block, and technical factors, such as the use of heart rate adjustment, to be significantly related to test accuracy.[44]

Accuracy in the Asymptomatic Population

The clinician who subjects an asymptomatic patient to exercise testing is effectively asking the following question: What is the probability that my patient has flow-limiting coronary artery disease given a positive test? To answer this question, one must know the pretest probability of disease and the likelihood ratio of a positive exercise test. The likelihood ratio is a function of a test's sensitivity and specificity. To determine the sensitivity and specificity of exercise ECG in asymptomatic subjects, one must design a study in which coronary arteriography is performed independent of the stress study results. Such a study, which would subject asymptomatic patients with negative exercise ECGs to coronary angiography, has not been performed. Thus, one must extrapolate data from the symptomatic population to this cohort. This may or may not be a valid approach.

A number of investigators, however, have defined the positive predictive value of an exercise test with respect to angiographic disease. Erikssen et al., in a study of Norwegian factory workers, performed coronary arteriography on 105 of 115 asymptomatic men who had positive exercise tests.[47] Seventy-two percent had significant coronary atherosclerosis (defined as >75% stenosis). Froelicher et al. showed the positive predictive value of an abnormal test among United States Air Force personnel to be 25%.[30] When clinical and additional exercise variables were included in a subsequent analysis, the predictive value increased to almost 90%.[48] Maneuvers to increase positive predictive value invariably decrease negative predictive value. In general, studies have shown that the greater the ischemic change, as demonstrated by the degree and persistence of ST depression as well as the blood pressure response to exercise, the greater the likelihood of severe disease in the asymptomatic patient.[49,50]

Prognostic Accuracy

A test that is 100% accurate with respect to prognosis would perfectly delineate those who are destined to develop clinical events from those who are not. Due to the capricious nature of coronary events, such a test will never be found. Patients with angiographic evidence of minimal disease may still develop clinical events, albeit at a lower rate than their more plaque-burdened counterparts. If the number of individuals with minimal disease is substantially larger than those with more extensive disease, the *absolute* number of events can be higher in the minimally diseased cohorts. Such has been the case with many populations studied using exercise ECG.[32,36,38,40] Even though a positive exercise test identified patients at higher risk for events in these studies, the absolute number of events was higher in those with negative test results.

Benefit of Identifying High-Risk Asymptomatic Subjects

In the context of these observations, one might question whether there is benefit in identifying higher risk subjects—we believe that there is. The Multiple Risk Factor Intervention Trial (MRFIT) study randomized a large group of asymptomatic men with multiple cardiac risk factors to a "usual care" or a "special intervention" group.[31] The special intervention group received counseling on smoking cessation, advice on dietary practices to lower blood cholesterol level, and stepped-care drug treatment for hypertension. There was a trend toward reduction in overall CHD mortality in the special intervention group, but this trend did not reach statistical significance. However, when subanalysis of the subjects with positive exercise tests was performed, special intervention dramatically reduced events. Thus, those identified through exercise testing as being at the highest risk for cardiac events substantially benefited from risk factor modification.

One of the earliest and largest studies to address the prognostic significance of a positive exercise test was the Seattle Heart Watch. Robert Bruce and colleagues reported the 5 year results of this study in 1980.[32] Of the 2,365 subjects who underwent symptom-limited exercise ECG testing, 47 sustained cardiac events, defined as angina, sudden cardiac death, or myocardial infarction. The relative risk of a cardiac event was 29:1 for the presence of any conventional risk factor and *two* exercise test findings: chest pain, exercise duration less than 6 minutes, failure to achieve greater than 90% age-predicted heart rate, or ST depression of a horizontal or downsloping nature and persisting for 1 minute or more into recovery. Ischemic ST depression alone carried a 3.4-fold higher risk for events. A total of three cardiac events occurred in patients with no conventional risk factors, and exercise testing was of no predictive value in this low risk cohort.

Summaries of some of the larger trials addressing the prognostic significance of exercise testing in asymptomatic subjects are depicted in Table 6-1. The relative risk for a coronary event associated with a positive exercise ECG varies from 1.2 (not significant) to 14. This wide variation can be attributed to several important differences in study design.

Multivariate Adjustment

A critical question is whether a positive exercise test provides prognostic information *independent* of conventional cardiac risk factors. To answer this question, multivariate adjustment, using conventional risk factors as confounders, must be performed. Giagnoni and colleagues, the first to employ this technique, followed 135 Italian factory workers who had positive exercise ECGs for cardiac events.[33] These subjects were matched for age, sex, work community, and coronary-risk factor index against 379 controls who had normal exercise responses. The relative risk for a cardiac event, defined as angina, myocardial infarction, or sudden cardiac death, was 5.5 after adjustment for confounders.

Other investigators, using multivariate adjustment, have shown similar results. Multivariate adjustment was performed in both the Lipid Research Clinic (LRC) and MRFIT studies. For the endpoint of 1 mm ST-segment depression and using an exercise protocol to achieve 90% maximum predicted heart rate, Gordon and colleagues reported a relative risk for coronary death of 4.6:1 in the LRC study.[34] Using an ST-segment integral of 16 μV-second as an endpoint, Rautaharjul and colleagues reported a relative risk for CHD death of 3.8 in the MRFIT study.[35] Thus, similar results were found in these two large-scale and well-conducted studies, both with excellent follow-up (<0.3% lost in follow-up).

Hard vs. Soft Endpoints

Most of the studies listed in Table 6-1 defined a cardiac event as angina, myocardial infarction, or sudden cardiac death. Clearly, angina carries different weight than the latter two events, and exercise testing would be of greater use if it could predict myocardial infarction and sudden coronary death as well as angina. In addition, angina, as reported by study participants, could clearly be affected by recall bias—patients who are told that their exercise test is positive may be more likely to report angina on follow-up questioning.

McHenry and colleagues,[36] using a maximal protocol and 1-mm horizontal or downsloping ST-segment depression as an endpoint, showed that the relative risk of a cardiac event on univariate testing to be 4.9:1. However, this difference was seen only for angina, and not for myocardial infarction or sudden cardiac death. In a subsequent editorial, Epstein and colleagues[51] attributed this result to the "protective effect" of ischemia. Patients with flow limiting lesions, they argued, develop protective collaterals; if the vessel occludes, it is less likely to precipitate acute myocardial infarction or sudden cardiac death.

Other larger studies, however, support the prognostic significance of a positive exercise ECG for hard endpoints.[33–35,37] Both the LRC[34] and MRFIT[35] studies found a correlation between a positive exercise ECG and the occurrence of coronary heart disease death. Data from Giagnoni et al. show a *stronger* association between a positive exercise ECG and myocardial infarction than angina pectoris (relative risk 13.4 vs. 3.4).[33] This association was also demonstrated in the Framingham offspring study (relative risk for myocardial infarction = 6.7, relative risk angina pectoris = 4.0).[37] In our opinion, these studies conclusively demonstrate the prognostic significance of the exercise test for hard endpoints.

Exercise Protocol and Criteria for Abnormality

Intuitively, the use of a maximal, as opposed to a submaximal, protocol should yield a higher relative risk for events. Three of the studies in Table 6-1 used submaximal testing with a target heart rate as an endpoint.[33–35] The relative risk for cardiac events in these three studies, after multivariate adjustment, ranged from 3.8 to 5.6. The two studies that adjusted for confounders and used symptom-limited protocols showed a relative risk of 2.4 and 1.2 (p = NS) for coronary heart disease events.[37,40] Thus, these data do not support a clear relationship between predictive value and level of stress.

Exercise Duration

Bruce et al. found that an exercise duration of less than 6 minutes on the Bruce protocol was associated with an unadjusted relative risk of 6.7 for cardiac events in men and 3.6 in women.[38] Allen and colleagues reported a relative risk of 5.6 for cardiac events given an exercise duration of less than 5 minutes on a maximal Ellestad protocol.[39] Women who could not complete 3 minutes on this protocol had a 14.7-fold higher risk. It is not clear if this finding is independent of patient age, since neither study adjusted for confounders. Flegg et al., after performing multivariate adjustment, reported exercise duration to be significantly associated with coronary events,[40] although they did not report the value obtained. Thus, exercise tolerance alone appears to have independent prognostic significance.

Criteria for ST Abnormality

Most investigators define a positive test by the presence of 1 mm or more of horizontal or downsloping ST-segment depression measured 80 ms after the J point. The LRC and MRFIT study both used the ST integral as a marker for ischemia.[34,35] Figure 6-1 shows the method used in the MRFIT study.[35] An ST-segment depression integral of 16 μV-seconds or more during peak exercise with a resting value of less than 6 μV-seconds was considered a positive response. Note that this endpoint is independent of the ST-segment slope. In the LRC study, a test was considered positive if ST depression or elevation of greater than 1 mm was determined visually, or a computer-determined ST integral fell or rose by at least 10 μV-second from its resting value.[34] In most

Table 6-1. Prognostic Significance of an Abnormal Exercise (ECG) in Asymptomatic Subjects[a]

Reference	Subjects	Women Included	Exercise Protocol	Criteria for Abnormality	Cardiac Events
Froelicher et al. (1974)[64]	1390	No	Master 2 step, max treadmill	ST depression (1)	AP + MI + SCD
Bruce et al. (1980)[32]	2365	No	Max Bruce	Chest pain Exercise duration <6 min MHR <90% predicted ST depression (1)	AP + MI + SCD
Cumming et al. (1975)[65]	510	No	Max bicycle	Not stated	AP + MI + SCD
McHenry et al. (1984)[36]	916	No	Max Mod Balke	ST depression (1)	AP + MI + SCD
Bruce et al. (1983)[38]	4158	Yes	Max Bruce	Exercise duration <6 min Chest pain MHR <90% predicted RPP <80% predicted ST depression (1)	AP + MI + SCD
Giagnoni et al. (1983)[33]	510[b]	Yes	Supine bike, 85% MPHR	ST depression (1)	MI AP AP + MI + SCD
Allen et al. (1980)[39]	1077	Yes	Max Ellestad	ST depression (1) R wave response (6) Exercise duration (7)	AP + MI + SCD
Gordon et al. (LRC) (1986)[34]	3260	No	Mod Bruce, 90% MPHR	ST response (2)	CHD death (8)
Rautaharju et al. (1986)[35] (MRFIT)	6438	No	Submax treadmill	ST depression (3)	CHD death (9) AP MI
Fleg et al. (1990)[40]	407	Yes	Max Balke	ST depression (1) Segmental thallium defect	AP AP + MI + SCD MI
Okin et al. (1991)[37] (Framingham)	3168	Yes	Max Bruce	ST depression (1) ST/HR index (4) Recovery loop (5)	AP + MI + SCD

Abbreviations: ECG, electrocardiograph; FU, follow-up; AP, angina pectoris; MI, myocardial infarction; SCD, sudden cardiac death; MHR, maximum heart rate; MPHR, maximum predicted heart rate; RPP, rate-pressure product; CHD, coronary heart disease; LRC, Lipid Research Clinic; MRFIT, Multiple Risk Factor Intervention Trial; ST/HR, ST-segment heart rate.

[a] (1) 1 mm horizontal or downsloping ST depression, 80 ms after J-point; (2) ST depression or elevation 1 mm or more or rise or fall in ST integral by 10 μV-second; (3) ST depression 16 μV-second or more with less than 6 μV-second at rest; (4) >16 μV/beat/min; (5) ST depression greater in early recovery than at corresponding exercise heart rate; (6) no change or increase; (7) men: 5 min or less, women: 3 min or less; (8) CHD death as determined by blinded panel of five cardiologists; (9) Documented MI, SCD within 60 min or between 1 and 24 hours of symptom onset without documented MI, congestive heart failure from CHD, death associated with surgery for CHD.
[b] 135 case, 375 control.
[c] Not significant.

cases, the visual and computer codes were in agreement. Both of these studies showed significant predictive values of these ST-integral endpoints.

Heart Rate Adjustment

Risk stratification in the Framingham Offspring study failed to demonstrate prognostic significance of ST depression alone for coronary events.[37] When the degree of ST depression was adjusted for heart rate and recovery, however, subjects could be separated into high, intermediate, and low risk groups. Heart rate adjustment has been extensively studied in *symptomatic* patients undergoing exercise testing.[52–57] As discussed by Pashkow, this method has been validated by some authors,[52–55] but not by others.[56,57]

Conversion to a Positive Test

McHenry and colleagues analyzed the results of serial maximal stress tests in asymptomatic male employees of the Indiana State Police department.[36] Over a mean follow up period of 12.7 years, 5.1% of

Relative Risk for Cardiac Events	Cardiac Events/1000 Patient Years	Multivariate Adjustment	Prevalence of ST Depression (%)	Years FU	% Lost to FU
14.3	5.2	No	13.8	6.3	Not stated
29 for two exercise criteria, 3.4 for ST depression	3.5	No	11.1	5.6	Not stated
10.3	17	No	11.9	3	None
4.9	5.6	No	2.5	12.7	Not stated
Exercise duration = 6.7 men, 3.6 women Chest pain = 3.5 men, 3.3 women MHR = 2.4 men, 1.8 women RPP = 2.4 men, 1.3 women ST = 2.6 men, 6.7 women	8	No	14.6	6.1	6.8
13.4 (univariate) 3.4 (univariate) 5.6 (adjusted)	n/a	Yes	1.3	6	None
ST depression = 2.4 men (>40 y), 1.9^c women R wave = 2.7 men (>40 y), 1.9^c women Exercise duration = 5.6 men (>40 y), 14.7 women	10.8	Yes	9.7	5	17.5
Strong positive = 5.0 All positive = 4.6	2.1	Yes	5.7	8.4	0.1
3.8 1.6 1.2^c	2.5 16.9 4.7	Yes	12.2	7	0.3
Both positive = 4.0 ST depression = 2.4 Segmental thallium defect = 1.4^c Both positive = 3.6 Both positive = 6.7	21	Yes	16.2	4.6	2.0
ST depression = 1.2^c ST/HR = 2.2 Recovery loop = 2.1 Combined = 3.6	4.7	Yes	14.6	4.3	0.0

the subjects experienced conversion to an abnormal test. The percentage of subjects with initially positive tests who developed cardiac events was similar to those who converted. Josephson and colleagues analyzed the results of serial stress tests in healthy men and women participating in the Baltimore Longitudinal Study of Aging.[58] The incidence of events was nearly identical between those who were initially positive and those who converted. Thus, in asymptomatic individuals, conversion from a negative to a positive stress test imparts the same risk as an initially positive test.

The High Risk Patient

The absolute risk of a cardiac event is a function of both conventional risk factors and the results of the exercise ECG. Patients at highest risk for events have several conventional risk factors, in addition to abnormal exercise ECG studies. Exercise ECG abnormalities, in the absence of conventional risk factors, however, have little predictive value.[32] In contrast, Bruce and colleagues identified a very high risk cohort on the basis of conventional risk factors and the presence of *two or more* exercise ECG abnormalities. These included ST depression, chest pain, failure to attain greater than 90% maximum predicted heart rate on a symptom limited study, and rate-pressure product less than 80% of predicted. In patients with at least one conventional risk factor, the presence of two or more exercise endpoints imparted a 30-fold higher risk for coronary events.

Other studies have shown a combination of exercise ECG abnormalities and conventional risk factors to indicate the highest risk. After multivariate adjust-

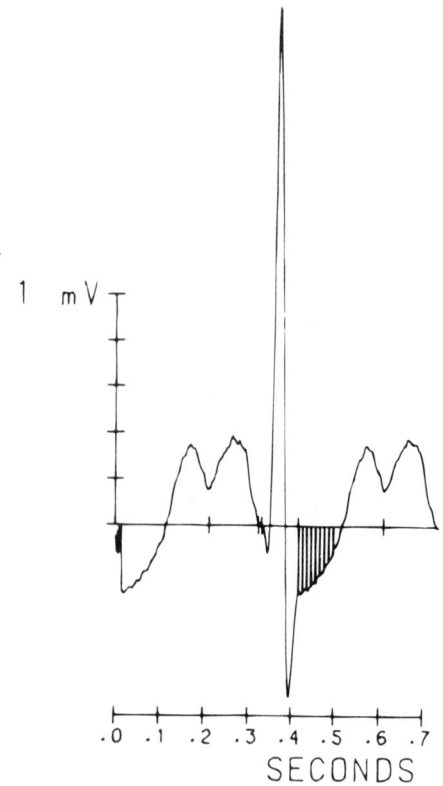

Fig. 6-1 The ST-depression integral: voltage-time integral (in microvolt-seconds) calculated from the end of the QRS complex (J point) to the zero crossing or to the time point corresponding to 7/16 of the total ST-T (J-T) duration, whichever occurs first. The value of the shown ST-depression integral with a high amplitude R wave in the CS_5 lead is 19.2 µV-seconds. Heart rate = 149/min. (From Rautaharju et al.,[35] with permission.)

ment, investigators in the MRFIT study determined a "strong positive," defined as 2 mm or more of ST depression or onset in the first 6 minutes of the modified Bruce protocol, to have a 5.0:1 relative risk for CHD death.[35] For the presence of ST depression alone, the result was 4.6:1. Thus, a strong positive test had additional prognostic significance.

Dealing with the Problem of False-Positive Results

The use of preexercise hypeventilation may unveil labile ST segment changes that might be associated with false-positive results. McHenry and colleagues found 37 of 916 subjects studied to have a positive exercise ST-segment response.[36] However, 14 of these demonstrated labile ST-T wave changes during pre-exercise hyperventilation or with postural maneuvers. Of those without labile changes, 39% sustained a coronary event, while none of those with labile changes had an event. The predictive value increased from 25.3% to 34.4% when those with labile changes were excluded. Despite the results of this study, a meta-analysis of exercise testing showed no improvement in specificity when pre-exercise hyperventilation was employed.[59]

Another strategy to define a "true positive" is to confirm the result with another, presumably more accurate test, such as angiography. However, since it is difficult to submit normal subjects without evidence of ischemia to angiography, investigators have used the results of the exercise thallium imaging as a surrogate. Flegg and colleagues performed maximal treadmill exercise ECG and thallium scintigraphy in 407 asymptomatic volunteers, and followed them for an average of 4.6 years.[40] ST-segment depression alone carried a relative risk of 2.4:1 for cardiac events. After multivariate adjustment, a subject with both a positive thallium and an ischemic ST-segment response had a 3.6:1 relative risk for an event. Thus, excluding the "false positives" or those with positive exercise ECG but negative thallium markedly increased the predictive value of the ECG test.

Screening for CAD in Women

As discussed in Chapters 1 and 7, the accuracy of exercise testing in women is controversial. Some investigators have reported lower specificity for exercise ECG in women than in men,[60] while others have found no difference.[61] Estrogen may have a role in the development of false-positive responses.[62] However, although estrogen has been shown to have vasoconstrictive properties,[63] the causal role for estrogen in false-positive exercise ECG has not been established.

From Table 6-1, most studies of prognosis in asymptomatic subjects have involved male subjects only.[32,34–36,64,65] Although the data are limited, they do support the prognostic importance of an exercise ECG in women. The first study to demonstrate this was the 10-year follow-up from the Seattle Heart Watch.[38] Bruce and colleagues analyzed 547 women and 3,611 men who underwent symptom-limited exercise testing. Univariate analysis revealed a number of exercise and ECG parameters to have prognostic significance for both men and women. Exercise duration of less than 6 minutes was associated with a relative risk of 3.6:1 for a cardiac event in men and 6.7:1 in women. Exercise-induced chest pain carried a relative risk of 3.5:1 in men and 3.3:1 in women. Failure to achieve greater than 90% age-predicted maximum heart rate and 80% predicted rate pressure product carried prognostic significance in both men and women. The prognostic significance of 1 mm ST depression was *higher* in women than in men (relative risk 2.6 men, 6.7 women). Unfortunately, these results were not subjected to multivariate adjustment. Since women tended to be older (30% over 55 years old, as opposed to 15% of the men), adjustment for age would tend to reduce the prognostic significance of the exercise ECG.

Several other studies of asymptomatic patients included women,[33,37,39,40] but separate analyses were not performed for this important subset. Of the 24,199 subjects from the 11 studies listed in Table 6-1, a total of 2,829 women were included (11.6%). Multivariate adjustment included gender as a confounder in the regression model for many of these studies.[33,37,40] However, no study analyzed men and women separately to determine the prognostic significance of exercise ECG with respect to gender.

The Prevalence of a Positive Test

The prevalence of exercise-induced ST depression in the asymptomatic population should reflect the pretest probability of disease. Figure 6-2 demonstrates the relationship between prevalence of positive exercise ECG responders and prevalence of disease (measured indirectly via cardiac event rate) among the different studies from Table 6-1. Despite methodologic differences among the various studies, a rough correlation between disease prevalence and ST depression is seen. The prevalence of exercise-induced ST depression ranges from 1.3% in the Giagnonni series[33] to 16.2% in the Flegg series.[40] Giagnonni and colleagues studied a relatively young, working population; Flegg analyzed subjects with a mean age of 60 years. Similarly, the high prevalence of positive ST responders in the MRFIT study (12.2%) can be attributed to the selection of men in the upper 10% to 15% of the risk score distribution based on Framingham data.[35]

Indications for Screening with Exercise ECG

Fitness Assessment

Fitness assessment determines whether an individual's exercise capacity is sufficient to meet expected physical demands. Maximum ventilatory oxygen uptake (VO_2 max) is a measure of functional capacity. It can be decreased by inactivity, bed rest,[66] anemia, vascular volume depletion, or heart or lung disease.[67] Maximum work capacity is a function of a patient's age, gender, and baseline level of activity.[68] Accurate measurement of VO_2 max requires expired gas analysis, but can be estimated from the maximum workload achieved.[69] Although it is useful to convert all exercise protocols to workload achieved (usually expressed as METS, 1 MET = 3.5 ml/kg/min of O_2), it is important to realize that performance using some protocols, such as supine ergometer, may be *highly* dependent on prior familiarity with the given protocol.[70] Age- and gender-specific capacities have been established for several of the protocols.[71]

The exercise test can be used to evaluate the safety of participating in an exercise program and can help formulate an exercise prescription.[72] Certain high risk individuals may be best evaluated in this controlled environment. For athletes in training, serial exercise testing can demonstrate improvement in performance, which can be an effective incentive and encouragement to such individuals.[73] Aerobic training can increase maximal oxygen uptake by approximately 25%.[74]

High Risk Professions

The American College of Cardiology/American Heart Association (ACC/AHA) Task Force identifies exercise testing in individuals in certain high risk professions (airline pilots, bus drivers, firemen, and policemen) as a Class II indication.[75] The rationale is that public safety may be jeopardized should these individuals sustain a sudden cardiac event. The U.S. Air Force screens all air crew over 35 years of age with resting ECGs. Subjects with "potential coronary artery disease" are referred for symptom-limited treadmill testing. Ninety-five percent of these individuals, in one report, were asymptomatic. Cardiac catheterization is mandatory if the exercise test is

134 Cardiac Stress Testing and Imaging

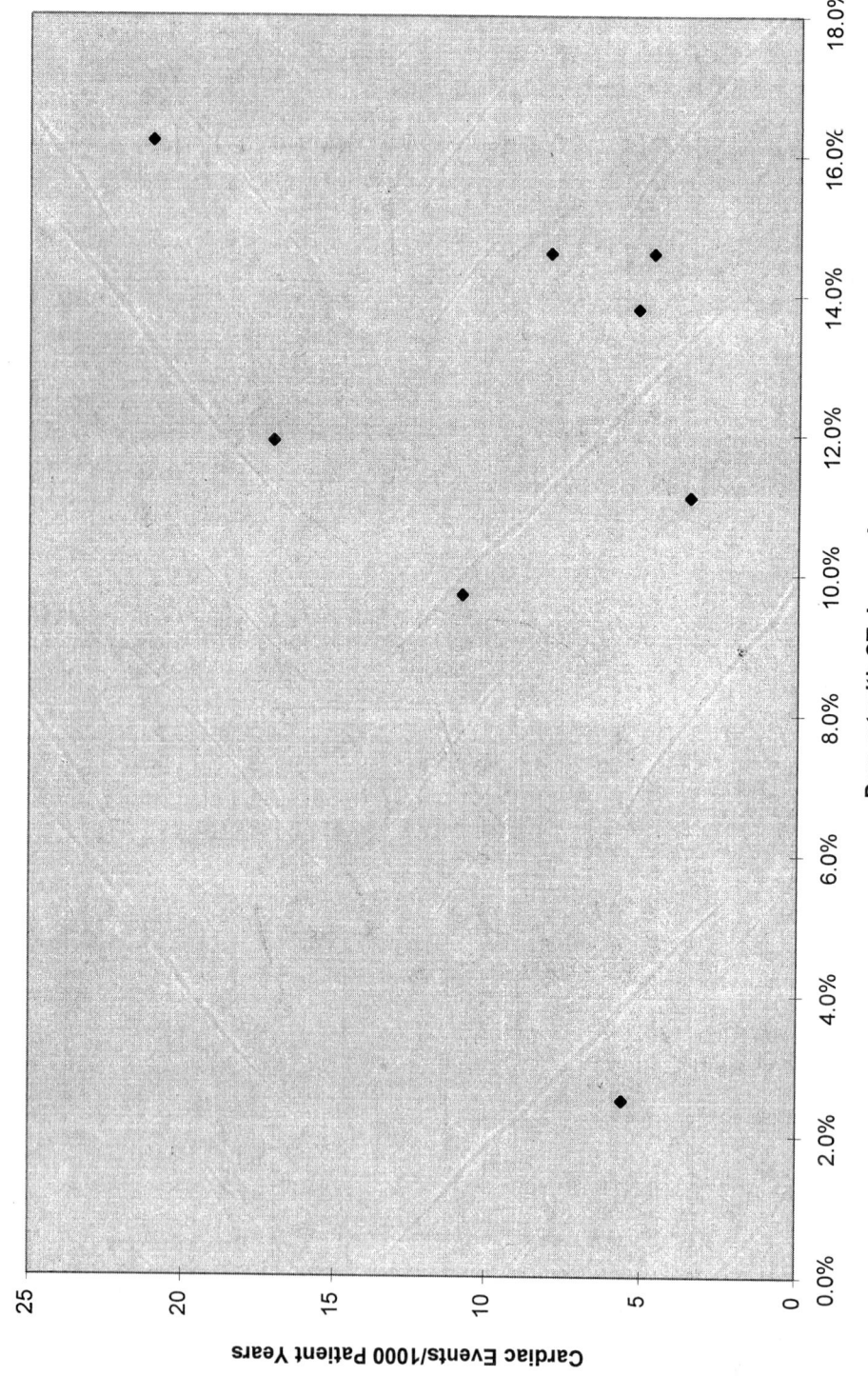

Fig. 6-2. Prevalence of ST depression in asymptomatic populations.

positive and the individual wishes to remain on flying status.[76]

Some police and fire departments require routine evaluation with exercise testing. In these physically demanding jobs, the test allows for fitness assessment as well as risk stratification for cardiac events. However, this routine testing may fail to account for conventional risk factors in determining the absolute risk for a coronary event. The probability of an event in a patient with multiple conventional risk factors for CAD but a negative exercise ECG may still be substantially higher than that of a low risk individual with a positive exercise ECG. Absolute risk of a coronary event can be calculated on the basis of conventional risk factors by using a probabilistic model such as the Framingham risk calculation algorithm.[77] Exercise ECG information can then be incorporated into this estimate. If risk determined in this manner exceeds a predetermined cut off, the individual in a high risk profession should either be excluded from activity or undergo further cardiac evaluation.

Selection of Other Patients for a "Screening" Exercise Test

Stress testing should only be used as a screening test for CAD in selected individuals. We agree with the ACC/AHA Task Force that exercise testing should *not* be used in asymptomatic individuals without conventional risk factors for CAD.[75] This is merely prudent application of Bayes' theorem, which states that positive studies in such individuals are most likely to represent false positives.

In subjects with one or more conventional risk factors for CAD, exercise testing can be justified based on its ability to further stratify risk. This information may then be used to

1. Determine target lipid levels.
2. Guide other risk factor modification such as smoking cessation, fitness and conditioning, and weight loss.
3. Guide medical and possibly surgical interventions.
4. Motivate patients to follow risk factor modification.
5. Evaluate the safety of starting a regular exercise program in a sedentary individual.
6. Evaluate the suitability for participation in high risk professions.

THE ANATOMIC APPROACH

It is evident that despite risk stratification with exercise testing, many acute cardiac events occur in subjects without evidence of flow limiting lesions.[32,36,38,40] Though a positive exercise ECG raises the relative risk of an event, its positive predictive value, especially in low risk populations, can be quite low. Why do so many patients with negative exercise tests have cardiac events? In part, this is due to the inherent inaccuracy of the test to detect flow-limiting disease. However, even if the test were 100% accurate in identifying flow limiting stenosis, the positive predictive value may not be substantially better. Plaque rupture is a highly unpredictable event, and may occur in non-flow-limiting as well as flow-limiting lesions.[78-81] A screening test that could identify both types of lesions could have greater prognostic importance.

Such a strategy is embodied in screening for coronary calcifications. Pathologic studies confirm the predictive value of calcification for coronary atherosclerosis.[82,83] Cinefluoroscopy has been used in asymptomatic individuals to identify the presence or absence of such calcifications.[76,84-92] The prevalence of calcification increases with age; by the ninth decade, it reaches 100%.[93] Detrano and colleagues performed cinefluoroscopy in a high risk, asymptomatic cohort.[84] At 1 year follow-up, the adjusted relative risk for a cardiac event due to the presence of coronary calcium was 2.4. This result is comparable to, but not better than, the prognostic significance of exercise testing. Electron beam computed tomography (CT) (Fig. 6.3), which is more specific for coronary calcium and can quantitate its extent,[94] may prove to be a more powerful prognostic tool. There is a theoretical limit, however, to the prognostic significance of any modality that can screen for the extent of atherosclerosis. A majority of Americans, by the end of their third decade, have pathologic evidence of atherosclerotic lesions.[9] Many of these individuals, however, will never have any coronary events. A test so sensitive that it could identify *any* atherosclerosis would have little predictive value.

Clearly, the extent of disease has been shown to correlate with the probability of events.[95,96] Exercise ECG is one method to measure extent of disease. Electron beam CT for identification of coronary cal-

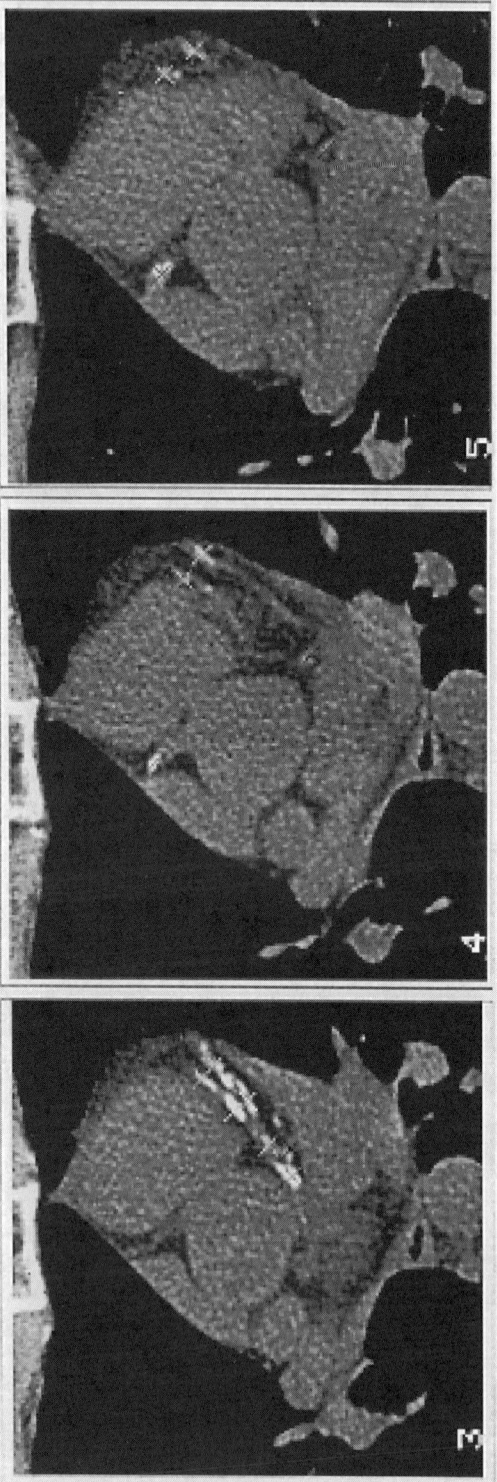

Fig. 6-3. Ultrafast computed tomography imaging. The three panels represent successive image levels from cardiac base to apex showing calcification in the three major coronary arteries. This patient also had severe two-vessel coronary disease and suffered a myocardial infarction within two years after this scan was done.

cium is another. Whether this, or other modalities such as cardiac magnetic resonance imaging (MRI) and positron emission tomography (PET) scanning can provide prognostic information beyond that of the exercise ECG remains to be determined.

CLINICAL DECISION-MAKING
Approach to Asymptomatic Patients with a Positive Study

While our recommendation is that stress testing be used only in patients with conventional risk factors, the physician may be referred individuals, both with and without risk factors, who have already undergone exercise testing. The approach to these two groups varies, and is illustrated in Figure 6-4.

The vast majority of positive studies in individuals without risk factors will be false positives. That is, most of these patients do not have flow limiting CAD, nor are they destined to develop clinical events. A positive study, however, labels the patient as "diseased," which can have negative psychologic impact and make it more difficult for the patient to obtain indemnity insurance. For this reason, we strongly advocate confirmation with a second study. Cinefluoroscopy or electron beam CT can be used to detect

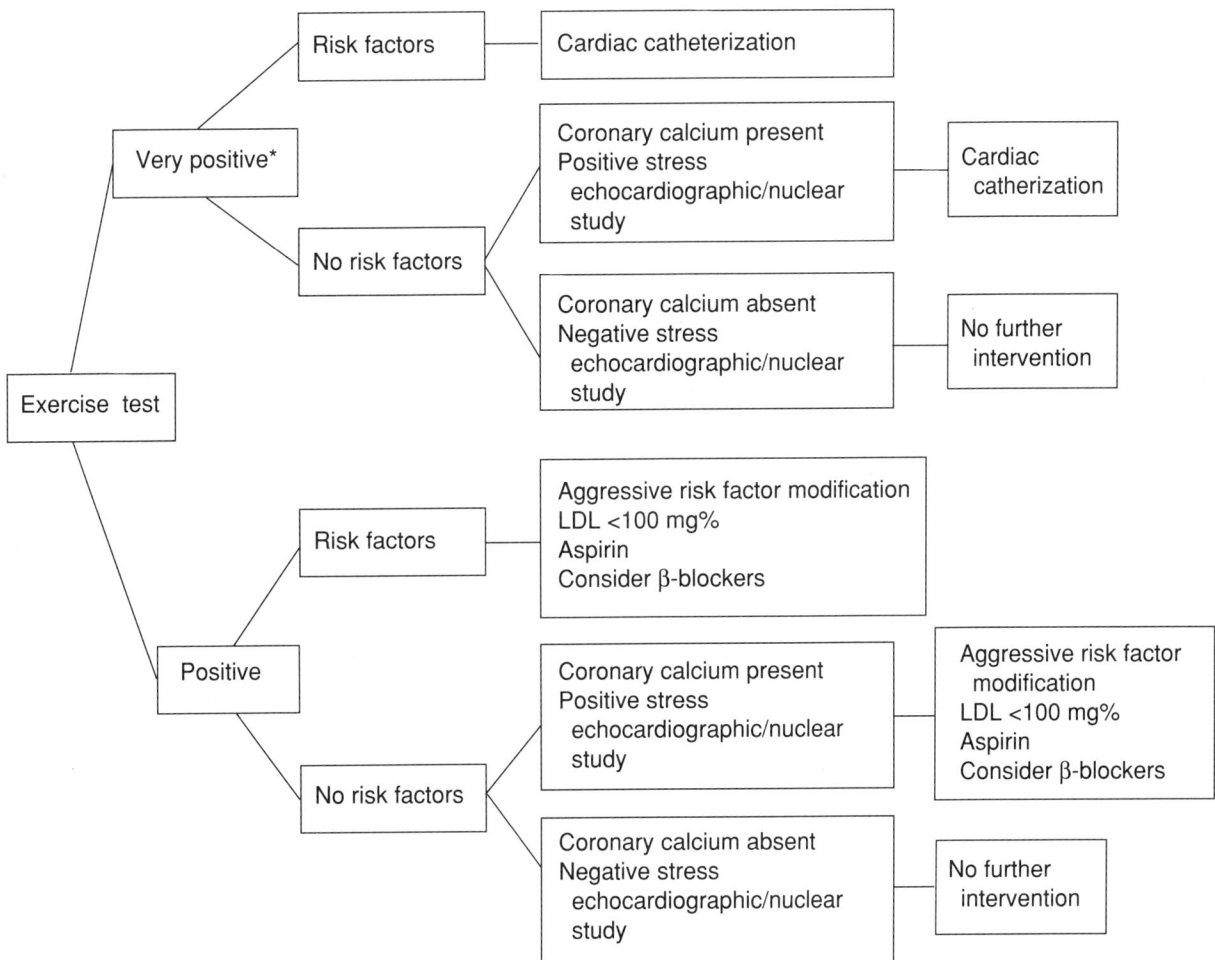

Fig. 6-4. Approach to the asymptomatic patient with a positive stress test (see text for details). LDL, low-density lipoprotein. *, Abnormal BP response, ST depression greater than 2 mm, occurring at less than 6 METS, or persisting for greater than 5 minutes into recovery, or sustained ventricular arrhythmia.

coronary calcium. The absence of calcification makes atherosclerosis much less likely.[83] Alternatively, exercise echocardiography or exercise radionuclide studies can be used to exclude false positives. If these follow-up studies confirm ischemia, the patient should be told of their increased risk, just as they would be informed of their increased risk on the basis of conventional risk factors. They should be encouraged to aggressively modify their risk factors, and we believe target lipid levels should be pursued that are similar to those advocated in patients with established CAD. Daily aspirin use is prudent,[97] and β-blocker therapy may also be of value.[98]

Low risk patients with "very positive" studies (abnormal blood pressure response, ST depression >2 mm occurring at less than 6 METS or persisting for >5 minutes into recovery, sustained ventricular arrhythmias) should be offered cardiac catheterization after confirming the presence of ischemia with stress echocardiographic or radionuclide study. The purpose of angiography is to identify patients with "life threatening" CAD (left main disease, triple-vessel disease with depressed left ventricular function), who may benefit from surgical revascularization.

A positive test in a patient with one or more conventional risk factors should prompt aggressive risk factor modification, with a targeting of low-density lipoprotein (LDL) levels to less than 100 mg/dl. Aspirin should be started, and strong consideration should be given to β-blocker therapy. Very positive studies should proceed to cardiac catheterization.

Options for Management of Patients with Positive Tests

A screening program can be defined as effective if it "identifies disease early in its natural course, which then alters the type or timing of treatment, which in turn must change health outcome."[99] Exercise ECG can identify asymptomatic patients at higher risk for coronary events. The next question becomes: What are our options for management in this higher risk population? Treatment options available for the asymptomatic patient at highest risk for coronary events include risk factor modification, medication, and revascularization with either percutaneous or surgical techniques.

Risk Factor Modification

Risk factor modification has clearly been shown to affect CHD events. This has been demonstrated for smoking cessation,[100] blood pressure control,[101] lipid lowering therapies,[102-104] and exercise.[105] A physician screening a patient with exercise ECG, however, would institute many of these modalities despite the results of the exercise ECG. Smoking cessation, an active lifestyle, and a low-fat, low-cholesterol diet would be *recommended* regardless of the results of the exercise study. The results of the test then do not necessarily alter the "timing" of the treatment. On the other hand, there is evidence that patients with positive exercise ECGs may be more motivated to pursue risk factor modification.[106] In addition, the results of testing might influence the aggressiveness of strategies employed by the physician. A more aggressive smoking cessation program, active encouragement to exercise and maintain ideal body weight, and a more stringent dietary program could be offered. A lower LDL level could be targeted, with a tendency to use medication earlier should dietary therapy fail. This strategy would be supported by recent secondary prevention trials,[103,107,108] which have clearly shown that those with the highest risk for near-term coronary events derive the most benefit from aggressive lipid lowering.

Medical Management

Medications of potential benefit to the asymptomatic, high risk patient include aspirin and β-blocker therapy. There is evidence from the Physicians' Health Study that aspirin therapy, particularly in high risk men, can reduce CHD events.[97] In this study, high risk was defined by clinical variables alone. Since a positive ECG also carries a poorer prognosis, it would be prudent to administer aspirin in this population as well.

β-Blockers clearly improve outcome when administered in the acute[109,110] and convalescent[111-113] period of a myocardial infarction as well as unstable angina.[114] The Atenolol Silent Ischemia Trial (ASIST),[98] a trial designed to assess the effects of treatment with either atenolol or placebo on outcome in 350 patients with silent ischemia, was recently terminated. After 306 patients were enrolled, the data and safety monitoring board discontinued the study because of a significant reduction in clinical events in patients receiving atenolol. All patients had angiographically documented coronary atherosclerosis and exercise and/or ambulatory ECG evidence of silent ischemia. Should these findings be validated in subsequent studies, there would be a compelling reason to identify asymptomatic patients with ischemia.

Revascularization

Potential benefits of revascularization in the asymptomatic population include improved survival and/or prevention of nonfatal infarction. However, randomized trials assessing the relative benefits of coronary artery bypass grafting (CABG) and medical therapy did not include asymptomatic patients. The Coronary Artery Surgery Study (CASS) showed that patients with left main disease[95] or triple-vessel disease with depressed left ventricular function had prolonged survival with revascularization.[96] Whether asymptomatic patients with similar coronary anatomy will derive the same benefit is not clear. In the recently completed Asymptomatic Cardiac Ischemia Pilot (ACIP) study, patients with documented coronary atherosclerosis and silent ischemia were randomized to revascularization versus medical therapy.[115] At 12 weeks, fewer patients in the revascularization group had silent ischemia or angina. At 1-year follow-up, significantly fewer deaths and nonfatal infarctions occurred in patients assigned to the revascularization strategy. This benefit was largely due to the result of bypass surgery. Of note, no randomized study has shown percutaneous revascularization to reduce the risk of "hard" CHD events: fatal and nonfatal infarction or sudden cardiac death.

In summary, the results of a screening exercise ECG could potentially alter the timing of treatment, which in turn could affect outcome. The nature of risk factor modification, the type of medication(s) prescribed, and the recommendation for revascularization may all be influenced by results of the test. In 1987, an ACC/AHA task force concluded that screening of asymptomatic males with two or more risk factors was frequently performed, but that there was a divergence of opinion with respect to its value and propriety.[75] Incorporation of newer data concerning risk factor modification and other treatment modalities could affect the consensus on this issue.

Cost and Cost Effectiveness

A screening program can be labeled effective if it leads to improvement in health outcome. To be cost effective, it must achieve this goal while minimizing costs. A formal cost-effective analysis of screening with exercise testing was performed by Sox and colleagues,[116] and a decision model was constructed to compare screening versus not screening (Fig. 6-5). Prognosis was determined by the extent of angiographically defined disease and left ventricular dysfunction. From the decision tree, it can be seen that patients with positive exercise studies proceeded to undergo coronary arteriography, and those found to have severe coronary disease were offered surgery. The authors assumed the benefits of surgery in this anatomically defined, but asymptomatic, high risk group were the same as the benefits seen in the symptomatic patients studied in the CASS trial. Costs included exercise ECG testing, coronary arteriography for those with positive studies, and surgical costs. Analysis showed that screening the average 60-year-old male would increase life expectancy by 12 days. Cost effectiveness was approximately $80,000 per year of life saved for a 40-year-old male, and $24,600 per year of life saved for a 60-year-old male. Many of the authors' assumptions, however, favored screening, so the actual cost effectiveness may be lower.

Whether revascularizing an asymptomatic individual with severe CAD will improve outcome is a matter of controversy. Most would agree that this is the case for left main disease or triple-vessel disease with left ventricular dysfunction, but this represents a small subset of screened individuals. A study of 298 asymptomatic aircrew who had arteriography because of ECG findings revealed none with left main disease or triple-vessel disease with depressed left ventricular function.[117] It is unlikely, then, that screening *solely* to identify patients with high risk anatomy who would then undergo CABG represents a cost-effective strategy. A more viable strategy might be to identify the high risk patient through use of a combination of conventional risk factors and exercise ECG findings. Patients with a probability of coronary events above a chosen cutoff could be targeted for aggressive risk factor modification. This strategy would be supported, at least in terms of effectiveness, by the findings in the MRFIT study.[31] As noted ear-

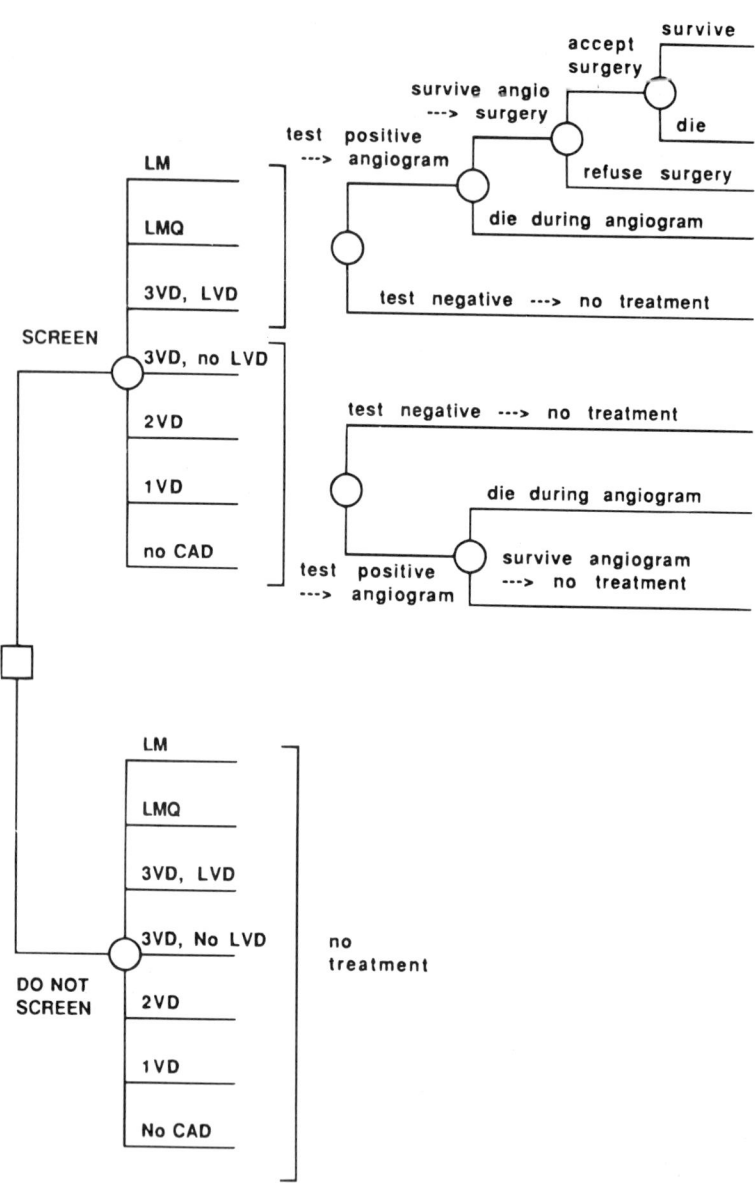

Fig. 6-5. Decision tree used in cost-effectiveness analysis by Sox and colleagues. This model is for screening in asymptomatic persons. Squares represent decision nodes, circles represent chance nodes. Surgery is offered only if the angiogram shows severe coronary artery disease (CAD). LM, stenosis of the left main coronary artery; LMQ, left main equivalent CAD; 3VD, 2VD, and 1VD, triple-vessel, double-vessel, and single-vessel CAD (without left main stenosis), respectively; LVD, left ventricular dysfunction (35% to 50% ejection fraction measured in patients at rest); angio, angiography. (From Sox et al.,[116] with permission.)

lier, high risk patients in this study, defined on the basis of their exercise ECG results, sustained a dramatic reduction in coronary events through a risk factor modification program. The costs associated with this program were not delineated, so cost-effectiveness cannot be determined. It has been shown that aggressive lipid lowering strategies applied to those at highest risk for coronary events is both effective[103,104] and cost effective.[118] Whether incorporating exercise testing into conventional risk assessment is also cost effective remains to be determined.

SUMMARY

Coronary atherosclerosis is extremely prevalent in Western populations. The majority of patients with atherosclerosis are asymptomatic. Exercise testing is a proven method to stratify these patients in terms of their risk for future coronary events. The absolute risk for future events is related to a combination of conventional risk factors and stress testing parameters. Stress testing may have value in individuals with one or more conventional risk factors to guide pharmacologic, nonpharmacologic, and, rarely, surgical therapies. However, a higher *absolute* number of events has been shown to occur in patients with normal exercise studies. This is due to the unpredictable nature of coronary events, a reflection of the fact that both flow-limiting and non-flow-limiting lesions can undergo plaque rupture. An anatomic approach using modalities that can detect both flow-limiting and non-flow-limiting disease may augment the prognostic value of exercise testing.

REFERENCES

1. Enos WF, Holmes RH, Beyer J. Coronary disease among United States soldiers killed in action in Korea: preliminary report. JAMA 152:1090, 1953
2. McNamara JJ, Molot MA, Stremple JF, Cutting RT: Coronary artery disease in combat casualties in Vietnam. JAMA 216:1185, 1971
3. Holman RL, McGill HC Jr, Strong JP et al: The natural history of atherosclerosis: The early aortic lesions as seen in New Orleans in the middle of the 20th century. Am J Pathol 34:209, 1958
4. Strong JP, McGill HC Jr: The natural history of coronary atherosclerosis. Am J Pathol 40:37, 1962
5. Strong JP, McGill HC Jr, Tejada C et al: The natural history of atherosclerosis: Comparisons of the early aortic lesions in New Orleans, Guatemala and Costa Rica. Am J Pathol 34:731, 1958
6. Stemmermann GN, Steer A, Rhoads GG et al: A comparative pathology study of myocardial lesions and atherosclerosis in Japanese men living in Hiroshima, Japan and Honolulu, Hawaii. Lab Invest 34:592, 1976
7. McGill HC Jr: The Geographic Pathology of Atherosclerosis. Williams & Wilkins, Baltimore, 1968
8. Strong JP, McGill HC Jr: Pediatric aspects of atherosclerosis. J Atheroscl Res 9:25, 1969
9. Strong JP: Coronary atherosclerosis in soldiers: a clue to the natural history of atherosclerosis in the young. JAMA 256:2863, 1986
10. The PDAY Research Group: Relationship of atherosclerosis in young men to serum lipoprotein cholesterol concentrations and smoking. JAMA 264:3018, 1990
11. Stary HC: Evolution of atherosclerotic plaques in the coronary arteries of young adults. Arteriosclerosis 3:471, 1983
12. Muller JE, Toffler GH, Stone PH: Circadian variation and triggers of onset of acute cardiovascular disease. Circulation 79:733, 1989
13. American Heart Association 1990 Heart Facts: American Heart Association National Center, Dallas, 1990
14. American Heart Association 1993 Heart and Stroke Facts and Statistics. American Heart Association, 1992
15. Zir LM, Miller SW, Dinsmore RE et al: Interobserver variability in coronary angiography. Circulation 53:627, 1976
16. Reiber JHC, Serruys PW, Kooijman CJ et al: Assessment of short-, medium-, and long-term variations in arterial dimensions from computer assisted quantitation of coronary cineangiograms. Circulation 71:280, 1985
17. Crouse JR, Thompson CJ: Evaluation of methods for quantifying lumen stenosis andatherosclerosis. Circulation, suppl. 2:17, 1993
18. Ambrose JA, Tannenbaum MA, Alexopoulos D et al: Angiographic progression of coronary artery disease and the development of myocardial infarction. J Am Coll Cardiol 12:56, 1988
19. Brown G, Albers JJ, Fisher LD et al: Regression of coronary artery disease as a result of intensive lipid-lowering therapy in men with high levels of apolipoprotein B. N Engl J Med 323:1289, 1990
20. Watts GF, Lewis B, Brunt JNH et al: Effects on coronary artery disease of lipid lowering diet, or diet plus cholestyramine, in the St. Thomas Atherosclerosis Regression Study (STARS). Lancet 339:563, 1992
21. Levine GN, Kearey JF, Vita JA. Cholesterol reduction

21. in cardiovascular disease: clinical benefits and possible mechanisms. N Engl J Med 332:512, 1995
22. Vita JA, Treasure CB, Nabel EG et al: Coronary vasomotor response to acetylcholine relates to risk factors for coronary artery disease. Circulation 81:491, 1990
23. Ludmer PL, Selwyn AP, Shook TL et al: Paradoxical vasoconstriction induced by acetylcholine in atherosclerotic coronary arteries. N Engl J Med 315:1046, 1986
24. Ellis S, Alderman E, Cain V et al: Prediction of risk of anterior myocardal infarction by lesion severity and measurement method of stenosis in the left anterior descending coronary distribution: a CASS Registry study. J Am Coll Cardiol 11:908, 1988
25. Mock MB, Ringqvist I, Fisher LD et al: Survival of medically treated patients in the Coronary Artery Surgery Study (CASS) Registry. Circulation 66:562, 1982
26. Weiner DA, Ryan TJ, McCabe CH et al: Prognostic importance of a clinical profile and exercise test in medically treated patients with coronary artery disease. J Am Coll Cardiol 3:772, 1984
27. Weiner DA, Ryan TJ, McCabe CH et al: Value of exercise testing in determining the risk classification and the response to coronary artery bypass grafting in three vessel coronary artery disease: a report from the CASS Registry. Am J Cardiol 60:262, 1987
28. Severi S, Orsini E, Marracini P et al: The basal electrocardiogram and the exercise stress test in assessing prognosis in patients with unstable angina. Eur Heart J 9:441, 1988
29. Froelicher VF, Perdue S, Pewer W, Risch M: Application of meta-analysis using an electronic spread sheet to exercise testing in patients after myocardial infarction. Am J Med 93:1045, 1987
30. Froelicher VF, Thompson AJ, Longo MR et al: Value of exercise testing for screening asymptomatic men for latent coronary artery disease. Prog Cardiovasc Dis 3:887, 1984
31. Risk Factor Intervention Trial Research Group: Exercise electrocardiogram and coronary heart disease mortality in the Multiple Risk Factor Intervention Trial. Am J Cardiol 55:16, 1985
32. Bruce RA, DeRouen TA, Hossack KF: Value of maximal exercise tests in risk assessment of primary coronary heart disease events in healthy men: five years experience of the Seattle Heart Watch Study. Am J Cardiol 46:371, 1980
33. Giagnoni E, Secchi MB, Wu SC et al: Prognostic value of exercise testing in asymptomatic normotensive subjects. a prospective matched study. N Engl J Med 309: 1085, 1983
34. Gordon DJ, Ekelund LG, Karon JM et al: Predictive value of the exercise tolerance test for mortality in North American men: the Lipid Research Clinics mortality follow-up study. Circulation 74:252, 1986
35. Rautaharju PM, Prineas RJ, Fifler WJ et al: Prognostic value of exercise electrocardiogram in men at high risk of future coronary heart disease: Multiple Risk Factor Intervention Trial experience. J Am Coll Cardiol 8:1, 1986
36. McHenry PL, O'Donell J, Morris SN, Jordan JJ: The abnormal exercise electrocardiogram in apparently healthy men: a predictor of angina pectoris as an initial coronary event during long-term follow-up. Circulation 70:547, 1984
37. Okin PM, Anderson KM, Levy D, Kligfield P: Heart rate adjustment of exercise-induced ST segment depression: improved risk stratification in the Framingham Offspring Study. Circulation 83:866, 1991
38. Bruce RA, Hossack KF, DeRouen TA, Hofer V. Enhanced risk assessment for primary coronary heart disease events by maximal exercise testing: 10 years' experience of Seattle Heart Watch. J Am Coll Cardiol 2:565, 1983
39. Allen WH, Aronow WS, Goodman P, Stinson P: Five-year follow-up of maximal treadmill stress test in asymptomatic men and women. Circulation 62:522, 1980
40. Fleg JL, Gerstenblith G, Zonderman AB et al: Prevalence and prognostic significance of exercise-induced silent myocardial ischemia detected by thallium scintigraphy and electrocardiography in asymptomatic volunteers. Circulation 81:428, 1990
41. Uren NG, Melin JA, De Bruyne B et al: Relation between myocardial blood flow and the severity of coronary artery stenosis. N Engl J Med 330:1782, 1994
42. Detrano R, Lyons KP, Marcondes G et al: Methodologic problems in exercise testing research: are we solving them? Arch Intern Med 148:1289, 1988
43. Philbrick JT, Horwitz RI, Feinstein AR: Methodologic problems of exercise testing for coronary artery disease: groups, analysis, and bias. Am J Cardiol 46:807, 1980
44. Detrano R, Gianrossi R, Mulvihill D, Lehmann K et al: Exercise-induced ST segment depression in the diagnosis of multivessel coronary disease: a meta analysis. J Am Coll Cardiol 14:1501, 1989
45. Ransohoff DF, Feinstein AR: Problems of spectrum and bias in evaluating the efficacy of diagnostic tests. N Engl J Med 299:926, 1978
46. Detrano R, Janosi A, Lyons K, Marcondes G et al: Factors affecting sensitivity and specificity of a diagnostic test: the exercise thallium scintigram. Am J Med 84:699, 1988

47. Erikssen J, Enge I, Forfang R, Storstein D: False positive diagnostic tests of coronary angiographic findings in 105 presumably healthy males. Circulation 54: 371, 1976
48. Hopkirck JA, Uhl GS, Hickman JR Jr et al: Discriminate value of clinical and exercise variables in detecting significant coronary artery disease in asymptomatic men. J Am Coll Cardiol 3:887, 1984
49. Hamby RI, Davison ET, Hilsenrath J et al: Functional and anatomic correlates of markedly abnormal stress tests. J Am Coll Cardiol 3:1375, 1984
50. Blumenthal DS, Weiss JL, Mellits ED, Gerstenblith G: The predictive value of a strongly positive stress test in patients with minimal symptoms. Am J Med 70: 1005, 1981
51. Epstein SE, Quyyumi AA, Bonow RO: Sudden cardiac death without warning: possible mechanisms and implications for screening asymptomatic populations. N Engl J Med 321:320, 1989
52. Simoons ML: Optimal measurements for detection of coronary artery disease by exercise ECG. Comput Biomed Res 10:483, 1977
53. Kligfield P, Ameisen O, Okin PM: Heart rate adjustment of ST segment depression for improved detection of coronary artery disease. Circulation 79:245, 1989
54. Haraphongse M, Kappagoda T, Tymchak W, Rossal RE: The value of sum of ST segment depression in 12 lead electrocardiogram in relation to change in heart rate during exercise to predict the extent of coronary artery disease. Cardiovasc Med 2:64, 1986
55. Deckers JW, Rensing BJ, Tijssen JGP et al: A comparison of methods of analyzing exercise tests for diagnosis of coronary artery disease. Br Heart J 62:438, 1989
56. Lachterman B, Lehmann KG, Detrano R et al: Comparison of ST segment/heart rate index to standard ST criteria for analysis of exercise electrocardiogram. Circulation 82:44, 1990
57. Thwaites BC, Quyyumi AA, Raphael MJ et al: Comparison of the ST/heart rate slope with the modified Bruce exercise test in the detection of coronary artery disease. Am J Cardiol 57:554, 1986
58. Josephson RA, Shefrin E, Flegg JL: Is conversion from negative to positive exercise ECG a specific marker for future coronary events in asymptomatic subjects?, abstracted. Circulation, suppl. 2:246, 1988
59. Detrano R, Gianrossi R, Froelicher V: The diagnostic accuracy of the exercise electrocardiogram: a meta-analysis of 22 years of research. Prog Cardiovasc Dis 32:173, 1989
60. Fletcher GF, Froehlicher VF, Hartley LH et al: Exercise standards: a statement for health professionals from the American Heart Association. Circulation 82: 2286, 1990
61. Tavel MB: Specificity of electrocardiogram stress test in women versus men. Am J Cardiol 70:545, 1992
62. Morise AP, Dalal JN, Devaul RD: Frequency of oral estrogen replacement therapy in women with normal and abnormal exercise electrocardiograms and normal coronary arteries by angiogram. Am J Cardiol 72:1197, 1993
63. Colucci WS, Gimbrone MA, McLaughlin MK et al: Increased vascular catecholamine sensitivity and alpha-adrenergic affinity in female and estrogen-treated male rats. Circ Res 50:805, 1982
64. Froelicher VF Jr, Thomas MM, Pillow C, Lancaster MC: Epidemiologic study of asymptomatic men screened by maximal treadmill testing for latent coronary artery disease. Am J Cardiol 34:770, 1974
65. Cumming GR, Samm J, Borysyk L, Kich L: Electrocardiographic changes during exercise in asymptomatic men: 3-year follow-up. CMA 112:578, 1975
66. Convertino V, Hung J, Goldwater D et al: Cardiovascular responses to exercise in middle-aged man after 10 days of bedrest. Circulation 65:134, 1982
67. Shepard RJ: Tests of maximum oxygen uptake—a critical review. Sports Med 1:99, 1984
68. Froelicher VF, Brammell H, Davis G et al: A comparison of the reproducibility and physiological response to three maximal treadmill protocols. Chest 65:512, 1974
69. Robinson S: Experimental studies of physical fitness in relation to age. Arbeitsphysiologie 10:251, 1939
70. Niederberger M, Kusumi BF, Whitkanack S: Disparities in ventilatory and circulatory responses to bicycle and treadmill exercise. Br Heart J 36:377, 1974
71. Wasserman K, Hansen JE, Sue DY, Whipp BJ: Principles of Exercise Testing and Interpretation. Lea & Febiger, Philadelphia, 1987
72. Detrano R, Froelicher VF: Exercise testing: uses and limitations considering recent studies. Prog Cardiovasc Dis 31:173, 1988
73. Patterson J, Naughton J, Pietra R: Treadmill exercise in the assessment of the functional capacity of patients with cardiac disease. Am J Cardiol 30:757, 1972
74. Astrand PO, Rodahl K: Testbook of Work Physiology: Physiological Bases of Exercise. McGraw-Hill, New York, 1977
75. ACC/AHA Task Force: Guidelines for exercise testing. J Am Coll Cardiol 8:725, 1986
76. Loecker TH, Schwartz RS, Cotta CW, Hickman JR: Fluoroscopic coronary artery calcification and associ-

ated coronary disease in asymptomatic young men. J Am Coll Cardiol 19:1167, 1992
77. US NHLBI. Framingham Study: An Epidemiological Investigation of Cardiovascular Disease. Section 37. U.S. Department of Commerce, National Bureau of Information Services, 1987
78. Davies MJ, Thomas A: Thombosis and acute coronary-artery lesions in sudden cardiac ischemic death. N Engl J Med 310:1137, 1984
79. Gorlin R, Fuster V, Ambrose JA: Anatomic-physiologic links between acute coronary syndromes. Circulation 74:6, 1986
80. Davies MJ, Thomas AC: Plaque fissuring—the cause of acute myocardial infarction, sudden ischaemic death, and crescendo angina. Br Heart J 53:363, 1985
81. Fuster V, Steele PM, Chesebro JH: Role of platelets and thrombosis in coronary atherosclerotic disease and sudden death. J Am Coll Cardiol 5:175B, 1985
82. Blankenhorn D: Coronary arterial calcification, a review. Am J Med Sci July:1, 1961
83. Arnett EN, Isner JM, Redwood DR et al: Coronary artery narrowing in coronary heart disease: comparison of cineangiographic and necropsy findings. Ann Intern Med 91:350, 1979
84. Detrano RC, Wong ND, Tang W et al: Prognostic significance of cardiac cinefluoroscopy for coronary calcific deposits in asymptomatic high risk subjects. J Am Coll Cardiol 24:354, 1994
85. Hamby R, Tabrah E, Wisoff K, Hartstein J: Coronary artery calcification: clinical implications and angiographic correlates. Am Heart J 87:565, 1974
86. Bartel A, Chen J, Peter R et al: The significance of coronary calcification detected by fluoroscopy: a report of 360 patients. Circulation 49:1247, 1974
87. Aldrich R, Brensike J, Battaglini J et al: Coronary calcifications in the detection of coronary artery disease and comparison with electrocardiographic exercise testing. Results from the NHLBI's Type II Coronary Intervention Study. Circulation 59:1113, 1979
88. Margolis J, Chen J, Kong Y et al: The diagnostic and prognostic significance of coronary artery calcification: a report of 800 cases. Radiology 137:609, 1980
89. Hung J, Chaitman B, Lam J et al: Noninvasive diagnostic test choices for the evaluation of coronary artery disease in women: a multivariate comparison of cardiac fluoroscopy, exercise ECG and exercise thallium myocardial perfusion scintigraphy. J Am Coll Cardiol 4:8, 1984
90. Carboni L, Celli M, D'Ermo A et al: Combined cardiac cinefluoroscopy, exercise testing and ambulatory ST-segment monitoring in the diagnosis of coronary artery disease: a report of 104 symptomatic patients. Int J Cardiol 9:91, 1985
91. Detrano R, Salcedo E, Hobbs R, Yiannikis J: Cardiac cinefluoroscopy as an inexpensive aid in the diagnosis of coronary artery disease. Am J Cardiol 57:1041, 1986
92. Uretsky B, Rifkin R, Sharma S, Reddy P: Value of fluoroscopy in the detection of coronary stenosis: influence of age, sex and number of vessels calcified on diagnostic efficacy. Am Heart J 115:323, 1988
93. Lie JT, Hammond PI: Pathology of the senescent heart: anatomic observations of 237 autopsy studies of patients 90 to 105 years old. Mayo Clinic Proc 63:552, 1988
94. Agatston AS, Janowitz WR, Hildner FJ et al: Quantification of coronary artery calcium using ultrafast computed tomography. J Am Coll Cardiol 15:827, 1990
95. Chaitman BP, Fisher LD, Bourassa MG: Effect of coronary bypass surgery on survival patterns in subsets of patients with left main coronary artery disease: report of the Collaborative Study in Coronary Artery Surgery (CASS). Am J Cardiol 48:765, 1981
96. Alderman EL, Bourassa MG, Cohen LS et al: Ten-year follow-up of survival and myocardial infarction in the randomized coronary artery surgery study. Circulation 82:1629, 1990
97. Steering Committee of the Physicians' Health Study Group: Final report on the aspirin component of the ongoing physicians' health study. N Engl J Med 321:129, 1989
98. Pepine CJ, Cohn PF, Deedwania PC et al: Effects of treatment on outcome in mildly symptomatic patients with ischemia during daily life: the Atenolol Silent Ischemia Study (ASIST). Circulation 90:762, 1994
99. Eddy DM: Assessing Health Practices and Designing Practice Policy: The Explicit Approach. American College of Physicians, Philadelphia, 1992
100. Kannel WB: Hypertension, blood lipids, and cigarette smoking as co-risk factors for coronary heart disease. Ann NY Acad Sci 304:128, 1978
101. Trap-Jensen J: Effects of smoking on the heart and peripheral circulation. Am Heart J 115:263, 1988
102. Manninen V, Elo MO, Frick L: Lipid alterations and decline in the incidence of coronary heart disease in the Helsinki Heart Study. JAMA 260:641, 1988
103. Scandinavian Simvastatin Survival Study Group: Randomised trial of cholesterol lowering in 4444 patients with coronary heart disease: The Scandinavian Simvastatin Survival Study (4S). Lancet 344:1383, 1994
104. Canner PL, Berge KG, Wenger NK et al: Fifteen year mortality in the Coronary Drug Project patients: long-

term benefit with niacin. J Am Coll Cardiol 8:1245, 1986
105. Blair SN, Kohl HW, Paffenberger RS Jr et al: Physical fitness and all-cause mortality. A prospective study of healthy men and women. JAMA 262:2395, 1989
106. Bruce RA, DeRouen TA, Hossack KF: Pilot study examining the motivational effects of maximal exercise testing to modify risk factors and health habits. Cardiology 66:111, 1980
107. Coronary Drug Project Research Group: Clofibrate niacin in coronary heart disease. JAMA 231:360, 175
108. Buchwald H, Varco RL, Matts JP et al: Effect of partial ileal bypass surgery on mortality and morbidity from coronary heart disease in patients with hypercholesterolemia: report of the Program on the Surgical Control of the Hyperlipidemic (POSCH). N Engl J Med 323:946, 1990
109. ISIS-1 (First International Study of Infarct Survival) Collaborative Group: Randomized trial of intravenous atenolol among 16,027 cases of suspected acute myocardial infarction. Lancet 2:57, 1986
110. Roberts R, Rogers WJ, Mueller HS et al: Immediate versus deferred B-blockade following thrombolytic therapy in patients with acute myocardial infarction: results of the Thrombolysis in Myocardial Infarction (TIMI) II-B Study. Circulation 83:422, 1991
111. Roberts R, Croft C, Gold HK, et al: Effect of propranolol on myocardial infarct size in a randomized blinded multicenter trial. N Engl J Med 311:218, 1984
112. Hjalmarson A, Herlitz J, Malek L et al: Effect on mortality of metroprolol in acute myocardial infarction. Lancet 2:823, 1981
113. Beta Blocker Heart Attack Study Group: The beta blocker heart attack trial. JAMA 246:2073, 1981
114. Hint Research Group: Early treatment of unstable angina in the coronary care unit: a randomized, double-blind, placebo-controlled comparison of recurrent ischaemia in patients treated with nifedipine or metroprolol or both. Br Heart J 56:400, 1986
115. Knatterud GL, Bourassa MG, Pepine CJ et al: Effects of treatment strategies to suppress ischemia in patients with coronary artery disease: 12-week results of the Asymptomatic Cardiac Ischemia Pilot (ACIP) Study. J Am Coll Cardiol 24:10, 1994
116. Sox HC, Littenberg B, Garber AM: The role of exercise testing in screening for coronary artery disease. Ann Intern Med 110:456, 1989
117. Froelicher VF Jr, Thompson AJ, Wolthuis R et al: Angiographic findings in asymptomatic aircrewman with electrocardiographic abnormalities. Am J Cardiol 39:32, 1977
118. Goldman L, Weinstein MC, Goldman PA, Williams LW: Cost-effectiveness of HMG-CoA reductase inhibition for primary and secondary prevention of coronary heart disease. JAMA 265:1145, 1991

Chapter 7

Diagnosis of CAD in Women: Multivariate Approaches to Stress Testing

Annie R. Robert

Exercise electrocardiographic (ECG) testing began with the observation of abnormal downsloping ST depression and T-wave inversion in the ECG of 3 male patients experiencing anginal attacks after climbing the stairs to a physician's office in 1928.[1] Despite innumerable controversies in the literature about its diagnostic value, this technique has stood the test of time. It remains the most widely used noninvasive diagnostic test for coronary artery disease (CAD) in patients referred for evaluation of chest pain.[2]

BAYES THEOREM AND THE INFLUENCE OF GENDER

The importance of pretest CAD probability on post-test probability in the presence of a positive or negative test result has been discussed by Pashkow in Chapter 1 on exercise ECG testing. The probabilistic approach to CAD diagnosis is based upon this relationship. However, the calculation of pretest probability is more accurate in men than women, due to the difficulties posed by symptom evaluation in this group. Thus, in the Framingham Study, the incidence of uncomplicated angina pectoris was disproportionately represented in women, being more frequent than myocardial infarction. Moreover, angiographic studies have shown that more than 50% of women presenting with chest pain and referred for catheterization have no significant coronary lesions. For these reasons, many clinicians believe that the symptom of chest pain in women is unreliable.

Clinicians also have less confidence in a positive stress test response in a woman than the same response in a man. This reflects the ambiguity of chest pain as a diagnostic guide in women, the lower prevalence of CAD, and the higher false-positive fraction observed with the use of male-specific noninvasive test criteria for CAD. The perceived low pretest CAD probability has been believed to be responsible for a sex-related bias in the management of women with suspected or even proven CAD.[3-6] However, recent studies[7,8] have suggested that the higher coronary heart disease mortality in women might be the result of a gender-based referral bias, since women are catheterized half as often as men with equivalent results of noninvasive tests and women are revascularized at a later stage in their disease than men.

ASPECTS OF EXERCISE TEST INTERPRETATION PERTINENT TO A MULTIVARIATE MODEL

The advent of computers and the statistical tools have allowed many refinements in the diagnostic criteria for exercise testing. While there has been some debate about the merits of automated interpretation, summarized previously, computer-assisted exercise ECG measurements had greater than 90% reliability in one study, while visual measurements had only about 70% reliability.[9]

Exercise variables other than the ST segment are of diagnostic value. The use of these data permits development of a multivariate score, which can enhance the diagnostic value of exercise stress testing in both men and in women. An important constituent of these scores is the ST-segment heart rate, (ST/HR) index, notwithstanding the debate about the diagnostic value of this in the current literature. The various available computerized measurements can be integrated in a gender-specific multivariate diagnostic algorithm in both men and women.

The use of a probabilistic approach formalizes the physician's use of non-ECG cues pertaining to test positivity. For example, the likelihood of disease can be expected to be greater if exercise-induced ST depression is 0.2 mV than if it is 0.1 mV. By combining this and other continuous variables, a score reflecting the global probability of coronary disease can be calculated. The main advantage of this approach is its reliability—because it is not observer dependent, there is no need for a clinician to be an expert in exercise stress testing interpretation. Moreover, these likelihood ratios depend only upon computerized exercise variables, which may be used irrespective of the clinical status of the patient, which only alter the physician's estimation of pretest probability. After combination of pretest likelihood with the likelihood ratio derived from the study, the choice to perform other noninvasive tests in a particular patient depends upon the physician's confidence in the assessment of post-test probability.

Exercise ST-Segment Analysis
Accuracy of ST-Segment Changes

Myocardial ischemia has traditionally been defined as the development of horizontal or downsloping ST-segment depression of at least 0.1 mV, 60 ms after the J point on the ECG at maximal exercise. Because myocardial ischemia is related to the presence of a reduced coronary flow reserve,[10,11] ECG evidence of ischemia has been used for predicting an anatomical stenosis of at least 50% in at least one coronary vessel, which is the definition of CAD.[12] The diagnostic value of this at least 0.1 mV stress-induced ST-segment depression has been studied by numerous investigators,[13] but, as discussed already by Pashkow (see Ch. 1) little agreement has been reached. Indeed, only 35% of the variability in the reported accuracy of ST analysis was explained by the data reported in the literature, mainly because of incomplete reporting of potentially important data (such as gender distribution). Nonetheless, the reported sensitivity of 68% in a prominent meta-analysis leads the relevance of conventional ST analysis for detecting CAD to be questioned.

Influence of Gender on the Accuracy of the Stress ECG

Most studies on the diagnostic value of exercise testing have reported the proportion of men in their population, but results are seldom split into subgroups of men and women. However, it is widely acknowledged that many ECG parameters differ between men and women, and, indeed, differentiation between the resting ECGs of normal male and female subjects begins quite early in life. In a study[14] of the quantitative computerized analysis of the Frank orthogonal ECG of 1,317 normal infants, children, and teenagers, sex-related differences were the most marked for ST-T amplitudes and orientations. In adults, the sex differences in normal ECG remain striking. Macfarlane and Lawrie[15] reported that all wave amplitudes were lower in women and repolarization abnormalities were more frequently observed in women, especially in the inferior leads and in the right precordial leads with the 12-lead ECG. Those differences were confirmed in the orthogonal ECG of normal women as compared to normal men[16] women had a more superiorly and posteriorly directed J point and ST segment.[17] Chapter 1 discusses the accuracy of exercise ECG testing in women—a trend toward higher frequency of ST depression in women has been demonstrated in large clinical trials and epidemiologic studies when sex-specific criteria were not considered.[18]

Some of the ST-T changes in women have been attributed to specific conditions that have been considered to be more prevalent in women, such as the hyperventilation syndrome (which can modify the whole repolarization process), or electrolyte and ionic disturbances. Changes in electrode position due to the breast has also been suspected to play a role. Sex-related differences in the exercise ECG have been described in healthy subjects.[19] With increasing heart rate and increasing age in women, ST-segment amplitude changes occurred more in the inferiorly oriented lead Y than in the lateral lead X, unrelated to changes in the QRS vectors in the same leads. In our own published data on healthy adults (Table 7-1),[20,21] maximal exercise ECG measurements were less depressed in women than in men, although this may have been influenced by a nonsignificantly lower peak heart rate or target heart rate in healthy women. These intrinsic differences between men and women in the ECG responses to exercise should lead to the conclusion that nonischemic factors are included in this response.

In our published data on patients undergoing coronary angiography,[20,21] presented in the first and second columns of Table 7-1, maximal exercise ECG measurements in CAD patients were compared with those of patients without CAD. The differences between men with and without CAD (expressed as a Z value, derived from the Student's t test), exceeded those between women with and without CAD, for example, the most abnormal ST_{60} segment was 0.09 mV more depressed in men with than men without CAD, while it was only 0.03 mV more depressed in women with than without CAD. These differences could not be explained by the extent of CAD, as multivessel disease had a comparable prevalence in men and women.

Our data also suggest that measurements in lead Y (equivalent to the inferior limb leads in the conventional 12-lead ECG system), and to a lesser degree, lead Z (corresponding to anterior leads), have no diagnostic value in women as compared with men. These observations are in concordance with our findings in healthy women. The most reliable ECG measurement for CAD diagnosis in women was the ST_{60} segment in lead X, whereas in men, this parameter was also relevant, but to the same extent as the most abnormal ST_{60} segment. The most relevant ECG measurement for predicting CAD in men was the ST_{20-60} slope of the most abnormal ST_{60} segment, but this ECG parameter had no diagnostic value in women. These results were explained by more negative exercise ECG measurements in women without significant stenoses than in men without CAD at similar cardiac workloads.

These results suggest that *studies including ECG measurements at rest and/or at exercise should not combine the results of men and women.* Horizontal or downsloping exercise-induced depression of 0.1 mV or greater is a male-specific criterion for predicting CAD. It is less accurate in women not only because of Bayesian considerations,[22] but mainly because of the intrinsic differences between men and women in rest and in exercise-induced ST-segment depression.

Exercise Non-ECG Factors with a Diagnostic Value for CAD

Exercise stress testing provokes the myocardial pathophysiologic sequelae of ischemia which are not limited to the electrical consequences manifest by ST-segment change. The limited diagnostic value of ST analysis reported by Gianrossi and colleagues[13] reflects the shortcomings of using only one of several ischemic markers. In response to this well-recognized problem, there have been attempts to improve the diagnostic value of exercise testing by including non-ST-segment variables in the interpretation of test results. These factors have been briefly mentioned in Chapter 1 and will be discussed in more detail in this section.[23–35]

The improvement of the diagnostic performance of exercise testing by inclusion of non-ECG may renew interest in standard stress testing. Unfortunately, these refinements in the diagnostic criteria for CAD have been derived from studies involving a high percentage of men. When applied to women, these global criteria yielded higher percentages of false-positive and false-negative responses than those expected by using gender-specific criteria.

ST/Heart Rate Relationship

The first non-ECG exercise factor with a diagnostic value for CAD reported in the literature was the exercise heart rate.[23] Through stress-strain diagrams (i.e., plots of ST displacements vs. heart rate during exercise), Bruce and McDonough showed that ST-segment evolution could not be related to the presence of CAD without accounting for the corresponding heart rate. The importance of chronotropic incompetence and the use of various heart rate-corrected criteria have been introduced by in Chapter 1.

In 1979, Barolsky and colleagues[24] observed that

Table 7-1 Maximal Bicycle Ergometer Exercise Data and Diagnostic Value in Catheterized Patients Only[a]

	CAD		No CAD		Z Test		Healthy	
	Men (N = 230)	Women (N = 56)	Men (N = 54)	Women (N = 79)	Men	Women	Men (N = 103)	Women (N = 76)
Maximal exercise ECG measurements								
ST_{60} segment in lead X (mV)	−0.14 ± 0.11	−0.14 ± 0.09	−0.04 ± 0.09	−0.10 ± 0.07	6.2[b]	3.0[c]	0.07 ± 0.13	−0.00 ± 0.08
ST_{60} segment in lead Y (mV)	−0.06 ± 0.07	−0.07 ± 0.06	−0.02 ± 0.07	−0.07 ± 0.08	3.7[b]	0.5	0.03 ± 0.08	−0.01 ± 0.07
ST_{60} segment in lead Z (mV)	0.04 ± 0.09	0.02 ± 0.09	0.06 ± 0.06	0.01 ± 0.05	2.7[c]	1.2	0.12 ± 0.11	0.05 ± 0.07
ST_{80} segment in lead X (mV)	−0.11 ± 0.13	−0.12 ± 0.11	0.01 ± 0.12	−0.08 ± 0.08	6.0[b]	2.8[c]	0.18 ± 0.18	0.08 ± 0.12
ST_{80} segment in lead Y (mV)	−0.04 ± 0.09	−0.06 ± 0.08	0.01 ± 0.09	−0.05 ± 0.07	3.4[b]	0.5	0.09 ± 0.11	0.04 ± 0.09
ST_{80} segment in lead Z (mV)	0.07 ± 0.11	0.04 ± 0.11	0.11 ± 0.10	0.02 ± 0.06	2.2[d]	1.5	0.17 ± 0.15	0.10 ± 0.09
Most abnormal ST_{60} segment (mV)	−0.15 ± 0.10	−0.14 ± 0.09	−0.06 ± 0.08	−0.11 ± 0.06	6.2[b]	2.6[c]	0.00 ± 0.08	−0.03 ± 0.07
Most abnormal ΔST_{60} segment (mV)	−0.13 ± 0.09	−0.11 ± 0.08	−0.04 ± 0.07	−0.08 ± 0.05	6.0[b]	2.9[c]	0.00 ± 0.08	−0.03 ± 0.07
Most abnormal ST_{20-60} slope (mV)	0.50 ± 0.75	0.35 ± 0.53	1.07 ± 0.76	0.72 ± 0.63	6.9[b]	0.5	1.83 ± 1.13	1.68 ± 1.05
Maximal exercise non-ECG measurements								
Work load (W)	147 ± 41	106 ± 30	193 ± 45	130 ± 23	7.1[b]	5.2[b]	243 ± 79	145 ± 28
Heart rate (beats/min)	133 ± 23	135 ± 24	154 ± 23	156 ± 22	6.2[b]	5.1[b]	176 ± 16	171 ± 20
Achieved heart rate (%)	79 ± 13	82 ± 13	90 ± 12	92 ± 13	5.4[b]	4.3[b]	99 ± 8	97 ± 11
Heart rate change (beats/min)	54 ± 19	52 ± 22	74 ± 22	69 ± 19	6.4[b]	4.7[b]	91 ± 20	84 ± 20
Systolic blood pressure (mm Hg)	184 ± 29	179 ± 31	194 ± 31	190 ± 29	1.9	1.7	218 ± 25	187 ± 28
Angina-limited exercise (%)	58	46	13	15	6.3[b]	4.2[b]	0	0

Abbreviations: CAD, coronary artery disease; ECG, electrocardiogram; SD, standard deviation.
[a] Values are mean ± SD.
[b] $p < 0.001$.
[c] $p < 0.01$.
[d] $p < 0.05$ CAD vs. no CAD.

even in patients with similar prevalence rates of CAD, the positive predictive value of ST-segment depression was significantly higher in men than in women (77% vs. 47%, $p < 0.05$). Authors, therefore, introduced an exercise score with different ST-segment weights for men and for women. Using simple algebraic calculations, the Barolsky score can be expressed as follows:

1. If the ST segment is greater than -0.1 mV, heart rate is considered regardless of the patient gender. If peak heart rate is less than 132 beats/min, the likelihood ratio for CAD is greater than 1, and CAD is more likely to be present if there is no prior (clinical) knowledge.
2. If the ST segment is less than -0.1 mV, a peak heart rate cut off is set to 199 beats/min for males and 167 beats/min for females. The likelihood ratio for CAD is greater than 1 for an observed peak heart rate lower than those gender-related cutpoints.

The distinction between ST-segment weights in men and in women also means that at the same peak heart rate, an ST-segment depression greater than 0.1 mV has a likelihood ratio for CAD lower in a woman than in a man. With a peak heart rate of 170 beats/min, for example, the likelihood ratio for CAD is greater than 1 if ST-segment depression is greater than 0.1 mV for a man but is less than 1 for a woman. These differences in ECG response to exercise of women and men were described as a "non-Bayesian factor" by Barolsky and colleagues.[24]

In 1980, Elamin and colleagues[25] proposed an exercise interpretation that could predict the severity of CAD, and the generation of "heart rate adjustment of ST-segment depression" was born. Two methods of heart rate adjustment of ST-segment depression have evolved. The simplest one is the ST/HR index[26] which is the ratio between the maximal exercise-induced ST-segment change from rest and the maximal exercise-induced heart rate change from rest. The second method, the ST/HR slope,[27] is based on linear regressions of ST segment on heart rate during exercise stages; from the end of exercise to progressively earlier intermediate stage data, linear regressions of ST on heart rate are computed and the highest (if the negative sign is ignored) significant slope is retained within each lead except aVR, aVL, and V_1. ST/HR slope is the maximum (if the negative sign is ignored) slope over all considered leads. Absolute ST/HR index should, theoretically, be less than absolute ST/HR slope if one assumes that the relationship between ST-segment depression and heart rate has a strictly positive curvature in all individuals. Cut-off points recommended by various authors are -1.6 mV/beat/min for ST/HR index and -2.4 mV/beat/min for ST/HR slope. A value lower than the cut-off point has a likelihood ratio greater than 1 for the presence of CAD.

Okin and Kligfield[28] compared the diagnostic value of those two methods in men and women. *Specificities* were assessed in 121 men and 29 women who had been referred for medical check-up and were clinically normal (cardiac catheterization was not used in this group). The specificity of the ST/HR index criterion was 97% in both men and women and that of the ST/HR slope criterion was 98% in men and 97% in women. However, the specificity of the standard criterion of additional (measured from rest rather than from isoelectric baseline) horizontal or downsloping ST segment less than -0.1 mV was 99% in men and 93% in women. *Sensitivities* were assessed in a group with clinical angina without catheterization, pooled with a group with CAD proven by catheterization. These comprised 187 men (including 68% with proven CAD) and 67 women (including only 39% with proved CAD). Sensitivities reported for ST/HR index criterion were 93% in men and 82% in women, and for the ST/HR slope criterion were 95% in men and 93% in women. Those for the standard criterion were significantly lower: 67% in men and 60% in women.

Unfortunately, the design of Okin's study overestimated sensitivity for at least two reasons. First, patients with clinical angina were supposed to have CAD, while with typical angina, a woman greater than 60 years old has a 9% chance of having no CAD according to Diamond and Forrester[29] and a 39-year-old woman with angina has a 74% chance of having no CAD; true positive results were, therefore, mixed with some false-positive results when computing sensitivities. It is unfortunate that the authors did not report sensitivities in the subgroup of patients with CAD proved by cardiac catheterization. Second, 52% of men and 43% of women were on β-

blocker therapy at the time of the treadmill exercise and could, therefore, not reach a high peak heart rate; because the two ST/HR criteria are inversely related to heart rate, the absolute values of the criteria will be greater than expected. Despite these problems, the lower sensitivity of ST/HR index than the ST/HR slope observed in women remains a finding that supports the use of the more complex ST/HR slope method for the detection of CAD in women. This benefit should be confirmed in a group of women with proven CAD, without β-blockade at the time of exercise, and without a history of myocardial infarction or left ventricular hypertrophy.

Morise and Duval[30] reported that ST/HR index was valuable in men, but not in women for the diagnosis of CAD, but ST/HR slope was not considered in their study, and no information about the performance of other exercise variables was reported for the subgroup of women. Women developed significantly less ST-segment depression than did men (-0.16 ± 0.08 mV vs. -0.22 ± 0.12 mV, $p < 0.01$), exercised to higher peak systolic blood pressures than did men (166 ± 21 mmHg vs. 156 ± 22 mmHg, $p < 0.05$), and exercised for a shorter period of time than men (7.3 ± 2.6 minutes vs. 9.9 ± 3.8 minutes, $p < 0.001$). If clinically normal subjects were compared with patients with known CAD in their study, differences between these groups were more marked in men than women with respect to exercise duration (Z test = 20.5 in men and 8.1 in women), peak heart rate (Z test = 27.7 in men and 8.8 in women), peak systolic blood pressure (Z test = 10.2 in men and 0.2 in women), and ST-segment change (Z test = 14.5 in men and 6.3 in women). These results indicate higher diagnostic values in men, as in our own published data (Table 7-1). Peak heart rate and exercise duration in this study had higher diagnostic relevance than ST segment in men and also in women, confirming data obtained using the bicycle ergometer in Table 7-1. Peak systolic blood pressure has no diagnostic relevance in women, while it was important in men. Important interactions between disease status and gender were also present in this study, but no distinct criteria were proposed for men and for women, perhaps because the estimated sensitivity of ST/HR slope was high in the studied women.

When myocardial oxygen demand increases, the severity of ischemia increases, but it remains unclear if increasing severity of ischemia is completely equilibrated with changing heart rate. Women, for example, can change their heart rate in the same way as men without increasing the severity of ischemia as much as men. Because many exogenous factors influencing coronary flow might have conflicting influences on ischemia and heart rate, the hypothesis of a constant of proportionality between ST changes and heart rate changes should be questioned in women, particularly. The slope of such a relationship may also be influenced by coronary stenosis severity—hence a man and a woman having similar anatomic changes in atherosclerotic coronary arteries should have the same ST_{60}-segment amplitude at the same heart rate level. The morphology of the ST-segment slope, chest pain during exercise, exercise duration, or workload has no additional diagnostic information with regard to ST_{60} segment:heart rate ratio, either in men or in women.

In a recent review, Okin and Kligfield[31] recommended the use of computerized ST-segment measurements of the total deviation below the isoelectric baseline, 60 ms after the J point, and computation of ST/HR slope rather than ST/HR index. They believe that the simple ST/HR index appears to approach the performance of the ST/HR slope for identification of coronary disease only, but not for assessment of its anatomic severity. It seems obvious today that ST depression alone cannot be directly related to the presence or extent of disease without adjustment for the corresponding myocardial work load.

Heart Rate

The peak heart rate attained during exercise is both predictive of the diagnosis of CAD and also the severity of the disease. Chae and colleagues[32] performed a stepwise discriminant analysis to identify parameters that could predict left main or three-vessel coronary disease in women (24% of severe CAD out of 243 studied women). The most significant predictor of severe CAD in their study was a multivessel abnormality at exercise single-photon emission computed tomographic thallium imaging. Peak heart rate was the only exercise variable that was an independent predictor of severe CAD in their results.

Based on peak heart rate and perfusion defect extent, a model may be developed that separated women into three risk groups. Despite the absence of differences between men and women in severity and extent of CAD, women had a shorter exercise duration (6.4 vs. 8.7 minutes, $p < 0.0001$) and lower exercise heart rate (140 vs. 144 beats/min, $p < 0.001$). Exercise duration was more different between men and women than was heart rate. Because no other data were reported on those patients, we cannot calculate the diagnostic value of exercise duration and compare it between men and women, with regard to heart rate diagnostic value in men and in women.

Exercise Duration

Exercise duration or exercise work load has been reported in a number of studies[21,33-35] as an important variable that should be considered when assessing the likelihood of a "positive" exercise result in a woman. In a study of 880 asymptomatic men and women without known coronary heart disease, Allen and colleagues[33] found that an exercise duration of less than 3 minutes was an important predictor of the presence of CAD in women. In 200 women with chest pain and greater than 0.1 mV exercise ST-segment depression, Pratt and colleagues[34] compared the exercise characteristics of 80 women with CAD (defined as 70% stenosis or more) and 120 women with angiographically confirmed normal or minimally diseased arteries (stenoses between 40% and 69% were excluded). Using stepwise logistic regression, the authors identified four independent variables associated with the likelihood of CAD: (1) time to ST normalization greater than 6 minutes, $p < 0.001$, (2) absence of mitral valve prolapse, $p < 0.003$, (3) exercise duration less than 5 minutes, $p < 0.02$, and (4) achieved target heart rate, $p < 0.03$, a less significant value than exercise duration. No multivariate score was presented by the authors and no results were presented in women without a positive ST-segment depression and in women with about 50% stenosis on a major coronary vessel.

Deckers and colleagues[35] reported exercise data of 73 catheterized women, of whom 51% had CAD. Maximal exercise work load was also the most significant variable distinguishing patients with CAD from those without CAD (93 ± 23 W vs. 129 ± 24 W, Z test = 5.3), replicating the data presented in Table 7-1. Other significant exercise variables were maximal ST_{80} segment in lead X (-0.08 ± 0.06 mV vs. -0.02 ± 0.06 mV, Z test = 3.6, $p < 0.001$), maximal ST_{60} segment in lead X (-0.08 ± 0.06 mV vs. -0.04 ± 0.05 mV, Z test = 3.2, $p < 0.001$), and angina during exercise (41% vs. 11%, Z test = 2.9, $p < 0.004$). Peak heart rate did not significantly differentiate patients with and without CAD in the study (118 ± 22 beats/min vs. 111 ± 19 beats/min, Z test = 1.5, $p = 0.13$), perhaps reflecting the high number of women treated with β-blockers at the time of exercise (76% in women with CAD and 67% in women without CAD).

As an indicator of cardiovascular conditioning or functional capacity, exercise duration or exercise work load has a diagnostic value at least as high as peak heart rate. Exercise duration should, therefore, be accounted for even if the heart rate is considered either directly or through an ST/HR relationship.

MAXIMAL EXERCISE MULTIVARIATE SCORES
Additive Diagnostic Value of Stress Test Variables

At the University of Louvain, we have used a large database of exercise tests to develop a multivariate analysis of the factors predicting CAD in a group of men (age 52 ± 7 years) and women (56 ± 8 years). Men and women with CAD achieved similar peak heart rate but at lower work load for women than for men. In both men and women, maximal work load achieved on the bicycle ergometer was the most relevant variable for discriminating between patients with and without CAD. In women, peak heart rate was the second predictive factor, with the Z test (between patients with and without CAD) clearly higher than all ECG measurements. Peak heart rate and work load reflected independent diagnostic information, as shown in Figure 7-1. In women undergoing catheterization, a work load less than 130 W (panels I and III on Fig. 7-1) had a sensitivity of 82% and a specificity of 51% (76% in healthy women): achievement of a high work load suggests that CAD is unlikely. A peak heart rate less than or equal to 140 beats/min (panels III and IV on Fig. 7-1) had a sensitivity of 60% and a specificity of 80% (90% in healthy women): failure to achieve an adequate heart rate is indicative of CAD. Work load has a higher negative predictive value and heart rate has a higher

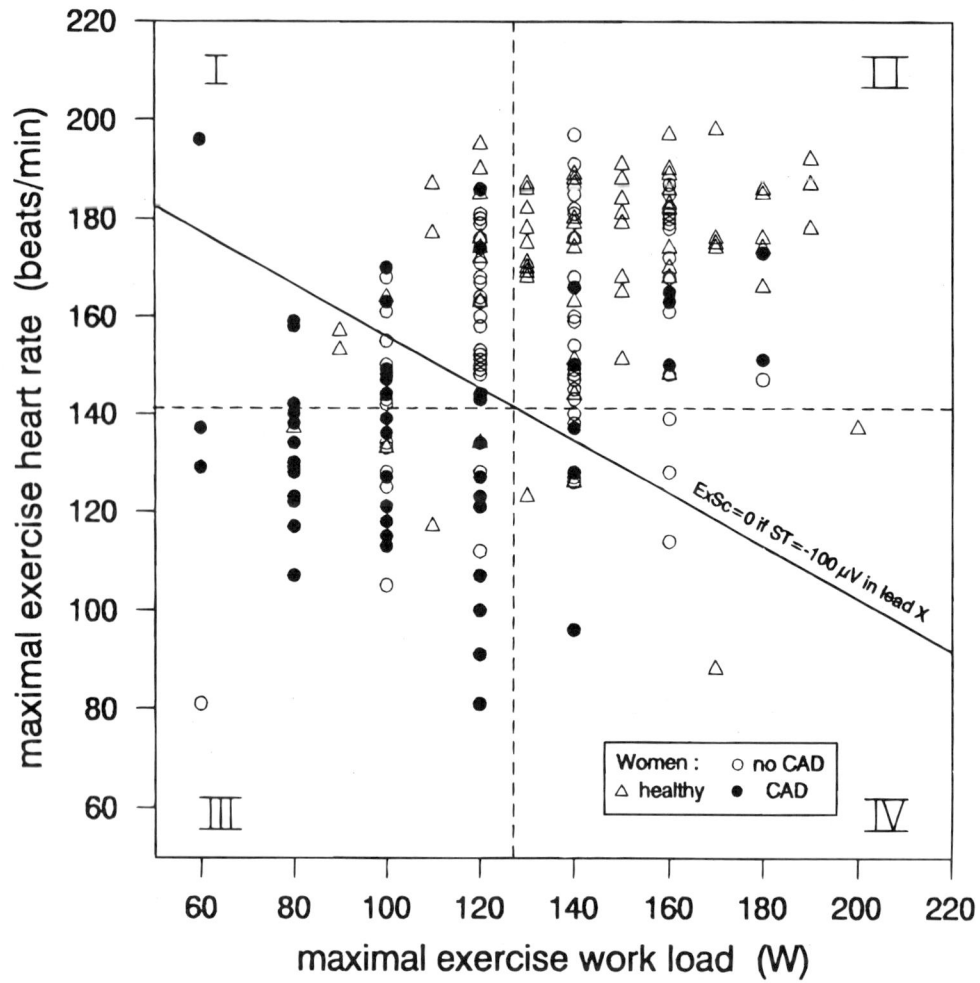

Fig. 7-1. Plot of maximal exercise heart rate versus maximal exercise work load in 76 healthy women, in 79 women without coronary artery disease (CAD) by cardiac catheterization, and in 56 women with CAD. The dashed lines indicate optimal decision cutpoint on either maximal exercise heart rate or maximal exercise work load for CAD diagnosis. The solid line corresponds to the optimal decision cutpoint (0) on the woman-specific exercise score projected for noninformative ST_{60} segment in lead X ($ST_{60}X = -0.1$ mV).

positive predictive value. The combination of those two variables can be considered as more informative than each one separately. Among the 40 catheterized women with *low heart rate and low work load* (panel III), 31 (78%) had CAD, including 18 out of 21 (86%) women with greater than 0.1 mV ST_{60}-segment depression in lead X (5% of healthy women were in panel III and none had an ST_{60} segment depression in lead X greater than -0.1 mV). Among the 40 catheterized women with *both high heart rate and high work load* (panel II), 33 (82%) had no CAD, including 15 of 16 (94%) women with greater than 0.1 mV ST_{60}-segment depression in lead X (71% of healthy women were in panel II, 59% without and 11% with greater than 0.1 mV ST_{60}-segment depression in lead X). Forty-five patients (and 18% of healthy women but only 3% with greater than 0.1 mV ST_{60}-segment depression in lead X) had a *high heart rate with a low work load* (panel I) and 15 of them (33%) had CAD, 12/28 (43%) with and 3/17 (18%)

without abnormal ST_{60}-segment depression in lead X. Ten patients (and 5% of healthy women but none with ST_{60}-segment depression in lead X) had a *low heart rate with a high work load* (panel IV) and 3 of them (30%) had CAD, 1/1 with ST_{60}-segment depression in lead X and 2/9 (22%) with no ST changes.

Discriminant Analysis

The above summary highlights the additive diagnostic value of peak heart rate, achieved work load, and ST_{60}-segment depression in the detection of CAD, but it also emphasizes how difficult it is to consider three variables together, even when they are expressed as binary variables (presence/absence). While the binary approach is necessary to define sensitivity and specificity, all decision cutpoints are arbitrary, and more information can be obtained from a continuous, quantitative measurement than a binary transformation of such a measurement. Discriminant analysis (either linear or logistic) is a complex but useful statistical tool that can help in diagnostic problems when there are a number of variables to integrate.

The result of a discriminant analysis is a single variable or allocator, usually called a diagnostic rule or a score in the medical literature (or a canonical axe or a discriminant axe in the statistical literature). Thus, multiple informative variables (multidimensional space) are combined to define a score (one-dimensional space), which is easier to handle. The score is a weighted sum of all informative variables, and an intercept is set to allow for a zero noninformative value (for example, [ST + 0.1] as a logical allocator taking more negative values in more diseased patients and more positive values in more normal patients). With statistical discriminant analysis, weights are calculated to maximize the distance between two "clouds" of points (the two groups that should be separated) while minimizing the variances and covariances within each cloud. Methods to compute those weights are based only on variations and covariations between the informative variables, not corrected for sample size ratio in linear models and corrected for in logistic models (these two models perform equally in large sample sizes and the logistic model performs better in smaller groups). These weightings have no physiologic meaning, and the allocator is a dimensionless measurement. Such an index can have a good diagnostic performance in one group of patients while yielding poor results in another group of patients, so that all allocators should be validated.

Multivariate Models in Men

Ten years ago, we created such an index for the diagnosis of CAD in men, using our own exercise data base.[20] Healthy men and men without CAD at heart catheterization were pooled to correct for the angiographic referral bias observed in our center.[36] The constituent variables and their associated weights are reported in the last column of Table 7-2. Peak heart rate was the most important factor, followed by the most abnormal ST_{60} segment, exertional angina, achieved work load, and ST_{20-60}-segment slope in lead X. After summation of these factors, more severely diseased patients should have a more negative score value because of a lower peak heart rate, a lower ST_{60} segment, appearance of angina, a lower achieved work load, and a less upsloping ST_{60} segment. In our experience in men, this score was negative in 82% of men with CAD and positive in 92% of men without CAD (giving a sensitivity of 82% and a specificity of 92% using a cutoff of 0). However, this specificity may have been overestimated, because the "no disease" group comprised 54 patients without CAD by catheterization, pooled with 103 healthy men.

The transportability of our discriminant score for men has been evaluated by Deckers and colleagues[37] in a group of 222 men who had undergone angiography (77% had CAD and 52% were taking β-blockers) and 123 healthy men. The authors built their own discriminant score for men (Table 7-2) and compared its diagnostic performance with six other diagnostic methods, including ST/HR index and our discriminant score. At a specificity of 90%, the ST/HR index had a sensitivity of 78% and our discriminant score had a sensitivity of 84%, close to the values reported in our own data. The authors concluded that ST/HR index and our discriminant score had excellent diagnostic value that were little affected by the concomitant use of β-blockers. In the top part of Table 7-2, we reported the weights of the Barolsky score,[24] of the ST/HR index[26] expressed in a form comparable to scores, and of the two discriminant scores[20,37] for men. The weights in the two discrimi-

Table 7-2 Maximal Exercise Variables and Associated Weights for Exercise Interpretations

	Score = Σ (Variable X_i × Weight β_i)			
	Barolsky Score[a] β_i	ST/HR Index β_i	Deckers Score β_i	Our Score β_i
In men: variables X_i				
Peak heart rate (beats/min)	+0.026	+0.016	+0.020	+0.022
[Rest heart rate (beats/min)]	0	−0.016	0	0
ST_{60} segment (mV)	0	+10.000	+7.000	+3.776
[Rest ST_{60} segment (mV)]	0	−10.000	0	0
[$ST_{60} \leq -0.1$ mV (no = 0, yes = 1)]	0	0	0	0
Angina-limited (no = 0, yes = 1)	0	0	−0.920	−0.782
Achieved work load (W)	0	0	+0.004	+0.004
ST_{20-60} slope in lead X (mV/sec)	0	0	+0.210	+0.156
Intercept	−3.443	0	−2.540	−3.473
In women: variables X_i				
Achieved work load (W)	0	0	+0.061	+0.021
Peak heart rate (beats/min)	+0.026	+0.016	0	+0.039
[Rest heart rate (beats/min)]	0	−0.016	0	0
ST_{60} lead X (mV)	0	+10.000	+18.000	+9.798
[Rest ST_{60} segment (mV)]	0	−10.000	0	0
ST_{60} lead X ≤ -0.1 mV (no = 0, yes = 1)	−0.913	0	0	0
Angina-limited (no = 0, yes = 1)	0	0	−7.660	0
Intercept	−3.443	0	−2.500	−6.979[b]

[a] Multiplied by −1 to have negative values indicating presence of coronary artery disease.
[b] ln(56/79) added because of a logistic discriminant model.

nant scores were close, and the peak heart rate weighting as well as the intercept in the Barolsky score were also close to those of the discriminant scores.

Multivariate Models in Women

In a study of 73 catheterized women and 116 healthy volunteers, Deckers and colleagues[35] also built a discriminant score for women (Table 7-2) and compared the diagnostic performance of their score, ST/HR index (with −1.2 mV/beat/min cutpoint), the Barolsky score (with −0.7 cutpoint), our discriminant score for men (using −0.75 cutpoint), and the standard ST-segment depression (≤0.1 mV). At a specificity of 90%, the sensitivities of those four allocators were, respectively, 73%, 77%, 60%, 70%, and 48%. At a specificity of 80%, the sensitivities were, respectively, 90%, 83%, 76%, 89%, and 60%. The lowest cutpoint reported for ST/HR index (−1.5 mV/beat/min) gave a specificity of 95% and a sensitivity of 54%. The authors concluded that the diagnostic yield of exercise testing in women could be improved by use of more sophisticated ECG and exercise variables.

We have also tried to build a female-specific exercise score for the diagnosis of CAD, using our own data.[21] In this series, women without CAD and healthy women were not pooled because, at our center, angiographic referral bias in women was mainly due to a history of β-blocker therapy and thallium scintigraphy results, rather than exercise results. Constituent variables and their associated weights are reported in the last column of Table 7-2 (bottom part). Fewer variables were selected than in men. Maximal exercise work load was the most discriminant variable in women, with a higher weighting than in men, followed by peak heart rate, and maximal ST_{60} segment in lead X. Using a cutoff of zero, the female-specific discriminant score was negative in 77% of diseased women and positive in 77% of women without CAD, and in 96% of healthy women. This diagnostic score has been validated in a consecutive group of 115 women studied over 4 years at our center.[21] The score was positive in 45 of 61 (74%)

women without CAD, and negative in 43 of 54 (80%) women with CAD. Even if the diagnostic gain was not as great as that observed in men for the male-specific exercise score, the female-specific exercise score yielded a better specificity than ST analysis in women, without a loss of sensitivity. Recovery variables such as time to ST normalization, development of ST-segment "sagging," and heart rate and systolic blood pressure 3 to 5 minutes after maximal exercise might further increase the diagnostic value of exercise stress testing in women, but they were not considered in our study.

In a group of 70 catheterized women (60 ± 9 years of age) studied by Williams and colleagues,[38] patients exercised to a work load of 108 ± 32 W, with a peak heart rate of 137 ± 23 beats/min (45% with target heart rate <85%), lower than in our group of slightly younger women. The authors compared the diagnostic accuracy of 0.1 mV or greater horizontal or downsloping ST_{60}-segment depression, our female-specific exercise score −0.34 or lower, and the echocardiographic development of a new or worsening wall motion abnormality criterion for the diagnosis of CAD (which was present in 47% of women). For these three criteria, authors reported sensitivities of 67% (22/33), 61% (20/33), and 88% (29/33) with specificities of 51% (19/37), 73% (27/37), and 84% (31/37), respectively. Thus, in comparison with conventional ST analysis, the female-specific exercise score yielded a better specificity without a loss of sensitivity, although it was less accurate than the imaging approach.

The Barolsky score, ST/HR index, and Deckers' score also had diagnostic merits in our population. Using a zero cutoff, sensitivities of those three allocators were, respectively, 79%, 77%, and 57% (compared with 66% for ≥0.1 mV ST_{60}-segment depression in lead X and 23% for ≥0.1 mV horizontal or downsloping ST_{60} segment in any lead). Specificities were 58%, 68%, and 84% (53% for ≥0.1 mV ST_{60}-segment depression in lead X and 76% for ≥0.1 mV horizontal or downsloping ST_{60}-segment depression in any lead) in women without CAD and specificities were 91%, 88%, and 100% (88% for ≥0.1 mV ST_{60}-segment depression in lead X and 96% for ≥0.1 mV horizontal or downsloping ST_{60}-segment depression in any lead) in healthy women. We did not investigate the diagnostic merit of ST/HR slope in our groups of women. Table 7-3 summarizes the mean values of these indices, within each subgroup of men and women. All the allocators had a higher Z test value in men than in women, reflecting their lower diagnostic power in women than in men. The four allocators were more negative in patients with CAD, and the highest values were observed in healthy subjects. Allocators with a higher standard deviation have a greater overlap between subgroup distributions, suggesting that distribution scores have to be taken into account in the interpretation of exercise stress tests.

Table 7-3 Maximal Exercise Scores and Diagnostic Value in Catheterized Patients[a]

	CAD		No CAD		Z Test[b]		Healthy	
	Men (N = 230)	Women (N = 56)	Men (N = 54)	Women (N = 79)	Men	Women	Men (N = 103)	Women (N = 76)
ST/HR index [$\Delta ST/\Delta HR$]	−2.86 ± 2.36	−3.32 ± 4.33	−0.92 ± 0.94	−1.41 ± 0.71	5.9	3.8	−0.35 ± 0.83	−0.64 ± 0.99
Barolsky's exercise score	−1.10 ± 1.01	−0.55 ± 0.68	0.08 ± 0.85	0.13 ± 0.60	8.0	6.1	0.93 ± 0.73	0.84 ± 0.62
Deckers' exercise score	−1.07 ± 1.19	−2.07 ± 5.51	0.66 ± 0.90	2.49 ± 3.56	10.0	5.8	2.21 ± 1.10	6.28 ± 2.59
Our exercise score	−0.95 ± 0.99	−0.88 ± 1.41	0.51 ± 0.79	0.80 ± 1.13	10.2	7.7	1.80 ± 0.77	2.65 ± 1.52

Abbreviations: CAD, coronary artery disease; ST/HR, ST-segment heart rate; SD, standard deviation.
[a] Values are mean ± SD.
[b] $p < 0.001$ for $Z > 3.3$, CAD vs no CAD.

Figures 7-2 to 7-4 are plots of peak exercise heart rate versus maximal most abnormal ST_{60}-segment in our subgroups of men (panel A), and versus maximal ST_{60} segment in lead X in our subgroups of women (panel B). In Figure 7-2, the zero level of the Barolsky score showed a greater separation of patients with and without CAD, more evident in men than in women, as compared with the conventional limit of greater than 0.1 mV ST_{60}-segment depression. It can also be seen that few men and women without CAD had an ST segment depression greater than 0.2 mV, and few men and women with CAD had no exercise ST-segment depression. Thus, even for the maximal exercise ST segment, taking into account the observed value rather than the binary positive or negative result improves the diagnostic accuracy. In Figure 7-3, the −1.6 mV/beat/min level of the ST/HR index also showed an important improvement in the separation of patients with and without CAD in both women and men, as compared to conventional ST analysis. The effect of a change in ST/HR limit level is illustrated in Figure 7-3B.

Because more than two variables are considered in our discriminant scores, projections were performed, as illustrated in Figure 7-4. In women, only three variables were needed to compute the score: the two variables defining the axes, and achieved work load. Three values for achieved work load have been used to draw lines on the lower plot of Figure 7-4: the noninformative achieved work load value (120 W), a lower value (80 W), and a higher value (160 W). The idea was to show the role of the third variable: if a woman has a peak heart rate of 180 beats/min and a maximal ST_{60} segment in lead X of −0.2 mV, her score will be more positive (more indicative of no CAD) if her achieved work load is 160 W than if it is 120 W, whereas her score will be negative (indicative of presence of CAD) if her achieved work load on the bicycle ergometer is only 80 W. Healthy subjects are more clustered in the upper right corner of the plots, and diseased patients are more concentrated in the lower left part of the plots. Patients without CAD proven by catheterization are more or less scattered along the noninformative line in the two plots, between the groups of healthy subjects and the patients with CAD. Whether more severely diseased patients are farther from the noninformative line remains a question that should be investigated.

Likelihood Assessment with Scores

As discussed previously, there is more diagnostic information in a quantitative measurement than in a dichotomization of this measurement. In our male population, we have shown[20] that the diagnostic information content of the exercise stress test was 25% greater if quantitative score values were considered rather than binary values (either positive or negative). Quantitative measurements are no more difficult to consider than binary measurements, if Bayes' theorem is well understood. Bayes' rule (or the "probability decomposition theorem") is a probabilistic law deduced from the elementary basic rules of probability calculus, which uses deductive reasoning on population samples, unlike statistical reasoning, which is inductive (from likelihoods in samples to probabilities in populations). Let us suppose that the diagnostic space is partitioned into two events: the presence of disease (D) and the absence of disease (NoD), so that the associated probabilities are nontrivial (neither 0 nor 1). Expressing the response of a test as T, Bayes' rule expresses the probability of disease in the setting of a positive test by re-evaluating prior knowledge (i.e., pretest disease probability) in light of new information (i.e., the test result):

$$P(D|T) = 1 / \left[1 + \frac{P(\text{No}D)}{P(D)} \frac{P(T|\text{No}D)}{P(T|D)} \right].$$

The ratio $P(D)/P(\text{No}D)$ is called the *prior risk ratio* (prior to the test); in populations in whom the prevalence of disease is known, it can be estimated by prevalence/(1 − prevalence). If prevalence is unknown, it may be estimated from other knowledge (e.g., age, gender, and symptoms for CAD), or approximated to 1 if there is no prior knowledge (i.e., prior probabilities are vague or noninformative). The ratio $P(T|D)/P(T|\text{No}D)$ is called the *conditional likelihood ratio* because it is usually estimated from observed data. If T takes two exclusive values (e.g., $T = 1$ if abnormal and $T = 0$ if normal), there are two possible likelihood ratios: (1) $P(T = 1|D)/P(T = 1|\text{No}D)$, which is well known in the medical literature as sensitivity/(1 − specificity), and (2) $P(T = 0|D)/P(T = 0|\text{No}D)$, which is also known as (1 − sensitivity)/specificity. Now, if T can take 10 exclusive values, there are 10 possible likelihood ratios. If T can take an infinite number of values (i.e., the test result is a

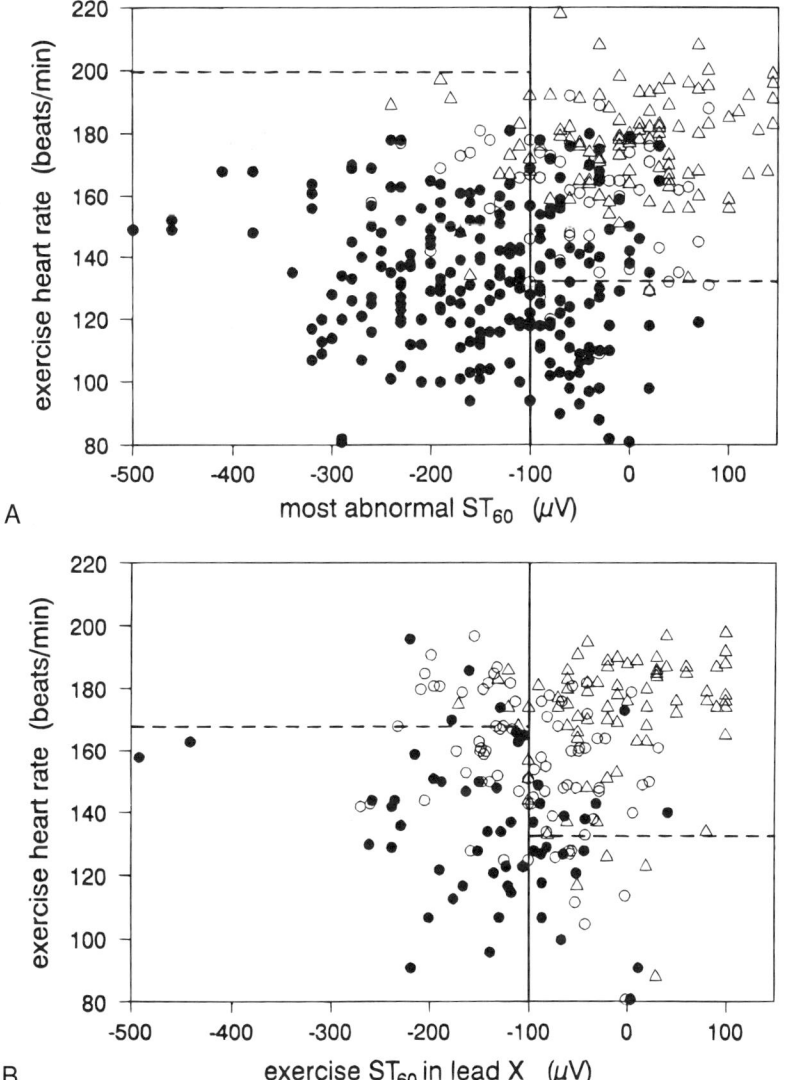

Fig. 7-2. Plot of peak exercise heart rate versus maximal most abnormal ST_{60} segment in men (**A**), and versus maximal ST_{60} segment in lead X in women (**B**). Solid lines, limit of ST segment less than or equal to -0.1 mV criterion; dashed lines, optimal cutpoint of the Barolsky score; triangles, healthy; open circles, no CAD; solid circles, CAD.

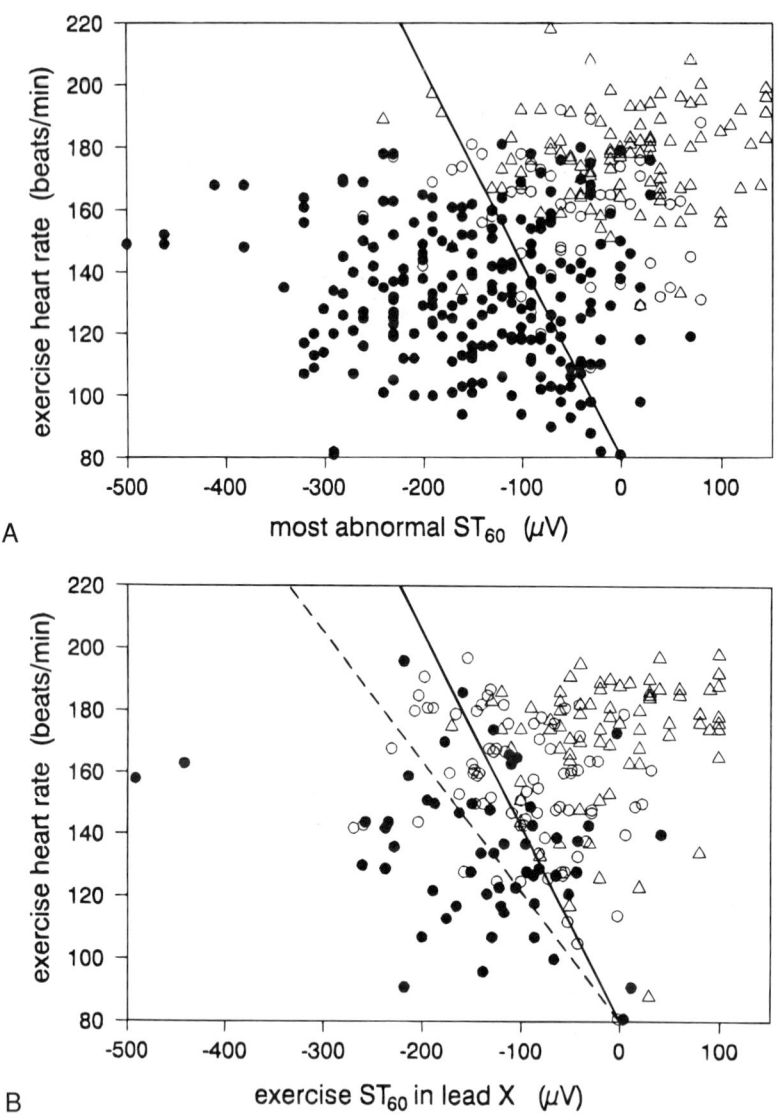

Fig. 7-3. Plot of peak exercise heart rate versus maximal most abnormal ST_{60} segment in men (**A**), and versus maximal ST_{60} segment in lead X in women (**B**). Solid lines, the limit of ST/HR index less than or equal to -1.6 μV/beat/min criterion; dashed line (in **B**), the limit of a ST/HR index less than or equal to -2.4 μV/beat/min criterion; triangles, healthy; open circles, no CAD; solid circles, CAD.

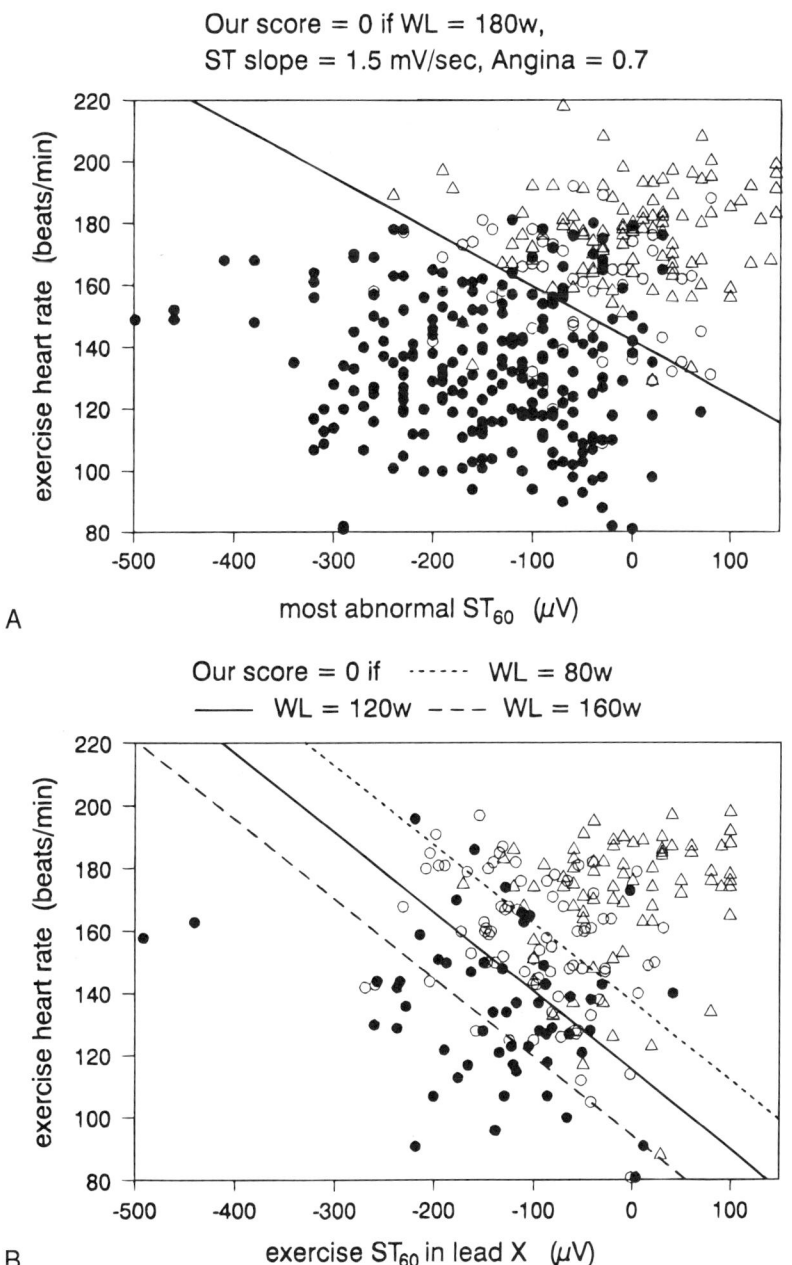

Fig. 7-4. Plot of peak exercise heart rate versus maximal most abnormal ST_{60} segment in men (**A**), and versus maximal ST_{60} segment in lead X in women (**B**). The lines correspond to optimal decision cutpoint for projected exercise score: the solid lines are noninformative projections, and the dashed lines on **B** correspond to projections when the work load is 80 W and when it is 160 W; triangle, healthy; open circle, no CAD; closed circle, CAD.

Table 7-4 Conditional Likelihoods and Likelihood Ratios Associated with the Woman-Specific Score

		Likelihood if CAD (%)	Likelihood if no CAD (%)	Likelihood ratio
Score value	≤ −1.6	32.1	1.3	24.91/1
in	[−1.6, −1.2]	14.3	1.9	7.38/1
in	[−1.2, −0.8]	7.1	1.9	3.68/1
in	[−0.8, −0.4]	10.7	4.5	2.37/1
in	[−0.4, +0.0]	12.5	3.9	3.23/1
in	[+0.0, +0.4]	7.1	5.8	1/1.23
in	[+0.4, +0.8]	5.4	11.6	1/2.17
in	[+0.8, +1.2]	3.6	8.4	1/2.35
in	[+1.2, +1.6]	3.6	9.0	1/2.53
	> +1.6	3.6	51.6	1/14.46

continuous variable), hypotheses on *T* distributions should be made (two Gaussian distributions with equal variance most of the time).

For our discriminant score for men, the Gaussian assumptions were not satisfied and we have reported the empirical likelihood ratios estimates in the published paper.[19] For our discriminant score for women, the empirical likelihood ratios are reported in Table 7-4 when a 0.4 interval length is used. The sum of the percents in the first five first-column entries corresponds to the 0 level sensitivity and the sum of the percents in the last five second-column entries corresponds to the 0 level specificity of our woman-specific exercise score. Even if greater than 1, the likelihood ratio of a negative but near-zero value is lower than the likelihood ratio of a negative but far-from-zero value: there is a gain in diagnostic performance with quantitative score values in common with binary score values. Of course, if the sample sizes were larger, the diseased and nondiseased women groups could have been split into subgroups according to age and clinical symptoms, in order to estimate likelihoods conditional not only to disease status but also to age and clinical symptoms (using values published by Diamond and Forrester[29] as prior probabilities). We have done this in men (unpublished study) and the results were that full-conditional likelihoods were unchanged or greater in diseased men with typical angina complaints when the score was negative, and unchanged or lower in nondiseased men without typical angina chest pain when the score was positive. Age had no statistical effect on conditional likelihoods in our groups of men. Therefore, the postexercise probabilities of CAD were underestimated in diseased men and overestimated in nondiseased men. Moreover, the age and clinical symptom repartition was close to Diamond and Forrester's table for men. Our conclusion was that probability of CAD can be calculated using the likelihood ratio estimates associated with our score, using Diamond and Forrester tables[29] to estimate prior risk ratios. We did not perform such a study in women because of the smaller samples. Data regarding oral estrogen replacement therapy was available in our data base at that time, but it has been described[39] as a clinical factor affecting the prevalence of CAD in women and also affecting the exercise stress test response in women with comparable CAD status.

On the basis of our data, the probability of CAD can be calculated using the likelihood ratio estimates associated with our score (Table 7-4), and using Diamond and Forrester tables[29] to estimate prior risk ratios.

ONGOING ROLE OF EXERCISE STRESS TESTING: WITH OR EXCHANGED FOR IMAGING APPROACHES?

Several reports elsewhere mentioned in this text[32,34,38] indicate that imaging approaches are superior to exercise stress testing for the diagnosis of CAD and the assessment of its severity in women. However, rather than comparing[38] these diagnostic tests, which study different manifestations of myocardial ischemia, there may be some benefit in looking at the problem from every angle and trying to organize the conflicting data from various sources.

A sequential diagnostic strategy has been reported as an efficient means of diagnosing CAD in women.[39] First, a prior risk ratio is obtained from the clinical symptoms and age of the patient.[29] After performance of an exercise stress test, the response is translated into a likelihood ratio and a postexercise stress test probability of CAD is computed. If the value is not high enough to justify cardiac catheterization, or if it is not low enough to be confident about the absence of CAD, an exercise imaging test can be requested to gain new information on the possible existence of myocardial ischemia. At this step, the postexercise stress test probability of CAD may be used as the preimaging test probability. The response to an exercise imaging test should also be translated into a new likelihood ratio, and reassessment of the post-test probability of CAD may be made. From a statistical point of view, such strategies lead to angiographic referral bias, because the test outcomes are used in the patient's management: women with a high probability of CAD will be referred more often for angiography than women with a low probability of CAD.

An alternative to these diagnostic strategies would be to develop multivariate scores that take into account all the various test results, and to correct associated likelihood ratios for center-specific angiographic referral bias when applied to the overall population of women addressed for evaluation of chest pain in a particular center. However, while this approach is attractive, large prospective data bases are needed to correct for catheterization decision variables.

CONCLUSION: PROBABILITY IS NOT CERTAINTY

Of 79 women in our series without significant coronary artery disease, two had an exercise score lower than -1.6. The first case was a 42-year-old woman with typical angina chest pain (prior probability of CAD of 55.2%). This woman achieved a work load of 100 W on the bicycle ergometer, with a peak heart rate of 142 beats/min (80% of target heart rate) and a horizontal ST_{60} segment in lead X of -0.27 mV, but without angina symptoms during the exercise test. Her exercise test score was therefore low, $0.021 \times (100) + 0.039 \times (142) + 9.798 \times (-0.27) - 6.979 = -2.0$. The corresponding likelihood ratio was 24.91/1 and her postexercise probability of CAD was $[1 + (44.8/55.2) \times (1/24.91)]^{-1} = 96.8\%$ or, a postexercise stress test risk ratio for CAD of 31 to 1. This woman had an ST/HR index of -4.2 mV/beat/min and her thallium scan was abnormal. However, all her coronary vessels had less than 25% stenosis at coronary angiography. The second case was a 58-year-old woman with typical angina chest pain (prior probability of CAD of 79.4%), who could not exercise to a work load greater than 60 W because of anginal symptoms. Her peak heart rate was 77 beats/min (48% of target heart rate) with a horizontal ST_{60} segment in lead X of -0.01 mV. The exercise test score for this women was, therefore, also low, $0.021 \times (60) + 0.039 \times (77) + 9.798 \times (-0.01) - 6.979 = -2.7$, which corresponds to a likelihood ratio of 24.91/1. Her postexercise probability of CAD was $[1 + (20.6/79.4) \times (1/24.91)]^{-1} = 99.0\%$, or a postexercise stress test risk ratio for CAD of 96 to 1. This woman had an ST/HR index of -0.9 mV/beat/min and her thallium scan was normal. The coronary angiography of this woman showed only a stenosis of 40% to 50% on the left main artery and no other stenosis greater than 25%.

Some studies[40,41] have also reported examples of women with a previous myocardial infarction, with a reduced regional coronary flow, but with normal coronary arteries. The reverse phenomen was also observed in our population of women. Of our 56 women with significant CAD, two had an exercise score greater than $+1.6$. The first case was a 45-year-old woman with typical angina chest pain (prior probability of CAD of 55.2%). Without developing symptoms, this woman achieved a work load of 160 W on the bicycle ergometer, with a peak heart rate of 165 beats/min (94% of target heart rate) and an upsloping ST_{60} segment in lead X of -0.10 mV at maximal exercise test. Her exercise test score was therefore high, $0.021 \times (160) + 0.039 \times (165) + 9.798 \times (-0.10) - 6.979 = +1.7$. The corresponding likelihood ratio was 1/14.46 and her postexercise probability of CAD was $[1 + (44.8/55.2) \times (14.46/1)]^{-1} = 7.9\%$ or, a postexercise stress test risk ratio for CAD of 1 to 12. This woman had an ST/HR index of -1.6 mV/beat/min and her thallium scan was normal. However, she had a 75% stenosis on the right coronary artery and 75% stenosis on the left anterior descending coronary artery at the angiography. The second case was a 42-year-old woman with atypical chest pain (prior probability of CAD of 13.3%). This woman exercised until a work load of 180 W, without anginal symptoms. Her peak heart rate was 173 beats/min (97% of target heart rate) with an upsloping ST_{60} segment in lead X of -0.03 mV. Her exercise test score was also high, $0.021 \times (180) + 0.039 \times (173) + 9.798 \times (-0.03) - 6.979 = +3.4$, which corresponds to a likelihood ratio of 1/14.46. Her postexercise probability of CAD was $[1 + (86.7/13.3) \times (14.46/1)]^{-1} = 1.0\%$, or a postexercise risk ratio for CAD of 1 to 96. This woman had an ST/HR index of -0.5 mV/beat/min and her thallium scan was normal. This woman coronary angiography showed a proximal stenosis of 99% on the left anterior descending artery and no other significant stenosis. Those four examples illustrate how patients can give different exercise stress test responses that reflect varying physiologic responses to an imbalance between available supply of oxygenated coronary blood flow and myocardial demands.

Despite those chosen examples, and even if the clinical definitions of CAD are somewhat fuzzy, it is the fuzziness that makes this disease so suitable to a probabilistic approach. This may be applied to the diagnosis of CAD, the assessment of its severity, and the prognostic assessment. A few years ago, George Diamond[42] posed the following question on John's postexercise probability of CAD, still true today for Jane's postexercise probability of CAD: "What, for instance, is the fundamental nature of the similarities and differences among the following clinically relevant statements?

> Jane has a 70 ± 20% chance of having CAD.
>
> Jane has a 70 ± 20% diameter stenosis on her coronary artery.
>
> Jane has a 70 ± 20% reduction in myocardial ischemic reserve.
>
> Jane has a 70 ± 20% chance of a coronary event over 30 years.
>
> Jane has a 70% chance of a coronary event over 30 ± 10% years."

Whether or not the multivariate ECG approaches find a persistent niche as an accurate and cost-effective tool for the assessment of CAD, their statistical methodology is translatable to other approaches and will not be outmoded.

REFERENCES

1. Feil H, Siegel ML: Electrocardiographic changes during attacks of angina. Am J Med Sci 175:235, 1928
2. Al-Joundi B, Chaitman BR: The use of electrocardiography as a diagnostic and prognostic tool in coronary artery disease. Curr Opin Cardiol 7:587, 1992
3. Ayanian JZ, Epstein AM: Differences in the use of procedures between men and women hospitalized for coronary artery disease. N Engl J Med 325:221, 1991
4. Steingart RM, Packer M, Hamm P, and the Survival and Ventricular Enlargement [SAVE] investigators: Sex differences in the management of coronary artery disease. N Engl J Med 325:226, 1991
5. Shaw LJ, Miller DD, Romeis JC et al: Gender differences in the noninvasive evaluation and management of patients with suspected coronary artery disease. Ann Intern Med 120:559, 1994
6. Mark DB, Shaw LJ, DeLong ER et al: Absence of sex bias in the referral of patients for cardiac catheterization. N Engl J Med 330:1101, 1994
7. Khan SS, Nessim S, Gray R et al: Increased mortality of women in coronary artery bypass surgery: evidence for referral bias. Ann Intern Med 112:561, 1990
8. Sans S: Coronary heart disease in women. Heart Beat 3:1, 1993
9. Caralis DG, Wiens G, Shaw LK et al: An off-line digital system for reproducible interpretation of the exercise ECG. J Electrocardiol 23:285, 1990
10. Wilson RF, Marcus ML, Christensen BV et al: Accuracy of exercise electrocardiography in detecting physiologically significant coronary arterial lesions. Circulation 83:412, 1991
11. Uren NG, Melin JA, De Bruyne B et al: Relation between myocardial blood flow and the severity of coronary-artery stenosis. N Engl J Med 330:1782, 1994
12. Gould KL, Lipscomb K: Effect of coronary stenoses on coronary flow reserve and resistance. Am J Cardiol 34:50, 1974
13. Gianrossi R, Detrano R, Mulvihill D et al: Exercise-induced ST depression in the diagnosis of coronary artery disease. A meta-analysis. Circulation 80:87, 1989
14. Brohet CR, Hoeven C, Robert AR et al: The normal pediatric Frank orthogonal electrocardiogram: variations according to age and sex. J Electrocardiol 19:1, 1986
15. MacFarlane PW, Lawrie TDV: The normal electrocardiogram and vectocardiogram. p. 407. In MacFarlane PW, Lawrie TDV (eds): Comprehensive Electrocardiol-

ogy. Theory and Practice in Health and Disease, Vol. 1. Pergamon Press, New York, 1989
16. Pipberger HV, Simonson E, Lopez EA et al: The electrocardiogram in epidemiologic investigations. A new classification system. Circulation 65:1456, 1982
17. Nemati M, Doyle JT, McCaughan D et al: The orthogonal electrocardiogram in normal women. Implication of sex differences in diagnostic electrocardiography. Am Heart J 95:12, 1978
18. Rautaharju PM: Electrocardiography in epidemiology and clinical trials. p. 1220. In MacFarlane PW, Lawrie TDV (eds): Comprehensive Electrocardiology. Theory and Practice in Health and Disease, Vol. 1. Pergamon Press, New York, 1989
19. Deckers JW, Vinke RVH, Simoons M: Changes in the electrocardiographic response to exercise in healthy women. Br Heart J 64:376, 1990
20. Detry JMR, Robert AR, Luwaert RJ et al: Diagnostic value of computerized exercise testing in men without previous myocardial infarction. A multivariate, compartmental and probabilistic approach. Eur Heart J 6: 227, 1985
21. Robert AR, Melin JA, Detry JMR: Logistic discriminant analysis improves the diagnostic accuracy of exercise testing for coronary artery disease in women. Circulation 83:1202, 1991
22. Sawada SG, Ryan T, Fineberg NS et al: Exercise echocardiographic detection of coronary artery disease in women. J Am Coll Cardiol 14:1440, 1989
23. Bruce RA, McDonough JR: Stress testing in screening for cardiovascular disease. Bull NY Acad Med 45:1288, 1969
24. Barolsky SM, Gilbert CA, Faruqui A et al: Differences in electrocardiographic response to exercise in women and men: a non-Bayesian factor. Circulation 60:1021, 1979
25. Elamin MS, Mary DASG, Smith DR, Linden RJ: Prediction of severity of coronary artery disease using slope of submaximal ST-segment/heart rate relationship. Cardiovasc Res 14:681, 1980
26. Detrano R, Salcedo E, Passalaqua M, Friis R: Exercise electrocardiographic variables: a critical appraisal. J Am Coll Cardiol 8:836, 1986
27. Kligfield P, Okin PM, Ameisen O, Borer JS: Evaluation of coronary artery disease by an improved method of exercise electrocardiography: the ST/HR slope. Am Heart J 112:589, 1986
28. Okin PM, Kligfield P: Identifying coronary artery disease in women by heart rate adjustment of ST-segment depression and improved performance of linear regression over simple averaging method with comparison to standard criteria. Am J Cardiol 69:297, 1992
29. Diamond GA, Forrester JS: Analysis of probability as an aid in the clinical diagnosis of coronary-artery disease. N Engl J Med 300:1350, 1979
30. Morise AP, Duval RD: Accuracy of ST/heart rate index in the diagnosis of coronary artery disease. Am J Cardiol 69:603, 1992
31. Okin PM, Kligfield P: Heart rate adjustment of ST-segment depression and performance of the exercise electrocardiogram: a critical evaluation. J Am Coll Cardiol 25:1726, 1995
32. Chae SC, Heo J, Iskandrian AS, Wasserleben V, Cave V: Identification of coronary artery disease in women by exercise single-photon emission computed tomographic (SPECT) thallium imaging. J Am Coll Cardiol 21:1305, 1993
33. Allen WH, Aranow WS, Goodman P, Stinson P: Five-year follow-up of maximal treadmill stress test in asymptomatic men and women. Circulation 62:522, 1980
34. Pratt CM, Francis MJ, Divine GW, Young JB: Exercise testing in women with chest pain: are there additional exercise characteristics that predict true positive test results? Chest 95:139, 1989
35. Deckers JW, Rensing BJ, Simoons ML, Roelandt JRTC: Diagnostic merits of exercise testing in females. Eur Heart J 10:543, 1989
36. Robert AR, Melin JA, Brohet CR et al: The bias of population referred to angiography: a method to control it for the interpretation of non-invasive tests. IEEE Computer Society Press 309, 1987
37. Deckers JW, Rensing BJ, Tijssen JG et al: A comparison of method of analysing exercise tests for diagnosis of coronary artery disease. Eur Heart J 62:438, 1989
38. Williams MJ, Marwick TH, O'Gorman D, Foale RA: Comparison of exercise echocardiography with an exercise score to diagnose coronary artery disease in women. Am J Cardiol 74:435, 1994
39. Melin JA, Wyns W, Vanbutsele R et al: Alternative diagnostic strategies for coronary artery disease in women: demonstration of the usefulness and efficiency of probability analysis. Circulation 71:535, 1985
40. Welch CC, Proudfit WL, Sheldon WC: Coronary arteriographic findings in 1000 women under age 50. Am J Cardiol 35:211, 1975
41. Engel HJ, Hundeschagen H, Lichtlen P: Transmural myocardial infarction in young women taking oral contraceptives. Evidence of reduced regional coronary flow in spite of normal coronary arteries. Br Heart J 39:477, 1977
42. Diamond GA: An optimistic interpretation of an optimistic bias. J Chron Dis 39:856, 1986

Chapter 8

Stress Echocardiography for the Diagnosis of CAD in Women

M. John Williams and Thomas H. Marwick

BACKGROUND

Results of Noninvasive Testing in Women

The accuracy of diagnostic tests has been defined from population-based studies, but there is a need to establish an individualized diagnostic strategy tailored to each subject. Tests should be selected based upon their performance under circumstances reflecting the characteristics of that patient. Extrapolation of results from one subgroup to another should be undertaken with attention to potential limitations. Variations in population characteristics may have an impact on test accuracy, and at least partly explain the spectrum of results reported with different noninvasive studies for the diagnosis of coronary artery disease (CAD).[1-7] This may be compounded by variations in disease criteria (e.g., definition of "significant" stenosis), differences in test methodology, and differences in the definition of an abnormal test.[8] Unfortunately, in individual studies, it is often difficult to elucidate the relative contribution of these factors due to inadequate characterization of the study groups, inadequate stratification of extent of coronary disease, excessive exclusion criteria, problems with posttest bias, and problems with review bias.[9,10]

The diagnosis of CAD in women is particularly relevant in this context. A preponderance of the early data with noninvasive testing was obtained in men, and it was assumed that these results would apply to women, but, as discussed in the previous chapter by Robert, this is not the case. Women differ from men in body composition, and exercise capacity and hemodynamic responses,[11-13] and the importance of obtaining data in women has been recognized.[14-16] These data will enable the development of specific diagnostic strategies in women.

Assessment of Coronary Disease Probability in Women

The diagnostic process begins with the formulation (either qualitative or quantitative) of a pretest likelihood of coronary disease, based on the patient's history and physical examination. However, the diagnosis of CAD on history and physical characteristics alone is difficult, especially in women, among whom the presence of chest pain may be deceptive. The resting electrocardiogram (ECG) is normal in up to 70% of cases presenting with a clinical determination of angina pectoris.[17] At best, therefore, the patient may be stratified into a low-, intermediate-, or high-risk group and further testing is often warranted.[18]

If the pretest likelihood of disease is high, the physician might proceed directly to coronary angiography without resorting to a functional test to confirm the diagnosis. However, in most cases either a functional evaluation might be desirable or a further test is performed to confirm a clinical suspicion. Posttest probability can be derived from pretest probability and test accuracy, by application of Bayes theorem of conditional probability.[19-21]

Multiple diagnostic tests are sometimes performed in the belief that the predictive accuracy of any one test applied in a population with low disease prevalence is low; it may be significantly enhanced with multiple testing if the results are concordant.[20,22] Unfortunately, results are frequently discordant, and the increased cost of multiple testing is difficult to justify in the current cost-conscious environment. The importance of defining an optimal diagnostic test and the shortcomings of the established literature for this purpose in women are presented in this chapter.

EXERCISE TESTING IN WOMEN

The standard treadmill exercise test (with electrocardiographic monitoring) is the simplest, most convenient, and "traditional" initial diagnostic test performed in the work-up of patients with suspected coronary disease. The basic principles of the stress test[23] have been dealt with in Chapter 1; conditions are best fulfilled by continuous graded treadmill exercise testing to maximal or near maximal heart rates with the protocol selected according to the patient's functional capacity. In some centers bicycle exercise is the preferred mode; issues regarding the hemodynamic and ECG parameters of treadmill and bicycle exercise have been dealt with in Chapters 1 and 3, as well as in the literature.[24]

Gender Differences in Exercise Performance

The structural and developmental differences between the sexes obviously influence exercise performance. Compared with men, women have a larger surface area to mass ratio, a greater fat to muscle ratio, a smaller thoracic cage (resulting in lower lung volumes), a lower oxygen carrying capacity, and also have a resting metabolic rate (RMR) that is 5% to 10% lower than that in men (presumably reflecting the relative metabolic demands of fat vs. muscle).[25]

The initial work examining the variation of VO_2max with age and sex was done in groups of highly trained men and women by Astrand in 1960.[26] In men and women matched for age, weight and physical training, men reach a higher VO_2max,[27] although habitual activity, nutrition, climate, occupation, and ethnic origin can affect VO_2max within the same sex and age group. However, the most important determinant of VO_2max is absolute fat free body weight, and the lower VO_2max in women is probably largely a function of this index.[27]

ST-Segment Analysis

As discussed in Chapter 1, ST-segment depression is not specific for coronary disease. Nonischemic ST-segment depression may be associated with metabolic changes, drug therapy, resting ST-segment abnormalities, or other structural heart diseases such as cardiomyopathies, and mitral valve prolapse.[23] Syndrome X results in exercise-induced ST-segment depression and may account for some "false-positive" findings.

The specificity of ST-segment changes is particularly problematic in women. However, while mitral valve prolapse[28] and syndrome X[29] are more prevalent in women than men, this is probably not sufficient to account for the overall difference. The female hormonal milieu could be implicated,[30-33] but the data are somewhat limited in this area. Some structural similarities exist between estrogen and digitalis, so it is possible that estrogen may contribute to the false-positive ST-segment response. Furthermore, the effects of estrogen on endothelial and vasomotor function may influence arteriolar function and microvascular flow,[34] directly provoking ST-segment shift perhaps in a similar manner to that involved in syndrome X. However, at this stage the role of estrogen as the main "perpetrator" in ST-segment deviation remains speculative and is beyond the scope of this review.

Standard treadmill testing shows a wide range of accuracy, with sensitivities from 20% to 80% and specificities from 32% to 100%, depending on the population studied, test protocols, and methodologies used for analysis.[1] Various factors contribute to this wide differential, including the type of exercise, the ECG leads recorded, criteria for a positive test, variability in patient selection, prevalence of CAD, and the absolute standard for defining CAD. Patient-specific factors affecting exercise ECG sensitivity include maximal exercise heart rate, extent of CAD, site of CAD, symptomatic status, age, and gender.[35]

Stress testing in females presents problems for both sensitivity and specificity of the exercise ECG. The lower sensitivity of exercise ECG testing in women is probably due to low exercise capacity.[36] However, the main problem is an increase in false-positive ST-segment responses, yielding a suboptimal specificity. A study by Barolsky et al.[37] has suggested that the higher false-positive rate in women was not only a reflection of Bayesian factors and disease prevalence, but also other intrinsic parameters that increased test positivity in women.

Many approaches have been followed to improve the suboptimal specificity of exercise ECG. These consist of either altering the diagnostic criteria for defining a positive test[38–40] or incorporating other exercise data into a multivariate score.[41–43] At its simplest, the former might comprise ignoring inferior ST depression (which is disproportionately represented in patients with false-positive responses[1,44]), or changes that are evident only during exercise and resolve rapidly after stress.[45] The predictive value of downsloping ST-segment depression is similar to that of horizontal depression and exclusion of slowly upsloping ST-segments did not improve specificity as opposed to the findings in male populations.[45] More complex multivariate approaches, including those of Deckers, Robert, and Barolsky, have been discussed in Chapter 7. While these data are promising, it would be realistic to say that the multivariate exercise techniques have not been widely accepted.

Exercise Thallium Scintigraphy

An alternative strategy to improve the diagnostic accuracy of routine exercise ECG is to combine it with an imaging modality, and this originally involved exercise thallium scintigraphy. Most of the early studies of thallium imaging (up to 1980) were performed in men; subsequent studies of thallium scintigraphy in women are discussed elsewhere in this volume.

Early reports of exercise thallium in women showed suboptimal sensitivity (31% and 71%) and specificity (82% and 67%), however, there were methodological problems in these studies as well as interpretative difficulties with respect to breast artifact. However, in a group of 60 women, Friedman et al.[46] reported the sensitivity and specificity of the exercise ECG to be 32% and 41%, respectively, compared with 75% and 97% by thallium imaging. Similary, in 92 symptomatic women without prior infarction, Hung et al.[47] reported the sensitivity and specificity of exercise electrocardiography to be 73% and 59%, respectively, compared with 75% and 91% for thallium scintigraphy. These studies showed that exercise thallium scintigraphy in females had an overall accuracy (slightly lower sensitivity) similar to the results obtained from predominantly male subgroups, provided that breast artifacts were recognized. The accuracy of thallium imaging exceeded that of the stress ECG, based upon avoidance of nondiagnostic ECG results, resting ECG abnormalities, and also a low prevalence of multivessel CAD.

However, in a group of 243 women with a high pretest probability of CAD, Chae et al.[48] found the sensitivity and specificity of exercise ECG (after exclusion of the nondiagnostic responses), to be 66% and 60%, respectively, compared with 71% and 65% for single photon emission computed tomography (SPECT) thallium imaging. In patients with single vessel disease, the sensitivity was 52%, compared with 82% for those patients with multivessel disease. Only multivessel thallium abnormality and peak exercise heart rate were independent predictors of left main or three-vessel coronary disease. The low sensitivity for single-vessel disease probably reflected an inadequate heart rate response to exercise in almost 50% of the women. They postulated that some perfusion defects were misinterpreted as attenuation artifacts in women, and it is possible that the newer technetium-labeled imaging agents might improve accuracy in this regard.

These limited data suggest that myocardial perfusion imaging may not be as accurate for the diagnosis of CAD in women as it is in men. Breast attenuation artifacts may compromise specificity, but in an effort to avoid this, underinterpretation of anterior defects may limit sensitivity.

STRESS ECHOCARDIOGRAPHY

The idea of obtaining echocardiographic images of the heart during exercise evolved as technological improvements made possible the ability to obtain readable images immediately post-treadmill exercise or during supine bicycle exercise. Exercise echocardiography was initially performed utilizing M-mode and basic two-dimensional (2D) imaging[49] and early progress was hampered by poor imaging related to technical inadequacies coupled with difficulties obtaining images in a moving patient with hyperventilation and tachycardia. Diagnostic images were obtained in a large percentage of cases with the further progress and development of 2D imaging.[50–52] Exercise echocardiography began to show favorable sensitivity and specificity for the detection of CAD, but these data were obtained in groups with a preponderance of male subjects.[53–56]

Exercise Echocardiography versus ECG in Women

The initial evaluation of stress echocardiography exclusively in women was performed by Sawada et al.[57] who evaluated 57 female subjects (CAD prevalence 49%) with exercise echocardiography and compared the results with coronary angiography. The exercise echocardiogram had a sensitivity and specificity of 86%, compared with a sensitivity of 29% and a specificity of 83% for the exercise ECG. When the nondiagnostic ECGs (which were present in 30% of patients) were removed from analysis, the sensitivity of exercise ECG was 47% and the specificity was 78%. The comparison was also colored by the use of only three bipolar ECG leads, which may have compromised the sensitivity of the exercise ECG.

Although the stress echocardiogram was more accurate than the conventional exercise test in women, the apparent superiority of the multivariate score over the exercise ECG suggested that a comparison should be performed between the exercise echocardiography and the multivariate score. We performed this comparison in 70 women (pretest CAD probability 53 ± 30%), who were stressed using a maximal symptom limited bicycle exercise protocol before proceeding to angiography.[58] The conventional stress test was defined as positive in the presence of significant ST-segment depression greater than 0.1 mV at 0.06 second after the J point *excluding inferior leads*.[44] The exercise score was calculated from ST response, heart rate, and workload, using the equation derived from the multivariate model of Robert et al.[43] We considered a positive stress echocardiogram to be defined in the standard manner by the development of a new or worsening wall motion abnormality. In this study, patients with CAD were older, more likely to have a history of angina, perform to a lower exercise capacity, and attain a lower heart rate than those without CAD. The findings of this study are summarized in Figure 8-1, which shows the sensitivity of exercise echocardiography (88%) to exceed that of the ST analysis alone (67%), and the exercise score (61%; both $p < 0.05$ vs. exercise echocardiography). While the specificity of exercise echocardiography (84%) and the multivariate score (73%) were comparable, both exceeded that of the ST analysis (51%) in 37 patients without CAD ($p < 0.01$). The accuracy of exercise echocardiography (86%) exceeded that of the exercise score (67%, $p = 0.01$) and ST analysis (59%, $p < 0.01$). Thus, we found exercise echocardiography to be more sensitive than the exercise score, and more sensitive and specific than ST-segment analysis for the diagnosis of CAD in women.

The superiority of exercise echocardiography for the detection of CAD was confirmed in a larger group of 161 women (age 60 ± 9 years, pretest CAD probability 44 ± 33%), without previous Q-wave infarction, cardiomyopathy, or prior revascularization, who underwent exercise echocardiography and coronary angiography.[59] Positive exercise echocardiography and exercise ECG were defined in the usual manner and although exercise ECG ST-segment analysis was deemed nondiagnostic in the presence of resting repolarization abnormalities ($n = 43$), all exercise echocardiograms were interpreted. The sensitivity of exercise echocardiography was 78 ± 3% in the overall 59 patients with significant coronary stenoses (diameter > 50%), including 32 with single-vessel disease. In the 48 patients with significant disease and interpretable ECGs, the sensitivity of exercise echocardiography was 81 ± 3% and that of the exercise ECG was 77 ± 3% ($p = $ NS). There was a small incremental improvement in the sensitivity of exercise echocardiography to 85 ± 3% after exclusion of negative submaximal tests. The overall specificity of exercise echocardiography was 81 ± 4% in 102 patients without coronary disease. In the group of 70 patients without significant disease and with interpretable ECG, the specificity of exercise echocardiography (80 ± 3%) exceeded that of the exercise ECG (56 ± 4%), $p < 0.0004$. The accuracy of exercise echocardiography was also greater than that of the exercise ECG (80 ± 5% vs. 64 ± 6%,

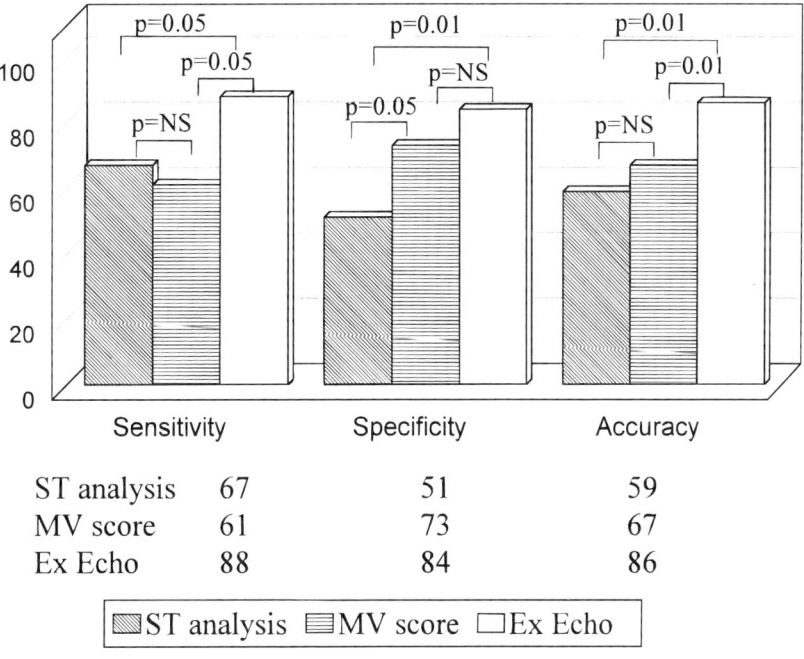

Fig. 8-1. Sensitivity, specificity, and accuracy of ST analysis (ST), multivariate exercise score (MV), and exercise echocardiography (Ex Echo) in 70 women investigated for chest pain symptoms. Ex Echo vs MV: sensitivity $p < 0.05$, specificity $p = $ NS, accuracy $p = 0.01$.

$p < 0.005$) in accordance with previous reported data.

Importance of Referral Bias

In contrast to these favorable findings, investigators from the Mayo Clinic reported a sensitivity of 85% and a specificity of 47% for the diagnosis of CAD in women.[60] The cause for this is unclear, but the pattern of a high sensitivity and low specificity reported in this study suggests the phenomenon of posttest referral bias. This entity occurs when the test under study has been used as a determinant for proceeding to angiography; as the test is usually positive for the patient to proceed to angiography, false negatives are poorly represented and false positives are overrepresented.[21,61]

In addition to posttest bias, pretest bias may also influence the results of these reports. A particular concern is that referral for an exercise echocardiogram may be provoked by a positive exercise ECG (especially if this were inconsistent with the clinical scenario). This might inflate the number of false-positive exercise ECGs, and inflate the benefit of exercise echocardiography, compared with the exercise ECG. To circumvent this, we examined a group of patients referred for exercise echocardiography as their primary test.[59] While the difference between the two tests was less marked in this subgroup than those with prior exercise ECG testing ("referral bias"), Figure 8-2 shows that exercise echocardiography remained superior to the exercise ECG (80 ± 3% vs. 64 ± 3%, $p = 0.05$).

The third form of bias involved in these studies reflects the original referral of patients for investigation. Obviously, studies of patients referred for angiography have a tendency for bias toward severe disease. If the specificity component of the study involves patients at low risk (e.g., patients undergoing angiography with valvular disease), the combination of the "sickest of the sick" and "wellest of the well" may lead to very misleading data. The assessment of pretest disease probability is a means of expressing these referral considerations. In our initial series of 70 patients, exercise echocardiography was

Table 8-1. Pretest and Posttest Probability of CAD in Women Studied by ST Analysis, Exercise Score, and Exercise Echocardiography

	HP (% with CAD)	IP (% with CAD)	LP (% without CAD)
Pretest	22 (64%)	32 (50%)	16 (81%)
Post-ST analysis	17 (65%)	38 (53%)	15 (87%)
Postmultivariate score	18 (67%)	38 (53%)	14 (93%)
Postexercise echocardiogram	26 (92%)	21 (29%)	23 (87%)

Abbreviations: CAD, coronary artery disease; HP, high probability group (>80%); IP, intermediate probability group (20% to 80%); LP, low probability group (<20%). (From Williams et al.,[58] with permission.)

more effective than either of the other tests for classifying patients into groups at high and low probability of CAD, and classified the smallest number into an intermediate (20% to 80%) probability of coronary disease (Table 8-1).

This posttest stratification is important and impacts significantly on subsequent management strategy. For example, an argument could be given to not investigate further those patients in a low probability group after testing and indeed this could be borne out by the good prognosis of patients with a negative stress echocardiogram.[62] Investigation is usually desirable in those stratified to the high probability group. Those patients in the intermediate probability group after testing are the ones where there are no firm guidelines for further management and we noted that exercise echocardiography effectively stratified patients out of this intermediate group, a clinically important result.[41,63]

Cost Effectiveness

The apparent underestimation and investigation of coronary disease in women has been a cause of concern,[14–16,64–68] and the limitations of exercise testing may be an important contributor to this process. Some have argued for a more aggressive referral to coronary angiography, but this is difficult to justify on the basis of cost, the frequency of normal angiograms, and procedure-related complications. While the superiority of stress imaging approaches over the exercise ECG has been shown in several studies, the cost implications of replacing the latter test by exercise echocardiography are an important consideration in the current medical economy. The additional

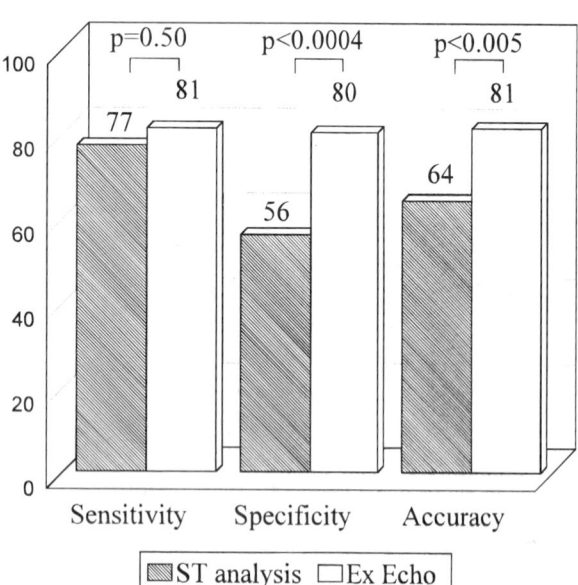

Fig. 8-2 Comparison of the sensitivity (sens) and specificity (spec) and accuracy of exercise electrocardiography and exercise echocardiography in women without (nonreferred) and with (referral) prior exercise tests. (From Marwick et al.,[59] with permission.)

Table 8-2. Clinical Features of Patients at High, Intermediate, and Low Probability of Coronary Artery Disease on Clinical Grounds ("Pretest Probability")

	High Probability	Intermediate Probability	Low Probability
n (patients)	32	72	57
Age (years)	67 ± 6	61 ± 8	55 ± 10
Typical angina	32	16	0
Atypical angina	0	55	10
Coronary artery disease	22	29	8

Table 8-3. Cost per Patient, Angiography Rate, Inappropriate (Negative) Angiography, and False-Negative Rate of Seven Diagnostic Strategies for the Diagnosis of Coronary Disease Using Exercise ECG and Exercise Echocardiogram[a]

Strategy	Cost/pt ($)	Angiography (%)	Inappropriate Angiography (%)	False Negative (%)
I—angiography	1,434	100	63	0
II—exercise ECG	1,023 ± 43	69 ± 3	56 ± 4	11 ± 3
III—exercise echo	828 ± 44	41 ± 3	29 ± 5	13 ± 4
IV—selective ECG/echo	836 ± 45	51 ± 3	44 ± 5	14 ± 4
V—stepwise ECG/echo	663 ± 36	31 ± 2	26 ± 4	22 ± 6
VI—Bayesian ECG	740 ± 29	50 ± 2	32 ± 2	29 ± 1
VII—Bayesian echo	641 ± 24	37 ± 2	25 ± 1	25 ± 1

Abbreviations: Cost/pt, cost per patient; ECG, electrocardiogram; echo, echocardiogram.
[a] See text for details.
(From Marwick et al.,[59] with permission.)

cost of incorporating the exercise echocardiogram as the primary diagnostic test instead of the exercise ECG might be balanced by the savings incurred by avoiding unnecessary angiograms.

With this in mind, we investigated the cost and diagnostic implications of several strategies involving exercise ECG testing, exercise echocardiography, and angiography in a multicenter study of 161 women—both in the group as a whole as well as after initial stratification into low, intermediate, and high probability subgroups[59] (Table 8-2). The standard diagnostic approaches are outlined in Table 8-3. These begin with the standard approach (*strategy II*) centered on the exercise ECG, with angiography in those with a positive or nondiagnostic test. Use of the exercise ECG with substitution of the exercise echocardiogram for nondiagnostic tests (*strategy IV*) led to an excessive number of inappropriate angiograms, and therefore high cost. An alternative strategy could propose exercise echocardiography in all patients, with angiography being limited to patients with a positive stress echocardiogram (*strategy III*) and this proved less expensive (because of the performance of fewer angiograms) but offered a similar level of accuracy to the standard approach. Many algorithms could be proposed for diagnostic strategies in this patient group depending on the relative bias between diagnostic accuracy and cost containment. The stepwise combination of exercise ECG with exercise echocardiography in patients with positive or nondiagnostic exercise tests (*strategy V*) led to the least number of angiograms and was least expensive, but resulted in an unacceptable number of false negatives. The utility of the Bayesian approaches was compromised by the limitations of clinical stratification of women into groups at high and low probability of coronary disease.

In this group, exercise echocardiography had the best balance between accuracy and cost for the diagnosis of CAD in women. However, the analysis neglects the true cost of a false-negative test result, although this is probably justifiable as outlined previously, given the favorable prognosis for a negative stress echocardiogram.[62] Again, the analysis also neglects issues related to ongoing diagnostic uncertainty, but it should be noted that the performance of coronary angiography is rarely effective in alleviating patients' symptoms.[69-71]

Pharmacologic Stress

The sensitivity of exercise echocardiography in women appears to be inferior to its sensitivity in men. This difference is attenuated after exclusion of nondiagnostic test results, reflecting the contribution of submaximal exercise to false negatives in women. As a consequence, the use of high dose dipyridamole stress has been examined in a group of 83 women, 39 of whom had CAD and 15 had previous myocardial infarction.[72] There appeared to be an advantage of dipyridamole over exercise echocardiography with respect to specificity (93% vs. 52%). The cause for this is unclear. Certainly, this level of specificity is inferior to that usually reported with exercise echocardiography (Ch. 3).

In 39 patients with CAD (15 single-vessel disease, 24 multiple vessel disease) there was no significant difference in sensitivity of dipyridamole and exercise echocardiography (79% vs. 72%). This does not support the contention that submaximal exercise contributes to the low sensitivity of exercise echocardiography, but this result may be colored by the low sensitivity of dipyridamole echocardiography in patients with mild disease.

CONCLUSION

Exercise ECG is the oldest, least expensive, and most widely utilized screening test for CAD; however its accuracy in women is suboptimal, often leading to more definitive testing. The accuracy of exercise ST-segment analysis has been enhanced by either incorporating exercise parameters or by ST-segment heart rate correction, but despite this improved accuracy these methods have not achieved widespread clinical acceptance.

What the clinician desires is an accurate, cost-effective test for evaluation of women presenting with chest pain syndrome. It is our contention that exercise echocardiography when used in conjunction with clinical evaluation of pretest probability can fulfill this need. It has shown an ability to stratify patients from an intermediate probability group into either high or low probability groups and therefore to streamline referral for angiography. Depending on the particular physician or institutional bias with respect to acceptable levels of accuracy and cost containment, a management algorithm may be designed to achieve the appropriate number of referrals for angiography.

Exercise echocardiography is in its relative infancy with respect to other imaging modalities such as thallium scintigraphy, but data have accumulated over recent years depicting a comparable accuracy of both techniques. Exercise echocardiography, however, can also provide ancillary structural and functional cardiac information, at a lower cost and without exposure to radiation. It is likely that once the technique becomes more widespread and clinicians feel more comfortable with image interpretation and the information provided, it will form an important part of the diagnostic armamentarium in the work-up of women with suspected CAD.

REFERENCES

1. Sketch MH, Mohiuddin SM, Lynch JD et al.: Significant sex differences in the correlation of electrocardiographic exercise testing and coronary arteriograms. Am J Cardiol 36:169, 1975
2. Cumming GR, Dufresne C, Kich L, Samm J: Exercise electrocardiogram patterns in normal women. Br Heart J 35:1055, 1973
3. Linhart JW, Laws JG, Satinsky JD: Maximum treadmill exercise electrocardiography in female patients. Circulation 50:1173, 1974
4. Profant GR, Early RG, Nilson KL et al.: Responses to maximal exercise in healthy middle-aged women. J Appl Physiol 33:595, 1972
5. Manca C, Dei Cas L, Albertini D et al.: Different prognostic value of exercise electrocardiogram in men and women. Cardiology 63:312, 1978
6. Detry JM, Kapita BM, Cosyns J et al.: Diagnostic value of history and maximal exercise electrocardiography in men and women suspected of coronary heart disease. Circulation 56:756, 1977
7. Weiner DA, Ryan TJ, McCabe CH et al.: Exercise stress testing: Correlations among history of angina, ST-segment response and prevalence of coronary-artery disease in the country artery surgery study (CASS). N Engl J Med 301:230, 1979
8. Detrano R, Janosi A, Lyons KP et al.: Factors affecting sensitivity and specificity of a diagnostic test: the exercise thallium scintigram. Am J Med 84:699, 1988
9. Philbrick JT, Horwitz RI, Feinstein AR: Methodologic problems of exercise testing for coronary artery disease: groups, analysis and bias. Am J Cardiol 46:807, 1980
10. Ransohoff DF, Feinstein AR: Problems of spectrum and bias in evaluating the efficacy of diagnostic tests. N Engl J Med 299:926, 1978
11. Higginbotham MB, Morris KG, Coleman RE, Cobb FR: Sex-related differences in the normal cardiac response to upright exercise. Circulation 70:357, 1984
12. Hanley PC, Zinsmeister AR, Clements IP et al.: Gender-related differences in cardiac response to supine exercise assessed by radionuclide angiography. J Am Coll Cardiol 13:624, 1989
13. Younis LT, Melin JA, Robert AR, Detry JM: Influence of age and sex on left ventricular volumes and ejection fraction during upright exercise in normal subjects. Eur Heart J 11:916, 1990
14. Khaw KT: Where are the women in studies of coronary heart disease? BMJ 306:1145, 1993
15. Manolio TA, Harlan WR: Research on coronary disease in women: political or scientific imperative? Br Heart J 69:1, 1993

16. Healy B: The Yentl syndrome. N Engl J Med 325:274, 1991
17. McHenry PL, Morris SN, Jordan JW: Stress testing in coronary heart disease. Heart Lung 3:83, 1974
18. Diamond GA: A clinically relevant classification of chest discomfort. J Am Coll Cardiol 1:574, 1983
19. Diamond GA, Forrester JS: Analysis of probability as an aid in the clinical diagnosis of coronary-artery disease. N Engl J Med 300:1350, 1979
20. Diamond GA, Forrester JS, Hirsch M et al.: Application of conditional probability analysis to the clinical diagnosis of coronary artery disease. J Clin Invest 65:1210, 1980
21. Sox HC Jr: Probability theory in the use of diagnostic tests. An introduction to critical study of the literature. Ann Intern Med 104:60, 1986
22. Epstein SE: Implications of probability analysis on the strategy used for noninvasive detection of coronary artery disease. Role of single or combined use of exercise electrocardiographic testing, radionuclide cineangiography and myocardial perfusion imaging. Am J Cardiol 46:491, 1980
23. Ellestad MH, Cooke BM, Jr., Greenberg PS: Stress testing: clinical application and predictive capacity. Prog Cardiovasc Dis 21:431, 1979
24. Klein J, Cheo S, Berman DS, Rozanski A: Pathophysiologic factors governing the variability of ischemic responses to treadmill and bicycle exercise. Am Heart J 128:948, 1994
25. Sanborn CF, Jankowski CM: Physiologic considerations for women in sport. Clinics Sports Med 13:315, 1994
26. Astrand I: Aerobic work capacity in men and women with special reference to age. Acta Physiol Scand, suppl. 49:169, 1960
27. Shvartz E, Reibold RC: Aerobic fitness norms for males and females aged 6 to 75 years: a review. Aviation Space Environ Med 61:3, 1990
28. Aufderheide S, Lax D, Goldberg SJ: Gender differences in dehydration-induced mitral valve prolapse. Am Heart J 129:83, 1995
29. Rosen SD, Uren NG, Kaski JC et al.: Coronary vasodilator reserve, pain perception, and sex in patients with syndrome X. Circulation 90:50, 1994
30. Clark PI, Glasser SP, Lyman GH et al.: Relation of results of exercise stress tests in young women to phases of the menstrual cycle. Am J Cardiol 61:197, 1988
31. Morise AP, Dalal JN, Duval RD: Frequency of oral estrogen replacement therapy in women with normal and abnormal exercise electrocardiograms and normal coronary arteries by angiogram. Am J Cardiol 72:1197, 1993
32. Morise AP, Dalal JN, Duval RD: Value of a simple measure of estrogen status for improving the diagnosis of coronary artery disease in women. Am J Med 94:491, 1993
33. Jaffe MD: Effect of oestrogens on postexercise electrocardiogram. Br Heart J 38:1299, 1976
34. Gilligan DM, Quyyumi AA, Cannon RO: Effects of physiological levels of estrogen on coronary vasomotor function in postmenopausal women. Circulation 89:2545, 1994
35. Hlatky MA, Pryor DB, Harrell FE, Jr. et al.: Factors affecting sensitivity and specificity of exercise electrocardiography. Multivariable analysis. Am J Med 77:64, 1984
36. Okin PM, Kligfield P: Gender-specific criteria and performance of the exercise electrocardiogram. Circulation 92:1209, 1995
37. Barolsky SM, Gilbert CA, Faruqui A et al.: Differences in electrocardiographic response to exercise of women and men: a non-Bayesian factor. Circulation 60:1021, 1979
38. Detrano R, Salcedo E, Passalacqua M, Friis R: Exercise electrocardiographic variables: a critical appraisal. J Am Coll Cardiol 8:836, 1986
39. Kligfield P, Ameisen O, Okin PM: Heart rate adjustment of ST segment depression for improved detection of coronary artery disease. Circulation 79:245, 1989
40. Guiteras P, Chaitman BR, Waters DD et al.: Diagnostic accuracy of exercise ECG lead systems in clinical subsets of women. Circulation 65:1465, 1982
41. Melin JA, Wijns W, Vanbutsele RJ et al.: Alternative diagnostic strategies for coronary artery disease in women: demonstration of the usefulness and efficiency of probability analysis. Circulation 71:535, 1985
42. Detry JM, Kapita BM, Cosyns J et al.: Diagnostic value of history and maximal exercise electrocardiography in men and women suspected of coronary heart disease. Circulation 56:756, 1977
43. Robert AR, Melin JA, Detry JM: Logistic discriminant analysis improves diagnostic accuracy of exercise testing for coronary artery disease in women. Circulation 83:1202, 1991
44. Deckers JW, Rensing BJ, Simoons ML, Roelandt JR: Diagnostic merits of exercise testing in females. Eur Heart J 10:543, 1989
45. Goldschlager N, Selzer A, Cohn K: Treadmill stress tests as indicators of presence and severity of coronary artery disease. Ann Intern Med 85:277, 1976
46. Friedman TD, Greene AC, Iskandrian AS et al.: Exer-

cise thallium-201 myocardial scintigraphy in women: correlation with coronary arteriography. Am J Cardiol 49:1632, 1982
47. Hung J, Chaitman BR, Lam J et al.: Noninvasive diagnostic test choices for the evaluation of coronary artery disease in women: a multivariate comparison of cardiac fluoroscopy, exercise electrocardiography and exercise thallium myocardial perfusion scintigraphy. J Am Coll Cardiol 4:8, 1984
48. Chae SC, Heo J, Iskandrian AS et al.: Identification of extensive coronary artery disease in women by exercise single-photon emission computed tomographic (SPECT) thallium imaging. J Am Coll Cardiol 21:1305, 1993
49. Morganroth J, Chen CC, David D et al.: Exercise cross-sectional echocardiographic diagnosis of coronary artery disease. Am J Cardiol 47:20, 1981
50. Robertson WS, Feigenbaum H, Armstrong WF et al.: Exercise echocardiography: a clinically practical addition in the evaluation of coronary artery disease. J Am Coll Cardiol 2:1085, 1983
51. Limacher MC, Quinones MA, Poliner LR et al.: Detection of coronary artery disease with exercise two-dimensional echocardiography. Description of a clinically applicable method and comparison with radionuclide ventriculography. Circulation 67:1211, 1983
52. Wann LS, Faris JV, Childress RH et al.: Exercise cross-sectional echocardiography in ischemic heart disease. Circulation 60:1300, 1979
53. Crouse LJ, Harbrecht JJ, Vacek JL et al.: Exercise echocardiography as a screening test for coronary artery disease and correlation with coronary arteriography. Am J Cardiol 67:1213, 1991
54. Armstrong WF, O'Donnell J, Dillon JC et al.: Complementary value of two-dimensional exercise echocardiography to routine treadmill exercise testing. Ann Intern Med 105:829, 1986
55. Marwick TH, Nemec JJ, Pashkow FJ et al.: Accuracy and limitations of exercise echocardiography in a routine clinical setting. J Am Coll Cardiol 19:74, 1992
56. Ryan T, Segar DS, Sawada SG et al.: Detection of coronary artery disease with upright bicycle exercise echocardiography. J Am Soc Echocardiog 6:186, 1993
57. Sawada SG, Ryan T, Fineberg NS et al.: Exercise echocardiographic detection of coronary artery disease in women [see comments]. J Am Coll Cardiol 14:1440, 1989
58. Williams MJ, Marwick TH, O'Gorman D, Foale RA: Comparison of exercise echocardiography with an exercise score to diagnose coronary artery disease in women. Am J Cardiol 74:435, 1994
59. Marwick TH, Anderson T, Williams MJ et al.: Exercise echocardiography is an accurate and cost-efficient technique for detection of coronary artery disease in women. J Am Coll Cardiol 26:335, 1995
60. Roger VL, Pellikka PA, Miller FA. Stress echocardiography for the detection of coronary artery disease in women, Abstracte. Circulation, suppl. 88(I): 403, 1993
61. Tavel ME: Specificity of electrocardiographic stress test in women versus men. Am J Cardiol 70:545, 1992
62. Sawada SG, Ryan T, Conley MJ et al.: Prognostic value of a normal exercise echocardiogram. Am Heart J 120: 49, 1990
63. Patterson RE, Horowitz SF: Importance of epidemiology and biostatistics in deciding clinical strategies for using diagnostic tests: a simplified approach using examples from coronary artery disease. [Review]. J Am Coll Cardiol 13:1653, 1989
64. Krumholz HM, Douglas PS, Lauer MS, Pasternak RC: Selection of patients for coronary angiography and coronary revascularization early after myocardial infarction: is there evidence for a gender bias? Ann Intern Med 116:785, 1992
65. Steingart RM, Packer M, Hamm P et al.: Sex differences in the management of coronary artery disease. Survival and Ventricular Enlargement Investigators. N Engl J Med 325:226, 1991
66. Bickell NA, Pieper KS, Lee KL et al.: Referral patterns for coronary artery disease treatment: gender bias or good clinical judgment? Ann Intern Med 116:791, 1992
67. Ayanian JZ, Epstein AM: Differences in the use of procedures between women and men hospitalized for coronary heart disease. N Engl J Med 325:221, 1991
68. Wenger NK: Coronary heart disease in women: gender differences in diagnostic evaluation. J Am Med Womens Assoc 49:181, 1991
69. Papanicolaou MN, Califf RM, Hlatky MA et al.: Prognostic implications of angiographically normal and insignificantly narrowed coronary arteries. Am J Cardiol 58:1181, 1986
70. Sullivan AK, Holdright DR, Wright CA et al.: Chest pain in women: clinical, investigative, and prognostic features. BMJ 308:883, 1994
71. Ockene IS, Shay MJ, Alpert JS et al.: Unexplained chest pain in patients with normal coronary arteriograms: a follow-up study of functional status. N Engl J Med 303:1249, 1980
72. Masini M, Picano E, Lattanzi F et al.: High dose dipyridamole-echocardiography test in women: correlation with exercise-electrocardiography test and coronary arteriography. J Am Coll Cardiol 12:682, 1988

Chapter 9

Perfusion Imaging for the Diagnosis and Risk Assessment of CAD in Women

Ami E. Iskandrian, Jaekyeong Heo, and Nasaraiah Nallamothu

DIAGNOSIS OF CORONARY DISEASE IN WOMEN

Coronary artery disease (CAD) is rare in women before the menopause. However, its incidence increases rapidly after menopause such that, at age 70, the prevalence is similar in women and men.[1,2] Several studies[3-5] have suggested a gender-related bias in the use of invasive testing and coronary revascularization (i.e., less cardiac catheterization and less coronary revascularization in women). The increased mortality in women after acute myocardial infarction has been attributed to older age and more unfavorable risk characteristics, including more advanced disease.[5]

Not only are the manifestations of heart disease different in women and men, but gender-related differences have been shown in exercise physiology. Higginbotham et al.[6] reported that during peak exercise the left ventricular (LV) ejection fraction (EF) is lower in women than men. Further, women responded to exercise by utilizing the Frank-Starling mechanism (LV dilation) whereas men utilized increased contractility (a decrease in end-systolic volume). Whether these represent true biological phenomena or technique-related changes is not entirely clear. We have recently shown, using the ambulatory nuclear detector which allows beat-to-beat assessment of LV function, that healthy women utilize both the Frank-Starling mechanism and increased contractility during exhaustive exercise and these changes are more pronounced at peak exercise than submaximal exercise.[7] Further, the type of exercise (Bruce protocol or individualized ramp protocol) did not affect the results.

The apparent underestimation of the problem of CAD in women may in part reflect difficulties in the diagnosis of CAD in women. The clinical prediction of CAD based on the symptom status of the patient is less accurate in women than in men. For example, the probability of CAD is less in women than men with typical angina pectoris, atypical angina pectoris, or nonanginal chest pain.[8] The clinical implications of these observations are that negative exercise electrocardiogram (ECG) results in women with a low pretest probability of CAD are likely to be true negative responses. We observed, for example, that only 6% of women with a low pretest probability of CAD and negative exercise ECGs had perfusion abnormalities on single-photon emission computed tomographic (SPECT) thallium-201 imaging.[9] The problem, however, is that the exercise ECG has a low diagnostic accuracy in women with intermediate or high pretest probability of CAD and is not useful in patients with nondiagnostic exercise results because of resting ECG abnormalities or submaximal exercise. The results of exercise ECG response in 637 men and 188 women with CAD, and 70 men

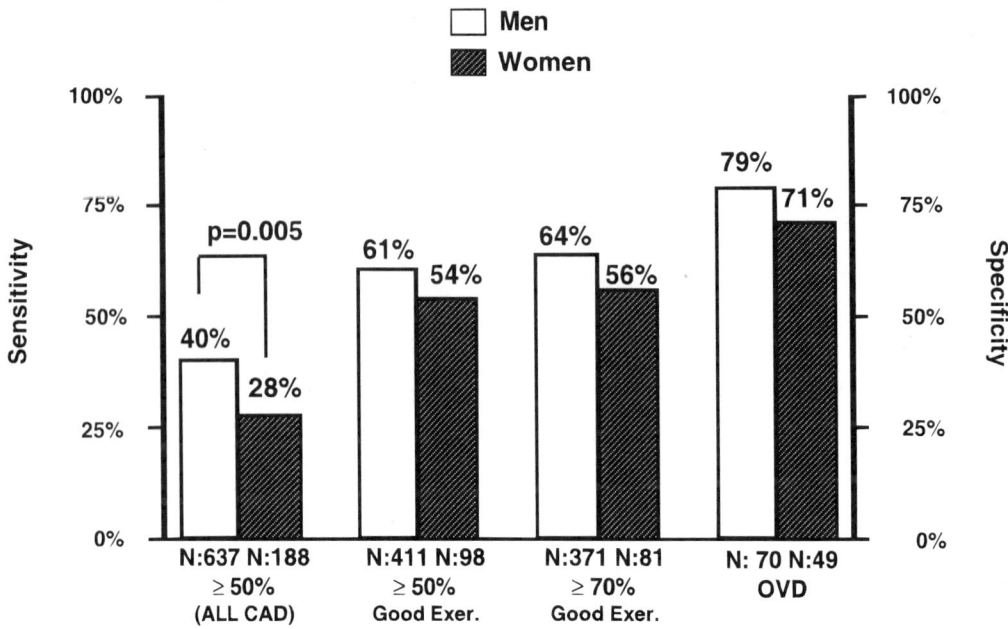

Fig. 9-1. The sensitivity and specificity of exercise electrocardiogram in women and men. (Data from The American Heart Association,[31] with permission.)

and 49 women with no CAD (by coronary angiography) are shown in Figure 9-1. The sensitivity was lower in women than men (28% vs. 40%, $p = 0.005$). The sensitivity in women increased if patients with submaximal exercise were excluded from (28% to 54%, $p = 0.001$) or if CAD was defined as greater or equal to 70% rather than greater or equal to 50% diameter stenosis from 28% to 56% ($p = 0.001$). The specificity was comparable in women and men (71% vs. 79%, p = NS). The use of multivariate analysis, based on the ability of other exercise variables to improve the diagnostic accuracy of the ST response, is discussed by Robert in Chapter 7. However, while modifications of the exercise ECG interpretation may be beneficial, many physicians rely on stress imaging techniques to improve the accuracy of noninvasive testing for CAD in women.

USE OF NUCLEAR CARDIOLOGY TECHNIQUES IN WOMEN

General Considerations

A detailed discussion of perfusion imaging techniques is beyond the scope of this chapter and is presented in Chapter 2. With particular attention to the diagnosis of CAD in women, it may be important to consider the type of stress, the type of radiotracer, and the type of imaging modality. The types of stress tests[10,11] include exercise, dipyridamole, adenosine, dobutamine, arbutamine, or a combination of these (for example, dipyridamole plus exercise). The types of radiotracers[12,13] include thallium-201 and technetium-99m-labeled compounds (sestamibi, teboroxime, tetrofosmin, and furifosmin). The imaging modalities[14] include planar and SPECT (with one or multiple detectors). Other issues of less importance include the imaging protocol, the use of gated imaging, simultaneous assessment of perfusion and function, attenuation and scatter correction, and quantitation.

Some data obtained from studies with predominant male populations are probably pertinent to the diagnosis of CAD in women. First, the sensitivity of perfusion imaging is lower at submaximal than maximal exercise.[10] Second, the sensitivity of perfusion imaging using coronary vasodilators (such as dipyridamole and adenosine) is better than that of submaximal exercise and is at least as good as that with maximal exercise.[11] Third, the sensitivity of perfusion imaging with SPECT is better than that of planar imaging, specially for detecting mild disease, one-vessel disease, and circumflex disease.[14] Fourth, the sensitivity of stress perfusion imaging using technetium agents is comparable to thallium-201 while specificity may be better.[12,13] Specificity also depends on experience, image quality, pretest and posttest biases in patient selection, and other factors. Finally, gated imaging or the combination of first-pass radionuclide angiography and SPECT perfusion imaging improves the diagnostic and prognostic information.[15]

Special Features of Perfusion Imaging in Women

Breast Attenuation

Breast attenuation artifacts may be seen both with planar and SPECT imaging using either thallium and technetium agents.[16] The degree and the site of attenuation are variable and may be dependent on the breast size, consistency, and shape. Taping the breast away from the cardiac silhouette, use of markers, experience, review of the cine display of the raw images, the use of gender-specific normal files, and the use of gated imaging or simultaneous perfusion and function studies are important in the recognition of breast attenuation artifacts. Most artifacts appear as fixed defects but a change in the breast position between the stress and rest study may give the appearance of a reversible defect. These defects are often seen in the anterior wall and, at times, they extend to the lateral wall and to the septum. In obese women, diaphragmatic attenuation may be seen in combination with breast attenuation; otherwise, in general, the count density in women in the inferior wall is greater than the anterior wall—which is the opposite of findings in men. It should be noted that in many large-scale clinical trials the readers were blinded as to the gender of the patient to meet federal regulatory requirements. This may contribute to the low specificity of early reports. Obviously, when these tests are used for clinical management the observer is not blinded to the gender of the patient.

Lung Thallium Uptake

Increased lung thallium uptake denotes LV dysfunction, which, in patients with CAD, indicates extensive ischemia, scar, or both. In our experience, increased lung thallium uptake is less common in women than men, regardless of the extent of CAD.[17] This observation may be due to several factors, including breast attenuation (which decreases the lung activity more than cardiac activity), smaller size of the myocardium at risk in women than men (hence causing less LV dysfunction), and lower myocardial blood flow and washout in women (possibly reflecting the lower workload and peak heart rate in women than men). The latter factor is important only if initial images are obtained 30 minutes or longer after thallium injection. There are no data on gender-related differences in lung sestamibi uptake.

MYOCARDIAL PERFUSION IMAGING FOR DIAGNOSIS OF CORONARY DISEASE IN WOMEN

Accuracy of Stress SPECT

Several studies have examined the accuracy of myocardial perfusion imaging for the detection of CAD in women;[9,18-22] published series are summarized in Table 9-1. The results of exercise SPECT thallium-201 imaging in women and men with angiographically defined CAD studied in our laboratory are compared in Figure 9-2. The sensitivity was 72% in 188 women and 92% in 637 men with greater than or equal to 50% diameter stenosis of one or more vessels ($p = 0.0001$). If patients with submaximal exercise were excluded, the sensitivity was 77% in women ($n = 98$) and 94% in men ($n = 411$) ($p = $

Table 9-1. Accuracy of Stress Myocardial Perfusion Imaging in Women

Author	Test Type	Number of Patients	CAD prevalence (%)	Sensitivity	Specificity
Friedman et al. (1982)[20]	Planar	60	47	75	97
Hung et al. (1984)[21]	Planar	92	30	75	91
Melin et al. (1985)[22]	Planar	93	26	71	91
Chae et al. (1993)[9]	SPECT	243	67	71	65

Abbreviations: CAD coronary artery disease; SPECT, single-photon emission computed tomography.

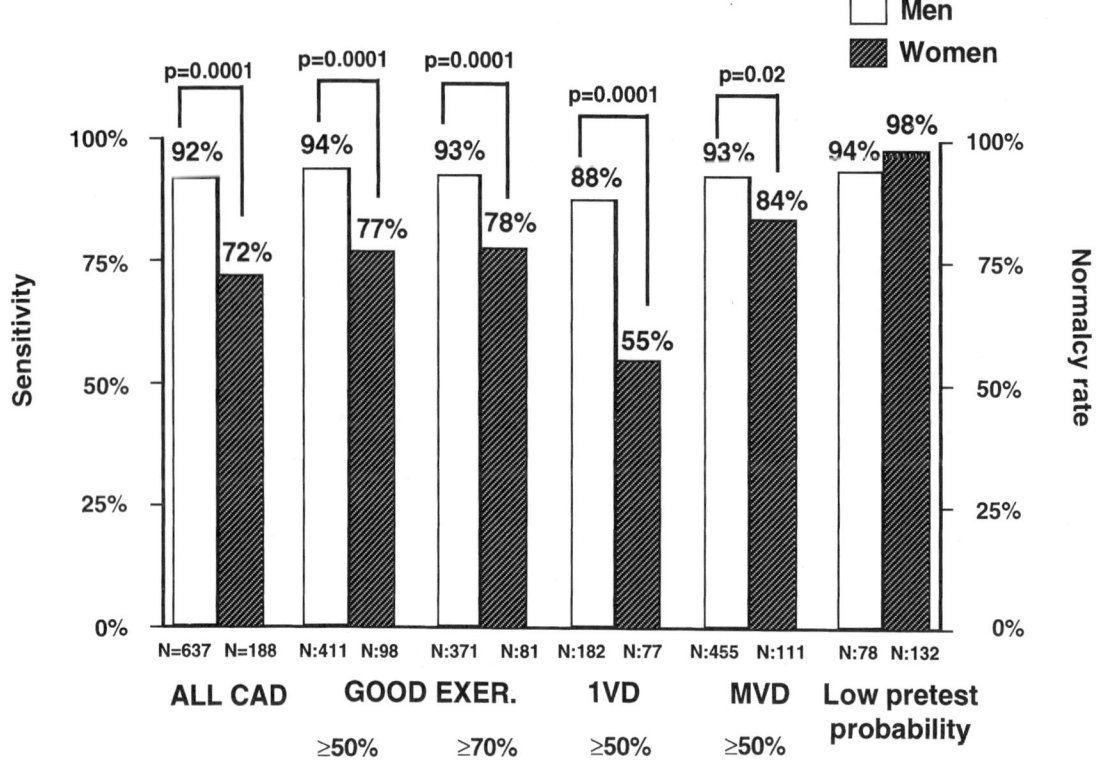

Fig. 9-2. The results of exercise single-photon emission computed tomograph thallium imaging in women and men. (From The American Heart Association,[31] with permission.)

0.0001). The sensitivity was slightly higher if CAD was defined as greater than or equal to 70% diameter stenosis (78% in women [$n = 159$] and 93% in men [$n = 58$], $p = 0.0001$). The difference in sensitivity between women and men was greater in patients with one-vessel disease (55% in women [$n = 77$] vs. 88% in men [$n = 182$], $p = 0.0001$) than multivessel disease (84% in women [$n = 111$] vs. 93% in men [$n = 455$], $p = 0.02$). The normalcy rate was comparable in women ($n = 132$) and men ($n = 78$) with low pretest probability of CAD (98% vs. 94%).

Preliminary data by Marwick et al.[18] in 97 women undergoing exercise SPECT thallium imaging and 107 women undergoing dipyridamole rubidium-82 positron emission tomographic PET imaging showed that the overall sensitivity of exercise SPECT thallium imaging was only 54%, compared to 88% with rubidium PET.[18] The sensitivity was 42% in 26 women with one-vessel disease undergoing exercise SPECT imaging and 77% in 35 women tested with PET imaging ($p = 0.006$). The respective sensitivities of SPECT and PET for multivessel CAD were 68% and 100% ($p = 0.001$). The specificity of SPECT was 63% compared to 79% with PET.

Taillefer et al.[19] compared the results of exercise thallium SPECT and exercise sestaMIBI SPECT in 85 women, 64 with and 19 without CAD ($\geq 50\%$ diameter stenosis). The sensitivity by thallium was 80% and by sestaMIBI 69% ($p = NS$). The specificity by thallium was 62% and by sestaMIBI was 86% ($p = NS$). The improved specificity by sestaMIBI was most likely due to less attenuation artifacts.

Our results with adenosine SPECT thallium imaging are shown in Figure 9-3. Overall, the sensitivity in women was higher with adenosine than with exercise but still slightly lower than the sensitivity of adenosine SPECT thallium imaging in men (82% vs. 95%, $p = 0.0001$). The sensitivity was higher in both men and women if the severity of the disease was defined as 70% or greater. Importantly, in women

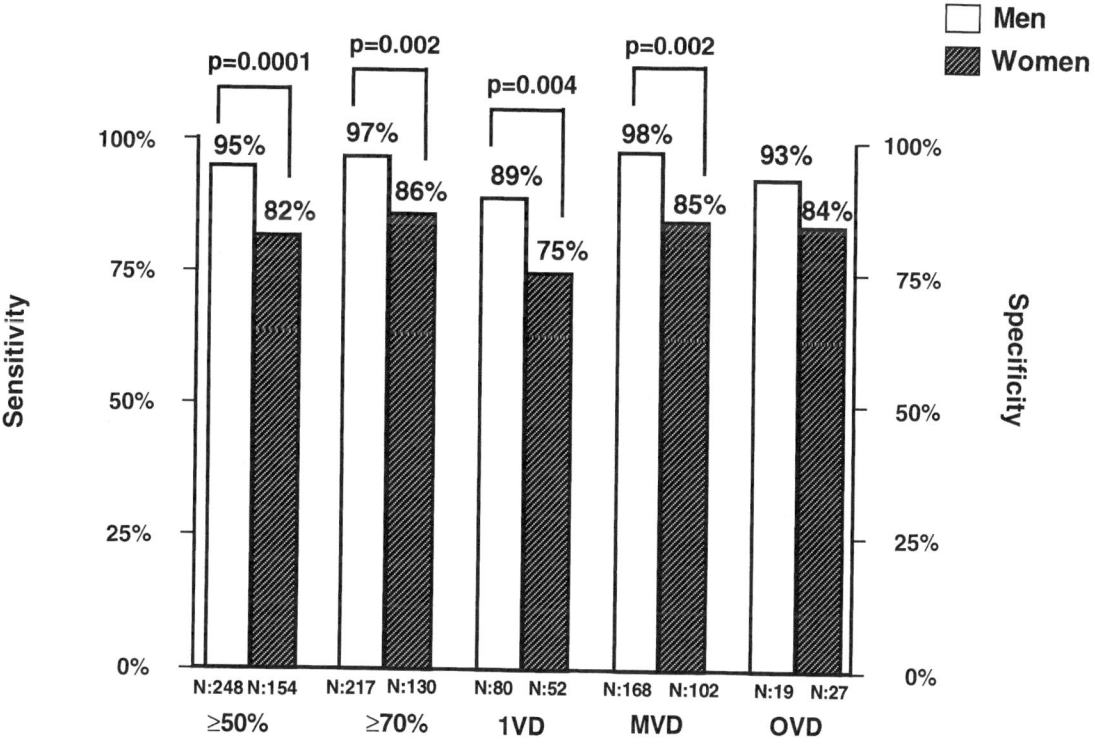

Fig. 9-3. The results of adenosine single-photon emission computed tomograph thallium imaging in women and men. (From The American Heart Assocation,[31] with permission.)

with one-vessel disease, the sensitivity of adenosine SPECT thallium imaging was 75%, which, although lower than the corresponding sensitivity in men (89%, $p = 0.004$), is higher than the corresponding results obtained with exercise imaging. In women with multivessel disease the sensitivity was 85% compared to 98% in men. The specificity of the test in patients with no CAD by angiography was 84% in women and 93% in men.

In general, these results suggest that the sensitivity for detecting any CAD and, especially, one-vessel disease is lower in women than men, but the sensitivity is greater with a higher level of exercise; higher with pharmacologic testing than exercise, and higher with more extensive or more severe CAD.

Possible Reasons for Gender Differences in the Accuracy of SPECT

The possible reasons for gender-related differences in the detection of CAD by perfusion imaging are shown in Table 9-2. It is possible that problems with

Table 9-2. Possible Reasons for Gender-Related Differences in Detection of CAD by Perfusion Imaging

1. Problems in image interpretation
2. Problems in assessing coronary angiography
3. Alteration in coronary blood flow after menopause
4. Left ventricular size
5. Level of exercise/type of stress
6. Extent of CAD

Abbreviation: CAD, coronary artery disease.

cautious image interpretation, such as misinterpretation of true defects as breast attenuation artifacts, might be responsible for decreasing the sensitivity of perfusion imaging.

Several differences may exist between women and men with respect to coronary physiology. Because of the smaller caliber of the vessels in women, it is possible that coronary angiographic results may be more difficult to interpret in women. Sambuceti et

Table 9-3. Global Alteration in Perfusion in One-Vessel Disease

Myocardial Blood Flow (ml/100 g/min)	Normal Subjects (n = 9)	One-Vessel Disease (n = 21)	
		Stenosis	Remote
Baseline	0.92 ± 0.13	0.68 ± 0.14	0.74 ± 0.18
Pacing	1.95 ± 0.64	0.92 ± 0.29	1.16 ± 0.40
Dipyridamole	3.59 ± 0.71	1.18 ± 0.34	1.77 ± 0.71

al.[23] reported on the presence of global alterations in myocardial blood flow in patients with single-vessel disease. In this study, myocardial blood flow during pacing or dipyridamole infusion was not only impaired in the territory of the diseased artery but also in the remaining arteries without stenosis. This effect was significantly different from normal subjects. Thus, the myocardial blood flow during dipyridamole infusion increased from 0.68 ± 0.14 to 1.18 ± 0.34 (ml/100 g/min) in the diseased artery, from 0.74 ± 0.18 to 1.77 ± 0.71 (ml/100 g/min) in the remote artery with no coronary stenosis, and from 0.92 ± 0.13 to 3.59 ± 0.71 (ml/100 g/min) in normal subjects (Table 9-3). Whether this response is more common in women than men is not clear, but such global reduction in flow, if indeed more common in women, may explain the lower sensitivity of perfusion results in women. It is also possible that abnormal hyperemic flow response in women may be more marked after menopause.[24,25] Studies have shown that treatment with estrogen increases the hyperemic flow in women, even in the absence of CAD, although a recent study suggested that this improvement is seen only with acute therapy and not with chronic therapy.[26]

Another factor possibly responsible for compromising the sensitivity of myocardial perfusion imaging in women may be related to LV size. Possibly, because LV size is smaller in women than men, the recognition of small defects may be more difficult. Using quantitative measurement of LV muscle mass with 2D echocardiography,[27] we found a significantly lower ventricular mass in women with CAD and normal scans compared to women with abnormal scans (Fig. 9-4). The impact of LV size would be more marked in patients with single-vessel disease because in these patients the size of the abnormality would be smaller.

Finally, lower levels of exercise in women may contribute to lower levels of sensitivity of myocardial perfusion imaging, as sensitivity is lower with submaximal than maximal exercise.[9] The improvement in sensitivity with pharmacologic testing discussed earlier supports these assumptions.

In summary, stress perfusion imaging is better than exercise ECG in detecting CAD in women. Comparison between PET and SPECT is difficult because PET is routinely done with pharmacologic testing, which, even with SPECT, provides a higher sensitivity. It is conceivable that in the subgroup of women with small hearts, the improved resolution of PET may offer an advantage. It is likely that stress echocardiography will have an intermediate sensitivity between exercise ECG and perfusion imaging.

PROGNOSTIC ASSESSMENT USING MYOCARDIAL PERFUSION IMAGING IN WOMEN

The use of myocardial perfusion imaging for prognostic evaluation is discussed in more detail in a subsequent chapter. We have examined the ability of exercise SPECT thallium imaging to identify high risk women with left main or three-vessel CAD using a stepwise discriminant analysis.[9] Exercise SPECT thallium imaging and coronary arteriography were performed for evaluation of chest pain in 243 women, who were divided into those with left-main or three-vessel coronary disease (Group 1, n = 58), and women with no, one-, or two-vessel disease (Group 2, n = 185). On univariate analysis, women in Group 1 were older ($p < 0.03$) and had a lower exercise workload ($p < 0.02$), lower exercise heart rate ($p < 0.004$), higher prevalence of diabetes mellitus ($p < 0.0003$), and more multivessel thallium abnormality ($p < 0.0001$) compared to women in Group 2 (Tables 9-4 and 9-5). On multivariate analy-

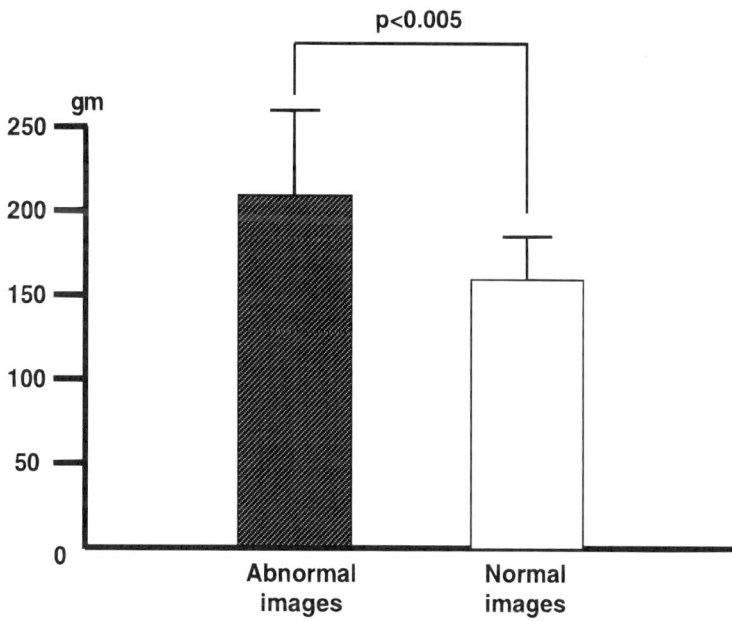

Fig. 9-4. The left ventricle mass in women with coronary artery disease and normal vs abnormal exercise single-photon emission computed tomograph thallium images.

Table 9-4. Exercise Results in Patients with Left Main or Three-Vessel Coronary Disease (Group 1) and Those with No, One-Vessel or Two-Vessel Disease (Group 2)[a]

	Group 1 (n = 58)	Group 2 (n = 185)	p-Value
Exercise duration (min)	5.8 ± 2.4	6.0 ± 2.6	NS
Exercise workload (METs)	5.3 ± 2.3	6.2 ± 2.5	0.02
Exercise heart rate (beats/min)	122 ± 25	132 ± 23	0.004
Exercise systolic BP (mmHg)	168 ± 25	172 ± 26	NS
Exercise ECG response			NS
Positive	18 (31)	43 (23)	
Negative	11 (19)	46 (25)	
Inconclusive	29 (50)	96 (52)	
Strongly positive ECG	11 (19)	27 (15)	NS
Early positive ECG	15 (26)	40 (22)	NS
Duration of ST depression (min)	6.3 ± 2.9	7.1 ± 4.3	NS
Angina during exercise	21 (36)	62 (34)	NS
Abnormal systolic BP response	11 (19)	21 (11)	NS

[a] Values are expressed as mean value ± SD or number (%) of patients.
Abbreviations: BP, blood pressure; ECG, electrocardiographic; NS, not significant.
(From Chae et al.,[9] with permission.)

Table 9-5. Results of Exercise Tomographic Thallium Imaging in Patients with Left Main or Three-Vessel Coronary Disease (Group 1) and Those with No Disease, One-Vessel or Two-Vessel Disease (Group 2)[a]

	Group 1 (n = 58)	Group 2 (n = 185)	p-Value
Abnormal thallium images	49 (84)	94 (51)	0.0001
Reversible perfusion defects	44 (76)	64 (35)	0.0001
Increased lung/heart ratio (%)	18 (31)	20 (11)	0.0002
Left ventricular cavity dilation	14 (24)	11 (6)	0.0002
Segments with perfusion defects (no.)	8.2 ± 5.7	3.8 ± 4.9	0.0001
Segments with reversible defects (no.)	6.3 ± 5.1	2.6 ± 4.3	0.0001
Extent of perfusion abnormality (%)	25 ± 9	15 ± 12	0.0001
Multivessel thallium abnormality	32 (55)	37 (20)	0.0001

[a] Values are expressed as mean value ± SD or number (%) of patients.
(From Chae et al,[9] with permission.)

sis, only multivessel thallium abnormality ($F = 43$) and exercise heart rate ($F = 6$) were independent predictors of left-main or three-vessel coronary disease. A model based on these two variables separated the women into three risk groups: 99 patients with a 9% prevalence of left-main or three-vessel disease, 70 patients with a 23% prevalence, and 74 patients with a 45% prevalence ($p < 0.0001$) (Fig. 9-5). These data confirm that high-risk women with left-main or three-vessel coronary disease can be identified by exercise SPECT thallium imaging.

The independent and incremental prognostic value of exercise SPECT thallium imaging[28] has also been examined in 212 women who had coronary angiography and a normal LVEF (mean 65 ± 15%). During a mean follow up of 40 months, 27 women had events (cardiac death or nonfatal myocardial infarction). Univariate Cox survival analysis showed several variables to be different between patients with events and those without events: age, exercise heart rate, the extent of CAD, reversible thallium defects, number of segments with reversible abnormality, and size of perfusion abnormality (Table 9-6 and Fig. 9-6). Multivariate survival analysis showed that a large perfusion abnormality and age were independent predictors of events. Actuarial life table analysis showed that women with a large thallium abnormality ($\geq 15\%$ of the myocardium) had significantly worse event-free survival than women with no or small abnormality (Mantel-Cox statistic = 16, $p = 0.0001$) (Fig. 9-7). The SPECT results had independent and incremental prognostic power compared to clinical, exercise, and catheterization data (Fig. 9-8). Thus, exercise SPECT thallium imaging provides independent and incremental prognostic information to clinical, exercise, and coronary angiographic results in women. The presence of a larger thallium abnormality identifies women at high risk of cardiac events.

In patients undergoing vascular surgery, Hendel et al.[29] observed sex differences in perioperative and

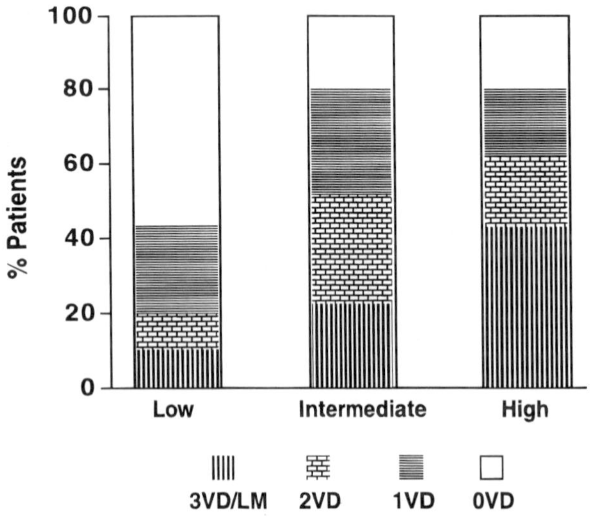

Fig. 9-5. Coronary anatomy in low, intermediate and high risk groups; 0VD, no significant coronary artery disease; 1VD, single-vessel disease; 2VD, two-vessel disease; 3VD/LM, three-vessel disease or left main coronary artery disease. (From Chae et al.,[9] with permission.)

Table 9-6. Comparison between Women with and without Events

	Events (n = 27)	No Events (n = 185)	p-Value
Exercise duration (min)	6.2 ± 2.7	6.5 ± 3.0	NS
Exercise workload (METs)	5.7 ± 2.6	6.2 ± 2.5	NS
Exercise heart rate (bpm)	124 ± 26	132 ± 23	0.07
Exercise systolic BP (mmHg)	170 ± 28	170 ± 24	NS
ST depression	4 (15%)	40 (22%)	NS
Abnormal BP response (blunted or hypotensive)	4 (15%)	23 (12%)	NS
Angina during exercise	10 (37%)	51 (28%)	NS
Abnormal images	23 (85%)	90 (49%)	0.001
Reversible abnormality	16 (59%)	64 (35%)	0.03
Extent abnormality (%)	20 ± 13	10 ± 12	0.0003
Number of abnormal segments	8 ± 5	4 ± 5	0.001
Number of reversible segments	5 ± 5	2 ± 4	0.01
Number of abnormal vascular territories	1.4 ± 0.8	0.8 ± 0.9	0.002
LV dilation	3 (11%)	16 (9%)	NS
Increased lung thallium uptake	3 (11%)	22 (12%)	NS
LVEF (%)	61 ± 17	66 ± 15	NS
Coronary anatomy			0.05
One-vessel disease	8 (30)	57 (31%)	
Two-vessel disease	6 (22)	30 (16%)	
Three-vessel disease	9 (33)	27 (15%)	
No significant disease	4 (15)	71 (38%)	

Abbreviations: BP, blood pressure, EF, ejection fraction; LV, left ventricular; NS, not significant.
(From Pancholy et al.,[28] with permission.)

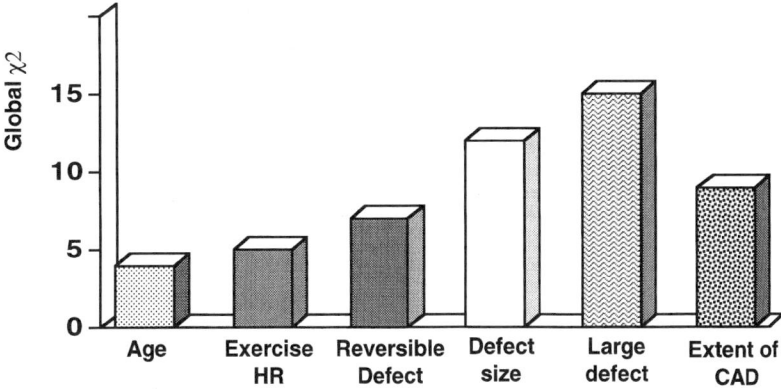

Fig. 9-6. Univariate predictors of cardiac events. (From Pancholy et al.,[28] with permission.)

186 Cardiac Stress Testing and Imaging

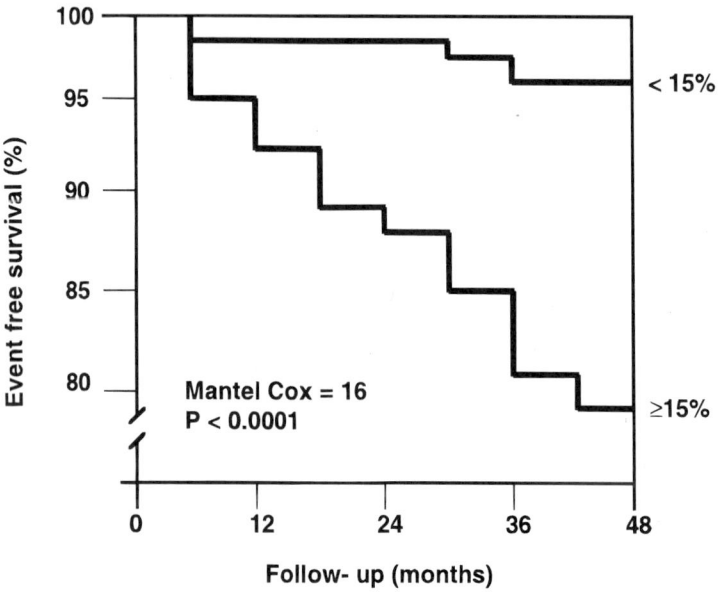

Fig. 9-7. Actuarial event-free survival curve. Patients are divided into two groups on the basis of large perfusion abnormality (≥15% of myocardium). (From Pancholy et al.,[2] permission.)

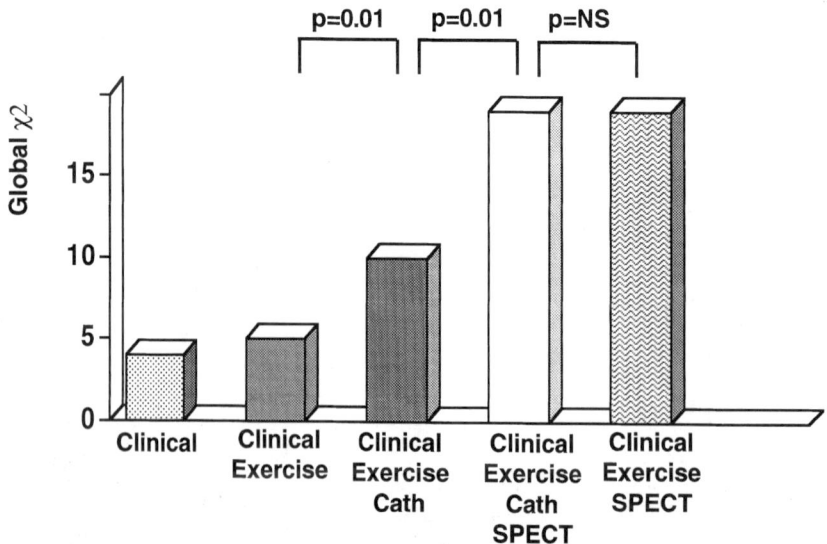

Fig. 9-8. Incremental prognostic value of clinical, exercise, catheterization, and single-photon emission computed tomography thallium variables (From Pancholy et al., [28] with permission.)

long-term cardiac event-free survival based on analysis of clinical and dipyridamole thallium variables. Thallium defects were more common in men than women; reversible defects were predictive of perioperative events in men and women while fixed defects were predictive of late events in women but not men.

Exercise SPECT thallium imaging is useful in management of women with known or suspected CAD. Although the test accuracy is lower in women than men, its prognostic performance appears just as robust in women as men.[28] Women with normal scans had a low event rate (1%/year) (high negative predictive value). It is therefore important to note that women with CAD and normal scans (false negatives) have a benign prognosis. It should also be noted that in women with large perfusion defects (as in men), although the risk of an event is higher, most do not suffer cardiac events (low positive predictive value). Thompson et al.[30] observed that in patients with angina pectoris the levels of fibrinogen, von Willebrand factor-antigen, and t-PA antigen (markers of impaired fibrinolysis, endothelial cell injury, and inflammatory activity) were independent predictors of events.[30]. This may explain the suboptimal positive predictive value of myocardial perfusion imaging; in addition to the extent of CAD, LV function, and ischemia, multiple factors affect prognosis, including markers of impaired fibrinolysis. Future studies should address these combined issues.

ACKNOWLEDGMENT

This project was funded in part by The Sidney Kimmel Cardiovascular Research Center.

REFERENCES

1. Wenger NK: Coronary disease in women. Ann Intern Med 36:285, 1985
2. Lerner DJ, Kannel WB: Patterns of coronary heart disease morbidity and mortality in the sexes. A 26-year follow-up of the Framingham population. Am Heart J 111:383, 1986
3. Steingart RM, Packer M, Mammul et al.: Sex differences in the management of coronary artery disease. N Engl J Med 325:226, 1991
4. Cowley MJ, Mullin SM, Kelsey SF et al.: Sex differences in early and long-term results of coronary angioplasty in the NHLBI PTCA registry. Circulation 71:90, 1985
5. Vaccarino V, Krumholz HM, Berkman LF, Horwitz RI: Sex differences in mortality after myocardial infarction: is there evidence for an increased risk for women? Circulation 91:1861, 1995
6. Higginbotham MB, Morris KG, Coleman E, Cobb FR: Sex-related differences in the normal cardiac response to upright exercise. Circulation 70:357, 1984
7. Bhadha K, Johnson J, Walter J et al.: Assessment of left ventricular performance during exercise in healthy women using the ambulatory nuclear detector: comparison of the Bruce and ramp protocols. Am J Cardiol 75:963, 1995
8. Diamond GA, Forrester JS: Probability as an aid in the diagnosis of coronary artery disease. N Engl J Med 14:1477, 1979
9. Chae SC, Heo J, Iskandrian AS, Wasserleben V, Cave V: Identification of extensive coronary artery disease in women by exercise single-photon emission computed tomographic (SPECT) thallium imaging. J Am Coll Cardiol 21:1305, 1993
10. Iskandrian AS, Heo J, Kong B, Lyons E: Effect of exercise levels on the ability of thallium-201 tomographic imaging in detecting coronary artery disease: analysis of 461 patients. J Am Coll Cardiol 14:1477, 1989
11. Iskandrian AS, Heo J: Pharmacologic stress testing. p 170. In Zaret B, Beller G (eds): Nuclear Cardiology. CV Mosby, St. Louis, 1993
12. Heo J, Iskandrian AS: Technetium-labelled myocardial perfusion agents. Cardiology Clinics 12:187, 1994
13. Iskandrian AS, Heo J, Kong B, Lyons E, Marsch S: Use of technetium-99m isonitrile (RP-30a) in assessing left ventricular perfusion and function at rest and during exercise in coronary artery disease and comparison with coronary arteriography and exercise thallium-201 SPECT imaging. Am J Cardiol 64:270, 1989
14. Iskandrian AS, Heo J, Askenase A, Segal BL, Helfant RH: Thallium imaging with single photon emission computed tomography. Am Heart J 114:852, 1987
15. Borges-Neto S, Coleman RE, Potts JM, Jones RH: Combined exercise radionuclide angiography and single-photon computed tomography perfusion studies for assessment of coronary artery disease. Sem Nucl Med 21:223, 1991
16. DePuey EG, Garcia EV: Optimal specificity of thallium-201 SPECT through recognition of imaging artifacts. J Nucl Med 30:441, 1989
17. Aksut S, Mallavarapu C, Russell J, Iskandrian AS: Lung thallium uptake by SPECT thallium imaging. Am Heart J 130:367, 1995
18. Marwick TH, Lauer MS, Neumann DR et al.: Diagnosis

of coronary artery disease in women using thallium-201 SPECT and rubidium-82 PET, abstracted. J Nucl Med 36:78P, 1995
19. Taillefer R, DePuey GE, Udelson J et al.: Comparison of thallium-201 and Tc-99m sestamibi (perfusion and gated SPECT) myocardial perfusion imaging in detection of coronary artery disease in women [abstract]. Circulation 92:129, 1995
20. Friedman TD, Greene AC, Iskandrian AS et al.: Exercise thallium-201 myocardial scintigraphy in women: Correlation with coronary angiography. Am J Cardiol 49:1632, 1982
21. Hung J, Chaitman BR, Lam J et al.: Noninvasive diagnostic test choices for the evaluation of coronary artery disease in women: a multivariate comparison of cardiac fluoroscopy, exercise electrocardiography and exercise thallium myocardial perfusion scintigraphy. J Am Coll Cardiol 4:8, 1984
22. Melin JA, Wijns W, Vanbusele RJ et al.: Alternative diagnostic strategies for coronary artery disease in women: Demonstration of the usefulness and efficacy of probability analysis. Circulation 71:535, 1985
23. Sambuceti G, Marzullo P, Giorgetti A et al.: Global alteration in perfusion response to increasing oxygen consumption in patients with single-vessel coronary artery disease. Circulation 90:1696, 1994
24. Gilligan DM, Badar DM, Panza JA et al.: Acute vascular effects of estrogen in postmenopausal women. Circulation 90(2):786, 1994
25. Gilligan DM, Badar DM, Panza JA et al.: Effects of estrogen replacement therapy on peripheral vasomotor function in postmenopausal women. Circulation 89:2545, 1994
26. Gilligan DM, Badar DM, Panza JA et al.: Effects of estrogen replacement therapy on peripheral vasomotor function in postmenopausal women. Am J Cardiol 75:264, 1995
27. Ghods M, Gioia G, Ren J-F, Heo J, Iskandrian AS: Effect of left ventricular muscle mass on the results of exercise SPECT thallium images in women with coronary artery disease [abstract]. J Nucl Med 35:99, 1994
28. Pancholy S, Fattah AA, Kamal AM et al.: Independent and incremental prognostic value of exercise SPECT thallium imaging in women. J Nucl Cardiol 2:110, 1995
29. Hendel RC, Chen MH, L'Italien J et al.: Sex differences in perioperative and long-term cardiac event-free survival in vascular surgery patients. An analysis of clinical and scintigraphic variables. Circulation 91:1044, 1995
30. Thompson SG, Kienast J, Pyke SDM et al.: Hemostatic factors and the risk of myocardial infarction on sudden death in patients with angina pectoris. N Engl J Med 332:635, 1995
31. American Heart Association Scientific Sessions. Circulation 92:1, 1995

Chapter 10

Diagnosis of CAD in the Presence of Left Ventricular Hypertrophy

Michael S. Lauer

BACKGROUND

Left ventricular hypertrophy (LVH) is a common condition that results from myocardial responses to overload.[1,2] Pressure overload, for example due to hypertension and aortic stenosis, is thought to stimulate parallel replication of myocardial sarcomeres, leading to concentric hypertrophy. Volume overload, which may be due to obesity or valvular regurgitation, leads to serial sarcomere replication and eccentric hypertrophy.[1] In these situations, hypertrophy acts as a successful short-term response to overload, but in the long run, this is deleterious and eventually leads to congestive heart failure. Katz[2] has emphasized the harmful effects of hypertrophy by describing the "cardiomyopathy of overload." Numerous epidemiologic and clinical studies have demonstrated that LVH is a powerful predictor of an adverse cardiovascular prognosis.[3–15]

The importance of accurate diagnosis of coronary artery disease (CAD) in the setting of LVH stems from two key clinical observations. First, LVH is an important, independent risk factor for CAD,[9] and second, LVH in combination with CAD is associated with very high risk for an adverse outcome.[12–15] Furthermore, LVH is a common finding, especially in elderly patients,[16] and is associated with two very common disorders, namely, hypertension[17] and obesity,[18,19] which are themselves important risk factors for CAD.

DEFINITION AND DIAGNOSIS OF LVH

Left ventricular hypertrophy is defined by the presence of an abnormally high left ventricular mass (LVM). While LVM can be estimated using left ventriculography, computed tomography, or magnetic resonance imaging (MRI), in standard clinical practice the two primary methods for detecting LVH are electrocardiography[20] (ECG) and echocardiography.[21,22]

ECG LVH suffers from a low sensitivity and a relatively low prevalence in population studies.[23] In the Framingham cohort of 4,684 subjects who had adequate echocardiograms, 755 met echocardiographic criteria for LVH. ECG criteria had sensitivity of only 6.9%; the corresponding specificity was 98.8%. Echocardiography is a more sensitive technique for detecting LVH, but is considerably more labor-intensive and expensive than ECG. The remainder of this section discusses each of these two techniques in detail.

Echocardiographic LVH

A number of M-mode and two-dimensional echocardiographic methods for estimating LVM have been proposed and validated against pathologic studies.[21,22,24] Common to all echocardiographic methods is an attempt to estimate left ventricular muscle volume by subtracting left ventricular cavity size from "total" (i.e., cavity plus walls) left ventricular size. This left ventricular muscle volume is then multiplied by the density of left ventricular muscle to obtain LVM. A particularly useful method for population studies, such as the Framingham Heart Study, is the "Penn Convention," which requires M-mode estimates of left ventricular chamber method and wall thickness.[21] According to this convention, estimated LVM in grams is

$$LVM = 1.04[(LVID\text{-}D + IVST + PFWT)^3 - (LVID\text{-}D)^3] - 13.6$$

where LVID-D is left ventricular internal dimension at end-diastole in centimeters, IVST is interventricular septal thickness in centimeters, and PWFT is posterior free wall thickness in centimeters (Fig. 10-1).

Considerable controversy exists as to how best to adjust estimated echocardiographic LVM for body size. While many authors have utilized a "left ventricular mass index" in which LVM is divided by body surface area, others have advocated adjusting by height.[9] As LVH may well be related to obesity,[18] as discussed below, using body surface area to adjust LVM for body size may result in inappropriate attenuation of the association between LVM and body mass.[9,25,26] One group[25] has advocated dividing LVM by height$^{2.7}$. Recent analysis of a young, healthy reference subset of the Framingham Study has suggested that adjustment by height$^{2.0}$ may best adjust LVM for body size.[26]

A major limitation of echocardiography for estimating LVM is the relatively high frequency of technically inadequate studies. For example, in the Framingham Study, nearly 21% of subjects studied had echocardiograms that were inadequate.[7] Compared to subjects with technically adequate studies, those with inadequate studies tended to be older.[7] Thus, clinical studies that rely on echocardiography for estimation of LVM are limited by an inherent selection bias.

Electrocardiographic LVH

Because of this and other limitations of echocardiography, there has been growing interest in using the ECG to estimate LVM and not just divide populations into those with and without LVH. Most classic

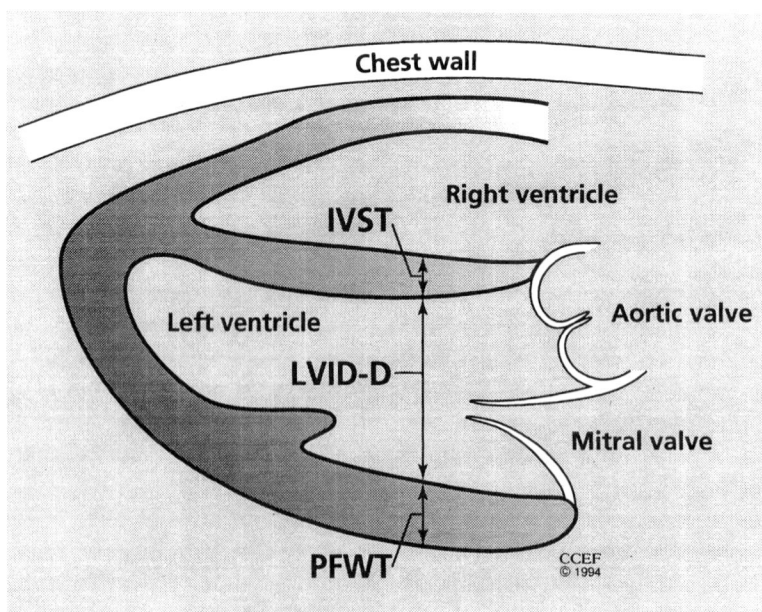

Fig. 10-1. Schematic of the heart as it would appear in an echocardiographic parasternal long-axis view, illustrating how left ventricular mass can be estimated from echocardiographic data. (Modified from Lauer,[3] with permission.)

methods of ECG interpretation are used to identify individuals likely to have LVH, rather than to estimate actual LVM. These classic methods include the Sokolow-Lyon voltage[27] (sum of amplitude of the S wave in lead V_1 and the R wave in lead V_5 or V_6 > 35 mm), Gubner-Ungerleider voltage[28] (sum of the amplitude of R wave in lead I and the amplitude of the S wave in lead III > 25 mm), Cornell voltage[29] (sum of the amplitude of the R wave in lead aVL and the amplitude of the S wave in lead V_3, with the addition of 800 μV for females, as described), the Romhilt-Estes point score,[30] which incorporates QRS voltage, QRS duration, QRS axis, P wave changes, and repolarization abnormalities, and most recently voltage–QRS duration products.[31,32]

Several studies have explored the accuracy of these different criteria for detecting LVH using autopsy and echocardiographic measures of LVM as reference standards. Casale and colleagues[33] prospectively studied 414 subjects who had both ECG and echocardiograms technically adequate for estimation of LVM. Using logistic regression, they determined that the strongest predictors of echocardiographic LVH were age, sex, the amplitude of the R wave in aVL, the amplitude of the S wave in lead V_3, and the amplitude of the T wave in lead V_1. From these data, the Cornell criteria were derived (LVH suggested if the sum of R in aVL and S in V_3 exceeds 35 mm in men or 25 mm in women; for adults under age 40 positive T-wave voltage in lead V_1 is also required). These criteria were then compared with other criteria in a prospective validation set of 129 subjects. The Cornell criteria had superior sensitivity (49%) and specificity (93%) compared to the Romhilt-Estes point score (sensitivity 31%, specificity 83%) or the Sokolow-Lyon index (sensitivity 20%, specificity 93%). The same group[34] also compared the Cornell criteria to the Sokolow-Lyon index in an autopsy series and again found superior sensitivity (42% vs. 22%) with similar high specificity (96% vs. 100%).

Recent work has explored actual estimation of LVM from the ECG. Rautaharju and colleagues[8] derived regression models relating ECG parameters to echocardiographic LVH. One such regression equation, which applies to white and black men, estimates LVM according to the Penn Convention as follows: LVM Index (g/m^2) = $-36.4 + 0.010 \times R(V_5) + 0.020 \times S(V_1) + 0.028 \times S(III) + 1.82 \times T_{neg}(V_6) - 0.148 \times T_{pos}(aVR) + 1.049 \times$ QRS duration. Another regression equation derived from the Framingham data base incorporating patient age and body mass index was recently described by Norman and colleagues; by receiver operating characteristic curve analyses this approach improved the ability of ECG to detect echocardiographic LVH.[35] The role such regression equations will play in epidemiologic research regarding LVH and in clinical practice remains to be explored.

LVH AND CAD: CLINICAL CONSIDERATIONS
LVH as a Risk Factor for CAD

Epidemiologic studies relating echocardiographic LVH to an increased risk for cardiovascular events are summarized in Table 10-1; a detailed discussion of these is beyond the scope of this chapter, but can be found elsewhere.[3] The impact of echocardiographic LVH on cardiovascular disease risk (Fig. 10-2) has been documented in healthy population-based cohorts, patients with asymptomatic hypertension, and patients with angiographically documented CAD. ECG LVH has also been found to be an important, independent predictor for development of CAD.[4,8,36]

The relevance of these data to the diagnosis of CAD is that LVH should be considered a risk factor for CAD when evaluating a patient suspected of having CAD. Thus, clinicians should have a higher pretest likelihood of suspecting CAD in a patient with LVH, just as they would in the setting of other traditional risk factors such as diabetes, hypercholesterolemia, smoking, and hypertension.

Prognostic Impact of LVH in Combination with CAD

Substantial data now indicate that the presence of LVH itself confers an adverse prognosis. Hence, clinicians should focus not only on whether or not CAD is present, but also the presence or absence of LVH, as the latter is associated with worse outcome in patients already diagnosed with CAD.

Galderisi and colleagues investigated echocardiographic determinants of prognosis in subjects of the Framingham Heart Study who had clinically identified CAD.[15] The population sample consisted of 185

Table 10-1 Summary of Epidemiologic Studies Relating Echocardiographic Left Ventricular Mass with Long-Term Prognosis

Reference	Type of Cohort (n)	Follow-up (years)	End-point	Total Events	RR with LVH	
Levy et al. (1989)[9]	GP (1911)	4	CHD	70	Men:	1.67[a]
					Women:	1.60[a]
Levy et al. (1990)[7]	GP (3220)	4	CVD	208	Men:	1.49[b]
					Women:	1.57[b]
			All death	124	Men:	1.73[b]
					Women:	2.12[b]
Casale et al. (1986)[10]	HTN (140)	4.8	CVD	14	Men:	3.83
Koren et al. (1991)[11]	HTN (280)	10.2	CVD	40	All:	2.17
			CVD death	11	All:	14.00
			All death	19	All:	3.50
Ghali et al. (1992)[12]	HTN, mostly black, had angio (785)	4	Cardiac death	NA	CAD:	2.73[c]
					No CAD:	2.80[c]
			All death	80	CAD:	2.14[c]
					No CAD:	4.14[c]

Abbreviations: RR, relative risk; LVH, echocardiographic left ventricular hypertrophy; GP, general population; CHD, coronary heart disease; CVD, cardiovascular disease; HTN, hypertensive patients; angio, coronary angiography.

[a] Relative risks for each increment of 50 g/m of left ventricular mass after adjusting for age, systolic blood pressure, smoking, and ratio of total to high-density lipoprotein cholesterol.
[b] Relative risks for each increment of 50 g/m of left ventricular mass after adjusting for age, blood pressure, antihypertensive treatment, ratio of total to high-density lipoprotein cholesterol, number of cigarettes smoked per day, diabetes, body mass index, and electrocardiographic LVH.
[c] Adjusted for age, gender, and hypertension.
(From Lauer,[3] with permission.)

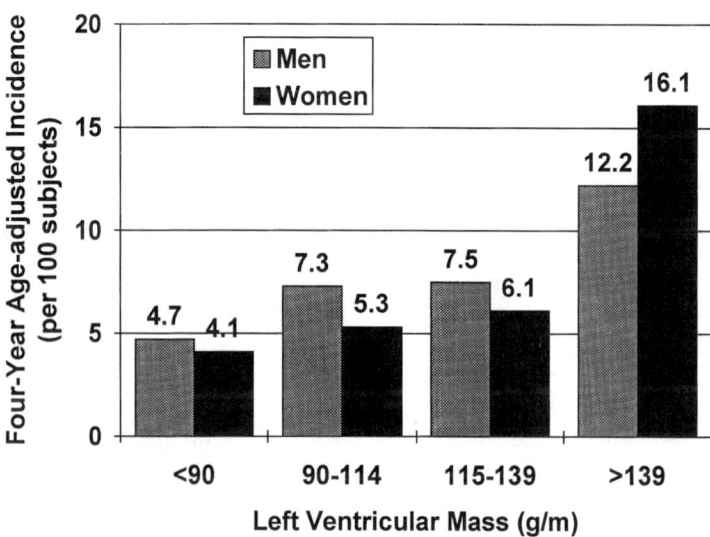

Fig. 10-2. Four-year age-adjusted incidence of cardiovascular disease according to left ventricular mass adjusted for height in the Framingham Heart Study. (Modified from Levy et al.,[7] with permission.)

men and 147 women who had overt CAD and technically adequate M-mode echocardiograms for the estimation of LVM. Echocardiographic LVH was quite common in this population, being noted in 76 (41%) men and 76 (52%) women. During 3.9 years of follow-up there were 99 new cardiovascular events in 60 men and 131 events in 58 women, including 22 myocardial infarctions in men and 16 in women. When considered as a continuous variable in Cox regression analyses, LVM adjusted for height was associated with a greater risk of cardiovascular events [for 50 g/m increment in men relative risk (RR) = 1.25, 95% confidence interval (CI) 1.01 to 1.55; for 43 g/m increment in women RR = 1.22, 95% CI 0.98 to 1.54]. Echocardiographic LVH, considered as a dichotomous variable, was also associated with an increased risk (in men RR = 1.30, 95% CI 0.78 to 2.17; in women RR = 2.30, 95% CI 1.29 to 4.12).

The impact of LVH on prognosis in patients with and without CAD as assessed angiographically was recently reported by Liao and colleagues[13] from the Cook County Heart Disease Registry. They studied a sample of 1,089 black adults who underwent coronary angiography and M-mode echocardiography. CAD was present in 568 patients; LVH was noted in 56% of patients with CAD and 44% of patients without CAD. There were 242 deaths during 5 years of follow-up, 67% from cardiac causes. Among all CAD subgroups (no CAD, single-vessel disease, multivessel disease), LVH was associated with a higher mortality rate (Fig. 10-3). Among all patients (with and without CAD), independent predictors of all-cause mortality in Cox regression analyses were LVH (RR = 2.4, 95% CI 1.7 to 3.2), single-vessel CAD (vs. normal coronaries, RR = 1.1, 95% CI 0.7 to 1.8), multivessel CAD (vs. normal coronaries, RR = 1.6, 95% CI 1.1 to 2.2), and low ejection fraction (RR = 2.0, 95% CI 1.4 to 2.7). It is noteworthy that LVH was a stronger predictor of death than the presence of CAD or left ventricular dysfunction. Among patients *with* CAD LVH was independently predictive of death in multivariable analyses (RR = 2.1, 95% CI 1.5 to 3.1). LVH was more predictive of death than angiographic severity of CAD (for multivessel vs. single-vessel RR = 1.4, 95% CI 1.0 to 2.2) and was as predictive of death as left ventricular systolic dysfunction (RR = 2.2, 95% CI 1.5 to 3.1).

Thus, existing evidence suggests that LVH is itself a marker of worse outcome in patients with diagnosed CAD, making it important for the clinician to identify high risk patients in whom both conditions coexist.

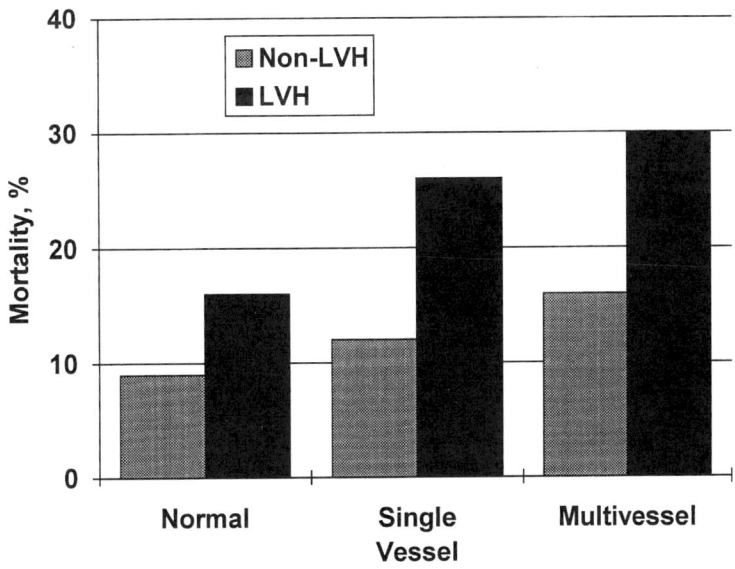

Fig. 10-3. Five-year cumulative mortality by left ventricular hypertrophy and severity of coronary artery disease. (Modified from Liao et al.,[13] with permission.)

IMPAIRED FLOW RESERVE IN LVH AND CAD

LVH is associated with a variety of anatomic and physiologic changes that may predispose to myocardial ischemia[37] in the presence or absence of epicardial coronary disease (Table 10-2). "False-positive" studies suggesting myocardial ischemia in the absence of CAD render the diagnosis of CAD difficult in the setting of LVH. Moreover, alterations of myocardial blood flow and responses to ischemia in patients with epicardial CAD may help explain the worse outcome associated with LVH in patients with CAD.

Impaired Flow Reserve in the Absence of Epicardial Coronary Disease

Experimental Studies

Investigations in animals and humans have shown that epicardial vessels do dilate in the setting of LVH, but not to a degree proportionate to the increase in LVM.[38–40] For example, Vassalli and colleagues recently reported a study of 30 patients with normal coronary arteries, among whom LVM was assessed using ventriculography.[40] Patients with LVH had a lesser increase in epicardial coronary circumference in response to nitroglycerin compared to patients with normal LVM. The authors suggest that this impaired vasodilator capacity may be due to vascular remodeling and "predilation" in the setting of chronic hypertrophy with its associated increase in resting coronary blood flow. There is considerable controversy, however, about anatomic changes in the microvasculature, with some suggesting that capillary luminal volume may be inadequately increased relative to LVM.[37,41]

To investigate anatomic and functional abnormalities of coronary flow in LVH, Bache and colleagues[42] induced pressure overload LVH in seven dogs and compared them to seven control animals. At rest, the dogs with LVH had a higher mean coronary perfusion pressure and a greater minimum coronary resistance. When the animals were paced at 250 beats/min, coronary flow, as assessed by radioactive microspheres, was redistributed away from the subendocardium in the dogs with LVH, but not in the control dogs, and addition of the vasodilator adenosine to rapid pacing did not change these observations. The authors concluded that pressure-overload LVH is associated with both anatomic and functional abnormalities of coronary flow, which predispose to subendocardial ischemia under conditions of stress. Similarly Harrison and colleagues[42] investigated coronary autoregulation in 12 conscious instrumented dogs with hypertension-induced LVH and in 11 control animals. At rest, coronary hemodynamics and flow (as assessed by radioactive microspheres) were similar in the two groups. A reduction of circumflex perfusion pressure from 100 to 75 mmHg did not result in any major changes in either group. When pressure was lowered further to 40 mmHg, subendocardial perfusion decreased markedly in the dogs with LVH, with a profound decrease in the subendocardial to subepicardial flow ratio; these changes were not seen in the control animals. Rembert and colleagues[43] also noted similar changes in coronary flow under stress

Table 10-2. Anatomical and Physiologic Changes in Hypertrophied Myocardium That May Affect Predisposition and Sensitivity to Myocardial Ischemia[a]

Site or Type of Abnormality	Description of Abnormality (References)
Anatomic abnormalities	
Epicardial coronary vessels	Coronary vessels enlarge, but not to the proportion expected for the increase in myocardial mass[37–40]
Smaller coronary vessels	Relative decrease in capillary density with reference to increased myocardial mass[41]
Cellular level	Reduced mitochondrial to myofibrillar volume ratio[41]
Physiologic abnormalities	
Vasodilator response	Decreased coronary flow reserve with attenuated response to vasodilators Resistance to flow may be increased at rest as well[37,42–45]
Heart rate response	Reduced ability to achieve 85% of age-predicted target heart rate[53]
Peak double-product (heart rate × blood pressure)	Increased with respect to work-load achieved[53]

[a] See text for details.

in a canine model, but also described decreased subendocardial to subepicardial flow ratios at rest.

One possible explanation for these findings is that hypertension, by itself, leads to functional abnormalities in the coronary microvasculature, rather than hypertrophy. To investigate this possibility, Mueller and colleagues[44] studied a canine model of renal hypertension induced LVH in which the hypertension was treated by restoring normal renal blood flow. These dogs were compared to others with both untreated animals with hypertension and LVH and with controls. During maximal vasodilation with adenosine, coronary vascular resistance was identical in all three groups, suggesting that the cross-sectional area of the coronary bed does not increase in the presence of hypertrophy, and implying that this is not due to a functional abnormality associated with hypertension.

Taken together, these animal studies suggest that pathologic hypertrophy is associated with alterations in the distribution of myocardial flow away from the endocardium, particularly under conditions of stress, and a failure to appropriately increase coronary flow proportional to the increase in left ventricular mass. Both anatomic and functional abnormalities may be operative.

Human Studies

The association of LVH with impaired coronary flow reserve in humans without CAD has been described by Houghton and colleagues.[45] They studied 48 patients who were referred to coronary angiography for suspected CAD and found to have normal or near normal coronary arteries. These patients also underwent Doppler flow studies under resting and hyperemic conditions to assess coronary flow reserve, in addition to echocardiography and dipyridamole thallium scintigraphy. Impaired coronary flow reserve was considered present if intravenous dipyridamole failed to increase mean coronary flow velocity by at least threefold. Patients with an abnormal thallium scan ($n = 11$) had a higher LVM (153 vs. 114 g, $p = 0.0007$) and lower coronary flow reserve; there was a nonsignificant trend relating a low coronary flow reserve to a higher LVM. Of note, with the exception of one patient with idiopathic cardiomyopathy, abnormal thallium scans were found only in patients with echocardiographic LVH. These data suggest that false-positive thallium scans may be expected in patients with LVH and impaired coronary flow reserve, even in the absence of epicardial CAD.

LVH and Vulnerability to Ischemia in the Presence of Epicardial CAD

The clinical observation that CAD is associated with a worse outcome in the setting of LVH suggests that the latter may increase the vulnerability of the myocardium to ischemia. Two animal studies support this hypothesis. Koyanagi and colleagues[46] assessed myocardial infarction size after occluding the circumflex coronary artery in 28 dogs with renal hypertension and LVH and 30 control dogs. The 48-hour mortality rate in the dogs with LVH was markedly increased compared to the control dogs (54% vs. 17%, $p < 0.01$). The ratio of the mass of the infarct area, as assessed pathologically, to the mass of the risk area was significantly higher in the LVH animals (0.54 vs. 0.31, $p < 0.05$) than in the control animals. The same group also described a higher rate of sudden death after acute coronary occlusion,[47] despite similar sizes of the occluded coronary beds. The authors concluded that LVH and its associated impaired flow reserve results in larger infarctions and higher mortality rates.

The association of thallium ischemia and LVH in humans with CAD was recently described by Salcedo and colleagues[48] in a study of 150 patients who underwent echocardiography, single-proton emission computed tomographic (SPECT) thallium-20 scintigraphy, and coronary angiography. Among the 11 patients who had both LVH and CAD, all (100%) had evidence of thallium ischemia, whereas only 78% of the 51 patients with CAD but no LVH had ischemia. In a multivariable model, both LVM and CAD were independent predictors of thallium ischemia; the authors concluded that LVH sensitizes the myocardium to ischemia from epicardial CAD.

ACCURACY OF DIAGNOSTIC TESTS FOR DETECTION OF CAD IN THE PRESENCE OF LVH

The above discussion suggests that LVH may predispose to ischemia even in the absence of epicardial CAD, and thus may present a serious diagnostic challenge to the clinician attempting to diagnose CAD noninvasively in the many patients who coinciden-

Table 10-3. Impact of LVH on the Accuracy of Noninvasive Modalities Used to Diagnose CAD

Noninvasive Test	Impact of LVH (Reference)
Stress ECG	Increased false positive rate[51,52]
	Impaired heart rate response, may affect sensitivity[53]
	No association with standard ST-segment response in population-based cohort, but increased rate of abnormal heart-rate indexed ST-segment response[53]
Ambulatory ST-segment monitoring	Increased false-positive rate[55-57]
Dipyridamole stress thallium scintigraphy	Increased false-positive rate[45,60]
Exercise stress thallium scintigraphy	Possibly no effect[57]
Dobutamine sestamibi scintigraphy	Increased false-positive rate[61]
Dobutamine echocardiography	Possibly no effect[61]
Exercise echocardiography	Possibly no effect[62]
Dipyridamole stress PET imaging	Decreased sensitivity and specificity[59]

Abbreviations: LVH, left ventricular hypertrophy; CAD, coronary artery disease; ECG, electrocardiography; PET, positron emission tomography.

tally have LVH. It is a well-accepted clinical axiom that ECG LVH precludes diagnosis of myocardial ischemia by stress ECG[49,50] and, therefore, great interest has developed in assessing the impact of LVH on the accuracy of other noninvasive modalities (Table 10-3), including ambulatory ST-segment monitoring, thallium scintigraphy, stress echocardiography, and positron emission tomography (PET).

Exercise Electrocardiography

Remarkably few data exist that describe the impact of ECG and echocardiographic LVH on the exercise ECG. In a frequently cited study, Harris and colleagues[51] identified patients who had undergone coronary angiography and had ECG LVH (by Sokolow-Lyon voltage criteria along with ST-segment changes and other evidence of LVH by either chest x-ray or left ventricular angiogram). Subjects were then identified who did not have significant CAD (defined as >50% stenosis) with 17 of 21 subjects having completely normal coronary angiograms. These patients were then recalled for a standard treadmill stress test. Of the 16 subjects who achieved at least 90% of their age-predicted heart rate, 6 (38%) had an abnormal exercise electrocardiogram with at least 1 mm of horizontal or downsloping ST-segment depression persisting at least 0.08 seconds after the J point. The authors concluded that ECG LVH may be a cause of false-positive exercise electrocardiograms.

A more recent study[52] evaluated 95 patients with a variety of ECG abnormalities who underwent both exercise ECG and thallium SPECT scintigraphy. Seventeen subjects had electrocardiographic LVH; of these five had false-positive studies while two had a false negative. Although the number of subjects studied was small, these results are consistent with reduced accuracy of exercise ECG in the setting of ECG LVH.

With the advent of echocardiography as a more accurate method of estimating LVM, interest has focused more recently on the impact of *echocardiographic LVH* on ST-segment responses to exercise. A preliminary study from the Framingham Heart Study[53] evaluated exercise ECG (Bruce protocol) in 1,408 men and 1,618 women who were free of clinical cardiac disease, were not on β-blockers, and underwent technically adequate echocardiography on the same day. Echocardiographic LVH was defined as a LVM of at least 143 g/m of height in men and 102 g/m in women. The exercise ST-segment response was evaluated in two ways: (1) the standard approach, which required at least 1 mm of horizontal or downsloping ST-segment depression at least 0.08 seconds after the J-point, and the (2) heart-rated indexed approach. The latter technique involves dividing the additional ST-segment depression that occurs with exercise by the exercise-induced increase in heart rate; in the Framingham population the heart-rate indexed ST-segment change has been found to be better than the standard approach for predicting coronary events.[54] The authors found that echocardiographic LVH was associated with a greater likelihood of an abnormal heart-rate indexed ST-segment response (in men 13% vs. 7%, odds ratio = 1.78, 95% CI 1.05 to 3.01,

$p = 0.02$; in women 16% vs. 8%, odds ratio = 2.13, 95% CI 1.31 to 3.44, $p = 0.002$), but not with an abnormal ST-segment response as assessed by the standard approach. Another potentially important finding was a markedly higher rate of failure to achieve at least 85% of the age-predicted maximum heart rate among subjects with echocardiographic LVH (in men 34% vs. 19%, $p = 0.001$; in women 35% vs. 22%, $p = 0.001$). Moreover, the peak heart rate blood pressure double product adjusted for work load in METs was increased in subjects with LVH, a finding that is consistent with an increased predisposition for ischemia. Further studies will be needed to determine the clinical significance of these findings.

Ambulatory ST-Segment Monitoring

Several small studies have found that ischemic ambulatory ST-segment changes occurring in the absence of significant epicardial CAD are common in patients with systemic hypertension and are associated with LVH.[55-57] For example, Massie and colleagues[55] studied 226 asymptomatic men with hypertension and no clinical evidence of CAD who then underwent echocardiography, exercise thallium scintigraphy, exercise ECG, and ambulatory ST-segment monitoring; 80 subjects had at least one positive study and of these 34 had coronary angiography performed. These 226 hypertensive men were compared to 54 age- and risk-factor-matched controls. Ischemic ST-segment changes occured in 15% of the hypertensive subjects, but in none of the controls ($p < 0.05$); they were also significantly more common in patients with echocardiographic LVH (23% vs. 12%, $p < 0.05$). Among the patients who underwent coronary angiography, ambulatory ST segment had both low sensitivity (50%, 95% CI 27% to 73%) and specificity (57%, 95% CI 29% to 82%) for predicting significant angiographic CAD. In comparison, thallium scintigraphy had markedly higher sensitivity (90%, 95% CI 68% to 99%) and specificity (79%, 95% CI 49% to 95%) (Fig. 10-4). Although this study suffers from effects of sequential work-up bias[58] and small sample size, it and others[56,57] suggest that echocardiographic LVH may adversely impact on the diagnostic accuracy of ambulatory ST-segment monitoring for predicting significant epicardial CAD.

Stress Thallium Scintigraphy

Animal and human studies have shown abnormal myocardial blood flow under resting and stress conditions in the setting of LVH.[39-53] This process may

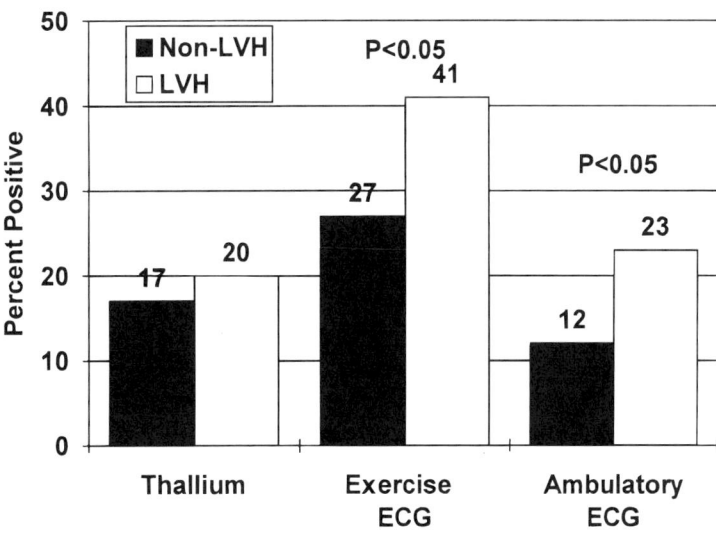

Fig. 10-4. Prevalence of positive tests in 113 hypertensive patients without echocardiographic left ventricular hypertrophy (LVH) (hatched bars) and with echocardiographic LVH (white bars). (Modified from Massie et al.,[55] with permission.)

be nonhomogeneous, causing regional perfusion abnormalities. In addition, LVH may sensitize the myocardium to ischemia, further increasing the likelihood of perfusion defects in the absence of critical disease. Thus, it is not surprising that "false-positive" perfusion defects limit the accuracy of myocardial perfusion techniques in patients with LVH. Moreover, a study using pharmacologic vasodilation with dipyridamole has shown that myocardial perfusion imaging is less sensitive for detecting epicardial CAD in the presence of LVH than in patients with normal LVM. This may be due to impaired vasodilator reserve in LVH, which conceals the difference between normal and ischemic regions. Whether the use of exercise rather than dipyridamole stress may lead to better accuracy of in this situation should be clarified.[59]

Likewise, in the study of Houghton and colleagues[45] in which 11 of 43 hypertensive patients without epicardial CAD had dipyridamole stress-induced thallium perfusion deficits, patients with thallium perfusion abnormalities had significantly higher echocardiographic LVM than those who did not (157 vs. 114 g/m^2, $p = 0.0007$). Similarly, DePuey and colleagues[60] compared 100 patients with hypertension due to end-stage renal disease with 35 normotensive controls; all underwent SPECT thallium scintigraphy (70 with exercise stress and 30 by dipyridamole). Echocardiography was performed in 12 patients and all had increased end-diastolic wall thickness. Among the hypertensive patients many had a decrease in the lateral-to-septal count density during both immediate and delayed imaging, thus mimicking lateral wall myocardial infarction. The authors found that stress thallium scintigraphy may, therefore, be less specific for predicting CAD in the lateral territory in patients with LVH than in patients without LVH (Plate 10-1).

On the other hand, Massie and colleagues[55] found a reasonably good test accuracy of exercise stress thallium scintigraphy (90% sensitivity and 79% specificity) among asymptomatic hypertensive patients; of note, there was no association between reversible thallium defects and echocardiographic LVH (17% vs. 20%, $p = NS$) (Fig. 10-4). These data are consistent with the suggestion that exercise stress would be inherently superior to dipyridamole stress for detecting epicardial CAD in the setting of LVH.[59]

Stress Echocardiography

There are relatively few data on the use of stress echocardiography for diagnosing CAD in the setting of LVH. Marwick and colleagues[61] compared dobutamine stress echocardiography with dobutamine stress sestamibi scintigraphy in 217 patients without prior myocardial infarction who had been referred for diagnostic coronary angiography. Significant CAD was present in 142 patients, of whom 74 had multivessel disease. Echocardiography and sestamibi scintigraphy had similar sensitivities for detecting significant CAD and multivessel disease, but echocardiography had a markedly higher specificity (83% vs. 67%, $p = 0.05$). When the authors explored the reasons for the higher false-positive rates with scintigraphy, they found that most of the discrepancy could be explained by the occurrence of false-positive studies among patients with LVH, which they defined as a left ventricular wall thickness of greater than 12 mm. These data suggest that echocardiography may be superior to scintigraphy for accurately assessing the presence of CAD in the setting of LVH.

More recently, Marwick and colleagues[62] studied 147 patients without prior myocardial infarction who underwent both exercise stress echocardiography and coronary angiography; 62 patients had significant (>50% stenosis) CAD. Echocardiographic LVH was defined as a left ventricular mass index of at least 131 g/m^2 in men and at least 100 g/m^2 in women. In the entire population sample, exercise echocardiography had a sensitivity of 71%, specificity of 91%, and overall accuracy of 82%. Among the patients with *echocardiographic* LVH ($n = 68$), exercise echocardiography had a sensitivity of 71%, specificity of 95%, and overall accuracy of 85%; thus, echocardiographic LVH did not appear to impact on the diagnostic accuracy of the stress echocardiogram. In contrast, even in patients with normal resting ECG, the specificity of exercise ECG was lower in patients with LVH. The authors also looked at "clinically suspected LVH" based on electrocardiographic LVH or a history of hypertension or aortic stenosis, and again found that exercise echocardiography had comparable diagnostic accuracy as in patients without *clinically* suspected LVH, and was again more accurate than the exercise ECG.

Positron Emission Tomography

There are few data that specifically address the question of whether LVH impacts on the diagnostic accuracy of PET imaging for predicting angiographic CAD. Marwick and colleagues[59] reported on 75 patients who underwent coronary angiography and rubidium-82 PET imaging after dipyridamole-induced stress. Echocardiographic LVH (again defined as greater than 131 g/m^2 in men and greater than 100 g/m^2 in women) was present in 25 subjects. Significant CAD was present in 54 patients, with no marked differences in CAD and multivessel prevalence among patients with and without echocardiographic LVH. The sensitivity of PET imaging was higher in patients with normal LVM (85% vs. 55%, $p = 0.03$) and the specificity was also higher (88% vs. 60%, p = NS). As discussed above, the authors argue that the lower sensitivity may have been due to impaired vasodilator reserve present in LVH. The numbers of patients with no CAD and negative scans was too small to allow meaningful analyses. Further studies will be needed to confirm and extend these results; for now, the accuracy of dipyridamole stress rubidium-82 PET imaging should be suspect in the setting of LVH.

Comparisons of Different Modalities

The preceding studies suggest that while LVH poses problems for the accuracy of both exercise ECG and myocardial perfusion imaging, stress echocardiography may not share these limitations. The impact of LVH on new technologies such as stress MRI remains undefined.

Few studies have performed head-to-head comparisons of different diagnostic methodologies for detecting epicardial CAD in the presence of LVH. Massie and colleagues[55] found that exercise stress thallium scintigraphy was superior to exercise ECG and ambulatory ST-segment monitoring in asymptomatic hypertensive patients, with these differences being more marked in the setting of echocardiographic LVH. As discussed above, Marwick and colleagues[61] found that the improved diagnostic accuracy of dobutamine echocardiography over dobutamine sestamibi scintigraphy primarily stemmed from results in patients with LVH. Using exercise stress, the presence of ECG "silent" LVH appears to compromise the accuracy of the exercise electrocardiogram in comparison with stress echocardiography.[62]

CONCLUSIONS

LVH, whether detected by electrocardiography or echocardiography, is an important and powerful predictor of an adverse cardiovascular prognosis, whether or not CAD is present. The combination of LVH and CAD may be a particularly hazardous one, due both to the increased risk from the two diseases themselves as well as from the diagnostic difficulties for detecting CAD discussed above. CAD is difficult to identify in patients with LVH with decreased sensitivities and specificities of the most commonly used noninvasive tests, although stress echocardiography may be promising.

All studies that attempt to associate findings of noninvasive studies with angiographic findings suffer from an inherent sequential work-up bias[58] that tends to inflate sensitivity and deflate specificity. As the relative impact of this bias may vary at different institutions, comparisons of test accuracies across different reports are problematic. Two potential approaches to this problem would include (1) multimodality comparisons in patients with and without LVH as part of one study or (2) defining clinical events (death, nonfatal myocardial infarction, hospital admission for congestive heart failure) rather than angiographic findings as primary study endpoints. At this time, there is a need for more data regarding prognosis of CAD and LVH when considered in combination.

As more data on noninvasive techniques, especially stress echocardiography, accrue, attention may turn to the opposite question, namely the accurate diagnosis of LVH in the setting of CAD. A recent study of patients presenting to an emergency room[63] with suspected acute myocardial ischemia found that physicians often did not accurately identify ECG LVH. These patients, while less likely to have acute myocardial ischemia, had equally high mortality rates and were more likely to have congestive heart failure. As LVH and CAD are independently predictive of survival,[12,13] it is incumbent on the clinician to accurately diagnose both conditions and target appropriate patients for aggressive treatment.

A key issue that remains unresolved is whether

regression of increased LVM improves clinical outcome. LVH regression has been documented with antihypertensive drugs[64] and with weight loss.[65] If a clinical strategy that specifically aims to regress increased LVM is found to be beneficial, then the accurate identification of LVH in patients with CAD will become even more paramount.

REFERENCES

1. Grossman W, Jones D, McClaurin LP: Wall stress and patterns of hypertrophy in the human left ventricle. J Clin Invest 56:56, 1975
2. Katz AM: Cardiomyopathy of overload; a major determinant of prognosis in congestive heart failure. N Engl J Med 322:100, 1990
3. Lauer MS: Left ventricular hypertrophy and cardiovascular prognosis. Cleve Clin J Med 62:169, 1995
4. Kannel WB, Gordon T, Castelli WP, Margolis JR: Electrocardiographic left ventricular hypertrophy and risk of coronary heart disease: the Framingham Study. Ann Intern Med 72:813, 1970
5. Kannel WB, Dannenberg AL, Levy D: Population implications of electrocardiographic left ventricular hypertrophy. Am J Cardiol 60:851, 1987
6. Aronow WS, Ahn Ch, Kronzon I, Koenigsberg M: Congestive heart failure, coronary events and atherothrombotic brain infarction in elderly blacks and whites with systemic hypertension and with and without echocardiographic and electrocardiographic evidence of left ventricular hypertrophy. Am J Cardiol 67:295, 1991
7. Levy D, Garrison RJ, Savage DD et al: Prognostic implications of echocardiographically determined left ventricular mass in the Framingham Heart Study. N Engl J Med 322:1561, 1990
8. Rautahrju PM, LaCroix AZ, Savage DD et al: Electrocardiographic estimate of left ventricular mass versus radiographic cardiac size and the risk of cardiovascular disease mortality in the epidemiologic follow-up study of the first National Health and Nutrition Examination Survey. Am J Cardiol 62:59, 1988
9. Levy D, Garrison RJ, Savage DD et al: Left ventricular mass and incidence of coronary heart disease in an elderly cohort: the Framingham Heart Study. Ann Intern Med 110:101, 1989
10. Casale PN, Devereux RB, Milner M et al: Value of echocardiographic measurement of left ventricular mass in predicting cardiovascular morbid events in hypertensive men. Ann Intern Med 105:173, 1986
11. Koren MJ, Devereux RB, Casale PN, Savage DD, Laragh JH: Relation of left ventricular mass and mortality in uncomplicated essential hypertension. Ann Intern Med 114:345, 1991
12. Ghali JK, Liao Y, Simmons B et al: The prognostic role of left ventricular hypertrophy in patients with or without coronary artery disease. Ann Intern Med 117:831, 1992
13. Liao Y, Cooper RS, McGee DL et al: The relative effects of left ventricular hypertrophy, coronary artery disease, and ventricular dysfunction on survival among black adults. JAMA 273:1592, 1995
14. Cooper RS, Simmon BE, Castaner A et al: Left ventricular hypertrophy is associated with worse survival independent of ventricular function and number of coronary arteries severely narrowed. Am J Cardiol 65:441, 1990
15. Galderisi M, Lauer MS, Levy D: Echocardiographic determinants of clinical outcome in subjects with coronary artery disease (the Framingham Heart Study). Am J Cardiol 70:971, 1992
16. Levy D, Anderson KM, Savage DD et al: Echocardiographically detected left ventricular hypertrophy: prevalence and risk factors. The Framingham Heart Study. Ann Intern Med 108:7, 1988
17. Lauer MS, Anderson KM, Levy D: Influence of contemporary versus 30-year blood pressure levels on left ventricular mass and geometry: the Framingham Heart Study. J Am Coll Cardiol 18:1287, 1991
18. Lauer MS, Anderson KM, Kannel WB, Levy D: The impact of obesity on left ventricular mass and geometry: the Framingham Heart Study. JAMA 266:231, 1991
19. Sasson Z, Rasooly Y, Bhesania T, Rasooly I: Insulin resistance is an important determinant of left ventricular mass in the obese. Circulation 88:1431, 1993
20. Chou TC: Electrocardiography in Clinical Practice, 3rd Ed. W. B. Saunders, Philadelphia, 1991, pp. 37–52
21. Devereux RB, Reichek N: Echocardiographic determination of left ventricular mass in man: anatomic validation of the method. Circulation 55:613, 1977
22. Schiller NB, Shah PM, Crawford M et al: Recommendations for quantitation of the left ventricle by two-dimensional echocardiography. J Am Soc Echo 2:358, 1989
23. Levy D, Labib SB, Anderson KM et al: Determinants of sensitivity and specificity of electrocardiographic criteria for left ventricular hypertrophy. Circulation 81:815, 1990
24. Devereux RB, Alonso DR, Lutas EM et al: Echocardiographic assessment of left ventricular hypertrophy: comparison to necropsy findings. Am J Cardiol 57:450, 1986

25. de Simone G, Daniels SR, Devereux RB et al: Left ventricular mass and body size in normotensive children and adults: assessment of allometric relations and impact of overweight. J Am Coll Cardiol 20:1251, 1992
26. Lauer MS, Anderson KM, Larson M, Levy D: A new method for indexing left ventricular mass for differences in body size. Am J Cardiol 74:487, 1994
27. Sokolow M, Lyon TP: The ventricular complex in left ventricular hypertrophy as obtained by unipolar precordial and limb leads. Am Heart J 37:161, 1949
28. Gubner R, Ungerleider HE: Electrocardiographic criteria of left ventricular hypertrophy. Arch Intern Med 72:196, 1943
29. Casale PN, Devereux RB, Alonso DR et al: Improved sex-specific criteria of left ventricular hypertrophy for clinical and computer interpretation of electrocardiograms: validation with autopsy findings. Circulation 75:565, 1987
30. Romhilt D, Bove KE, Norris RJ et al: A critical appraisal of the electrocardiographic criteria for the diagnosis of left ventricular hypertrophy. Circulation 40:185, 1969
31. Molloy TJ, Okin PM, Devereux RB, Kligfield P: Electrocardiographic detection of left ventricular hypertrophy by the simple QRS voltage-duration product. J Am Coll Cardiol 20:1180, 1992
32. Okin PM, Roman MJ, Devereux RB, Kligfield P: Electrocardiographic identification of increased left ventricular mass by simple voltage-duration products. J Am Coll Cardiol 25:417, 1995
33. Casale PN, Deverux RB, Kligfield P et al: Electrocardiographic detection of left ventricular hypertrophy: development and prospective validation of improved criteria. J Am Coll Cardiol 6:572, 1985
34. Casale PN, Devereux RB, Alonso DR et al: Improved sex-specific criteria of left ventricular hypertrophy for clinical and computer interpretation of electrocardiograms: validation with autopsy findings. Circulation 75:565, 1987
35. Norman JE Jr., Levy D, Campbell G, Bailey JJ: Improved detection of echocardiographic left ventricular hypertrophy using a new electrocardiographic algorithm. J Am Coll Cardiol 21:1680, 1993
36. Sutherland SE, Gazes PC, Keil JE et al: Electrocardiographic abnormalities and 30-year mortality among white and black men of the Charleston Heart Study. Circulation 88:2685, 1993
37. Marcus ML, Harrison DG, Chillian WM et al: Alteration in the coronary circulation in hypertrophied ventricles. Circulation 75(suppl I):I-19, 1987
38. Stack RS, Rembert JC, Schirmer B, Greenfield JC: Relation of left ventricular mass to geometry of the proximal coronary arteries in the dog. Am J Cardiol 51:1728, 1983
39. Paulsen S, Vetner M, Hagerup LM: Relationship between heart weight and the cross-sectional area of the coronary ostia. Acta Pathol Microbiol Scand 83:429, 1975
40. Vassalli G, Kauffmann P, Villari B et al: Reduced epicardial coronary vasodilator capacity in patients with left ventricular hypertrophy. Circulation 91:2916, 1995
41. Anversa P, Ricci R, Olivetti G: Quantitative structural analysis of the myocardium during physiologic growth and induced cardiac hypertrophy: a review. J Am Coll Cardiol 7:1140, 1986
42. Harrison DG, Florentine MS, Brooks LA et al: The effect of hypertension and left ventricular hypertrophy on the lower range of coronary autoregulation. Circulation 77:1108, 1988
43. Rembert JC, Kleinman LH, Fedor JM et al: Myocardial blood flow distribution in concentric left ventricular hypertrophy. J Clin Invest 62:379, 1978
44. Mueller TM, Marcus ML, Kerber RE et al: Effect of renal hypertension and left ventricular hypertrophy on the coronary circulation in dogs. Circ Res 42:543, 1978
45. Houghton JL, Frank MJ, Carr AA et al: Relations among impaired coronary flow reserve, left ventricular hypertrophy and thallium perfusion defects in hypertensive patients without obstructive coronary artery disease. J Am Coll Cardiol 15:43, 1990
46. Koyanagi S, Eastham CL, Harrison DG, Marcus ML: Increased size of myocardial infarction in dogs with chronic hypertension and left ventricular hypertrophy. Circ Res 50:55, 1982
47. Koyanagi S, Easthan CL, Marcus ML: Effects of chronic hypertension and left ventricular hypertrophy on the incidence of sudden cardiac death after coronary artery occlusion in conscious dogs. Circulation 65:1192, 1982
48. Salcedo EE, Marwick TH, Korzick DH et al: Left ventricular hypertrophy sensitizes the myocardium to the development of ischemia. Eur Heart J 11:G72–8, 1990
49. Harris CN, Aronow WS, Parker DP, Kaplan MA: Treadmill stress test in left ventricular hypertrophy. Chest 63:353, 1973
50. Meyers DG, Bendon KA, Hankins JH, Stratbucker RA: The effect of baseline electrocardiographic abnormalities on the diagnostic accuracy of exercise-induced ST segment changes. Am Heart J 119:272, 1990
51. Harris CN, Aronow WS, Parker DP, Kaplan MA: Treadmill stress test in left ventricular hypertrophy. Chest 63:353, 1973

52. Meyers DG, Bendon KA, Hankins JH, Stratbucker RA: The effect of baseline electrocardiographic abnormalities on the diagnostic accuracy of exercise-induced ST segment changes. Am Heart J 119:272, 1990
53. Lauer MS, Okin PM, Anderson KM, Levy D: The impact of echocardiographic left ventricular mass on exercise testing parameters. Am J Cardiol 76:952, 1995
54. Okin PM, Anderson KM, Levy D, Kligfield P: Heart rate adjustment of exercise-induced ST segment depression: improved risk stratification in the Framingham Offspring Study. Circulation 83:866, 1991
55. Massie BM, Szlachcic Y, Tubau J et al: Scintigraphic and electrocardiographic evidence of silent coronary artery disease in asymptomatic hypertension: a case-control study. J Am Coll Cardiol 22:1598, 1993
56. Yurenev AP, DeQuattro V, Devereux RB: Hypertensive heart disease: relationship of silent ischemia to coronary artery disease and left ventricular hypertrophy. Am Heart J 120:928, 1990
57. Pringle SD, Dunn FG, Tweddel AC, et al: Symptomatic and silent myocardial ischemia in hypertensive patients with left ventricular hypertrophy. Br Heart J 67:377, 1992
58. Choi BCK: Sensitivity and specificity of a single diagnostic test in the presence of work-up bias. J Clin Epidemiol 45:581, 1992
59. Marwick TH, Cook SA, Lafont A et al: Influence of left ventricular mass on the diagnostic accuracy of myocardial perfusion imaging using positron emission tomography with dipyridamole stress. J Nucl Med 32:2221, 1991
60. DePuey EG, Guertler-Krawczynska E, Perkin JV et al: Alterations in myocardial thallium-201 distribution in patients with chronic systemic hypertension undergoing single-photon emission computed tomography. Am J Cardiol 62:234, 1988
61. Marwick TH, D'Hondt AM, Baudhuin T et al: Optimal use of dobutamine stress for the detection and evaluation of coronary artery disease: combination with echocardiography or scintigraphy, or both? J Am Coll Cardiol 22:159, 1993
62. Marwick TH, Harjai K, Haluska B et al: Influence of left ventricular hypertrophy on detection of coronary artery disease using exercise echocardiography. J Am Coll Cardiol 26:1180, 1995
63. Larsen GC, Griffith JL, Beshansky JR et al: Electrocardiographic left ventricular hypertrophy in patients with suspected acute cardiac ischemia—its influence on diagnosis, triage, and short-term prognosis: a multicenter study. J Gen Intern Med 9:666, 1994
64. Georgiou D, Brundage BH: Regression of left ventricular mass in systemic hypertension. Clin Cardiol 15:5, 1992
65. MacMahon SW, Wilcken DEL, MacDonald GJ: The effect of weight reduction on left ventricular mass: a randomized controlled trial in young, overweight hypertensive patients. N Engl J Med 314:334, 1986

Chapter 11

Noninvasive Diagnosis of CAD in Patients with End-Stage Renal Disease

Charles A. Herzog

CLINICAL IMPORTANCE OF CAD IN PATIENTS WITH END-STAGE RENAL FAILURE

Magnitude of the Problem

Cardiovascular mortality is the predominant cause of death in patients with end-stage renal disease (ESRD), accounting for 43% of combined dialysis and transplant deaths.[1] In chronic hemodialysis patients, cardiac disease is the major cause of death and approximately 40% of all-cause mortality is attributable to ischemic heart disease.[2] About one-fourth of these deaths in dialysis patients are ascribed to acute myocardial infarction (MI), predominantly in older patients and patients with diabetic nephropathy.

Not only is cardiac disease common in patients with renal disease, but the effects of this association are being magnified by the increasing prevalence of ESRD. From 1988 to 1990, the number of patients with treated ESRD increased by 9.9% *per year* in patients ages 65 to 74, 14% *per year* in patients older than 75 years of age,[3] and approximately 12% *per year* in patients with diabetic nephropathy. Over the same period, the increase in treated ESRD was even greater in Native Americans (nearly 17% per year),[3] among whom diabetic nephropathy is the commonest etiology (64% of Native Americans, compared to 34% of all patients).[3] Thus, as the number of older ESRD patients and those with diabetic nephropathy continues to rise, it will become increasingly important to accurately identify patients with ischemic heart disease for the purposes of risk stratification and treatment in both chronic dialysis and transplantation groups. Furthermore, as the number of cardiac interventions increases in both dialysis patients and in patients followed after successful renal transplantation, accurate noninvasive techniques will be important for assessment of the long-term adequacy of therapeutic coronary interventions in patients with ESRD.

Angiographic Evidence of CAD

The prevalence of coronary artery disease (CAD) in diabetic renal transplant candidates and selected nondiabetic ESRD patients with other CAD risk factors has been remarkably consistent in angiographic series. Although some variation in this association derives from different definitions of "significant" fixed coronary artery stenosis severity (ranging from 50% to 70% by qualitative visual estimation), about one-third (25% to 40%) of patients undergoing coronary angiography have been found to have "significant" disease. Using a cutoff of greater than 70% stenosis in at least one vessel, Braun et al. reported significant CAD in 27 of 70 nondiabetics (38%) and 9 of 29 diabetic patients (31%), most of whom were undergoing transplant evaluation.[4] In a subsequent

Cleveland Clinic series of 100 diabetic renal transplant candidates, 25 of 100 patients (25%) had significant CAD (>70% stenosis).[5] Lorber et al. reported "serious" CAD in 25 of 77 diabetic renal transplant candidates (32%).[6] The largest series of diabetic renal transplant candidates, mostly Type 1 diabetes mellitus (DM), undergoing angiography was reported from the University of Minnesota by Manske et al.[7,8] Forty-eight of 151 (32%) had a greater than 70% stenosis in at least one coronary artery.

Reduction of Cardiac Risk by Intervention
Renal Transplantation Candidates

In older series, the 2-year mortality rate was at least 50% for diabetic ESRD patients who did not receive coronary artery revascularization for significant CAD. Manske and colleagues prospectively randomized diabetic renal transplant candidates (atypical or no chest pain) with left ventricular (LV) ejection fraction greater than 35% and at least one coronary artery stenosis of greater than 75%, to medical therapy (calcium-channel blocker plus aspirin) or coronary artery revascularization (percutaneous transluminal coronary angioplasty [PTCA] or coronary artery bypass grafting [CABG]).[7] Thirty-one of the 151 patients studied were eligible for randomization, and 26 agreed to study entry. Ten of 13 medically treated and 2 of 13 revascularized patients reached a cardiac endpoint (unstable angina, MI, or cardiac death) at a median time of 8.4 months ($p = 0.002$). This prospective coronary interventional trial in diabetic renal transplant candidates is noteworthy for several reasons. First, there was an improved outcome with coronary revascularization compared to medical therapy in diabetic renal transplant candidates without angina. Second, identification of "significant" CAD leading to treatment randomization was entirely based on coronary angiographic findings, and functional noninvasive assessment of CAD was *not* performed.[7] This latter point deserves emphasis, because most reports on the diagnostic accuracy of noninvasive testing for detection of significant CAD in renal transplant candidates have relied on post-testing clinical cardiac event rates as a surrogate for CAD severity. If noninvasive diagnostic testing is to be used as a screening test identifying diabetic ESRD patients as appropriate potential candidates for prophylactic coronary revascularization before renal transplantation, then the noninvasive diagnostic modality must be validated against an angiographic standard. As routine coronary angiography is not an appealing strategy when only one-third of patients have "significant" CAD, the goal of all noninvasive diagnostic testing strategies should be the accurate identification of that one-third of the patient population needing angiography.

Patients on Hemodialysis

Although several series have focused on the detection of significant CAD in predominantly diabetic renal transplant candidates, this represents only a subset of ESRD patients at risk for cardiovascular mortality. Death rates due to all causes, including cardiovascular, are higher for dialysis patients as a group than for the transplant population, the latter being younger and relatively healthier. Indeed, identification of significant CAD may be potentially more important in the chronic dialysis population in terms of disease prevalence, yet the clinical outcome of this group has not been well studied after noninvasive or angiographic detection of significant CAD or subsequent coronary revascularization.

The outcome of coronary artery revascularization procedures (PTCA and CABG) in dialysis patients has been reviewed in several small series. Opsahl et al. compared the outcome of dialysis patients who underwent CABG from 1976 to 1988 with medically treated ESRD patients, matched for factors influencing cardiovascular mortality.[9] Although the perioperative mortality was 3%, the 2-year survival of the surgical group was 92%, compared with 51% in the medically treated control group. Other small series have confirmed the efficacy of CABG in relieving angina pectoris in dialysis patients,[10-14] with 2-year survivals of 66% to 85%,[11,13,14] at the cost of a perioperative mortality of 8 to 9%,[15] but as high as 20%.[10,11]

Scant data exist regarding the outcome of dialysis patients after PTCA. Kahn reported procedural success in 47 of 49 vessels in 17 chronic hemodialysis patients, but angina returned within 6 months in 12 patients, among whom restenosis was demonstrated in 26 of 32 PTCA sites (81%).[16] In another series of retrospectively matched cohorts undergoing PTCA[17] (13 hemodialysis patients with 13 patients not on dialysis), procedural success was similar in each group, but at 2 years, 7 of 13 (54%) dialysis patients had experienced a cardiac event (angina recurrence, MI, CABG, or cardiac death), compared to 15% of controls. Ahmed et al.[18] reported a less favorable picture; PTCA was successful in 57% of patients, and in-hospital complications occurred in 38% (including three deaths, four MI, and one emergency CABG). After 27 ± 15 months of follow-up, 4 patients (27%) had death from cardiac causes, 9 had recurrent angina (60%), and 7 had repeat angiography (all of whom had restenosis of the previous PTCA site). Of the original cohort of 21 patients, only two (10%) remained alive and free of recurrent angina at follow-up.

The largest series of chronic hemodialysis patients undergoing coronary artery revascularization (24 PTCA and 60 CABG) was reported by Rinehart et al. from our institution.[19] In this study, more diabetics were in the PTCA group, and more severe CAD was present in the CABG group. Thirty-day perioperative CABG mortality was 3.2%, versus 0% procedure-related mortality in the PTCA group. However, more patients undergoing CABG were free of a cardiac event (angina, MI, or cardiovascular death) at follow-up than patients undergoing PTCA, in both patients with or without diabetic ESRD. By 6 months, 23% of CABG patients and 60% of the PTCA group had experienced a cardiac event. Figure 11-1 shows the cumulative event curves and highlights the dismal long-term outcome of the PTCA group. Fourteen of 24 PTCA patients experienced recurrent angina, and restenosis was found in 9 of 13 patients restudied (69%). The 2-year cumulative survival rate for the CABG and PTCA patients was 66% and 51%, respectively. The 5-year cumulative survival rate was 40% for CABG patients and 14% for PTCA patients. The trend favoring improved survival of the CABG patients was not statistically significant.

Clinical Significance

The patient on chronic dialysis following PTCA presents a distinct challenge to the clinician. The clinical recognition of restenosis is difficult, as these patients have a high prevalence of left ventricular hypertrophy (LVH) and can experience similar symptoms (i.e., angina and/or dyspnea) from either myocardial ischemia due to restenosis or volume overload. Hence, provocative noninvasive stress testing may

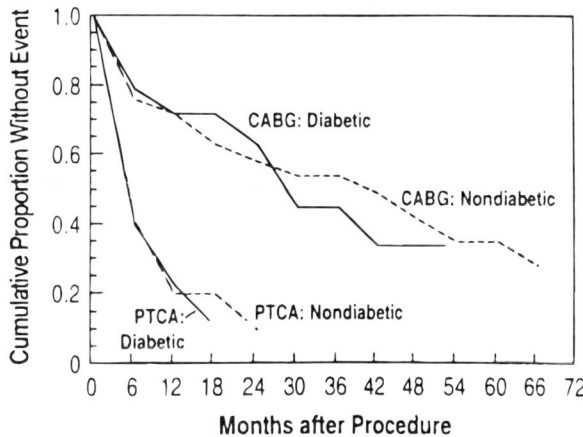

Fig. 11-1. Cumulative proportion of chronic dialysis patients free of angina, myocardial infarction, or cardiovascular death after coronary artery bypass grafting (CABG) or percutaneous transluminal coronary angioplast (PTCA). The two upper curves represent CABG patients with (solid line) and without (dashed line) diabetes mellitus. The two lower curves represent PTCA patients with (solid line) and without (dashed line) diabetes mellitus. The log-rank test for differences between CABG (with or without diabetes mellitus) and PTCA (with or without diabetes mellitus) curves is significant at $p < 0.0001$. (From Rinehart,[19] with permission.)

be performed in response to symptoms, or for surveillance at time intervals after PTCA when restenosis is most likely to occur. With the lesion remodeling that can occur after PTCA (and perhaps postprocedure alterations in coronary vasomotor function) a reasonable time for initial noninvasive provocative testing would be 5 weeks post-PTCA with the second test performed 12 to 16 weeks post-PTCA. However, the optimal frequency of subsequent follow-up is unclear. Pharmacologic stress imaging is the favored approach in many chronic dialysis patients because of the high prevalence of peripheral vascular disease and other comorbidity limiting the utility of exercise stress testing in dialysis patients, and the potential morbidity and expense of routine follow-up coronary angiography.

DIAGNOSTIC STRATEGIES USING NONINVASIVE APPROACHES

For reasons discussed in the previous section, the identification of CAD by noninvasive techniques is an important part of the clinical management of

ESRD patients being considered for renal transplantation or those followed on chronic dialysis. Although coronary angiography can be performed in these patients, a noninvasive surrogate offers the advantage of lower cost, avoidance of angiographic morbidity (such as cholesterol emboli and contrast nephropathy[20]), and relative ease of serial outpatient studies in selected patients. *If* noninvasive testing could accurately identify "clinically important" CAD, then coronary angiography could be reserved for the subset of patients who are likely candidates for coronary revascularization, based on their initial noninvasive clinical assessment.

Nuclear Stress Perfusion Imaging

The noninvasive cardiac evaluation of renal transplant candidates with diabetic nephropathy has been the major focus of studies utilizing stress nuclear scintigraphy (Table 11-1). Morrow et al.[21] at the University of Minnesota performed exercise planar thallium stress testing in 85 type 1 DM patients, 24 of whom had clinical evidence for pre-existing CAD. Only 6 of 85 (7%) were able to exercise to 85% of predicted maximal heart rate (HR), with a mean peak HR of 127 ± 22. Eighteen of 85 patients (21%) had a stress perfusion defect or abnormal stress electrocardiogram (ECG). Over a mean follow-up of 30 months, 31 of the 85 study patients had a cardiovascular event; thallium stress testing had a 44% sensitivity and 82% specificity for prediction of future events. Seven patients died of fatal MI, four with positive imaging tests. In this study, an abnormal resting ECG or history consistent with pre-existing CAD was as predictive for subsequent events as thallium testing. The performance of the latter may have been compromised by the exclusion of fixed defects from their definition of a positive test, as well as poor treadmill exercise performance (which may be less prevalent in the current era, due to the widespread use of erythropoietin [EPO]).

Philipson et al.[22] used exercise planar thallium imaging to evaluate 60 Type 1 DM patients awaiting renal transplantation at the University of Pittsburgh. Seven patients attaining greater than 85% predicted HR without angina, ischemic ECG changes, or perfusion defects received cardiovascular clearance for transplant, and the remaining 53 with positive or nondiagnostic testing underwent coronary angiography. Over a follow-up of 8 to 15 months, patients with insignificant CAD and normal left ventricular function (LVF) had a "good" outcome (2 deaths in 26 patients, both noncardiac). Patients with multivessel CAD or significant LV dysfunction had a worse outcome with 10 of 27 deaths (5 cardiac) in follow-up. Unfortunately, the estimation of sensitivity and specificity is problematic in this study, since 7 patients had normal studies and no angiography, and positive and nondiagnostic tests were lumped together (and only 12 of 60 attained target HR). Twenty-six of 53 patients with positive or nondiagnostic tests had visually estimated insignificant CAD, for a "51% test specificity."

Brown et al.[23] at the University of Vermont reported on 65 "high risk" renal transplant candidates (36 with insulin-dependent DM, 29 patients >40 years old with >1 CAD risk factor) evaluated with dipyridamole-planar thallium imaging and radionuclide ventriculography. Thirty-one of 36 (86%) patients with DM and 26 of 29 (90%) patients without DM had a normal dipyridamole thallium study. Patients were followed for 23 ± 11 months and 16 (25%) died, including six cardiac deaths (but no nonfatal MI). Five of 6 patients with cardiac death had a reversible thallium defect or left ventricular ejection fraction (LVEF) less than 55%. Five of 23 (22%) patients with reversible defects or LVEF less than 55% suffered a fatal cardiac event, compared with one of 42 (2%) with neither. All three (100%) patients with transient thallium defects had a cardiac event in follow-up, compared with only 3 of 62 (5%) without transient defects. Although in this study, patients with a normal dipyridamole thallium result had a low cardiac death rate, the study population showed an unexpectedly low prevalence of CAD (only 12% of patients had a fixed or reversible perfusion defect). Depending on the definition of "significant CAD" used, a prevalence of 25% to 40% would be anticipated for a "high-risk" population. Unfortunately, it is unclear as to how many results were false negatives, as coronary angiography was not performed. An alternative hypothesis is that significant numbers of patients with occult CAD were misclassified by dipyridamole–thallium stress imaging. These results may, therefore, be difficult to apply in other populations of high-risk renal transplant candidates.

Marwick et al.[24] at the Cleveland Clinic studied

45 "high-risk" dialysis patients referred for renal transplant evaluation with dipyridamole single photon emission computed tomographic (SPECT) thallium and coronary angiography. Evaluation was prompted by diabetic nephropathy (25 of 45, 56%), chest pain (60%), or age older than 40. Nineteen of 45 (42%) of patients had at least one coronary stenosis greater than 50% and 14 of 45 (31%) of patients had at least one stenosis greater than 70% by visual estimation. Thirteen of 45 patients had abnormal thallium images (12 reversible, one fixed defect). In patients with CAD greater than 50% stenosis, 7 of 19 had a positive thallium scan (37% sensitivity); for CAD greater than 70% stenosis, only 4 of 14 patients had positive thallium studies (29% sensitivity). In 10 patients with multivessel CAD, seven had negative thallium studies (30% sensitivity). Seven of 26 patients without CAD (<50% stenosis) had a false-positive scan (specificity 73%). Because of the unexpectedly poor diagnostic accuracy of dipyridamole SPECT thallium imaging, the authors retrospectively matched the ESRD cohort to a non-ESRD control group of 19 patients from the Cleveland Clinic database on dipyridamole SPECT thallium sensitivity (matching for CAD severity). The sensitivity of dipyridamole SPECT thallium was 95% in the control group, compared to 37% in the ESRD patients. Study patients were followed for 26 ± 14 months. Twelve died, six due to cardiac causes. All patients dying from cardiac causes had significant CAD by coronary angiography, but five of these six had normal thallium imaging.

The latter data[24] are unsettling because it suggests that ESRD patients may be a qualitatively different population. The poor accuracy of dipyridamole SPECT thallium imaging was not attributable to the institution, based on the control group. The poor sensitivity of dipyridamole stress imaging may relate to an altered response to this stressor in ESRD patients. Marwick et al.[24] have implicated abnormally high resting adenosine levels (blunting the effect of adenosine-mediated vasodilator stress by dipyridamole) in dialysis patients secondary to decreased lymphocyte adenosine deaminase activity.[25] Another explanation may relate to the abnormal, blunted vasodilator response to adenosine in coronary artery flow measured with Doppler flow probes in diabetic patients. Nahser et al.[26] found that maximal pharmacologic coronary flow reserve was depressed in diabetic patients (2.8 ± 0.2) compared to nondiabetic patients (3.7 ± 0.2, $p < 0.001$). Nitenberg et al.[27] also showed an abnormal coronary vasomotor response in diabetic patients. In the ESRD population referred for transplant evaluation, abnormal coronary flow reserve and blunted responses to vasodilator stress may also occur as a consequence of LVH. Ross et al.[28] measured the change in left anterior descending coronary artery diameter with high-frequency transthoracic echocardiography after nitroglycerin in normal patients, patients with nonischemic cardiomyopathy, and hypertensive dialysis patients. Coronary diameter increased by 55% in normals, 27% in patients with nonischemic cardiomyopathy, and only 10% in the dialysis patients after sublingual nitroglycerin. It is conceivable that other mechanisms may play a role in affecting coronary artery flow regulation and response to vasodilator stress in ESRD patients. An intriguing question is whether SPECT perfusion imaging would be more accurate using inotropic, rather than vasodilator stress. In a non-ESRD population Marwick et al.[29] found similar accuracy comparing dobutamine stress echocardiography to dobutamine technetium-99m sestamibi SPECT imaging in 217 patients. In the subset of patients with LVH, dobutamine stress echocardiography was more accurate, predominantly due to decreased specificity of positive dobutamine MIBI-SPECT (technetium-99m methoxyisobutyl isonitrilet [MIBI] studies in patients with LVH.

Boudreau et al.[30] at the University of Minnesota used oral or intravenous dipyridamole planar thallium imaging to evaluate 80 type 1 DM renal transplant candidates, 10 of whom (13%) had a previous MI by history. A scan was judged abnormal ($n = 44$) if fixed or reversible perfusion defects were present, but all abnormal scans were judged to have at least partial reversibility of perfusion defects. Significant CAD, defined as a greater than 70% reduction in cross-sectional area (i.e., >45% stenosis) using quantitative coronary angiography, was present in 42 patients (53%). The pooled negative predictive value for dipyridamole stress thallium imaging in this study was 83% (6 of 36 patients with normal scans had "significant" CAD by quantitative coronary angiography). The sensitivity and specificity of oral dipyridamole stress imaging were both 85%; in the

Table 11-1. Stress Nuclear Imaging in ESRD

Reference	Patient Population	Stress	Validation	Findings	Comments
Morrow et al. (1983)[21]	85 Type I DM transplant candidate	Exercise planar thallium	Clinical event rate (30 month FU)	44% Sensitivity 82% Specificity (36% event rate)	Only 6/85 patients reached target HR Resting ECG and history were of equal predictive value
Gelber et al. (1984)[49]	10 chronic hemodialysis	Rest planar thallium at end of hemodialysis	None	10/10 (+) reversible defects	Difficult to interpret
Dudczak et al. (1984)[50]	33 chronic dialysis (7 DM)	Dipyridamole planar thallium RNV	Clinical event rate	55% (+) thallium (+) scan—39% mortality (−) scan—23% mortality	Article written in German
Philipson et al. (1986)[22]	60 Type 1 DM transplant candidate	Exercise planar thallium	Coronary angiography (53/60) Clinical event rate (8–15 month mean FU)	Normal—(0 cardiac death) MVD/ << LVF— 5/27 cardiac deaths	Unknown sensitivity (+) and equivocal scans lumped together 51% specificity
Krawczynska et al. (1988)[51]	305 transplant candidate	Exercise (200) Dipyridamole (105) SPECT thallium	Clinical event rate Coronary angiography in 46/305	155/305 (+) thallium (+) thallium—9 died (6 cardiac) (−) thallium—7 died (0 cardiac)	Preliminary report 100% sensitivity 30% specificity based on 8 normals mean FU?
Marcen et al. (1989)[52]	29 chronic hemodialysis	Dipyridamole planar thallium	4 yr FU for death	13/29 (+) thallium 4/6 cardiac death (+) thallium	Age >50 only predictor of (+) thallium
Brown et al. (1989)[23]	65 transplant candidate (36 DM; 29 high-risk non-DM)	Dipyridamole planar thallium RNV	Clinical event rate (23 month mean FU)	88% normal thallium (+) predictive value 22% (−) predictive value 98%	Unusually low of (+) thallium
Marwick et al. (1990)[24]	45 chronic dialysis (high risk) Transplant candidate (25 DM)	Dipyridamole SPECT thallium	Coronary angiography Clinical event rate (26 month mean FU)	13/45 (+) thallium 19/45 CAD ≥50% 14/45 CAD ≥70% 37% sensitivity vs. ≥50% 73% specificity vs. ≥70% stenosis 29% sensitivity vs. ≥70%	Poor accuracy of dipyridamole SPECT thallium only in ESRD as matched cohort had 95% sensitivity

Study	Population	Test	Endpoint	Results	Comments
Boudreau et al. (1990)[30]	80 Type 1 DM transplant candidate	40 oral dipyridamole planar thallium / 40 IV dipyridamole planar thallium	QCA	42/80 (53%) CAD Oral: 85% sensitivity/ 85% specificity IV: 86% sensitivity/72% specificity	Only study of thallium vs. QCA in ESRD (CAD ≥70% reduction in cross-sectional area) Short clinical FU
Camp et al. (1990)[31]	40 DM transplant candidate	Dipyridamole planar thallium	Clinical event rate (11 month mean FU) Coronary angiography in 8	17/40 (+) thallium 8 fixed defects/9 reversible defects 6 events in reversible group	
Holley et al. (1991)[32]	189 DM transplant candidate	Exercise planar thallium	Perioperative event rate Coronary angiography for 34/41 (+) tests 27/36 inadequate tests	17/34 patients had (+) tests CAD <50%	Sensitivity ? (no angioplasty in normals) Referral bias—44 patients had only coronary angiography and worse survival Low event rate regardless of thallium
Trochu et al. (1991)[53]	25 Type 1 DM transplant candidate	20 exercise and 5 pharm planar thallium	Perioperative event rate	11/25 (+) thallium	No perioperative MI
Derfler et al. (1991)[33]	36 chronic dialysis 23 Transplant	Dipyridamole planar thallium	Clinical event rate (6 yr survival)	Dialysis—18/36 (+) thallium Transplant—9/23 (+) thallium (+) thallium: 11% survival (dialysis) (−) thallium: 39% survival (dialysis)	(+) thallium: 12%/yr fatal cardiac events (dialysis) (−) thallium: 1.9%/yr fatal cardiac events (dialysis) (+) thallium: 7.4%/yr fatal cardiac events (transplant) (−) thallium: 2.4%/yr fatal cardiac events (transplant)
Brown et al. (1993)[34]	103 "high risk" asymptomatic transplant candidate	Exercise planar thallium	Clinical event rate (4 yr FU) Coronary angiography in 30	60/103 (+) thallium 15 fatal cardiac events 70% specificity, 88% sensitivity	Prospective Fixed defects outcome not better than reversible defects

(Continues)

Table 11-1. (Continued).

Reference	Patient Population	Stress	Validation	Findings	Comments
Le et al. (1994)[35]	196 transplant candidate stratified to 96 low or 100 high risk (57 DM)	Exercise planar thallium in 89 Dipyridamole stress in 6 No stress imaging in low risk group	Clinical event rate (47 ± 16 months FU) Coronary angiography in 21 patients	53/95 (+) thallium (14 fix., 39 reversible defects Low risk—1% cardiac mortality High risk—17% cardiac mortality with (−) thallium 5% with (+) thallium 25%	Fixed and reversible thallium defects had similar outcomes Prior coronary revascularization in 11 patients (+ thallium in 10) Sensitivity? (no angiography in normals) 11/19 (42%) false (+) thallium vs. angiography
Singh et al. (1994)[46]	10 chronic dialysis	Nuclear vest ECG Sestamibi on dialysis	None	9/10 <LVF 7/10 perfusion defects	Small sample size
Legallicier et al. (1994)[40]	40 chronic asymptomatic high risk hemodialysis	Simultaneous exercise Dipyridamole thallium	Coronary angiography	12/40 (+) thallium 3/12 false (+) thallium 1/28 false (−) thallium	Preliminary report 88% sensitivity 90% specificity

Abbreviations: ESRD, end-stage renal disease; DM, diabetes mellitus; MI, myocardial infarction; CAD, coronary artery disease; FU, follow-up; HR, heart rate; ECG, electrocardiogram; RNV, radionuclide ventriculography; MVD, multivessel disease; LVF, left ventricular function; SPECT, single photon emission computed tomography; IV, intravenous, QCA, quantitative coronary angiography.

intravenous (IV) stress group the sensitivity was 86% and specificity 72%.

Camp et al.[31] used dipyridamole planar thallium imaging to study 40 patients awaiting transplantation for end-stage renal failure from diabetic nephropathy (including 8 with a history of MI or chest pain), and followed the patients over an average of 11 months. Twenty-three of 40 patients had normal thallium scans (8 with fixed defects and 9 with reversible defects). Eight of nine patients with reversible defects had coronary angiography (the ninth died suddenly before planned angiography): three had insignificant CAD and five had one artery with greater than 70% stenosis. Six of 40 patients had cardiac events, including two deaths. All cardiac events occurred in patients with reversible defects. The authors' discussion included an interesting comment relating to test interpretation and institutional learning curve effects: "We also found that thallium defects which we originally described as minor were of diagnostic significance in this population."

Holley et al.[32] at the University of Pittsburgh reviewed exercise planar thallium studies performed in 141 diabetic renal transplant candidates at 31 different centers. A thallium study was considered adequate if 70% of age-predicted HR was attained, and normal if the patient had no chest pain, no ischemic ECG changes with exercise, and no perfusion defects. Seventeen of 34 patients with abnormal thallium studies had insignificant CAD by coronary angiography (<50% by visual estimation). In the 27 patients having angiography for inadequate tests, nine (33%) had significant CAD. In the 44 patients referred directly for angiography, 20 (45%) had significant CAD. On follow-up of 41 ± 19 months for the normal scan group, 47 ± 22 months for the abnormal or inadequate scan group, and 32 ± 21 months for the angiography only group, there was no difference in survival between patients with normal or abnormal exercise stress thallium tests. Both groups had a low incidence of myocardial events within 2 weeks after transplantation, the difference in event rates being insignificant (1 of 48 [2%] patients with a normal study had an MI, 3 of 53 [6%] with abnormal or inadequate tests had an MI). In contrast, patients referred directly to angiography had a significantly shorter survival (approximately 60% at 30 months vs. 80% in the groups studied noninvasively), probably due to referral bias. The authors concluded that exercise planar thallium stress testing was not cost-effective.

Derfler et al.[33] at the University of Vienna examined the prognostic value of dipyridamole planar thallium imaging in 36 chronic hemodialysis patients and 23 with renal transplants and calculated 6-year cumulative survival. Twelve of 36 (33%) dialysis and 4 of 23 (17%) transplant patients had a chest pain history, and 17% of each group had DM. Eighteen of 36 (50%) dialysis patients had perfusion defects (fixed in 2, reversible in 16), and 9 of 23 transplant patients had abnormal studies. The 6-year event-free survival of dialysis patients with abnormal scans was 11% versus 39% for patients with normal studies ($p < 0.05$). For transplant patients with abnormal studies the 6-year cumulative survival was 56%, versus 64% for normal scans ($p = ns$). Figure 11-2 contrasts the survival of each group by thallium result. Dipyridamole thallium imaging was even a better predictor of *fatal* cardiac events. Hemodialysis patients with positive scans had a 12% per year occurrence of fatal cardiac events (MI, congestive heart failure [CHF]) versus 1.9% per year for those with normal perfusion scans. For transplant patients with abnormal scans the fatal cardiac event rate was 7.4% per year and 2.4% per year for those with normal scans. Interestingly, asymptomatic dialysis patients with abnormal scans had a worse survival than symptomatic patients (15.8 ± 13 months vs. 24.8 ± 19 months, $p < 0.005$). In a logistic regression model, dipyridamole thallium imaging was the only predictor for fatal cardiac events. The study of Derfler et al. provides valuable prognostic data for a select population of older, symptomatic, and predominantly nondiabetic ESRD patients who did not receive coronary revascularization.[33]

Brown et al.[34] in Manchester, England prospectively followed 103 asymptomatic ESRD patients eligible for renal transplant who were at "high risk" for ischemic heart disease, including 27% with DM. Twenty-three were on hemodialysis, 45 received continuous ambulatory peritoneal dialysis (CAPD), and 35 were dialysis-independent. Bicycle exercise planar thallium imaging was performed and 60 of 103 (58%) patients had positive studies (44 reversible and 16 with fixed defects). Patients were followed for 4 years, and their clinical outcome is summarized

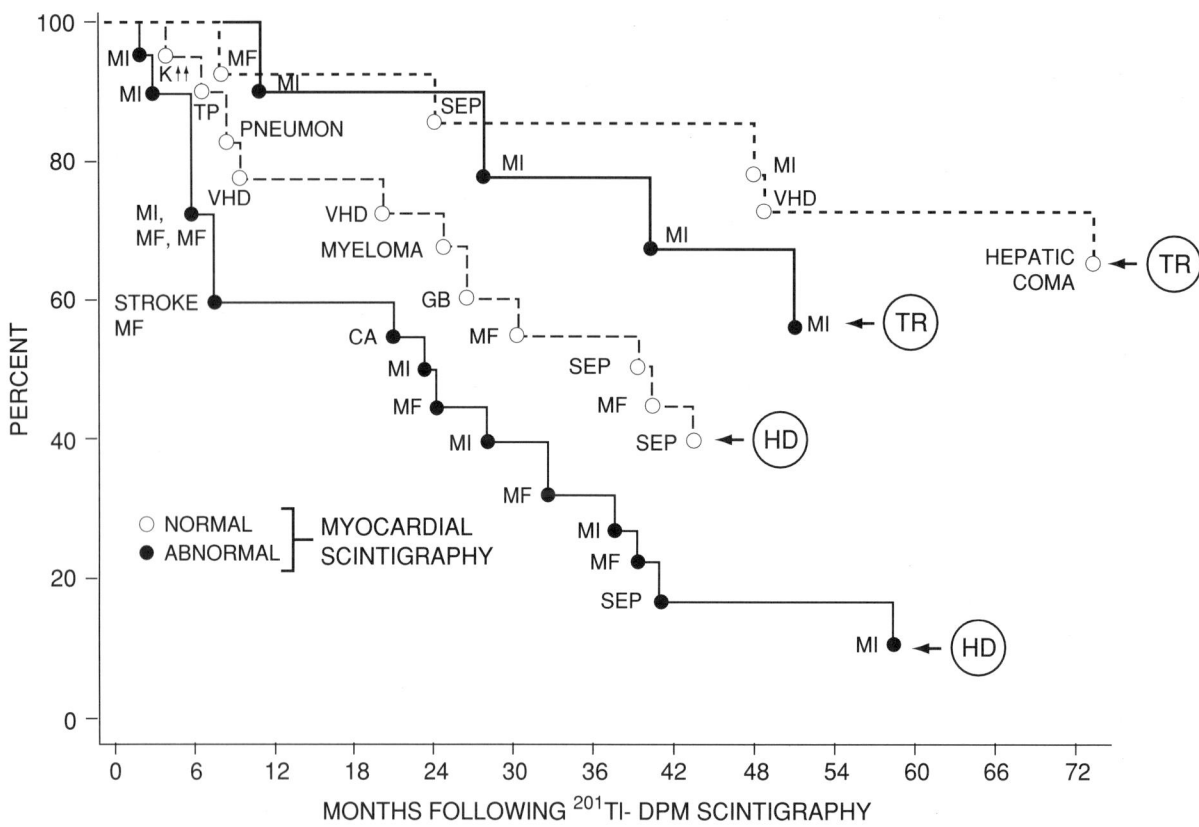

Fig. 11-2. Probability of survival in HD (hemodialysis patients) and TRs (renal transplant recipients) following ^{201}Tl-DPM scintigraphy. Causes of death are indicated: MI, myocardial infarction; MF, myocardial failure; VHD, valvular heart disease; K, hyperkalemia; GB, gastrointestinal bleeding; SEP, sepsis; CA, carcinoma; PNEUMON, pneumonia. (From Derfler,[33] with permission.)

in Figure 11-3. Twenty-eight (27%) patients died from cardiac causes and another 19 had nonfatal cardiac events (MI, CHF, angina, or stroke). A positive perfusion study was 88% sensitive and 70% specific for the occurrence of a cardiac event. The predictive value of a positive test was 73%. In the diabetic subgroup, 50% had a positive test, and 10 of 14 (71%) experienced a cardiac event, compared to 2 of 14 with negative scans. For DM patients, the sensitivity of the test for future event occurrence was 83%, specificity 75%, and the predictive value of a positive test was 71%. In a subgroup of 30 patients undergoing angiography, 23 (77%) had at least one stenosis greater than 50%, and 22 had positive thallium tests (two of whom had insignificant CAD). Of eight patients with negative studies, three had significant disease, including two with three-vessel CAD. In this subgroup new angina was 77% specific for "significant CAD" and a positive thallium was 91% specific. The sensitivity of thallium testing was 87%, but the predictive value of a negative test was only 64%.

The work of Brown et al.[34] raises interesting questions, as it is one of the best-designed "natural history" studies published. In contrast to other studies, fixed or reversible perfusion defects were both associated with adverse outcomes: 9 of 16 (56%) with fixed defects and 16 of 44 with reversible defects (36%) suffered fatal cardiac events. In their asymptomatic cohort of 103 patients, 16 had fixed perfusion defects at study entry, suggesting prior history of silent MI. This study details the natural history of

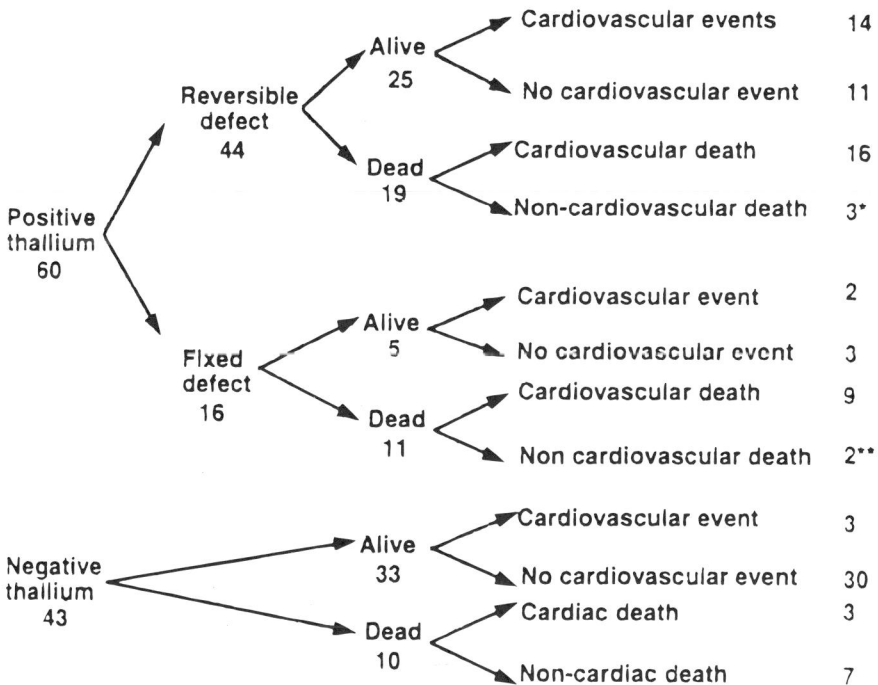

Fig. 11-3. Results of thallium test and eventual outcome in all 103 patients. *Two patients developed nonfatal cardiac events. **One patient developed a nonfatal cardiac event. (From Brown,[34] with permission.)

ESRD patients with CAD who apparently did not receive coronary revascularization. There is also an issue of unavoidable selection bias, as all 103 patients (selected from a larger group of 380 entering a renal replacement therapy program) were able to perform bicycle exercise; 56% exercised to an impressive greater than 120 W/min, and this study was performed in the pre-EPO era.

Le et al.[35] at the University of Oregon performed an interesting tiered study of 196 renal transplant candidates who were prospectively entered into a risk-stratification algorithm. Risk factors considered were older than 50, presence of insulin-dependent DM, anginal history, CHF, or abnormal ECG (excluding LVH). The 96 patients with none of these cardiac risk factors underwent no further cardiac evaluation. In the remaining "high risk" 100 patients (57 DM), 89 had exercise planar thallium imaging, and six had dipyridamole stress. Patients with reversible thallium defects "were advised that further cardiac evaluation would be required," implying an unstated assumption at the time of study inception that reversible and fixed defects have a different clinical significance. Ninety-four of the low risk group and 95 in the high risk group were available for 47 ± 16 month follow-up; respectively, 65 and 41 of the patients were transplanted. The cardiac mortality rate was only 1% in the low-risk group and 17% in the high-risk group. Fifty-three of 95 high-risk patients (56%) had abnormal thallium scans (39 reversible, 14 fixed defects), and these patients showed a 25% cardiac mortality, compared with 5% for normal studies ($p < 0.02$). The cardiac mortality for patients with fixed or reversible defects was similar (29% and 23%, respectively). In patients with DM, 13 of 32 with abnormal thallium studies died (8 from cardiac causes), compared to 7 of 25 with normal scans (none cardiac). Only 21 of 39 patients with reversible thallium defects had cardiac catheterizations; in 19 patients with positive scans, eight (42%) had greater than 50% stenoses, and 11 had stenoses less than 50%. The low specificity of thallium testing in this group is similar to the results of Holley et al.[32]

The identification of a low-risk group of renal transplant candidates on clinical grounds is an important goal, as it may avoid provocative testing of all subjects. However, the assumption of Le et al.[35] that all insulin-dependent diabetics are at high risk has been refuted by Manske et al.[36] Coronary angiography was performed in 141 consecutive type 1 diabetic renal candidates at the University of Minnesota from 1987 to 1991. In patients older than 45, 88% (14 of 16) had a coronary artery stenosis greater than 50% by visual estimation. In 125 patients younger than 45, 90 were studied to develop a clinical model for prediction of CAD (>50% stenosis definition), and the prediction algorithm was tested in the remaining 35 patients younger than 45 years old and in 35 subsequent consecutive asymptomatic diabetic transplant candidates. Patients with previous MI or coronary bypass were excluded. In a logistic regression analysis, only abnormal ST-T segments on the resting ECG and duration of diabetes were significant, and smoking greater than 5 pack years was of borderline significance ($p = 0.08$). Thus, the clinical combination of type 1 diabetic renal transplant candidates younger than 45 years old with abnormal ST-T segments on ECG, smoking greater than 5 pack years, or diabetes for at least 25 years was associated with the presence of CAD in 33 patients and incorrectly predicted CAD in 14. The combination correctly predicted the absence of CAD in 22 patients and incorrectly in 1 patient. The sensitivity and negative predictive accuracy of the algorithm were respectively an impressive 97% and 96%, but the specificity and positive predictive accuracy were only 61% and 70%, respectively. In their patient population of predominantly young Caucasian Type 1 diabetic renal transplant candidates, this clinical algorithm identified a group of *diabetic* patients who were at low risk for CAD (defined angiographically). The authors are correct to point out that transplant candidates with differing demographics (e.g., African-Americans or Native Americans with Type 2 DM) may not be suitable for this algorithm.

Stress Echocardiography

Accuracy

As discussed in prior chapters, stress echocardiography is most commonly performed with either exercise or dobutamine stress. Dobutamine stress echocardiography (DSE) is favored in patients with renal disease because they frequently are unable to exercise maximally. Chronologically, stress echocardiography is a younger technique than myocardial perfusion imaging, and this is reflected in the paucity of studies using this technique for the detection of CAD in ESRD patients (Table 11-2).

Reis et al.[37] performed DSE without atropine administration in 97 chronic dialysis patients (38 CAPD, 59 hemodialysis) as part of their preoperative evaluation before renal transplantation. A significant proportion had clinical evidence for CAD (30%) including MI in 18%; 62 (64%) had DM. All patients completed the DSE protocol, but only 11 patients (14% of those with available data) reached target HR. Twenty-nine of 97 patients had abnormal studies. Of 27 patients with abnormal resting LV function (10 global, 17 regional wall motion abnormalities), 20 had inducible ischemia. In 30 patients, coronary angiography was performed for "clinical indictions" (including abnormal DSE in 23) within 4 months of DSE; 23 (77%) had at least one greater than 50% stenosis by visual estimation. A sensitivity of 95% and specificity of 86% were obtained, but as only 7 with normal studies had coronary angiography, a significant referral bias is likely. Patients were followed for 12 ± 6 months; 6 died during follow-up, but none due to MI (1 post-CABG, 3 sepsis, and 2 cerebrovascular accident [CVAs]). DSE had a positive predictive value of 14% and a negative predictive value of 97% for 1-year survival. Coronary revascularization was performed in four patients before transplant, and none of the 25 suffered perioperative cardiac complications. The paucity of cardiac events (MI, sudden cardiac death) occurring in these 97 ESRD patients during follow-up is interesting and perhaps unexpected. There were no fatal MIs, but there was no discussion of nonfatal MIs. With the short clinical follow-up in this study, the use of only fatal endpoints may provide an unrealistic estimate of test accuracy.

As a direct response to the work of Manske and others at the University of Minnesota,[7,8] we designed a prospective study testing the accuracy of dobutamine stress echocardiography compared to quantitative coronary angiography for the detection of clinically significant CAD in renal transplant candidates.[38] Our study group was comprised primarily of patients with diabetic nephropathy without

Table 11-2. Stress Echocardiography in ESRD

Reference	Patient Population	Stress	Validation	Findings	Comments
Herzog et al. (1993)[38]	29 transplant candidate (22 DM)	DSE (with atropine)	QCA + visual estimate	13/29 (+) DSE 13/29 QCA >50% 8/29 QCA >70% 10/29 visual estimate >75% QCA >50% 69% sensitivity; 69% specificity QCA >70% 100% sensitivity; 62% specificity Visual estimate >75% 90% sensitivity; 69% specificity	Preliminary report Prospective design Only study comparing DSE in ESRD to QCA
Nally et al. (1993)[54]	30 transplant candidate 30 matched controls	DSE (no atropine)	Coronary angiography CAD >50%	14/30 CAD 86% sensitivity 94% specificity	Preliminary report Accuracy of DSE similar in ESRD and control: No. DM?
Albanese et al. (1994)[55]	45 ESRD	DSE (no atropine)	Clinical event rate (mean FU 22 ± 9 month) 33/45 coronary angiography	16/33 CAD>50% DSE vs. angiography 69% sensitivity 94% specificity; cardiac event 7/45 patients (DSE predicted 4/7)	Preliminary report
Reis et al. (1995)[37]	97 chronic dialysis transplant candidate (64% DM) CAD history in 30%	DSE (no atropine)	Clinical event rate (mean FU 12 ± 6 month) 30/97 coronary angiography (CAD>50%)	29/97 (+) DSE 23/30 CAD 6 deaths in FU (+) predictive value for death at 1 yr 14%, (−) predictive value 97%	Short clinical FU Referral bias for coronary angiography No MI deaths

Abbreviations: ESRD, end-stage renal disease; DM, diabetes mellitus; DSE, dobutamine stress echo; QCA, quantitative coronary angiography; CAD, coronary artery disease; MI, myocardial infarction; FU, follow-up.

clinical evidence of CAD, to validate the accuracy of DSE for noninvasive selection of patients requiring coronary angiography and possible revascularization. A second smaller group of patients was included who were unable to perform treadmill exercise and had CAD risk factors or some clinical evidence for CAD (high risk nondiabetics). The preliminary findings of this and similar studies are summarized in Table 11-2.

Feasibility

For patients on hemodialysis, stress imaging studies are simplest to schedule on nondialysis days. Most hemodialysis patients receive dialytic therapy 3 times per week (Monday, Wednesday, Friday, or Tuesday, Thursday, Saturday). The typical hemodialysis patient experiences 1 day per week of increased volume stress, and may be markedly hypertensive following the long weekend between dialysis runs. Patients receiving CAPD therapy do not experience the large nonphysiologic volume shifts present with hemodialysis. In the CAPD patient, normotensive blood pressure is probably the best indication of optimal volume status. Following hemodialysis, orthostatic hypotension is not unusual when the patient has been brought down to his "dry weight." It may be prudent for the noninvasive laboratory to contact the patient's dialysis unit before scheduling stress testing to ascertain that patient's particular pattern of blood pressure response in relation to dialytic therapy. Exercise and pharmacologic stress imaging tests should not be scheduled at times when the patient is known to be significantly hypertensive or hypotensive.

In the normotensive patient, there is frequently a biphasic blood pressure response with dobutamine administration: initial rise in blood pressure at lower doses followed by a plateau, and than fall of blood pressure at higher doses. This phenomenon has been attributed predominantly to vasodilation, vagally mediated reflexes (i.e., Bezold–Jarisch), and (to a lesser extent) dynamic intracavitary obstruction. Hypovolemic patients with LVH are likely candidates for severe hypotension with dobutamine stress and the baseline echocardiogram showing a hyperdynamic hypertrophied LV with a tiny intracavitary volume should identify the patient at risk. Even in dialysis-dependent patients, small amounts of normal saline (e.g., 250 ml) can be infused to attenuate the hypotensive response when it occurs.

Hypertensive patients present a different set of problems. Some dialysis patients demonstrate an "accelerated" hypertensive response to very low levels of dobutamine, necessitating test termination prematurely before a significant HR increase occurs. DSE should not be performed if the patient's resting systolic blood pressure exceeds 180 mmHg after 30 minutes of waiting quietly. Even in patients with baseline blood pressures of below 180 mmHg, blood pressures in excess of 240 mmHg at a dobutamine dose of 10 μg/kg/min have occurred in our laboratory. Because of this, prescribed antihypertensive agents are not withheld before stress testing, including β-blockers.

A standard dobutamine infusion protocol (5, 10, 20, 30, 40 μg/kg/min administered in 3-minute stages) is used. If 85% of target HR is not attained (220 − age × 0.85) a total of up to 1.0 mg IV atropine is administered. Dobutamine infusions are terminated before target HR is attained for intolerable side effects, systolic blood pressure greater than 240, or diastolic blood pressure greater than 120 (diastolic pressure nearly always drops), silent myocardial ischemia in more than one vascular territory, symptomatic myocardial ischemia with objective findings, or repetitive sustained or nonsustained tachyarrhythmia. Although atrial fibrillation is a relatively rare occurrence with dobutamine stress in the non-ESRD population (0.5% frequency), this appears to be 5 to 10 times more prevalent in the dialysis population, probably reflecting the high prevalence of LVH and the common occurrence of atrial tachyarrhythmias in this group. In nearly all of our patients, there has been a premonitory burst of nonsustained atrial tachycardia followed by sustained atrial fibrillation or flutter. These atrial tachyarrhythmias have not always terminated spontaneously with discontinuation of dobutamine. Our preferred treatment of this complication in this setting has been esmolol, since it functions as a dobutamine antagonist and atrioventricular (AV)-nodal blocker simultaneously. Two dialysis patients have required prolonged esmolol infusions before conversion to normal sinus rhythm (34 minutes and 6 hours). To date, no ESRD patient has experienced a life-threatening complication during DSE.

Not all ESRD patients require pharmacologic stress to obtain an adequate peak HR. Table 11-3 summarizes our laboratory's experience. Exercise stress has several advantages. It is less expensive to perform, and avoids the time and effort that can be expended in an attempt to obtain adequate venous access, particularly in institutions where an arteriovenous fistula is a privileged site not to be used by nondialysis personnel. Despite the better image quality with DSE, exercise stress may avoid the interpretive difficulties posed by the small intracavitary volume obscuring the detection of small wall motion abnormalities, and probably affords a greater stress on the heart.[39] Figure 11-4 documents

Table 11-3. Stress Echo in ESRD Patients (Hennepin County Medical Center)

	Number of Studies	Attained ≥85% HR	<85% HR	Test Stopped for Other Endpoint
Dialysis				
Exercise	74 (31%)[a]	39 (44%)	34 (15%)	1 (100%)
Dobutamine	114 (32%)	58 (31%)	42 (24%)	14 (64%)
Transplant				
Exercise	31 (35%)	15 (33%)	16 (44%)	
Dobutamine	11 (18%)	8 (25%)	1 (0%)	2 (0%)

[a] Percentage positive studies.

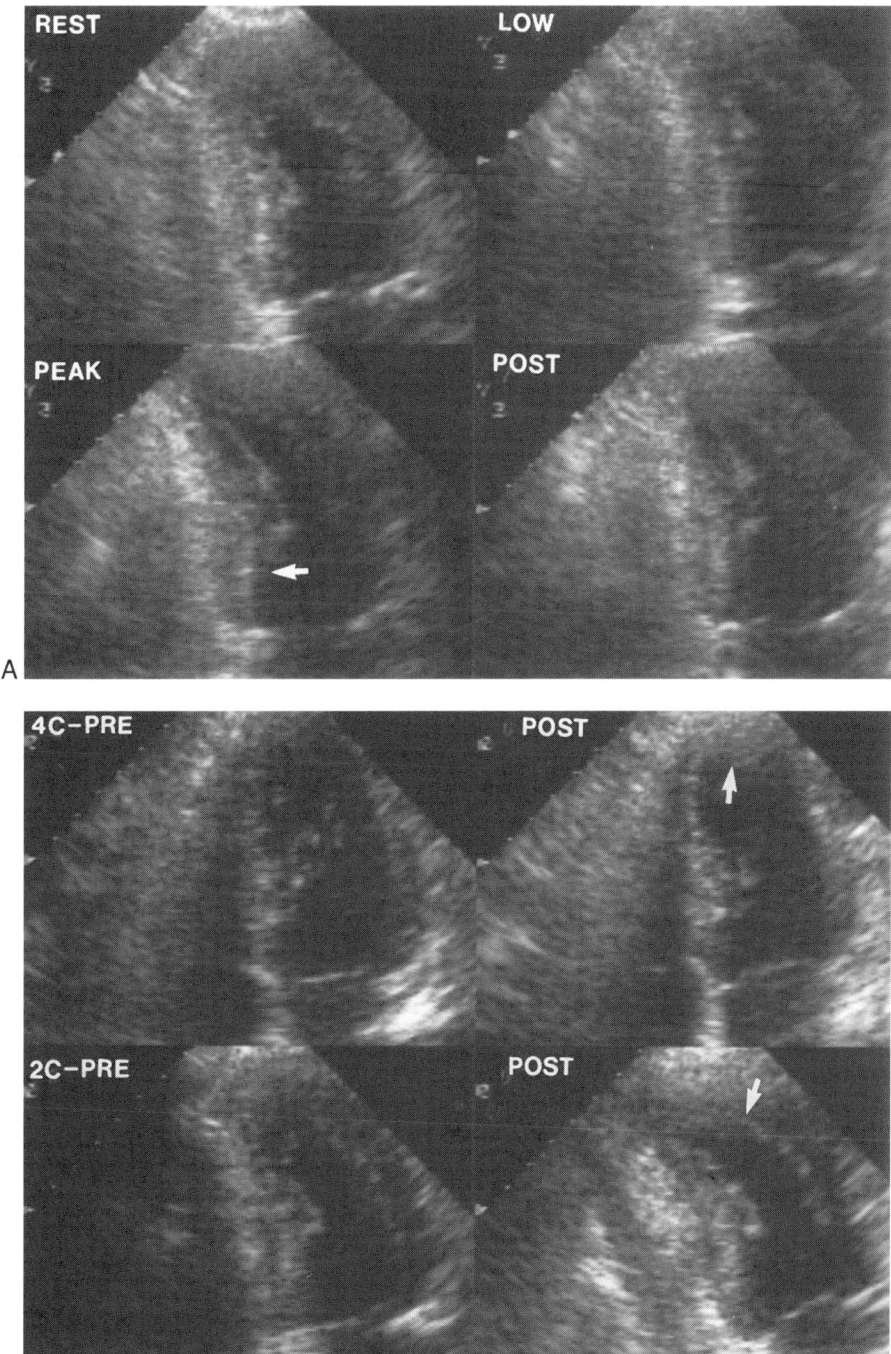

Fig. 11-4. (A) Dobutamine stress echocardiogram (peak heart rate [HR] 141) of a 65-year-old renal transplant candidate with hypertensive nephropathy. Apical two-chamber view shows a "pseudo-wall motion abnormality" of the basal inferior segment (*arrow*). The anterior wall is normal. **(B)** Exercise echocardiogram (peak HR 163) of the same patient: apical four- and two-chamber views. Note the anterior-apical wall motion abnormalities (*arrows*).

the importance of maximum HR in stress echocardiographic imaging. This 65-year-old transplant candidate with hypertensive nephropathy and degenerative musculoskeletal disease had a negative DSE (peak HR 141, systolic blood pressure 178 at 30 µg/kg/min) (Fig. 11-4A). He subsequently underwent symptom-limited exercise stress imaging (with the examiner standing on the back end of the treadmill), attaining a HR of 163 and systolic blood pressure of 220 after exercising 6 minutes on a standard Bruce protocol, and developed an anterior apical wall motion abnormality (Fig. 11-4B). With both stress imaging tests, there were no symptoms or ischemic ECG changes. Coronary angiography revealed a 90% stenosis in the midportion of the left anterior descending coronary artery distal to a large diagonal branch. Repeat exercise stress imaging after successful PTCA was normal.

With the widespread use of EPO and the attendant improvement in exercise capacity, exercise stress imaging is a viable option in many patients. The patient's reporting of exercise capacity is an unreliable screen for triaging of stress modality in our laboratory. An unscientific but useful strategy is to perform a ministress test before the patient is brought into the noninvasive laboratory. The patient is asked to walk briskly (approximately 4 km/h) for a distance of 40 to 50 m, stop, turn abruptly, and walk quickly back to the examiner. If the patient can perform this minitest and is not receiving β-blockers, he or she can usually be encouraged to reach target HR. In patients receiving β-blockers, DSE with atropine will probably be more successful. In our laboratory, we have not attempted the simultaneous performance of exercise and pharmacologic stress imaging.[40]

Assessment of ischemia involving the basal inferior segment on the apical two-chamber view is difficult,[41] particularly in patients with marked LVH. In our ESRD patients with LVH, we require at least half of the inferior wall to be scored as abnormal to be interpreted as positive on the apical two-chamber view (i.e., basal inferior segment plus half of the ad-

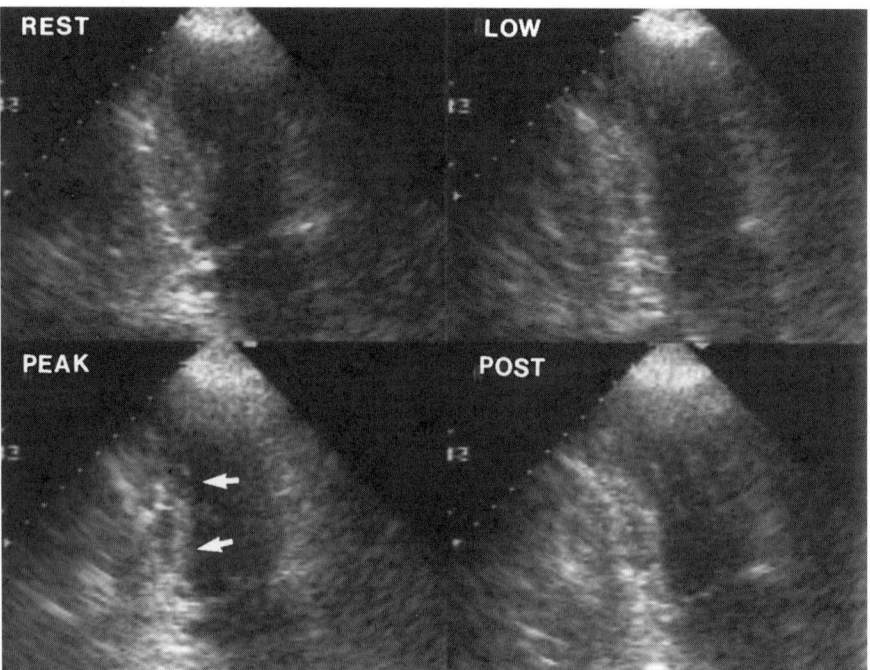

Fig. 11-5. Dobutamine stress echocardiogram, apical two-chamber view of a 65-year-old renal transplant candidate with diabetic nephropathy. Note the inferior wall motion abnormality at peak stress involving both the basal inferior and mid-inferior segments (*arrows*). Subsequent coronary angiography demonstrated a 95% stenosis of the mid right coronary artery.

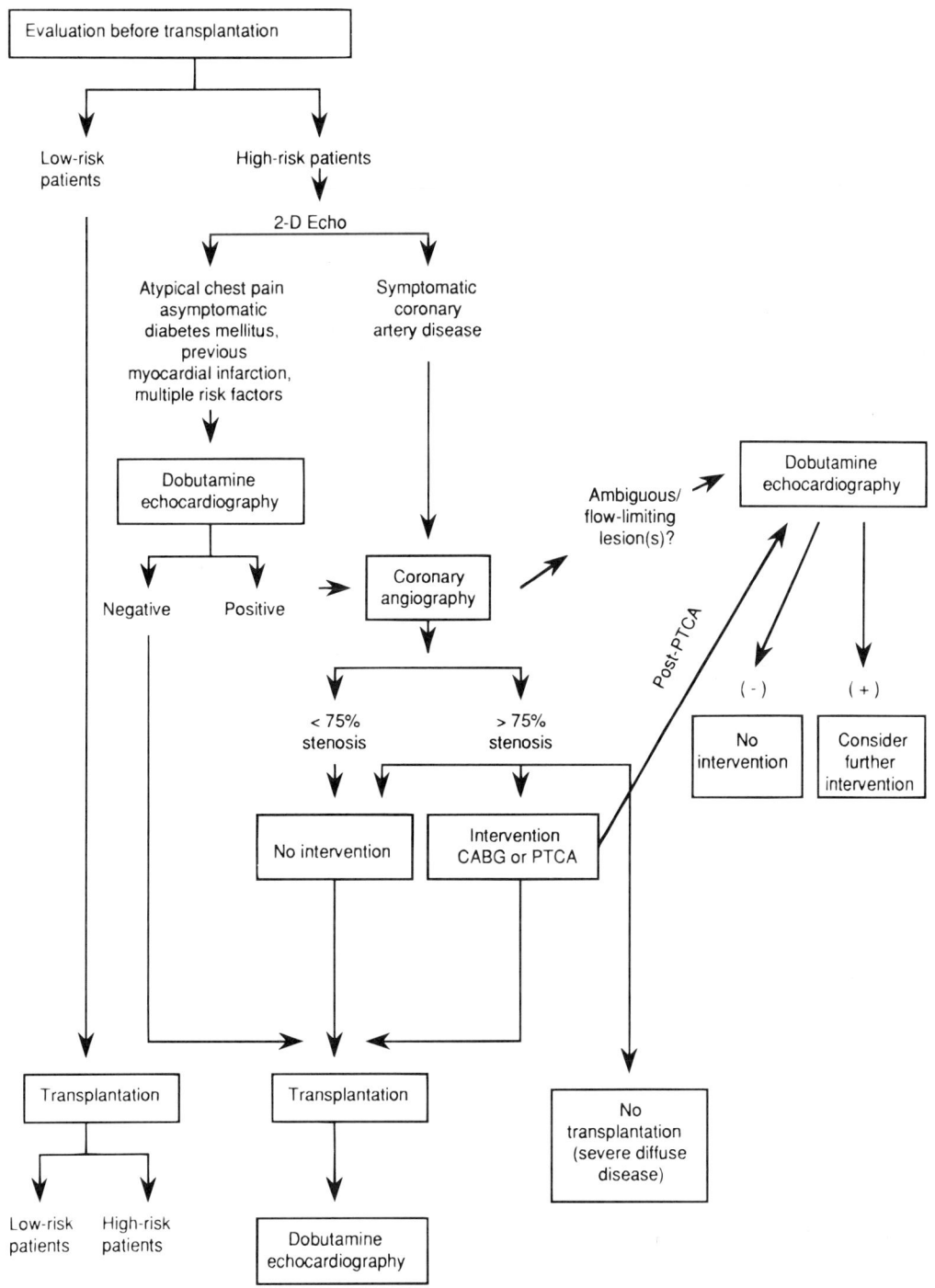

Fig. 11-6. Algorithm for management of coronary artery disease in renal transplant candidates. (Modified from Braun,[42] with permission.)

joining midinferior segment). Figure 11-5 shows abnormal systolic thickening of the basal inferior and midinferior segments with dobutamine stress (apical two-chamber view) in a 65-year-old transplant candidate with diabetic nephropathy and no previous cardiac history. The abnormal segments comprise at least two-thirds of the inferior wall. In contrast, Figure 11-4A demonstrates a "pseudo-wall motion abnormality" of the basal-inferior segment (apical two-chamber view) due to LVH.

OTHER NONINVASIVE MODALITIES AND FUTURE DIRECTIONS

This chapter has focused predominantly on radionuclide perfusion imaging techniques and stress echocardiographic imaging for the noninvasive detection of CAD. Even without considering other modalities such as magnetic resonance imaging (MRI) noninvasive imaging is constantly evolving, rapidly outdating studies. For example, most studies of radionuclide techniques in ESRD patients have utilized planar thallium imaging, leading to the suspicion that MIBI-SPECT would be better. Similarly, combinations of exercise and dipyridamole stress imaging or new inotropic stress agents (e.g., arbutamine) may offer potential improvements in diagnostic accuracy.[40] The newer generations of myocardial contrast agents should allow for better imaging, and perhaps permit the realization of a reliable automated edge detection program for quantitative measurement of regional systolic thickening.

The issue of CAD detection is important only if it affects prognosis or triggers therapeutic interventions altering clinical outcomes. If only prognosis were of interest, risk stratification strategies including noninvasive imaging would be justified based on published data. Figure 11-6 summarizes the algorithm we use for cardiac management of CAD in renal transplant candidates.[42]

A variety of other noninvasive techniques for detection of CAD have attracted the attention of investigators. Ambulatory ECG has been attempted in ESRD patients without adequate validation by other techniques.[43] We are skeptical of its value, as electrolyte shifts may make dialysis-related ECG changes a poor diagnostic test for painless myocardial ischemia.[44] With the combination of LVH and exercise intolerance in the ESRD population, stress electrocardiography is problematic as a solo diagnostic test. Hemodynamic alterations during dialysis have been measured by impedance cardiography[45] and the ambulatory nuclear vest,[46] but neither directly assesses myocardial ischemia.

A more promising technique that has its roots in older clinical studies is ultrafast electron beam CT. Coronary calcification on fluoroscopy was advocated as a screening test for CAD years ago. Indeed, Marwick et al. examined the accuracy of digital subtraction fluorography compared to coronary angiography for the detection of CAD in 86 high-risk renal transplant candidates on chronic dialysis.[47] Thirty-six (42%) had significant CAD (>50% stenosis) and 45 patients (52%) had coronary artery calcification. The sensitivity of detected calcification for CAD diagnosis was 78% and the specificity was 66%. In a preliminary report, ultrafast CT was shown to quantitatively measure coronary calcification,[48] but it has not been systematically validated for the detection of significant CAD in ESRD patients.

In conclusion, end-stage renal disease represents but a small fraction of the general population developing CAD. However, as a population at particularly high risk for the complications of ischemic heart disease, it is one worthy of concentrated future efforts in the areas of prevention, diagnosis, and treatment.

Since the submission of this chapter, two additional reports have appeared on the evaluation of renal transplant candidates with DSE.[56,57] The preliminary communication of Costello et al.[56] prospectively compared DSE in 40 high-risk renal transplant candidates to visually estimated coronary angiography. Bates et al.[57] retrospectively compared the results of DSE in 53 diabetic transplant candidates to cardiac event rates. Both support the role of DSE in the cardiac evaluation of high-risk renal transplant patients.

REFERENCES

1. United States Renal Data System: USRDS 1995 Annual Data Report. National Institute of Diabetes and Digestive and Kidney Diseases, Bethesda, Maryland, 1995, pp 79–90
2. United States Renal Data System: USRDS 1993 Annual Data Report. National Institute of Diabetes and Digestive and Kidney Diseases, Bethesda, Maryland, 1993, pp 49–54

3. United States Renal Data System: USRDS 1993 Annual Data Report. National Institute of Diabetes and Digestive and Kidney Diseases, Bethesda, Maryland, 1993, pp 19–28
4. Braun WE, Phillips D, Vidt DG et al: Coronary arteriography and coronary artery disease in 99 diabetic and nondiabetic patients on chronic hemodialysis or renal transplantation programs. Transplant Proc 13:128, 1981
5. Braun WE, Phillips DF, Vidt DG et al: Coronary artery disease in 100 diabetics with end-stage renal failure. Transplant Proc 16:603, 1984
6. Lorber MI, Van Buren CT, Flechner SM et al. Pretransplant coronary arteriography for diabetic renal transplant recipients. Transplant Proc 19:1539, 1987
7. Manske CL, Wang Y, Rector TS et al: Coronary revascularisation in insulin-dependent diabetic patients with chronic renal failure. Lancet 340:998, 1992
8. Manske CL, Wang Y, Wilson RF et al: Coronary revascularization may improve short term survival in insulin-dependent diabetics considered for renal transplantation. Circulation, Suppl II, 84:II-516, 1991
9. Opsahl JA, Husebye DJ, Helseth HK et al: Coronary artery bypass surgery in patients on maintenance dialysis: long-term survival. Am J Kidney Dis 12:271, 1988
10. Rostand SG, Kirk KA, Rutsky EA et al: Results of coronary artery bypass grafting in end stage renal disease. Am J Kidney Dis 12:266, 1988
11. Batiuk T, Kurtz SB, Oh JK et al: Coronary artery bypass operation in dialysis patients. Mayo Clinic Proc 66:45, 1991
12. Deutsch E, Bernstein RC, Addonizio P et al: Coronary artery bypass surgery in patients on chronic hemodialysis. Ann Intern Med 110:369, 1989
13. De Meyer M, Wynns W, Dion R et al: Myocardial revascularization in patients on renal replacement therapy. Clin Nephrol 36:147, 1991
14. Kaul TK, Fields BL, Reddy MA et al: Cardiac operations in patients with end-stage renal disease. Ann Thorac Surg 57:691, 1994
15. Ko W, Kreiger KH, Ison OW: Cardiopulmonary bypass procedures in dialysis patients. Ann Thorac Surg 55:677, 1993
16. Kahn JK, Rutherford BD, Mcconahay DR et al: Short- and long-term outcome of percutaneous transluminal coronary angioplasty in chronic dialysis patients. Am Heart J 19:44, 1990
17. Reusser LM, Osborn LA, White HJ et al: Increased morbidity after coronary angioplasty in patients on chronic hemodialysis. Am J Cardiol 73:965, 1994
18. Ahmed WH, Shubrooks SJ, Gibson CM et al: Complications and long-term outcome after percutaneous coronary angioplasty in chronic hemodialysis patients. Am Heart J 128:252, 1994
19. Rinehart AL, Herzog CA, Collins AJ et al: A comparison of coronary angioplasty and coronary artery bypass grafting outcomes in chronic dialysis patients. Am J Kidney Dis 25:281, 1995
20. Manske CL, Sprafka JM, Strony J et al: Acute renal failure after radio-contrast exposure in azotemic, insulin-dependent diabetics. Am J Med 89:615, 1990
21. Morrow CE, Schwartz JS, Sutherland DER et al: Predictive value of thallium stress testing for coronary and cardiovascular events in uremic diabetic patients before renal transplantation. Am J Surg 146:331, 1983
22. Philipson JD, Carpenter BJ, Itzkoff J et al: Evaluation of cardiovascular risk for renal transplantation in diabetic patients. Am J Med 81:630, 1986
23. Brown KA, Rimmer J, Haisch C: Noninvasive cardiac risk stratification of diabetic and nondiabetic uremic renal allograft candidates using dipyridamole-thallium-201 imaging and radionuclide ventriculography. Am J Cardiol 64(16):1017, 1989
24. Marwick TH, Steinmuller DR, Underwood DA et al: Ineffectiveness of dipyridamole spect thallium imaging as a screening technique for coronary artery disease in patients with end-stage renal failure. Transplantation 49:100, 1990
25. Melissinos K, Delidou A, Grammenou S et al: Study of the activity of lymphocyte adenosine deaminase in chronic renal failure. Clin Chim Acta 135:9, 1983
26. Nahser PJ, Brown RE, Oskarsson H et al: Maximal coronary flow reserve and metabolic coronary vasodilation in patients with diabetes mellitus. Circulation 91:635, 1995
27. Nitenberg A, Valensi P, Sachs R et al: Impairment of coronary vascular reserve and ACh-induced coronary vasodilation in diabetic patients with angiographically normal coronary arteries and normal left ventricular systolic function. Diabetes 2:1017, 1993
28. Ross JJ, Ren JF, Land W et al: Transthoracic high frequency (7.5 MHz) echocardiographic assessment of coronary vascular reserve and its relation to left ventricular mass. J Am Coll Cardiol 16(6):1393, 1990
29. Marwick T, D'Hondt A, Baudhuin T et al: Optimal use of dobutamine stress for the detection and evaluation of coronary artery disease: combination with echocardiography or scintigraphy, or both? J Am Coll Cardiol 22:159, 1993
30. Boudreau RJ, Strony JT, duCret RP et al: Perfusion thallium imaging of type I diabetes patients with end stage renal disease: comparison of oral and intravenous dipyridamole administration. Radiology 175:103, 1990
31. Camp AD, Garvin PJ, Hoff J et al: Prognostic value of intravenous dipyridamole thallium imaging in patients with diabetes mellitus considered for renal transplantation. Am J Cardiol 65(22):1459, 1990

32. Holley JL, Fenton RA, Arthur RS: Thallium stress testing does not predict cardiovascular risk in diabetic patients with end-stage renal disease undergoing cadaveric renal transplantation. Am J Med 90:563, 1991
33. Derfler K, Kletter K, Balcke P et al: Predictive value of thallium-201-dipyridamole myocardial stress scintigraphy in chronic hemodialysis patients and transplant recipients. Clin Nephrol 36:192, 1991
34. Brown JH, Vites NP, Testa HJ et al: Value of thallium myocardial imaging in the prediction of future cardiovascular events in patients with end-stage renal failure. Nephrol Dial Transplant 8(5):433, 1993
35. Le A, Wilson R, Douek K et al: Prospective risk stratification in renal transplant candidates for cardiac death. Am J Kidney Dis 24:65, 1994
36. Manske CL, Thomas W, Wang Y et al: Screening diabetic transplant candidates for coronary artery disease: identification of a low risk subgroup. Kidney Int 44:617, 1993
37. Reis G, Marcovitz PA, Leichtman AB et al: Usefulness of dobutamine stress echocardiography in detecting coronary artery disease in end-stage renal disease. Am J Cardiol 75:707, 1995
38. Herzog CA, Dick CD, Anderson RC et al: Dobutamine stress echocardiography for the detection of significant coronary artery disease in patients undergoing renal transplant evaluation. Circulation, Suppl. II, 88:I-557, 1993
39. Paulsen PR, Pavek T, Crampton M et al: Which stress is best? Exercise dobutamine, dipyridamole and pacing in an animal model. J Am Coll Card 21(2):90A, 1993
40. Legallicier B, Siohan P, Dahan M et al: Diagnostic value of coupled stimulation myocardic thallium tomoscintigraphy for the diagnosis of coronary artery disease in chronic haemodialysis patients. J Soc Nephrol 5(3):518, 1994
41. Bach DS, Muller DWM, Gros BJ et al: False positive dobutamine stress echocardiograms: characterization of clinical echocardiographic and angiographic findings. J Am Coll Cardiol 24:928, 1994
42. Braun WE, Marwick TH: Coronary artery disease in renal transplant recipients. [Review]. Cleve Clin J Med 61(5):370, 1994
43. Pochmalicki G, Jan I, Fouchard I et al: Frequency of painless myocardial ischemia in 50 patients with end stage renal failure undergoing dialysis. Arch Mal Coeur 83:1671, 1990
44. Kremastinos D, Paraskevaidis I, Voudiklari S et al: Painless myocardial ischemia in chronic hemodialysed patients: a real event? Nephron 60:164, 1992
45. Albertazzi A, Del Rosso G, Di Paolo B et al: Computerised non-invasive monitoring of cardiovascular stress in haemodialysis patients. Nephrol Dial Transplant, suppl 1:133, 1990
46. Singh N, Langer A, Freeman MR et al: Myocardial alterations during hemodialysis: insights from new noninvasive technology. Am J Nephrol 14:173, 1994
47. Marwick TH, Hobbs R, Vanderlaan RL et al: Use of digital subtraction fluorography in screening for coronary artery disease in patients with chronic renal failure. Am J Kidney Dis 14(2):105, 1989
48. Akiba T, Takamoto T, Sakamoto H et al: Non-invasive detection of coronary artery stenosis in end-stage renal disease (ESRD). J Soc Nephrol 4:329, 1993
49. Gelber CM, Diskin CJ, Claunch BC et al: Thallium-201 myocardial imaging in patients on chronic hemodialysis. Nephron 36:136, 1984
50. Dudczak R, Derfler K, Kletter K et al: Scintigraphic procedures in hemodialysis patients, Tl 201 myocardial perfusion scanning after dipyridamol for diagnosing coronary artery disease. Wiener Klin Wochenschrift 96(9):332, 1984
51. Krawczynska EG, DePuey EG, Whelchel JD: Tl-201 cardiac spect to evaluate pre-renal transplant patients. J Nucl Med 29:950, 1988
52. Marcen R, Lamas S, Orofino L et al: Dipyridamole thallium-201 perfusion imaging for the study of ischemic heart disease in hemodialysis patients. Int J Artif Organs 12(12):773, 1989
53. Trochu JN, Cantarovich D, Renaudeau J et al: Assessment of coronary artery disease by thallium scan in type-I diabetic uremic patients awaiting combined pancreas and renal transplantation. Angiol J Vasc Dis 42:302, 1991
54. Nally J, Mairesse G, Grimm R et al: Dobutamine echocardiography (DbE) is an effective screening tool for coronary artery disease (CAD) in ESRD. J Soc Nephrol 4:255, 1993
55. Albanese J, Nally J, Marwick T et al: Dobutamine echocardiography is effective in the non-invasive detection of prognostically important coronary artery disease in patients with end-stage renal disease. J Soc Nephrol 5(3):322, 1994
56. Costello JM Jr, Butcher JR, Nassef LA et al: Prospective comparison of routine cardiac catheterization versus dobutamine stress echocardiography for assessing the need for coronary revascularization prior to renal transplantation. Circulation, suppl. I, 92:I-336, 1995
57. Bates JR, Sawada SG, Segar DS et al: Evaluation using dobutamine stress echocardiography in patients with insulin-dependent diabetes mellitus before kidney and/or pancreas transplantation. Am J Cardiol 77:175, 1996

Chapter 12

Diagnosis of CAD in Patients with Left Bundle Branch Block

Georges H. Mairesse

The currently accepted electrocardiographic (ECG) criteria for complete left bundle branch block (LBBB), initially delineated by Wilson et al. in the early 1930s,[1] include QRS interval prolongation greater or equal to 120 ms, delayed intrinsicoid deflection in lead V_6, absent Q-waves and slurred broad R-waves in leads I, aVL, and V_6, rS, or QS deflections in leads V_1 and V_2, and an ST- and T-wave vector 180° discordant to the QRS vector.[2] These ECG changes, together with their counterpart abnormalities of myocardial perfusion and function, pose diagnostic challenges for the detection of coronary artery disease (CAD) using any of the noninvasive techniques. Indeed, the majority of studies designed to specifically evaluate the sensitivity, specificity, and predictive values of various diagnostic tests have usually excluded patients with LBBB from their patient population. The present chapter will emphasize first the importance and relevance of the diagnosis of CAD in these patients, second, the anatomic, physiologic, and metabolic correlates of LBBB, and finally the different pitfalls of traditional CAD detection methods and alternative techniques to avoid these limitations.

CLINICAL AND PROGNOSTIC SIGNIFICANCE OF LBBB

Resting LBBB

A number of studies have examined the clinical features associated with LBBB. In 1951, Johnson et al.[3] reported an average survival time of 3.3 years in a follow-up study of 555 patients who were diagnosed between 1937 and 1948, at the Massachusetts General Hospital. Patients with the largest QRS complexes had the shortest survival, and the prognosis was strongly dependent on the nature of the underlying heart disease. In this study, most patients were over 50 years old, and although men predominated, the prognosis was somewhat better in women.

More recently, the influence of the presence or absence, and degree of associated cardiovascular disease on the prognosis of patients with bundle branch block was determined in different patient populations.[4-6] In patients with myocardial infarction, preexisting bundle branch block or its development during the acute infarction was associated with a greater incidence of peri-infarction "pump" failure and a higher mortality rate.[7] To assess the prognostic significance of newly acquired LBBB in the general population, cardiovascular abnormalities were prospectively identified in the 55 persons who developed an LBBB during the 18 years of follow-up of the Framingham cohort.[8] In men, the presence of LBBB was associated with a significantly greater prevalence of cardiac enlargement and congestive heart failure, and there was also a trend suggesting a higher mortality rate from cardiovascular disease in these patients.

Exercise-induced LBBB

Exercise-induced LBBB is rarer. However, a strong association with CAD has also been reported.[9] Exercise-induced LBBB was found by Williams et al. in

50 of 10,176 (0.5%) consecutive patients referred for exercise testing. Significant CAD was diagnosed in 70% of them, with an 85% prevalence of proximal left anterior descending coronary artery stenoses. Furthermore, subsequent development of permanent LBBB in patients with exercise-induced LBBB was also shown to be related to the presence of underlying CAD.[10]

ANATOMIC, PHYSIOLOGIC, AND METABOLIC CORRELATES

Permanent complete LBBB is usually caused by microscopic lesions in the left bundle branch. In transient bundle branch blocks, the specific underlying electrophysiological mechanism may be more difficult to determine. Asynchrony of conduction in the bundles, nonuniformity of refractoriness, changes in membrane responsiveness, or a decrease in the magnitude of phase 4 of the transmembrane action potential may, singly or in combination, cause block of conduction in the bundle branches.[2] While CAD may be associated with the development of LBBB, no relation has been identified between the specific coronary artery anatomy and the presence of LBBB.[11]

Abnormal interventricular septal motion has been well recognized in patients with complete LBBB,[12] and three types of abnormal septal motion have been described.[13] In types A and B, early and abrupt posteriorly directed motion of the septum occurs during the pre-ejection period (Fig. 12-1). After this early abnormal motion, the septum moves anteriorly in type A and posteriorly in type B. Type C exhibits akinetic or dyskinetic septal motion throughout systole. The onset of posterior wall contraction is delayed in all patients with complete LBBB. Types A and B were also observed during right ventricular (RV) pacing, thus suggesting that these types of abnormal septal motion could be explained by asynchronous contraction of the left ventricle. The septal motion of type C is almost the same as that seen in patients with extensive septal infarction, suggesting sufficient septal damage to prevent the early posterior motion seen in type A and B patients. These data have been confirmed by studies using either qualitative visual inspection or computer-assisted quantitative assessment of biplane cineangiograms.[14] Segmental wall motion abnormalities were present in 83% patients, mainly in the septum, but wall motion abnormalities were also reported in anterior, inferior, or lateral segments even in the absence of CAD.

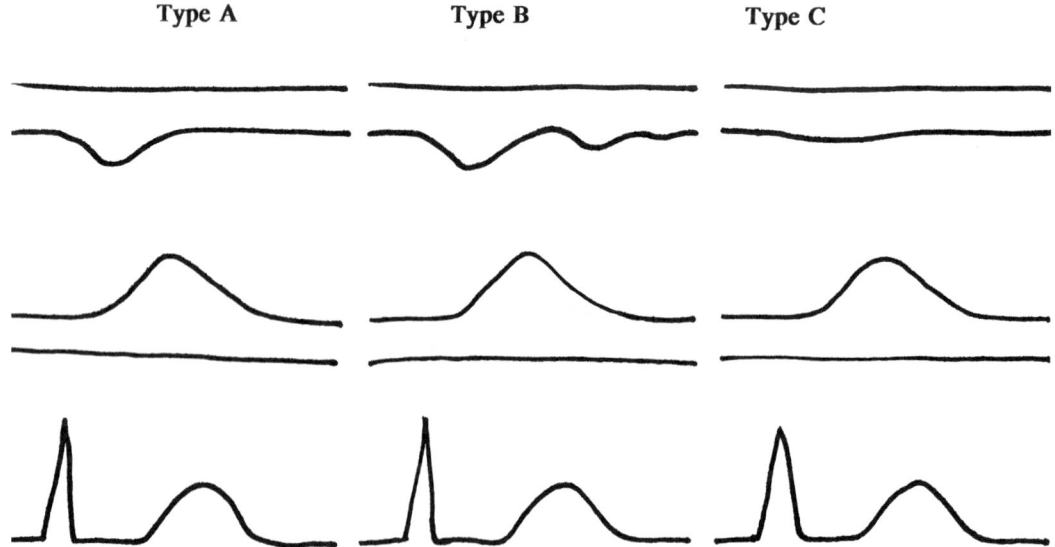

Fig. 12-1. Schematic representation of M-mode wall motion types A, B, and C in patients with left bundle branch block. Note, electrocardiogram (ECG) on bottom.

To determine whether these wall motion abnormalities observed in patients with LBBB were due to abnormal myocardial perfusion or even ischemia, Ono et al.[15] studied an in vivo canine model, in which LBBB was simulated by RV pacing in open-chest dogs. Regional blood flow (measured with microspheres), myocardial perfusion (assessed by thallium-201), metabolism (calculated from 18-fluorodeoxyglucose uptake), and systolic thickening (assessed by echocardiography) were reduced in the septum. However, mean aortic pressure, left anterior descending Doppler flow velocity, and lactate extraction rate showed no significant change. It was, therefore, concluded that LBBB was able to alter myocardial perfusion and metabolism in the septum, but that this reduction was not necessarily followed by septal ischemia. However, these conclusions apply only to types A and B septal motion, which can be reproduced by RV pacing, while type C motion has not been reproduced experimentally.

DETECTION OF CAD IN PATIENTS WITH LBBB

The association of LBBB with CAD has been shown to be a strong predictor of cardiovascular mortality. However, the noninvasive diagnosis of CAD in these patients has been disappointing.

Stress-Induced Angina and ECG Changes

The first systematic study to determine the effect of the exercise test on the ECG of patients with LBBB was undertaken in the early 1950s,[16] and treadmill exercise testing was further assessed by Orzan et al.[17] In 57 patients with LBBB, exercise-induced ST-segment changes were comparable in the presence or absence of significant CAD. This remained true irrespective of the criteria selected; with additional ST-segment depression of either 1 or 2 mm below the baseline value, the predictive accuracy was only 53% to 49%. Even the combination of exertional chest pain and 1 mm ST-segment depression did not significantly increase the predictive value of exercise testing (Table 12-1).

Several factors are probably responsible for the nondiagnostic nature of the ECG response. Because of the altered sequence of depolarization, repolarization also follows different routes. In LBBB, the left ventricle is activated late, and the spread of depolarization also changes from centrifugal (from endocardium to epicardium) to tangential. During repolarization, the same phenomenon may result in unexpected ST-segment or T-wave abnormalities.[18] Moreover, changes in the sequence of excitation can also affect local recovery properties of the myocardium, probably by way of electronic interaction.[19]

Recently developed techniques have allowed continuous computerized digital analysis of the ST segment that can be zeroed to the patient's own baseline ECG even if that baseline was abnormal. In a study of 30 patients undergoing balloon coronary angioplasty using this approach,[20] ST-segment deviation was comparable in patients with and without LBBB, suggesting a reasonable sensitivity for the detection of CAD. However, as specificity has not been assessed, digital self-referenced ST-segment analysis should be considered a promising technique for the monitoring of myocardial ischemia, rather than for the diagnosis of CAD.

Myocardial Perfusion Scintigraphy
Conventional Scintigraphic Approaches

False-positive perfusion defects have been repeatedly reported in patients with LBBB and no

Table 12-1. Diagnosis of Coronary Artery Disease in Patients with LBBB Using Exercise ECG

Reference	Criteria	Sensitivity	Specificity	Accuracy
Feil and Brofman (1952)[16]	0.5-mm ST depression	4/9 (44%)	8/11 (73%)	12/20 (60%)
Orzan et al. (1978)[17]	2-mm ST depression	7/30 (23%)	21/27 (78%)	28/57 (49%)
Orzan et al. (1978)[17]	1-mm ST depression	23/30 (77%)	7/27 (26%)	30/57 (53%)
Orzan et al. (1978)[17]	Chest pain	13/30 (43%)	20/27 (74%)	33/57 (58%)
Orzan et al. (1978)[17]	ST elevation	5/30 (17%)	27/27 (100%)	32/57 (56%)
Orzan et al. (1978)[17]	1-mm ST depression + chest pain	10/30 (33%)	23/27 (85%)	33/57 (58%)

Abbreviations: LBBB, left bundle branch block; ECG, electrocardiography.

Table 12-2. Diagnosis of Coronary Artery Disease in Patients with LBBB Using Planar Myocardial Scintigraphy

Reference	Stress	Isotope	CAD	Sensitivity	Specificity	Accuracy
McGowan et al. (1976)[21]	Exercise	Rb/K	Global	5/5 (100%)	0/11 (0%)	5/16 (25%)
Hirzel et al. (1984)[22]	Exercise	^{201}Tl	Global	4/4 (100%)	0/15 (0%)	4/19 (21%)
Jazmati et al. (1991)[24]	Exercise	^{201}Tl	LAD	4/4 (100%)	0/2 (0%)	4/6 (67%)
Delonca et al. (1992)[25]	Exercise	^{201}Tl	LAD	16/17 (94%)	14/43 (33%)	30/60 (50%)
Total				29/30 (97%)	14/71 (20%)	43/101 (42%)

Abbreviations: LBBB, left bundle branch block; CAD, coronary artery disease diagnosed globally or restricted to the left anterior descending coronary artery territory (LAD); Rb/K, rubidium-81 and potassium-43; ^{201}Tl, thallium-201

CAD.[21–31] This observation was first described by McGowan et al.,[21] who found anteroseptal perfusion defects at rest, which were sometimes amplified after exercise testing even in the absence of CAD, in 27 patients with LBBB who were imaged using potassium-43 and rubidium-81 myocardial imaging. Using planar thallium-201 scintigraphy for the noninvasive diagnosis of CAD in 19 patients, Hirzel et al. confirmed the presence of significant anteroseptal perfusion defects on exercise scintigrams in all patients, although only four of these patients had CAD involving the left anterior descending coronary artery.[22] Other studies have confirmed that despite acceptable sensitivity, overall specificity and accuracy remained unacceptably low for the noninvasive diagnosis of CAD in patients with LBBB (Table 12-2).

More recent studies of perfusion imaging in patients with LBBB have been performed using single photon emission computed tomography (SPECT) (Table 12-3).[26–31] As discussed in Chapter 2, SPECT is now well established as being superior to planar imaging for the detection and sizing of perfusion defects, due to the higher image contrast resolution and improved definition of individual vascular territories afforded by tomography.[32] However, the use of this technique may even have increased the number of false-positive septal or anteroseptal perfusion defects. These studies confirmed a similar sensitivity in all vascular territories, ranging from 70% to 100%. Specificity was satisfactory in the left circumflex and right coronary artery territory, ranging from 50% to 100%, while specificities as low as 10% have been reported regarding left anterior descending CAD.[26]

Various mechanisms have been proposed to explain these false-positive myocardial perfusion defects. First, a reduction of myocardial blood flow within the interventricular septum has been observed during rapid pacing and artificial induction of LBBB in dogs.[15,22] This phenomenon is thought to be related to increased systolic and reduced diastolic time in the septum due to the conduction de-

Table 12-3. Diagnosis of Coronary Artery Disease in Patients with LBBB Using Single Photon Emission Computed Tomography

Reference	Stress	Isotope	CAD	Sensitivity	Specificity	Accuracy
DePuey et al. (1988)[20]	Exercise	^{201}Tl	LAD	4/4 (100%)	1/10 (10%)	5/14 (36%)
Burns et al. (1991)[27]	Exercise	^{201}Tl	LAD	5/6 (83%)	3/10 (30%)	8/16 (50%)
Matzer et al. (1991)[28]	Exercise	^{201}Tl	LAD	18/18 (100%)	2/14 (14%)	20/32 (62%)
Larcos et al. (1991)[30]	Exercise	^{201}Tl	LAD	26/38 (68%)	15/45 (33%)	41/83 (49%)
Krishman et al. (1993)[31]	Exercise	^{201}Tl	LAD	16/19 (84%)	5/13 (38%)	21/32 (66%)
Mairesse et al. (1995)[39]	Dobutamine	MIBI	LAD	12/12 (100%)	0/12 (0%)	12/24 (50%)
O'Keefe et al. (1993)[46]	Exercise	^{201}Tl	LAD	11/15 (73%)	7/16 (44%)	18/31 (58%)
Total				92/112 (82%)	33/120 (27%)	125/232 (54%)

Abbreviations: LBBB, left bundle branch block; CAD, coronary artery disease diagnosed globally or restricted to the left anterior descending coronary artery territory (LAD); MIBI, technetium-99m methoxyisobutylisonitrile; ^{201}Tl, thallium-201.

fect, although this hypothesis has been contested.[33] Second, imaging and quantification factors including partial volume effect, camera field nonuniformity, breast attenuation, patient motion during imaging, or incorrect definition of the long axis of the left ventricle can all contribute to produce false-positive septal perfusion defects.[29,34] Other considerations include a possible role of exaggerated septal or apical thinning, microvascular problems,[35] myocardial cell dysfunction,[36] or myocardial fibrosis,[37] which have been observed in patients with complete LBBB.

The same factors may explain a high proportion of the reversible thallium-201 defects demonstrated in the septum of patients with exercise-induced LBBB without any evidence of CAD at angiography or coronary spasm at ergonovine testing.[37,38]

Alternative Scintigraphic Approaches

Alternative interpretative criteria have been proposed to try to decrease this high proportion of false-positive scintigraphic defects in the left anterior descending coronary artery territory.

First, as most of these false-positive results are *fixed* defects, it has been suggested that *reversible* septal defects are more likely to correspond to myocardial ischemia due to CAD than to the LBBB (Table 12-4).[23,30] We have recently compared the diagnostic accuracy of fixed and reversible perfusion defects for the diagnosis and localization of CAD in 24 patients with LBBB.[39] In all patients, septal perfusion defects were detected on the poststress scan. In 12 patients with left-anterior descending CAD, 9 true-positive defects were partially reversible, while in patients with normal left anterior descending coronary arteries, all but one false-positive septal perfusion defects were found to be fixed. The use of this interpretive criterion thus significantly increased specificity and accuracy in comparison with conventional analysis.

Second, quantitative approaches have also been proposed to improve the diagnostic accuracy of scintigraphy in patients with LBBB. In a comparison of qualitative analysis of myocardial perfusion scintigrams with a quantitative computer-assisted analysis,[30] segmental perfusion defects were considered pathological if myocardial thallium-201 uptake was greater than 2.5 standard deviations below normal limits in more than 3% of the myocardium. Although highly sensitive, this method was neither specific nor accurate. Septal abnormality scores were also computed based on comparison of each subject's short-axis circumferential profile with a normal reference curve.[29] This method improved the discrimination between patients with LBBB and significant left anterior descending CAD from those with LBBB alone, but due to selection bias, sensitivity, specificity, and predictive accuracy could not be determined in the study cohort.

Third, to avoid isolated septal defects as a possible source of false-positive tests, Matzer et al. suggested that abnormal apical thallium-201 uptake should be present in addition to septal defects to indicate left anterior descending CAD in the presence of LBBB.[28] In this study, left anterior descending CAD was considered present only when the stress polar map contained a perfusion defect greater than 12% and the stress defect involved greater than 50% of the apex. This approach improved specificity from 14% to 79% ($p < 0.001$) by visual analysis and from 14% to 64% ($p < 0.01$) by quantitative analysis. We also tested this method and confirmed an improved specificity from 0% to 50% in 12 patients without left anterior descending CAD, together with an increase

Table 12-4. Diagnosis of Coronary Artery Disease in Patients with LBBB by Requiring Reversible Defects at Myocardial Scintigraphy

Reference	Stress	Isotope	Scintigraphy	CAD	Sensitivity	Specificity	Accuracy
Braat et al. (1985)[23]	Exercise	^{201}Tl	Planar	Global	14/16 (88%)	7/8 (86%)	21/24 (87%)
Larcos et al. (1991)[30]	Exercise	^{201}Tl	SPECT	LAD	23/38 (61%)	19/45 (42%)	42/83 (51%)
Mairesse et al. (1995)[39]	Dobutamine	MIBI	SPECT	LAD	9/12 (75%)	11/12 (92%)	20/24 (83%)
Total					44/66 (70%)	37/65 (57%)	83/131 (63%)

Abbreviations: LBBB, left bundle branch block; CAD, coronary artery disease diagnosed globally or restricted to the left anterior descending coronary artery territory (LAD); MIBI, technetium-99m methoxyisobutylisonitrile; SPECT, single photon computed emission tomography.

Table 12-5. Diagnosis of Left Anterior Descending CAD in Patients with LBBB by Requiring Apical Defects at Myocardial Scintigraphy

Reference	Stress	Isotope	Scintigraphy	Sensitivity	Specificity	Accuracy
Delonca et al. (1992)[25]	Exercise	^{201}Tl	Planar	7/17 (35%)	39/43 (85%)	46/60 (77%)
Matzer et al. (1991)[28]	Exercise	^{201}Tl	SPECT	17/18 (94%)	11/14 (79%)	28/32 (87%)
Larcos et al. (1991)[30]	Exercise	^{201}Tl	SPECT	30/38 (79%)	17/45 (38%)	47/83 (57%)
Mairesse et al. (1995)[39]	Dobutamine	MIBI	SPECT	11/12 (92%)	6/12 (50%)	17/24 (71%)
Total				65/85 (76%)	73/114 (64%)	138/199 (69%)

Abbreviations: CAD, coronary artery disease; LBBB, left bundle branch block; MIBI, technitium-99m methoxyisobutylisonitrile; SPECT, single photon computed emission tomography; ^{201}Tl, thallium-201.

in accuracy from 50% to 71% compared with the conventional approach.[39] However, this improvement failed to reach statistical significance. Other studies have also described this improved specificity by restricting the diagnosis of left anterior descending CAD to patients with apical defects.[25] However, this was accompanied by a slightly reduced sensitivity, so that the overall accuracy failed to achieve 70% (Table 12-5).

Radionuclide Ventriculography

Wall motion abnormalities are common at rest in patients with LBBB. Using nuclear ventriculography to examine regional and global left ventricular (LV) function, neither exercise-induced wall motion abnormalities nor an impaired ejection fraction response to exercise could be related to the presence of additional CAD.[40] Thus, using the usual criteria for the diagnosis of CAD by radionuclide ventriculography (i.e., failure to increase ejection fraction by 5 points with exercise and/or development of a wall motion abnormality), Rowe reported a sensitivity of 100%, with a specificity of only 15%.[40] Similarly, in patients with rate-dependant LBBB, the development of the conduction defect coincides with changes in global and regional LV function, mainly in the lower septum or inferoapical segments, that may be confused with development of LV ischemia during exercise.[41]

Stress Echocardiography

Two-dimensional echocardiography differs from nuclear ventriculography in respect of its high temporal and spatial resolution, and its ability to document myocardial thickening. These aspects facilitate recognition of the typical asynchronous septal contraction due to the LBBB,[12,13] together with the presence of normal or nearly normal myocardial thickening in the absence of CAD. This preservation of wall thickening in LBBB has been confirmed experimentally, in which RV pacing (corresponding to types A and B septal wall motion abnormalities) has been shown to induce septal thickening greater than 80% of that normally defined by two-dimensional echocardiography.[15] This does not apply to the septal motion of type C, in which diffuse dyskinetic septal motion is characteristic.

During stress echocardiography, a normal response can be defined by an enhancement of wall thickening with stress. Heterogeneity of endocardial motion is disregarded as a possible marker of CAD, while an ischemic response is identified by stress-induced impairment of wall thickening, including failure to improve wall thickening relative to hyperkinetic response to maximal stress. Infarction is characterized by failure of wall thickening (akinesia or dyskinesia) at rest. Preliminary data have indicated that stress echocardiography using these criteria may increase the diagnostic specificity for the noninvasive identification of CAD in patients with complete LBBB.[42]

We recently compared the accuracy of dobutamine stress two-dimensional echocardiography with that of SPECT for the detection of left anterior descending CAD in 24 patients with LBBB, and further evaluated the diagnostic accuracy of dobutamine stress echocardiography in the other vascular territories.[39] Using the above criteria, the sensitivity for left anterior descending CAD was 83%, the specificity was 92%, and the diagnostic accuracy was 87%. Sensi-

Table 12-6. Diagnosis of CAD in Patients with LBBB Using Dobutamine Stress Two-Dimensional Echocardiography[39]

Coronary Artery	Sensitivity	Specificity	Accuracy
Left anterior descending	10/12 (83%)	11/12 (92%)	21/24 (87%)
Left circumflex and/or right	11/13 (85%)	8/11 (73%)	19/24 (79%)

Abbreviations: CAD, coronary artery disease; LBBB, left bundle branch block.

tivity for left circumflex and/or right CAD was 85%, the specificity was 73%, and the accuracy was 79% (Table 12-6). There was no significant difference between these two vascular territories. However, both the specificity and diagnostic accuracy of dobutamine stress echocardiography were significantly superior to that of the conventional scintigraphic interpretation, and comparable with that of alternative scintigraphic interpretations either requiring reversible defects or apical defects to indicate left anterior descending CAD. Despite these encouraging results, several limitations should be considered. First, inclusion of patients with previous myocardial infarction into the study may color the results because the interpretation of ischemia in the left anterior descending coronary artery territory is based on failure to develop myocardial wall thickening in the septum. In this respect, scar is more easily identified than myocardial ischemia, possibly provoking an overestimation of sensitivity. Nonetheless, both imaging modalities were tested in the same patients, and the same limitations thus similarly affected both imaging techniques. Second, patients with idiopathic cardiomyopathy were not included in that series. In these patients, failure to improve wall thickening with stress may produce false-positive diagnosis of ischemic cardiomyopathy. Accordingly, further studies in larger patients population would thus be needed to clarify the role of stress echocardiography in the noninvasive diagnosis of CAD in patients with LBBB.

New Imaging Modalities

New technologies, including contrast echocardiography, Doppler tissue imaging, magnetic resonance imaging, or ultrafast computed tomography scanning have been proposed for the noninvasive diagnosis of CAD. None has yet found a routine clinical role, and no specific data exist to date to assess their respective diagnostic accuracy in patients with LBBB.

Alternative Stress Modalities

The vast majority of the above-cited studies were conducted during exercise stress testing. However, increasing interest has been given to pharmacologic stress testing, for patients unable to exercise, and because these approaches may offer specific benefits for the accurate detection of coronary disease in patients with LBBB.

Vasodilator Agents

Dipyridamole thallium-201 SPECT has been assessed in several studies of patients with LBBB (Table 12-7).[27,43,44] In the first published report by Burns et al.,[27] 16 patients were evaluated using both exercise and dipyridamole stress tests, and SPECT was scored either qualitatively or quantitatively. The sensitivity for the detection of left anterior descending CAD was 83% for exercise, and 100% for dipyridamole. The specificity was 30% qualitatively and 20% quantitatively for exercise, and 80% qualitatively and 90% quantitatively for dipyridamole. This enhancement of specificity may be related to the mechanism responsible for the false-positive scintigraphic defects during exercise. Dipyridamole produces a smaller increase in heart rate than exercise, and thus less shortening of diastolic time—consequently, septal hyperemia during stress is less likely to be blunted than during exercise.

Similar results were also reported by O'Keefe et al. in 121 patients studied with adenosine thallium-201 scintigraphy.[45,46] The predictive accuracies of adenosine thallium-201 imaging for identifying and localizing ischemia to a specific coronary distribution were 88% in the left anterior descending coronary artery territory, 84% for the left circumflex, and 88% for the right coronary artery territory. In a separate patient population with LBBB, the overall predictive accuracy was significantly higher when adenosine was compared with exercise thallium-201 (91% vs. 71%, $p < 0.05$).

Table 12-7. Diagnosis of Left Anterior Descending CAD in Patients with LBBB Using Myocardial Scintigraphy During Vasodilator Stress

Reference	Stress	Isotope	Scintigraphy	Sensitivity	Specificity	Accuracy
Burns et al. (1991)[27]	Dipyridamole	^{201}Tl	SPECT	6/6 (100%)	8/10 (80%)	14/16 (87%)
Larcos et al. (1991)[44]	Dipyridamole	^{201}Tl	SPECT	12/16 (75%)	5/8 (63%)	17/24 (74%)
O'Keefe et al. (1992)[45]	Adenosine	^{201}Tl	SPECT	108/110 (98%)	7/11 (64%)	115/121 (95%)
O'Keefe et al. (1993)[46]	Adenosine	^{201}Tl	SPECT	23/24 (96%)	13/18 (72%)	36/42 (88%)
Total				149/156 (96%)	33/47 (70%)	182/203 (90%)

Abbreviations: CAD, coronary artery disease; LBBB, left bundle branch block; SPECT, single photon computed emission tomography; ^{201}Tl, thallium-201.

Dobutamine

Dobutamine stress echocardiography and scintigraphy have been extensively validated as sensitive and specific methods for detecting CAD and identifying disease in individual coronary arteries.[47–49] In patients who are able to exercise, however, dobutamine usually produces smaller amounts of ischemia in fewer patients than does exercise, and exercise is believed to be of superior diagnostic accuracy.[51]

In patients with LBBB, false-positive reversible defects during dobutamine stress thallium-201 imaging have been reported by Tighe et al.[52] It was postulated that due to similar physiologic effects of increased contractility and increased heart rate, the prevalence of septal perfusion abnormalities would parallel that observed during exercise. However, the presence of septal perfusion abnormalities during exercise is particularly seen in patients achieving very high peak heart rates (>170 beats/min),[23] which are infrequent with dobutamine.[53] It might be expected that false-positive perfusion defects would be smaller or fewer during the dobutamine test. However, no data exist to date to compare dobutamine and exercise in the same patients.

We have compared the diagnostic value of the dobutamine stress test using either perfusion scintigraphy or stress echocardiography.[39] False-positive dobutamine-induced septal perfusion defects were noted in a proportion of patients similar to that previously reported with exercise (Table 12-3). However, dobutamine stress echocardiography (using wall thickening criteria as described) showed very acceptable sensitivity, specificity, and diagnostic accuracy. As the dobutamine test is performed in the supine position and without patient motion artifacts, better image quality may allow easier interpretation of myocardial wall thickening than can be obtained with exercise echocardiography. This may favor the sensitivity and specificity of dobutamine compared with exercise stress echocardiography in patients with LBBB.[54]

CONCLUSIONS AND FUTURE PERSPECTIVES

LBBB is known to be a strong predictor of cardiovascular mortality. However, the ability of noninvasive tests to diagnose and localize CAD in these patients has been disappointing. Exercise-induced changes in the ECG are nondiagnostic in the presence of LBBB, and several scintigraphic studies have reported a high prevalence of false-positive anteroseptal and septal perfusion defects. This high prevalence can be significantly reduced by use of alternative scintigraphic interpretation techniques, or by use or vasodilator agents. Dobutamine stress echocardiography, using myocardial thickening impairment as the diagnostic criterion, may also significantly improve specificity for the detection of left anterior descending CAD. Further studies in larger populations of patients without previous myocardial infarction are needed to confirm the relative sensitivities of these approaches.

REFERENCES

1. Wilson FN, MacLeod AG, Barker PS: The order of ventricular excitation in human bundle branch block. Am Heart J 7:305, 1932
2. Josephson ME: Intraventricular conduction disturbances. p. 117. In: Clinical Cardiac Electrophysiology. Techniques and Interpretation. Lea & Febiger, Philadelphia, 1992
3. Johnson RP, Messer AD, Shreenivas, White PD: Prog-

nosis in bundle branch block. Factors influencing the survival period in left bundle branch block. Am Heart J 41:225, 1951
4. Lamb LE, Kable KD, Averill KH: Electrocardiographic findings in 67,375 asymptomatic subjects. Left bundle branch block. Am J Cardiol 6:130, 1960
5. Smith S, Hayes WL: The prognosis of complete left bundle branch block. Am Heart J 70:157, 1965
6. Rotman M, Triebwasser JH: A clinical and follow-up study of right and left bundle branch block. Circulation 51:477, 1975
7. Hindman MC, Wagner GS, JaRo M et al.: The clinical significance of bundle branch block complicating acute myocardial infarction. Clinical characteristics, hospital mortality, and one-year follow-up. Circulation 58:679, 1978
8. Schneider JF, Thomas HE, Sorlie P et al.: Comparative features of newly acquired left and right bundle branch block in the general population: The Framingham Study. Am J Cardiol 47:931, 1981
9. Williams MA, Esterbrooks DJ, Nair CK et al.: Clinical significance of exercise-induced bundle branch block. Am J Cardiol 61:346, 1988
10. Heinsimer JA, Irwin JM, Basnight LL: Influence of underlying coronary artery disease on the natural history and prognosis of exercise-induced left bundle branch block. Am J Cardiol 60:1065, 1987
11. De Mots H, Rosch J, Rahimtoola SH: Coronary anatomy in left bundle branch block. Circulation 48:605, 1973
12. Abbasi AS, Eber LM, MacAlpin RN, Kattus AA: Paradoxical motion of the intraventricular septum in left bundle branch block. Circulation 49:423, 1974
13. Fujii J, Watanabe H, Watanabe T et al.: M-mode and cross sectional echocardiographic study of the left ventricular wall motions in complete left bundle-branch block. Br Heart J 42:255, 1979
14. Williams RS, Behar VS, Peter RH: Left bundle branch block: angiographic segmental wall motion abnormalities. Am J Cardiol 44:1046, 1979
15. Ono S, Nohara R, Kambara H et al.: Regional myocardial perfusion and glucose metabolism in experimental left bundle branch block. Circulation 85:1125, 1992
16. Feil H, Brofman BL: The effect of exercise on the electrocardiogram of bundle branch block. Am Heart J 45: 665, 1952
17. Orzan F, Garcia E, Mathur VS, Hall RJ: Is the treadmill exercise test useful for evaluating coronary artery disease in patients with complete left bundle branch block? Am J Cardiol 42:36, 1978
18. Spach MS, Barr RC: Analysis of ventricular activation and repolarization from intramural and epicardial potential distributions for ectopic beats in the intact dog. Circ Res 37:830, 1975
19. Abildskov JA: Effects of activation sequence on the local recovery of ventricular excitability in the dog. Circ Res 38:240, 1976
20. Stark KS, Krucoff MW, Schryver B, Kent KM: Quantification of ST-segment changes during coronary angioplasty in patients with left bundle branch block. Am J Cardiol 67:1219, 1991
21. McGowan RL, Welch TG, Zaret BL et al.: Noninvasive myocardial imaging with potassium-43 and rubidium-81 in patients with left bundle branch block. Am J Cardiol 38:422, 1976
22. Hirzel HO, Senn M, Nuesch K et al.: Thallium-201 scintigraphy in complete left bundle branch block. Am J Cardiol 53:764, 1984
23. Braat SH, Brugada P, Bar FW et al.: Thallium-201 exercise scintigraphy and left bundle branch block. Am J Cardiol 55:224, 1985
24. Jazmati B, Sadaniantz A, Emaus SP, Heller GV: Exercise thallium-201 imaging in complete left bundle branch block and the prevalence of septal perfusion defects. Am J Cardiol 67:46, 1991
25. Delonca J, Camenzind E, Meier B, Righetti A: Limits of thallium-201 exercise scintigraphy to detect coronary disease in patients with complete and permanent bundle branch block: a review of 134 cases. Am Heart J 123:1201, 1992
26. DePuey EG, Guertler-Krawczynska E, Robbins WL: Thallium-201 in coronary artery disease patients with left bundle branch block. J Nucl Med 29:1485, 1988
27. Burns RJ, Gallighan L, Wright LM et al.: Improved specificity of myocardial thallium-201 single-photon emission computed tomography in patients with left bundle branch block by dipyridamole. Am J Cardiol 68:504, 1991
28. Matzer L, Kiat H, Friedman JD et al.: A new approach to the assessment of tomographic thallium-201 scintigraphy in patients with left bundle branch block. J Am Coll Cardiol 17:1309, 1991
29. Civelek AC, Gozukara I, Durski K et al.: Detection of left anterior descending coronary artery disease in patients with left bundle branch block. Am J Cardiol 70: 1565, 1992
30. Larcos G, Gibbons RJ, Brown ML: Diagnostic accuracy of exercise thallium-201 single-photon computed tomography in patients with left bundle branch block. Am J Cardiol 68:756, 1991
31. Krishman R, Lu J, Zhu YY et al.: Myocardial perfusion scintigraphy in left bundle branch block: a perspective on the issue from image analysis in a clinical context. Am Heart J 126:578, 1993

32. Ritchie J, Williams DL, Harp G et al.: Transaxial tomography with thallium-201 for detecting remote myocardial infarction. Comparison with planar imaging. Am J Cardiol 50:1236, 1982
33. Nozawa T, Sasayama S, Takabatake H: Usefulness of thallium-201 scintigraphy during right ventricular pacing for detecting myocardial ischemia with angiographically normal coronary arteries. Am J Cardiol 59:1222, 1987
34. Gerwitz H, Grotte GJ, Strauss HW et al.: The influence of left ventricular volume and wall motion on myocardial images. Circulation 59:1172, 1979
35. Rothbart RM, Beller GA, Watson DD et al.: Diagnostic accuracy and prognostic significance of quantitative thallium-201 scintigraphy in patients with left bundle branch block. Am J Noninvasive Cardiol 1:197, 1987
36. Master AM, Dack S, Jaffe HL: Bundle branch and intraventricular block in acute coronary artery occlusion. Am Heart J 16:283, 1938
37. Kurata C, Terada H, Fujii T et al.: A ^{201}Tl perfusion defect in a case with rate-dependent left bundle branch block. Eur J Nucl Med 10:169, 1985
38. LaCanna G, Giubbini R, Metra M et al.: Assessment of myocardial perfusion with thallium-201 scintigraphy in exercise-induced left bundle branch block: diagnostic value and clinical significance. Eur Heart J 13:942, 1992
39. Mairesse GH, Marwick TH, Arnese M et al.: Improved identification of coronary artery disease in patients with left bundle branch block by use of dobutamine stress echocardiography and comparison with myocardial perfusion scintigraphy. Am J Cardiol 76:321, 1995
40. Rowe DW, DePuey EG, Sonnemaker RE et al.: Left ventricular performance during exercise in patients with left bundle branch block: evaluation by gated radionuclide ventriculography, Am Heart J 105:66, 1983
41. Bramlet DA, Morris KG, Coleman RE et al.: Effects of rate-dependent left bundle branch block on global and regional left ventricular function. Circulation 67:1059, 1983
42. Mairesse GH, Marwick T, DHondt AM et al.: How reliable is stress 2D echocardiography to detect coronary artery disease in patients with complete left bundle branch block? A comparison with Tc99m-MIBI SPECT scintigraphy, abstracted. Eur Heart J, suppl. 14:454, 1993
43. Rocket JF, Wood WC, Moinuddin M et al.: Intravenous dipyridamole thallium-201 SPECT imaging in patients with left bundle branch block. Clin Nucl Med 15:401, 1990
44. Larcos G, Brown ML, Gibbons RJ: Role of dipyridamole thallium-201 imaging in left bundle branch block. Am J Cardiol 68:1097, 1991
45. O'Keefe JH Jr, Bateman TM, Silvestri R, Barnhart CS: Safety and diagnostic accuracy of adenosine thallium-201 in patients unable to exercise and those with left bundle branch block. Am Heart J 124:614, 1992
46. O'Keefe JH Jr, Bateman TM, Barnhart CS: Adenosine thallium-201 is superior to exercise thallium-201 for detecting coronary artery disease in patients with left bundle branch block. J Am Coll Cardiol 21:1332, 1993
47. Mertens H, Sawada GS, Ryan T et al.: Symptoms, adverse effects, and complications associated with dobutamine stress echocardiography. Experience in 1118 patients. Circulation 88:15, 1993
48. Marwick T, DHondt AM, Baudhuin T et al.: Optimal use of dobutamine stress for the detection and evaluation of coronary artery disease: combination with echocardiography or scintigraphy, or both? J Am Coll Cardiol 22:159, 1993
49. Forster T, McNeill AJ, Salustri A et al.: Simultaneous dobutamine stress echocardiography and 99m-technetium isonitrile single photon emission computed tomography in patients with suspected coronary artery disease. J Am Coll Cardiol 21:1591, 1993
50. Pennell DJ, Underwood SR, Swanton RH et al.: Dobutamine thallium myocardial perfusion tomography. J Am Coll Cardiol 18:1471, 1991
51. Marwick T, DHondt AM, Mairesse GH et al.: Relative ability of dobutamine and exercise stress to induce ischemia in active patients. Br Heart J 10:74, 1994
52. Tighe DA, Hutchinson HG, Park CH et al.: False-positive reversible perfusion defect during dobutamine-thallium imaging in left bundle branch block. J Nucl Med 35:1989, 1994
53. Mairesse GH, Marwick TH, Wijns W et al.: Evidence for different pathophysiological mechanisms underlying dobutamine- and exercise-induced wall motion abnormalities, abstracted. J Am Coll Cardiol 22:16A, 1994
54. Pellika PA, Roger VL, Oh JK, Seward JB: Accuracy of stress echocardiography in patients with left bundle branch block, abstracted. Circulation 88:I-557, 1993

Chapter 13

Pharmacologic Stress Testing

Thomas H. Marwick

INDICATIONS FOR PHARMACOLOGIC AND NONEXERCISE STRESS TESTING

Inability to Exercise

Autoregulation of flow in the coronary circulation prevents the myocardium from developing ischemia until coronary stenoses are very severe.[1,2] The identification of coronary disease is therefore dependent upon examination of cardiac function under situations of stress, where the vasodilator reserve (or contractile reserve) of territories supplied by a stenosed vessel will be exhausted before the reserve of normal territories. The stress techniques discussed in the previous chapters have assumed that the patient is able to exercise maximally, to exploit this difference in flow or contractile reserve between normal and stenotic segments.

Patients presenting to a stress testing laboratory at a referral institution fall broadly into four categories: those who can exercise maximally with and without an interpretable electrocardiogram (ECG), and those who either cannot exercise or are only able to exercise submaximally.[3] The latter two groups account for 30% to 40% of patients (Fig. 13-1). It has been shown with exercise ECG testing, stress echocardiography, and thallium scintigraphy, that performance of submaximal exercise is associated with a reduction of test sensitivity.[4,5] Causes of submaximal exercise performance include

peripheral vascular disease,

cerebrovascular disease (history of stroke),

orthopedic problems (arthritis and musculoskeletal pain),

chronic lung disease,

general debility (limitation by fatigue),

medical therapy (e.g., β-blockers), and

poor motivation.

Patients Able to Exercise

As discussed in Chapter 1, exercise testing offers many other physiologically and prognostically important data as well as ST-segment response. These include exercise capacity, workload on the heart, the hemodynamic response to exercise, and the presence or absence of dysrhythmias. Moreover, exercise mimics the normal provoking circumstances of chest discomfort, and this may be of value in assessing the degree of functional compromise. For these reasons, if a patient is able to exercise maximally, exercise is a more attractive form of stress than the pharmacologic techniques, in which these data are either not available (e.g., exercise capacity) or less meaningful (e.g., rhythm changes, hypotension). Additionally,

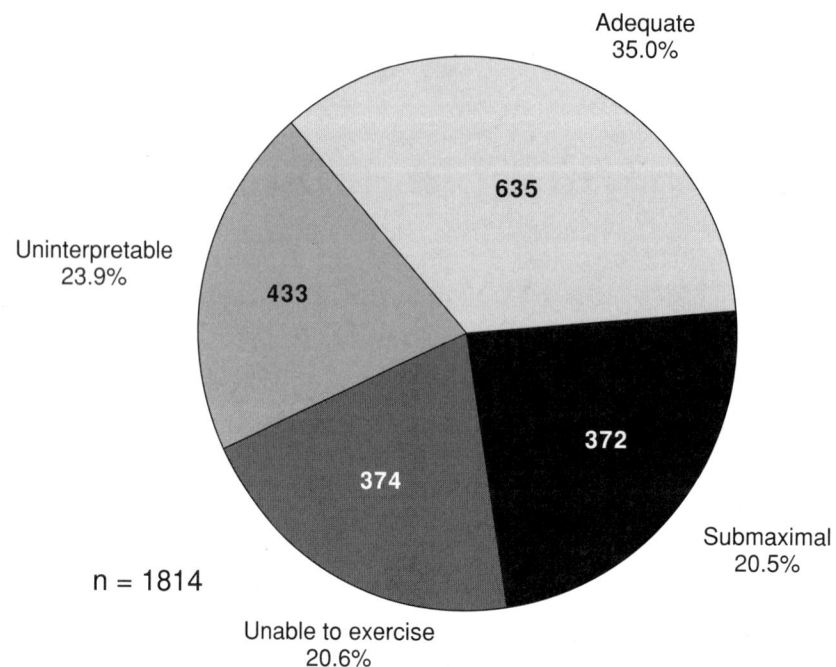

Fig. 13-1. Distribution of patients presenting to a stress laboratory, based on interpretability of the electrocardiogram and exercise capacity. (From Marwick,[3] with permission.)

for tests that depend on the provocation of ischemia by increasing cardiac workload (e.g., stress ECG, stress echocardiography), maximal exercise appears to be a more potent stress than the pharmacologic stressors.[6,7]

Nonetheless, the performance of stress under nonexercise conditions is attractive from a number of standpoints. As the patient is not mobile or hyperventilating, image degradation, which may occur with either echocardiography or perfusion scintigraphy,[8,9] may be avoided. Moreover, the use of pharmacologic stress is attractive in situations where patients are unable to exercise (e.g., during magnetic resonance imaging, or in the angiography laboratory or operating room), but where stressing the heart may be useful to clinical decision making. Specific pharmacologic agents may offer data unobtainable with exercise testing, for example, the use of ergonovine in the detection of coronary spasm[10] or dobutamine for the detection of myocardial viability.[11–13] Finally, the avoidance of a hyperventilating and mobile patient is attractive for the application of new technical developments in stress echocardiography, including tissue doppler imaging,[14] contrast echocardiography (Fig. 13-2),[15,16] and acoustic quantitation methodologies including color kinesis. Finally, like bicycle exercise, the use of pharmacologic stress may enable an assessment to be made of the workload at the onset of ischemia, which is important prognostically.

This chapter will focus on the use of nonexercise techniques for the diagnosis of coronary artery disease (CAD). Other aspects of pharmacologic stress, such as the use of these techniques for the diagnosis of myocardial viability, will be dealt with in later sections.

RATIONALE OF NONEXERCISE STRESS TESTING TECHNIQUES

Use of Coronary Vasodilators

The use of vasodilators for stress testing was initially based upon their ability to produce maximum coronary vasodilation. Using myocardial perfusion imag-

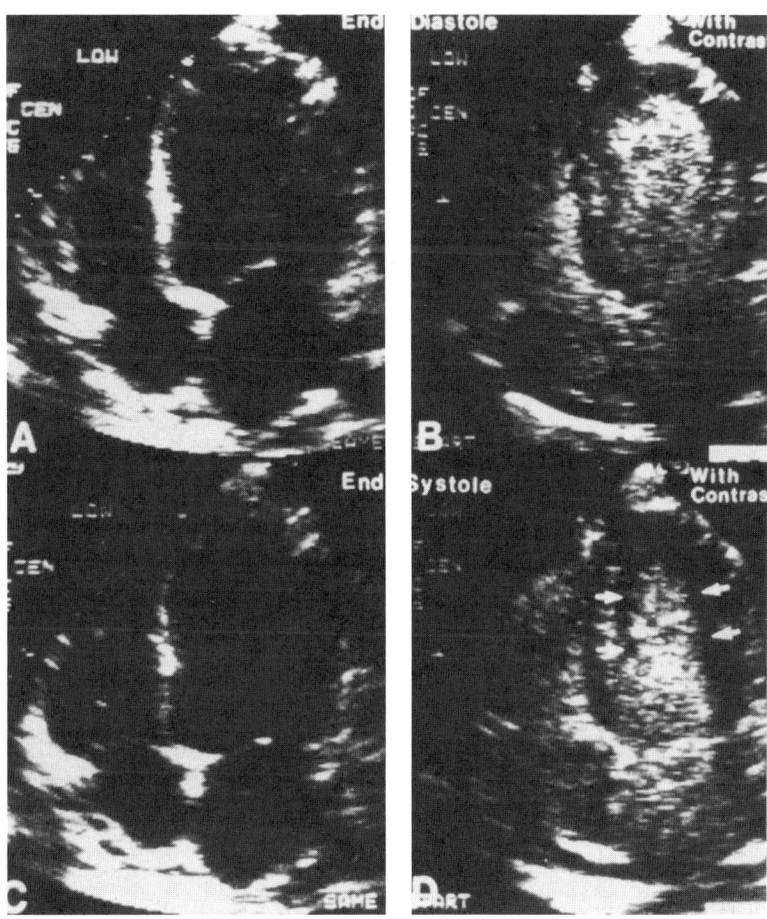

Fig. 13-2. Combination of contrast echocardiography with dobutamine stress echocardiography. Low dose (10 μg/kg/min) are shown (**A,C**) without and (**B,D**) with contrast, during diastole (**A,B**) and systole (**C,D**). Contrast enhances delineation of the lateral wall in diastole, and both septal and lateral walls during systole. (From Porter,[16] with permission.)

ing, coronary flow is compared in normal segments and those supplied by a stenosed coronary artery; the consequence of coronary stenosis is failure to achieve the same level of coronary hyperemia as in a normal segment. A relative perfusion defect is detected scintigraphically in the presence of a twofold difference in count activity between these segments.[17] This coronary vasodilator response may be provoked by adenosine, dipyridamole, or papaverine (the latter in the angiography laboratory). These stressors appear to be of comparable efficacy in most patients (increasing coronary flow by four or five times),[18] although up to 25% of patients fail to generate this response. As discussed in subsequent chapters, myocardial perfusion imaging examines relative coronary flow reserve, which is relatively independent of hemodynamic variables in hypertrophy. Nonetheless, under conditions of maximal coronary hyperemia, driving pressure does influence coronary flow, with the consequence that the development of hypotension may influence the development of differences in flow between normal and ischemic territories. This problem may be circumvented by combination of dipyridamole with other stressors (e.g., handgrip), which maintain the blood pressure.[19]

Adenosine induces coronary vasodilation by a direct effect on coronary smooth muscle relaxation, as well as inhibition of norepinephrine release.[20,21] Secondary effects of the drug include a negative inotropic effect, and reduction of atrioventricular (AV) node conduction. As this agent is actively metabolized in the vessel wall; its half-life is very short, of the order of 10 seconds. Dipyridamole acts as a prodrug, increasing the serum levels of adenosine by blocking cellular uptake of this molecule.[22] Dipyridamole has a longer half-life, of the order of 6 hours, and is metabolized by the liver.

In addition to inducing flow heterogeneity, the coronary vasodilators may induce myocardial ischemia through a steal phenomenon.[22] If an area is supplied by collaterals from a patent coronary artery, vasodilation of the distal bed of this normal coronary will reduce the pressure available to drive flow through collateral vessels. In such a situation, the normal segment is said to be "stealing" blood from the territories supplied by a stenotic artery. These phenomena may occur between endocardial and epicardial vascular territories of a single coronary segment (vertical steal) or, less commonly, may involve multiple coronary segments (horizontal steal). For steal to occur, the supplying vessel must be severely stenosed, and the collateral circulation well developed. Therefore, coronary steal is a correlate of severe and extensive ischemia. Nonetheless, this mechanism is the main explanation for the development of ischemic wall motion abnormalities in patients undergoing dipyridamole stress echocardiography.

Ergonovine may also be useful for noninvasive stress testing. This drug may induce coronary spasm, leading to both heterogeneity in myocardial perfusion and regional left ventricular function.

Rationale of Exercise Simulating Approaches

Various alternatives have been used for the purpose of simulating exercise, including dobutamine and arbutamine stress, as well as pacing stress, handgrip, and the cold pressor test. With the exception of the latter, which works partly through the induction of coronary spasm, these techniques increase myocardial oxygen requirements by increasing the cardiac workload. Dobutamine[23] and arbutamine[24-26] exert this effect by stimulation of cardiac β-receptors, which increase the force and frequency of contraction. Secondarily, these agents induce coronary vasodilation, largely by increasing cardiac work. The development of functional ischemia may also be accentuated by an oxygen wasting effect.[27]

In the presence of a fixed coronary stenosis, myocardial oxygen demand in response to these increased workloads may exceed myocardial oxygen supply. The consequent development of ischemia may be detected as a wall motion abnormality on stress echocardiography or nuclear ventriculography. In addition, the secondary development of regional coronary hyperemia may lead to local variations in the extent of hyperemia in a fashion similar to the vasodilators.[25,28,29] This process may be accentuated by the reduction of subendocardial blood flow, particularly with pacing.

The involvement of different pathways to the development of myocardial ischemia with these stressors has led to their combination. Unfortunately, combinations of dipyridamole and dobutamine lead to an excessively long protocol.[30] However, the addition of atropine to either dobutamine[31,32] or dipyridamole[33] has been shown to increase the level of stress on the heart, and commensurately increase the sensitivity of wall motion imaging techniques. Similarly, the combination of dipyridamole stress with a small amount of exercise, including isotonic exercise, has the effect of maintaining blood pressure and, therefore, preserving the difference in coronary hyperemia between ischemic and nonischemic territories.[19,34-37]

In summary, the rationale and mechanism of action of the vasodilators most favor their use in combination with myocardial perfusion scintigraphy. While wall motion imaging may be performed for the detection of myocardial ischemia, this is not a uniform occurrence in patients with coronary disease who are exposed to vasodilator stress, and could be expected to occur with more severe disease. In contrast, the increase of myocardial oxygen requirements in response to dobutamine favors its use in combination with techniques that identify myocardial ischemia. The association of these changes with alterations of coronary blood flow allows the combination of this test with myocardial perfusion imaging.

METHODOLOGY OF PHARMACOLOGIC AND NONEXERCISE STRESS TECHNIQUES

Although pharmacologic stress tests are less onerous to the patient than exercise stress, they nonetheless provoke various degrees of ischemia, and carry a small risk of significant side effects. Thus, the patient should be prepared and monitored in the same way as for exercise stress. In addition to the usual equipment for resuscitation, specific antagonists to the various stressors should be available (intravenous [IV] aminophylline for dipyridamole and IV β-blockers for dobutamine). Generally, two to three personnel are required: a nuclear medicine technician or sonographer to acquire the images (and inject radionuclide or contrast), a nurse or physician to insert the intravenous line, administer drugs, and monitor the ECG and hemodynamics, and (if a nurse is administering the test) a physician close by to assist with any problems.

Dipyridamole Stress

Dipyridamole was the first pharmacologic agent to be widely used for stress testing. Its development arose from two sources: first, the application of data derived from the coronary blood flow laboratory, for which purpose it was used to induce coronary hyperemia as described above; and second, its use as an agent to induce metabolic and functional evidence of ischemia arose from the accidental development of ischemia when the drug was used as an antianginal agent.[38] These two approaches led to different administration protocols.

Dipyridamole is a strongly alkaline compound, which induces venous irritation, and should be flushed briskly into a proximal arm vein. Following the work of Gould et al.,[39] the most commonly administered dose is 0.56 mg/kg intravenously, over 4 minutes,[39] this being chosen largely because greater doses were associated with patient intolerance. Perfusion tracers are usually injected at about 8 minutes from the start of the test, which corresponds to the time of peak vasodilation. Subsequent protocols have incorporated handgrip or mild physical exercise to avoid hypotension, which may adversely effect coronary flow during maximal hyperemia, as discussed above. More recently, the use of a higher dose of dipyridamole has been advocated in the hope of avoiding dipyridamole nonresponsiveness, but while some favorable results have been reported,[40] the use of higher doses appears to be of limited benefit for perfusion imaging.[41]

Application of the standard dose of dipyridamole (0.56 mg/kg) to stress echocardiography did not commonly provoke myocardial ischemia, especially in the setting of mild coronary disease.[42] However, a higher dose dipyridamole protocol, involving the administration of half of the initial dose, 4 minutes after the conclusion of the initial injection (Fig. 13-3), has been more effective for stress echocardiography.[43] Subsequent developments of the protocol have included the administration of atropine[33] or dobutamine,[30] to induce ischemia through both coronary steal and increased myocardial work. Using a standard quad-screen display, we digitize resting images (upper left), low dose (i.e., before administration of second dose, upper right), high dose (lower left), and dipyridamole + atropine (lower right).

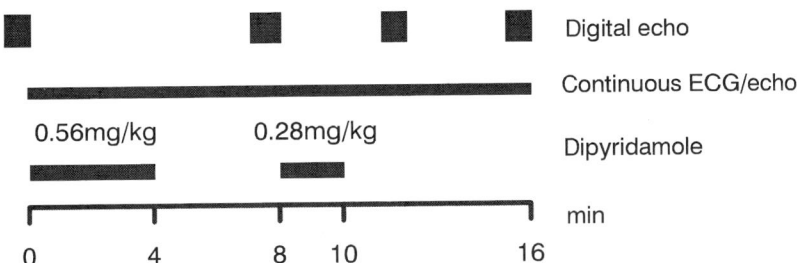

Fig. 13-3. Dipyridamole administration protocol. The standard protocol for myocardial perfusion imaging involves the initial dose only. Dobutamine may be added in preference to or instead of atropine. (From Marwick T: Stress Echocardiography—Its Role in the Diagnosis and Evaluation of Coronary Artery Disease. Kluwer Academic, Dordrecht, 1994, with permission.)

As the effect of adenosine and its augmentation in response to dipyridamole are both blocked by the presence of xanthines, patients should abstain from caffeine for a day prior to the test, and also should not take theophylline or aminophylline for five half-lives prior to the test.[44,45] Patients should be studied in the fasting state, both to reduce gut hyperemia, which can interfere with myocardial perfusion imaging, and also because gastrointestinal side effects may be provoked by dipyridamole. The stress protocol is performed under the usual circumstances of ECG and hemodynamic monitoring. Some centers routinely administer aminophylline at the conclusion of the dipyridamole stress to antagonize its side effects and reverse the development of ischemia. Paradoxically, ischemia may be induced by this agent due to the development of coronary spasm.[22]

Adenosine Stress

In comparison with dipyridamole, adenosine has the benefit of direct action, with rapid onset and offset. Adenosine administration protocols vary—some incorporate an incremental dose schedule. Some centers use a single dose of 0.14 mg/kg/min; we have used an incremental protocol from 0.10, to 0.14, and then 0.18 mg/kg,[20,46,47] digitizing these in separate quadrants of the quadscreen display. The very short half-life of adenosine leads side effects to be of short duration (although they may appear quite intense), with the consequence that aminophylline is rarely required for reversal of its effect. Similarly, atropine could be administered in association with adenosine, but the latter has not developed wide acceptance in combination with stress echocardiography.

Dobutamine Stress

Protocols for the administration of dobutamine have been derived empirically, and wide variations of the duration and peak administered dose have been described.[29,48-51] The most widely utilized protocol involves initial administration of 5 μg/kg/min of dobutamine, increasing to 10, 20, 30, and 40 μg/kg/min at 3 minute intervals. Atropine (1 to 2 mg IV) may be administered over the subsequent few minutes, usually in increments of 0.25 mg (Fig. 13-4). For *diagnostic* studies, we usually organize the quadscreen display with rest, one low-dose (10 μg/kg/min), and two peak dose (usually 40 μg/kg/min and dobutamine + atropine) images and focus on the comparison of resting and peak images (Fig. 13-5). Other centers record one peak and one poststress image, as the latter may show new or more readily recognizable abnormalities after the hyperkinesis, small ventricular cavity, and tachycardia induced by dobutamine have resolved. For *viability* studies, we digitize rest, two low-dose (5 and 10 μg/kg/min) and one set of peak dose images; this is discussed in more detail in Chapter 21. Echo imaging may also be performed using the transesophageal approach,[52-54] which has the benefit of offering excellent endocardial resolution (Fig. 13-6A). However, apart from obvious limitations with respect to feasibility, the visualization of the apex may be problematic with this approach (Fig. 13-6B), even using a multiplane transducer.

When combined with myocardial perfusion imaging, the tracer is injected at peak dose—20 and 40 μg/kg/min have been used. Magnetic resonance imaging has been performed with both dobutamine[55] and dipyridamole stress,[56,57] and has briefly been discussed by Ryan, in Chapter 3. Though accurate, these stress-imaging combinations are not currently used clinically, reflecting problems of cost and availability.

Shorter protocols have been designed, starting at 10 μg/kg/min, as ischemia is rarely induced at low doses. However, these protocols have the disadvantage of failing to incorporate low dose administra-

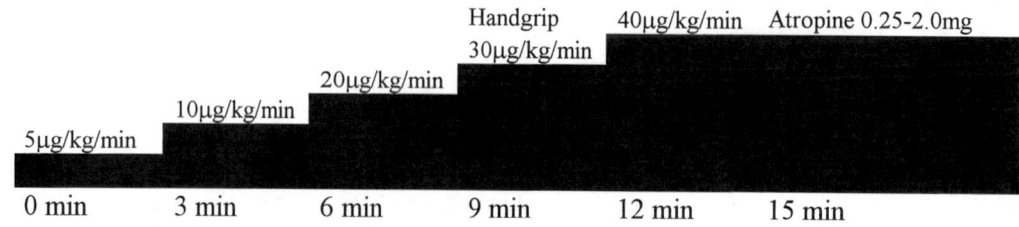

Fig. 13-4. Standard dobutamine–atropine protocol used for stress echocardiography. Lower doses have been used with perfusion imaging.

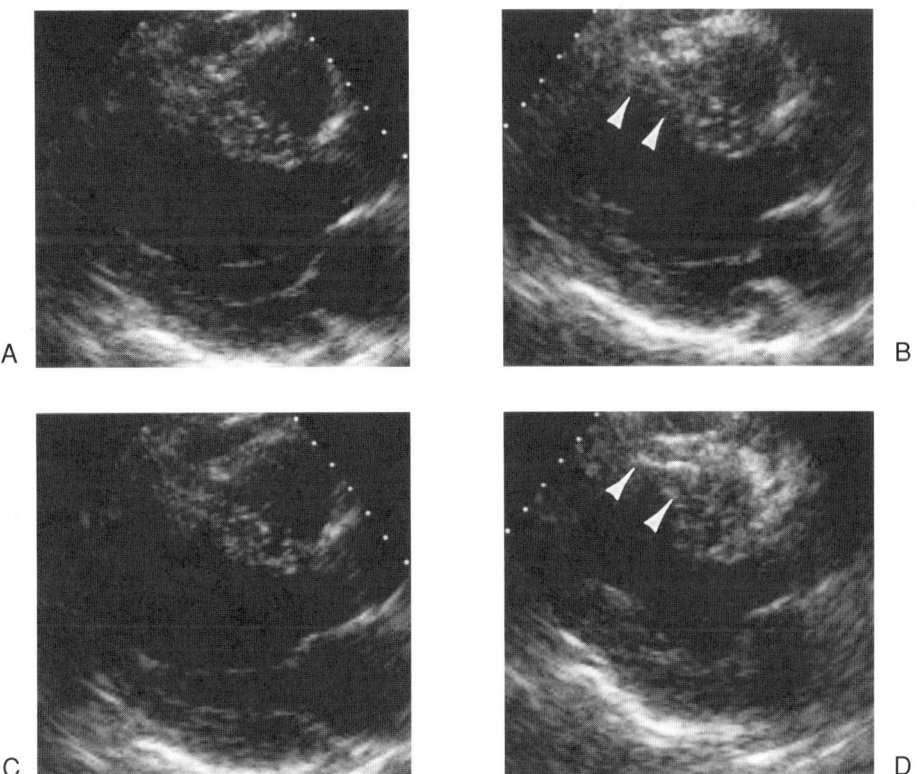

Fig. 13-5. Dobutamine stress echocardiography. **(A,B)** Resting and **(C,D)** peak end-diastolic **(A,C)** and end-systolic **(B,D)** images. A hinge-point develops in the midanteroseptal wall at peak stress, suggesting midanteroseptal ischemia (arrows).

tion, which may be useful for the identification of viable myocardium. Similarly, other protocols have used lower peak doses of dobutamine, for example to 20 μg/kg/min. While this approach has produced lower levels of sensitivity in some studies, Picard has suggested that this has similar efficacy to higher doses when the administration intervals are longer (e.g., 5 rather than 3 minutes per stage).[58]

As with any form of stress testing, the patient is best studied in the fasting state. Unlike dipyridamole and adenosine, xanthines do not counter the effect of dobutamine, and may be administered to the patient prior to the test if necessary. However, anti-ischemic medications (especially β-blockers) may preclude the development of wall motion abnormalities in response to dobutamine,[59] just as they may prevent the development of ischemia in response to dipyridamole or even exercise. The decision to test the patient on or off therapy should be individualized—generally, diagnostic testing should be performed off therapy, but testing on therapy may be useful for defining the efficacy of therapy.

Arbutamine Stress

Arbutamine is a dobutamine analog. It is unique among the pharmacologic stressors in that it was developed specifically as a stress agent, as well as its administration by an automated feedback device, so that no standardized dosage schedule is followed.[24–26] This device automatically senses the hemodynamic response to the agent (Fig. 13-7), and augments its delivery in accordance with the response of the patient. The rate of increase of heart rate as well as the target heart rate may be determined by the supervising physician. Deviations from the closed loop protocol and combination with other

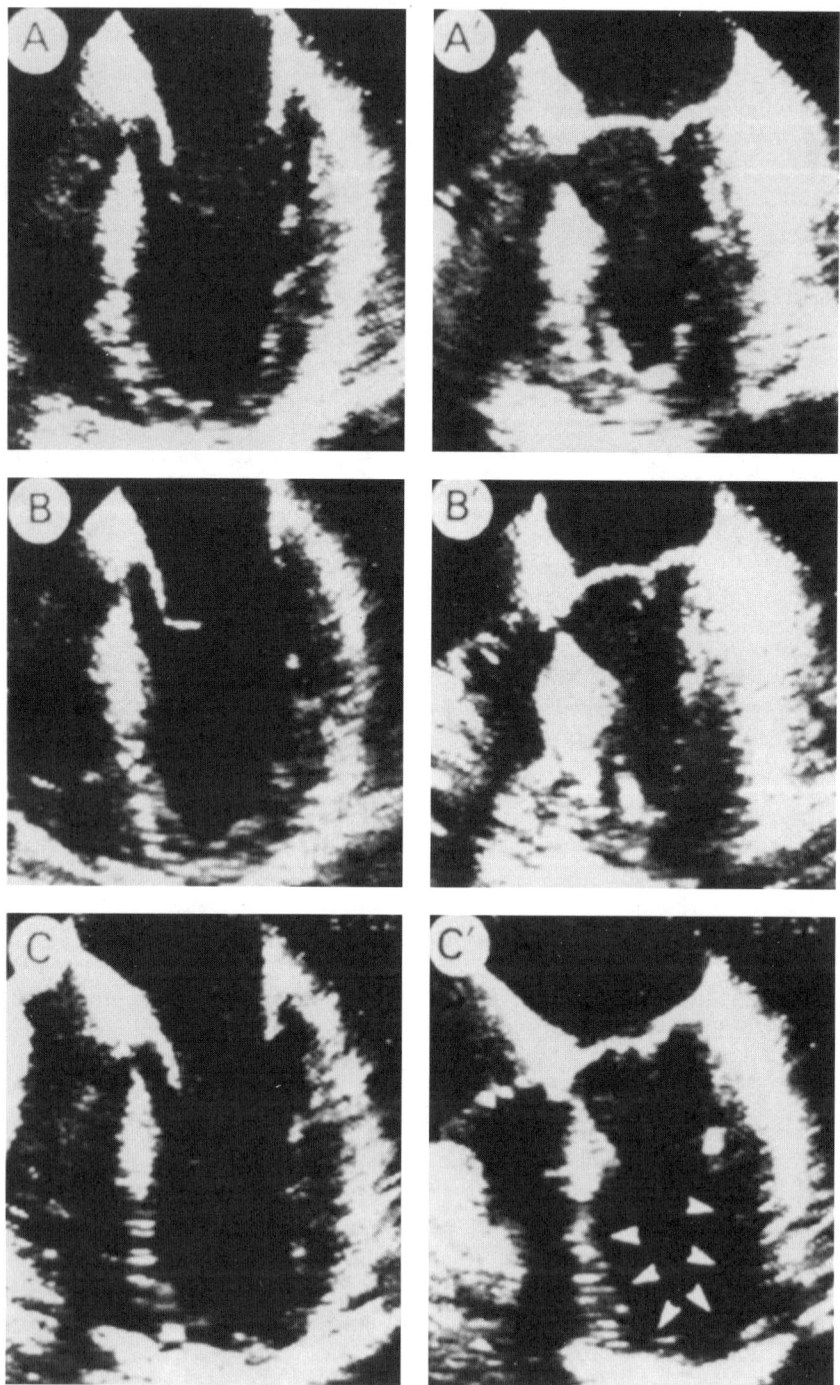

Fig. 13-6. Dobutamine transesophageal echocardiography. **(A)** Diastolic (A–C) and systolic (A'–C') freeze-frames at rest (A & A'), low-dose (B & B'), and peak (20 μg/kg/min) (C & C'). After an initially normal response, akinesia of the apical septal and lateral wall develops (arrows), together with left ventricular cavity enlargement. (*Figure continues.*)

Pharmacologic Stress Testing 241

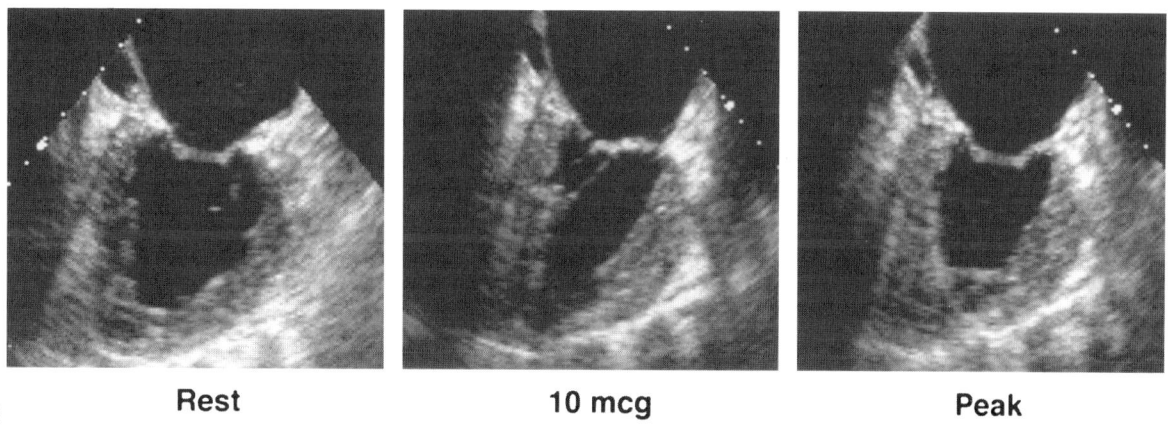

Fig. 13-6. (Continued). **(B)** Limitation of the transesophageal approach. Equivalent orientation of this two-chamber-equivalent view is obtained at each dose (note the location of the coronary sinus). However, the true apex is not visualized at peak stress, causing an apparent alteration of left ventricular contour. (Fig. **A** From Panza et al.,[54] with permission.)

stress agents have not been thus far examined. The use of the closed loop device may reduce the number of personnel required for administration of this stress, but as this usually involves only two personnel, it is unlikely that this can be reduced further. Another benefit may be the duration of the test—as the heart rate increment may be programmed, the time required to attain the desired heart rate may be reduced. Whether the total duration of the test will be shortened is unclear, as the longer half-life of arbutamine (compared with dobutamine) may lengthen the recovery phase.

Echocardiographic images are recorded throughout the test; we digitize images at rest, submaximal

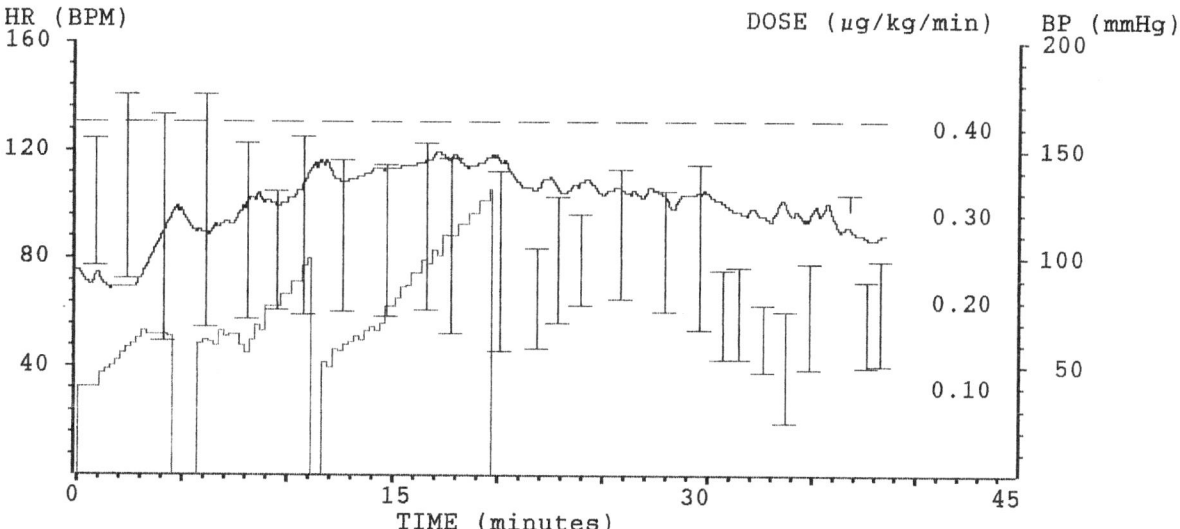

Fig. 13-7. Hemodynamic response to arbutamine, using a closed-loop delivery system. Note, the cessation of administration twice during the protocol (lower line) as a response to an excessively rapid increment the heart rate response. Blood pressure is portrayed by vertical lines.

heart rate (usually about 100/min) and two peak images. Perfusion tracers are injected at peak stress.

Pacing Stress

Pacing stress has been utilized using a variety of protocols, which have incorporated both invasive (transvenous) pacing as well as esophageal techniques.[60–63] The latter usually require some degree of sedation and topical anesthesia, although both of these steps may become unnecessary in the light of future hardware developments. As the development of Wenckebach type AV block is a frequent consequence of increasing pacing rates, atropine is almost always administered in combination with pacing. The standard pacing protocol usually commences at 100 beats/min, and increases in 2 minute stages by 20 beats/min to an eventual target heart rate of 140 to 160 beats/min, depending on the patient's age. Echocardiographic imaging is usually performed at each stage, and if combined with perfusion imaging, the isotope is injected at peak stress.

A major difference between pacing and the other stressors is the ability to terminate the stress very rapidly, which enhances the safety of the procedure, as well as facilitating observation of the consequences of ischemia in the absence of tachycardia. This may be of value in the identification of changes of diastolic function with Doppler.[64]

Other Stress Techniques

Other nonexercise stressors, such as the cold pressor test, have been superceded by the above approaches, which are better tolerated and more effective. Mental stress and ergotamine stress may be useful in specific circumstances (especially when the question of coronary spasm arises), but are rarely performed.

Finally, while some pharmacologic techniques have recently been combined (Fig. 13-8), this approach has the disadvantage of producing a long period of stress, which is unattractive from the standpoint of clinical practice.

Thus, a range of nonexercise stresses may be used in combination with various imaging techniques for the identification of coronary disease. Most of these protocols are of an acceptable duration, a period of about 10 minutes being looked upon as being optimal for this purpose. The simplest protocols involve dipyridamole and arbutamine, although the efficacy of the latter in relation to the others remains to be defined.[65]

HEMODYNAMIC RESPONSES TO PHARMACOLOGIC STRESS

Vasodilators

While the aim of vasodilator administration is to produce changes in the coronary vasculature, the effects of these agents are not specific to this vascular territory. Consequently, the hemodynamic responses to dipyridamole and adenosine reflect the presence of systemic vasodilation, producing decreases in blood pressure and increases of heart rate. Indeed, the tachycardia reported by Rossen et al.[18] in response to 0.14 mg/kg/min of adenosine was comparable to that of a standard dose of 0.56 mg/kg of dipyridamole over 4 minutes, both increasing the heart rate by 11 beats/min. The hypotensive effect of adenosine was slightly more marked than that of dipyridamole (-16 ± 5 vs. -10 ± 3 mmHg, $p < 0.01$). Using an incremental dose protocol, however, hypotension developed in response to adenosine only at at peak dose of 0.14 mg/kg/min,[66] although the develop-

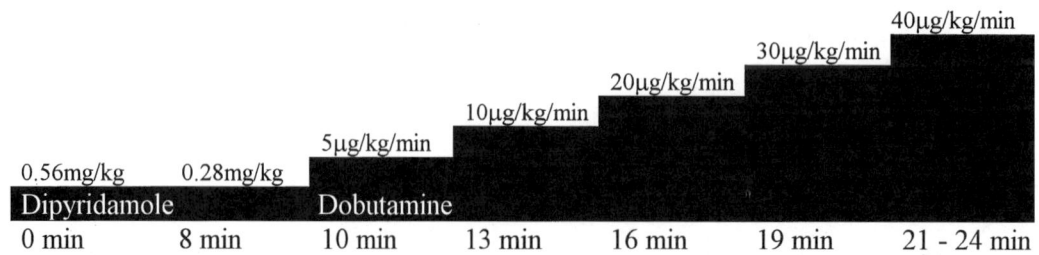

Fig. 13-8. Dipyridamole–dobutamine protocol. This recently designed protocol for stress echocardiography combines low- and high-dose dipyridamole with dobutamine stress.

ment of a mild increase of heart rate was noted at low doses, beginning at 0.05 mg/kg/min. The minor reduction of blood pressure in response to adenosine is offset, however, by the reduction of peripheral resistance, such that cardiac output in response to a dose of 0.14 mg/kg/min increases from an average of 6 L/min at rest to 8 to 10 L/min during stress.[46] Despite this, however, pulmonary wedge pressure has been reported to increase in normal subjects in response to adenosine administration, possibly reflecting reduction of left ventricular compliance in response to vascular engorgement.[67]

Exercise-Simulating Agents

Dobutamine was initially designed as an agent to support the hemodynamics of patients in the intensive care environment. Consequently, at low doses, dobutamine enhances left ventricular contractility, usually without the development of tachycardia.[23] At doses greater than 20 μg/kg/min, tachycardia and hypertension develop. Using a standard administration protocol to a peak of 40 μg/kg/min, Hayes et al.[28] and Cohen et al.[68] reported peak heart rates of the order of 120 beats/min, reflecting an increment of 40 to 50 beats/min. Similarly, the eventual blood pressure increment is 30 to 40 mmHg, producing a peak systolic blood pressure of 170 mmHg in normotensive patients (Fig. 13-9). While initial reports suggested that a hypotensive response was associated with severe disease, this has been shown to be a nonspecific finding. The most common cause of a reduction of blood pressure at peak dose is the vasodilator effect of dobutamine. Left ventricular outflow tract

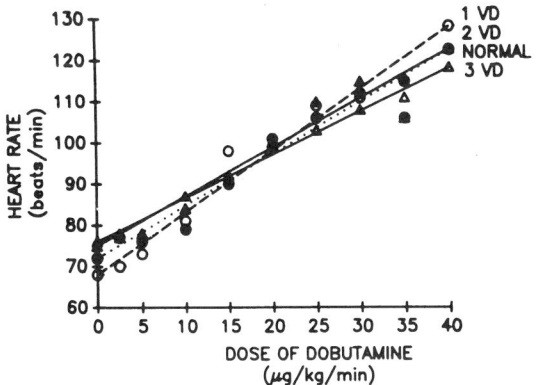
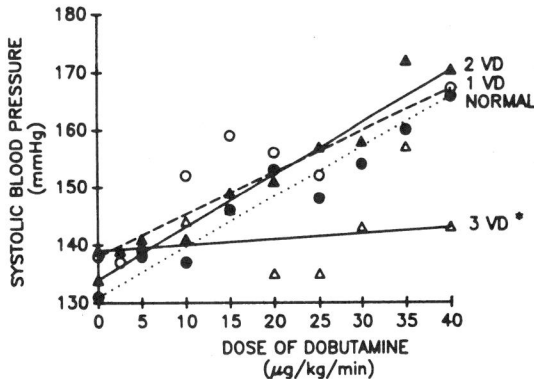
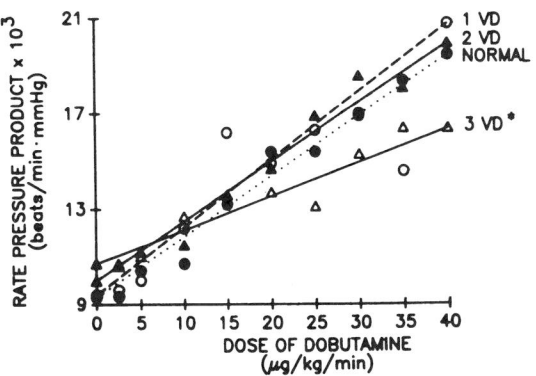
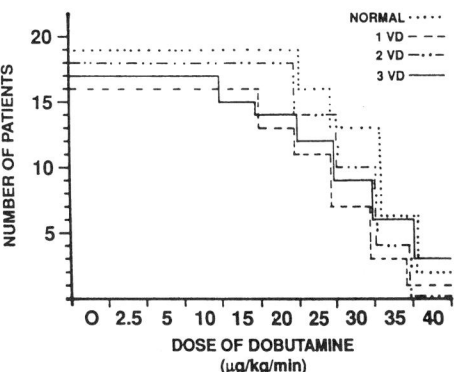

Fig. 13-9. Hemodynamic response to dobutamine. The blunted hemodynamic response in the setting of three-vessel disease is unfortunately nonspecific (see text). (From Cohen et al.,[68] with permission.)

obstruction is another (but an uncommon) cause of this response.[69,70] Conversely, in hypertensive patients the systolic blood pressure response may be augmented. The diastolic blood pressure often falls in response to dobutamine, reflecting vasodilation. In response to this augmentation of heart rate and systolic blood pressure, the peak rate pressure product increases to the range of 16,000 to 20,000.

Significant inter-individual variations in hemodynamic responses have been reported. An attenuated response occurs in the presence of β-blockers,[59] with a peak heart rate of 90 to 100 beats/min, and a rate pressure product of around 14,000. The addition of atropine may circumvent this problem.[32] It is important to note that even in the absence of medical therapy, the peak heart rate and the rate product response to dobutamine alone are significantly less than during exercise stress. This may have important consequences in respect of the relative efficacy of dobutamine and exercise stress for provoking ischemia.

In contrast to dobutamine, arbutamine was developed primarily as a stress agent, and the development of tachycardia in response to this drug is seen at low doses. This is not, however, readily apparent during administration, as the rate of drug delivery is variable, depending on the hemodynamic response of the patient. In other respects the peak stress on the heart obtained with arbutamine appears to be comparable to that attainable with dobutamine. Interestingly, ischemia has been reported at lower cardiac workload (i.e., rate pressure product) during arbutamine than exercise,[71] a finding concordant with comparisons of dobutamine and exercise, but somewhat more marked. Possibly this reflects an additional oxygen wasting effect.

A maximal heart rate response can virtually be guaranteed with atrial pacing, provided that atrioventricular block does not occur, and capture is maintained. However, in contrast to the other exercise-simulating agents, the blood pressure response to pacing is limited, and to obtain a maximal stress on the heart, the conjunction of pacing with low doses of pharmacologic stress may be of benefit.

The different mechanisms of action of vasodilator and exercise simulating agents translate into different hemodynamic effects. Protocols which are used in combination with myocardial perfusion imaging generally require smaller stresses on the heart, provided that adequate levels of coronary vasodilation are achieved by other means. The requirement of ischemia in combination with stress echocardiography would suggest that the greatest possible workload increment is desirable, and this can probably be obtained with a dobutamine–atropine combination.

SIDE EFFECTS OF PHARMACOLOGIC STRESS
Vasodilator Stress

As dipyridamole acts as a prodrug for the release of adenosine, it is not surprising that the side effects of these agents are qualitatively similar (Table 13-1). Probably because of the rapid response to the drug, side effects appear to be more intense with adenosine, but on the other hand these side effects are of brief duration, reflecting the shorter half-life of this agent.

The side effect profile of dipyridamole in *standard doses* (0.56 mg/kg IV) of have been reported by Ranhosky et al.[72] Some side effect occurred in 47% of these patients, the commonest being chest pain, headache, and dizziness. In all, 12% of patients required aminophylline for the treatment of side effects, of whom 97% had complete symptomatic relief with this agent. Serious side effects occurred in only four patients (<1%), comprising two fatal and two nonfatal myocardial infarctions.

The safety profile of *high dose* dipyridamole has been reported by Picano et al.[73] in a multicenter study of over 10,000 patients. Again, major side effects occurred in under 1% of patients, and included myocardial infarctions, ventricular tachycardia, asystole, heart failure, and death. Other significant side effects included hypotension, bradycardia, bronchospasm, and nonsustained tachyarrhythmias. Flushing and headache are frequent in patients studied with high-dose dipyridamole. In the light of these findings, dipyridamole stress should be contraindicated in patients with untreated atrioventricular block and asthma. Decisions to use the agent in the face of chronic obstructive airways disease should be based upon the degree of a bronchospastic and reversible component. Caution should be applied in the use of dipyridamole in patients with hypotension or bradycardia. Obviously, patients with unstable coronary syndromes should not be stressed, irrespective of the nature of the stress.

Table 13-1. Side Effects of Pharmacologic Stress Protocols in Four Studies

Variable	Dipyridamole 0.54 mg/kg Ranhosky et al. (1990)[72]	Dipyridamole 0.81 mg/kg Picano et al. (1992)[73]	Adenosine Cerqueira et al. (1994)[74]	Dobutamine 40 µg/kg/m ± atropine Mertes et al. (1993)[76]
n	3911	10,451	9256	1118
Total S/E	47%	—	81%	35% (cardiac)
Major S/E	0.26%	0.07%	<0.10%	0%
Fatal MI	0.05%	0.01%	0	0%
Nonfatal MI	0.05%	0.02%	0.01%	0%
Bronchospasm	0.15%	0.05%	0.07%	0%
Anxiety	—	—	—	6%
Chest pain	20%	—	35%	19%
Dizziness	12%	—	9%	—
Dyspnea	3%	—	35%	5%
Flushing	3%	—	37%	—
Headache	12%	—	14%	4%
Hypotension	5%	0.50%	—	3%
Nausea	5%	—	15%	8%
Palpitations	3%	—	7.6% (AVB)	35% (arrh)
Paresthesia	1%	—	—	—
ST changes	8%	—	6%	9%

Abbreviations: AVB, atrioventricular; MI, myocardial infarction; S/E, side effects; arrh, arrhythmia.

Studies of large groups of patients stressed with adenosine[74,75] have shown side effects to occur in over 80% of patients. The most common of these side effects are headache, dizziness, and chest pain, similar to the pattern observed with dipyridamole. However, in this series, no major cardiac events were reported. Surprisingly, atrioventricular block is rarely reported. The contraindications to adenosine are similar to those for dipyridamole. In view of the shorter duration of action of this agent, some authorities have felt that these contraindications should be applied less stringently. However, bronchospasm may be initiated by this agent, and may continue even after the resolution of this stress, so that use of this agent in patients with asthma is inadvisable.

Exercise-Simulating Agents

Both dobutamine and arbutamine produce intense adrenergic stimulation, and the side effects of these agents parallel this mechanism of action. Serious side effects are rare during dobutamine stress testing, with no major events being reported by Mertes et al.[76] in a study of over 1,000 patients. Similarly, Poldermans et al.[77] reported no patients who died or suffered myocardial infarction after stress with either dobutamine or dobutamine–atropine combinations. Cardiac arrhythmias occurred no more frequently in patients with pre-existing ventricular arrhythmias or left ventricular dysfunction. In the largest multicentric study reported to date, Picano et al.[78] described nine major cardiac events in nearly 3,000 examinations, including five with serious ventricular arrhythmias, ischemia, and myocardial infarction in three and one patient with hypotension. Surprisingly, atropine psychosis was observed in five patients, a complication that has not been reported in other studies. Dobutamine stress thus has a favorable safety record, but its use is contraindicated in patients with serious arrhythmias, or patients with previous allergies to dobutamine.

Apart from these serious complications, dose-limiting side effects have occurred in 5% of patients, although some form of side effect has been reported in greater than 80% of patients. Some variability in the definition of these side effects has led to variations in their reported frequency, particularly hypotension, which in the initial years of dobutamine usage was identified on the basis of a greater than 20 to 30 mmHg drop during the test or a greater than 50 mmHg fall from baseline, and is now identified only if the systolic blood pressure falls to less than 100 mmHg.

The side effects experienced with arbutamine are qualitatively similar to those described with dobutamine.[24-26] Most side effects are mild and resolve after cessation of the agent, although with the longer half-life of arbutamine in comparison with dobutamine, the duration of side effects may be longer. Some form of side effect has been reported in 80% of patients. Arrhythmias occur in about 8% of patients, this possibly being slightly greater in frequency than with dobutamine, possibly reflecting the use of higher doses of the agent. The relative frequency of side effects with dobutamine and arbutamine awaits comparison in the same patients.

Side Effects of Pacing Stress

The most troublesome side effects of pacing derive from instrumentation of the patient rather than the nature of the stress,[79] but these aspects nonetheless reduce the overall feasibility of the test compared with pharmacologic techniques.[80,81] Using transesophageal pacing, esophageal discomfort, particularly at higher stimulation thresholds, gagging, and nausea are frequent. Esophageal injury is a theoretical concern that has not been reported in practice. Atrial flutter or fibrillation may be precipitated by transesophageal pacing, but are unusual complications. As in the case of all stressors, angina may be provoked during the protocol.

Summary

All forms of nonexercise stress pose potential problems with respect to side effects. In general, side effects occurring in response to vasodilators (breathlessness, headache, flushing) are more of a concern to the patient than the physician. In contrast, side effects occurring in response to dobutamine (dysrhythmias, blood pressure disturbances) are often more of a concern to the physician than the patient. As dipyridamole exerts its effects indirectly, the onset of side effects is delayed usually until after completion of the dose administration, and, therefore, the side effects rarely interfere with the completion of the test, unless they are particular severe and warrant treatment with aminophylline. This may not be the case with adenosine, where side effects can develop abruptly, and the test may need to be terminated due to patient intolerance. Serious side effects are uncommon with all pharmacologic stressors, and the selection between them is rarely dependent on contraindications alone.

PHARMACOLOGIC STRESS ECG

Vasodilator Stress

In our experience, significant ST-segment depression, defined by greater or equal 0.01 mV deviation from the rest or the isoelectric line measured at 0.08 seconds after the J point, occurs in less than 25% of patients stressed with dipyridamole. The frequency of this finding depends on the nature of the study group, and is more often reported in older patients, or those with ischemic findings. In the study of Chambers and Brown,[82] the rate pressure product at the time of peak dipyridamole effect and the presence of coronary collaterals were independent predictors of ST-segment depression. These are interesting findings, as the former would suggest ST depression to reflect cardiac workload, while the latter is more consistent with a steal mechanism. Villanueva et al.[53] reported thallium redistribution in 64% of patients with ST-segment depression, and only 38% of those without ST depression. In agreement with ischemic cascade, the number of ischemic segments was the most important predictor of ST depression (χ^2 16.8, $p \leq 0.001$). In accordance with the report of Chambers and Brown,[82] Vilanueva et al.[83] also reported the heart rate at the time of thallium injection was a predictor of ST depression, as was the presence of angina and increasing age.

Similar data have been reported with adenosine,[84] the correlates of ST depression in the experience reported by Nishimura et al.[84] included coronary collaterals and angina. In the latter study, the sensitivity of ST-segment depression for the prediction of significant coronary disease was 77%, and the specificity was 95%. These results exceed the previously reported levels of sensitivity for vasodilator stress ECG testing, which have been more in the range of 50%.

Exercise-Simulating Agents

The frequency of significant ST-segment depression in patients during dobutamine testing in our experience is also less than 25%, again depending on the nature of the constituent population. Considerable variation has been reported in the sensitivity of dobutamine stress ECG testing for coronary disease. In initial reports focusing on patients with a high probability of disease, the sensitivity was reported to be favorable.[85] However, in later reports involving unselected populations, the sensitivity has been less than 50%.[86,87] In contrast, the specificity of dobutamine ECG testing has been more favorable. The presence of a discrepancy between low sensitivity and high specificity implies the cut off for a positive test to be inappropriate. However, even after modification of these criteria, based on the use of receiver operating curve analysis, use of the optimal ECG criteria (0.5 mm ST-segment depression) produced a limited increment in the accuracy of dobutamine ECG testing, the best obtainable sensitivity being 42%.[86]

ACCURACY OF VASODILATOR STRESS TESTING

Oral Dipyridamole Stress

Prior to regulatory approval of intravenous dipyridamole in the United States, several studies of dipyridamole stress were performed using oral administration. Although the reported sensitivity of this approach was reasonably favorable, using planar and single-photon emission computed tomography (SPECT) imaging[88–91] as well as echocardiography,[92] the absorption of oral dipyridamole is fairly erratic,[93,94] and large oral doses of the drug often provoke patient discomfort, including nausea and vomiting. Moreover, the sensitivities in these studies may have been influenced by the prevalence of myocardial infarction and multivessel coronary disease. Now that intravenous dipyridamole is readily available, we believe that oral administration should be looked upon as a historical curiosity.

Dipyridamole and Adenosine Perfusion Scintigraphy

A large experience has now been accumulated with the use of intravenous dipyridamole (Table 13-2). Using both planar and SPECT imaging, sensitivities have been reported in the range of 80 to 90%, with

Table 13-2. Accuracy of Vasodilator Stress Myocardial Perfusion Scintigraphy

Author	n	Stress	Imaging	CAD Definition (%)	CAD n (%)	Sensitivity (%)	Specificity (%)
Albro et al. (1978)[39]	62	IV dipyridamole	Planar	50	51 (82)	67	91
Leppo et al. (1982)[95]	60	IV dipyridamole	Planar	50	40 (67)	93	80
Francisco et al. (1982)[97]	86	IV dipyridamole	SPECT	70	51 (59)	92	96
Schmoliner et al. (1983)[96]	60	IV dipyridamole	Planar	70	60 (100)	95	—
Okada et al. (1983)[99]	30	IV dipyridamole	Planar	50	23 (77)	91	100
Sochor et al. (1984)[98]	194	IV dipyridamole	Planar	70	149 (77)	92	81
Taillefer et al. (1986)[101]	50	IV dipyridamole	Planar	70	39 (78)	82	91
Ruddy et al. (1987)[100]	80	IV dipyridamole	Planar	50	53 (66)	85	93
Lam et al. (1988)[102]	132	IV dipyridamole	Planar	70	101 (77)	85	71
Huikuri et al. (1988)[105]	93	IV dipyridamole	SPECT	70	81 (87)	96	75
Nguyen et al. (1990)[107]	60	IV adenosine	SPECT	50	53 (88)	92	100
Verani et al. (1990)[66]	45	IV adenosine	SPECT	50	29 (64)	83	94
Iskandrian et al. (1991)[106]	148	IV adenosine	SPECT	50	132 (89)	92	88
Nishimura et al. (1991)[108]	101	IV adenosine	SPECT	50	70 (69)	87	90
Kong et al. (1992)[103]	114	IV dipyridamole	Planar	50	94 (82)	91	60
Mendelson et al. (1992)[104]	79	IV dipyridamole	SPECT	70	76 (100)	89	—

Abbreviations: CAD, coronary artery disease; IV, intravenous; SPECT, single-photon emission computed tomography.

somewhat lower specificities, particularly with SPECT imaging.[39,66,95–108] As in all stress imaging tests for the diagnosis of coronary disease, the inclusion of patients with prior myocardial infarction tends to enhance the sensitivity. Similarly, the presence of multivessel coronary disease facilitates detection of ischemia.

Studies of dipyridamole and adenosine in combination with myocardial perfusion imaging have demonstrated the results of these tests to be comparable, with respect to both feasibility and accuracy. In a comparison of 1,000 patients studied with dipyridamole with another 1,000 studied with adenosine, Johnston et al.[109] reported side effects to be less common with the former, but when present, these were much more troublesome and time consuming to control.

Comparisons of dipyridamole and exercise perfusion imaging[105,110] have shown that the stressors have similar sensitivity and specificity. Indeed, the avoidance of tachycardia with vasodilator stress may be of value in evaluating patients with left bundle branch block.[111,112] These patients commonly have false-positive septal perfusion defects, as flow is com-

Table 13-3. Sensitivity and Specificity of Echocardiography with Vasodilator Stress

Author	n	Stress	CAD Definition (%)	n (CAD)	Multivessel (% all CAD)	Myocardial (% all CAD)	Infarction Sensitivity (%)	Specificity (%)
Picano et al. (1985)[42]	66	Dipyridamole 0.56 mg/kg	>70	50	20 (40)	9 (18)	56	100
Picano et al. (1986)[43]	93	Dipyridamole 0.84 mg/kg[a]	>70	72	48 (67)	17 (24)	74	100
Masini et al. (1988)[117]	83	Dipyridamole 0.84 mg/kg[a]	>70	39	24 (62)	15 (38)	79	93
Cohen et al. (1989)[92]	50	Dipyridamole 400 mg PO	>70	36	28 (78)	16 (44)	81	93
Massa et al. (1989)[118]	52	Dipyridamole 0.84 mg/kg[a]	>70	52	12 (23)	9 (17)	90	—
Zoghbi et al. (1991)[119]	73	Adenosine 0.14 µg/kg/min[a]	>75	54	24 (44)	38 (70)	85	92
Picano et al. (1991)[120]	445	Dipyridamole 0.84 mg/kg[a]	>50	256	119 (46)	0 (0)	96	96
Mazeika et al. (1992)[121]	55	Dipyridamole 1.00 mg/kg[a]	>70	40	30 (75)	18 (45)	40	93
Marwick et al. (1993)[47]	97	Adenosine 0.18 µg/kg/min[a]	>50	59	28 (47)	0 (0)	58	87
Picano et al. (1993)[33]	130	Dipyridamole 0.84 mg/kg + atrophine	>50	94	—	—	87	94
Previtali et al. (1993)[122]	80	Dipyridamole 0.84 mg/kg[a]	>50	57	33 (58)	15 (26)	60	96
Beleslin et al. (1994)[6]	136	Dipyridamole 0.84 mg/kg[a]	>50	119	11 (9)	41 (34)	74	94
Ostojic et al. (1994)[30]	150	Dipyridamole 0.84 mg/kg[a]	>50	131	16 (12)	38 (29)	71	89
Marangelli et al. (1994)[81]	60	Dipyridamole 0.84 mg/kg[a]	>75	35	19 (54)	—	43	92
Dagianti et al. (1995)[123]	60	Dipyridamole 0.84 mg/kg[a]	>50	25	15 (60)	41 (39)	52	97

Abbreviations: CAD, coronary artery disease.
[a] Low dose positivity permits conclusion of study before stated "peak" dose.

promised by shortening of the diastolic filling period due both to tachycardia and delayed septal activation. In comparisons between adenosine and exercise stress, agreement between the stressors was 86% by quantitative analysis[113] with comparable levels of sensitivity and specificity.[114–116] Indeed, it is inevitable that some discrepancies would arise between exercise and nonexercise stress, given the importance of attaining adequate heart rate to obtain reliable exercise stress data.

Dipyridamole and Adenosine Stress Echocardiography

Studies examining the accuracy of vasodilator stress echocardiography are summarized in Table 13-3.[6,30,33,42,43,47,81,92,117–123] Although the specificity of the technique is high in almost all studies, the sensitivity demonstrates wide variation, from the 50% to the 90% range. This variation probably reflects differences in the population studied. As illustrated in Table 13-3, studies demonstrating a high degree of sensitivity with dipyridamole echocardiography have generally involved patients with multivessel disease and prior myocardial infarction, as well as a higher cutoff for defining significant disease (e.g., 70% vs. 50% coronary stenosis). Picano et al.[124] have shown that coronary flow reserve is compromised slightly more in patients with significant stenoses who have a positive dipyridamole echocardiogram than in those with a negative dipyridamole echocardiogram (Fig. 13-10).

As discussed in a previous section, the dose of vasodilator is an important determinant of sensitivity in combination with stress echocardiography. Use of the standard dose used for perfusion imaging (0.56 mg/kg), has been associated with low levels of sensitivity, and more favorable results have been obtained using a two-step high-dose (0.84 mg/kg) protocol, as previously described.[42,43] The addition of atropine has further enhanced the sensitivity of dipyridamole stress echocardiography;[33] the same is true of the combination of dobutamine with dipyridamole testing, the protocol for which is described above. Combination stresses may be particularly important in patients taking antianginal therapy.

Most adenosine stress echocardiography data have been obtained using a dose of 0.14 μg/kg/min.[119] Higher doses have been attempted, but are often not tolerated.[47]

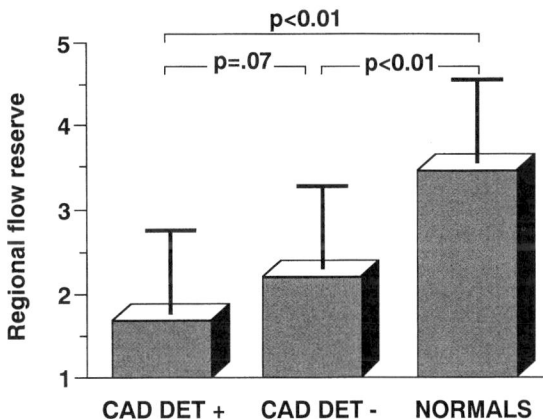

Fig. 13-10. Coronary flow reserve in normals, and patients with coronary artery disease with and without ischemia at the dipyridamole echocardiography test (DET). The presence of ischemia was associated with functionally more significant stenoses, evidenced by lower regional flow reserve. (From Picano et al.,[124] with permission.)

Which Is the Optimal Methodology for Combination with Vasodilator Stress?

Considerable variability is seen with respect to the accuracy of vasodilator stress echocardiography. On the other hand, the sensitivity of a vasodilator stress myocardial perfusion scintigraphy has been reproducibly in the range of 85%. Of course, the optimal circumstances for comparison of the methodologies involve a paired comparison, which has been reported in a number of studies.[47,125–127] As discussed in Chapter 4, these studies have shown perfusion scintigraphy to be the best choice for combination with vasodilator stress, with few exceptions.[128]

Side effects are probably more common with adenosine, as discussed previously, but they are also more transient. Generally, comparisons between dipyridamole stress echo and exercise stress ECG[122,129–131] have shown the former to be more sensitive, as would be expected of an imaging test. However, comparisons of dipyridamole and exercise stress echocardiography have shown exercise echocardiography to be more difficult (less feasible) but more sensitive,[6,81,123] presumably reflecting a greater stress on the heart. Studies suggesting comparable levels of sensitivity[132] may be colored by the nature of patient selection.

ACCURACY OF DOBUTAMINE STRESS TESTING

Dobutamine and Arbutamine Perfusion Scintigraphy

When dobutamine stress is combined with perfusion scintigraphy, the effect of the stress is to produce coronary hyperemia by increasing cardiac work. It is unclear as to whether this is as efficacious an approach as direct vasodilation, but if a perfusion approach is desired (e.g., because of local expertise), and the patient is unsuitable for use of a coronary vasodilator (e.g., because of asthma or AV conduction disturbances), dobutamine is a reasonable alternative.

The accuracy of studies of stress perfusion scintigraphy using exercise simulating agents is summarized in Table 13-4.[25,28,29,47,133–135] It is readily apparent that this technique is sensitive, and that this level of sensitivity may be attained with the use of smaller doses of dobutamine than are required for echocardiography. This observation is concordant with the theory of the ischemic cascade,[136] that flow heterogeneity should develop at a lesser level of stress than ischemia. Exercise and dobutamine stress scintigraphy have comparable levels of sensitivity, provided that adequate stress is provided by each agent.[7]

Dobutamine and Arbutamine Stress Echocardiography

In view of the failure of vasodilators to induce ischemia, stress echocardiography has largely been combined with dobutamine, or more recently arbutamine, when a pharmacologic stress is required. Data from the Thoraxcenter have shown that the presence of wall motion abnormalities during a dobutamine–atropine stress test may be predicted by a stenosis of greater than 52% diameter, greater than 75% area, or less than 1.07 mm diameter (Fig. 13-11).[137] Studies addressing the accuracy of regional dysfunction during dobutamine and arbutamine stress echocardiography are summarized in Table 13-5.[6,30,31,49,50,52,54,68,122,135,138–142] These findings have indicated the specificity of these approaches to be very favorable. As usual, there is some variation in the reported levels of sensitivity—Table 13-5 illustrates how this reflects differences in patient selection, especially the impact of prior myocardial infarction and multivessel disease. The addition of Doppler evaluation of mitral inflow velocity probably does not materially benefit the accuracy of either dobutamine[143] or dipyridamole stress.[144] This is probably because although the development of ischemia produces delayed ventricular relaxation[145] (and, hence, lower E wave velocity—Fig. 13-12), this is often balanced by an increase in the left atrial pressure, which tends to pseudonormalize the E wave.

Additionally, some of the variation in sensitivity between studies may be accounted for by differences in the protocol; transesophageal imaging may enhance accuracy, and more recent, high dose protocols, especially in association with atropine,[31] have generated high levels of sensitivity. As discussed in the section on hemodynamics, dobutamine is not a particularly potent stress, and the sensitivity of dobutamine stress echocardiography may be compromised in patients on anti-ischemic medication, and

Table 13-4. Accuracy of Stress Myocardial Perfusion Scintigraphy Using Exercise-Simulating Agents

Author	n	Stress	Imaging	CAD definition (%)	CAD n (%)	Sensitivity (%)	Specificity (%)
Mason et al. (1984)[133]	24	Dobutamine 20 μg/kg/m	Planar	>50	16 (67)	94	87
Pennell et al. (1991)[29]	50	Dobutamine 20 μg/kg/m	SPECT[a]	>50	40 (80)	96	80
Hays et al. (1993)[28]	84	Dobutamine 40 μg/kg/m	SPECT	>50	57 (68)	76	90
Pennell et al. (1993)[134]	20	Dobutamine 40 μg/kg/m	SPECT	>50	11 (55)	91	78
Marwick et al. (1993)[47]	97	Dobutamine 40 μg/kg/m	SPECT	>50	59 (61)	80	74
Marwick et al. (1993)[135]	217	Dobutamine 40 μg/kg/m	SPECT	>50	142 (65)	80	67
Kiat et al. (1995)[25a]	184	Arbutamine	SPECT	>50	122 (66)	87	90

Abbreviations: CAD, coronary artery disease; SPECT, single-photon emission computed tomography.
[a] Normalcy used instead of specificity in this study.

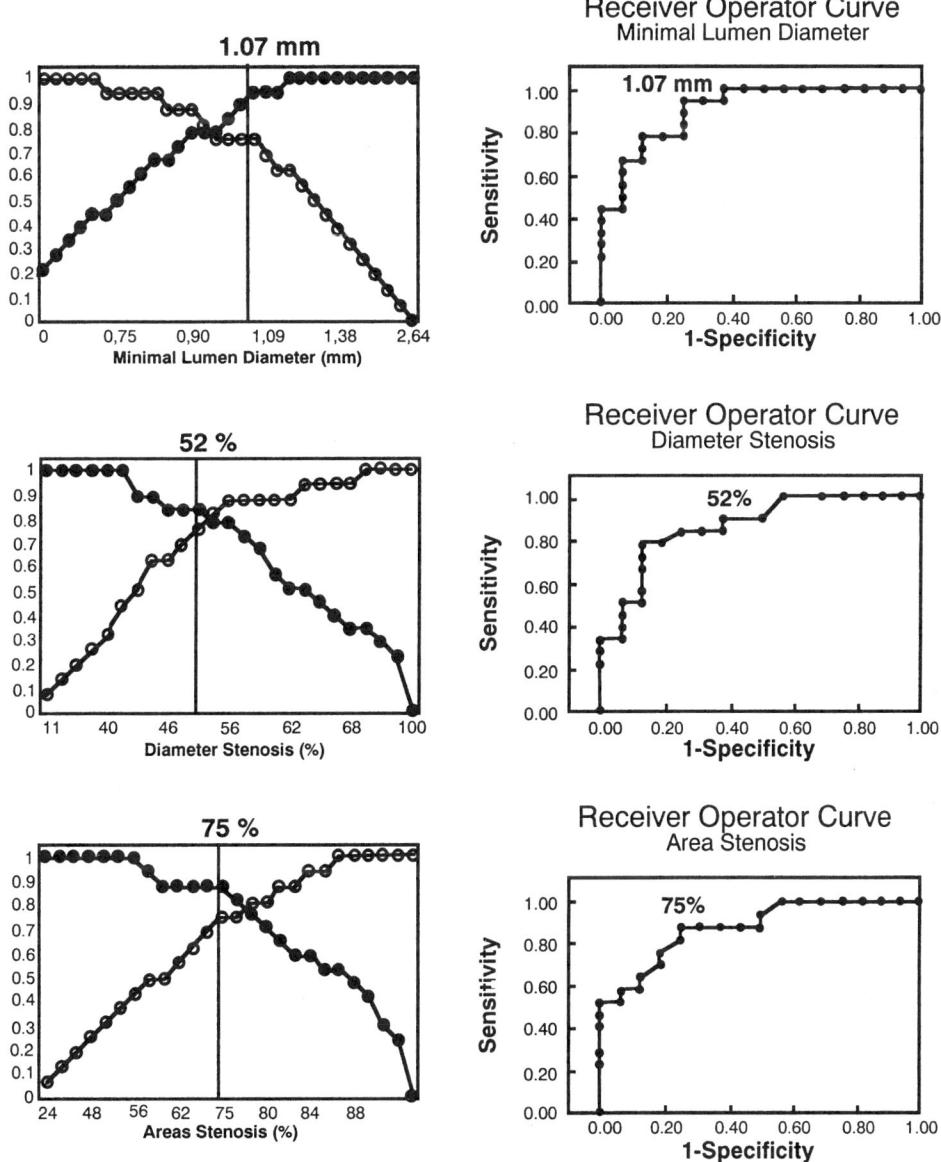

Fig. 13-11. Relation between sensitivity and specificity of the dobutamine–atropine stress test, and cutoff values of stenosis severity. The graphs on the left chart sensitivity (filled circles) and specificity (open circles) using various cutoffs for "significant" coronary artery disease. Receiver operating curves for each angiographic variable are presented on the right. (From Baptista et al.,[137] with permission.)

Table 13-5. Sensitivity and Specificity of Echocardiogrpahy with Dobutamine Stress

Author	n	Dobutamine Protocol	CAD definition (%)	n (CAD)	Multivessel (% all CAD)	Myocardial Infarction (% all CAD)	Sensitivity (%)	Specificity (%)
Sawada et al. (1991)[49]	103	30 μg/kg/min	>50	81	14 (40)	35 (43)	95	77
Cohen et al. (1991)[68]	70	40 μg/kg/min	>70	51	35 (69)	19 (37)	86	95
Salustri et al. (1992)[138]	52	40 μg/kg/min	>50	37	17 (46)	14 (38)	54	80
Marcowitz and Armstrong (1992)[139]	141	30 μg/kg/min	>50	109	47 (43)	—	96	66
Mazeika et al. (1992)[121]	50	20 μg/kg/min	>70	36	24 (67)	13 (36)	78	93
McNeill et al. (1992)[31]	80	40 μg/kg/min + atropine	>50	47	15 (32)	28 (60)	70	88
Marwick et al. (1993)[135]	217	40 μg/kg/min	>50	142	74 (52)	0 (0)	72	83
Hoffmann et al. (1993)[140]	66	40 μg/kg/min	>70	50	21 (42)	0 (0)	79	87
Previtali et al. (1993)[122]	80	40 μg/kg/min	>50	57	33 (58)	15 (26)	79	83
Prince et al. (1994)[52]	81	40 μg/kg/min + TEE	>70	21	16 (76)	7 (33)	90	94
Panza et al. (1994)[54]	76	40 μg/kg/min + TEE	>70	62	37 (60)	23 (37)	89	100
Takeuchi et al. (1994)	120	30 μg/kg/min	>50	74	37 (50)	62 (84)	85	93
Beleslin et al. (1994)[6]	136	40 μg/kg/min	>50	119	11 (9)	41 (34)	82	77
Ostojic et al. (1994)[30]	150	40 μg/kg/min	>50	131	16 (12)	38 (29)	75	79
Ostojic et al. (1994)[30]	55	40 μg/kg/min + dipyridamole	>50	131	16 (12)	38 (29)	92	89
Ho et al. (1995)[142]	54	40 μg/kg/min	>50	43	36 (84)	22 (51)	93	73

Abbreviations: CAD, coronary artery disease; TEE, transesophageal echocardiography.

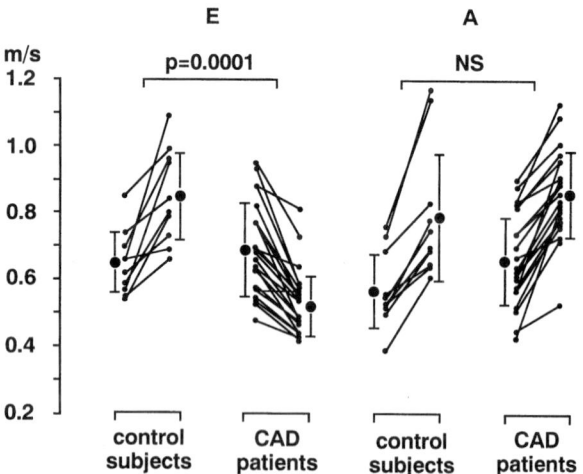

Fig. 13-12. Dobutamine-induced changes in diastolic function. Controls demonstrate an increase of passive (E-wave) and active (A-wave) filling velocities with stress. Patients with coronary artery disease develop delayed relaxation due to ischemia. (From El-Said,[155] with permission.)

those who fail to complete the dobutamine protocol due to the development of side effects.

Dobutamine and vasodilator stress echocardiography have been compared in several studies (Table 13-6). Although two of these papers showed the sensitivities to be comparable,[30,138] the remainder showed dobutamine stress echocardiography to be a more sensitive test for CAD,[6,47,146,147] especially in patients with single-vessel disease. This finding is concordant with the greater hemodynamic stress provided by dobutamine than dipyridamole, as discussed previously. As the diagnosis of CAD at myocardial perfusion imaging is based upon the detection of relative hyperemia, and both stressors induce coronary vasodilation, it is not surprising that their results are comparable with myocardial perfusion imaging.[47]

Dobutamine echocardiography has been compared with exercise echocardiography in several studies. These data have shown some variability, with three studies showing exercise provides higher levels

Table 13-6. Studies Comparing Sensitivity and Specificity of Dobutamine and Vasodilator Stress Echocardiography

Author	n	CAD n (%)	Multivessel (% all CAD)	Myocardial Infarction (% all CAD)	Sensitivity Dobutamine (%)	Sensitivity Dipyridamole (%)	Specificity Dobutamine (%)	Specificity Dipyridamole (%)
Martin et al. (1992)[146]	40	25 (63)	18 (72)	—	76	56	60	67
Salustri et al. (1992)[138]	46	18 (39)	18 (64)	15 (83)	79	82	78	89
Marwick et al. (1993)[47a]	97	59 (61)	28 (47)	0 (0)	85	58	82	87
Previtali et al. (1993)[122]	80	57 (71)	33 (58)	15 (26)	79	60	83	96
Beleslin et al. (1994)[6]	136	119 (88)	11 (9)	41 (34)	82	74	77	94
Ostojic et al. (1994)[30]	150	131 (87)	16 (12)	38 (29)	75	71	79	89

Abbreviations: CAD, coronary artery disease.
[a] Adenosine used instead of dipyridamole.

of sensitivity,[6,7,123] and two suggesting dobutamine is more sensitive.[48,140] The relative accuracy of the tests is probably dependent on whether the patients are able to stress maximally. In patients who have the dobutamine infusion terminated prematurely due to the development of side effects, the sensitivity of this technique can be expected to be less than that of exercise echocardiography.[7] Conversely, patients who are unable to exercise maximally will have better results with dobutamine imaging. Detection of a deterioration of pre-existing wall motion abnormalities may be difficult during exercise stress, but the ability to examine both low-dose and peak-dose responses may have improved the sensitivity of dobutamine stress for ischemia in this circumstance.[148]

Arbutamine and dobutamine stress appear to have similar levels of sensitivity. To date, these have not been compared on a head-to-head basis in a study of significant size. Such a study is likely to show that the tests are equivalent with respect to accuracy, but the relative feasibility and tolerability of these different stresses need to be defined.

Combination of Echocardiography or Scintigraphy with Dobutamine?

Several studies have compared stress echocardiography and perfusion scintigraphy on a head-to-head basis in patients undergoing dobutamine stress.[135,149,150] These have generally shown the echocardiographic techniques to be more specific, but to have slightly lower levels of sensitivity. The combination of both tests does enhance the prediction of CAD in a statistical sense,[151] but this increment of sensitivity is at the cost of specificity, and the combination is not justifiable apart from patients who are stressed submaximally with dobutamine.[135] In patients who are on antianginal therapy, scintigraphy may prove somewhat more sensitive, as the attainment of peak stress may be less important in the demonstration of flow heterogeneity than it is for the demonstration of ischemia. These issues have been discussed further in Chapter 4.

One of the limitations of a head-to-head study design in patients undergoing angiography is that there is a selection of patients toward those with a higher pretest probability of disease and more severe coronary disease. In a comparative study of patients who did not proceed to angiography, Simek et al.[152] demonstrated ischemia to be more frequently detected using perfusion imaging than stress echocardiography. Unfortunately, however, the disadvantage of such a study design is the fact that it is indeterminant whether this ischemia represents a true or false positive. In the context of recent data indicating a lower specificity of perfusion scintigraphy compared with echocardiography, it is probable that at least some of these discrepancies may have arisen because of false-positive perfusion images rather than false-negative stress echocardiograms.

PACING STRESS

Pacing stress has been combined with echocardiography, mainly using the transesophageal technique. The sensitivity of this approach has been reported to be in the range of 90%, with similar levels of specificity.[62,63,80,81,153] In a comparison with the exercise ECG, pacing stress echocardiography produced an increment of sensitivity, and appears to be comparable to myocardial perfusion scintigraphy.[154] To date, no large study has reported on the combination of transesophageal pacing with myocardial perfusion scintigraphy. Similarly, there is a dearth of comparitive data between pacing and pharmacologic stressors. Pacing stress appears to provide higher sensitivity than dipyridamole,[81] although with the current generation of equipment, it is probably less feasible.

While the technique has attractive features with respect to safety, due to the ability to suddenly terminate the stress, it is clearly more invasive and more uncomfortable than the other nonexercise alternatives, and offers no specific benefit at present.

CONCLUSION: WHICH IS THE OPTIMAL PHARMACOLOGIC STRESS AGENT?

The data summarized in this chapter offer evidence that pharmacologic stress agents of both the vasodilator and exercise-simulating type are feasible, well-tolerated, safe, and efficacious. The choice of an agent is highly dependent on the selection of a particular imaging modality. If the local expertise is greater in stress echocardiography, and the patient is unable to exercise, dobutamine or arbutamine appears to be the best choice, at least for diagnostic purposes. No data are currently available to rationalize a selection between dobutamine and arbutamine. If on the other hand the local expertise is more in the realm of perfusion imaging than stress echocardiography, a vasodilator stress will be the better choice. In patients who are unsuitable for this, such as those with asthma or conduction disturbances, dobutamine may be combined with perfusion imaging. Although the results of dobutamine and vasodilator stress perfusion scintigraphy are fairly comparable, we do not recommend dobutamine perfusion imaging as a routine because of the wealth of experience obtained with vasodilator stress perfusion imaging, and because of the factors that may limit the production of a satisfactory level of stress with dobutamine.

In patients who are able to exercise, there is no convincing data to suggest that a pharmacologic technique is the better option, apart from in patients with left bundle branch block. Indeed if such a course is chosen, much useful information that would be obtainable from the exercise test, relating to exercise capacity, symptom significance, rhythm evaluation, and ST-segment changes, will be neglected—all of which have potential prognostic as well as diagnostic importance.

REFERENCE

1. Gould KL, Lipscomb K: Effects of coronary stenoses on coronary flow reserve and resistance. Am J Cardiol 34:48, 1974
2. Gould KL, Kirkeeide RL, Buchi M: Coronary flow reserve as a physiologic measure of stenosis severity. J Am Coll Cardiol 15:459, 1990
3. Marwick TH: Current status of non-invasive techniques for the diagnosis of myocardial ischemia Acta Clin Belg 47:1, 1992
4. Iskandrian AS, Heo J, Kong B, Lyons E: Effect of exercise level on the ability of thallium-201 tomographic imaging in detecting coronary artery disease: analysis of 461 patients. J Am Coll Cardiol 14:1477, 1989
5. Marwick TH, Nemec JJ, Pashkow FJ et al.: Accuracy and limitations of exercise echocardiography in a routine clinical setting. J Am Coll Cardiol 19:74, 1992
6. Beleslin BD, Ostojic M, Stepanovic J et al.: Stress echocardiography in the detection of myocardial ischemia. Head-to-head comparison of exercise, dobutamine, and dipyridamole tests. Circulation 90:1168, 1994
7. Marwick TH, D'Hondt AM, Mairesse GH et al.: Comparative ability of dobutamine and exercise stress in inducing myocardial ischaemia in active patients. Br Heart J 72:31, 1994
8. Friedman J, Berman DS, Van Train K et al.: Patient motion in thallium-201 myocardial SPECT imaging. An easily identified frequent source of artifactual defect. Clin Nucl Med 13:321, 1988
9. Friedman J, Van Train K, Maddahi J et al.: "Upward creep" of the heart: a frequent source of false-positive reversible defects during thallium-201 stress-redistribution SPECT. J Nucl Med 30:1718, 1989
10. Previtali M, Ardissino D, Barberis P et al.: Hyperventilation and ergonovine tests in Prinzmetal's variant angina pectoris in man. Am J Cardiol 63:17, 1989
11. Pierard LA, De Landsheere CM, Berthe C et al.: Identification of viable myocardium by echocardiography during dobutamine infusion in patients with myocardial infarction after thrombolytic therapy: comparison with positron emission tomography. J Am Coll Cardiol 15:1021, 1990
12. Smart SC, Sawada S, Ryan T et al.: Low-dose dobutamine echocardiography detects reversible dysfunction after thrombolytic therapy of acute myocardial infarction. Circulation 88:405, 1993
13. Watada H, Ito H, Oh H et al.: Dobutamine stress echocardiography predicts reversible dysfunction and quantitates the extent of irreversibly damaged myocar-

dium after reperfusion of anterior myocardial infarction. J Am Coll Cardiol 24:624, 1994
14. Sutherland GR, Stewart MJ, Groundstroem KW et al.: Color Doppler myocardial imaging: a new technique for the assessment of myocardial function. J Am Soc Echocardiogr 7:441, 1994
15. Schroder K, Agrawal R, Voller H et al.: Improvement of endocardial border delineation in suboptimal stress-echocardiograms using the new left heart contrast agent SH U 508 A. Int J Card Imag 10:45, 1994
16. Porter TR, Xie F, Kricsfeld A et al.: Improved endocardial border resolution during dobutamine stress echocardiography with intravenous sonicated dextrose albumin. J Am Coll Cardiol 23:1440, 1994
17. Gould KL: Noninvasive assessment of coronary stenoses by myocardial perfusion imaging during pharmacologic coronary vasodilation. 1. Physiologic basis and experimental validation. Am J Cardiol 41:267, 1978
18. Rossen JD, Quillen JE, Lopez AG, et al.: Comparison of coronary vasodilation with intravenous dipyridamole and adenosine. Am J Cardiol 18:485, 1991
19. Brown BG, Josephson MA, Peterson RB, et al.: Intravenous dipyridamole with isometric handgrip for near maximal acute increase in coronary flow in patients with CAD. Am J Cardiol 48:1077, 1981
20. Verani MS, Mahmarian JJ: Myocardial perfusion scintigraphy during maximal coronary artery vasodilation with adenosine. Am J Cardiol 67:12D, 1991
21. Knabb RM, Gidday JM, Ely SW et al.: Effects of adenosine on myocardial adenosine and active hyperemia. Am J Physiol 247:H804, 1994
22. Picano E: Dipyridamole-echocardiography test: historical background and physiologic basis Eur Heart J 10:365, 1989
23. Tuttle RR, Mills J: Dobutamine: development of a new catecholamine to selectively increase cardiac contractility. Circ Res 36:185, 1975
24. Dennis CA, Pool PE, Perrins EJ et al.: Stress testing with closed loop arbutamine as an alternative to exercise. J Am Coll Cardiol 26:1151, 1995
25. Kiat H, Iskandrian AS, Villegas BJ et al.: Arbutamine stress thallium-201 single photon emission computed tomography using a computerized closed loop delivery system: Multicenter trial for evaluation of safety and diagnostic accuracy. J Am Coll Cardiol 26:1159, 1995
26. Cohen JL, Chan KL, Jaarsma W et al.: Arbutamine echocardiography: efficacy and safety of a new pharmacologic stress agent to induce myocardial ischemia and detect coronary artery disease. J Am Coll Cardiol 26:1168, 1995
27. Vanoverschelde JL, Wijns W, Essamri B et al.: Hemodynamic and mechanical determinants of myocardial O_2 consumption in normal human heart: effects of dobutamine. Am J Physiol 265:H1884, 1993
28. Hays JT, Mahmarian JJ, Cochran AJ, Verani MS: Dobutamine thallium-201 tomography for evaluating patients with suspected coronary artery disease unable to undergo exercise or vasodilator pharmacologic stress testing. J Am Coll Cardiol 21:1583, 1993
29. Pennell DJ, Underwood SR, Swanton RH et al.: Dobutamine thallium myocardial perfusion tomography. J Am Coll Cardiol 18:1471, 1991
30. Ostojic M, Picano E, Beleslin B et al.: Dipyridamole-dobutamine echocardiography: a novel test for the detection of milder forms of coronary artery disease. J Am Coll Cardiol 23:1115, 1994
31. McNeill AJ, Fioretti PM, el-Said SM et al.: Enhanced sensitivity for detection of coronary artery disease by addition of atropine to dobutamine stress echocardiography. Am J Cardiol 70:41, 1992
32. Fioretti PM, Poldermans D, Salustri A et al.: Atropine increases the accuracy of dobutamine stress echocardiography in patients taking beta-blockers. Eur Heart J 15:355, 1994
33. Picano E, Pingitore A, Conti U et al.: Enhanced sensitivity for detection of coronary artery disease by addition of atropine to dipyridamole echocardiography. Eur Heart J 14:1216, 1993
34. Stein L, Burt R, Oppenheim B et al.: Symptom-limited arm exercise increases detection of ischemia during dipyridamole tomographic thallium stress testing in patients with coronary artery disease. Am J Cardiol 75:568, 1995
35. Verzijlbergen JF, Vermeersch PH, Laarman GJ, Ascoop CA: Inadequate exercise leads to suboptimal imaging. Thallium-201 myocardial perfusion imaging after dipyridamole combined with low-level exercise unmasks ischemia in symptomatic patients with nondiagnostic thallium-201 scans who exercise submaximally. J Nucl Med 32:2071, 1991
36. Ignaszewski AP, McCormick LX, Heslip PG et al.: Safety and clinical utility of combined intravenous dipyridamole/symptom-limited exercise stress test with thallium-201 imaging in patients with known or suspected coronary artery disease [see comments]. J Nucl Med 34:2053, 1993
37. Stern S, Greenberg ID, Corne R: Effect of exercise supplementation on dipyridamole thallium-201 image quality. J Nucl Med 32:1559, 1991
38. Wilcken DEL, Paolini HJ, Eickens E: Evidence for intravenous dipyridamole producing a "coronary steal" effect in the ischaemic myocardium. Aust N Z J Med 1:8, 1971
39. Albro PC, Gould KL, Westcott RJ et al.: Non-invasive

assessment of coronary stenoses by myocardial imaging during pharmacologic coronary vasodilation. III Clinical trial. Am J Cardiol 42:751, 1978
40. Fleming RM, Rose CH, Feldmann KM: Comparing a high-dose dipyridamole SPECT imaging protocol with dobutamine and exercise stress testing protocols. Angiology 46:547, 1995
41. Casanova R, Patroncini A, Guidalotti L et al.: Dose and test for dipyridamole infusion and cardiac imaging early after uncomplicated acute myocardial infarction. Am J Cardiol 70:1402, 1992
42. Picano E, Distante A, Masini M et al.: Dipyridamole-echocardiography test in effort angina pectoris. Am J Cardiol 56:452, 1985
43. Picano E, Lattanzi F, Masini M et al.: High dose dipyridamole echocardiography test in effort angina pectoris. J Am Coll Cardiol 8:848, 1986
44. Jacobson AF, Cerqueira MD, Raisys V, Shattuc S: Serum caffeine levels after 24 hours of caffeine abstention: observations on clinical patients undergoing myocardial perfusion imaging with dipyridamole or adenosine. Eur J Nucl Med 21:23, 1994
45. Smits P, Corstens FH, Aengevaeren WR et al.: False-negative dipyridamole-thallium-201 myocardial imaging after caffeine infusion. J Nucl Med 32:1538, 1991
46. Ogilby JD, Iskandrian AS, Untereker WJ et al.: Effect of intravenous adenosine infusion on myocardial perfusion and function. Hemodynamic/angiographic and scintigraphic study [see comments]. Circulation 86:887, 1992
47. Marwick T, Willemart B, D'Hondt AM et al.: Selection of the optimal nonexercise stress for the evaluation of ischemic regional myocardial dysfunction and malperfusion. Comparison of dobutamine and adenosine using echocardiography and 99mTc-MIBI single photon emission computed tomography. Circulation 87:345, 1993
48. Cohen JL, Ottenweller JE, George AK, Duvvuri S: Comparison of dobutamine and exercise echocardiography for detecting coronary artery disease. Am J Cardiol 72:1226, 1993
49. Sawada SG, Segar DS, Ryan T et al.: Echocardiographic detection of coronary artery disease during dobutamine infusion. Circulation 83:1605, 1991
50. Mazeika PK, Nadazdin A, Oakley CM: Dobutamine stress echocardiography for detection and assessment of coronary artery disease. J Am Coll Cardiol 19:1203, 1992
51. Pellikka PA, Roger VL, Oh JK et al.: Stress echocardiography. Part II. Dobutamine stress echocardiography: techniques, implementation, clinical applications, and correlations. Mayo Clinic Proc 70:16, 1995
52. Prince CR, Stoddard MF, Morris GT et al.: Dobutamine two-dimensional transesophageal echocardiographic stress testing for detection of coronary artery disease. Am Heart J 128:36, 1994
53. Baer FM, Voth E, Deutsch HJ et al.: Assessment of viable myocardium by dobutamine transesophageal echocardiography and comparison with fluorine-18 fluorodeoxyglucose positron emission tomography. J Am Coll Cardiol 24:343, 1994
54. Panza JA, Laurienzo JM, Curiel RV et al.: Transesophageal dobutamine stress echocardiography for evaluation of patients with coronary artery disease. J Am Coll Cardiol 24:1260, 1994
55. van Rugge FP, van der Wall EE, de Roos A, Bruschke AV: Dobutamine stress magnetic resonance imaging for detection of coronary artery disease. J Am Coll Cardiol 22:431, 1993
56. Pennell DJ, Underwood SR, Ell PJ et al.: Dipyridamole magnetic resonance imaging: a comparison with thallium-201 emission tomography. Br Heart J 64:362, 1990
57. Baer FM, Smolarz K, Jungehulsing M et al.: Feasibility of high-dose dipyridamole-magnetic resonance imaging for detection of coronary artery disease and comparison with coronary angiography. Am J Cardiol 69:51, 1992
58. Weissman NJ, Nidorf SM, Guerrero JL et al.: Optimal stage duration in dobutamine stress echocardiography. J Am Coll Cardiol 25:605, 1995
59. Weissman NJ, Levangie MW, Newell JB et al.: Effect of beta-adrenergic receptor blockade on the physiologic response to dobutamine stress echocardiography. Am Heart J 130:248, 1995
60. Pasternac A, Gorlin R, Sonnenblick EH et al.: Abnormalities of ventricular motion induced by atrial pacing in coronary artery disease. Circulation 45:1195, 1972
61. Matthews RV, Haskell RJ, Ginzton LE, Laks MM: Usefulness of esophageal pill electrode atrial pacing with quantitative two-dimensional echocardiography for diagnosing coronary artery disease. Am J Cardiol 64:730, 1989
62. Iliceto S, Sorino M, D'Ambrosio G et al.: Detection of coronary artery disease by two-dimensional echocardiography and transesophageal atrial pacing. J Am Coll Cardiol 5:1188, 1985
63. Lambertz H, Kreis A, Trumper H, Hanrath P: Simultaneous transesophageal atrial pacing and transesophageal two-dimensional echocardiography: a

64. Iliceto S, Amico A, Marangelli V et al.: Doppler echocardiographic evaluation of the effect of atrial pacing-induced ischemia on left ventricular filling in patients with coronary artery disease. J Am Coll Cardiol 11: 953, 1988
65. Marwick T: Arbutamine stress testing with closed loop drug delivery: Toward the ideal or just another pharmacologic stress technique?. J Am Coll Cardiol 26: 1176, 1995
66. Verani MS, Mahmarian JJ, Hixson JB et al.: Diagnosis of coronary artery disease by controlled coronary vasodilation with adenosine and thallium-201 scintigraphy in patients unable to exercise. Circulation 82:80, 1990
67. Vogel WM, Apstein CS, Briggs LL et al.: Acute alterations in left ventricular diastolic chamber stiffness. Role of the "erectile" effect of coronary arterial pressure and flow in normal and damaged hearts. Circ Res 51:465, 1982
68. Cohen JL, Greene TO, Ottenweller J et al.: Dobutamine digital echocardiography for detecting coronary artery disease. Am J Cardiol 67:1311, 1991
69. Mazeika PK, Nadazdin A, Oakley CM: Clinical significance of abrupt vasodepression during dobutamine stress echocardiography. Am J Cardiol 69:1484, 1992
70. Pellikka PA, Oh JK, Bailey KR et al.: Dynamic intraventricular obstruction during dobutamine stress echocardiography. A new observation. Circulation 86: 1429, 1992
71. Bach DS, Armstrong WF: Adequacy of low-stress arbutamine to provoke myocardial ischemia during echocardiography. Am J Cardiol 76:259, 1995
72. Ranhosky A, Kempthorne-Rawson J: The safety of intravenous dipyridamole thallium myocardial perfusion imaging. Intravenous Dipyridamole Thallium Imaging Study Group. Circulation 81:1205, 1990
73. Picano E, Marini C, Pirelli S et al.: Safety of intravenous high-dose dipyridamole echocardiography. The Echo-Persantine International Cooperative Study Group. Am J Cardiol 70:252, 1992
74. Cerqueira MD, Verani MS, Schwaiger M et al.: Safety profile of adenosine stress perfusion imaging: results from the Adenoscan Multicenter Trial Registry. J Am Coll Cardiol 23:384, 1994
75. Abreu A, Mahmarian JJ, Nishimura S et al.: Tolerance and safety of pharmacologic coronary vasodilation with adenosine in association with thallium-201 scintigraphy in patients with suspected coronary artery disease. J Am Coll Cardiol 18:730, 1991
76. Mertes H, Sawada SG, Ryan T et al.: Symptoms, adverse effects, and complications associated with dobutamine stress echocardiography. Experience in 1118 patients. Circulation 88:15, 1993
77. Poldermans D, Fioretti PM, Boersma E et al.: Safety of dobutamine-atropine stress echocardiography in patients with suspected or proven coronary artery disease. Am J Cardiol 73:456, 1994
78. Picano E, Mathias W Jr, Pingitore A et al.: Safety and tolerability of dobutamine-atropine stress echocardiography: a prospective, multicenter study. Lancet 344:1190, 1994
79. Zabalgoitia M, Gandhi DK, Abi-Mansour P, Rosenblum J: Feasibility and safety of transesophageal stress echocardiography. Am J Med Sci 303:90, 1992
80. Kamp O, De Cock CC, Kupper AJ et al.: Simultaneous transesophageal two-dimensional echocardiography and atrial pacing for detecting coronary artery disease. Am J Cardiol 69:1412, 1992
81. Marangelli V, Iliceto S, Piccinni G et al.: Detection of coronary artery disease by digital stress echocardiography: comparison of exercise, transesophageal atrial pacing and dipyridamole echocardiography. J Am Coll Cardiol 24:117, 1994
82. Chambers CE, Brown KA: Dipyridamole-induced ST segment depression during thallium-201 imaging in patients with coronary artery disease: angiographic and hemodynamic determinants. J Am Coll Cardiol 12:37, 1988
83. Villanueva FS, Smith WH, Watson DD, Beller GA: ST-segment depression during dipyridamole infusion, and its clinical, scintigraphic and hemodynamic correlates. Am J Cardiol 69:445, 1992
84. Nishimura S, Kimball KT, Mahmarian JJ, Verani MS: Angiographic and hemodynamic determinants of myocardial ischemia during adenosine thallium-201 scintigraphy in coronary artery disease. Circulation 87:1211, 1993
85. Coma-Canella I: Dobutamine stress test to diagnose the presence and severity of coronary artery lesions in angina. Eur Heart J 12:1198, 1991
86. Mairesse GH, Marwick TH, Vanoverschelde JL et al.: How accurate is dobutamine stress electrocardiography for detection of coronary artery disease? Comparison with two-dimensional echocardiography and technetium-99m methoxyl isobutyl isonitrile (mibi) perfusion scintigraphy. J Am Coll Cardiol 24:920, 1994
87. Daoud EG, Pitt A, Armstrong WF: Electrocardiographic response during dobutamine stress echocardiography. Am Heart J 129:672, 1995
88. Gould KL, Sorenson SG, Albro P et al.: Thallium-201

myocardial imaging during coronary vasodilation induced by oral dipyridamole. J Nucl Med 27:31, 1986

89. Jain A, Mahmarian JJ, Borges-Neto S et al.: Clinical significance of perfusion defects by thallium-201 single photon emission tomography following oral dipyridamole early after coronary angioplasty. J Am Coll Cardiol 11:970, 1988

90. Borges-Neto S, Mahmarian JJ, Jain A et al.: Quantitative thallium-201 single photon emission computed tomography after oral dipyridamole for assessing the presence, anatomic location and severity of coronary artery disease. J Am Coll Cardiol 11:962, 1988

91. Taillefer R, Lette J, Phaneuf DC et al.: Thallium-201 myocardial imaging during pharmacologic coronary vasodilation: comparison of oral and intravenous administration of dipyridamole. J Am Coll Cardiol 8:76, 1986

92. Cohen JL, Greene TO, Alston JR et al.: Usefulness of oral dipyridamole digital echocardiography for detecting coronary artery disease. Am J Cardiol 64:385, 1989

93. Lattanzi F, Picano E, Frugoli A et al.: Oral vs intravenous dipyridamole echocardiography for detecting coronary artery disease. Chest 102:1189, 1992

94. Stringer KA, Branconi JM, Abadier R et al.: Disposition of oral dipyridamole in patients undergoing thallium 201 myocardial imaging. Pharmacotherapy 57:503, 1986

95. Leppo J, Boucher CA, Orada RD et al: Serial thallium-201 myocardial imaging after dipyridamole infusion: diagnostic utility in detection of coronary stenoses and relation to regional wall motion. Circulation 66:649, 1982

96. Schmoliner R, Dudczak R, Kronik G et al.: Thallium-201 imaging after dipyridamole in patients with coronary multivessel disease. Cardiology 70:145, 1983

97. Francisco DA, Collins SM, Go RT et al.: Tomographic thallium-201 myocardial perfusion scintigrams after maximal coronary artery vasodilation with intravenous dipyridamole. Comparison of qualitative and quantitative approaches. Circulation 66:370, 1982

98. Sochor H, Pachinger O, Ogris E et al.: Radionuclide imaging after coronary vasodilation: myocardial scintigraphy with thallium-201 and radionuclide angiography after administration of dipyridamole. Eur Heart J 5:500, 1984

99. Okada RD, Lim YL, Rothendler J et al.: Split dose thallium-201 dipyridamole imaging: a new technique for obtaining thallium images before and immediately after an intervention. J Am Coll Cardiol 1:1302, 1983

100. Ruddy TD, Dighero HR, Newell JB et al.: Quantitative analysis of dipyridamole-thallium images for the detection of coronary artery disease. J Am Coll Cardiol 10:142, 1987

101. Taillefer R, Lette J, Phaneuf DC et al.: Thallium-201 myocardial imaging during pharmacologic coronary vasodilation: comparison of oral and intravenous administration of dipyridamole. J Am Coll Cardiol 8:76, 1986

102. Lam JY, Chaitman BR, Glaenzer M et al.: Safety and diagnostic accuracy of dipyridamole-thallium imaging in the elderly. J Am Coll Cardiol 11:585, 1988

103. Kong BA, Shaw L, Miller DD, Chaitman BR: Comparison of accuracy for detecting coronary artery disease and side-effect profile of dipyridamole thallium-201 myocardial perfusion imaging in women versus men. Am J Cardiol 70:168, 1992

104. Mendelson MA, Spies SM, Spies WG et al.: Usefulness of single-photon emission computed tomography of thallium-201 uptake after dipyridamole infusion for detection of coronary artery disease. Am J Cardiol 69:1150, 1992

105. Huikuri HV, Korhonen UR, Airaksinen J et al.: Comparison of dipyridamole-handgrip test and bicycle exercise test for thallium tomographic imaging. Am J Cardiol 61:264, 1988

106. Iskandrian AS, Heo J, Nguyen T et al.: Assessment of coronary artery disease using single-photon emission computed tomography with thallium-201 during adenosine-induced coronary hyperemia. Am J Cardiol 67:1190, 1991

107. Nguyen T, Heo J, Ogilby JD, Iskandrian AS: Single photon emission computed tomography with thallium-201 during adenosine-induced coronary hyperemia: correlation with coronary arteriography, exercise thallium imaging and two-dimensional echocardiography [see comments]. J Am Coll Cardiol 16:1375, 1990

108. Nishimura S, Mahmarian JJ, Boyce TM, Verani MS: Quantitative thallium-201 single-photon emission computed tomography during maximal pharmacologic coronary vasodilation with adenosine for assessing coronary artery disease. J Am Coll Cardiol 18:736, 1991

109. Johnston DL, Daley JR, Hodge DO et al.: Hemodynamic responses and adverse effects associated with adenosine and dipyridamole pharmacologic stress testing: A comparison in 2,000 patients. Mayo Clinic Proc 70:331, 1995

110. Josephson MA, Brown BG, Hecht HS et al.: Noninvasive detection and localization of coronary stenoses in patients: comparison of resting dipyridamole and

exercise thallium-201 myocardial perfusion imaging. Am Heart J 103:1008, 1982
111. Burns RJ, Galligan L, Wright LM et al.: Improved specificity of myocardial thallium-201 single-photon emission computed tomography in patients with left bundle branch block by dipyridamole. Am J Cardiol 68:504, 1991
112. Jukema JW, van der Wall EE, van der Vis-Melsen MJ, Kruyswijk HH: Dipyridamole thallium-201 scintigraphy for improved detection of left anterior descending coronary artery stenosis in patients with left bundle branch block. Eur Heart J 14:53, 1993
113. Nishimura S, Mahmarian JJ, Boyce TM, Verani MS: Equivalence between adenosine and exercise thallium-201 myocardial tomography: a multicenter, prospective, crossover trial. J Am Coll Cardiol 20:265, 1992
114. Gupta NC, Esterbrooks DJ, Hilleman DE, Mohiuddin SM: Comparison of adenosine and exercise thallium-201 single-photon emission computed tomography (SPECT) myocardial perfusion imaging. The GE SPECT Multicenter Adenosine Study Group. J Am Coll Cardiol 19:248, 1992
115. Coyne EP, Belvedere DA, Vande Streek PR et al.: Thallium-201 scintigraphy after intravenous infusion of adenosine compared with exercise thallium testing in the diagnosis of coronary artery disease [see comments]. J Am Coll Cardiol 17:1289, 1991
116. O'Keefe JH Jr, Bateman TM, Barnhart CS: Adenosine thallium-201 is superior to exercise thallium-201 for detecting coronary artery disease in patients with left bundle branch block. J Am Coll Cardiol 21:1332, 1993
117. Masini M, Picano E, Lattanzi F et al.: High dose dipyridamole-echocardiography test in women: correlation with exercise-electrocardiography test and coronary arteriography. J Am Coll Cardiol 12:682, 1988
118. Massa D, Pirelli S, Gara E et al.: Exercise testing and dipyridamole echocardiography test before and 48 h after successful coronary angioplasty: prognostic implications. Eur Heart J, suppl. G, 10:13, 1989
119. Zoghbi WA, Cheirif J, Kleiman NS et al.: Diagnosis of ischemic heart disease with adenosine echocardiography. J Am Coll Cardiol 18:1271, 1991
120. Picano E, Severi S, Lattanzi F: The diagnostic and prognostic value of echo-dipyridamole in patients with suspected coronary disease. Giorn Ital Cardiol 21:621, 1991
121. Mazeika P, Nihoyannopoulos P, Joshi J, Oakley CM: Uses and limitations of high dose dipyridamole stress echocardiography for evaluation of coronary artery disease. Br Heart J 67:144, 1992
122. Previtali M, Lanzarini L, Fetiveau R et al.: Comparison of dobutamine stress echocardiography, dipyridamole stress echocardiography and exercise stress testing for diagnosis of coronary artery disease. Am J Cardiol 72:865, 1993
123. Dagianti A, Penco M, Agati L et al.: Stress echocardiography: comparison of exercise, dipyridamole and dobutamine in detecting and predicting the extent of coronary artery disease. J Am Coll Cardiol 26:18, 1995
124. Picano E, Parodi O, Lattanzi F et al.: Assessment of anatomic and physiological severity of single-vessel coronary artery lesions by dipyridamole echocardiography. Comparison with positron emission tomography and quantitative arteriography. Circulation 89:753, 1994
125. Heinle S, Hanson M, Gracey L et al.: Correlation of adenosine echocardiography and thallium scintigraphy. Am Heart J 125:1606, 1993
126. Amanullah AM, Bevegard S, Lindvall K, Aasa M: Assessment of left ventricular wall motion in angina pectoris by two-dimensional echocardiography and myocardial perfusion by technetium-99m sestamibi tomography during adenosine-induced coronary vasodilation and comparison with coronary angiography. Am J Cardiol 72:983, 1993
127. Perin EC, Moore W, Blume M et al.: Comparison of dipyridamole echocardiography with dipyridamole thallium scintigraphy for the diagnosis of myocardial ischemia. Clin Nucl Med 16:417, 1991
128. Jain A, Suarez J, Mahmarian JJ et al.: Functional significance of myocardial perfusion defects induced by dipyridamole using thallium-201 single-photon emission computed tomography and two-dimensional echocardiography. Am J Cardiol 66:802, 1990
129. Severi S, Picano E, Michelassi C et al.: Diagnostic and prognostic value of dipyridamole echocardiography in patients with suspected coronary artery disease. Comparison with exercise electrocardiography. Circulation 89:1160, 1994
130. Pirelli S, Danzi GB, Alberti A et al.: Comparison of usefulness of high-dose dipyridamole echocardiography and exercise electrocardiography for detection of asymptomatic restenosis after coronary angioplasty. Am J Cardiol 67:1335, 1991
131. Pirelli S, Massa D, Faletra F et al.: Exercise electrocardiography versus dipyridamole echocardiography testing in coronary angioplasty. Early functional evaluation and prediction of angina recurrence. Circulation 83:III38, 1991
132. Picano E, Lattanzi F, Masini M et al.: Comparison of the high-dose dipyridamole-echocardiography test and exercise two-dimensional echocardiography for

diagnosis of coronary artery disease. Am J Cardiol 59: 539, 1987
133. Mason JR, Palac RT, Freeman ML et al.: Thallium scintigraphy during dobutamine infusion: nonexercise-dependent screening test for coronary disease. Am Heart J 107:481, 1984
134. Pennell DJ, Mavrogeni S, Anagnostopoulos C et al.: Thallium myocardial perfusion tomography using intravenous dipyridamole combined with maximal dynamic exercise. Nucl Med Commun 14:939, 1993
135. Marwick T, D'Hondt AM, Baudhuin T et al.: Optimal use of dobutamine stress for the detection and evaluation of coronary artery disease: combination with echocardiography or scintigraphy, or both?. J Am Coll Cardiol 22:159, 1993
136. Nesto RW, Kowalchuk GJ: The ischemic cascade: temporal sequence of hemodynamic, electrocardiographic and symptomatic expressions of ischemia. Am J Cardiol 59:23C, 1987
137. Baptista J, Arnese M, Roelandt JRTC et al.: Quantitative coronary angiography in the estimation of the functional significance of coronary stenosis: Correlations with dobutamine-atropine stress test. J Am Coll Cardiol 23:1434, 1994
138. Salustri A, Fioretti PM, McNeill AJ et al.: Pharmacological stress echocardiography in the diagnosis of coronary artery disease and myocardial ischaemia: a comparison between dobutamine and dipyridamole. Eur Heart J 13:1356, 1992
139. Marcovitz PA, Armstrong WF: Accuracy of dobutamine stress echocardiography in detecting coronary artery disease. Am J Cardiol 69:1269, 1992
140. Hoffmann R, Lethen H, Kleinhans E et al.: Comparative evaluation of bicycle and dobutamine stress echocardiography with perfusion scintigraphy and bicycle electrocardiogram for identification of coronary artery disease. Am J Cardiol 72:555, 1993
141. Takeuchi M, Araki M, Nakashima Y, Kuroiwa A: Comparison of dobutamine stress echocardiography and stress thallium-201 single-photon emission computed tomography for detecting coronary artery disease. J Am Soc Echocardiogr 6:593, 1993
142. Ho FM, Huang PJ, Liau CS et al.: Dobutamine stress echocardiography compared with dipyridamole thallium-201 single-photon emission computed tomography in detecting coronary artery disease. Eur Heart J 16:570, 1995
143. Mazeika PK, Nadazdin A, Oakley CM: Influence of haemodynamics and myocardial ischaemia on Doppler transmitral flow in patients undergoing dobutamine echocardiography. Eur Heart J 15:17, 1994
144. Lattanzi F, Picano E, Masini M et al.: Transmitral flow changes during dipyridamole-induced ischemia. A Doppler-echocardiographic study. Chest 95:1037, 1989
145. el-Said ES, Roelandt JR, Fioretti PM et al.: Abnormal left ventricular early diastolic filling during dobutamine stress Doppler echocardiography is a sensitive indicator of significant coronary artery disease. J Am Coll Cardiol 24:1618, 1994
146. Martin TW, Seaworth JF, Johns JP et al.: Comparison of adenosine, dipyridamole, and dobutamine in stress echocardiography. Ann Intern Med 116:190, 1992
147. Previtali M, Lanzarini L, Ferrario M et al.: Dobutamine versus dipyridamole echocardiography in coronary artery disease. Circulation 83:III27, 1991
148. Senior R, Lahiri A: Enhanced detection of myocardial ischemia by stress dobutamine echocardiography utilizing the "biphasic" response of wall thickening during low and high dose dobutamine infusion. J Am Coll Cardiol 26:26, 1995
149. Forster T, McNeill AJ, Salustri A et al.: Simultaneous dobutamine stress echocardiography and technetium-99m isonitrile single photon emission computed tomography in patients with suspected coronary artery disease. J Am Coll Cardiol 21:1591, 1993
150. Gunalp B, Dokumaci B, Uyan C et al.: Value of dobutamine technetium-99m-sestamibi SPECT and echocardiography in the detection of coronary artery disease compared with coronary angiography. J Nucl Med 34:889, 1993
151. Senior R, Sridhara BS, Anagnostou E et al.: Synergistic value of simultaneous stress dobutamine sestamibi single-photon-emission computerized tomography and echocardiography in the detection of coronary artery disease. Am Heart J 128:713, 1994
152. Simek CL, Watson DD, Smith WH et al.: Dipyridamole thallium-201 imaging versus dobutamine echocardiography for the evaluation of coronary artery disease in patients unable to exercise. Am J Cardiol 72:1257, 1993
153. Stempfle HU, Kruger TM, Brandl BC et al.: Simultaneous transesophageal echocardiography and atrial pacing: assessment of the functional significance of coronary artery disease before surgical treatment of an abdominal aneurysm. Clin Invest 72:206, 1994
154. Norris LP, Stewart RE, Jain A et al.: Biplane transesophageal pacing echocardiography compared with dipyridamole thallium-201 single-photon emission computed tomography in detecting coronary artery disease. Am Heart J 126:676, 1993
155. El-Said EM, Roelandt JRTC, Fioretti P et al.: Abnormal left ventricular early diastolic filling during dobutamine stress Doppler echocardiography is a sensitive indicator of significant coronary artery disease. J Am Coll Cardiol 24:1618, 1994

Chapter 14

Can Coronary Angiography Provide Functional Data?

Neal G. Uren and Paolo G. Camici

PHYSIOLOGIC CONSIDERATIONS IN THE CORRELATION OF STENOSIS SEVERITY WITH FLOW

Coronary Vasodilator Reserve

The coronary flow reserve (or the coronary vasodilator reserve) has been proposed as an objective measurement to evaluate the vasodilator capacity of the coronary resistive vessels. This was defined as the ratio of maximal coronary blood flow to basal coronary blood flow, ideally for a given perfusion pressure, by Gould et al. in 1974.[1] Its validity has been confirmed and applied using different techniques such as coronary sinus thermodilution,[2] Doppler catheterization,[3] and positron emission tomography (PET),[4] using a pharmacological vasodilator stress such as intravenous dipyridamole or intracoronary papaverine. This index has been widely used as a physiologic measurement of the severity of a coronary artery stenosis, including all of its geometric characteristics.[5] The ultimate effect of a coronary stenosis depends on the degree to which the increased impedance to flow is compensated for by vasodilatation at the level of the resistive vessels—the "reserve." Thus, the coronary vasodilator reserve may be seen as an expression of the autoregulatory capacity of the coronary microcirculation. From this depends the ability of the coronary vascular bed to maintain an adequate flow for a given oxygen demand despite a decrease in coronary perfusion pressure (Fig. 14-1).[6]

In man, under conditions of a normal aortic pressure, the coronary vasodilator reserve, measured during pharmacologically induced vasodilatation, has a maximum of around 5 to 6 times.[7] It has been estimated from extensive animal studies that the coronary vasodilator reserve starts to diminish in the presence of a diameter stenosis greater than 40%. The reserve would be completely "exhausted" in the presence of a greater than 85% diameter stenosis when basal coronary flow starts to decline, at which point autoregulatory vasodilatation is maximal.[1,8]

The coronary vasodilator reserve, whether used to describe the functional significance of an epicardial stenosis or as an objective measure of the vasodilator capacity of a given myocardial territory, may be altered by many different factors. When used to measure functional stenosis severity, because of the nonlinear relationship between transstenotic pressure gradient and stenosis severity, a progressive nonlinear reduction in vasodilator reserve has been described (Fig. 14-2). There are three variables that need to be taken into further consideration when measuring the coronary vasodilator reserve at a given point in time: (1) the coronary perfusion pressure, (2) the basal flow, and (3) the pressure–flow relationship during maximal vasodilatation.

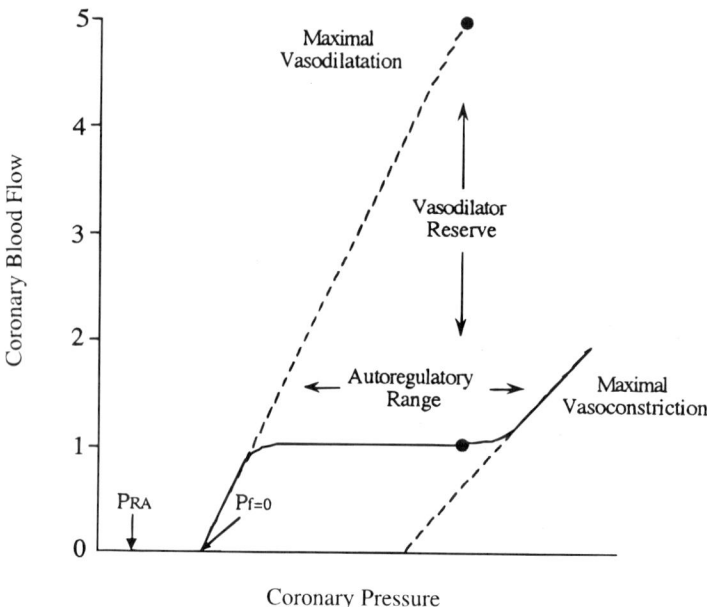

Fig. 14-1. Steady-state relationship between coronary flow and coronary arterial pressure in the left ventricle. The solid line describes the normal relationship. At a constant level of myocardial metabolic demand, coronary blood flow is maintained constant over a wide range of coronary perfusion pressure, between the boundaries of maximal vasodilatation and vasoconstriction. The black circles represent the basal state and maximal coronary blood flow under normal conditions, giving a coronary vasodilator reserve of 5.0. P_{RA}, right atrial pressure, $P_{f=0}$, pressure at zero flow (the back pressure opposing coronary flow). (Modified from Nanto et al.,[18] with permission.)

1. Modest changes in aortic pressure can have a significant effect on maximal flow because of the steepness of the pressure–flow relationship during maximal vasodilatation. Alternatively, small dynamic changes at the site of a severe stenosis (or passive collapse of the stenosis due to distal vasodilatation) leading to a reduction in perfusion pressure may reduce the reserve to a significant degree. However, under normal conditions the basal flow is changed very little due to autoregulation between mean arterial pressures of 40 and 130 mmHg.[6a]
2. Basal flow varies directly with myocardial oxygen demand (largely dependent on heart rate, contractility and myocardial wall tension), and as the denominator of coronary vasodilator reserve, a small increase in basal flow may reduce the derived value of vasodilator reserve accordingly. *This may lead to the estimation of erroneously low values of flow reserve* (Fig. 14-1).
3. The pressure–flow relationship during maximal dilation may be altered by several additional factors. Pathological left ventricular hypertrophy may reduce the slope of this relationship considerably (Fig. 14-3), such that a 30% increase in left ventricular mass may lead to a 60% reduction in vasodilator reserve.[6] This is probably due to a combination of factors, which include increased extravascular resistance and microvascular remodeling. Furthermore, changes in hemodynamic parameters may affect the coronary vasodilator capacity. An increase in left ventricular end-diastolic pressure (LVEDP) can reduce maximal vasodilatation. This effect is accentuated at low coronary perfusion pressures: for instance, at a perfusion pressure of 30 mmHg an elevation of LVEDP from 10 to 15 mmHg, would result in a 30% reduction in maximal flow. Tachycardia may reduce maximal dilatation by reducing diastolic filling time, notwithstanding the increase in myocardial oxygen demand and thus basal flow. It has also been shown that the effect of heart rate on

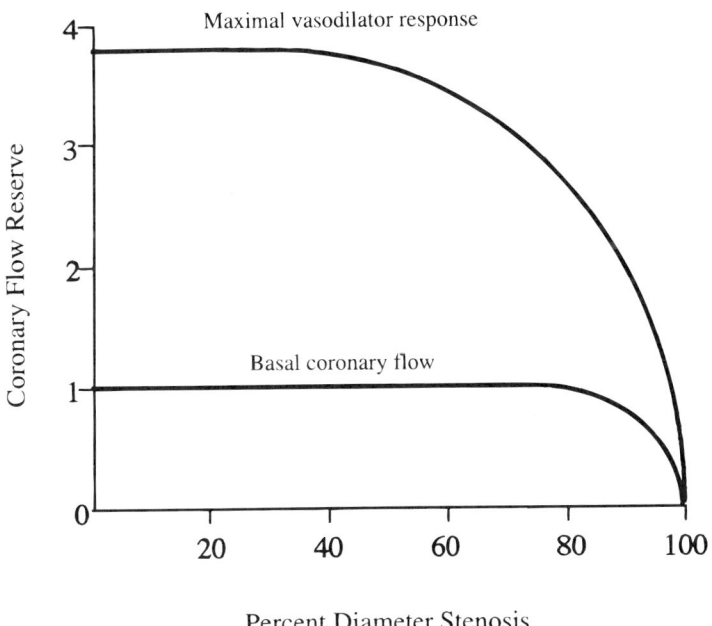

Fig. 14-2. The relationship between basal coronary blood flow and maximal coronary blood flow in dogs. With progressive acute epicardial coronary stenosis, basal flow did not change until the coronary stenosis diameter exceeded 80% stenosis. Maximal coronary blood flow decreased from the development of a 50% stenosis. (Modified from McGinn et al.,[10] with permission.)

maximal dilatation is greatest in the subendocardium because of the greater compressive effect of systolic contraction in the inner layers.[9] Other factors affecting coronary vasodilator reserve through an effect on maximal vasodilatation are blood viscosity and the extent of collateral flow, which is difficult to quantify, but which may be recruited by pharmacological agents.[6] In coronary artery disease, (CAD), the theoretical relationship between basal and maximal myocardial flow is complicated by increasing severity of coronary stenosis (Fig. 14-4).

Coronary vasodilator reserve remains highly reproducible in the same subjects studied several months apart using intracoronary Doppler catheterization, with any differences between studies being related to changes in heart rate rather than mean arterial pressure.[10] In this study investigating the hemodynamic determinants of the coronary vasodilator reserve, atrial pacing led to a rate-related increase in basal flow but with no reduction in maximal flow at a rate of 120 beats/min. A similar increase in basal flow was seen with volume expansion (an increase in preload), but with no effect on maximal flow. Increasing mean arterial pressure with handgrip caused a proportionate rise in basal and hyperemic flow and a maintenance of the coronary vasodilator reserve.[10] This confirms the importance of interpreting coronary vasodilator reserve measurements taking into account the hemodynamic conditions at the time of study.

It is often assumed in clinical studies that the coronary vasodilator reserve is a globally homogeneous measurement with regional differences that occur perhaps as a consequence of epicardial disease or altered myocardial function. Animal studies have suggested that there is marked spatial heterogeneity between different small regions of myocardium both under basal conditions and during maximal vasodilatation.[11] Regional coronary vasodilator reserve to adenosine may vary from 1.8 to 21.9, unexplained by different levels of basal and maximal flow. However, in this study using microspheres, basal coronary flow, and reserve appeared to be locally continuous, perhaps defining functional zones of vascular

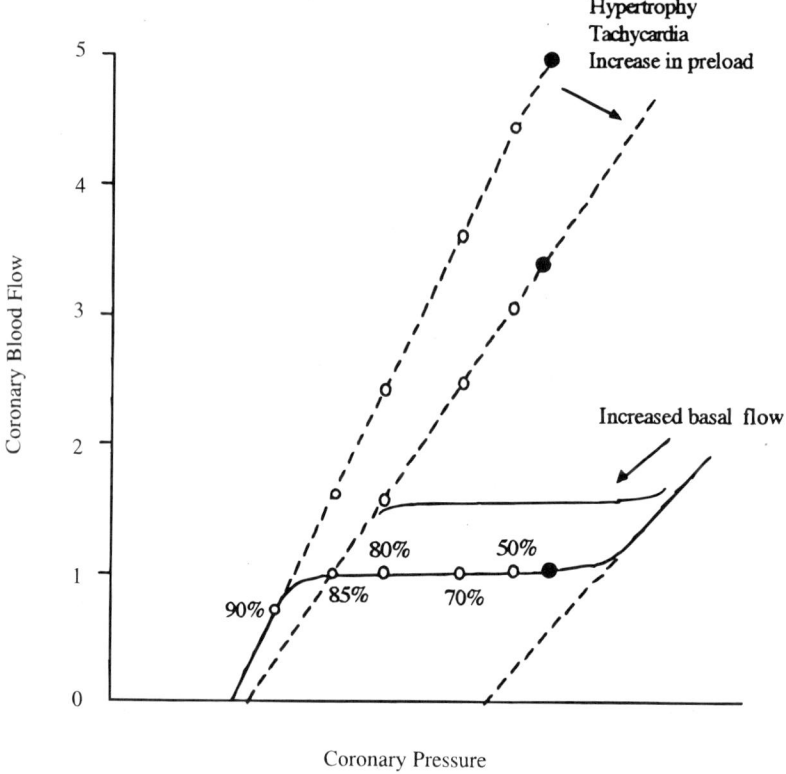

Fig. 14-3. Mechanisms whereby the coronary vasodilator reserve may be altered. The basal coronary flow may increase with an increase in myocardial metabolic demand. Maximal vasodilation may be reduced by an increase in heart rate or contractility, increased blood viscosity, and by resistive vessel dysfunction (in this case from 5.0 to just over 3.0). With hypertrophy, if coronary blood flow is measured as total flow (ml/min), then maximal vasodilation may be approximate to control values but with an increase in basal flow because of the increase in muscle mass. If measured as flow per unit mass (ml/min/g), then maximal vasodilation is reduced and basal flow per unit mass is the same as controls.[3] With a reduction in perfusion pressure, usually caused by epicardial disease, a third variable is introduced. Coronary artery stenoses are the open circles expressed as percent diameter stenoses. The horizontal distance along the autoregulatory range from control to stenosis is the transstenotic pressure gradient, which has a nonlinear relationship with diameter stenosis. Thus, resistive vessel dysfunction due to epicardial disease may compound an already compromised vasodilator reserve. (Modified from Nanto et al.,[18] with permission.)

control and vulnerability to ischemia.[11] With improvement in techniques used to measure myocardial perfusion in clinical studies, these observations may have implications in determining the control of regional microvascular function.

Absolute and Relative Coronary Flow Reserve

Conventionally, with the development of proximal coronary disease to a significant degree, coronary resistance would be determined by the geometry of the lesion, with compensatory vasodilatation in the resistive vessels to maintain basal myocardial perfusion and the increased perfusion in response to increased myocardial demand.[1] However, percent diameter stenosis is often poorly related to the functional severity of the coronary obstruction at quantitative angiography,[12] or the coronary vasodilator reserve at Doppler catheterization.[13] Cardiac workload (and thus myocardial oxygen consumption) may be affected by changes in aortic pressure (coronary perfusion pressure) and heart rate leading to changes in the basal coronary flow and ultimately

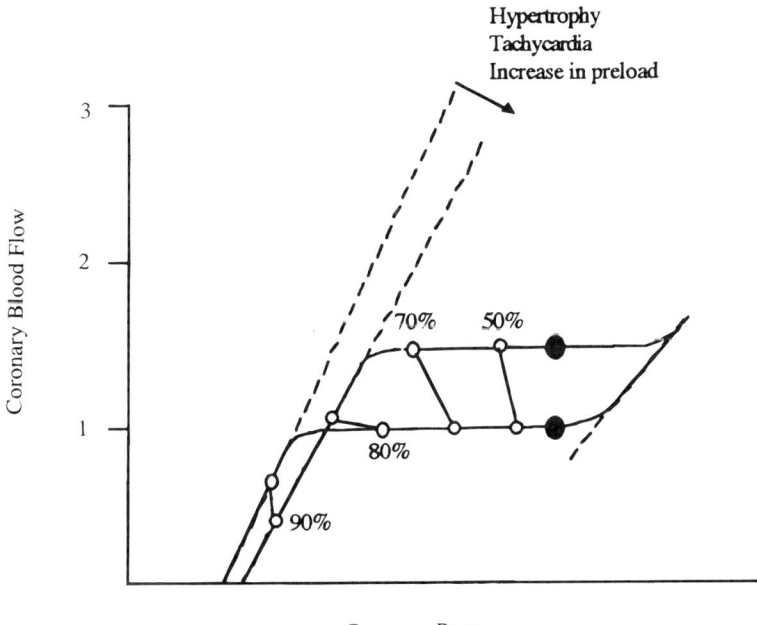

Fig. 14-4. The presence of coronary artery disease adds to the complexity of the coronary vasodilator reserve as a concept. Increasing myocardial oxygen demand, e.g., with atrial pacing, increases basal flow vertically in control subjects for a given perfusion pressure. With epicardial disease, the increase in flow leads to an increased pressure gradient across the lesion, as transstenotic gradients vary with flow (as well as with the degree of stenosis). With greater stenosis severity, the increase in basal flow is progressively limited, such that in the example, there is little increase in flow with an 80% stenosis, i.e., "exhaustion of reserve." With a 90% stenosis, flow is reduced. This is caused by the shift in the lowermost part of the pressure–flow relationship to the right. An increased heart rate does this by reducing diastolic filling time and increasing time-averaged compressive forces, the latter also augmented by increased contractility and hypertrophy. Increased preload increases pressure at zero flow ($P_{f=0}$) and right atrial pressure (P_{RA}). (Modified from Bergmann et al.,[4] with permission.)

maximal vasodilatation.[7] Thus, the absolute coronary vasodilator reserve may be affected by these determinants, independent of stenosis geometry. This may diminish the value derived under varying physiologic conditions and make it difficult to make comparisons between different patients.

The influence of these variables on absolute flow reserve has led to the concept of the relative coronary vasodilator reserve, which is the maximal coronary flow in the index artery/region divided by the maximal coronary flow in the control artery/region. As this ratio cancels out the effect of the prevailing physiologic conditions on coronary flow in both regions, this relative value reflects geometric stenosis severity, as long as there is maximal vasodilatation in the control region.

The ability to measure absolute and relative coronary vasodilator reserve is one of the major advantages of positron emission tomography. The quantitation of myocardial blood flow at basal and during maximal vasodilatation in the region subtended by the stenotic artery allows calculation of the absolute vasodilator reserve. In addition, the comparison with the reserve simultaneously measured in a control region determines the relative vasodilator reserve, thus providing complementary information in the same study.

Until the development of positron emission tomography, all methods used to measure basal and maximal coronary blood flow, and thus the coronary vasodilator response, were invasive. This often led to an interference with basal flow due either to the instrumentation of the patient or the injection of contrast medium, resulting in an underestimation of the ratio. It has also been argued that the coronary vasodilator reserve may appear diminished due to an increased basal flow in certain conditions such as left ventricular hypertrophy or valvular disease where it is argued that "vascular function" is normal.[14] This argument has led to the proposal that it is maximal myocardial blood flow alone that determines the functional status of the coronary circulation,[15] and that it is independent of other confounding variables. However, basal flow may change significantly after coronary interventions, which argues against the use of maximal flow as the solitary measurement of resistive vessel function.[16–19]

Variability of Myocardial Blood Flow

Although the overall relationship between the anatomic and functional measurements of stenosis severity is significant, for the same coronary stenosis severity, maximal myocardial blood flow and vasodilator reserve can vary appreciably in different patients. This may reflect either a true variability or may be due to the limitations of the assessment of stenosis severity and myocardial perfusion, or both. The former may occur through a differential responsiveness of individuals to pharmacological vasodilatation with adenosine and dipyridamole.[20,21]

Despite correcting for the rate-pressure product as an index of myocardiac oxygen consumption variability (particularly in the vasodilator response) may still occur because of different loading conditions and coronary perfusion pressures in individual patients.[6,10,22] However, a similar relationship is seen using coronary resistance to correct for coronary perfusion pressure.[23,24] Although patients were selected without extensive collateralization, individual variations in intramyocardial wall tension and resistive vessel function may have accounted for differences in regional myocardial perfusion.

To separate coronary stenosis severity assessment from coronary driving pressure, myocardial fractional flow reserve (FFR_{myo}) has been described to determine the functional significance of a coronary stenosis.[15] FFR_{myo} is the maximal achievable flow in a stenosis-related artery, divided by normal maximal flow if there were no stenosis. Thus, after a hyperemic stimulus, $FFR_{myo} = P_d - P_v/P_a - P_v$, where P_a is mean arterial pressure, P_d is distal coronary pressure, and P_v is central venous pressure. By also measuring coronary wedge pressure (P_w), which is distal coronary pressure at the time of balloon occlusion, it is possible to measure the component of myocardial flow that is coronary (i.e., through an epicardial stenosis—FFR_{cor}), and collateral flow (FFR_{coll}), with both expressed as a percentage of normal maximally achievable myocardial blood flow.[15] The derivation and validation of this approach are discussed in Chapter 15.

TECHNIQUES FOR MEASUREMENT OF CORONARY FLOW

Conventional Coronary Angiography

The anatomic significance of epicardial coronary artery disease may be documented by analysis of coronary arteriograms. However, it has been well-established for over 20 years that large intraobserver and interobserver variability exist with visual inspection of arteriograms.[25] Despite the use of computer-assisted edge-detection methods,[26] to reduce the error and inaccuracy of visual assessment,[27,28] poor correlations still exist with postmortem evaluation of coronary stenoses.[29,30] Furthermore, in the past, there has been a poor correlation between anatomic estimate of the severity of a coronary stenosis and any physiologic measurement of the functional significance of the stenosis.[13,31] This is particularly true for lesions in the 50% to 90% range of diameter stenoses, which are those of most interest in determining functional significance.[28]

Many of the problems relating to anatomic assessment occur because of the limitations of arteriography in reconstructing a three-dimensional lesion. Thus, the orientation of the vessel to the X-ray planes, stenoses at curvatures of the native vessel, and asymmetrical narrowing lead to inaccuracy. Because the effective resistance at the site of the stenosis is proportional to the fourth power of the radius, small changes in radius beyond the resolution of arteriographic assessment may cause disproportionately larger changes in resistance, particularly in more severe stenoses. Problems also arise when describing the stenosis as a percentage of normal as many adjacent "normal" segments are affected by diffuse disease, leading to an underestimation of stenosis severity. The use of intravascular ultrasound to document early atherosclerotic changes may indicate disease in "normal" adjacent segments or the presence of disease where not expected,[32] but the problem still remains of predicting functional significance of lesions. There is a complex nonlinear relationship between pressure gradient across a stenosis and flow through the stenosis which becomes accentuated with the increase in the severity of the stenosis.[1] Because of this, the effective resistance of even a rigid stenosis (without a dynamic component) increases with an increase in myocardial oxygen demand (i.e. flow requirement).

Quantitative Coronary Angiography

Minimal lumen diameter is an absolute measurement but does not take into account the large variability in coronary artery diameter in normal subjects. Moreover, the eccentricity and irregularity of a lesion will determine the transstenotic pressure drop for a given luminal diameter due to flow separation and shear stress,[33,34] causing much variability for the same absolute diameter. Estimates of the minimal cross-sectional area are complicated by uncertainty over the predicted reference area at the same point in a nondiseased artery, particularly in eccentric lesions, notwithstanding the process of arterial remodeling whereby the overall cross-sectional area of the artery may reduce as part of the restenosis process.[35]

The use of computer-assisted systems for quantitative coronary arteriography (QCA) has been developed as the final angiographic arbiter of coronary stenosis severity. Multicenter studies on the short- and long-term angiographic outcomes of patients undergoing interventional procedures or pharmacological restenosis prevention depend on the accuracy and reproducibility of such exact measurements of minimal lumen diameter. However, even with such advanced technology, comparing standardized cine films of either phantom stenoses,[36] or in patients before and after angioplasty,[37] by different automated QCA systems indicates significant variability in performance between systems. These findings argue for standardization of meta-analyses by adjusting for the precision of different QCA systems.

Despite its automation, QCA continues to have the limitation of two-dimensional projection of the vessel. As discussed in Chapter 16, in a direct comparison between intravascular ultrasound and quantitative arteriography in patients before and after angioplasty as well as in normal reference segments, cross-sectional areas measured by intravascular ultrasound were consistently larger.[38] Although there was a reasonable correlation between the two techniques in reference segments ($r = 0.73$), the correlation was poor at lesions before angioplasty ($r = 0.62$), deteriorating after angioplasty ($r = 0.47$). This emphasizes the inherent inaccuracy of the derived value of cross-sectional area from two isolated diameter measurements, even allowing for the extent of lumen eccentricity at the lesion site.

Quantitative coronary arteriography also fails to account for variables other than epicardial coronary diameter that determine myocardial perfusion. These include mean aortic pressure (coronary perfusion pressure), venous pressure (right atrial pressure), collateral blood flow, resistive vessel function in the distal vascular bed, and intraventricular wall tension.[5] These variables assume even greater importance in the presence of significant epicardial stenosis with progressive vasodilatation of the vascular bed distal to the obstruction to compensate for the proximal flow limitation.[6] Thus, new methods have been developed to allow an accurate and reproducible measure of the functional significance of an epicardial coronary stenosis.

Coronary Flow Measurement using PET

A number of techniques are available for measuring coronary or myocardial blood flow in man including Doppler catheterization, quantitative coronary arteriography, thermodilution, and measurement of the clearance of inert tracers.[39] Among radionuclide imaging techniques with single-photon emitters, thallium-201 perfusion scintigraphy is widely used to assess regional distribution of nutritive tissue perfusion. However, due to the intrinsic limitations of single-photon emission and to the physical constraints of the imaging systems, absolute quantification of blood flow using these techniques is not possible.

As discussed in Chapter 2, the physical properties of PET, coupled to coincidence detection and accurate attenuation correction, can overcome the limitations of single-photon imaging.[40] Dynamic PET imaging using later generation scanners, coupled with appropriate tracers and kinetic models (including corrections for underestimations of radiotracer concentration due to the partial volume effect and spillover from the left ventricular chamber[40]), permits the noninvasive quantitation of absolute regional myocardial blood flow.

Various positron-labeled tracers have been evaluated, including oxygen-15-labeled water ($H_2^{15}O$),[41–44] nitrogen-13-labeled ammonia ($^{13}NH_3$),[45–48] rubidium-82 (^{82}Rb),[49,50] and ^{62}Cu-PTSM.[51] Several clinical PET studies have used ^{82}Rb[52–54] to provide qualitative assessments of regional myocardial blood flow. Although models have been proposed for quantification of regional myocardial blood flow using ^{82}Rb,[50] these are limited by the critical dependence of the myocardial extraction of this tracer on the prevailing flow rate and myocardial metabolic state,[49] which makes quantification of blood flow under hyperemic conditions problematic. Furthermore, the high positron energy of this radionuclide results in relatively poor image quality and in a reduced spatial resolution due to the long positron track of ^{82}Rb. The accuracy of PET measurements with $^{13}NH_3$[45,47,48] and $H_2^{15}O$[42,43] (or both[55]) has been compared to radioactive microspheres in animals, over a wide range of flow values. As a consequence, the latter two tracers are currently the methodologies of choice for quantitative perfusion studies. Further details about coronary flow measurements with $^{13}NH_3$[45–48,55,51] and $H_2^{15}O$[41–44,56,57] are presented in Chapter 2.

It is important to realize that although inhalation of $C^{15}O_2$ provides a convenient means of generating an arterial supply of $H_2^{15}O$ avoiding both the sterility issue of intravenous infusion and the handling of high dose of radioactivity by the investigators, a slight overestimation of septal myocardial blood flow can be expected with $C^{15}O_2$ inhalation. This is probably due to inaccurate correction for spillover of activity from the right ventricular chamber in the presently available model. This kinetic model requires the following assumptions to be made.[43,44] (1) uptake of $H_2^{15}O$ is a nondiffusion limited process over a wide range of flows; (2) the partition coefficient of $H_2^{15}O$ between tissue and blood is constant; (3) the tissue within the region of interest is homogeneously perfused by $H_2^{15}O$. Therefore, in a myocardial region consisting of an admixture of normal and necrotic tissue, flow measurements with $H_2^{15}O$ will depend predominantly on activity coming from well perfused, residual normal myocardium.[58,59] The flow images obtained with $H_2^{15}O$ do not equal the quality of those with $^{13}NH_3$, due to lower counting statistics and the current lack of appropriate methods to generate voxel by voxel fitting of kinetic data. In a recent study comparing $H_2^{15}O$ and $^{13}NH_3$ in normal volunteers,[60] both tracers provided comparable estimates of myocardial blood flow, confirming previous animal data.[55] Whether this holds true under pathologic conditions is not known. The choice of the tracer and its way of administration will depend ultimately on a compromise based on experience, tracer availability, dosimetry, and convenience.

COMPARISON OF ANGIOGRAPHIC SEVERITY AND ALTERATIONS IN FLOW AND FLOW RESERVE

Relationship of PET Flow Measurements to Coronary Stenosis Severity

Effect of Defect Severity

In a study using rubidium-82 and nitrogen-13 ammonia, the relative perfusion reserve (the ratio of maximal to basal radioactivity in the stenosis-related region over that in a remote region) correlated well with percent diameter or area stenosis described by a curvilinear relationship.[46] A relationship with cross-sectional area was also preserved comparing lesions in the same index artery, and also with arteriographic-predicted stenosis flow reserve. However, not all patients had single-vessel disease and some had previous myocardial infarction or coronary angioplasty, which is known to affect myocardial blood flow in the stenosis-related regions,[19,51] and in the remote regions.[61] The subjective severity of perfusion defects at PET in the stenosis-related region correlates with the arteriographic-predicted stenosis flow reserve.[34] However, there is a wide variability in stenosis flow reserve in patients with diameter stenosis of 50% to 60%; 38% of patients with greater than 50% diameter stenoses have only a mild reduction in or even a normal estimated coronary flow reserve. This confirms the problem of defining myocardial perfusion in terms of the stenosis severity alone, despite the estimated stenosis flow reserve being independent of prevailing hemodynamic conditions.[62]

The demonstration of relative perfusion defects after exercise or pharmacological stress, using conventional nuclear cardiology testing, is a routine investigation to select patients who should undergo coronary arteriography. These procedures, however, give only an "all or nothing" picture on the presence or absence of CAD. The ability to make quantitative measurements of myocardial blood flow with PET allows determination of the functional significance of epicardial coronary lesions. In patients with single-vessel CAD, chronic stable angina, and no previous history of myocardial infarction, coronary flow reserve in response to a standard dose of dipyridamole was found to be markedly reduced in the myocardial regions supplied by the stenosed coronary artery compared with those regions supplied by angiographically normal vessels.[63]

Effects of Stenosis Severity

More recent work has evaluated the relationship between stenosis severity, measured by quantitative coronary angiography, and myocardial blood flow assessed by PET with $H_2^{15}O$ (Figs. 14-5 and 14-6).[23,24] In contrast with the canine model,[1,64] these studies showed that in humans, basal myocardial blood flow was preserved for greater than 90% diameter stenosis. Similar to the studies in dogs, the hyperemic response to dipyridamole and adenosine became attenuated at greater than 40% diameter stenosis and was abolished at greater than 80% stenosis.[23,24,65] Although the inverse relation between stenosis severity and coronary vasodilator reserve was highly significant, a certain degree of variability was observed, mainly at stenoses of intermediate severity. Variability was significantly less when minimal coronary resistance was plotted against stenosis severity, indicating the importance of accounting for interindividual differences in perfusion pressure.[23,24]

Relation to Other Indices of Ischemia

The relationship between regional myocardial blood flow, measured with $^{13}NH_3$ and PET, and regional wall motion, assessed by echocardiography, has also been investigated in patients with single-vessel CAD (> 50% diameter stenosis) without previous infarction following dipyridamole infusion.[66] Dipyridamole flow in regions subtended by a stenotic vessel was lower in the presence of inducible wall motion abnormalities (1.1 ± 0.3 ml/min/g) compared to regions without dysfunction (2.0 ± 0.4 ml/min/g, $p < 0.01$). In the former group with inducible wall motion abnormalities, the regional coronary flow reserve correlated well with the time to development of dyssynergy with dipyridamole ($r = 0.87$), and the reduction in flow reserve was greatest in those with most dyssynergy. Patients with inducible wall motion abnormalities had more severe cross-sectional area stenosis, 94 ± 8%, than those without change, 77 ± 10%. Thus, dipyridamole echocardiography not only has high specificity for coronary disease but the severity of the stenosis and impairment of coronary reserve were greater with earlier dyssynergy, indicating an objective measure of functional impairment.

Lessons from Intravascular Ultrasound

Angiographic visualization of atherosclerosis reflects luminal encroachment by plaque, which occurs when a sufficient plaque load is achieved, to cause a wall irregularity or even a stenosis in relation to another part of the vessel wall. In contrast, the evaluation of arterial wall architecture and circumferential dimensions by intravascular ultrasound allows for a more precise quantitation of atherosclerotic "plaque load" in vivo in the intact human coronary circulation, as well as plaque morphology. The reduction in cross-sectional luminal area may be accurately measured with intravascular ultrasound. Over the past 7 years, in addition to the accurate assessment of vessel wall morphology, clinical intravascular ultrasound has also developed as a adjunct to interventional therapies.[67] The following observations illustrate the limitations of quantitative angiography for the assessment of lesion significance; a more extensive discussion of intravascular ultrasound is presented in Chapter 16.

Intravascular ultrasound has been used to study epicardial arteries in 25 recently transplanted hearts from young donors (mean age 28 years).[32] In this unique study group, all donors aged under 25 years had a homogeneous nonlayered vessel wall. Another group of donors of mean age 32 years manifested

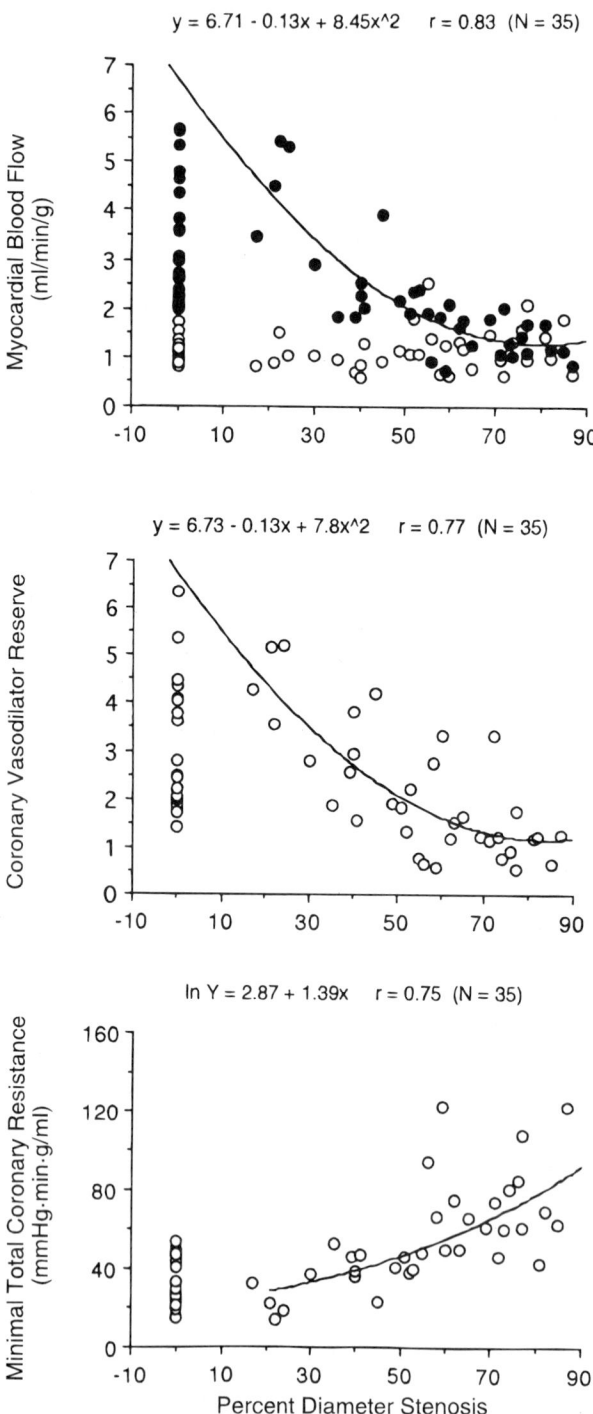

Fig. 14-5. (a) There was no significant correlation between corrected basal flow (white circles) and percent diameter stenosis. A significant fall of hyperemic blood flow (black circles) was observed with increasing percent diameter stenosis (top panel). Similarly, there was a significant fall in corrected coronary vasodilator reserve with increasing percent diameter stenosis (middle panel). Minimal total coronary resistance increased significantly with the severity of the stenosis (lower panel). For comparison, the values of corrected basal and hyperemic blood flow, coronary vasodilator reserve, and minimal total coronary resistance in normal controls are shown at zero percent diameter stenosis on the left of each panel. (From Ureu et al.,[23] with permission.) *(Figure continues.)*

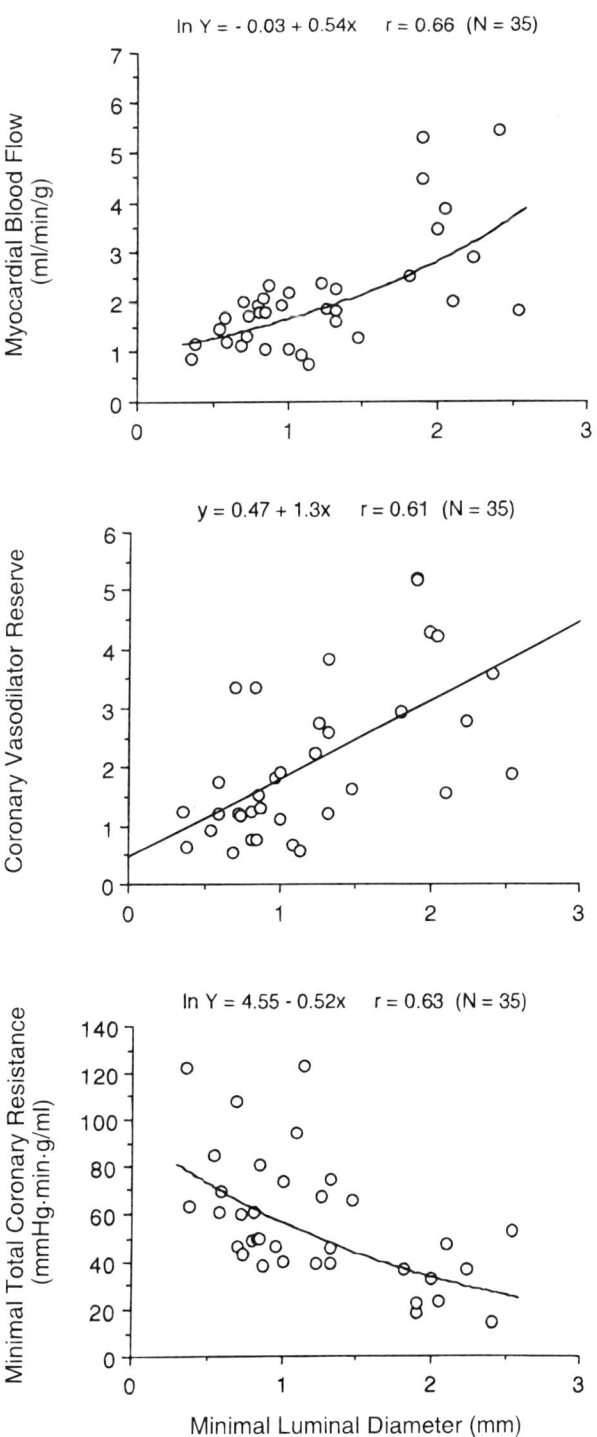

Fig. 14-5. *(Continued).* **(b)** There was a significant relationship between minimal lumen diameter and myocardial blood flow during hyperemia (top panel). Similarly, there was a significant relationship between minimal lumen diameter and coronary vasodilator reserve, with exhaustion of the coronary vasodilator reserve at a diameter of 0.5 mm (middle panel). Minimal total coronary resistance increased significantly with the progressive reduction in minimal lumen diameter (lower panel). (From Ureu et al.,[23] with permission.)

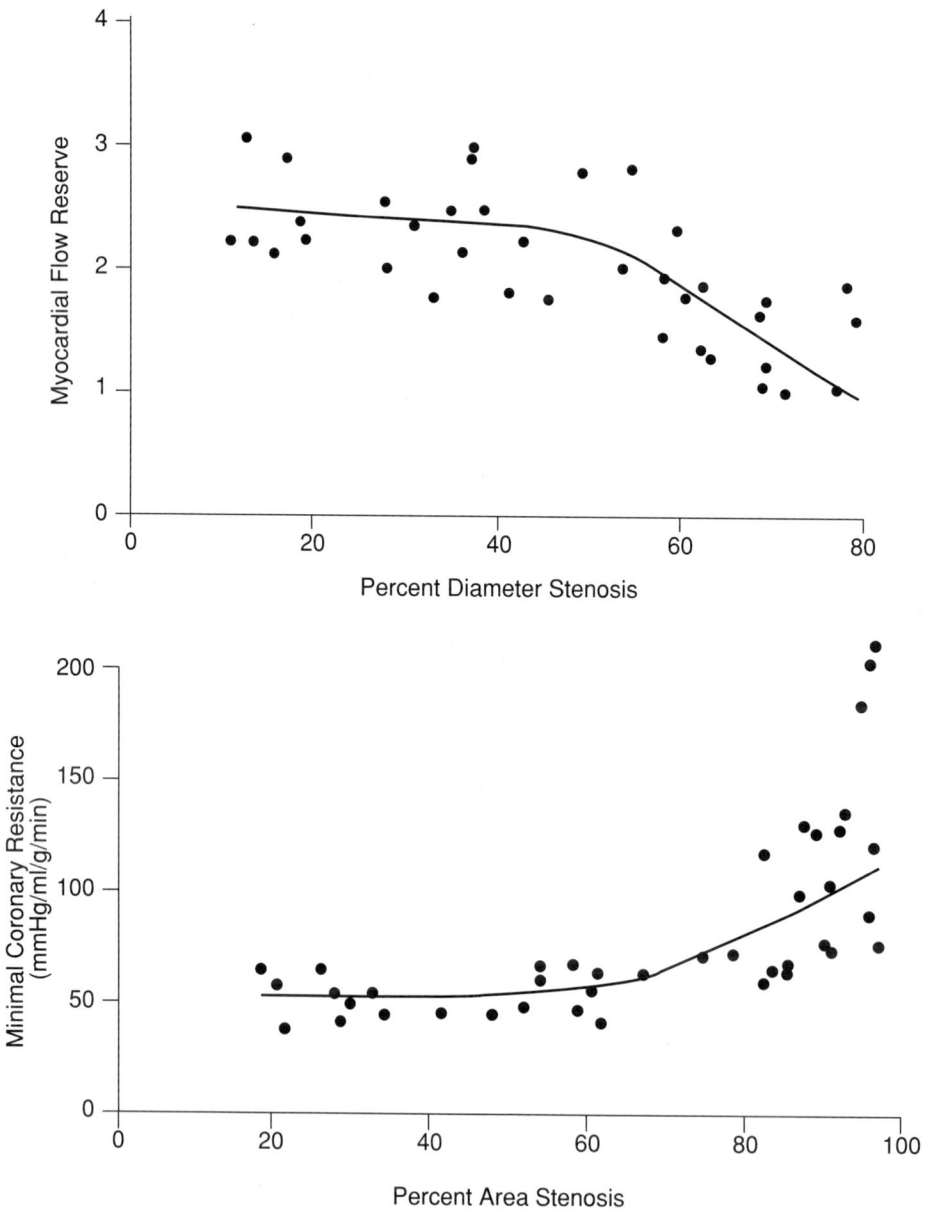

Fig. 14-6. (a) Scatterplot of relation between myocardial flow reserve and quantitative coronary angiographic measurements of percent diameter stenosis ($r = 0.77$, $p < 0.00001$). **(b)** Scatterplot of relation between minimal coronary resistance and quantitative coronary angiographic measurements of percent area stenosis ($r = 0.78$, $p < 0.00001$). (From Di Carli et al.,[24] with permission.)

a three-layered appearance. In 5 hearts, significant eccentric intimal thickening greater than 500 μm was shown in donors with risk factors for coronary disease, implying early coronary disease in the presence of angiographically normal arteries. Subsequent work by the same group in a larger group of transplant recipients over a period of long-term follow-up has shown that all 60 hearts had variable degree of concentric intimal thickening after 1 year, 42 of whom had normal coronary arteries at angiography.[68] This work confirms the inability of angiography to identify accurately the presence of early atherosclerosis.

Similarly, comparison of lumen volumes derived from examination of a vessel with either manual planimetry of two-dimensional images or three-dimensional intravascular ultrasound produced comparable values, $r = 0.97$ in both cases.[69] In contrast, a lesser correlation coefficient was obtained when the vessel was compared with volume derived from quantitative angiography in vivo studies.

The accurate measurement of epicardial cross-sectional area with intravascular ultrasound may be used in conjunction with the Doppler flow-wire to assess the response to various vasoactive agents, for example, adenosine, nitroglycerin, and ergonovine. In a study of normal coronary arteries of dogs,[70] adenosine induced resistive vessel dilatation alone, whereas nitroglycerin caused an increase in epicardial artery diameter and compliance as well as an increase in flow. Ergonovine constricted the epicardial artery studied to a small extent without change in blood flow velocity indicating a purely conduit effect. This study confirmed that the intravascular ultrasound catheter may be deployed on the Doppler guidewire. In physiologic terms, it also demonstrated that when extrapolating coronary blood flow from coronary blood flow velocity, it is imperative that accurate measurement of intraluminal diameter is achieved.

Comparison with Doppler and Pressure Catheter Approaches

Doppler Catheter Measurements

An angiographically obtained index derived from all the geometric characteristics of a coronary stenosis including percent stenosis, cross-sectional area, and stenosis length has been derived in dogs with acute experimental epicardial stenoses.[71] This study demonstrated a strong correlation between the arteriographic-predicted flow reserve and the value measured with an epicardial Doppler probe.

In man, intracoronary Doppler catheterization (which is discussed in detail in Chapter 15) has been used to measure blood flow velocity.[72,73] Absolute blood flow can be estimated from flow velocity if cross-sectional diameter is known. There is a significant inverse relationship between coronary stenosis severity and absolute myocardial blood flow during maximal vasodilatation. In man, basal flow remains constant with increasing stenosis severity and maximal myocardial blood flow starts to diminish progressively for stenoses greater than 40%. This is consistent with the preservation of basal flow to collateral-dependent myocardium seen in patients with complete coronary occlusion and normal regional wall motion.[74]

Measurement of the coronary vasodilator reserve using the Doppler catheter correlates reasonably well with the stenosis severity whether described as percent diameter stenosis ($r = 0.82$), percent area stenosis ($r = 0.85$), or minimum cross-sectional area ($r = 0.79$) determined from orthogonal planes.[3] Despite these reasonable correlations in a highly selected group, there was substantial scatter on individual vasodilator reserve values at any level of stenosis. This variability emphasizes the additional factors affecting coronary flow in the presence of an epicardial stenosis. These include failure of the Doppler technique to take into account collateral flow, flow to side branches proximal to the stenosis, and expansion of the distal vascular bed during vasodilatation. Consequently, Doppler approaches do not measure nutritive perfusion,[33] in contrast to PET, which assesses the functional severity of CAD.[74-76]

Measurement Using the Doppler Flow-Wire

The coronary vasodilator reserve may also be assessed with the flow-wire and, as such, is a composite measure of the ability of conduit vessels to deliver flow to the distal vasculature and of coronary resistive vessel function. The coronary vasodilator reserve remains highly reproducible in the same subjects studied several months apart using intracoronary Doppler catheterization, with interstudy differences related to changes in heart rate rather than mean arterial pressure.[10] With the flow-wire, it is possible to measure the above parameters of flow velocity and correlate them with coronary artery compliance and, ultimately, epicardial atherosclerotic bulk measured by intravascular ultrasound.

The use of the Doppler wire permits measurement of blood flow before and after a stenosis, and may therefore escape some of the limitations of the Doppler catheter, which is positioned more proximally in the vessel. As discussed in Chapter 16, Kern et al. proposed an impaired phasic pattern of coronary flow on passing the wire distal to an intermediate stenosis, and impaired distal hyperemia (i.e., a coronary flow reserve of <2.0) as flow-wire-derived parameters indicating an epicardial stenosis of functional severity.[77] In the left coronary artery, for example, the diastolic component of flow velocity is greater than 1.8 times that of the systolic component, this ratio being reduced with increasing stenosis severity. Furthermore, values of the coronary flow reserve when measured proximal to a significant stenosis may approach normal values due to side branch hyperemia. Placing a wire distal to the lesion obviates this effect, giving a significantly impaired value at the time of vasodilator stress.

Transstenotic Pressure Measurement

A direct relationship exists between pressure and flow when coronary resistance is kept constant (as is the case at the time of maximal coronary vasodilatation). Thus, transstenotic pressure measurements may be used as an indication of stenosis severity. Earlier attempts to equate the transstenotic pressure gradient (ΔP) with functional stenosis severity were relatively inaccurate because the smallest balloon catheters used were sufficiently large to obstruct the lumen significantly at the lesion site, and measurements were done in the basal state (where there is a constant change in epicardial and myocardial resistance due to myocardial oxygen demand, arterial pressure, and resistive vasomotion). A new approach, using a fluid-filled guidewire of 0.015 in. (0.38 mm) diameter, is discussed in Chapter 15. This is now validated both with respect to its feasibility, and its direct effect on stenosis hemodynamics.[78]

Using the fractional flow reserve (FFR) as a new gold standard for functional severity, a curvilinear relationship has been reported with the pressure gradient and percent area stenosis ($r^2 = 0.67$) or obstruction area ($r^2 = 0.72$).[79] Despite a wide spread of values, characteristic of previous studies with QCA, a high degree of concordance has been shown between a myocardial FFR of less than 0.72 and a minimum luminal diameter of less than 1.5 mm or diameter stenosis of greater than 50%. This suggests the ability of QCA-derived indices of stenosis severity to correlate broadly with a physiologic variable such as myocardial FFR, but not to allow accurate prediction particularly between different individuals.

Methodologic Comparisons among QCA, Doppler Wire Parameters, and FFR

The accuracy of quantitative coronary angiography in determining the functional severity of coronary stenoses has been compared with translesional pressure gradient measurement and the Doppler flowwire.[80] In this study, 28 large coronary arteries with a mean diameter stenosis ranging from 29% to 73% were studied using all three techniques. As described, the Doppler-tipped angioplasty guidewire was used to measure coronary blood flow velocity distal to a coronary stenosis, thus accurately determining the functional significance of a stenosis.[73] Subsequently, a 2.2F infusion catheter was positioned across the lesion in question and the translesional pressure gradient measured on pull-back. With quantitative angiography, the predicted pressure gradient (ΔP) was determined by the equation: $\Delta P = fQ + sQ^2$, where Q is the volume of flow, f the coefficient of pressure loss through viscous friction, and s the coefficient of pressure loss due to exit separation (both f and s are determined by the length, three-dimensional shape, and diameters of reference artery and stenosis and an average flow of 20 cm/s is usually assumed).[5] The stenosis flow reserve is derived from quantitative angiogram and assures standard physiological conditions such as a mean arterial pressure of 100 mmHg and a "normal" flow reserve of 5 times. No correlation was shown between the QCA-derived pressure gradient and that measured directly at baseline or at hyperemia. Similarly, the *QCA-derived stenotic flow reserve bore no relation to either the directly measured coronary flow reserve by Dopp-*

ler flow-wire or the translesional pressure gradient. Furthermore, comparisons between either coronary flow reserve or translesional pressure gradient with the simpler measurements of minimal luminal area or cross-sectional area were not significant.

The existing literature is split with respect to the accuracy of QCA-defined measurements of coronary flow reserve: some argue against it,[13] or demonstrate wide confidence intervals,[81] whereas others concur with a direct relationship, with translesional pressure gradient.[34,81,82] Certainly, wide confidence intervals exist in predicting coronary flow reserve from angiography.[23,24,82] Some variation may be accounted for by assumptions regarding coronary flow when estimating the pressure gradient at QCA, as wide variations in distal coronary flow velocity may occur,[80] perhaps through resistive vessel dysfunction and variable intramyocardial pressure. Stenosis flow reserve is also limited as it is a lesion-specific measure and takes neither the aforementioned variables nor collateral flow and true myocardial perfusion pressure into account. Nonetheless, allowing for the technical limitations of a sizable infusion catheter for measuring translesional gradient and assuming planar angiographic projections, even when using the simple direct measure of minimal luminal diameter, there was a poor correlation with direct measures of functional severity.

CONCLUSIONS

Coronary angiography is the most readily available means of assessing the extent and apparent severity of CAD. Quantitative coronary arteriography has been the gold standard of anatomical assessment against which other methodologies have been compared. However, the physiologic severity of coronary stenosis, particularly in the intermediate range, is less reproducibly defined by this technique. Angiographically defined values such as the stenosis flow reserve may be determined, albeit making several assumptions regarding loading conditions. However, many variables (including hemodynamic status, intramyocardial wall tension, presence of side branches, extent of collateralization, and resistive vessel function) determine myocardial perfusion. These influences reduce the accuracy of arteriography to determine functional severity.

Quantitative imaging techniques such as PET allow regional assessment of myocardial blood flow and coronary vasodilator reserve and have led to a greater understanding of myocardial perfusion in the presence and absence of epicardial coronary stenoses. The development of the Doppler-tipped guide wire to complement coronary interventional procedures has improved the ability to assess functional significance of coronary stenoses in the catheter laboratory. The derivation of the fractional flow reserve from translesional pressure gradient measurement also allows accurate determination of functional stenosis severity, and is much less affected by the prevailing hemodynamic conditions than is the Doppler wire approach. These latter techniques combined with coronary angiography remain the best readily available techniques for determining stenosis severity. Their use will continue in the immediate future until an accurate, readily-available, noninvasive imaging modality such as "one-stop" magnetic resonance imaging is validated to measure regional myocardial blood flow and stenosis severity at the same time.

REFERENCES

1. Gould KL, Lipscomb K, Hamilton GW: Physiologic basis for assessing critical coronary stenosis. Am J Cardiol 33:87, 1974
2. Ganz W, Tamura K, Marcus HS et al.: Measurement of coronary sinus blood flow by continuous thermodilution in man. Circulation 44:181, 1971
3. Wilson RF, Laughlin DE, Ackell PH et al.: Transluminal, subselective measurement of coronary artery blood flow velocity and vasodilator reserve in man. Circulation 72:82, 1985
4. Bergmann SR, Fox KAA, Geltman EM, Sobel BE: Positron emission tomography of the heart. Prog Cardiovasc Dis 28:165, 1985
5. Kirkeeide RL, Gould KL, Parsel L: Assessment of coronary stenoses by myocardial perfusion imaging during pharmacologic coronary vasodilation. VIII. Validation of coronary flow reserve as a single integrated functional measure of stenosis severity reflecting all its geometric dimensions. J Am Coll Cardiol 7:103, 1986
6. Klocke FJ: Measurements of coronary flow reserve: defining pathophysiology versus making decisions about patient care. Circulation 76:1183, 1987

6a. Canty JM: Coronary pressure function and steady-state pressure from relations during autoregulation in the unanesthetized dog. Circ Res 63:821, 1988
7. Gould KL, Kirkeeide RL, Buchi M: Coronary flow reserve as a physiologic measure of stenosis severity. J Am Coll Cardiol 15:459, 1990
8. Gould KL, Lipscomb K: Effects of coronary stenoses on coronary flow reserve and resistance. Am J Cardiol 34:48, 1974
9. Bache RJ, Cobb FR: Effect of maximal coronary vasodilatation on transmural myocardial perfusion during tachycardia in the awake dog. Circ Res 41:648, 1977
10. McGinn AL, White CW, Wilson RF: Interstudy variability of coronary flow reserve. Influence of heart rate, arterial pressure, and ventricular preload. Circulation 81:1319, 1990
11. Austin RE, Aldea GS, Coggins DL et al.: Profound spatial heterogeneity of coronary reserve. Discordance between patterns of resting and maximal myocardial blood flow. Circ Res 67:319, 1990
12. Demer LL, Gould KL, Goldstein RA et al.: Assessment of coronary artery disease severity by positron emission tomography. Comparison with quantitative arteriography in 193 patients. Circulation 79:825, 1989
13. White CW, Wright CB, Doty DB et al.: Does visual interpretation of the coronary arteriogram predict the physiologic importance of a coronary stenosis? N Engl J Med 310:819, 1984
14. Hoffman JIE: A critical review of coronary reserve. Circulation, suppl. I, 75:I6, 1987
15. Pijls NHJ, van Son JAM, Kirkeeide RL et al.: Experimental basis of determining maximum coronary, myocardial, and collateral blood flow by pressure measurements for assessing functional stenosis severity before and after percutaneous transluminal coronary angioplasty. Circulation 86:1354, 1993
16. Zijlstra F, Reiber JC, Juilliere Y, Serruys PW: Normalization of coronary flow reserve by percutaneous transluminal coronary angioplasty. Am J Cardiol 61:55, 1988
17. Kern MJ, Deligonul U, Vandormael M et al.: Impaired coronary vasodilator reserve in the immediate postcoronary angioplasty period: analysis of coronary artery flow velocity indexes and regional cardiac venous efflux. J Am Coll Cardiol 13:860, 1989
18. Nanto S, Kodama K, Hori M, Mishima M et al.: Temporal increase in resting coronary blood flow causes an impairment of coronary flow reserve after coronary angioplasty. Am Heart J 123:28, 1992
19. Uren NG, Crake T, Lefroy DC et al.: Delayed recovery of coronary resistive vessel function after coronary angioplasty. J Am Coll Cardiol 21:612, 1993
20. Wilson RF, White CW: Intracoronary papaverine: an ideal coronary vasodilator for studies of the coronary circulation in conscious humans. Circulation 73:444, 1986
21. Rossen JD, Simonetti I, Marans ML, Winniford MD: Coronary dilation with standard dose dipyridamole and dipyridamole combined with handgrip. Circulation 79:556, 1989
22. Gould KL, Kirkeeide RL, Buchi M: Coronary flow reserve as a physiologic measure of stenosis severity. Part I. Relative and absolute coronary flow reserve during changing aortic pressure and cardiac workload. Part II. Determination from arteriographic stenosis dimensions under standardized conditions. J Am Coll Cardiol 15:459, 1990
23. Uren NG, Melin JA, De Bruyne B et al.: Myocardial blood flow as a function of coronary stenosis severity in man. N Engl J Med 330:1782, 1994
24. Di Carli M, Czernin J, Sherman T et al.: Relationship between stenosis severity, hyperemic blood flow, flow reserve, and coronary resistance in patients with coronary artery disease. Circulation 91:1944, 1995
25. Zir LM, Miller SW, Dinsmore RE et al.: Interobserver variability in coronary angiography. Circulation 53:627, 1976
26. Brown BG, Bolson E, Frimer M, Dodge HT: Quantitative coronary angiography. Estimation of dimensions, hemodynamic resistance, and atheroma mass of coronary artery lesions using the arteriogram and digital computation. Circulation 55:329, 1977
27. Hoffman JIE: Maximal coronary flow and the concept of coronary vascular reserve. Circulation 70:15, 1984
28. Klocke FJ, Ellis AK, Canty JM: Interpretation of changes in coronary flow that accompany pharmacologic interventions. Circulation, suppl. V, 75:434, 1987
29. Grondin CM, Dyrda I, Pasternac A et al.: Discrepancies between cineangiography and postmortem findings in patients with coronary artery disease and recent revascularization. Circulation 49:703, 1974
30. Marcus ML, Armstrong ML, Heistad DD et al.: Comparison of three methods of evaluating coronary obstructive lesions: postmortem arteriography, pathologic examination and measurement of regional myocardial perfusion during maximal vasodilation. Am J Cardiol 49:1699, 1982
31. Harrison DG, White CW, Hiratzka LF et al.: The value of lesion cross-sectional area determined by quantitative coronary angiography in assessing the physiologic significance of proximal left anterior descending coronary arterial stenoses. Circulation 69:1111, 1984
32. St Goar FG, Pinto FJ, Alderman EL et al.: Detection

of coronary atherosclerosis in young adult hearts using intravascular ultrasound. Circulation 86:756, 1992
33. Sibley DH, Millar HD, Hartley CJ, Whitlow PL: Subselective measurement of coronary blood flow velocity using a steerable Doppler catheter. J Am Coll Cardiol 8:1332, 1986
34. Wilson RF, Marcus ML, White CW: Prediction of the physiologic significance of coronary arterial lesions by quantitative lesion geometry in patients with limited coronary artery disease. Circulation 75:723, 1987
35. Mintz GS, Kovach JA, Pichard AD et al.: Geometric remodelling is the predominant mechanism of clinical restenosis after coronary angioplasty. J Am Coll Cardiol 23:138A(abstr.), 1994
36. Keane D, Haase J, Slager CJ et al.: Comparative validation of quantitative coronary angiography systems. Circulation 91:2174, 1995
37. Desmet W, De Scheerder I, Beatt KJ et al.: In vivo comparison of different quantitative edge detection systems used for measuring coronary arterial diameters. Cath Cardiovasc Diag 34:72, 1995
38. Haase J, Ozaki Y, di Mario C et al.: Can intracoronary ultrasound correctly assess the luminal dimensions of coronary artery lesions? A comparison with quantitative angiography. Eur Heart J 16:112, 1995
39. Marcus ML, Wilson RF, White CW: Methods of measurement of myocardial blood flow in patients; a critical review. Circulation 76:245, 1987
40. Huang S-C, Phelps ME: Principles of tracer kinetic modelling in PET and autoradiography. p. 287. In Phelps ME, Maziotta JC, Schelbert HR (eds): Positron Emission Tomography and Autoradiography: Principles and Applications for the Brain and Heart. Raven Press, New York, 1986
41. Bergmann SR, Fox KAA, Rand AL et al.: Quantification of regional myocardial blood flow in vivo with $H_2^{15}O$. Circulation 70:724, 1984
42. Bergmann SR, Herrero P, Markham J et al.: Noninvasive quantification of myocardial blood flow in human subjects with O-15 labelled water and positron emission tomography. J Am Coll Cardiol 14:639, 1989
43. Araujo LI, Lammertsma AA, Rhodes CG et al.: Noninvasive quantification of regional myocardial blood flow in normal volunteers and patients with coronary artery disease using oxygen-15 labeled carbon dioxide inhalation and positron emission tomography. Circulation 83:875, 1991
44. Iida H, Rhodes CG, De Silva R et al.: Use of a left ventricular time-activity curve as a noninvasive input function in $H_2^{15}O$ dynamic positron emission tomography. J Nucl Med 33:1669, 1992

45. Bellina CR, Parodi O, Camici P et al.: Simultaneous in vitro and in vivo validation of nitrogen-13 ammonia for the assessment of regional myocardial blood flow. J Nucl Med 31:1335, 1990
46. Hutchins GD, Schwaiger M, Rosenspire KC et al.: Noninvasive quantification of regional blood flow in the human heart using N-13 ammonia and dynamic positron emission tomographic imaging. J Am Coll Cardiol 15:1032, 1990
47. Kuhle WG, Porenta G, Huang SC et al.: Quantification of regional myocardial blood flow using N13-ammonia and reoriented dynamic positron emission tomographic imaging. Circulation 86:1004, 1992
48. Muzik O, Beanlands RSB, Hutchins GD et al.: Validation of nitrogen 13 ammonia tracer kinetic model for quantification of myocardial blood flow using PET. J Nucl Med 34:83, 1993
49. Herrero P, Markham J, Shelton ME et al.: Noninvasive quantification of regional myocardial perfusion with rubidium-82 and positron emission tomography. Exploration of a mathematical model. Circulation 82:1377, 1990
50. Herrero P, Markham J, Shelton ME, Bergmann SR: Implementation and evaluation of a two-compartment model for quantification of myocardial perfusion with rubidium-82 and positron emission tomography. Circ Res 70:496, 1992
51. Herrero P, Markham J, Weinheimer CJ et al.: Quantification of regional myocardial perfusion with generator-produced ^{62}Cu-PTSM and positron emission tomography. Circulation 87:173, 1993
52. Selwyn AP, Allan RM, L'Abbate A et al.: Relation between regional myocardial uptake of rubidium-82 and perfusion: absolute reduction of cation uptake in ischemia. Am J Cardiol 50:112, 1982
53. Camici P, Araujo LI, Spinks T et al.: Increased uptake of ^{18}F-fluoro-deoxyglucose in postischemic myocardium of patients with exercise-induced angina. Circulation 74:81, 1986
54. Gould KL, Goldstein RA, Mullani N et al.: Noninvasive assessment of coronary stenoses by myocardial imaging during coronary vasodilation. VIII: feasibility of 3D cardiac positron imaging without a cyclotron using generator-produced Rb-82. J Am Coll Cardiol 7:775, 1986
55. Bol A, Melin JA, Vanoverschelde J-L et al.: Direct comparison of [^{13}N] ammonia and [^{15}O] water estimates of perfusion with quantification of regional myocardial blood flow by microspheres. Circulation 87:512, 1993
56. Bergmann SR, Hack S, Tewson T et al.: The depen-

dence of accumulation of $^{13}NH_3$ by myocardium on metabolic factors and its implications or the quantitative assessment of perfusion. Circulation 6:34, 1980
57. West JB, Holland RAB, Dollery CT, Matthews CME: Interpretation of radioactive gas clearance rates in the lung. J Appl Physiol 17:14, 1962
58. Iida H, Rhodes CG, De Silva R et al.: Myocardial tissue fraction: Correction for partial volume effects and measure of tissue viability. J Nucl Med 32:2169, 1991
59. Herrero P, Weinheimer CJ, Toeniskoetter PD et al.: Does perfusible tissue index (PTI) reflect tissue that can exchange water or flow heterogeneity? J Nucl Med 34:87(abstr.), 1993
60. Nitzsche E, Choi Y, Czernin J et al.: Comparison of O–15 water and N–13 ammonia PET measurement of myocardial blood flow in humans. Circulation 88: I–274(abstr.), 1993
61. Uren NG, Crake T, Lefroy DC et al.: Reduced coronary vasodilator function in infarcted and normal myocardium after myocardial infarction. N Engl J Med 331: 222, 1994
62. Goldstein RA, Kirkeeide RL, Demer LL et al.: Relation between geometric dimensions of coronary artery stenoses and myocardial perfusion reserve in man. J Clin Invest 79:1473, 1987
63. Sambuceti G, Parodi O, Marcassa C et al.: Alteration in regulation of myocardial blood flow in one vessel coronary artery disease determined by positron emission tomography. Am J Cardiol 72:538, 1993
64. Lipscomb K, Gould KL: Mechanism of the effect of coronary artery stenosis on coronary flow in the dog. Am Heart J 89:60, 1975
65. Beanlands RS, Muzik O, Sutor R et al.: Noninvasive determination of regional perfusion reserve in coronary artery disease using N–13 ammonia PET. J Nucl Med 33:826(abstr.), 1992
66. Picano E, Parodi O, Lattanzi F et al.: Assessment of anatomic and physiologic severity of single vessel coronary artery lesions by dipyridamole echocardiography: comparison with positron emission tomography and quantitative arteriography. Circulation 89:753, 1994
67. Waller BF, Pinkerton CA, Slack JD: Intravascular ultrasound: a histological study of vessels during life: the new "gold standard" for vascular imaging. Circulation 85:2305, 1992
68. St Goar FG, Pinto FJ, Alderman EL et al.: Intracoronary ultrasound in cardiac transplant recipients: in vivo evidence of "angiographically silent" intimal thickening. Circulation 85:979, 1992
69. Matar FA, Mintz GS, Douek P et al.: Coronary artery lumen volume measurement using three-dimensional intravascular ultrasound: validation of a new technique. Cath Cardiovasc Diag 33:214, 1994
70. Sudhir K, MacGregor JS, Barbant SD et al.: Assessment of coronary conductance and resistance vessel reactivity in response to nitroglycerin, ergonovine and adenosine: in vivo studies with simultaneous intravascular two-dimensional and Doppler ultrasound. J Am Coll Cardiol 21:1261, 1993
71. Gould KL, Kelley KO, Bolson EL: Experimental validation of quantitative coronary arteriography for determining pressure-flow characteristics of coronary stenosis. Circulation 66:930, 1982
72. Wilson RF, Laughlin DE, Ackell PH et al.: Transluminal, subselective measurement of coronary artery blood flow velocity and vasodilator reserve in man. Circulation 72:82, 1985
73. Doucette JW, Corl PD, Payne HM et al.: Validation of a Doppler guidewire for intravascular measurement of coronary artery flow velocity. Circulation 85:1899, 1992
74. Vanoverschelde JL, Wijns W, Deprè C et al.: Mechanisms of chronic regional postishemic dysfunction in humans: new insights from the study of noninfarcted collateral-dependent myocardium. Circulation 87: 1513, 1993
74a. Schelbert HR, Wisenberg G, Phelps ME et al.: Noninvasive assessment of coronary stenoses by myocardial imaging during pharmacologic coronary vasodilation. VI. Detection of coronary artery disease in man with intravenous $^{13}NH_3$ and positron computed tomography. Am J Cardiol 49:1197, 1982
75. Gould KL, Goldstein RA, Mullani A et al.: Noninvasive assessment of coronary stenoses by myocardial imaging during pharmacologic coronary vasodilation. VIII. Clinical feasibility of positron cardiac imaging without a cyclotron using generator-produced rubidium-82. J Am Coll Cardiol 7:775, 1986
76. Gould KL: Identifying and measuring severity of coronary artery stenosis: quantitative coronary arteriography and positron emission tomography. Circulation 78:237, 1988
77. Kern MJ, Donohue TJ, Bach RG et al.: Clinical applications of the Doppler coronary flow velocity guidewire for interventional procedures. J Intervent Cardiol 6: 345, 1993
78. De Bruyne B, Pijls NHJ, Paulus WJ et al.: Transstenotic coronary pressure gradient measurement in humans: in vitro and in vivo evaluation of a new pressure monitoring angioplasty guide wire. J Am Coll Cardiol 22: 119, 1993
79. Bartunek J, Sys SU, Hendrickx GR et al.: Quantitative

coronary angiography in predicting functional significance of coronary stenoses in unselected patients. Eur Heart J 16:1432(abstr.), 1995
80. Tron C, Kern MJ, Donohue TJ et al.: Comparison of quantitative angiographically derived and measured translesion pressure and flow velocity in coronary artery disease. Am J Cardiol 75:111, 1995
81. Zijlstra F, Van Omeren J, Reiber JHC, Serruys PW: Does the quantitative assessment of coronary artery dimensions predict the physiologic significance of a coronary stenosis? Circulation 75:1154, 1987
82. Zijlstra F, Fioretti P, Reiber JHC, Serruys PW: Which cine-angiographically assessed anatomic variable correlates best with functional assessments of stenosis severity? A comparison of quantitative analysis of the coronary cineangiogram with measured coronary flow reserve and exercise/redistribution thallium-201 scintigraphy. J Am Coll Cardiol 12:686, 1988

Chapter 15

Coronary Pressure Measurements in Evaluation of Coronary Stenoses

Bernard de Bruyne, Jozef Bartunek, and Nico HJ Pijls

ANATOMIC VERSUS FUNCTIONAL INDICES OF CORONARY STENOSES

In daily clinical practice, coronary angiography still remains the ultimate diagnostic test to prove the presence and to evaluate the extent and location of epicardial coronary narrowings. Quantitative analysis of the coronary arteriogram has drastically limited variability in the measurement of coronary stenoses, enabling the quantification and comparison of different therapeutic strategies.[1] However, it is increasingly appreciated that a refined understanding of the atherosclerotic lesion and its consequences on the perfusion of the underlying myocardium requires much more than the silhouette of the arterial lumen provided by contrast angiography.[2] Furthermore, in routine clinical practice the most common problem is not to assess the progression of a lesion over time (which has been favored by improvements in reproducibility), but to determine whether a given coronary narrowing can be flow limiting and thus responsible for the complaints of the patient.

The usefulness of quantitative coronary angiography for clinical decision making in lesions of intermediate severity remains controversial because the capability of even the most accurate geometric depiction of a coronary stenosis is limited to reflect its physiological repercussions on the underlying myocardium. Studies reporting close correlations between angiographic and functional assessments have been carried out in highly selected patients, who are not really representative for routine patients posing a problem for clinical decision making in everyday practice.[3,4] Therefore, the majority of therapeutic decisions in patients with documented coronary artery disease continue to be based on inferences about the adequacy or inadequacy of myocardial perfusion—based upon the patient's complaints as well as stress testing. Given the fact that the restenosis rate after coronary angioplasty exceeds 20%, that acute coronary occlusion after stenting and angioplasty remains a matter of concern, and that coronary bypass surgery is not without morbidity and mortality, it seems highly desirable to demonstrate the hemodynamic significance of a lesion to justify a revascularization procedure. However, examination of a large insurance database showed that in only 30% of patients was a stress test of any kind available at the time of angioplasty,[5] and as more and more diagnostic and therapeutic catheterizations are performed during the same session, information on the functional importance of the lesions should be available in the catheterization laboratory.

Over the last few years, three invasive techniques

have been proposed and have gained some clinical applications: myocardial videodensitometry, Doppler flow velocitometry, and coronary pressure measurements. The present chapter focuses on the technique and the clinical usefulness of coronary pressure measurements.

RATIONALE OF CORONARY PRESSURE MEASUREMENTS

Physiology of the Coronary Microcirculation

Under baseline conditions, coronary and myocardial flow are mainly controlled by the resistance of the microcirculation ("resistance vessels" and capillaries). The regulation of coronary resistance is, in turn, influenced by myocardial oxygen consumption or pharmacologic stimuli so that wide variations in coronary resistance may induce a fourfold to sixfold increase in myocardial blood flow. The extent to which coronary resistance can decrease is termed "resistance reserve." This reserve is needed to ensure normal myocardial metabolism during maximal exercise.

Pathophysiology of the Microcirculation

According to the theory of fluid dynamics, the transstenotic pressure gradient reflects the total amount of energy lost when a fluid traverses a narrowing. The underlying physiological rationale can be summarized as follows: when blood flows from the proximal to the distal part of a normal epicardial coronary artery, almost no energy is lost, and, therefore, the pressure remains constant throughout this "conductance vessel."[6] Data derived from the fluid-filled lumen in the first generation of balloon catheters supported the acceptance of the translesional pressure gradient as a straightforward index of the physiological consequences of a lesion on the flow to the subtended myocardium.

In the presence of an epicardial coronary narrowing, potential energy is transformed into kinetic energy and heat when blood traverses the lesion. The resultant pressure drop reflects the total loss of energy. To maintain resting myocardial perfusion at a constant level, a decrease in myocardial resistance will compensate for the increased resistance due to the epicardial narrowing. Therefore, the degree to which arteriolar resistance can decrease further to maintain myocardial flow is diminished (decreased resistance reserve). The decrease in myocardial resistance exactly reflects to what extent the myocardium has adapted its resistance to attune blood supply to metabolic demand. Furthermore, the progressive development of collateral circulation will contribute to myocardial flow and perfusion pressure. Hence, distal coronary pressure and transstenotic pressure gradient represent ideal indices of the physiological consequences of a given coronary narrowing on the perfusion of the underlying myocardium.

Thus far, two problems have hampered the use of coronary pressure measurements as a clinical tool for evaluating the severity of coronary stenoses: *first*, distal coronary pressure has been measured through the angioplasty balloon catheters inducing a major and unpredictable overestimation of the pressure gradient[7] (Fig. 15-1); *second*, translesional pressure gradient has been measured under baseline conditions when myocardial flow is autoregulated. Yet, it is impossible to relate precisely the extent of the pressure gradient to the severity of the epicardial narrowing unless translesional flow is known or at least maximum (i.e., during maximum vasodilatation).

The following sections summarize how these two problems have been solved.

MEASUREMENTS OF TRANSLESIONAL PRESSURE GRADIENT

The use of the transstenotic pressure gradient measured through the balloon catheter as a guide to the progress of coronary dilation was originally described by Grüntzig et al.[8] A marked reduction in coronary flow often accompanies the placement of the deflated balloon across the lesion, and the size of the angioplasty catheter (even with the presently available ultra-low-profile balloons) may cause a marked overestimation of the gradient. While the development of monorail angioplasty catheters[9] (which precluded pressure measurements) further prompted the trend away from measuring distal pressures during coronary angioplasty, the development of two types of pressure monitoring guidewires has revived interest in coronary pressure measurements.

High-Fidelity Pressure Monitoring Guidewires

The first guidewire equipped with a pressure sensor was reported by Emanuelsson et al.[10] The diameter of this sensor is 0.45 mm and it is positioned 3 cm

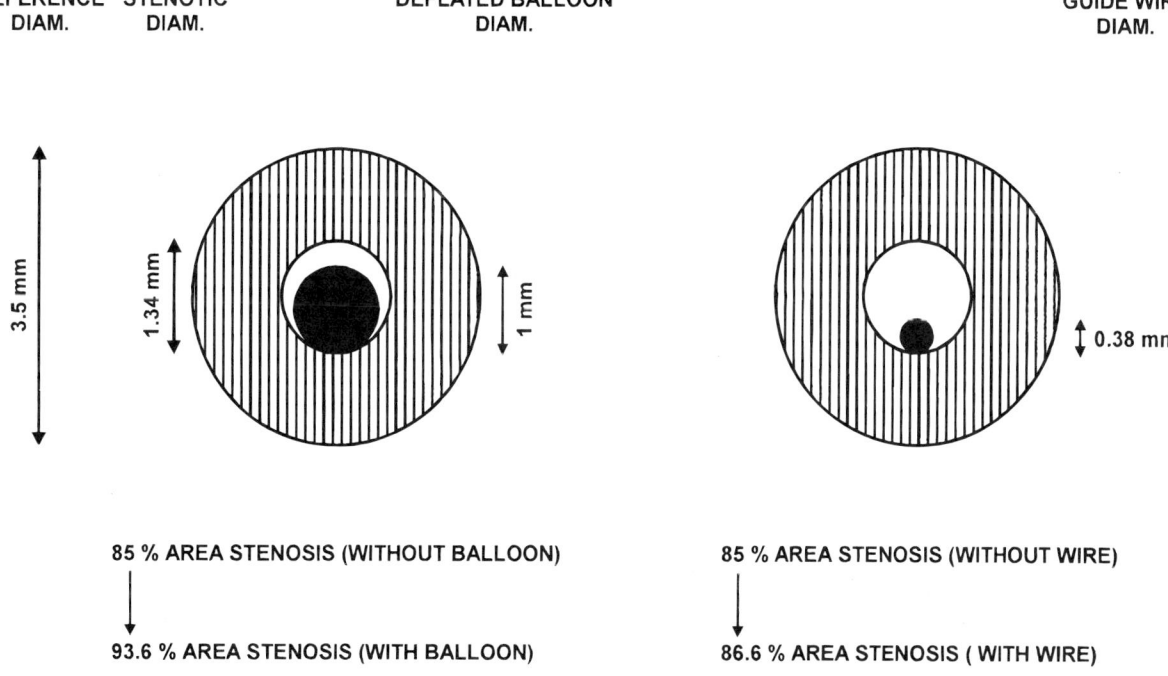

Fig. 15-1. Scale drawing illustrating the space occupied by a balloon catheter and by a guidewire passed through a coronary stenosis.

proximal to the tip of a 0.018-in. or 0.014-in. guidewire (Pressure Guide, RadiMedical Systems, Sweden). Light emitted from a diode is transmitted through a beam splitter to the sensor element. After modulation of the light intensity by a pressure-induced deflection of a mirror, the signal is transmitted back through the same optical fiber. In the control unit, the intensity of the reflected wave is analyzed and the pressure derived. This high-fidelity pressure monitoring guidewire has been used in the clinical setting of interventional cardiology,[11,12] but its steerability within the coronary tree is limited, due to connection of the device to the control unit with a fiberoptic cable (which cannot be detached). Nonetheless, the pressure wire provides the opportunity to record high-quality phasic pressure tracings in distal coronary arteries without obstructing the vessel.

Fluid-Filled Pressure Monitoring Guidewires

In contrast to the high-fidelity pressure monitoring guidewires, the fluid-filled guidewires are basically steerable angioplasty guidewires, with pressure transmitted through a fluid column.[13] Two types of fluid-filled guidewires have been developed thus far. The first (Advanced Cardiovascular Systems) consists of a 129-cm-long tube with an external diameter of 0.015 in., attached to a second tube of 45 cm, which is coaxial to a core wire. These two hypotubes communicate via ten 0.002-in.-diameter ports. A second series of ten 0.002-in.-diameter pressure monitoring ports is located 3 cm from the tip, at the junction of the nonradiopaque portion and the radiopaque tip, which is radiopaque, flexible, and shapable. The second fluid-filled pressure-monitoring guidewire (Schneider Europe) consists of a hollow, 0.014-in. nickel-titanium wire. Four entry ports are located 3 cm from the tip, at the junction of the nonradiopaque portion and the radiopaque flexible and shapable tip. The inner lumen is flushed with heparinized saline and attached via a small screwable valve and a three-way high-pressure stopcock to the pressure transducer and a high-pressure syringe filled with heparinized saline to flush the wire (Fig. 15-2).

Because of their thin lumen, fluid-filled pressure-monitoring guidewires produce very damped pres-

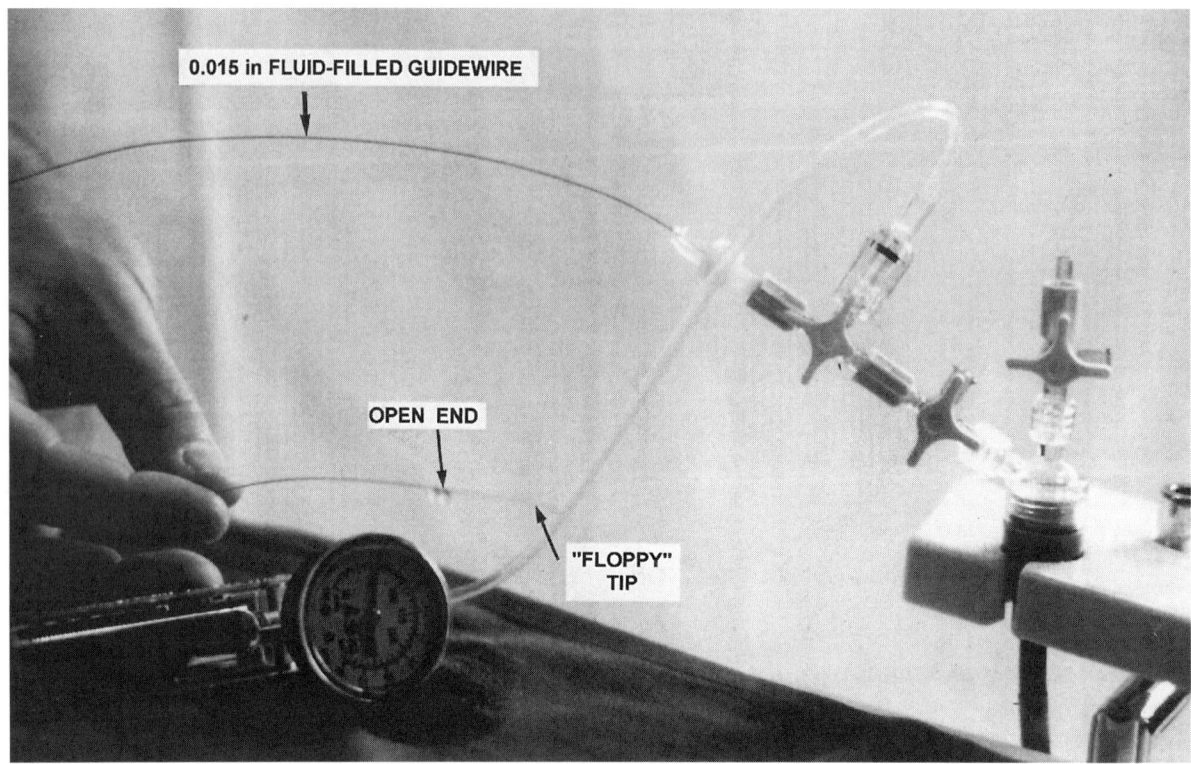

Fig. 15-2. Fluid-filled pressure-monitoring guidewire. The wire is connected to a conventional pressure transducer and can be easily disconnected to improve its responsiveness to manipulation. (From de Bruyne et al.,[13] with permission.)

sure tracings that preclude the separate assessment of systolic and diastolic gradients. To evaluate the hemodynamic impact of a lesion on the underlying myocardium, the mean transstenotic gradient of the whole cardiac cycle is considered. The advantages of the fluid-filled pressure-monitoring guidewires are to be detachable (and thus easily steerable in the coronary tree), and not to require any equipment other than a conventional pressure transducer.

Assessment of Translesional Pressure Using Guidewires

The influence of the presence of the guidewire in the stenosis has been investigated in an in vitro model using seven levels of stenoses (from 50% to 90% area stenosis) and five levels of constant flow rates (from 0.5 to 5 ml/s). For each level of stenosis severity, the pressures were recorded proximally and distally to the stenosis for the different flow rates. Each measurement was performed successively without and with the guidewire through the narrowing. The overestimation of pressure gradient induced by the presence of a 0.015-in. guidewire in a lesion was found to be negligible for mild and moderate stenoses and became significant only at high flow rates (larger than 4 ml/s) through very tight lesions (larger than 80% *area* reduction), a condition in which functional assessment would not be required in clinical practice (Fig. 15-3).

In contrast, comparative data of translesional pressure gradients measured in humans with pressure-monitoring guidewires versus angioplasty balloon catheters confirm that a uniform overestimation is induced by the presence of the balloon catheter in the lesion.[7] Moreover, it has been demonstrated that even after angioplasty, when an angiographically satisfactory result is achieved, a signifi-

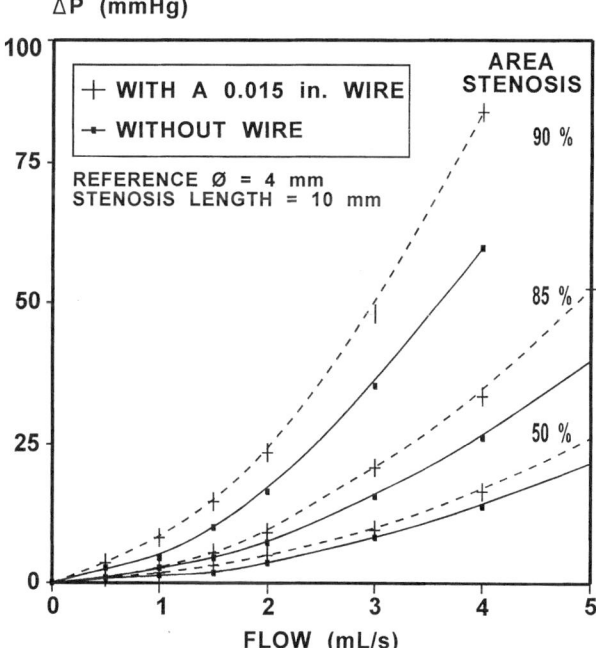

Fig. 15-3. Plot of the in vitro measured pressure gradient (ΔP) for varying stenosis severities (50%, 85%, and 90% area stenosis) at incremental flow rates. Each measurement was obtained with (continuous lines) and without (broken lines) a 0.015-in. guidewire through the stenosis. (From de Bruyne et al.,[13] with permission.)

cant overestimation of the pressure gradient is still present when measured with the angioplasty balloon catheter (Fig. 15-4).

In summary, in contrast to balloon catheters, newly developed pressure-monitoring guidewires enable us to measure coronary pressure distal to stenoses without significant additional obstruction to antegrade flow even at flow rates that prevail during maximal vasodilatation. Thus, the pressure-monitoring guidewire may play a dual role as part of both the diagnostic and the therapeutic procedure.

PRESSURE-DERIVED FRACTIONAL FLOW RESERVE

Definitions: Absolute, Relative, and Fractional Flow Reserve

The extent to which coronary (or myocardial) flow can increase in response to vasodilation is generally referred to as coronary (or myocardial) flow reserve.

The concept of *absolute* flow reserve, defined as the ratio of hyperemic to resting flow, was initially proposed by Gould et al.[14] The normal fourfold to sixfold increase in flow after a maximal vasodilatory stimulus identifies a normal coronary flow reserve. Since the development of Doppler flow velocity catheters, coronary flow velocity reserve has been used as a surrogate for coronary flow reserve in the catheterization laboratory.[15,16] However, several factors such as heart rate, blood pressure, and left ventricular hypertrophy will affect the level of resting flow and need to be taken into account.

In contrast, *relative* flow reserve, defined as the maximal flow in a stenotic artery divided by maximal flow in an adjacent normal artery, has been shown to be more independent of variations in baseline flow caused by changing cardiac workload and myocardial oxygen consumption.[17] This concept of relative flow reserve is referred to in relation to myocardial perfusion scintigraphy, although this measurement requires the presence of a territory perfused by a normal epicardial vessel and cannot be applied in case of "balanced" three vessel disease.

The concept of *fractional* flow reserve was introduced by Pijls et al.[18] to circumvent the major drawbacks of absolute flow reserve (i.e., dependence on the level of resting flow) and of relative flow reserve (i.e., need for an adjacent normal territory). Fractional flow reserve is defined as the ratio of the maximal achievable flow in a stenotic territory to the maximal achievable flow in case of normal epicardial vessel. Thus, maximal coronary or myocardial blood flow is expressed as a percent (fraction) of its normal value. By definition, basal coronary and myocardial flow is not taken into account. Moreover, each artery or myocardial region serves as its own control. Thus, fractional flow reserve exactly indicates to what extent coronary or myocardial flow is affected by the presence of an epicardial narrowing.

Calculation of Fractional Flow Reserve

The concepts of absolute, relative and fractional flow reserve are defined in Table 15-1 and illustrated in Figures 15-5 and 15-6. In Figure 15-5, the coronary circulation is represented schematically as an arrangement of resistances in parallel and in series. Mean arterial pressure (P_a), central venous pressure (P_v), and coronary pressure distal to the stenosis (P_d)

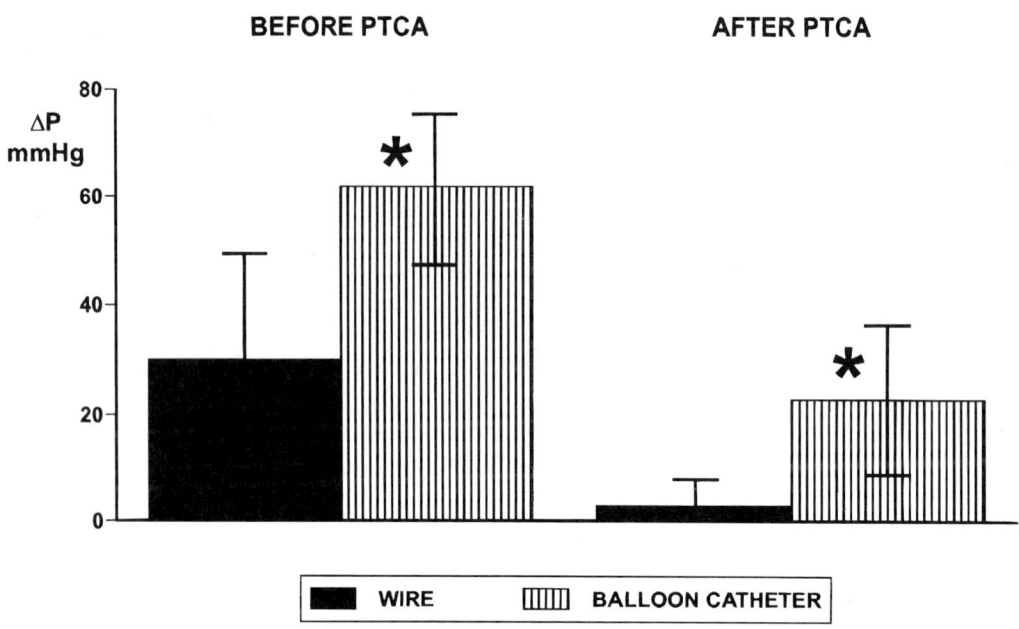

Fig. 15-4. Transstenotic pressure gradient as assessed with a pressure-monitoring guidewire or with an angioplasty balloon catheter before and after angioplasty.

Table 15-1. Definitions, Applications, and Limitations of Absolute, Relative, and Fractional Flow Reserve

	Absolute Flow Reserve	Relative Flow Reserve	Fractional Flow Reserve
Definition	Ratio of hyperemic to resting blood flow	Ratio of hyperemic flow in the stenotic region to hyperemic flow in a contralateral normal region	Ratio of hyperemic flow in the stenotic region to hyperemic flow in that same region if no lesion were present
Independent of driving pressure	No	Yes	Yes
Easily applicable in humans	Yes (flow velocity measurements, positron emmission tomography)	Yes (perfusion scintigraphy, positron emission tomography)	Yes (coronary pressure measurements)
Applicable to three-vessel disease	Yes	No	Yes
Assessment of collateral flow	No	No	Yes
Unequivocal reference value	No (=3 to 6)	Yes (=1)	Yes (=1)

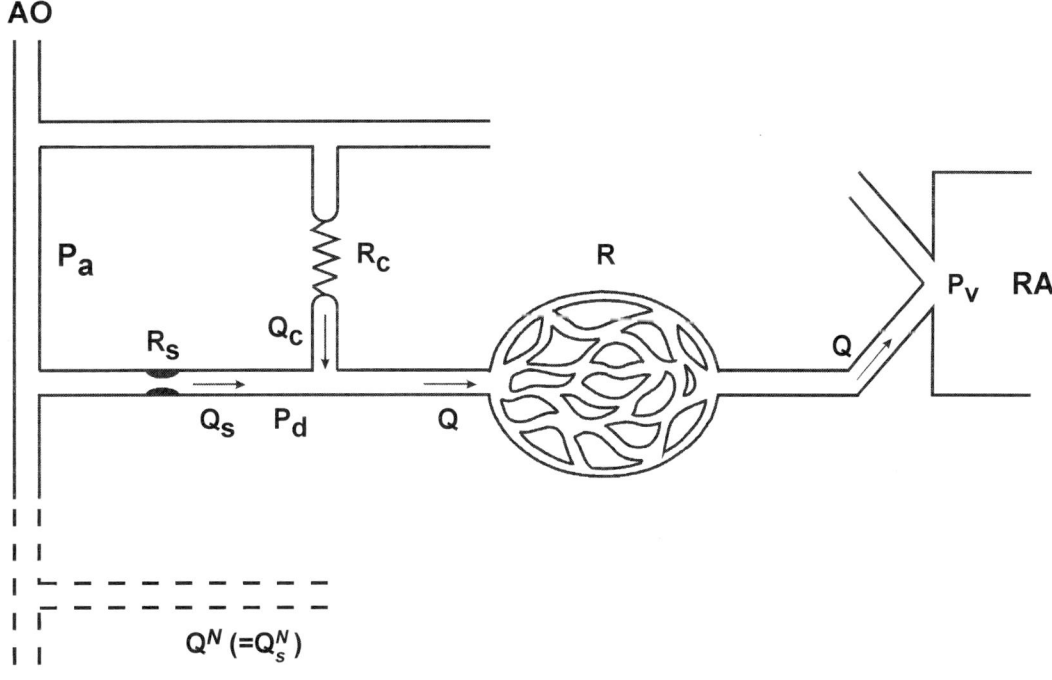

Fig. 15-5. Schematic model representing the coronary circulation. AO, aorta; P_a, arterial pressure; P_d, distal coronary pressure; P_v, venous pressure; Q, blood flow through the myocardial vascular bed; Q_c, collateral blood flow; Q^N, blood flow in the hypothetical case the epicardial vessel were normal; Q_s, blood flow through the supplying epicardial coronary artery; R, resistance of the myocardial vascular bed; R_c, resistance of the collateral circulation; R_s, resistance of the stenosis in the supplying epicardial coronary artery; RA, right atrium. (Modified from Pijls et al.,[18] with permission.)

are defined in the usual way, whereas coronary wedge pressure (P_w) is defined as the pressure distal to the stenosis during coronary occlusion. The difference between P_a and P_d represents the transstenotic pressure gradient (ΔP). During maximal vasodilatation, the resistances of the myocardial capillary bed (R) and the collateral circulation (R_c) are minimal and, therefore, the stenosis resistance (R_s) is maximal. The total blood flow through the myocardial bed (Q) is the sum of the blood flow through the supplying, stenotic artery (Q_s, coronary artery flow) and collateral flow (Q_c). When no stenosis is present, Q and Q_s are called Q^N and Q_s^N respectively and are assumed to be equal. In other words, during vasodilatation, Q^N and Q_s^N represent maximal myocardial and coronary flow, respectively, in case of normal epicardial artery.

Based on this model we can calculate separately the fractional flow reserve for the myocardium (FFR_{myo}), the stenotic epicardial vessel (FFR_{cor}), and the collateral circulation (FFR_{coll}) during maximal vasodilatation as follows:

Myocardial fractional flow reserve (FFR_{myo}):

$$FFR_{myo} = \frac{Q}{Q^N} = \frac{(P_d - P_v)/R}{(P_a - P_v)/R}$$

$$= \frac{P_d - P_v}{P_a - P_v} = 1 - \frac{\Delta P}{P_a - P_v}$$

$$\boxed{FFR_{myo} \sim \frac{P_d}{P_a}}$$

Coronary fractional flow reserve (FFR_{cor}):

$$FFR_{cor} = \frac{Q_s}{Q_s^N} = \frac{Q - Q_c}{Q^N - Q_c^N}$$

Because $Q_c^N = 0$

$$= \frac{Q - Q_c}{Q^N}$$

$$= \frac{(P_d - P_v)/R - (P_a - P_d)/R_c}{(P_a - P_v)/R}$$

$$= \frac{(P_d - P_v) - (P_a - P_d) R/R_c}{(P_a - P_v)}$$

$$= \frac{(P_d - P_v)(P_a - P_w) - (P_a - P_d)(P_w - P_v)}{(P_a - P_v)(P_a - P_w)}$$

$$= \frac{P_d - P_w}{P_a - P_w}$$

$$\boxed{FFR_{cor} = 1 - \frac{\Delta P}{P_a - P_w}}$$

Collateral fractional flow reserve (FFR_{coll}):

$$FFR_{coll} = \frac{Q_c}{Q^N}$$

Because $Q_c = Q - Q_s$

$$= \frac{Q}{Q^N} - \frac{Q_s}{Q^N}$$

Because $Q^N = Q_S^N$

$$= \frac{Q}{Q^N} - \frac{Q_s}{Q_S^N}$$

$$\boxed{FFR_{coll} = FFR_{myo} - FFR_{cor}}$$

These pressure-derived fractional flow reserve calculations were validated in an open-chest dog model by comparison with Doppler velocitometric assessment of coronary blood flow.[18]

Advantages and Limitations of Pressure-Derived Fractional Flow Reserve

This concept is unique in its ability to enable the calculation of a flow index solely from pressure measurements. As it does not account for basal pressure and flow, the variability induced by changes in baseline parameters is limited. Since it incorporates mean aortic pressure it should be independent from hemodynamic changes that are likely to occur during catheterization. Finally, each myocardial territory serving as its own control, calculations of fractional flow reserve are possible in case of multivessel disease since no normal adjacent myocardial region is required. Moreover, the normal value unequivocally equals 1 (or 100%) for any patient and for any vessel under study.

A theoretical limitation of fractional flow reserve involves its reliance on minimal, and therefore negligible, myocardial resistance during maximal arterio-

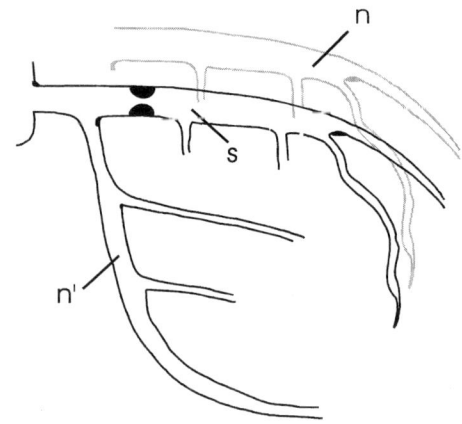

ABSOLUTE Flow Reserve : $AFR = \dfrac{Q_{max,s}}{Q_{rest,s}}$

RELATIVE Flow Reserve : $RFR = \dfrac{Q_{max,s}}{Q_{max,n'}}$

FRACTIONAL Flow Reserve : $FFR = \dfrac{Q_{max,s}}{Q_{max,n}}$

Fig. 15-6. Schematic drawing illustrating the respective definitions of absolute, relative, and fractional flow reserve. In the particular model of an isolated lesion in the proximal left anterior descending coronary artery, relative and fractional flow reserve should be identical (when normalized for tissue mass). (From de Bruyne et al.,[19] with permission.)

lar vasodilatation. Unfortunately, minimal myocardial resistance is often *not* negligible since resistive vessel dysfunction is frequently present in patients with diffuse coronary atherosclerosis. In case of small vessel disease, myocardial fractional flow reserve represents the ratio of maximal myocardial blood flow in the presence of an epicardial stenosis to maximal myocardial blood flow in the absence of that lesion, which may still be abnormal because of the presence of microvascular disease. Thus, myocardial fractional flow reserve takes into account only the contribution of the *epicardial* lesion to the decrease in maximal myocardial perfusion. Hence, it appears that myocardial fractional flow reserve is a lesion-specific index of the influence of a coronary stenosis on myocardial perfusion. Thus, the value of myocardial fractional flow reserve for clinical decision making is not affected by this limitation. Stated another way, the clinical question: "are we going to improve the patient by a revascularization procedure?" can be answered on the basis of fractional flow reserve measurements whether or not microvascular disease is present. In this respect, what appears to be a theoretical limitation turns out to be a practical advantage.

To be applied in clinical practice pressure-derived fractional flow reserve measurements should still prove to be meaningful in humans, to be reproducible, and to be useful for clinical decision making.

CLINICAL APPLICATION OF FRACTIONAL FLOW RESERVE IN HUMANS

Validation of Fractional Flow Reserve

To validate the calculation of pressure-derived myocardial fractional flow reserve in humans, we studied 22 patients with an isolated, discrete lesion of the proximal or midleft anterior descending coronary artery and normal left ventricular function.[20] Calculations of myocardial fractional flow reserve derived from intracoronary pressure measurements were compared to the values of relative flow reserve as assessed by oxygen-labeled water and positron emission tomography obtained within 24 hours before catheterization. Figure 15-7 illustrates a pressure recording enabling the calculation of myocardial fractional flow reserve.

A wide range of stenosis severity was studied (from 22% to 77% diameter stenosis) as calculated by quantitative coronary angiography. The main results of this validation study are summarized in Figure 15-8. Relative flow reserve in the anterior segment assessed by positron emission tomography varied from 0.27 to 1.23 and myocardial fractional flow reserve as calculated from pressure measurements for the same region ranging from 0.36 to 0.98. Myocardial fractional flow reserve assessed by pressure measurements correlated closely with relative flow reserve by positron emission tomography. The mean difference between myocardial fractional flow reserve values and relative flow reserve was -0.049 ± 0.092. the correlation remained unchanged when, in the equation for calculating myocardial fractional flow reserve, central venous pressure was neglected. These data confirm the feasibility of fractional flow reserve calculation, and demonstrate that myocardial fractional flow reserve as calculated from coronary pressure measurements during maximal hyperemia indeed represents a fraction of maximal myocardial blood flow in humans.

Reproducibility of Fractional Flow Reserve Calculations

During catheterization, and even more during coronary angioplasty, fluctuations occur in heart rate, blood pressure, and contractile state. Therefore, to avoid any ambiguity in the interpretation of the results, the evaluation of the coronary circulation should rely on methodologies that are independent of these hemodynamic changes. To investigate the reproducibility of the measurements of myocardial fractional flow reserve in humans, we studied 10 patients (12 stenoses) with normal left ventricular function. Distal coronary pressure was recorded with a pressure-monitoring guidewire as described above and the aortic pressure was recorded through the guiding catheter. Maximal coronary hyperemia was induced by intracoronary adenosine. To investigate the effects of hemodynamic changes on the measurements of fractional flow reserve, hyperemic pressures were taken in the four following pairs of conditions: (1) twice under baseline conditions at 3 minutes interval without any intervention, (2) during atrial pacing at 80 beats per minute (bpm) and at

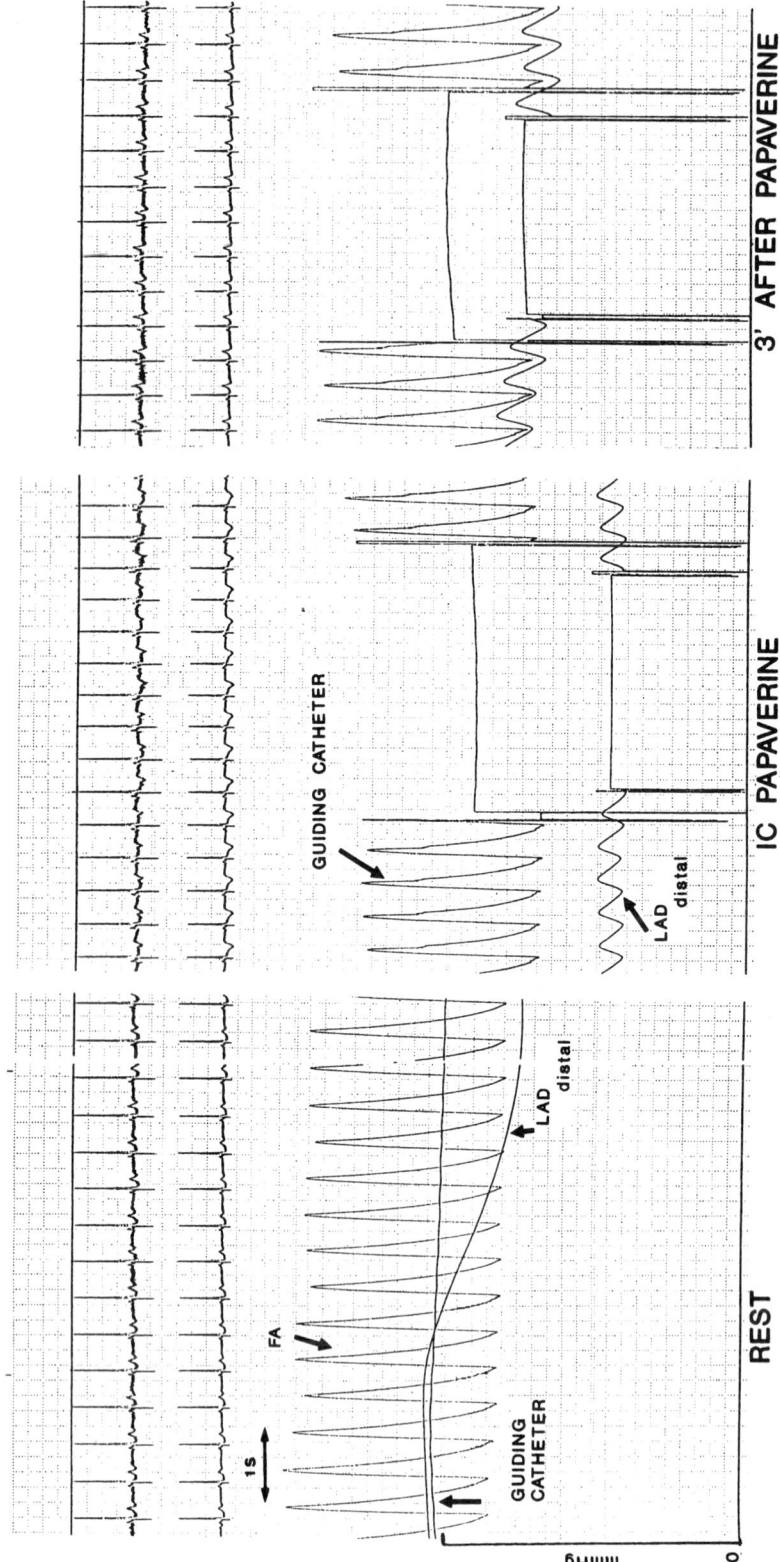

Fig. 15-7. Example of pressure tracing recorded under resting conditions (**A**), during papaverine-induced maximal vasodilatation (**B**), and 3 minutes after intracoronary (IC) papaverine (**C**). During maximal hyperemia myocardial fractional flow reserve can be calculated as the ratio of distal coronary pressure (45 mmHg) to mean aortic pressure (92 mmHg), i.e., 0.49. This means that in this particular patient the hyperemic myocardial flow is only 49% of the expected maximal value in the hypothetical case the epicardial vessel were normal. FA, femoral artery; LAD distal, mean pressure in the distal left anterior descending coronary artery.

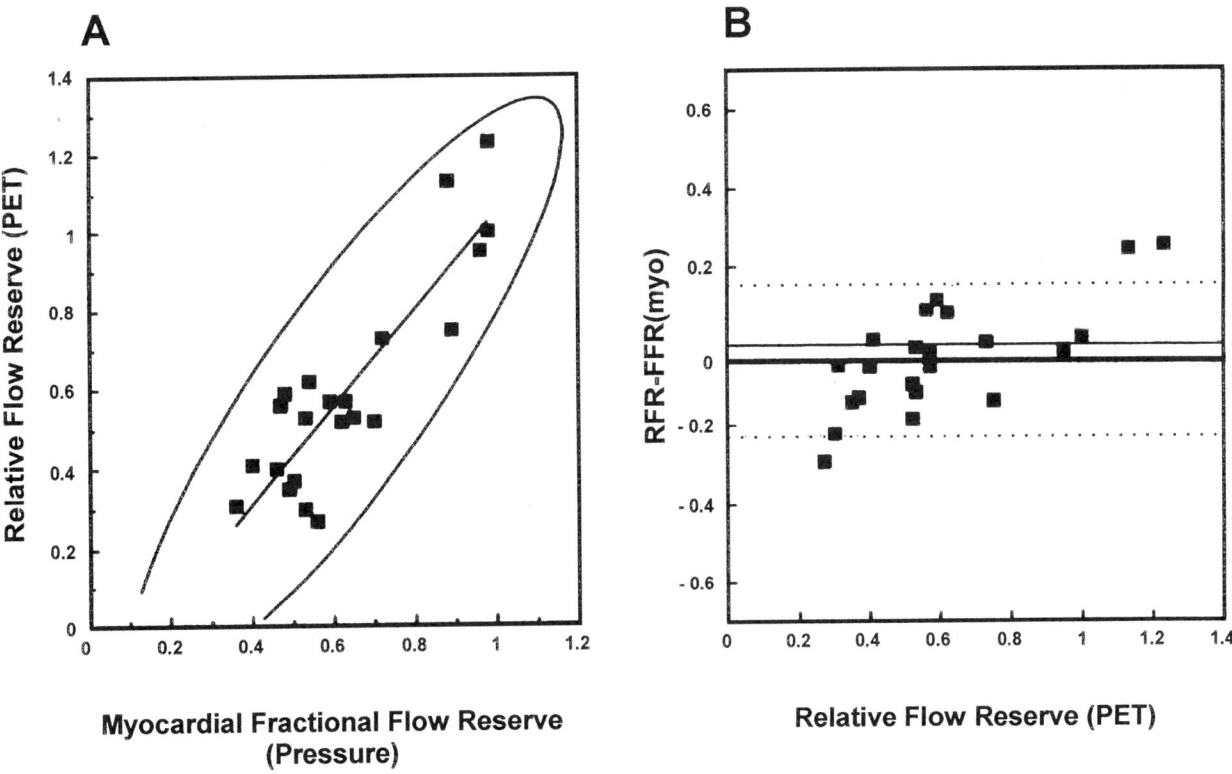

Fig. 15-8. (**A**) Relationship between relative myocardial flow reserve as assessed by positron emission tomography in the anterior region and myocardial fractional flow reserve as calculated from pressure measurements in the distal left anterior descending coronary artery. The regression line as well as the 95% tolerance ellipse are given. (**B**) Plots of the difference between relative flow reserve and myocardial fractional flow reserve values. The solid line represents the mean difference and the dashed lines represent 2 standard deviations from this mean. (From de Bruyne et al.,[20] with permission.)

110 bpm, (3) under basal blood pressure and during intravenous infusion of nitroprusside titrated to reach a decrease in systolic blood pressure of at least 20 mmHg, and (4) in basal contractile state and after 5 minutes intravenous infusion of 10 μg/kg/min of dobutamine to increase myocardial contractility. After each intervention heart rate, mean aortic pressure and distal coronary pressure were allowed to return to their baseline values after the next pair of recordings.

Figure 15-9 shows a very close correlation between the pairs of values of myocardial fractional flow reserve under baseline conditions and during manipulation of heart rate, blood pressure, and myocardial contractility. The present study demonstrates the hemodynamic independence of myocardial fractional flow reserve measurements. This is probably related to the combination of the following factors: (1) myocardial fractional flow reserve is unaffected by changes in resting conditions, (2) the index incorporates mean arterial pressure, therefore correcting for the changes in driving coronary pressure, (3) the mean coronary pressure as recorded in this study through a thin fluid-filled column appears to be an extremely stable signal, and (4) distal coronary pressure integrates all possible changes in vessel diameter that could accompany changes in coronary blood flow.[21]

The measurements of pressure-derived myocardial fractional flow reserve therefore provide similar results whatever the prevalent hemodynamic conditions.[22]

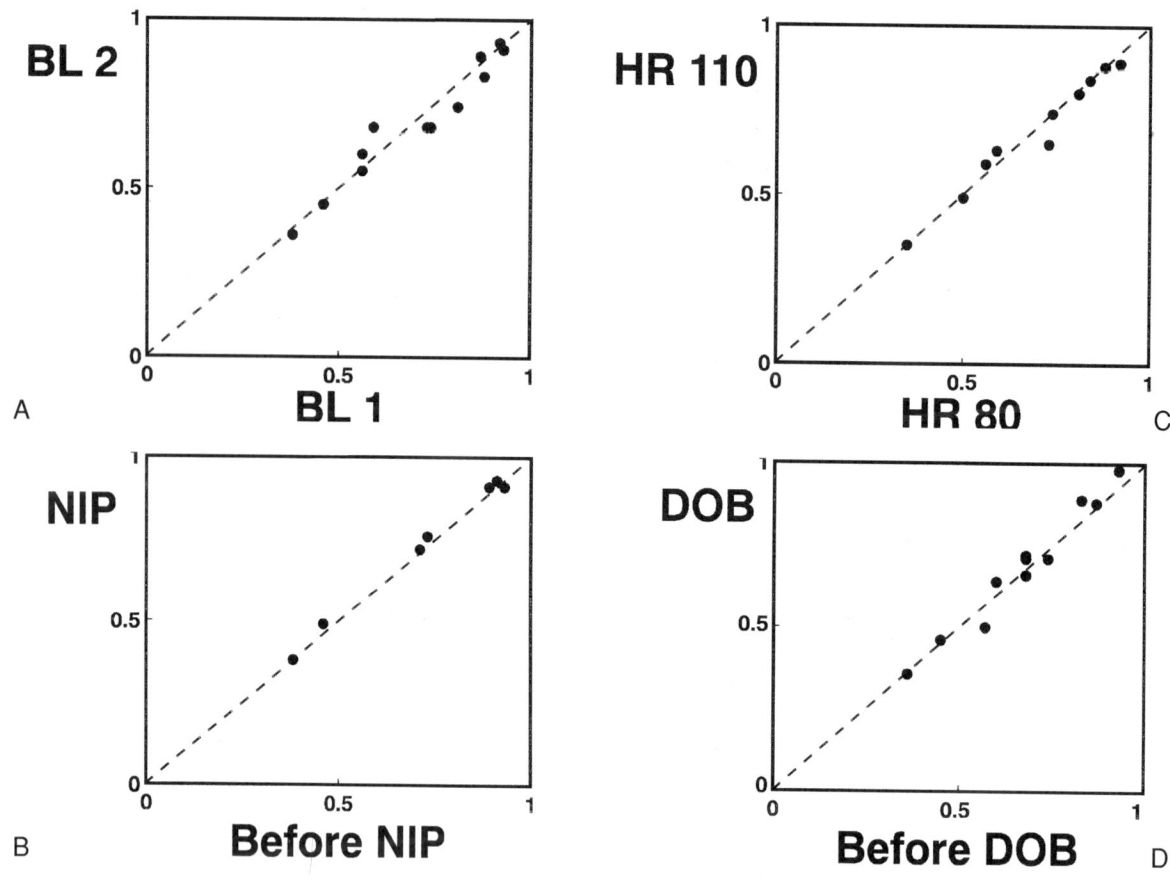

Fig. 15-9. Plots of relation between the pairs of value of myocardial fractional flow reserve measured twice under baseline conditions (**A**), at different heart rates (**B**), at different level of blood pressure (**C**) and before and during dobutamine infusion (**D**). bpm, beats per minute; DOB, dobutamine; NIP, Nipride; BL, baseline; FFR_{myo}, myocardial fractional flow reserve.

RELATION BETWEEN MYOCARDIAL FRACTIONAL FLOW RESERVE AND EXERCISE-INDUCED MYOCARDIAL ISCHEMIA

Coronary stenoses that induce compensatory arteriolar vasodilatation can be regarded as physiologically significant and will induce a pressure gradient during hyperemia. However, not all lesions responsible for a trans-stenotic pressure gradient during maximal hyperemia will induce clinical signs of myocardial ischemia during a maximal stress test (diastolic or systolic left ventricular function abnormalities, electrocardiographic [ECG] changes, anginal chest pain). Thus far, however, practical guidelines for the use of pressure-derived indices (resting pressure gradient, hyperemic pressure gradient, and pressure-derived fractional flow reserve) for clinical decision making have not yet been proposed. Therefore, we studied prospectively 60 patients referred for coronary angioplasty on the basis of a recently performed coronary angiogram and clinical complaints of chest pain suggestive of stable angina.[21] All of these patients had a normal ECG, normal left ventricular function, normal transthoracic echocardiogram, and an isolated lesion in the proximal or midleft anterior descending coronary artery or an isolated lesion in the right coronary artery or the circumflex coronary artery with a reference diameter larger than 2.6 mm. Within 24 hours the patients underwent a maximal exercise ECG (reaching a heart rate of at least 85% of the maximal predicted rate, unless limited by obvious

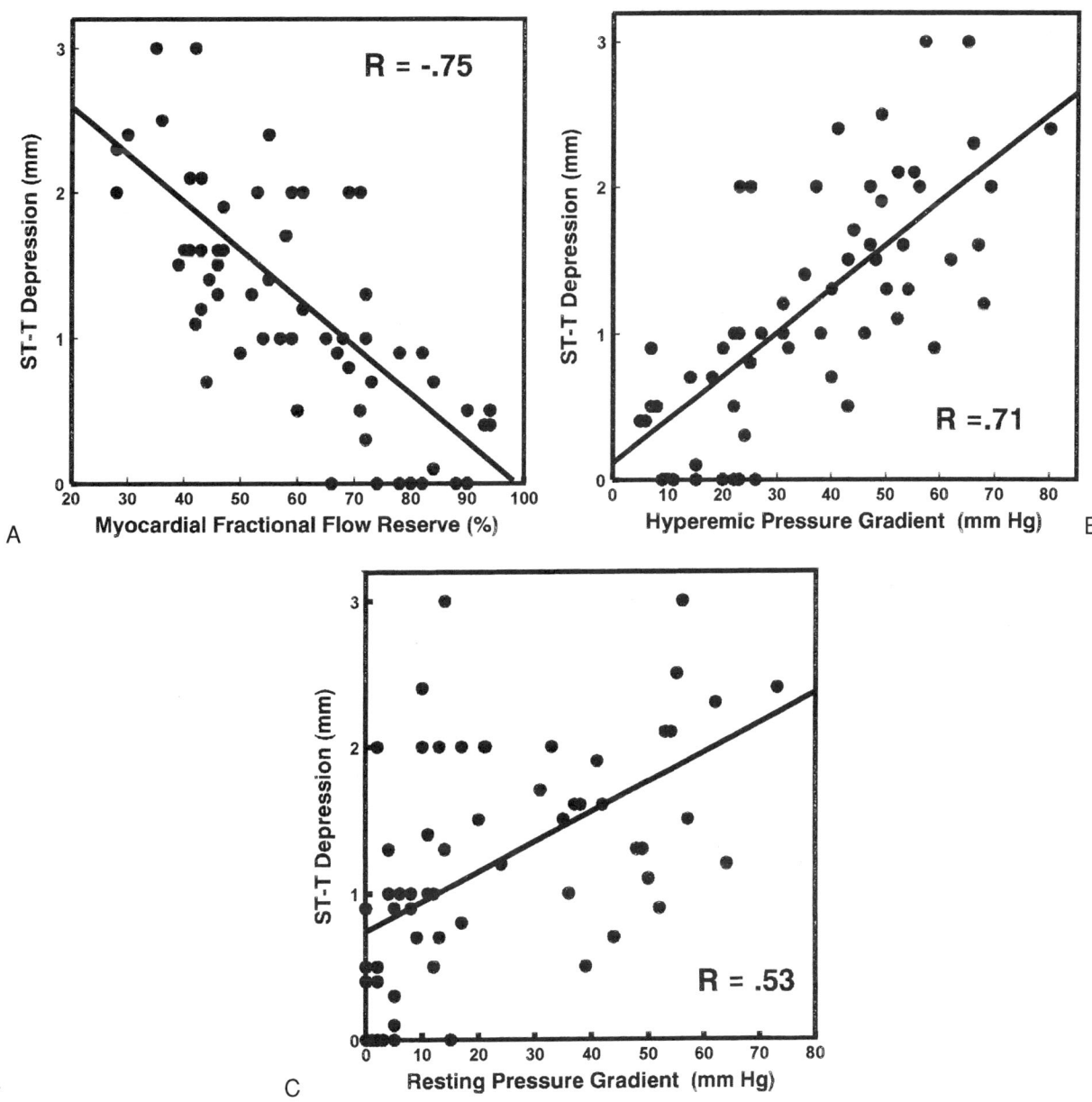

Fig. 15-10. Relationship between (**A**) myocardial fractional flow reserve, (**B**) hyperemic translesional pressure gradient, and (**C**) resting translesional pressure gradient and the magnitude of ST depression during peak exercise. (From de Bruyne et al.,[23] with permission.)

signs of myocardial ischemia) and had intracoronary pressure measurements during maximal hyperemia to calculate myocardial fractional flow reserve as previously described.

Thirty-seven patients had an abnormal and 23 patients a normal exercise ECG. Figure 15-10 shows the individual values of myocardial fractional flow reserve, hyperemic translesional pressure gradient, and resting translesional pressure gradient in patients with a normal and in patients with an

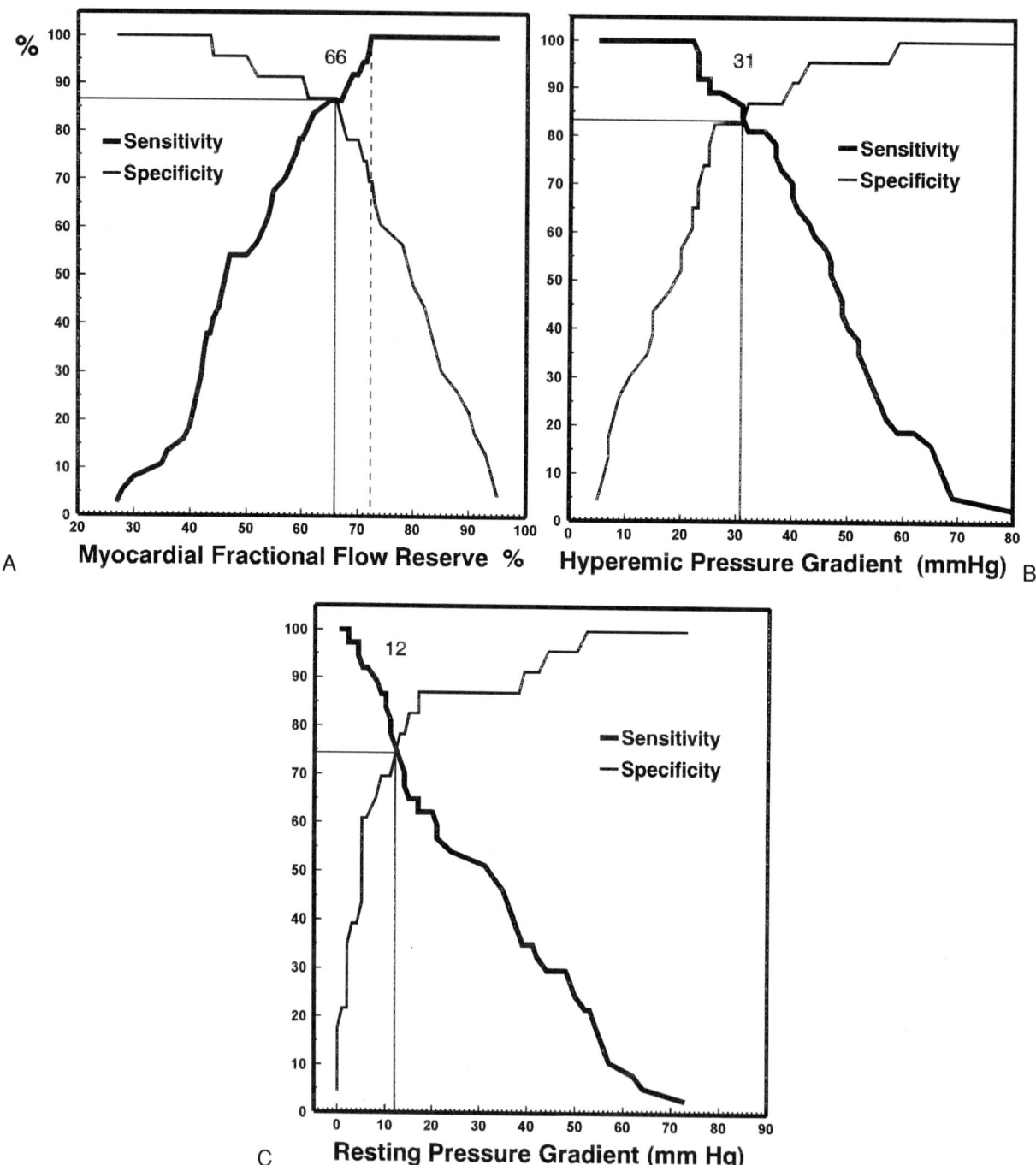

Fig. 15-11. Percent correct classification of an abnormal exercise ECG (sensitivity, %) and percent correct classification of a normal ECG (sensitivity, %) as a function of the different pressure-derived indices: **(A)** myocardial fractional flow reserve (FFR_{myo}, %), **(B)** hyperemic translesional pressure gradient (ΔP_{max}, mmHg), and **(C)** resting translesional pressure gradient (ΔP_{rest}, mmHg). The cutoff value of the different indices providing the highest diagnostic accuracy is located at the point of intersection of the two curves. The corresponding value is indicated above this point of intersection. (From de Bruyne et al.,[23] with permission.)

abnormal stress test. As could be expected, the mean value of myocardial fractional flow reserve was significantly higher and the values of hyperemic gradient and resting gradient significantly lower in patients with a normal exercise ECG as compared to patients with a normal exercise ECG. Furthermore, a significant inverse correlation was found between the value of myocardial fractional flow reserve and the magnitude of ST depression, suggesting that the intensity of ischemia within a given vascular bed plays a major role in producing the clinical range of ST depression. As shown in Figure 15-11, a myocardial fractional flow reserve of 66% offers the best compromise between sensitivity and specificity for predicting an abnormal exercise ECG. More importantly, for clinical decision making, no patients were found to have a abnormal exercise ECG when the myocardial fractional flow reserve was greater than 72% (this level offering a sensitivity of 100%). Figure 15-12 illustrates that indices obtained during hyperemia (namely, myocardial fractional flow reserve and hyperemic translesional pressure gradient) are superior in predicting the results of the exercise ECG than the resting translesional gradient.

CONCLUSIONS

Translesional pressure gradient measurements have been considered intuitively as the most straightforward method for assessing the functional significance of coronary lesions. Their underutilization is due to the fact that until recently, no optimal measurement tool was available. The recent development of pressure-monitoring guidewires should revive the clinical use of this simple index. Since the guidewire does not produce any additional resistance to coronary blood flow, distal coronary pressure can be accurately measured in the setting of both diagnostic and therapeutic catheterization.

The myocardial fractional flow reserve, which can be calculated from intracoronary pressure measurements during maximal hyperemia, provides a lesion-specific index of the consequence of the narrowing on the perfusion of the underlying myocardium. This functional information can be obtained without additional costs, within a few minutes and the very small risk of introducing a guidewire in a coronary

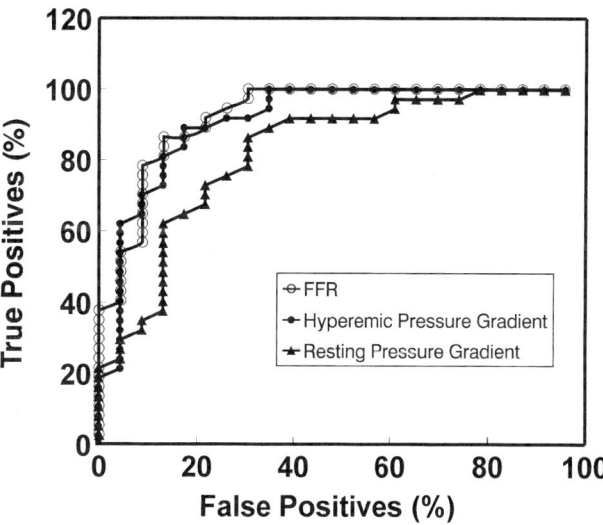

Fig. 15-12. Receiving operator characteristic curves for comparison of the diagnostic accuracy of myocardial fractional flow reserve (FFR), hyperemic translesional pressure gradient, and resting translesional pressure gradient for predicting the results of the exercise electrocardiogram. (From de Bruyne et al.,[23] with permission.)

artery is largely counterbalanced by the accurate information gained by this technique.

We have shown that pressure-derived calculations of myocardial fractional flow reserve do indeed correspond to the fraction of maximal myocardial perfusion including the contribution of the collateral circulation, and that the values of myocardial fractional flow reserve are independent of the prevailing hemodynamic conditions. Finally, it was demonstrated that coronary lesions with a myocardial fractional flow reserve value greater than 0.72 were uniformly associated with normal maximal exercise ECGs.

Based on these data, we believe that intracoronary pressure measurements and fractional flow reserve calculation could be proposed as a surrogate for a stress test for on-line clinical decision making in the catheterization laboratory when an objective proof of the functional significance of an epicardial lesion is lacking. A threshold-value of myocardial fractional flow reserve of 0.72 may be proposed to warrant percutaneous coronary interventions. Conversely, the finding of a myocardial fractional flow value larger than 0.72 could avoid unnecessary coronary interventions as illustrated in Figure 15-13.

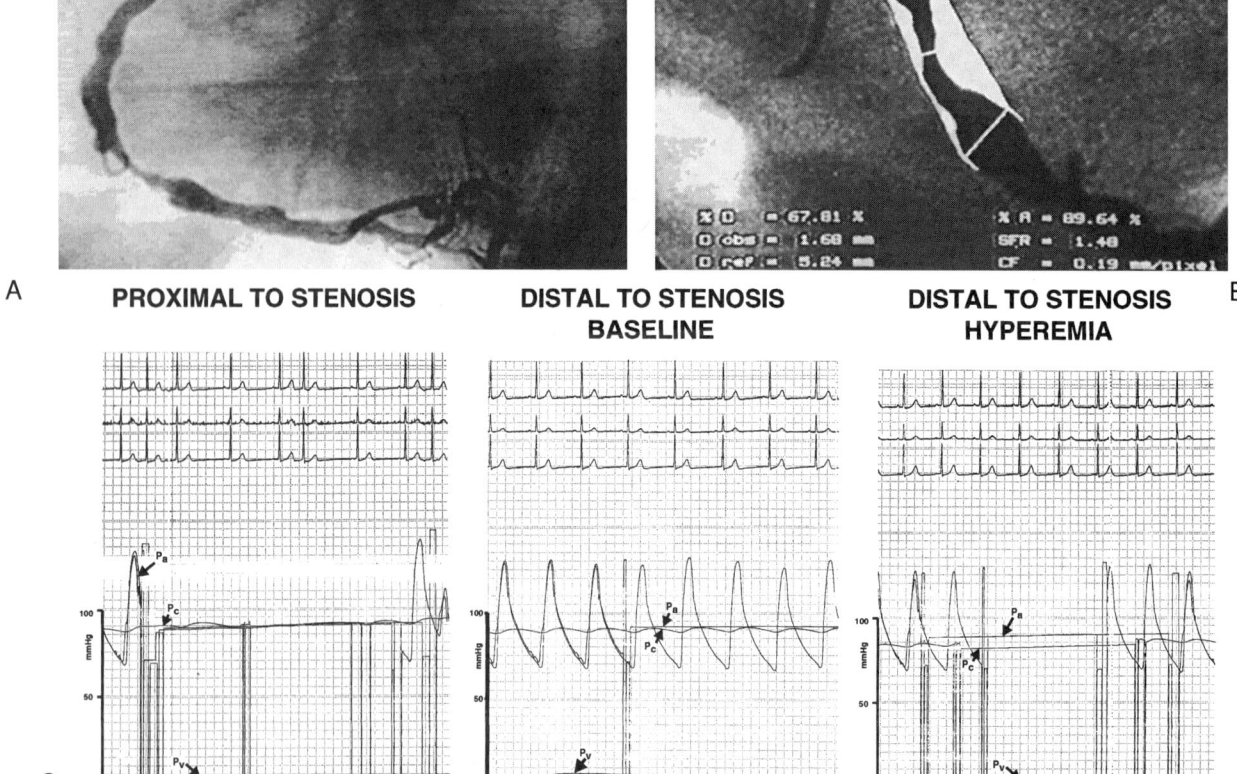

Fig. 15-13. Coronary angiography and transstenotic pressure gradient measurements in a 52-year-old patient admitted with unstable angina and ST-T changes at rest in the lateral leads. At coronary angiography, a critical lesion was found in the left circumflex coronary artery with TIMI 2 flow. The right coronary artery was diffusely ectatic and presented a long narrowing (**A**). The culprit lesion in the left circumflex coronary artery was successfully dilated. (**B**) By quantitative coronary angiography, the lesion in the right coronary artery was described as follows: minimal luminal diameter: 1.68 mm, area stenosis: 89.6% and stenosis flow reserve: 1.48 (**C**) Distal coronary pressure measurements were taken with a fluid-filled pressure-monitoring guidewire; at rest, there was virtually no transstenotic pressure gradient. During maximal vasodilation, a pressure drop of 7 mmHg appeared, corresponding to a myocardial fractional flow reserve of 0.92. No revascularization of this lesion was performed. A stress test performed 2 weeks later was negative. P_a aortic pressure; P_c, coronary pressure; P_v, right atrial pressure. (From de Bruyne et al.[19] with permission.)

REFERENCES

1. de Feyter PJ, Serruys PW, Davies MJ et al.: Quantitative coronary angiography to measure progression and regression of coronary atherosclerosis: value, limitations and implications for clinical trials. Circulation 84: 412, 1991
2. Libby P: Lesion versus lumen. Nature Med 1:17, 1995
3. Wilson RF, Marcus ML, White CW: Prediction of the physiological significance of coronary arterial dimensions by quantitative lesion geometry in patients with limited coronary artery disease. Circulation 75:723, 1987

4. Zijlstra F, van Ommeren J, Reiber JHC, Serruys PW: Does quantitative assessment of coronary artery dimensions predict the physiological significance of a coronary stenosis? Circulation 75:1154, 1987
5. Topol EJ, Ellis SE, Cosgrove DM et al.: Analysis of coronary angioplasty practice in the United States with an insurance-claims data base. Circulation 87:1489, 1993
6. Pijls NHJ, van de Voorde P, El Gamal MIH et al.: Fractional flow reserve: A useful ideal index to evaluate the influence of a coronary artery stenosis on myocardial blood flow. Circulation 92:3183, 1995
7. de Bruyne B, Sys SU, Heyndrickx GR: Percutaneous transluminal coronary angioplasty catheters versus fluid-filled pressure monitoring guidewires for coronary pressure measurements and correlation with quantitative coronary angiography. Am J Cardiol 72:1101, 1993
8. Grüntzig AR, Jenning A, Siegenthaler WE: Nonoperative dilatation of coronary artery stenosis. N Engl J Med 301:61, 1979
9. Bonzel T, Wollschläger H, Kasper W et al.: The sliding rail system (monorail): description of a new technique for intravascular instrumentation and its application to coronary angioplasty. Z Kardiol 76:119, 1987
10. Emanuelsson H, Dohnal M, Lamm C, Tenerz J: Initial experiences with a miniaturized pressure transducer during coronary angioplasty. Cath Cardiovasc Diagn 24:137, 1991
11. Serruys PW, Di Mario C, Meneveau N et al.: Intracoronary pressure and flow velocity from sensor tip guidewires. A new methodological comprehensive approach for the assessment of coronary hemodynamics before and after interventions. Am J Cardiol 71:41D, 1993
12. Di Mario C, Krams R, Gil R, Serruys PW: Slope of the instantaneous hyperemic diastolic coronary flow velocity-pressure relation. A new index for assessment of the physiological significance of coronary stenosis in humans. Circulation 90:1215, 1994
13. de Bruyne B, Pijls NHJ, Paulus WJ et al.: Transstenotic coronary pressure gradient measurement in humans: in vitro and in vivo evaluation of a new pressure monitoring angioplasty guidewire. J Am Coll Cardiol 22:119, 1993
14. Gould KL, Lipscomb K, Hamilton GW: Physiological basis for assessing critical coronary stenosis: instantaneous flow response and regional distribution during coronary hyperemia as measures of coronary flow reserve. Am J Cardiol 33:87, 1974
15. Wilson RF, Laughlin DE, Ackell PH et al.: Transluminal, subselective measurement of coronary artery blood flow velocity and vasodilator reserve in man. Circulation 72:82, 1985
16. Segal J, Kern MJ, Scott NA et al.: Alterations of phasic coronary artery flow velocity in humans during percutaneous coronary angioplasty. J Am Coll Cardiol 20:276, 1992
17. Gould KL, Kirkeeide RL, Buchi M: Coronary flow reserve as a measure of stenosis severity. J Am Coll Cardiol 15:459, 1990
18. Pijls NHJ, van Son AM, Kirkeeide RL et al.: Experimental basis of determining maximum coronary, myocardial and collateral blood flow by pressure measurements for assessing functional stenosis severity before and after percutaneous transluminal coronary angioplasty. Circulation 87:1354, 1993
19. de Bruyne B, Paulus J, Piljs NHJ: Rationale and application of coronary transstenotic pressure gradient measurements. Cathet Cardiovasc Diagn 33:250, 1994
20. de Bruyne B, Baudhuin T, Melin JA et al.: Coronary flow reserve calculated from pressure measurements in humans. Validation with positron emission tomography. Circulation 89:1013, 1994
21. Drexler H, Zeilher AM, Wollschläger H et al.: Flow-dependent artery dilatation in humans. Circulation 80:466, 1989
22. de Bruyne B, Barunek J, Sys SU et al: Simultaneous coronary pressure and flow velocity measurements in humans. Circulation, to be published, 1996
23. de Bruyne B, Bartunek J, Sys SU, Heyndrickx GR: Relation between myocardial fractional flow reserve calculated from coronary pressure measurements and exercise-induced myocardial ischemia. Circulation 92:39, 1995

Chapter 16

Intravascular Ultrasound and Coronary Doppler Flow Measurements

E. Murat Tuzcu, Anthony C. De Franco, Sorin J. Brener, and Steven E. Nissen

An expertly performed coronary angiogram is often sufficient to diagnose coronary atherosclerosis or the lack thereof. However, in some patients unanswered questions may remain even after a thorough radiographic examination. Ambiguous lesions may elude accurate characterization by angiography. Stenoses may be well characterized by angiography, but fall into the category of uncertain physiologic significance with a diameter stenosis of 50% to 70%. Coronary angiography may be completely normal in some patients after an apparent ischemic event. Similarly, angiography may remain unremarkable for years, despite progression of allograft vasculopathy in cardiac transplant recipients.

Some of these uncertainties can be resolved by performing an additional noninvasive test, but this has the disadvantage of prolonging the hospital stay and increasing the cost of patient care. Moreover, functional studies are not always accurate in discriminating the severity of stenosis involving multiple coronary arteries. Discrepancies between the patient's symptoms, clinical presentation, and functional tests may further complicate the problem. Two new technologies—intravascular ultrasound imaging and coronary blood flow measurements with Doppler technology—have improved the diagnostic capability of the angiographer and may solve the need for functional evaluation in the angiography laboratory. This chapter will discuss the role of these new methods in the diagnosis of coronary artery disease (CAD).

RATIONALE FOR INTRALUMINAL IMAGING
Limitations of Angiography

Although angiography is the commonly accepted "gold standard" for the evaluation of CAD, this procedure has important and clinically relevant limitations. In necropsy studies, significant discrepancies have been detected between the angiographic severity of lesions and postmortem findings.[1-5] The accuracy of visual assessment of coronary obstructions has been questioned by intraobserver and interobserver variability studies.[6] Although the development of quantitative coronary angiography has overcome some of these inconsistencies, it has not eliminated all the potential sources of error.[7,8] In addition to differences in the measurement of luminal diameter and percent stenosis, recent reports have demonstrated inconsistencies between the angiographic severity of lesions and physiologic measurements.[9]

Planar versus Tomographic Imaging

Many of the limitations of coronary angiography are inherent to the technique. Coronary vessels, particularly those affected by atherosclerosis, are complex

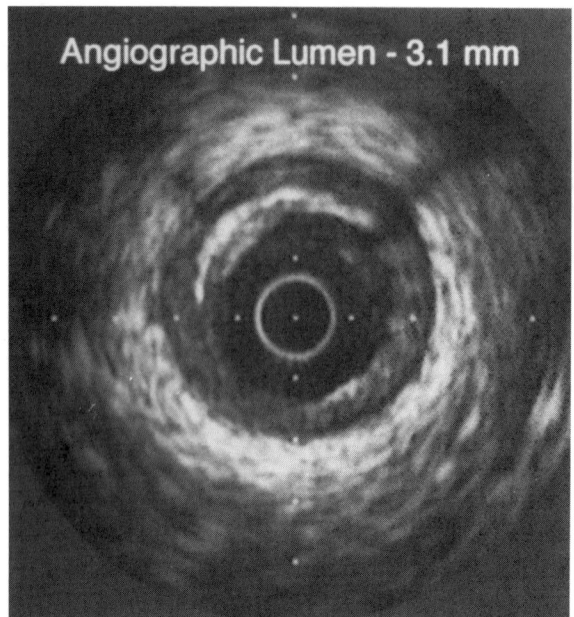 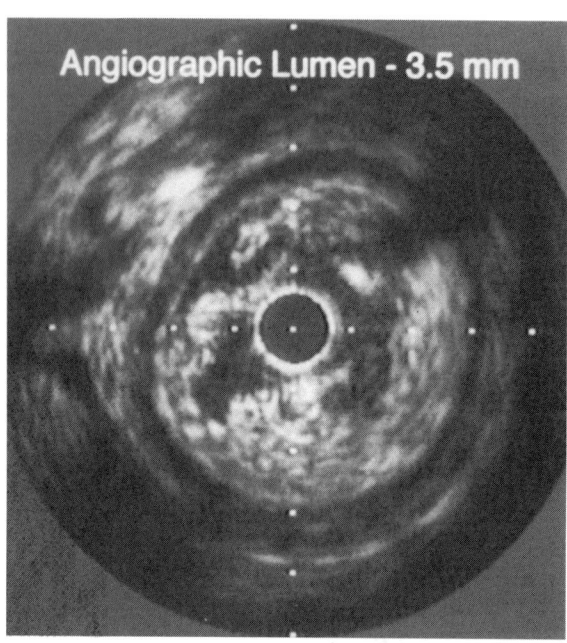

Fig. 16-1. (**A**) Concentric atherosclerotic plaque occupies the entire circumference of the vessel. Part of the plaque (9 o'clock to 1 o'clock) has brighter echoes compared with the rest of the plaque, suggesting fibrotic elements. Luminal diameter was determined as 3.1 mm on angiogram. (**B**) A very complex plaque occupying most of the lumen. The lumen is very irregular due to dissections. Angiographic measurement revealed a luminal diameter of 3.5 mm, which is larger than the lumen seen in **A**. These pictures illustrate the limitation of angiography in assessing the coronary lumen.

three-dimensional structures. Angiography depicts an artery as a silhouette of the contrast-filled lumen on a two-dimensional plane. However, the planar image cannot faithfully represent the irregular and complex lumen shapes of atherosclerotic arterial segments. For example, in patients with unstable angina, angiography may show only an ill-defined irregular narrowing, because contrast fills the crevices of the ruptured plaque. Percutaneous interventions often further exaggerate the complex, three-dimensional structure of coronary arteries.[10,11] With angiography, these vessels appear enlarged, although frequently they are described as "hazy" in appearance. The advantage of intravascular ultrasound is its *tomographic* orientation, which can reveal the irregular shape of the atheroma and its impact on the lumen size and shape (Fig. 16-1). Due to these differences in orientation, it is not surprising to find poor correlation between angiographic and ultrasound measurements following coronary interventions.[12]

Even in stable chronic coronary disease, angiography provides information about atherosclerotic changes only when the atheroma encroaches into the lumen; conclusions about the actual extent of disease can be made only inferentially.

Remodeling and Eccentricity

Necropsy studies have demonstrated that human atherosclerotic arteries can maintain lumen size despite the growth of atheroma within the arterial wall. This process has been called "compensatory enlargement" (because of the increase in the total size of the arterial wall) or "remodeling."[13] Intravascular ultrasound studies have also demonstrated this phenomenon invivo (Fig. 16-2).[14] Because coronary angiography can reveal only the effects of atheroma on the lumen, it cannot identify the presence of plaque until it starts to impinge upon the lumen. This is another advantage of the tomographic perspective of intravascular ultrasound, because the lo-

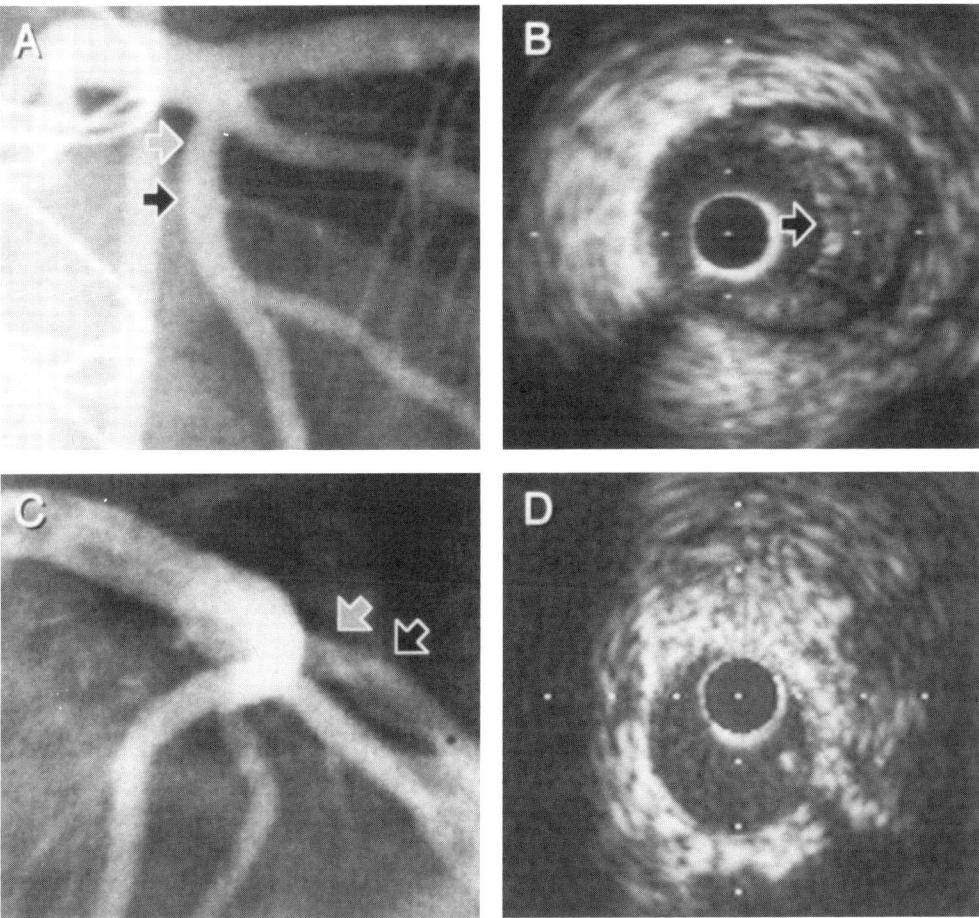

Fig. 16-2. (A & C) Coronary angiogram of the left coronary artery in the right anterior oblique and in the left anterior oblique projection respectively. The black arrows indicate the imaging sites shown in B. The white arrows indicate imaging sites shown in D. (B) The intravascular ultrasound image exhibits a large eccentric plaque; however, the large circular lumen of the proximal circumflex was not compromised. (D) The circular lumen is identical in area to the lumen in B. This figure illustrates how vascular remodeling accommodates the growing atheroma while preserving the lumen area in even advanced atherosclerosis.

cation and extent of even the smallest atheroma can be measured precisely.

In addition to remodeling, small eccentric atheroma may also escape angiographic detection by the same mechanism. This phenomenon is another important mechanism responsible for false-negative angiography. Even an unlimited number of angiographic projections may not allow the operator to identify small eccentric plaques that occupy only a portion of the vessel circumference. Nevertheless, small atheroma can rupture and cause unstable angina or myocardial infarction.

Reference Segment Atherosclerosis

Angiography is often used to assess the severity of an individual coronary lesion, however, the visual interpretation of the coronary angiogram has been shown to be an inadequate predictor of the physiologic significance of coronary lesions.[15] This limitation is inherent in the method of assessment of an-

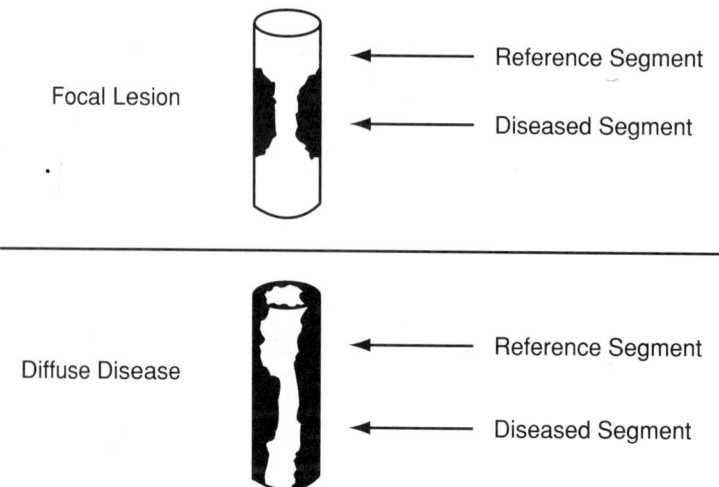

Fig. 16-3. The impact of diffuse atherosclerosis on the accuracy of coronary angiographic measurements. (**A**) The severity of the focal lesions is accurately determined by comparing the lumen diameter at the narrowed site with the lumen diameter at the reference site, which is truly normal. (**B**) Angiographically determined percent diameter stenosis underestimates the true severity of this lesion because the luminal diameter at the site of stenosis is compared with a reference diameter, which does not represent the true lumen diameter because of diffuse atherosclerosis.

giographic lesion severity. The angiographer calculates lesion severity by comparing the most severe portion of a stenosis to a "normal" reference segment in the vicinity of the lesion. However, atherosclerosis is known to be a diffuse rather than a focal process.[14] The diffusely diseased vessel often contains no truly normal segment from which to calculate percent diameter stenosis (Fig. 16-3). In this common situation, the calculated percent diameter stenosis often underestimates the true lesion severity due to the underestimation of the reference segment diameter. Diffuse atherosclerotic involvement may also have implications for interventional procedures, because reference segment disease may effect the assessment of vessel size and thus device selection, device sizing, and the assessment of results.[16,17]

Physiologic Significance of Coronary Stenoses

Although intravascular ultrasound overcomes many shortcomings of angiography, it cannot precisely determine the physiologic significance of a particular lesion. When a coronary stenosis is "borderline" angiographically (between 50% and 70% narrowed with respect to the reference diameter), it may or may not cause myocardial ischemia depending upon the length of the narrowing, the amount of myocardium supplied by the vessel, oxygen demand, and many other factors. Although ultrasound can precisely measure the actual lumen area at this lesion site, this morphological assessment is often not adequate to determine the effect of the lesion on myocardial perfusion. In these circumstances, intracoronary blood velocity measurements with Doppler techniques can provide valuable incremental information about the physiologic significance of a coronary narrowing.

INTRAVASCULAR ULTRASOUND TECHNOLOGY
Equipment

Intravascular ultrasound imaging systems consist of catheter-mounted transducers and dedicated scanners that reconstruct the electronic signal into images of the artery that are displayed on a video screen. Ultrasound technology has advanced to where currently available systems use miniaturized transducers, allowing the use of catheters as small as 2.9 to 3.5 French (0.96 to 1.7 mm). These small catheters can be advanced safely in most coronary segments. Despite their small size, current catheters consistently produce high-quality images.

There are two fundamentally different technologies employed in the design of intravascular ultrasound transducers: single element mechanical systems and multielement electronic systems. In the mechanical system, a single ultrasound transducer placed at or near the catheter tip emits and receives the ultrasound signals. To obtain images from the complete 360° circumferential arc of the vessel, an external motor (outside the body) rotates the transducer (or a mirror) via a drive shaft. Although current mechanical systems provide high-resolution images, the need to rotate the system creates the potential for artifacts and other difficulties. In contrast to mechanical systems, multielement electronic systems do not have moving parts. Instead, multiple transducer elements are placed circumferentially around the catheter. Various combinations of individual transducers operate sequentially to send and receive signals from the 360° circumference.

Delivery Systems

Intracoronary ultrasound catheters are placed into the coronary arteries in a fashion similar to balloon angioplasty catheters. As with angioplasty equipment, there are different delivery systems for ultrasound catheters. Whereas most mechanical catheters use a monorail design in electronic systems, over-the-wire catheters with coaxial lumens are available. Newer catheters have a unique sheath design with an ultrasound-transparent sheath at the distal portion, which is used as a common path for the guidewire and transducer.

Although the safety of ultrasound imaging in various patient populations has been demonstrated, the potential for complications still exists.[18] Intravascular ultrasound imaging should be performed by operators who are experts in intracoronary manipulation and in managing potential complications.

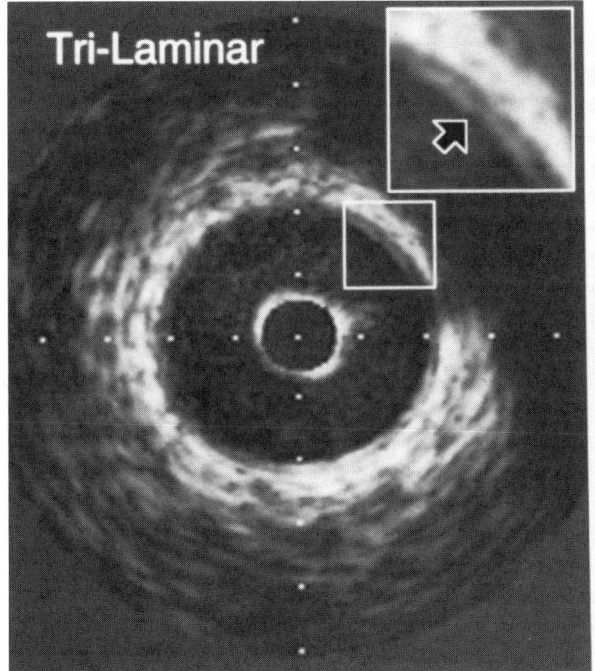
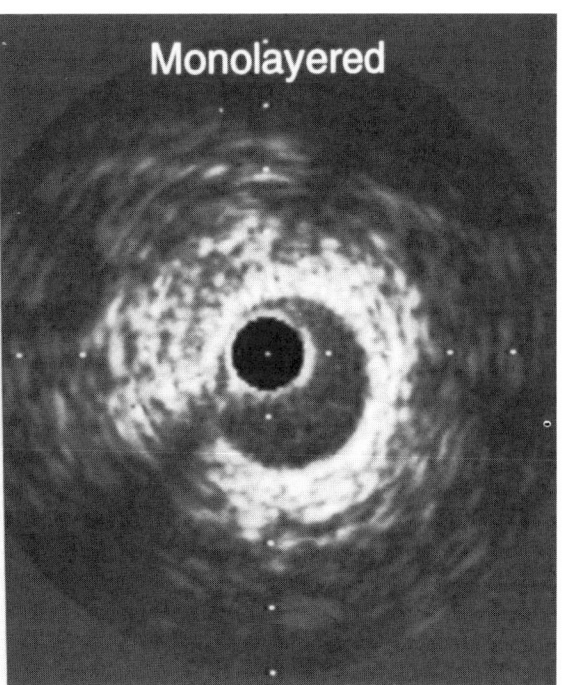

Fig. 16-4. Normal coronary morphology by intravascular ultrasound. (**A**) Ultrasound exhibits a triluminal structure. The magnified view of the vessel wall is shown in the insert at the upper right-hand corner. The thin innermost layer represents the intima, a thin sonolucent zone that corresponds to the media and echogenic third layer shows the adventitia. (**B**) None of the layers of the vessel wall is seen. The monolayer appearance of the vessel wall is common in children and young adults.

IMAGE INTERPRETATION

Normal Coronary Anatomy

Usual Appearance

In an intravascular ultrasound image, the catheter appears as a dark circle in the center of the picture surrounded by the sonolucent lumen, which often contains "speckles" that originate from ultrasonic reflections from flowing blood. The appearance of the vessel wall beyond the lumen depends on the thickness of the layers, the frequency of the transducer, and the proximity of the transducer to the wall (Fig. 16-4). In children and young adults, the arterial wall appears as a single layer when imaged by a 30-MHz tranducer. In middle aged and older adults, it appears as a trilayer structure.[19] Postmortem studies have shown that intimal thickness increases with age.[20] In a normal vessel the intima, the inner-most layer of the arterial wall, is depicted as a thin echogenic circle. The media appears as a thin sonolucent layer behind the intima. The outermost layer, the adventitia, is recognized by its relative echogenicity.

Artifacts

The intravascular ultrasonographer must always be alert to the potential for errors in image interpretation, because artifacts are common. To minimize this potential, care must be taken at every step of the procedure. For example, in mechanical transducers the speed of driving motor and the transducer must be identical; tortuous vessels, equipment errors, or poor technique can restrict the movement of the flexible drive shaft. In obvious cases the resulting images are distorted and uninterpretable; in other cases, the operator may be unaware of the significant distortion and may make erroneous conclusions about vessel anatomy (Fig. 16-5). In contrast, multielement systems are not susceptible to rotational artifacts. Another potential imaging difficulty is a circle of artifact around the catheter commonly called transducer "ring-down." This is a zone devoid of ultrasound information caused by high amplitude signals from the oscillation of the transducer. Although this area is small and infrequently interferes with interpretation, in some cases the ring-down obscures the tissues in the very near field, such as in small arteries.

Ultrasound transducers image the artery with

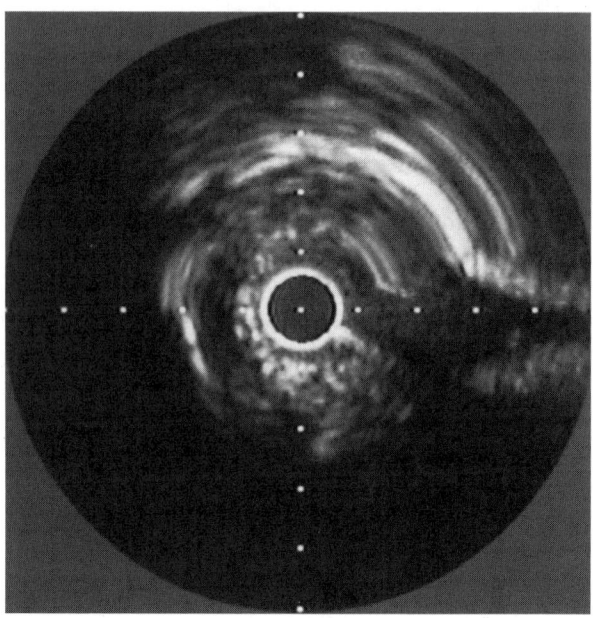

Fig. 16-5. Distorted intravascular ultrasound image of an atherosclerotic coronary artery. Image distortion is due to nonuniform rotational artifact. The image between 10 o'clock and 4 o'clock is uninterpretable due to this artifact.

beams nearly perpendicular to the vessel wall, but this is possible only if the catheter remains coaxial to the long axis of the vessel. If the catheter is not coaxial (such as in curved segments) the images may not represent the true morphology and measurements of the vessel wall and the lumen may be inaccurate.

Abnormal Morphology

Plaque Content

Morphology of the atheroma is an important determinant of the prognosis and natural history of CAD. Rupture of the atherosclerotic plaque with superimposed thrombus represents the principal mechanism underlying the conversion of stable clinical pictures to unstable coronary syndromes, including myocardial infarction. The atherosclerotic plaque, which is not appreciated fully by coronary angiography, comprises the target lesion for interventions designed to prevent or reverse progression of atherosclerosis. Recent studies suggest that morphology and content of the plaque are important determinants of the outcome following coronary interven-

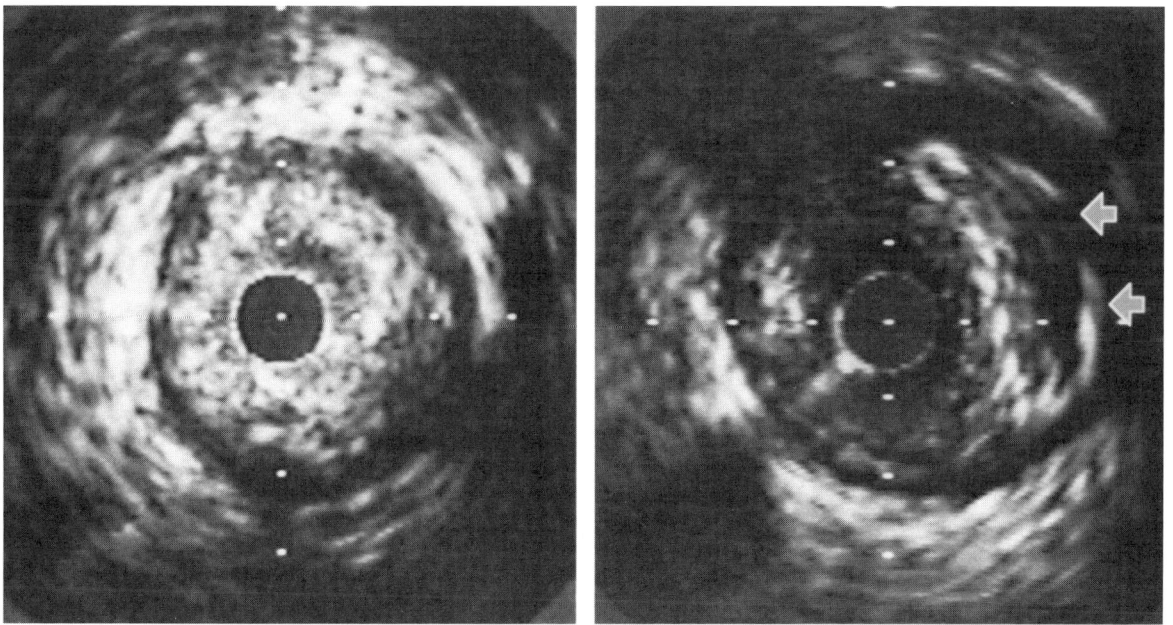

Fig. 16-6. (**A**) A "hard" plaque characterized by echoes as bright as the adventitia without acoustic shadowing occupies the entire lumen outside the catheter in a concentric manner. (**B**) A "soft" plaque in this artery has an echolucent core, indicated by arrows, suggesting a large lipid pool or a necrotic core.

tions.[14,21–23] Studies that have compared ultrasound images with actual histology have shown that ultrasound can give a reasonable approximation of plaque content.[14–26] Plaques that are less echogenic than the adventitia (denoted as "soft" plaque) often represent lipid-rich atheroma, although identical images can also originate from layered thrombi. Plaques that have echoes as bright as the adventitia are termed "hard" or "fibrotic" and often represent a high concentration of fibrotic elements (Fig. 16-6). Many plaques have a "mixed" appearance with both echolucent and echodense segments. It is important to remember that "fibrotic" and "lipid-laden" plaque are not distinct categories but rather part of a continuum of morphologic types. In the future, higher frequency transducers and radio frequency analysis of the ultrasound signals may allow more precise tissue characterization and lead to a better understanding of atheroma contents.

Calcified Atheroma

Intravascular ultrasound is more accurate than either fluoroscopy or angiography in the detection and quantification of coronary calcification. With ultrasound, calcium appears as bright echoes that are more echogenic than the surrounding adventitia. When "shadowing" of structures occurs deep to the bright echoes, the probability of heavy calcification increases further because current ultrasound devices cannot penetrate the calcification to reach the deeper structures (Fig. 16-7). The presence, location, and extent of calcification are important lesion characteristics that can strongly influence the strategies for percutaneous revascularization; therefore, an assessment of vessel and target calcification should often be included in preintervention planning. In addition to the detection of calcification, ultrasound is an excellent tool for determining the precise location of calcium in the vessel wall (Fig. 16-8). Ultrasound can determine whether calcium is superficial or deep and can quantify the arc of calcified vessel wall. For example, extensive superficial calcium at or near the intimal surface makes tissue removal by directional atherectomy difficult or impossible; rotational ablation may be preferred for these lesions. In a series of 185 patients imaged before a percutaneous coronary intervention, we found that the sensitivity of angiography in detecting target

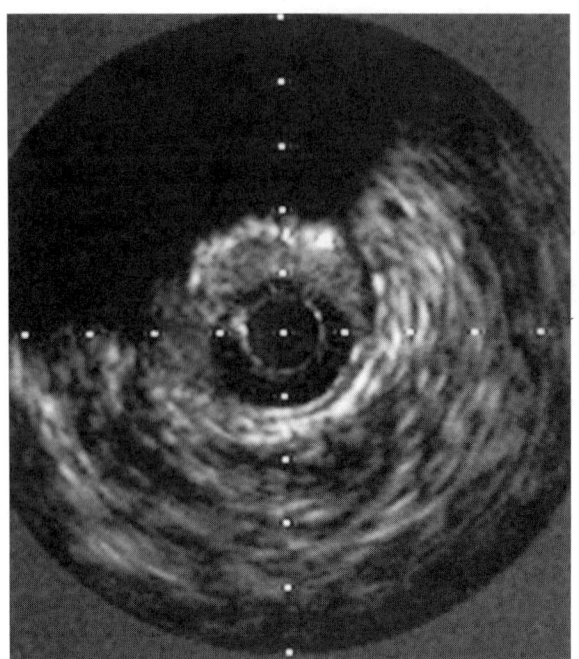 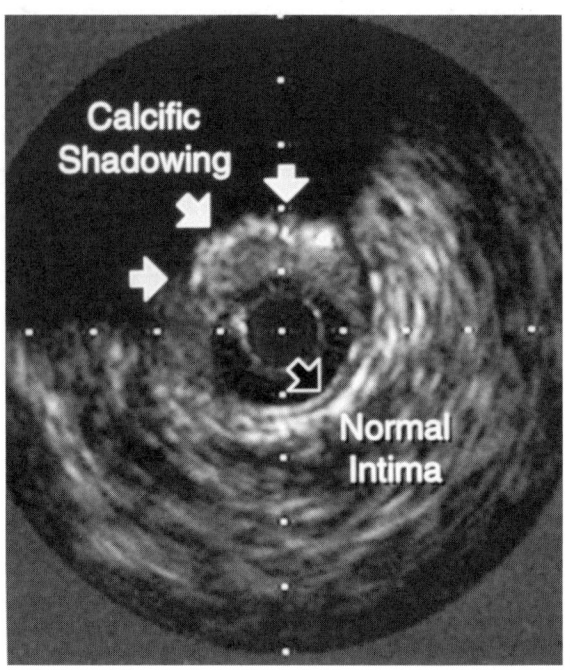

Fig. 16-7. (A & B) Example of a calcified atheroma that occupies two-thirds of the vessel wall, starting at 7 o'clock and ending at 3 o'clock. The remaining arc of the vessel is free of disease. There is calcification deep in the plaque with a characteristic shadowing behind it.

lesion calcification was only 45%.[27] When calcification was visible angiographically, it tended to be extensive and superficial. Although angiography was inaccurate in localizing calcification with respect to the luminal surface, the presence of calcium at any site on the coronary tree indicated a high probability of target lesion calcification, even when the lesion itself was free of angiographic calcification. Mintz et al.[28] reported similar findings from a large series of patients undergoing coronary interventions.

Extent and Location of Atherosclerotic Plaque

In addition to calcification, other arterial features are also better defined by intravascular ultrasound. For example, the absolute extent of atherosclerosis along the length of the vessel and the location of atheroma relative to the vessel circumference (plaque eccentricity) are better defined by ultrasound (Fig. 16-9). This additional information can assist the operator in planning an interventional strategy. For example, emerging evidence suggests that balloon selection according to the reference segment size, as measured by ultrasound, may lead to a better procedural result than the conventional method of angiographic measurement.[29] Plaque eccentricity (the location of the maximum plaque thickness with respect to the circumference of arterial wall) is determined more accurately by ultrasound than by angiography.[30,31] Precise knowledge of atheroma eccentricity is particularly important for optimizing directional atherectomy procedures.

INTRACORONARY DOPPLER

Coronary Physiology

The human cardiac capillary bed can dilate dramatically in response to increased metabolic demands (such as exercise) or to a decreased supply of oxygen (such as with a fixed epicardial coronary artery stenosis). However, this capacity to vasodilate is finite and depends upon the density of capillaries per unit of myocardial mass. When capillary vasodilatation occurs to compensate for a fixed epicardial coronary stenosis, evidence of vasodilatation can often be detected

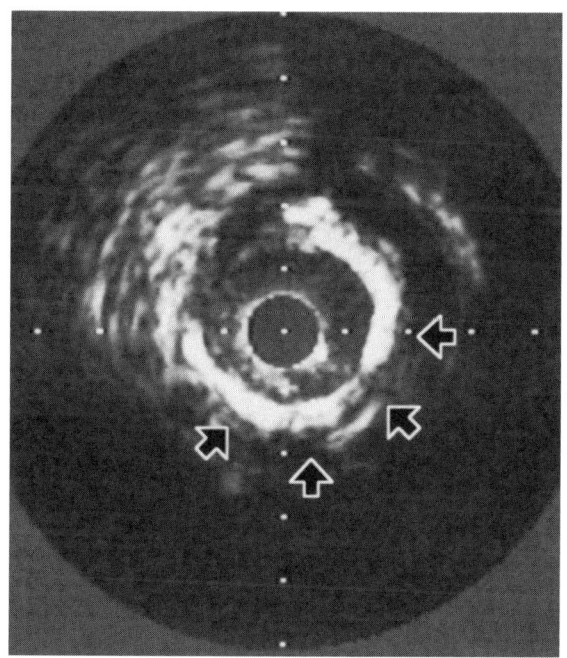 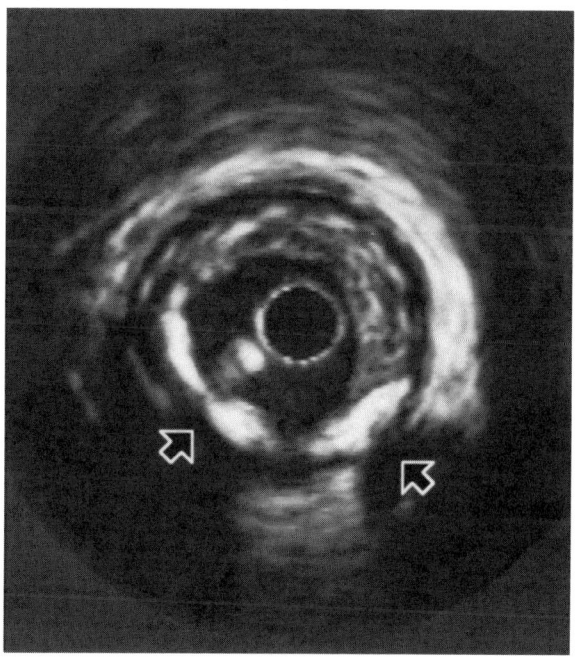

Fig. 16-8. Two examples of dense calcified atheroma. (**A**) A single piece of calcium covering the 270° arc of the vessel is shown by black arrows. (**B**) Two separate, relatively small, calcium deposits are seen with their characteristic shadowing.

at rest when the diameter of the epicardial coronary artery is reduced by 30% or more.[32] This compensatory mechanism, which attempts to preserve coronary blood flow at rest, is often exhausted when the stenosis reaches 90%. However, the potential for further increases in flow with exercise is diminished due to the reduced vasodilatory reserve. When the stenosis is greater than 90%, coronary flow is impeded even at rest, resulting in myocardial ischemia.

Doppler Measurements

The Doppler Principle

In the early 1800s Christian Johann Doppler described the shift in frequency that occurs when a sound source and sensor are in relative motion to each other. This phenomenon (the Doppler effect) has been widely applied in echocardiography, using the movement of red cells relative to the Doppler transducer to measure the velocity of blood flow.

Equipment

The in vivo physiological assessment of coronary stenoses started with the Judkins-style catheters equipped with an ultrasound Doppler transducer placed at the catheter tip. Further refinements led to the development of miniaturized catheters, which were placed into the proximal epicardial coronary arteries selectively over an angioplasty guidewire. However, these catheters with approximately 1 mm^2 cross-sectional area were limited by their size relative to the severely stenotic segments, small sampling volume, and low repetition frequency (62.5 kHz), which caused aliasing in high velocity areas. Furthermore, signal analysis was performed by *zero-crossing* method (ZC), based on measuring the interval between two adjacent ZCs of the frequency shift axis.

Development of a thin wire with a Doppler transducer at the tip (FloWire, Cardiometrics Inc., Mountain View, CA) overcame most of these limitations. The Doppler guidewire resembles a regular steerable angioplasty guidewire (0.014 or 0.018 in. in diameter) in its handling characteristics. It has a piezoelectric ultrasound transducer mounted at the distal end, that samples at 5.2 mm beyond the wire tip, at an angle of 28° around the centerline of flow. The wire is connected to a console (FloMap, Cardiometrics Inc., Mountain View, CA) that provides on-

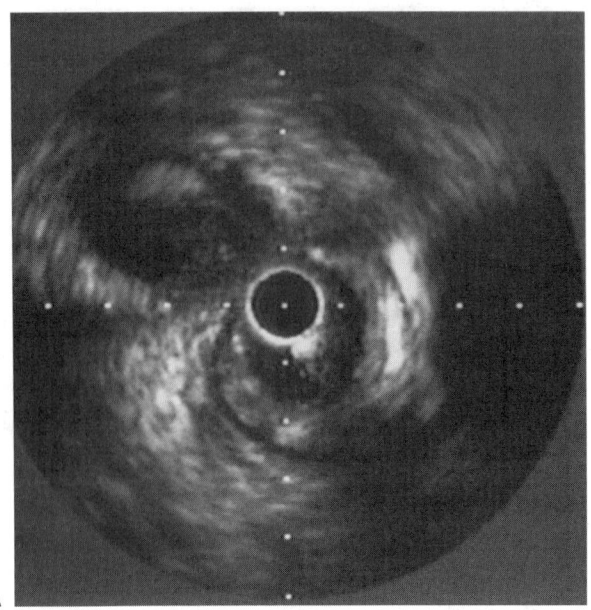 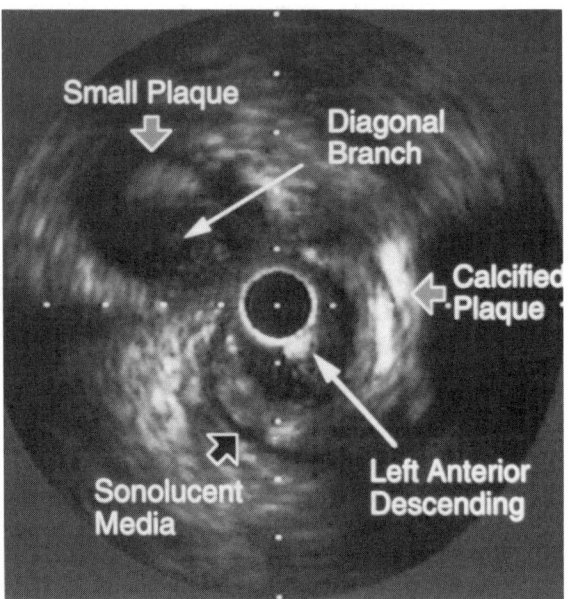

Fig. 16-9. (A & B) Intravascular ultrasound appearance of an eccentric, partially calcified atheroma in the proximal left anterior descending coronary artery. The plaque is located typically opposite to the flow-dividing wall at the major bifurcation site. A small eccentric plaque is seen in the far field in the diagonal branch as well.

line graphic display of average peak blood flow velocity, utilizing the *fast Fourier transformation* for spectral analysis (90 spectra per second). The Doppler wire can be advanced through coronary stenosis without creating flow disturbances because of its low profile (0.164 mm^2). Larger sampling volume and higher repetition frequency capacity (16 to 94 kHz) assure consistent velocity measurements. Spectral analysis is superior to the zero-crossing method in the evaluation of average and peak velocities as well as in near-laminar flow.[33,34]

Flow Velocity Measurements

The velocity and pattern of coronary flow vary according to the segment of the coronary tree and time in the cardiac cycle.[35] In 55 angiographically normal coronary arteries, the resting peak velocities during diastole were 37 ± 12 and 49 ± 20 m/s in the proximal right coronary artery and left anterior descending artery respectively. The measured peak diastolic velocities in the distal segments of the same arteries were 28 ± 8 and 35 ± 16 m/s, respectively. The hyperemic diastolic peak velocities created by intracoronary adenosine administration were 72 ± 13 and 104 ± 28 m/s, respectively. The proximal to distal velocity ratio in these 55 angiographically normal coronary arteries was 1.4:1.

The flow in the coronary arteries is dictated by the pulsatile nature of left ventricular ejection. The majority of flow in the left coronary system occurs during diastole, when the wall tension is minimal. The right coronary artery is not subjected to high right ventricular wall tension (unless pulmonary hypertension exists), resulting in a more evenly distributed flow between the two phases of the cardiac cycle. Thus, the diastolic to systolic velocity ratio was 1.5 ± 0.5 in the right coronary artery, 1.8 ± 0.7 in the lateral circumflex, and 2.0 ± 0.5 in the left anterior descending artery. The systemic arteries demonstrate a clear systolic preponderance of flow, as a result of left ventricular ejection. Saphenous bypass grafts and internal mammary artery bypass grafts exhibit flow characteristics intermediate between those of the coronary arteries and systemic arteries.[36]

The absolute (volume) blood flow can be calculated with the following formula if the flow velocity and the area of the blood vessel are known using a constant (k) that adjusts for mean velocity:[37]

$$\text{Volume (ml/s)} = k \times \text{area (cm}^2\text{)} \times \text{average peak velocity (cm/s)}$$

Using this equation, the volume of pulsatile flow through different size tubes (0.79 to 4.76 mm in diameter) assessed by Doppler wire correlated well with measurements obtained by electromagnetic flow meters ($r > 0.98$).[38] Doppler measurements were less accurate in larger or tortuous tubes. Similar results were obtained with the canine circumflex artery model.[38]

The reproducibility of Doppler measurements was evaluated by Di Mario et al.[39] in a comparative analysis of 31 patients studied 4 to 7 months apart. The resting flow parameters correlated with those measured at the time of follow-up angiogram ($r = 0.39$ to 0.46). The hyperemic flow velocity values correlated even more consistently ($r = 0.65$ to 0.70). In this study, differences in resting flow velocities that were observed in some patients were attributed to differences in arterial pressure, coronary resistance, and volumetric blood flows between the two measurements.

Intracardiac Doppler Parameters

The Proximal to Distal Velocity Ratio (P/D)

When a coronary artery has a stenosis distal to a branch, blood flow will be diverted preferentially into the branch. The severity of the obstruction determines the magnitude of this shift. Beyond the stenosis, blood will flow at a lower velocity than in the proximal vessel and in the proximal branch. The ratio of these two velocities (proximal and distal to the obstruction) is an easily obtainable and clinically useful parameter. A ratio of more than 1.7 (proximal to distal) is indicative of a hemodynamically significant obstruction (Figs. 16-10 and 16-11).[40,41] However, this measurement is not useful in nonbranching arteries (such as the proximal right coronary artery) since conservation of mass dictates that the same volume will be present proximal and distal to the lesion, at the expense of increased turbulence and time of transit.

The Diastolic to Systolic Velocity Ratio

As stenoses become more severe, the pressure gradient across the stenosis in diastole becomes insufficient to overcome the resistance to flow. The diastolic component of flow is diminished and a larger proportion of blood flow occurs in systole. A diastolic to systolic velocity ratio (DSVR) less than 1.8 measured distal to the lesion indicates a hemodynamically significant obstruction (Figs. 16-10 and 16-11).[40] There are limitations to the clinical application of these principles, however. For example, lesions in the proximal and midright coronary artery segments are not subject to the high wall tension created by left ventricular systole. Thus DSVR in these segments does not reflect the abnormality of coronary blood blow.

Coronary Flow Reserve

During exercise, coronary blood flow is dramatically increased to as much as six times the resting value. Approximately two-thirds of this increase is due to capillary vasodilatation and one-third is due to enhanced chronotropy. The ratio of the peak blood flow to the resting blood flow is defined as the coronary flow reserve (CFR). As a surrogate for the measurement of actual blood flow volume, the Doppler wire measures blood *velocity*. Adenosine is used to cause capillary vasodilatation to simulate increased metabolic demands. This compound occurs naturally as a purine metabolite and has a biologic half-life of 10 to 30 seconds. It causes vasodilatation independently of the endothelium. However, this vasodilatation has little effect on epicardial coronary arteries after these vessels have reached maximal diameter following intracoronary nitroglycerin. Thus, by maintaining constant epicardial cross-sectional area, increased flow velocity following administration of adenosine reflects the augmented blood flow that accompanies capillary vasodilatation. A CFR less than 2.0^{40} measured distal to the stenosis is abnormal and indicates a hemodynamically significant obstruction (Figs. 16-10 and 16-11).

However, a number of pitfalls limit the clinical utility of coronary flow reserve. An infarcted territory cannot usually respond with capillary vasodilatation due to the destruction or scarring of the capillary bed. In acute myocardial infarction the vasodilatory response is also often limited due to tissue edema,

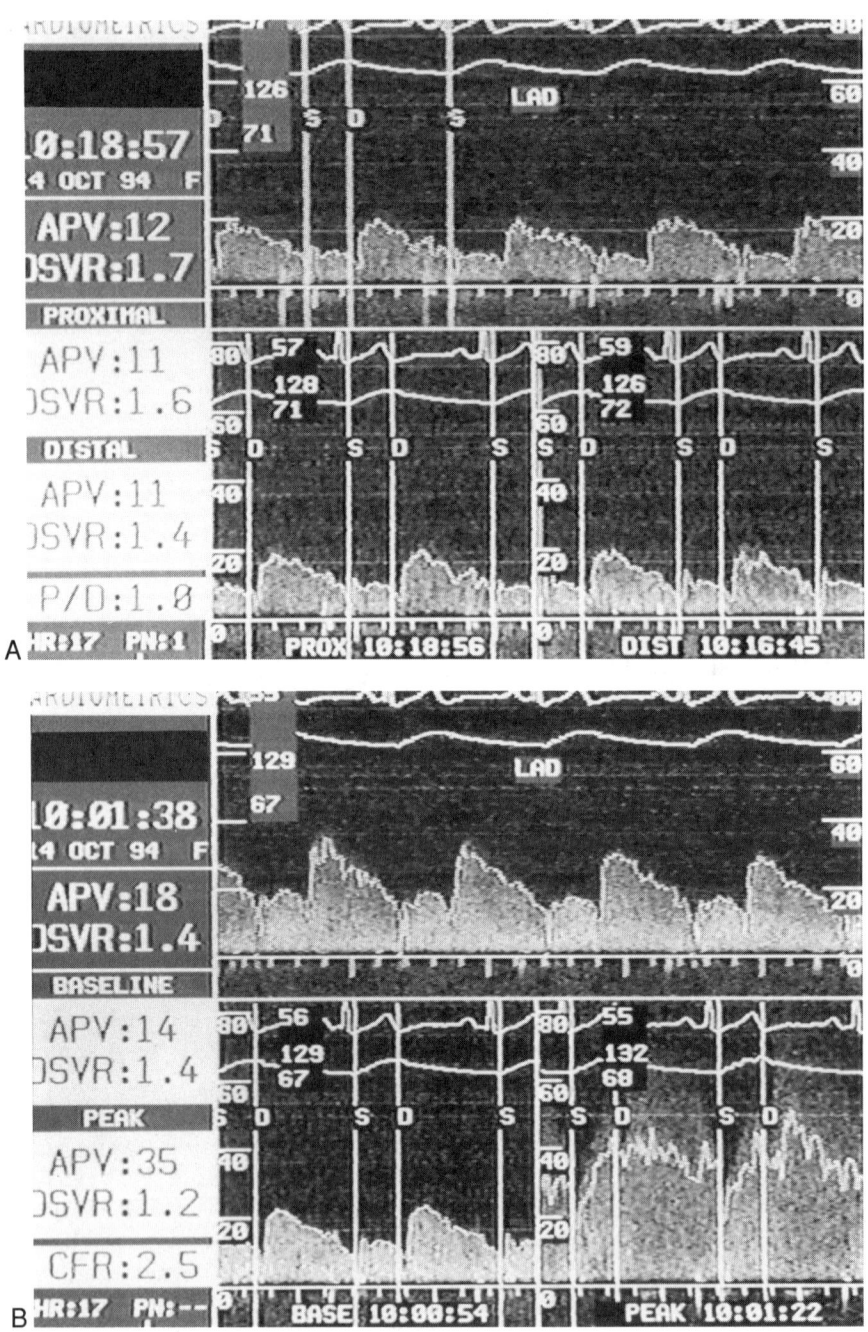

Fig. 16-10. The spectral display of coronary blood flow velocity and the derived Doppler flow parameters in the left anterior descending coronary artery with a lesion of indeterminate severity. (**A**) The average peak velocity (APV) is 11 cm/s proximal and distal to the lesion; diastolic–systolic velocity ratio (DSVR) is 1.6 and 1.4, respectively. The APV proximal and distal to the lesion is identical, giving a P/D of 1.0. (**B**) The average peak velocity distal to the lesion is 14 cm/s at baseline and increases to 35 cm/s after adenosine administration giving a coronary flow reserve (CFR) of 2.5. These measurements demonstrate normal coronary flow velocity profile and CFR.

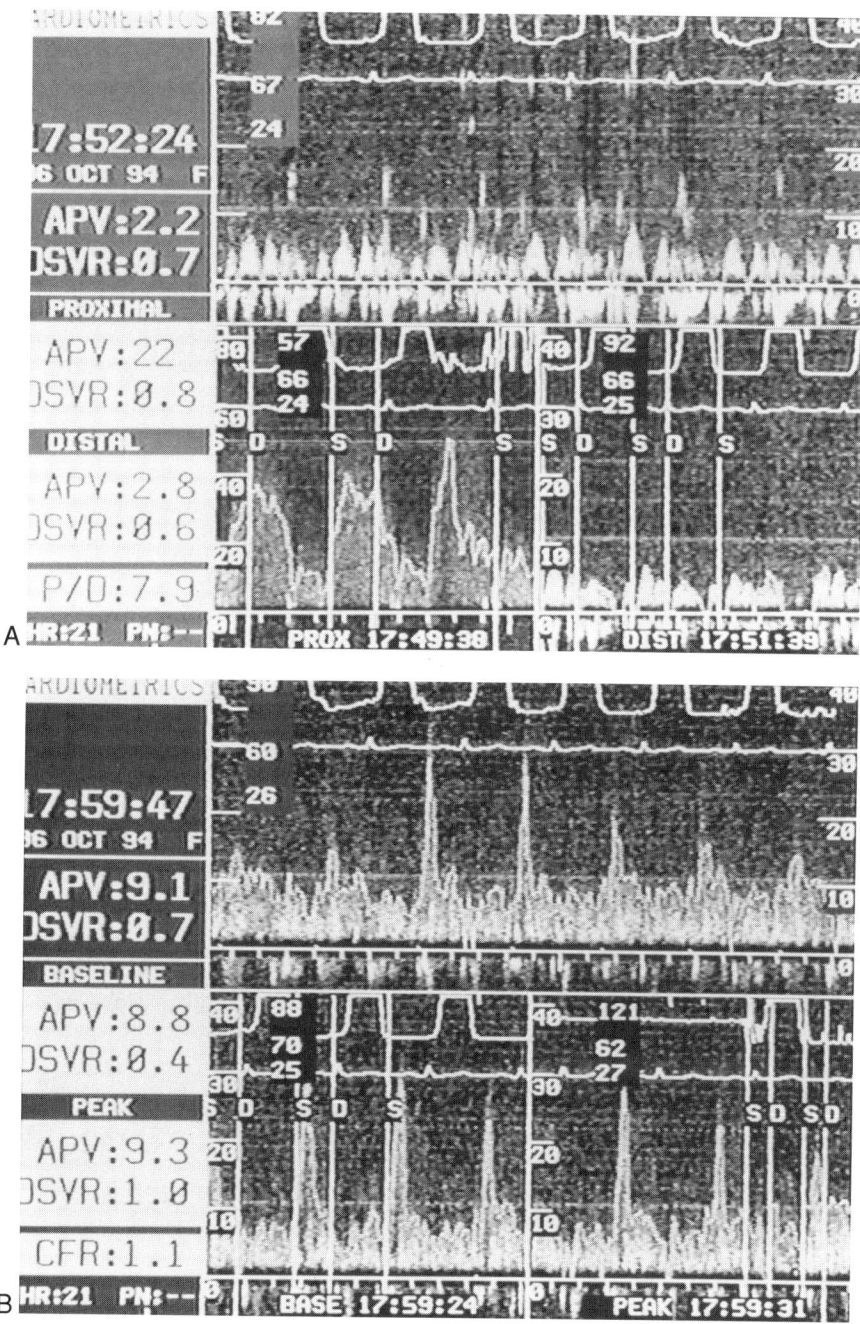

Fig. 16-11. Doppler flow measurements from another patient with a left anterior descending lesion of indeterminate severity. (**A**) The average peak velocity (APV) is 22 cm/s, but diminishes to 2.8 cm/s distal to the lesion; diastolic–systolic velocity ratio (DSVR) is 0.8 and 0.6, respectively. The average peak velocity proximal and distal to the lesion is 7.9. (**B**) The average peak velocity distal to the lesion is 8.8 cm/s at baseline and increases to only 9.3 cm/s after adenosine administration giving a coronary flow reserve (CFR) of only 1.1. These measurements demonstrate an abnormal velocity profile and coronary flow reserve as indicated by high proximal-to-distal ratio, low diastolic–systolic velocity ratio, and low CFR.

so the CFR may be abnormal despite widely patent epicardial arteries. Left ventricular hypertrophy can interfere with accurate CFR measurements, because the increased myocardial mass causes an augmented resting capillary flow, thus diminishing the reserve that can be recruited during exercise or adenosine administration. Thus, severe hypertrophy will result in an abnormally low CFR, whether or not a flow-obstructing epicardial stenosis is present. To some extent, this limitation can be circumvented by measuring the CFR in an artery free of any epicardial lesions. If the CFR is normal in the uninvolved vessel, then the low CFR in the diseased vessel probably reflects a hemodynamically significant stenosis.

Flow Turbulence in Lesions

The Doppler wire is also capable of estimating the degree of coronary stenosis by analyzing changes in velocity of flow in the obstruction itself. In the funnel created by the atherosclerotic lesion, blood flow must accelerate to cross the narrowed passage. Using the continuity equation, the ratio of flow in the narrowed and referenced segments can be calculated by measuring the respective velocities in the two areas, because the same volume of blood must be present proximal to and within the stenosis.[42] Therefore,

$$\text{Percent area stenosis} = [1 - APV_r/APV_s)]100$$

where APV is the average peak velocity in centimeters per second, r is the reference segment, and s denotes the stenotic segment. The result can be translated into percent diameter stenosis by assuming a cylindrical arterial segment. However, this measurement is time consuming and more difficult to obtain and reproduce than the P/D ratio, the CFR, and the DSVR. As a result, its use is often limited to research.

Doppler Measurement Technique

After routine coronary angiography, the area of interest is identified. After heparin is administered, the Doppler wire is advanced within the vessel using fluoroscopic guidance. Diagnostic coronary catheters are usually sufficient for the procedure. To avoid turbulent flow, the wire is first positioned at least 1 cm proximal to the lesion and, if possible, preferably proximal to a branch, and intracoronary nitroglycerin is given to assure maximal epicardial vasodilatation. The proximal average peak velocity (APV) is recorded. Then, the wire is advanced 1 to 2 cm beyond the lesion and the APV is again recorded. The P/D ratio is calculated using these values. The pulsatile nature of flow can then be assessed by the DSVR distal to the lesion. Finally, intracoronary adenosine (12 to 18 μg) is administered and the rise in APV is monitored. The maximum APV is detected and the CFR (the ratio of APV before and after adenosine) is calculated. These measurements can usually be performed in a short period of time. However, it is critical to invest the time necessary to obtain stable and clear Doppler signals to avoid inaccurate measurements. Slight changes in wire position, to avoid contact with the vessel wall and to eliminate noise from adjacent coronary veins, can improve the accuracy of this diagnostic procedure.

CLINICAL APPLICATION OF INTRACORONARY STUDIES

General Indications

Even after a complete examination, the angiographer may be unsure of the hemodynamic significance of the lesion and remain undecided whether revascularization is indicated. Examples of this situation include the symptomatic patient who undergoes coronary angiography without a preceding stress test and the patient whose coronary anatomy do not match the clinical data. Although it is possible to perform a stress test after the angiographic study, this strategy adds substantial cost and delay. Furthermore, in patients with multivessel CAD radioisotope stress imaging can underestimate total ischemic burden. Stress echocardiography also has limitations in the evaluation of multiple ischemic areas, particularly when the resting ventricular function is impaired. In other patients, angiographic images may be inadequate for a definitive diagnosis due to the limitations discussed above. Although intravascular ultrasound and Doppler measurements do not overcome all of these limitations, these procedures can provide critical incremental information and improve the accuracy of diagnosis. In addition to these general considerations, the techniques have specific application in a number of circumstances.

Specific indications

Coronary Ostia

Angiography is often inadequate in delineating the severity of disease at the coronary artery ostia, particularly as ostial lesions can cause inadequate catheter engagement. Sometimes the catheter becomes deeply seated beyond the stenosis, causing subselective contrast injection; or it does not engage the stenosis and opacification of the sinus of Valsalva obscures the ostium. Severe but eccentric ostial stenoses can be completely missed despite multiple projections, and origins of branches and overlapping vessels exacerbate this problem. In these situations, intravascular ultrasound can easily determine the extent of atherosclerosis and whether or not it involves the ostium.

Nevertheless, anatomic data from intravascular ultrasound images may be insufficient in some clinical situations. The physiologic effect of a coronary narrowing on myocardial perfusion can be investigated with Doppler flow measurements. For example, Kern et al.[43] confirmed severe stenoses in three ostial lesions that were difficult to assess angiographically using Doppler flow. The Doppler study revealed high velocities in the ostium of the grafts, up to 120 cm/s, predominantly systolic and markedly reduced coronary flow reserve. All Doppler parameters improved significantly after angioplasty. However, one must interpret Doppler data cautiously unless a stable signal is obtained.

Left Main Lesions

Angiography of left main coronary artery may be inconclusive due to angulation, inadequate angiographic projections, diffuse atherosclerotic involvement, and the inability to achieve selective cannulation. Failure to diagnose a significant left main stenosis can have dire clinical consequences. Postmortem studies have demonstrated the insensitivity of coronary angiography in detecting left main coronary atherosclerosis.[6] Intravascular ultrasound provides valuable incremental information in the assessment of such poorly defined but critical arterial segments. When a large plaque burden and small lumen area are seen in this situation the patient is usually referred for revascularization. Conversely, if a small amount of atheroma and a large lumen are seen, the patient is spared multiple costly tests or, worse, unnecessary surgery.

In addition to ostial disease, intravascular ultrasound is also useful in assessing the rest of the left main coronary artery (Fig. 16-12). In a study of 104 patients undergoing coronary intervention, De Franco et al.[44] demonstrated a high prevalence of atherosclerosis in angiographically normal left main coronary arteries. In another study, intravascular imaging discovered unrecognized left main coronary artery atherosclerosis in 45% of patients.[45] In our laboratory we routinely use ultrasound to evaluate ambiguous left main coronary lesions. In a small series of 10 patients who were initially referred for bypass surgery but in whom the clinical and angiographic data were (in our opinion) inconclusive, ultrasound was useful in determining the need for revascularization. In 4 of 10 patients ultrasound revealed only minimal atherosclerosis in the left main coronary artery and surgery was canceled. In the remaining six patients, ultrasound confirmed severe disease and coronary bypass surgery was carried out.[46]

All cardiologists encounter the angiographically "small" left main coronary artery that does not have an apparent focal stenosis. A recent ultrasound study suggests that many of these vessels actually contain significant or critical amounts of atherosclerotic plaque. Elliott et al.[47] measured the size of the left main, left anterior descending, and circumflex arteries with both angiography and intravascular ultrasound. The ratio between the diameter of the left main coronary artery and the sum of the diameters of its branch vessels were calculated, and a new index for left main coronary artery was proposed.[47] An abnormal left main ratio was defined as less than 0.58. This threshold value was 2 standard deviations less than the mean value of 0.67 in 30 patients with normal coronary arteries. This index was prospectively validated in 64 consecutive patients with coronary disease and found to have a specificity of 93% and sensitivity of 44%. Thus, patients with a left main ratio of less than 0.58 may warrant further investigation for possible unrecognized left main atherosclerosis.

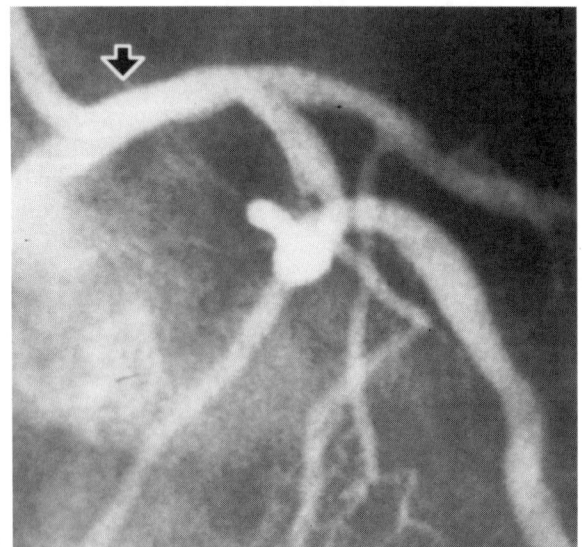 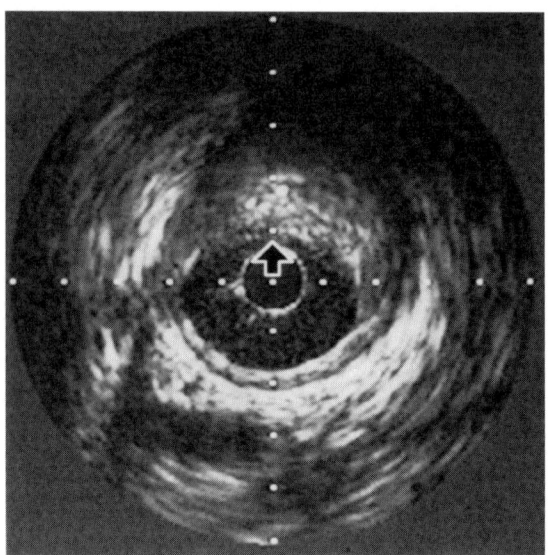

Fig. 16-12. **(A)** Left coronary angiogram in right anterior oblique projection. The left main coronary artery appears minimally irregular, but is free of significant obstruction. **(B)** The ultrasound section taken from the proximal left main coronary artery shows a large eccentric atherosclerotic plaque occupying almost half of the lumen (black arrow). This figure illustrates the insensitivity of angiography in detecting left main atherosclerosis.

Myocardial Bridging

Myocardial bridging is reported in 0.5% to 2.5% of patients undergoing angiography,[48] but its clinical significance not well understood. Erbel et al.[49] studied the morphological and physiological aspects of this dynamic obstruction, using intravascular ultrasound and Doppler flow measurements. They reported a higher incidence of myocardial bridging by demonstrating an alteration in the blood flow patterns, and trans-stenotic gradients accompanying changes in the lumen shape at the site of bridging. The same group of investigators documented a characteristic prominence of peak flow velocity in the early diastole that corresponds to the delayed relaxation of the bridged segment observed by intravascular ultrasound. Nitroglycerin or inotropic agents provoke bridging and lead to a high velocity flow in early diastole due to continuing compressions. This flow pattern may explain the reduced coronary flow reserve in the involved vessels. During these careful studies, atherosclerotic changes were found in 80% of all patients with myocardial bridging.[50] As our understanding of the relationship between myocardial bridging and clinical ischemic syndromes improves, intravascular ultrasound and Doppler measurements will help us in the identification of clinically significant cases.

Ambiguous Coronary Lesions

At times, the coronary angiogram may reveal a site that is abnormal but does not allow quantitative assessment. Haziness, napkin ring appearance, dynamic narrowing resembling kinking, or bridging may be very difficult to quantify. Haziness in a coronary segment may be due to various abnormalities: eccentric atheroma, thrombus, dissection, calcified plaque, bend in an artery, or artifact due to tissue overlap. Napkin ring lesions may be due to very discrete but severe obstructions, or severe angulations. Intravascular ultrasound is very effective in clarifying these ambiguous lesions.

Ischemic Syndromes and "Normal Coronary Arteries"

Patients who present with typical angina pectoris or acute coronary stenosis, but "normal coronary angiography" constitute a challenging problem. The finding of occult atherosclerosis or lack thereof by intravascular ultrasound can have therapeutic implications in such patients. Intravascular ultrasound may reveal a significant stenosis requiring intervention undetected by angiography or mild atherosclerotic changes or completely normal appearance.

In patients with syndrome X, defined as angina, positive stress test, and angiographically normal coronary arteries, the cause and effect association between atherosclerotic changes and the clinical syndrome is not well known. The relationship between mild atherosclerosis of the major epicardial coronary arteries and microcirculation is currently under investigation. In a recently published study, 50 patients with syndrome X were studied by intravascular ultrasound during peak exercise. Patients with intimal thickening greater than 0.25 mm had an abnormal (constrictive) vasomotor response to exercise, while those with ultrasonically normal arteries had a normal (vasodilatory) response.[51] Others have studied the capillary vasodilatation in the coronary and peripheral arterial systems in patients with syndrome X, utilizing the Doppler FloWire.[52] The endothelium-independent vasodilatation created by adenosine or nitroprusside was compared with the endothelium-dependent vasodilatation produced by acetylcholine in 23 patients. They found concordant endothelial dysfunction in the peripheral and coronary circulation, implying the presence of a diffuse anatomic defect or a circulating substance with vasoconstrictor properties.

Lesions of Uncertain Severity

Although intravascular ultrasound may be helpful in the delineation of some lesions of uncertain severity, in many cases it does not provide the necessary information (Fig. 16-13). Coronary blood flow measurements are most useful in the assessment of borderline coronary stenosis. The accuracy of the Doppler-derived parameters to differentiate physiologically significant and insignificant lesions has been evaluated in a comparative study in 30 patients who also underwent thallium single-photon emission computed tomography (SPECT).[53] Coronary flow reserve was abnormal in 15 patients, and thallium scans revealed defects in the corresponding myocardial segments. The sensitivity, specificity, and predictive values of Doppler flow measurements for

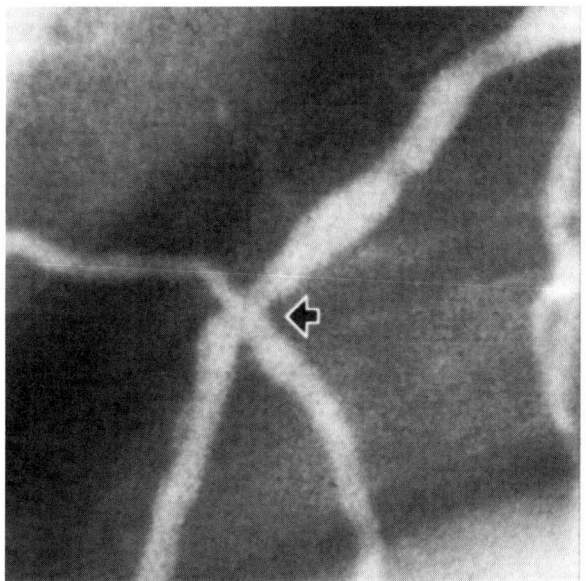
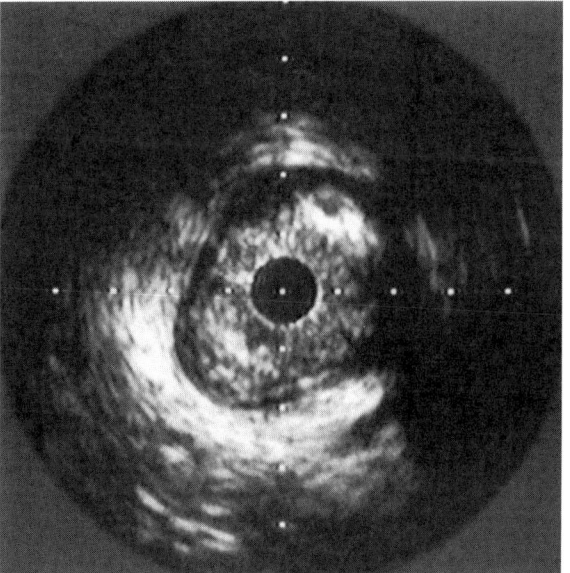

Fig. 16-13. (**A**) Right coronary angiogram in right anterior oblique projection showing a moderate stenosis. (**B**) The ultrasound image taken from the site indicated by a black arrow shows a severe obstruction with a concentric plaque, occupying the lumen outside the catheter. Although angiography shows only moderate narrowing with uncertain significance, ultrasound demonstrates a severe obstruction.

thallium defects were greater than 90%. In these patients, exercise tolerance was proportional to the coronary flow reserve. The normalized exercise time for age and gender correlated with coronary flow reserve ($r = 0.70, p < 0.001$) but not with the angiographic severity of the stenosis. These data suggest that exercise-induced ischemia and ischemia threshold can be predicted by Doppler flow measurements.

The pressure gradient across a coronary stenosis reflects its severity. Doppler-derived parameters such as proximal-to-distal velocity ratio correlate well with translesional gradients. In a recent study involving 84 patients with varying severity of coronary stenoses, translesional gradients and coronary blood flow velocities were measured.[54] Proximal-to-distal velocity ratio correlated with the translesional gradients ($r = 0.8, p < 0.001$). A ratio of greater than 1.7:1 was strongly associated with the presence of a greater than 30 mmHg gradient.

The safety of decision making based upon Doppler measurements was evaluated by Kern et al.[55] In 88 patients with coronary stenosis of uncertain severity, the decision to defer coronary intervention was made according to prespecified Doppler flow parameters. At follow-up, mortality and late target vessel revascularization were 2% and 8%, respectively, indicating that patients with borderline coronary stenosis and normal coronary flow parameters can be managed conservatively.

Percutaneous Coronary Interventions

The mechanisms of various coronary interventions in different plaque morphologies are better appreciated by intravascular ultrasound. Preprocedural ultrasound examination provides valuable information regarding the severity and extent of atherosclerosis, plaque content, and reference segment disease. This information helps in selecting the type and size of the interventional device and the plan of the procedure.[56] Imaging following initial intervention allows interim evaluation, which is particularly valuable in directional atherectomy and stent cases.[57-61] Ultrasound imaging after the intervention offers a comprehensive evaluation of the size, shape, and surface characteristics of the lumen, and the extent and depth of dissections.[45, 62] Post-

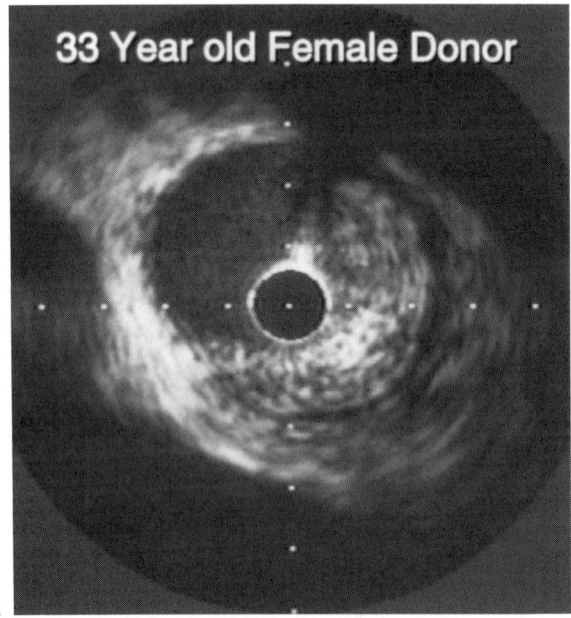 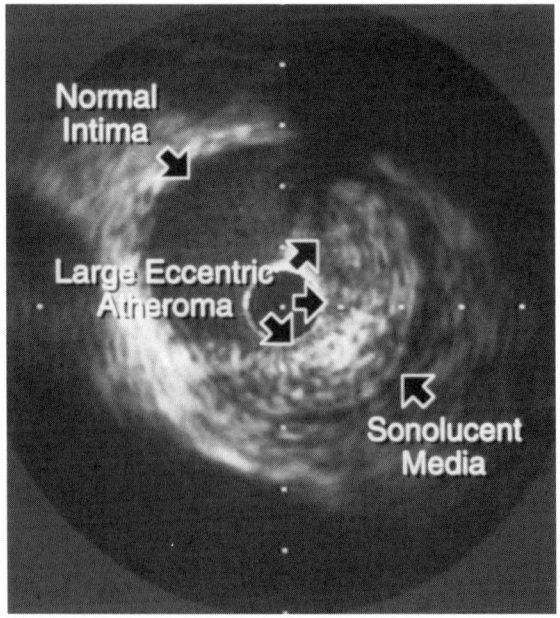

Fig. 16-14. (A & B) Ultrasound appearance of a coronary artery from a cardiac transplant recipient, who received a heart from a 33-year-old female donor. Intravascular ultrasound imaging, which was performed 3 weeks after transplantation, revealed a large eccentric atheroma despite a completely normal angiogram.

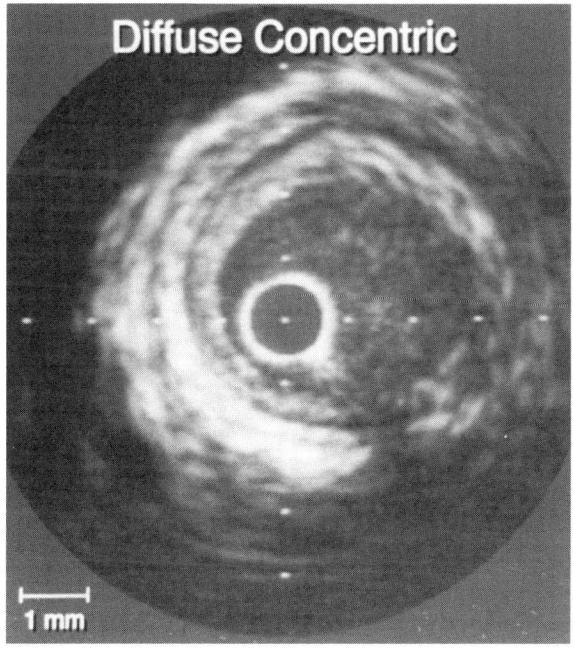 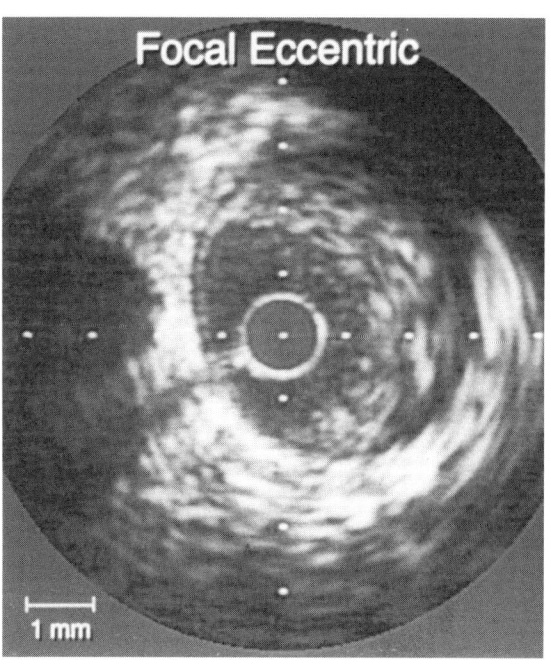

Fig. 16-15. Two distinct patterns of atherosclerosis in the same patient. (**A**) A concentric and diffuse atherosclerosis is thought to be due to allograft vasculopathy. (**B**) Focal and eccentric plaque located near a branching point in the proximal coronary artery is thought to be due to native atherosclerosis that came with the donor heart.

procedure assessment helps the operator to decide if further intervention is necessary. Doppler flow measurements at baseline provide valuable information regarding the physiologic significance of the stenosis.

Emerging data suggest postprocedure velocity parameters distal to the lumen may be helpful in the assessment of the intervention's outcome.[63] Recent reports suggest that residual plaque burden and lumen area determined by ultrasound are predictors of restenosis.[64,65] If these findings are confirmed, intravascular ultrasound and Doppler flow measurements may assume a larger role in the interventional catheterization laboratory.

Coronary Atherosclerosis in Cardiac Transplant Recipients

The early stages of coronary atherosclerosis are frequently missed at angiography. Ultrasound studies involving cardiac transplant recipients have demonstrated this point very clearly. Atherosclerosis (defined as 0.5 mm intimal thickness) was present in 28 of the 50 cardiac transplant recipients (mean donor age 31 years) that were imaged 4.6 ± 2.6 weeks after transplantation.[66] Angiography was slightly abnormal in 43% of patients with ultrasonographically evident atherosclerosis. Similar findings were reported by other investigators.[67] The distribution of atherosclerosis in these patients who underwent imaging shortly after cardiac transplantation was typical of conventional atherosclerosis: almost all atherosclerotic plaques were located in the proximal segments; more than 85% were focal and eccentric and half were located near bifurcations (Fig. 16-14). These characteristics are typical of patients with conventional atherosclerosis and distinctly different from immune-mediated allograft vasculopathy.

In patients who were imaged one or more years after transplantation, the prevalence of atherosclerosis was higher.[68,69] The distribution of atherosclerosis in 132 patients who were imaged 1 to 9 years after transplantation was different than the pattern observed within a few weeks of transplantation.[69] In most of these patients, the pattern of atherosclerosis was heterogeneous (Fig. 16-15). Diffuse and concentric disease was more frequent than focal and eccentric plaques, particularly in mid and distal segments. Focal and eccentric plaques were observed more commonly in the proximal segments. These findings suggest that the atherosclerotic changes that are observed years after cardiac transplantation have multiple etiologies including donor-transmitted conventional atherosclerosis and allograft vasculopathy. Ongoing serial ultrasound studies in cardiac transplant recipients will shed more light on the natural history of transplant CAD and allow us to design more effective and timely interventions for this difficult problem.

Even before anatomic evidence of transplant vasculopathy is evident, physiologic perturbation may already exist. To assess the endothelial function of transplanted hearts, Pinto et al.[70] measured endothelium-dependent vasodilatation with the Doppler wire in 15 cardiac transplant patients. The degree of vasodilatation was inversely related to intimal thickness, assessed by intravascular ultrasound. Five of six segments with normal intimal thickness demonstrated vasoconstriction in response to acetylcholine. Similarly, others have observed endothelial dysfunction without detectable intimal thickening.[71] In this study, there was no relation between the degree of intimal thickening and magnitude of endothelium-dependent response to acetylcoline. Thus, physiologic abnormalities appear to precede the presently quantifiable morphologic defects.

CONCLUSIONS

While angiography remains the most common invasive method for the anatomic detection of CAD, in particular clinical situations intravascular ultrasound and Doppler flow can contribute significant incremental information in the evaluation of the patient with CAD.

Ultrasound imaging presents a unique opportunity to visualize the complex morphologic aspects of coronary lesions, substantiates the angiographic appearance of the vessel with respect to the extent, distribution, and characteristics of atherosclerosis, or even detects obstructions not apparent by angiography. It also assists in the choice of the device with the best potential to treat the specific stenosis and guides the cardiologist in the evaluation of therapy results. Yet, the understanding of coronary anatomy and lesion morphology does not necessarily obviate the need to characterize the functional significance of the stenosis. A given lumen size as assessed by intravascular ultrasound, has different functional consequences, based upon the reference size and the amount and integrity of myocardium supplied. Measurement of flow parameters in these circumstances promises to shed light on the physiologic significance of such a stenosis and to assist in delivering optimal therapy.

It is important to stress that these newer technologies will not replace noninvasive functional testing or angiography; rather, they *complement* these methodologies by clarifying ambiguities and discrepancies between the clinical assessment and coronary angiogram. Furthermore, neither ultrasound nor Doppler can be used as the *sole* test to determine the need for revascularization. The data obtained by these modalities must be interpreted in the context of a comprehensive clinical evaluation.

REFERENCES

1. Arnett EN, Isner JM, Redwood DR et al.: Coronary artery narrowing in coronary heart disease: comparison of cineangiographic and necropsy findings. Ann Intern Med 91:350, 1979
2. Grodin C, Dydra I, Pastgernac A et al.: Discrepancies between cineangiographic and post-mortem findings in patients with coronary artery disease and recent myocardial revascularization. Circulation 49:703, 1974
3. Isner J, Kishel J, Kent K: Accuracy of angiographic determination of left main coronary arterial narrowing. Circulation 63:1056, 1981
4. Roberts W, Jones A: Quantitation of coronary arterial narrowing at necropsy in sudden coronary death. Am J Cardiol 44:39, 1979
5. Vlodaver Z, Frech R, van Tassel RA, Edwards JE: Correlation of the antemortem coronary angiogram and the postmortem specimen. Circulation 47:162, 1973
6. Keane D, Haase J, Slager C et al.: Comparative validation of quantitative coronary angiographic systems: results and implications from a multicenter study using standardized approach. Circulation 91:2174, 1995
7. Goldberg RK, Kleiman NS, Minor ST et al.: Compari-

son of quantitative coronary angiography to visual estimates of lesion severity pre and post percutaneous transluminal coronary angioplasty. Am Heart J 1:178, 1990
8. Fortin DF, Spero LA, Cusma JT et al.: Pitfalls in the determination of absolute dimensions using angiographic catheters as calibration devices in quantitative coronary angiography. Am J Cardiol 68:1176, 1991
9. Vogel RA: Assessing stenosis severity by coronary arteriography. Are the best variables good enough? J Am Coll Cardiol 12:692, 1988
10. Tobis JM, Mahon DJ, Moriuchi M et al.: Intravascular ultrasound imaging following balloon angioplasty. Int J Cardiol Imag 6:191, 1991
11. Honye J, Mahon DJ, White CJ et al.: Morphological effects of coronary balloon angioplasty in vivo assessed by intravascular ultrasound imaging. Circulation 85:1012, 1992
12. De Franco AC, Tuzcu EM, Abdelmeguid A et al.: Intravascular ultrasound assessment of percutaneous transluminal coronary angioplasty results: insights into the mechanisms of balloon angioplasty. J Am Coll Cardiol 21:485A, 1993
13. Glagov S, Weisenberg E, Zarins C et al.: Compensatory enlargements of human coronary arteries. N Engl J Med 316:1371, 1987
14. Pasterkamp G, Borst C, Gussenhoven EJ et al.: Remodeling of de novo atherosclerotic lesions in femoral arteries: impact of mechanism of balloon angioplasty. J Am Coll Cardiol 26:422, 1995
15. White CW, Wright CB, Doty BD et al.: Does visual interpretation of the coronary arteries predict the physiologic importance of a coronary stenosis? N Engl J Med 310:819, 1984
16. Nissen SE, De Franco AC, Raymond RE et al.: Angiographically unrecognized disease at normal reference sites: a risk factor for sub-optimal results after coronary interventions. Circulation 88:I-412, 1993
17. Mintz GS, Painter JA, Pichard AD et al.: Atherosclerosis in angiographically "normal" coronary artery reference segments: an intravascular ultrasound study with clinical correlations. J Am Coll Cardiol 25:1479, 1995
18. Hausmann D, Erbel R, Alibelli-Chemarin M-J et al.: The safety of intracoronary ultrasound. A multicenter survey of 2207 examinations. Circulation 91:623, 1995
19. Fitzgerald PJ, St. Goar FG, Connolly AJ et al: Intravascular ultrasound imaging of coronary arteries. Is three layers the norm? Circulation 86:154, 1992
20. Velican D, Velican C: Comparative study on age related changes and arteriosclerosis involvement of the coronary arteries of male and female subjects up to 40 years of age. Arteriosclerosis 38:39, 1981
21. Hodgson JMcB, Reddy KG, Suneja R et al.: Intravascular ultrasound imaging: correlation of plaque morphology with angiography, clinical syndrome and procedural results in patients undergoing coronary angioplasty. J Am Coll Cardiol 21:35, 1993
22. Fitzgerald PJ, Ports TA, Yock PG: Contribution of localized calcium deposits to dissection after angioplasty in vivo assessed by intravascular ultrasound imaging. Circulation 86:64, 1992
23. De Franco AC, Nissen S, Tuzcu E et al.: Ultrasound plaque morphology predicts major dissections following stand-alone and adjunctive balloon angioplasty, abstracted. Circulation 90:I59, 1994
24. Di Mario C, The SH, Madretsma S et al.: Detection and characterization of vascular lesions by intravascular ultrasound: an in vitro study correlated with histology. J Am Soc Echocardiogr 5:135, 1992
25. Gussenhoven EJ, Essed CE, Lancee CT et al.: Arterial wall characteristics determined by intravascular ultrasound imaging: an in vitro study. J Am Coll Cardiol 14:947, 1989
26. Tobis JM, Mallery J, Mahon D et al.: Intravascular ultrasound imaging of human coronary arteries in vivo. Analysis of tissue characterization with comparison to in-vitro histological specimens. Circulation 83:913, 1991
27. Tuzcu EM, Berkalp B, De Franco AC et al.: The dilemma of diagnosing coronary calcification: angiography vs. intravascular ultrasound. J Am Coll Cardiol 27:832, 1996
28. Mintz GS, Douek P, Pichard AD et al.: Target lesion calcification in coronary artery disease: an intravascular ultrasound study. J Am Coll Cardiol 20:1149, 1992
29. Hodgson J McB, Stone GW, St Goar et al.: Can intravascular ultrasound improve percutaneous transluminal coronary angioplasty results? Preliminary core lab ultrasound analysis from the CLOUT pilot study. J Am Coll Cardiol 25:143A, 1995
30. Hausmann D, Lundkvist JS, Friedrich G et al.: Lumen and plaque shape in atherosclerotic coronary arteries assessed by in vivo intravascular ultrasound. Am J Cardiol 74:857, 1994
31. De Franco AC, Tuzcu EM, Moliterno DJ et al.: "Directional" coronary atherectomy removes atheroma more effectively from concentric than eccentric lesions: intravascular ultrasound predictors of lesional success. J Am Coll Cardiol 137, 1995
32. Gould KL, Lipscomb K, Hamilton GW: Physiologic basis for assessing critical coronary stenoses. Am J Cardiol 33:87, 1974
33. Tanouchi J, Kitabatake A, Ishihara K et al.: Experimental validation of Doppler catheter technique using

fast Fourier spectrum analysis for measuring coronary flow velocity. Circulation 80:S(II)566, 1989
34. Tadaoka S, Kigiyama M, Hiramatsu O et al.: Accuracy of 20 MHz Doppler catheter coronary artery velocimetry for measurement of coronary flow velocity. Cathet Cardiovasc Diagn 19:205, 1990
35. Ofili EO, Labovitz AJ, Kern MJ: Coronary flow velocity dynamics in normal and diseased arteries. Am J Cardiol 71:3D, 1993
36. Bach RG, Kern MJ, Donohue T et al.: Comparison of arterial and venous coronary bypass conduits: analysis of intravessel blood flow characteristics. Circulation 86:118A, 1992
37. Labovitz AJ, Anthonis DM, Cravens TL et al.: Validation of volumetric flow measurements by means of a Doppler-tipped coronary angioplasty guide wire. Am Heart J 126:1465, 1993
38. Doucette JW, Douglas CP, Payne HP et al.: Validation of a Doppler guide wire for intravascular measurement of coronary artery flow velocity. Circulation 85:1899, 1992
39. Di Mario C, Gil R, Serruys PW: Long-term reproducibility of coronary flow velocity measurements in patients with coronary artery disease. Am J Cardiol 75:1177, 1995
40. Kern MJ, Donohue TJ, Aguirre FV et al.: Assessment of angiographically intermediate coronary artery stenosis using the Doppler Flowire. Am J Cardiol 71:26D, 1993
41. Di Mario C, Slager CJ, Linker DT, Serruys PW: Quantitative assessment of coronary artery stenosis by intravascular Doppler catheter technique. Circulation 86:2016, 1992
42. Nakatani S, Yamagishi M, Tamai J et al.: Quantitative assessment of coronary artery stenosis by intravascular Doppler catheter technique. Circulation 85:1786, 1992
43. Kern MJ, Flynn MS, Aguirre FV et al.: Application of intracoronary flow velocity for detection and management of ostial saphenous vein graft lesions. Cathet Cardiovasc Diagn 30:5, 1993
44. De Franco AC, Tuzcu EM, Eaton G et al.: Detection of unrecognized LMCA disease by intravascular ultrasound in patients undergoing interventions: prevalence and severity. Circulation 88:I-411, 1993
45. Gerber TE, Erbel R, Gorge G et al.: Extent of atherosclerosis and remodeling of the left main coronary artery determined by intravascular ultrasound. Am J Cardiol 73:666, 1994
46. Goodhart DM, Nissen SE, DeFranco AC et al.: Diagnosis of angiographically elusive left main and ostial left anterior descending lesions by intravascular ultrasound. Circulation 90:I-450, 1994
47. Elliott JM, Tuzcu EM, DeFranco AC et al.: The left main diameter ratio: a specific index of left main coronary artery disease as validated by intravascular ultrasound, abstracted. J Am Coll Cardiol 24:210A, 1994
48. Nobel J, Bourassa MG, Petitelere R, Dyrda I: Myocardial bridging and milking effect of the left anterior descending coronary artery: normal variant or obstruction? Am J Cardiol 37:993, 1976
49. Erbel R, Rupprecht HJ, Ge J et al.: Coronary artery shape and flow changes induced by myocardial bridging. Echocardiography 10:71, 1993
50. Ge J, Erbel R, Rupprecht HJ et al.: Comparison of intravascular ultrasound and angiography in the assessment of myocardial bridging. Circulation 89:1725, 1994
51. Weidermann JG, Schwartz A, Apfelbaum M: Anatomic and physiologic heterogeneity in patients with syndrome X: an intravascular ultrasound study. J Am Coll Cardiol 25:1310, 1995
52. Quyyumi AA, Dakak N, Gilligan DM et al.: Peripheral vascular endothelial dysfunction in syndrome X patients with endothelial dysfunction of the coronary microvasculature. Circulation 88:S1978, 1993
53. Joye JD, Schulman DS, Lasorda D et al.: Intracoronary Doppler guide wire versus single-photon emission computed tomographic thallium-201 imaging in assessment of intermediate coronary stenoses. J Am Coll Cardiol 24:940, 1994
54. Donohue TJ, Kern MJ, Aguirre FV et al.: Assessing the hemodynamic significance of coronary artery stenoses: analysis of translesional pressure-flow velocity relations in patients. J Am Coll Cardiol 22:449, 1993
55. Kern MJ, Donohue TJ, Aguirre FV et al.: Clinical outcome of deferring angioplasty in patients with normal translesional pressure-flow velocity measurements. J Am Coll Cardiol 25:178, 1995
56. Mintz GS, Pichard AD, Kovach JA et al.: Impact of preintervention intravascular ultrasound imaging on transcatheter treatment strategies in coronary artery disease. Am J Cardiol 73:423, 1994
57. Tenaglia AN, Buller CE, Kisslo BK et al.: Mechanisms of balloon angioplasty and directional coronary atherectomy as assessed by intracoronary ultrasound. J Am Coll Cardiol 20:685, 1992
58. Bauman RP, Morris KG, Krucoff MW et al.: Maximizing plaque removal with directional coronary atherectomy: a new method using ultrasound guidance. J Am Coll Cardiol 23:386A, 1994
59. Nakamura S, Colombo A, Gaglione et al.: Intracoronary ultrasound observations during stent implantation. Circulation 89:2026, 1994
60. Goldberg SL, Colombo A, Nakamura S et al.: Benefit

of intracoronary ultrasound in the deployment of Palmaz-Schatz stents. J Am Coll Cardiol 24:996, 1994
61. Colombo A, Hall P, Nakamura S et al.: Intracoronary stenting without anticoagulation accomplished with intravascular ultrasound guidance. Circulation 91:1676, 1995
62. Berkalp B, Nissen SE, DeFranco AC et al.: Intravascular ultrasound demonstrates marked differences in surface and lumen shape following interventional devices. Circulation 90:I-58A, 1994
63. Serruys PW, Di Mario C, Kern MJ: Textbook of Interventional Cardiology, 2nd Ed. Saunders, Philadelphia, 1994
64. Mintz GS, Pichard AD, Satler LF et al.: Intravascular ultrasound predictors of angiographic restenosis. Circulation 90:I-163A, 1994
65. The GUIDE Trial Investigators: Intravascular ultrasound-determined predictors of restenosis in percutaneous transluminal coronary angioplasty and directional coronary atherectomy: an interim report from the GUIDE Trial, Phase II. Circulation 90:I-23A, 1994
66. Tuzcu EM, Hobbs RE, Rincon G et al.: Occult and frequent transmission of atherosclerotic coronary disease with cardiac transplantation: insights from intravascular ultrasound. Circulation 91:1706, 1995
67. St. Goar FG, Pinto FJ, Alderman et al.: Intracoronary ultrasound in cardiac transplant recipients: in vivo evidence of "angiographically silent" intimal thickening. Circulation 85:979, 1992
68. Richenbacher PR, Pinto FJ, Chenzbraun A et al.: Incidence and severity of transplant coronary artery disease early and up to 15 years after transplantation as detected by intravascular ultrasound. J Am Coll Cardiol 25:171, 1995
69. Tuzcu EM, De Franco AC, Goormastic M et al.: Dichotomous pattern of coronary atherosclerosis 1 to 9 years after transplantation: Insights from systematic intravascular ultrasound imaging. J Am Coll Cardiol 27:839, 1996
70. Pinto FJ, Chenzbrun A, Drexler H et al.: Coronary endothelial function and vascular structure in cardiac transplant recipients. J Am Coll Cardiol 21:S119A, 1993
71. Anderson TJ, Meredith IT, Uehata A et al.: Functional significance of intimal thickening as detected by intravascular ultrasound early and late after cardiac transplantation. Circulation 88:1093, 1993

Chapter 17

Functional Testing in Patients with Previous Coronary Interventions

Anthony C. De Franco and Eric J. Topol

Soon after the initial development of coronary angioplasty, many investigators stressed the importance of performing an exercise stress test on essentially all patients within several months of the procedure because functional testing was assumed to give an indication of immediate and long-term clinical outcome. However, the clinical value of *routine* stress testing after successful percutaneous coronary intervention has been questioned, particularly because of its expense and the ever-increasing demand for cost-effective care.

There are two broad strategies of functional testing soon after coronary intervention, routine and selective. Proponents of the routine approach emphasize that restenosis can result in silent ischemia even in many patients who *had* symptoms before intervention; because silent ischemia worsens prognosis to the same degree as symptomatic ischemia, these clinicians argue that routine functional testing is *always* indicated. On the other hand, proponents of the *selective* use of functional testing after coronary intervention argue that the data on the prognostic effect of silent ischemia is still incomplete, and that symptomatic status along with consideration of the clinical, anatomic, and procedural variables, although imperfect, can nevertheless be used as a guide to selecting the patients at highest risk for functional testing.

Rational arguments can be assembled to support both the routine and selective strategies of functional testing after coronary intervention. This chapter will first review recent advances in our knowledge about the physiology of the restenotic process after coronary intervention, the differences between angiographic and clinical restenosis, and the relationship between symptomatic status and recurrent ischemia, because these concepts affect the indications, timing, and predictive accuracy of functional testing. We then review the rationale for the routine and the selective approaches to functional testing. An understanding of the selective approach requires a review of the variables that can be used to select patients at highest risk for recurrent ischemia. Whether one elects the routine or the selective strategy, a variety of functional tests are possible; we review the available data to compare their predictive accuracy. Finally, we discuss several new developments in interventional cardiology, such as platelet glycoprotein IIb/IIIa inhibitors and coronary stents, which may reduce the incidence of restenosis and thereby modify the indications for functional testing.

RESTENOSIS: IMPLICATIONS FOR FUNCTIONAL TESTING AFTER ANGIOPLASTY

Restenosis Is the Major Current Limitation to Percutaneous Intervention

Although nearly 500,000 percutaneous coronary interventions are performed annually in the United States, restenosis of the treated site remains the major limitation of angioplasty. In the past, necropsy and animal studies suggested that most of the restenotic process was due to a characteristic intimal hyperplasia that encroached upon the vessel lumen during the weeks to months after angioplasty. However, in the contemporary paradigm of restenosis, all angioplasty procedures are considered a form of arterial injury, and restenosis is considered to be a complex *set* of responses to this injury.[1] Although these responses occur to some extent in all patients after percutaneous intervention,[2] in some cases they are excessive, resulting in recurrence of the angiographic stenosis, of clinical ischemia, or both. These events are usually evident within 6 months of the procedure.

The set of responses that compose restenosis can be divided conceptually into three components: recoil of the residual atheroma, thrombus deposition and organization, and vascular remodeling. All interventional devices (including atherectomy procedures) enlarge the target vessel to some extent by stretching of the arterial wall. Vessel *recoil* refers to the rapid loss of the arterial cross-sectional area gained by the intervention,[2,3] occurring within minutes to hours after successful procedure. In most cases recoil is modest; however, in some it is so substantial that a narrowing of 50% or more occurs within 24 hours. Abnormal vasoconstriction can also contribute to recoil.[4] Although the amount of restenosis attributable to recoil is uncertain, some reports using serial intravascular ultrasound have suggested that it accounts for between 40% to 80% of the late lumen loss after coronary intervention (Fig. 17-1).[5,6]

After angioplasty-induced vessel injury, thrombus is the second factor associated with vessel renarrowing. In its extreme presentation it can result in abrupt vessel closure,[7,8] which usually occurs within hours to days of the procedure. Most percutaneous interventions expose subendothelial collagen and tissue factor, thereby stimulating platelet adhesion and accumulation within the first 24 hours.[9–12] These events are primarily mediated by the platelet glycoprotein IIb/IIIa receptor, which couples adjacent platelets.[11] These activated platelets release several substances that result in vasoconstriction, mitogenesis, chemotaxis, and thrombus formation. The amount of thrombus formed at the site also depends on injury, and to some extent restenosis may also be related to extent of deep-wall injury. The third component of restenosis is arterial remodeling,

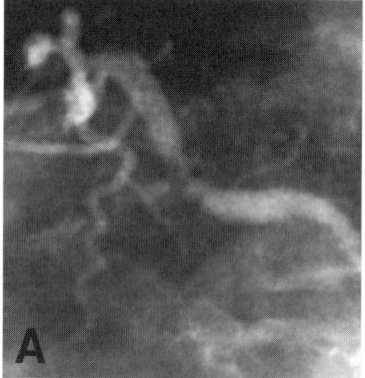 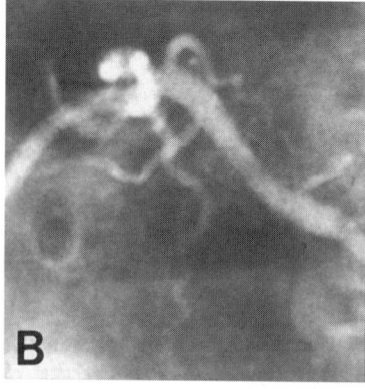 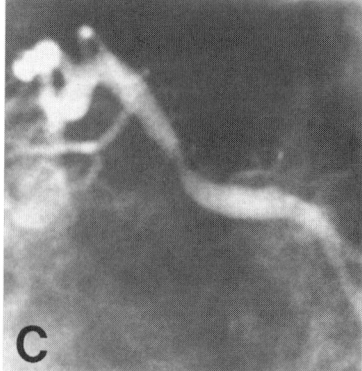

Fig. 17-1. A typical example of vessel recoil soon after successful balloon angioplasty. **(A)** Preprocedural angiogram. **(B)** Postprocedural angiogram demonstrating angiographic success. **(C)** An angiogram performed at 24 hours as part of a research protocol demonstrates significant vessel recoil. Although angiographically there is still some luminal enlargement when the 24-hour study is compared to the baseline examination, patients such as this may have recurrences of angina or a positive functional test soon after the "successful" intervention.

which refers to the process by which the injured arterial wall repairs itself over time. In the days after arterial injury, smooth muscle cells migrate to and proliferate in the injured arterial area and are transformed into cells that produce an extracellular matrix of connective tissue.[1,13] If this process is robust, it can so encroach upon the lumen that recurrent stenosis of the lesion site occurs. However, whereas remodeling after angioplasty was always assumed to result in a decrease in the size of the lumen, recent evidence from intravascular ultrasound suggests that remodeling can also result in an *increase* in vessel cross-sectional area (Fig. 17-2). As we will discuss, these concepts have important implications for the timing and interpretation of functional testing.

Angiographic Versus Clinical Restenosis

Restenosis can be defined either angiographically or clinically, and angiographic restenosis can be defined in a binary or continuous fashion. The binary definition of angiographic restenosis is usually taken as a 50% or more recurrent luminal narrowing when compared with a reference vessel diameter. Using this somewhat arbitrary definition, registry studies and clinical trials have demonstrated restenosis rates after balloon angioplasty and atherectomy of approximately 30% to 50% at 6 months.[14-16] Nevertheless, difficulties with procedural techniques, visual assessment,[17] and interobserver variability[18,19] confound this assessment; these problems are only partially remedied by computer-assisted quantitative angiography systems. Furthermore, the biology of restenosis is not a binary event; rather, the complex set of responses to arterial injury produces a continuum of luminal renarrowing that occurs to some extent in most patients after intervention. As a result, recent clinical trials have employed continuous measures of restenosis (Fig. 17-3) to avoid the problems inherent with an arbitrarily defined, binary definition. Using either a binary or a continuous approach, an angiographic endpoint assumes that the change in luminal diameter between the procedure and the follow-up study is the best assessment of restenosis and of the success of an interventional strategy.

Although the absolute amount of angiographic late lumen loss may be vitally important for a research trial comparing two interventional devices, the clinician is more concerned with the effects of the lesion on the patient's sense of well being and prognosis. Therefore, clinical restenosis refers to whether the patient is symptomatic, and more importantly, whether the loss of lumen area results in ischemia (symptomatic or not).

Although the results of functional testing are frequently included as secondary endpoints, they are rarely used as primary endpoints because of concerns about interobserver variability and because angiography is assumed to be the "gold standard." Research trials of interventional devices have, for the most part, avoided using the "hard" clinical endpoints of death, subsequent infarction, or the need for emergent revascularization because of the larger sample sizes needed (and the vastly increased costs of using these endpoints).

Symptomatic Status Is an Unreliable Indicator of Angiographic Restenosis

In many published studies the predictive value of recurrent angina as a marker of restenosis is difficult to assess because the timing and completeness of angiographic follow-up have often been determined by the patient's symptomatic status. In studies with a high rate of angiographic follow-up, the positive predictive value of symptoms ranges from 48% to 92%, whereas the negative predictive value of symptoms ranges from 70% to 98% (Table 17-1). The low positive predictive value found in many of these studies may be due, in part, to the presence of other mechanisms for chest pain, such as incomplete revascularization, progression of disease in other vessels, or a noncardiac source of pain. Thus, although an improvement in angina after angioplasty is a desirable clinical endpoint, symptomatic status is neither sensitive nor specific in determining the angiographic status of the index vessel treated with transcatheter intervention.

When angina does recur, the time between the angioplasty procedure and the recurrence of symptoms can be a clue to identify the most likely cause.[20] In the first week after angioplasty, between 5% and 8% of patients will experience recurrent angina or myocardial infarction, usually resulting from threatened or abrupt vessel closure, respectively. This is most often the result of underlying high-risk anatomy and subsequent thrombotic occlusion, occlusive dissection, or both. The incidence of this complica-

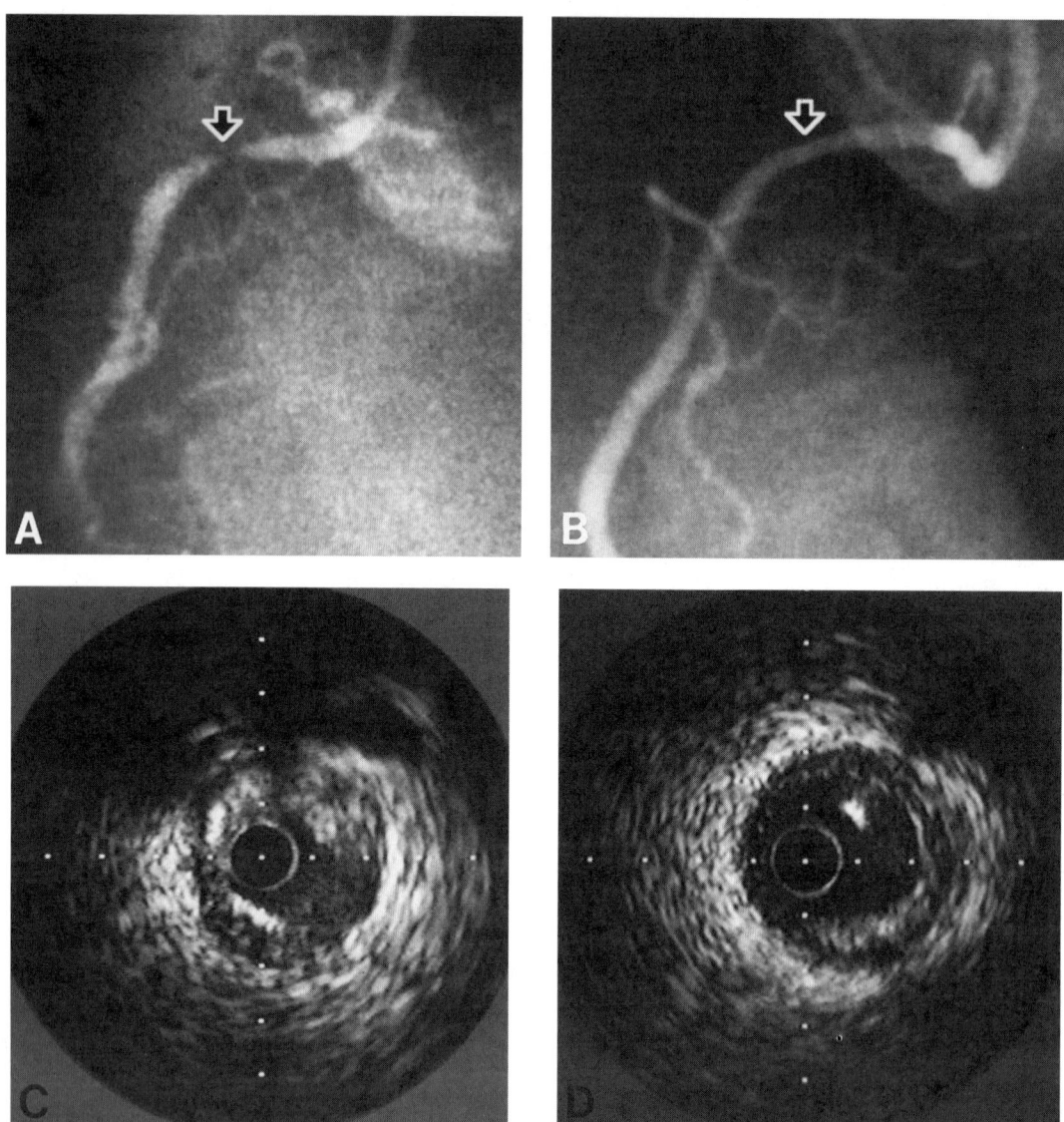

Fig. 17-2. An example of favorable remodeling occurring after angioplasty. **(A)** Preprocedural angiogram. **(B)** Postprocedural angiogram. Comparing the postprocedure intravascular ultrasound **(C)** with that obtained at follow-up **(D)**, the lumen area has increased significantly at the target site. The angiogram, however, (not shown) was unchanged at follow-up. The implication of favorable remodeling is that in some patients a positive or equivocal functional test soon after intervention may actually become negative during the following months. Thus, the "discordant" results between the two tests may actually represent an accurate assessment of the state of the vessel.

tion can be reduced to some extent by procedural factors and by the appropriate use of glycoprotein IIb/IIIa inhibitors;[21] when it is suspected, prompt repeat angiography is indicated. When symptoms recur within 1 month, the differential diagnosis includes incomplete revascularization (i.e., other untreated coronary lesions) or extensive "elastic" recoil of the treated site. Between 1 and 4 months (and in some cases as late as 6 months), the more gradual, healing responses collectively called restenosis are

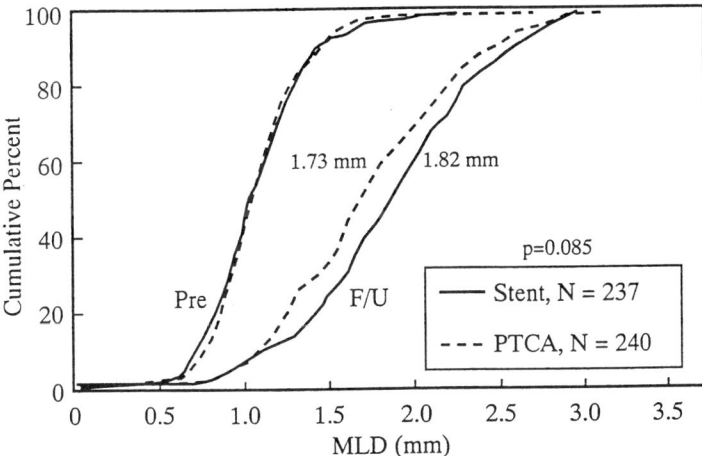

Fig. 17-3. Examples of a cumulative frequency distribution curves of minimum luminal diameters (MLD) before intervention and at 6 month follow-up for patients undergoing coronary stent deployment (solid line) or balloon angioplasty (dashed line). In patients who received a stent, a significantly larger postprocedural MLD was attained compared to patients treated with a balloon alone. This angiographic difference diminished during the six month follow-up period and was no longer statistically significant at follow-up. However, when a dichotomous definition of restenosis was used (defined as a 50% diameter stenosis at follow-up), patients assigned to stent implantation had a statistically significant reduction in restenosis, from 30% to 20%. The implications for functional testing is that any angiographic definition of restenosis is to some degree arbitrary, and the restenosis "rate" will be determined by the definition used as well as the precise angiographic techniques used to determine its incidence. (Adapted with permission from Serruys et al.,[111] with permission.)

Table 17-1. Sensitivity and Specificity of Anginal Symptoms in Identifying Restenosis after Coronary Angioplasty

Author	Angiographic Follow-up (%)	Restenosis (%)	Symptoms	
			NPV (%)	PPV (%)
Renkin et al. (1990)[113]	83	31	70	83
Bengtson et al. (1990)[34]	92	36	80	80
Simonton et al. (1988)[53]	90	35	75	48
Califf et al. (1990)[114]	100	38	85	60
Zaidi et al. (1985)[115]	100	49	69	66
Mabin et al. (1985)[116]	55	32	86	71
Levine et al. (1985)[117]	92	40	96	76
Jutzy et al. (1982)[118]	88	47	83	92
Gruentzig et al. (1987)[86]	93	31	98	92
Roth et al. (1994)[119]	100	28	78	38

Abbreviations: NPV, negative predictive value; PPV, positive predictive value.
(Modified from Califf et al.,[114] with permission.)

most likely. The time course of this healing process has implications for the timing of functional testing, as exemplified in Figures 17-1 and 17-2. Finally, the development of new coronary lesions are often responsible for angina that recurs 6 months or more after angioplasty. Rosing et al.[22] demonstrated that restenosis later than 12 months after conventional balloon angioplasty is uncommon and that the anatomic and functional success (measured by exercise time) were maintained during 3 years of follow-up. However, restenosis may present 12 months or more after angioplasty; for example, coronary stenting may shift this chronologic profile.

Fortunately, with the exception of abrupt closure soon after angioplasty, restenosis rarely presents with myocardial infarction or death. Unlike the lipid-laden lesion with a thin fibrous cap associated with acute myocardial syndromes, the restenotic lesion usually consists of smooth muscle cells and extracellular matrix.[1] As a result, recurrent angina or a positive functional test are far more frequent presentations of restenosis. Although clinical trials of devices or drugs to reduce restenosis will continue to use different definitions to measure restenosis and different methods to determine its incidence, we believe that the most relevant definition of restenosis is one that provides the most information about the patient's clinical outcome, specifically, the probability of survival free from recurrent angina, provokable ischemia, myocardial infarction, and death. Future clinical trials may adopt clinical endpoints (such as the persistence or recurrence of ischemia) because they are clinically more relevant than angiographic restenosis to judge the relative benefit of coronary revascularization procedures, although larger sample sizes will be required. Angiographic restenosis can still be measured in a predefined subset of patients to study procedural and technical aspects of the intervention.

The Dissociation of Angiographic and Clinical Restenosis

The dissociation of clinical symptoms and angiographic restenosis is an example of the general dissociation between angiographic and clinical restenosis.[23–28] Some authors have assumed that this discrepancy merely reflects the inaccuracy of functional testing. Nevertheless, it is the functional significance of the final, long-term result with which the clinician is most concerned.

Although many clinical trials report angiographic restenosis rates of 30% to 50%, the same trials frequently report evidence of ischemia and a need for repeat revascularization in only 20% to 30% (Fig. 17-4). This dissociation of angiographic and clinical restenosis underscores the fundamental difference of measuring the *artery* versus assessing the *patient*, and, to a large degree, is an artifact of the binary definition of restenosis. Because many vessels with a 50% to 60% stenosis (and even some with greater degrees of angiographic severity) produce neither ischemia nor symptoms, it is not unexpected that the binary angiographic definition will overestimate the clinical significance of intermediate lesions. In these cases, it is important for the clinician to be guided by the functional significance of the lesion, rather than a knee-jerk reaction to a restenotic but intermediate narrowing.

The "Gold Standard"—Angiogram or Functional Test?

When symptoms, the results of functional testing, and the coronary arteriogram do not agree in a particular patient, clinicians have often resorted to several conventional explanations.[29] For example, the territory distal to the stenosis may be nonviable, such as in a patient with a significant (>70%) stenosis and a completed myocardial infarction. Alternatively, adequate coronary collateral flow may prevent ischemia, or an adequate anti-ischemic medical regimen may prevent ischemia at the achieved workload. If none of these explanations fit the clinical situation, the functional test is often assumed to be incorrect. For example, there are several conventional explanations for a symptomatic, postangioplasty patient who has ischemia on functional testing but in whom the coronary angiogram (the gold standard) does not demonstrate restenosis. These explanations include vasospasm, disease in other coronary vessels, or the conclusion that the functional test is false positive. Conversely, the conventional explanation for a patient without symptoms and a *negative* functional test but who *has* angiographic restenosis have included nonviability, psychological factors, or the conclusion that the functional test is false negative.

Recent developments in our understanding of the limitations of angiography have revealed that many patients with discordant findings on history, functional testing, and coronary angiography have been

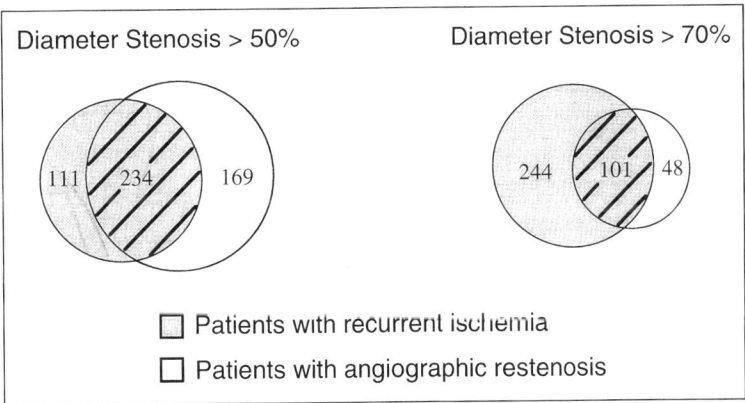

Fig. 17-4. The dissociation of angiographic and clinical restenosis underscores the fundamental difference of measuring the artery versus assessing the patient, and, to a large degree, is an artifact of the binary definition of restenosis. Although many clinical trials report angiographic restenosis rates of 30% to 50%, the same trials frequently report evidence of ischemia and a need for repeat revascularization in a much smaller percentage, typically 20 to 30%. These data are combined from three multicenter clinical trials; both the angiographic and functional test data were adjudicated by core laboratories blinded to the treatment strategy and clinical outcome. When restenosis was defined as the recurrence of a 50% diameter stenosis (left diagram), 403 (234 + 169) patients met the criteria for restenosis; but of these patients, 169 (41%) did not have evidence of recurrent ischemia. Conversely, 111 who did not have a 50% diameter stenosis did have evidence of recurrent ischemia. Similar findings were found when a 70% minimum luminal diameters (MLD) definition of restenosis was used. (right diagram). These data highlight the discordance between angiographic and clinical restenosis. The implication for functional testing is that presence of ischemia rather than an absolute "degree of stenosis" should guide the selection of patients for repeat interventional procedures. (See also Fig. 17-5 and 17-6.) (Adapted from Duerr et al,[135] with permission.)

misclassified; several important limitations of angiography must be acknowledged before using this technique to assess the accuracy of functional testing for the determination of restenosis. First, the incidence of angiographic restenosis can vary depending on the definition used (binary or continuous), as we have discussed. Second, the incidence of angiographic restenosis can vary depending on the method of measuring it (visual vs. computerized quantitative coronary angiography). There are several well-recognized methodological problems of quantitative coronary angiography. For example, meticulous attention is required to perform follow-up angiography under the same conditions as the index study, so as to match projection angles, the magnification of the image intensifier, and other procedural factors; there is also controversy regarding whether the worst projection is more relevant than an average of two (or more) views.

Third, the incidence of restenosis can vary depending on the rate at which follow-up angiography is performed. All trials with angiographic endpoints have some degree of attrition; the reported angiographic restenosis rate will be affected substantially by the rate of angiographic follow-up and the assumptions made about patients who do not undergo arteriography.[30] Patients who are asymptomatic and who do not undergo arteriography presumably have a lower rate of angiographic restenosis; however, the rate of restenosis in asymptomatic patients ranges from 10% to 35% (vide infra). Conversely, symptomatic patients who do not undergo arteriography presumably have a higher rate of angiographic restenosis. Similar problems occur for patients who die or who are lost to follow-up examination. The implication for the validity of functional testing is that the rate of follow-up for angiography affects the accuracy of the gold standard (angiography) to which functional testing is compared.

Finally, recent insights from intravascular ultrasound have revealed that the accuracy of angiography in measuring lumen size (and hence the effects

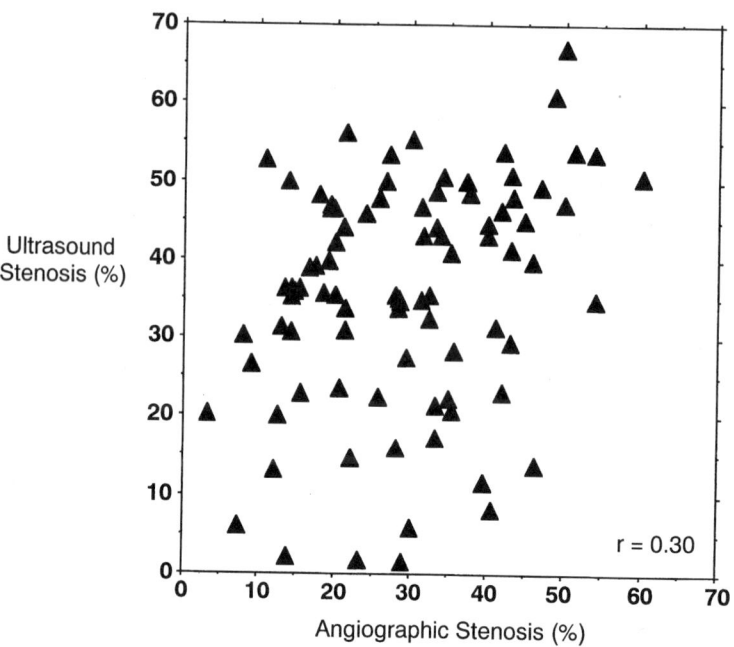

Fig. 17-5. There is a poor correlation between the residual stenosis determined by angiography and the actual lumen area planimetered by intravascular ultrasound. In this series[136] of patients treated exclusively with balloon angioplasty, the final percent diameter stenosis as measured by angiography was compared with the final percent diameter stenosis as measured directly by ultrasound. The correlation coefficient was only 0.30 Thus, a tomographic method of vessel assessment yields a different (and presumably more accurate) measure of lumen dimensions. The implication for functional testing is that some patients with an excellent angiographic result may still have a hemodynamically significant stenosis, whereas other patients with only a modest improvement angiographically may have achieved a significant improvement in lumen gain.

of a stenosis on distal perfusion) is particularly suspect in a coronary vessel after angioplasty. The tomographic orientation of intravascular ultrasound more accurately assesses lumen cross-sectional area (Figs. 17-5 and 17-6). An understanding of the limitations of angiography and the new insights from intravascular ultrasound has critical implications for an assessment of the accuracy of functional testing after coronary intervention. In the past, a functional test indicating clear-cut ischemia in a postintervention patient with an insignificant lesion on angiography was often labeled as false positive. In fact, many such patients have a hemodynamically significant stenosis that is simply undetected or underestimated using even the best angiographic techniques. A functional test can change a borderline angiographic lesion to a significant one (Fig. 17-7), and intravascular ultrasound can provide morphologic evidence to support the interpretation of the functional result. Conversely, a functional test that does *not* indicate ischemia in a postintervention patient with angiographic restenosis was often labeled as false negative (especially if an arbitrary, binary definition of 50% was used). In many of these patients angiography may overestimate the hemodynamic significance of an intermediate lesion, whether using conventional visual assessment[17] or state-of-the-art quantitative coronary artery systems. In many cases, intravascular ultrasound can provide morphologic evidence that the functional test, rather than the angiogram, is providing more accurate information about the hemodynamic effects of the lesion (Fig. 17-7). Other new modalities, such as Doppler flow[31,32] and fractional flow reserve[33] can also clarify discordant data from functional testing and angiography.

In summary, neither the functional test, nor the

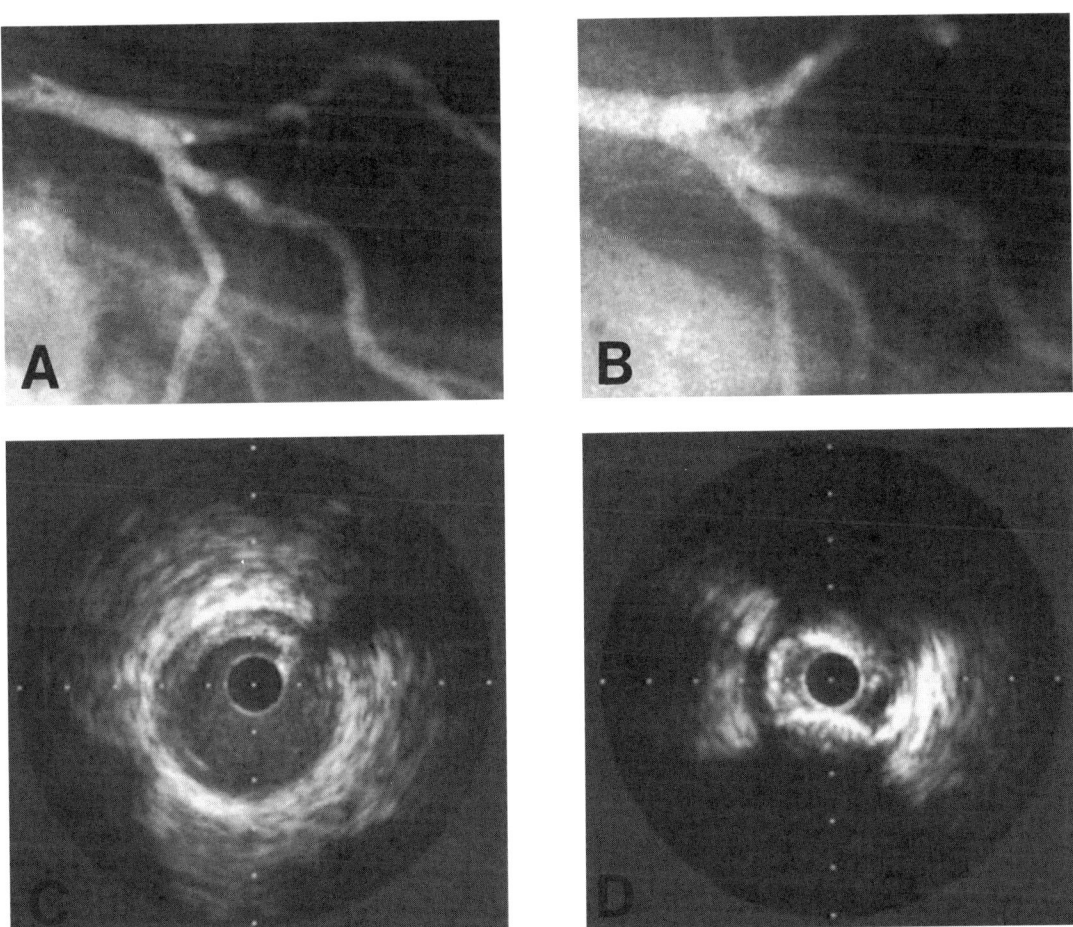

Fig. 17-6. In some circumstances, angiography is not a reliable "gold standard." This patient initially presented with new-onset exertional angina, Canadian functional class III. He was initially studied angiography **(A)**, in which the only coronary lesion was a 50%, slightly "hazy" area in a large obtuse marginal branch; the lesion was completely not apparent in other views **(B)**. After cardiac catheterization, however, exercise stress testing provoked the patient's symptoms and thallium scintigraphy demonstrated a large area of lateral wall ischemia. At repeat angiography, intravascular ultrasound demonstrated only a minimal amount of atheroma at the reference site **(C)**, but within the "hazy" area **(D)** a "napkin ring" of calcium nearly near obliterated the lumen. Presumably, even a small amount of calcification placed strategically can impair the ability of angiography to measure accurately a stenosis. After rotational ablation and adjunctive balloon angioplasty, ultrasound demonstrated a significant increase in lumen area (not shown), and the subsequent follow-up thallium exercise test was negative for ischemia. The implication for functional testing is that even a high-quality angiogram can underestimate the true lesion severity and its functional significance. In such cases, the functional test may provide more reliable assessment, rather than being "false positive."

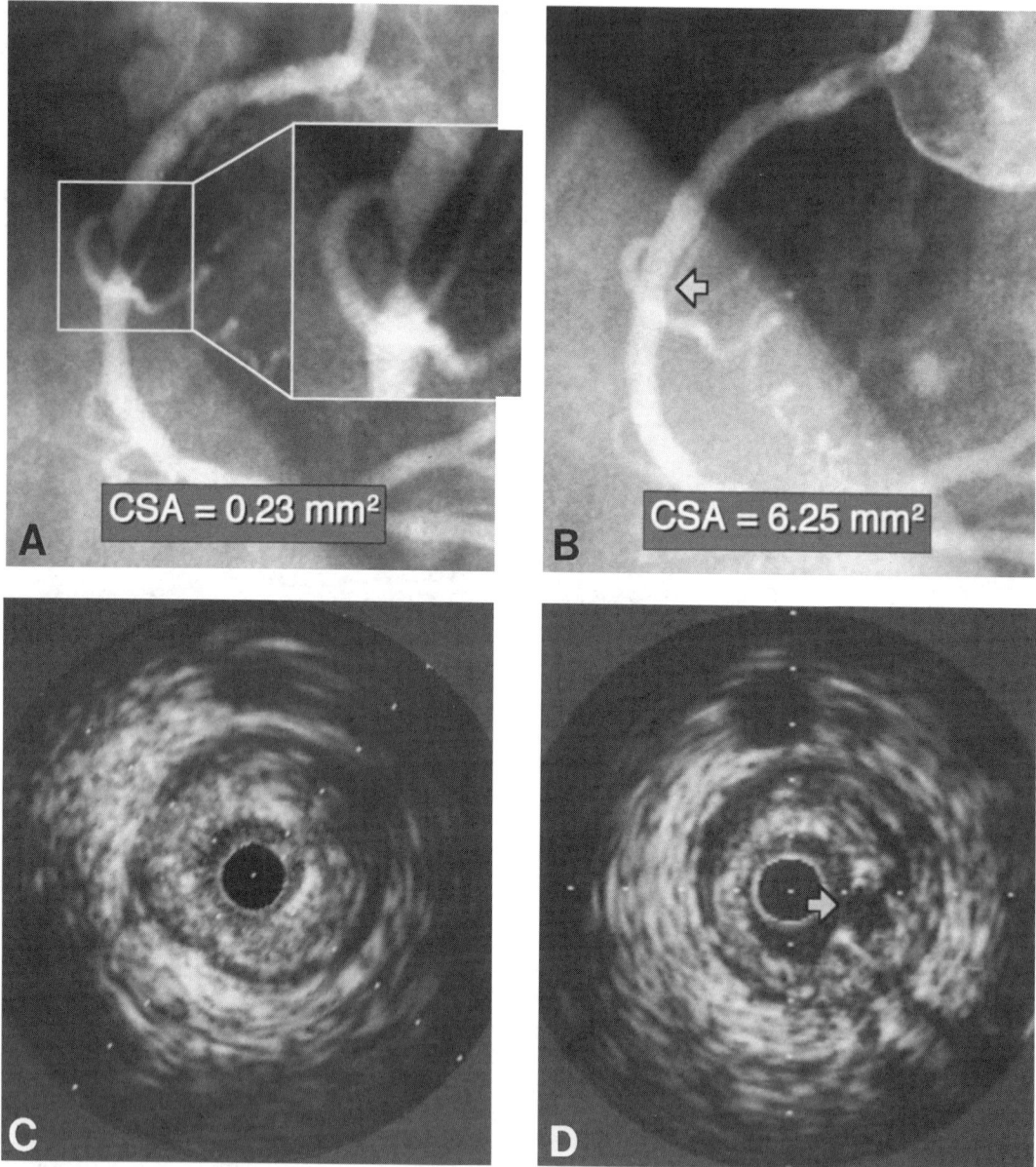

Fig. 17-7. Preprocedural **(A)** and postprocedural **(B)** angiograms of a patient with a midright coronary lesion. Although the postprocedural result suggests a 20-fold increase in lumen area, the intravascular ultrasound demonstrates a far more modest increase in lumen area. The implication for functional testing is that given the large size of the myocardial bed supplied by this vessel, a functional test performed after intervention may still indicate ischemia despite the dramatic angiographic success. Also, relatively little cellular proliferation would be required to remodel this result in an unfavorable fashion, resulting in angiographic restenosis. (Modified from Topel and Nissen,[137] with permission.)

Table 17-2. Variables Associated With an Increased Risk of Restenosis

Clinical Variables	Anatomic Variables	Procedural Variables
Diabetes mellitus	Lesion length >10 mm	Multivessel angioplasty
Unstable angina	Lesion severity before and after procedure	Type of interventional device (e.g., stent vs. balloon angioplasty)
? Uremia	Bifurcation lesions	
	Saphenous vein grafts	
	Ostial lesions	

angiogram, nor any new modality *alone* is the true gold standard for the determination of myocardial ischemia; rather, the gold standard is the cognitive *assembly* of clinical information from all sources—the history and physical examination, the results of the functional study, and the angiogram—using newer, specialized techniques to explain the discordance of results in selected patients. Unfortunately, many studies examining the predictive accuracy of functional testing have, by necessity, used a binary angiographic definition of restenosis by which to judge the results of the functional test; in many categories, these are the only data available. Similarly, although clinical events (death, myocardial infarction, or ischemia) are more relevant endpoints than angiographic restenosis to judge the predictive merit of functional tests, few studies provide these data. Having enumerated these limitations, we will proceed with a review of the available data.

RATIONALE FOR ROUTINE FUNCTIONAL TESTING AFTER CORONARY INTERVENTION

Symptomatic Status Is an Unreliable Indicator of Clinical Restenosis

Although the discordance between angiographic estimation of lumen size and ultrasound measurement of lumen area may account for some cases of discordance between angiographic and clinical restenosis, unfortunately, symptomatic status is also inaccurate for the prediction of ischemia on functional testing. Table 17-2 summarizes some of the studies with a high rate of follow-up after angiography that have examined the positive and negative predictive value of anginal symptoms. The positive predictive value averages only 70%. Thus, even in patients who had symptoms before the index angioplasty, the absence of symptoms during follow-up does not rule out either significant provokable ischemia on functional testing, angiographic restenosis, or both. For example, among the studies that examined whether objective evidence of ischemia was present in asymptomatic patients after intervention (rather than a binary angiographic endpoint) Bengtson et al.[34] reported that 25% of asymptomatic patients demonstrated evidence of ischemia on exercise electrocardiography.

Ischemia, Even If Silent, Worsens Prognosis

Considerable evidence supports the hypothesis that patients with ischemia have a less favorable prognosis than patients without ischemia, and that the absence of symptoms in ischemic patients does not lessen this risk. Using data from the Coronary Artery Surgery Study (CASS) databank, Falcone et al.[35] and Kent et al.[36] reported that patients without angina or ST-segment depression on exercise electrocardiography had a higher 7-year survival rate (88%) than patients who had silent exercise-induced ST-segment depression (survival rate, 76%), angina alone (77%), or both (78%). Weiner et al.,[37] reporting on 880 patients from the CASS registry, concluded that patients with silent ischemia (documented by exercise testing) had a risk of subsequent infarction or sudden death identical to patients with symptoms. Other studies have reported similar results.[38] Of course, it is now appreciated that no functional test can predict the probability of plaque rupture, the most common cause of myocardial infarction.

The documentation of asymptomatic ischemia in patients with coronary atherosclerosis has been associated with an increased risk for adverse outcome.

For example, the Atenolol Silent Ischemia (ASIST)[39] study was a multicenter, double-blind, placebo-controlled trial that randomized 306 patients with minimal or no angina but both ambulatory and exercise-induced ischemia to atenolol or placebo. Although the trend for fewer serious events in atenolol-treated patients (death, resuscitation from ventricular tachycardia or ventricular fibrillation, nonfatal myocardial infarction, or hospitalization for unstable angina) did not reach statistical significance, it is noteworthy that the most powerful predictor of event-free survival was the absence of ischemia on ambulatory monitoring at 4 weeks. Whereas the ASIST study was not designed to compare the relative efficacy of various therapies, the Asymptomatic Cardiac Ischemia Pilot (ACIP) study[40] did examine this issue. The ACIP was a multicenter trial designed to test the feasibility of performing a larger, prospective trial to determine whether suppression of silent ischemia improves clinical outcome. After 12 weeks, revascularization (with either bypass surgery or angioplasty) eliminated silent ischemia in 55% of patients compared with only 41% of patients prescribed medical therapy guided by ambulatory electrocardiographic (ECG) recordings and in only 39% of patients prescribed medical therapy guided by symptoms alone. Although the results of the final ACIP study will not be available until 1997, in aggregate these data suggest that the prognosis for patients with ischemia, whether silent or symptomatic, can be improved by medical therapy or revascularization.

Arguments for Routine Functional Testing

As a result of the data on the prognostic importance of silent ischemia, some investigators have argued that functional testing after coronary intervention should be routine (assuming that the initial angioplasty was appropriately performed to alleviate ischemia). Proponents of routine functional testing after coronary intervention argue that because 15% to 60% of patients with angina before angioplasty will develop restenosis and ischemia on functional testing *without* recurrent symptoms, functional testing should be routine. These investigators contend that there is no reason to assume that patients with silent ischemia caused by restenosis are fundamentally different from patients who have silent ischemia *without* a preceding coronary intervention. The "logic train" is that functional testing should be routine because (1) silent ischemia worsens prognosis to the same degree as symptomatic ischemia; (2) the severity of angiographic restenosis and amount of ischemic myocardium are similar in both groups;[41] and (3) data from several small series[34,42–44] suggest that the prognosis of patients with asymptomatic restenosis is the same as for patients with symptomatic restenosis (although the latter are more likely to undergo additional angioplasty).[45] It should be stressed that the purpose of these studies is to detect and to treat *ischemia*, rather than to detect angiographic restenosis in the absence of ischemia.

RATIONALE AND PRACTICAL APPLICATION FOR SELECTIVE FUNCTIONAL TESTING AFTER CORONARY INTERVENTION

Proponents of the selective use of functional testing after coronary intervention argue that the data on the prognostic effect of silent ischemia is still incomplete, that symptomatic status, although imperfect, can still be used as a guide to performing functional testing, and that a knowledge of the clinical and procedural variables that result in a higher risk of restenosis and recurrent ischemia can be used to select those at highest risk for functional testing.

To apply a selective strategy of functional testing, four sources of data are required to determine whether functional testing is indicated in an individual patient: first, an estimate of the probability of restenosis based on clinical, anatomic, and procedural variables; second, a knowledge of the patient's overall coronary anatomy; third, the symptomatic status both before intervention and at follow-up examination; and fourth, an estimate of the clinical implications of restenosis, if it occurs. We will consider each of these sources of data individually.

The Probability of Restenosis

A variety of clinical, anatomic, and procedural variables have been reported to increase the risk of restenosis (Table 17-2). Unfortunately, many of the studies reporting these were small retrospective analyses that were not substantiated in larger, prospective clinical trials. Several recent trials of new devices and pharmacologic adjuncts with high rates of angiographic follow-up have improved our understanding of factors that increase the risk of restenosis, which can be analyzed separately as relating to the patient, the lesion, or the procedure.

Clinical Variables

Of the multitude of clinical variables that have been studied, only diabetes mellitus and unstable angina have been consistently associated with an increased incidence of restenosis following successful coronary angioplasty.[46] On average, diabetics have a 30% greater risk of developing restenosis[14,47–49] and clearly have an increased incidence of adverse events after coronary intervention. For example, in the recently completed EPIC Trial, diabetics had a much higher incidence of repeat revascularizations within 180 days than did nondiabetics (38% vs. 28%).[21] Whether blood insulin level or the severity of hyperglycemia affects the risk of restenosis is unclear.

Compared with patients without chest pain or those with chronic stable angina, unstable angina preceding the index angioplasty is associated with a relative risk of 1.2 to 1.4 for the development of restenosis. Data from angiographic, necropsy, and angioscopy studies have demonstrated that ruptured coronary atheromata—the usual cause of unstable angina—commonly contain thrombus, whereas chronic, stable coronary lesions are much less likely to do so. In the setting of a recent plaque rupture, additional disruption by angioplasty may, in some cases, further stimulate thrombus propagation, organization, and loss of lumen size. Several potent mitogens that promote cellular proliferation and extracellular matrix formation are stimulated by clot-bound thrombin. Although there are diverse definitions of unstable angina, an increased incidence of restenosis has been reported for patients with angina at rest,[50] recent onset angina (<2 months),[14,51] and accelerating angina.[52]

Patients who undergo primary angioplasty for acute myocardial infarction are a unique subset. Thrombus is present by definition in the setting of acute coronary thrombosis; therefore, it is not surprising that these patients have a risk of restenosis at least as high as those undergoing angioplasty for chronic stable angina.[53] Almost no data is available regarding the relative risk of restenosis in this group of patients; therefore, the rationale for functional testing in this group is the same as for patients undergoing elective angioplasty.

Other factors known to promote atherosclerosis development or progression—such as gender, age, and hyperlipidemia—have *not* been proven to increase the risk of restenosis. Neither male gender nor age have been associated with a higher risk. Although several small series reported an association between restenosis and almost every lipoprotein fraction,[54–56] subsequent studies failed to demonstrate an increased risk.[57,58] For example, a single report suggested that lovastatin reduced the incidence of restenosis; this series included only 157 patients and had less than 50% angiographic follow-up.[59] This claim was not validated in the Lovastatin Restenosis Trial, in which a 44% reduction of low-density lipoproteins-cholesterol did not affect the incidence of restenosis,[60] nor in an analysis of data pooled from the PARK, CARPORT,[61] MERCATOR,[62] and MARCATOR[63] studies. It is likely that other patient-related variables will become evident in the future. For example, a specific form of acetylcholinesterase gene (the ACE-DD genotype) has been associated with a higher risk of restenosis,[64] implicating genetic factors.

Anatomic Variables

Lesion length, particular anatomic locations, and chronic total occlusions are associated with an increased risk of restenosis. Bourassa et al.[52] reported an increase in the angiographic restenosis rate from 38% to 52% for lesions greater than 10 mm in length. Other studies have reported similar results when lesions were stratified by length greater than 4.6 mm[65] or 6.8 mm.[66] Lesion location is also an important variable to consider when assessing the risk of restenosis. Angioplasty of saphenous vein grafts (in the absence of stent deployment), particularly of lesions located at the ostium or within the shaft, is associated with a much higher incidence of restenosis than distal anastomotic lesions or lesions within native coronary arteries. Similarly, specific lesion locations within native coronary vessels are often reported to be associated with higher rates of restenosis. Bifurcation lesions, lesions within 5 mm of the left anterior descending (LAD) origin, and true ostial lesions of any coronary artery are all associated with an increased risk of restenosis,[65,67] perhaps caused by recoil of displaced tissue, which is often observed (either angiographically or with intravascular ultrasound) within minutes to hours of a successful procedure. In addition to a lower procedural success rate, the incidence of restenosis is at least 45% for chronic occlusions, especially in those occluded for more than 3 months.[68–70]

Angiographic preprocedural lesion severity has been shown to be a strong predictor of lesion recurrence in many clinical studies. The M-HEART investigators[65] reported that when the preintervention stenosis severity was greater than 73% (by quantitative angiography), the angiographic restenosis rate increased from 25% to 40%. Similar findings were reported in the recent CARPORT study.[61]

The incidence of angiographic restenosis appears to be the same for *de novo* and restenotic lesions.[71–73] Additionally, restenotic lesions treated with a *third* angioplasty for a second episode of restenosis appear to have an angiographic restenosis rate of approximately 40%.[73–76] However, when patients develop recurrent symptoms within three months of the previous procedure, the risk of subsequent restenosis (after the next attempt at balloon angioplasty) exceeds 50%.[76] Finally, for patients treated with interventional procedures at different coronary sites at different times, restenosis at one site has correlated with a higher risk of restenosis at other sites in some studies[77–79] but not in others.[80]

In summary, lesion location, length, and preprocedural severity appear to increase the relative risk of restenosis, and this information can be useful in determining the indications and timing of functional testing. Data regarding the relative risk of restenosis for other angiographic features, such as lesion eccentricity or angulation, and postprocedural thrombus have been inconclusive. Unfortunately, recent data suggest that angiography is insensitive to many of the morphologic characteristics of coronary lesions; as we will discuss, intracoronary ultrasound and Doppler flow performed at the time of the initial coronary intervention may improve our ability to predict the likelihood of restenosis.

Procedural Variables

Although several recent trials of multivessel angioplasty versus bypass surgery have demonstrated comparable rates of survival and subsequent infarction, these trials have also demonstrated a higher rate of repeat revascularization procedures in patients randomized to percutaneous transluminal coronary angioplasty (PTCA). The greater the number of lesions treated with angioplasty, the greater the probability of restenosis at one or more sites. This has important implications for functional testing during follow-up, because patients treated with multivessel angioplasty may require more frequent functional testing.

Although many "new" interventional devices have been investigated with a hope of reducing restenosis when compared with conventional balloon angioplasty, only coronary stents have been shown to reduce the incidence of restenosis, both angiographic and clinical. Although clinical trials[15,81] comparing the directional atherectomy catheter and balloon angioplasty have demonstrated a modest reduction (approximately 55% vs. 49% in one trial) in angiographic restenosis with this new device, the restenosis rate remains exceedingly high and is the procedure associated with a higher rate of complications. In a single center trial that randomized 620 patients to one of three treatment strategies, rotational ablation was associated with fewer acute complications, and both rotational atherectomy and excimer laser atherectomy were associated with increased acute gain compared with balloon angioplasty alone. Nevertheless, there were no significant differences at clinical and angiographic follow-up, with angiographic restenosis rates exceeding 50% in all three treatment groups. Several trials are investigating whether technical refinements in the use of these new devices can result in lower rates of restenosis.

Post-Procedural Coronary Anatomy

Residual Stenosis After Intervention

Several studies have suggested that the angiographic postprocedural residual stenosis correlates with the risk of restenosis. Bourassa et al.[52] reported that a post-angioplasty diameter stenosis of 30% or more (by quantitative coronary angiography) was associated with a restenosis rate of 40%, whereas a diameter stenosis less than 30% was associated with a rate of 28%. Similarly, the M-HEART investigators[65] reported that a residual stenosis greater than 21% had a restenosis rate of greater than those with a residual stenosis of less than 21%. These data have led Kuntz et al.[82] to develop a statistical model of restenosis. According to this model, the larger the acute gain in angiographic luminal diameter after the initial angioplasty, the larger the lumen at angiographic follow-up, regardless of interventional device. However, even if this theory is validated from a theoretical standpoint, attempts to achieve larger luminal dimensions must be accomplished without an increase in periprocedural risk.

Completeness of Revascularization

Patients with incomplete revascularization at the initial angioplasty procedure have a higher rate of cardiac events during follow-up. Whether a follow-up exercise test will uncover myocardial ischemia depends not only on whether restenosis has occurred but also on the extent of coronary disease at the time of the index angioplasty and whether revascularization was complete. Bourassa et al.[83] demonstrated that incomplete revascularization is common after angioplasty in patients with multivessel disease, often because not all lesions are amenable to percutaneous intervention or because lesions are of intermediate severity (50% to 69%).

The Symptomatic Status of the Patient at Follow-up

Symptomatic status is, at best, an unreliable sign of both the angiographic and perfusion status of the patient, whether the patient has typical angina, atypical symptoms, or is asymptomatic. Nevertheless, in clinical practice, the relationship of symptoms after angioplasty to symptoms before the intervention is often cited as useful in determining the status of the coronary artery. Table 17-1 summarizes the data on the sensitivity and specificity of anginal symptoms in identifying restenosis after coronary angioplasty. In aggregate, these data lead to the conclusion that for the majority of patients, angina status is neither sensitive nor specific enough to eliminate the need for routine functional testing after coronary intervention. To support this conclusion, we will first consider patients without symptoms and then those with symptoms.

If one considers only patients with typical angina pectoris before intervention, it is remarkable that among those who develop *overt ischemia* on exercise thallium scintigraphy (along with angiographic restenosis), between 15% and 60% will not develop recurrent symptoms. Hecht et al.[41] studied 116 patients for suspected restenosis after coronary angioplasty. Restenosis occurred in 61% of asymptomatic and in 59% of symptomatic patients. Importantly, 76% of the patients with asymptomatic restenosis had chest pain before intervention. In another report, Pfisterer et al.[45] studied a consecutive series of 490 patients at 6 months after angioplasty with exercise thallium scintigraphy. Ischemia was documented by thallium in 112 patients (and by angiography in 107); importantly, 60% of these patients were asymptomatic during the 6-month interval and during exercise testing. Furthermore, the clinical characteristics, angioplasty procedural variables, and angiographic severity of restenosis were similar for patients with and without symptoms, as was the incidence of subsequent ischemic events (not counting repeat angioplasty). Thus, these data suggest that restenosis and recurrent ischemia may occur without angina, even when angina is present before the initial intervention. Other studies support these findings (Table 17-1).

The importance of functional testing after coronary intervention is underscored by the fact that the presence of ischemia on functional testing, rather than symptomatic status, predicts the risk of subsequent cardiac events. In the same study, Pfisterer et al.[45] demonstrated that patients with silent ischemia who did not undergo repeat revascularization immediately after its documentation had a higher rate of subsequent symptomatic ischemia (such as myocardial infarction and admission for unstable angina) and subsequent revascularization procedures, although there was no detectable difference in mortality. Other studies[29,42] have suggested that the midterm outcome of patients with asymptomatic restenosis is good; however, it must be noted that these studies used an *angiographic* definition of restenosis, rather than the recurrence of ischemia on functional testing. As in patients with chronic stable angina, it is the presence or absence of ischemia rather than the angiographic presence of an individual lesion that has the greatest effect on prognosis. Thus, in the study by Hernandez et al.,[29] asymptomatic patients with a positive functional test had a rate of angina recurrence twice that of asymptomatic patients with a negative functional test. These data also support the recommendations of the American College of Cardiology/American Heart Association

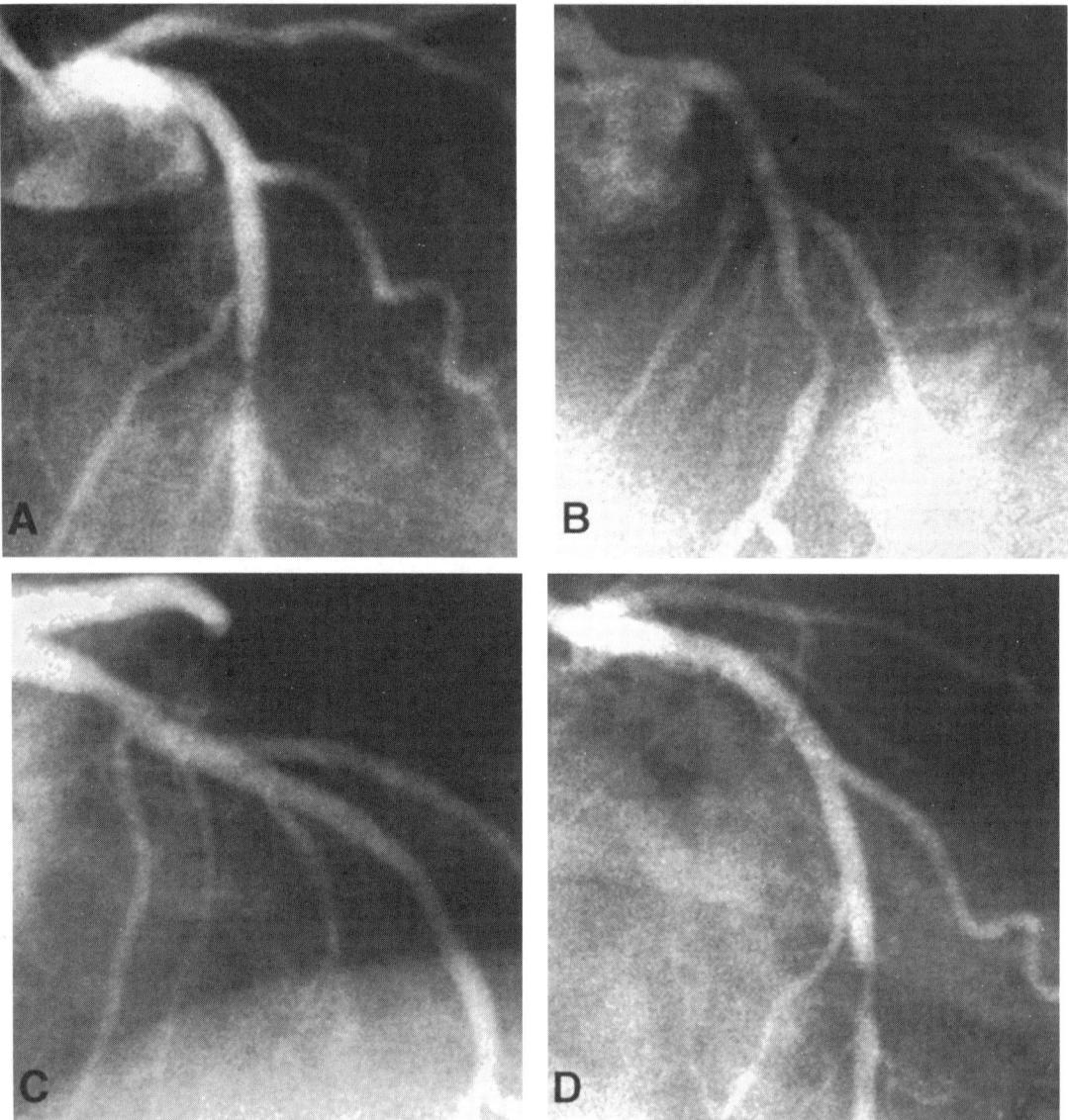

Fig. 17-8. Even in patients with "obvious" ischemia on the basis of symptoms, functional testing can be critical to determine the strategic approach in coronary intervention. In this patient who had class III angina, the lesion in the circumflex **(A)** was clearly the most severe in the coronary system, but the less severe, intermediate lesion in the left anterior descending **(B)** left anterior oblique ([LAO] cranial projection) was more consistent with the large anterior perfusion defect on thallium scintigraphy. As a result, the left anterior descending (LAD) lesion was successfully treated with angioplasty **(C)** posterior anterior ([PA] cranial projection) and the circumflex was deferred. Repeat exercise stress testing at six months was entirely negative for ischemia. However, one year later the patient again developed angina. At this time, however, the exercise test revealed ischemia in the distribution of the circumflex; at angiography, the circumflex appeared essentially unchanged **(D)** and the LAD remained patent **(E)**. The circumflex was successfully treated with angioplasty, and because the patient was enrolled in a randomized trial of a platelet antagonist, six months later a final exercise thallium test was negative for ischemia and an angiogram demonstrated an excellent long-term result in the circumflex **(F)** and in the LAD (not shown). The implications for functional testing are twofold: First, the most "severe" lesion angiographically may not be the most critical from a perfusion standpoint; functional testing preintervention can be invaluable to prioritize lesions for intervention. Second, a lesion may not produce ischemia at one point in time and clearly do so thereafter despite an identical (or nearly identical) angiographic appearance, as in the circumflex in this example (compare **A** and **D**). *(Figures continues.)*

(ACC/AHA) Task Force[84] that the results of functional testing, rather than the angiographic appearance of the lesion, be the determinant of the need for repeat coronary intervention.

On the other hand, patients with typical angina before the initial angioplasty who then redevelop the same symptoms have a relatively high probability of restenosis. As seen in Table 17-1, the positive predictive value of angina recurrence ranges from 70% to 92%. (A single study,[53] which included only patients undergoing primary angioplasty for myocardial infarction, reported the lowest positive predictive value of 48%.) Thus, although 10% to 30% of patients with a recurrence of angina after successful angioplasty will not require further mechanical intervention, the remainder have a high probability of restenosis, and a negative functional test in this setting will often warrant repeat angiography. As a result, many of these patients are referred directly to angiography rather than for functional testing. Nevertheless, in this setting selected patients can *still* benefit from functional testing. For example, for patients who had multivessel disease at the time of the initial angioplasty (whether or not multivessel angioplasty was performed), a functional test can quantify the amount of ischemia in each territory; this information can be invaluable in planning the repeat interventional procedure (Fig. 17-8). This is particularly true in patients with a history of myocardial infarction, in which the vessel with a more severe angiographic stenosis or the largest caliber may not be the most likely cause of the ischemia. In other situations, the extent of ischemia is considerably greater or less than expected; this may triage some patients to bypass surgery or medical therapy rather than to repeat angioplasty.

Clinical Implications of Restenosis

Clearly, certain clinical situations are associated with a very high risk of adverse outcome if restenosis occurs and is undetected and untreated. For example, patients who undergo angioplasty of a vessel supplying a very large amount of myocardium (such as proximal left anterior descending lesions), those undergoing angioplasty of a vessel supplying the only remaining viable myocardium, and those undergoing angioplasty of the only remaining coronary vessel or vein graft (who presumably are not candidates for surgery because of concomitant illnesses or other contraindications) are at inherently higher risk and should be considered for routine evaluation, after angioplasty, whether by functional testing or repeat angiography. Finally, some recommend careful follow-up in patients whose initial pre-

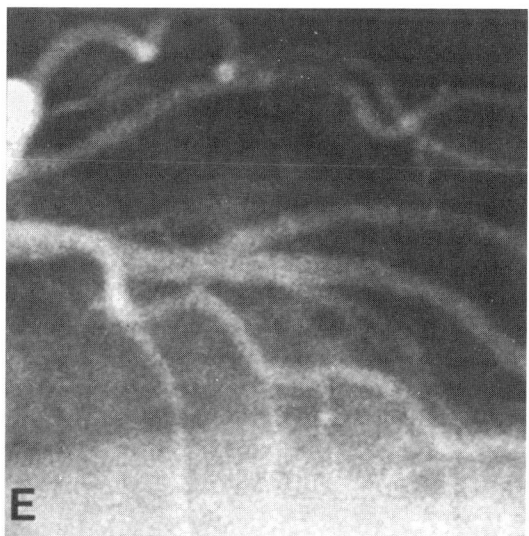 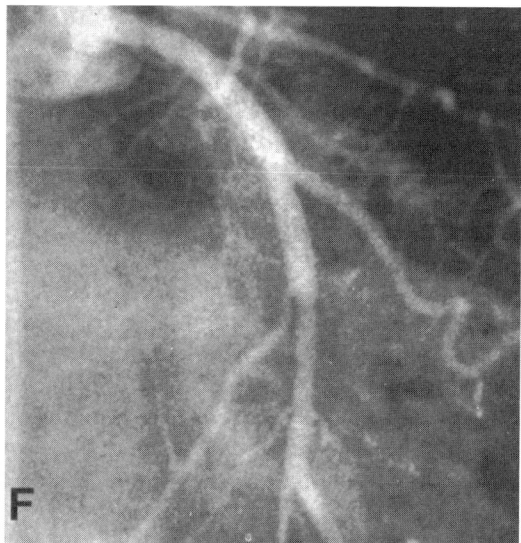

Fig. 17-8. *(Continued).*

sentation was a ventricular dysrhythmia or sudden cardiac death before index angioplasty.

WHICH STRATEGY: ROUTINE OR SELECTIVE FUNCTIONAL TESTING?

Using the data presented above, one can argue rationally for either selective or routine functional testing after coronary intervention. In applying the selective strategy, the clinician estimates the probability of restenosis based on the clinical, anatomic, and procedural variables and adjusts the threshold for ordering a follow-up functional test on the basis of a knowledge of the rest of the coronary anatomy at the time of angioplasty, the patient's symptomatic status at follow-up, and the clinical implications of restenosis, if it occurs. On the other hand, proponents of the routine approach argue that any attempt to select the highest risk patient is at best arbitrary and at worst leaves undetected many individuals who have restenosis and whose prognosis could be improved by repeat revascularization or intensification of medical therapy.

In clinical practice, few clinicians take a dogmatic stance regarding one strategy or another. Even those who recommend a selective strategy agree that some subgroups of patients should *always* undergo functional testing. Regardless of which strategy one advocates, it is critical to recognize those patients in whom functional testing is *always* indicated. For example, the patient who presents with a lesion at high-risk for restenosis in a vessel that supplies a large area of myocardium should always undergo follow-up functional testing, particularly if their symptoms were difficult to assess either before or after the intervention. The patient whose lesion is at an average risk of restenosis and which is in a vessel that supplies a moderate or a small amount of myocardium is more controversial. In our opinion, assuming the initial angioplasty was indicated because of ischemia, the potential benefits of routine functional testing to diagnose and treat provokable ischemia outweigh the increase in cost.

FOLLOW-UP AFTER ANGIOPLASTY: WHICH FUNCTIONAL TEST?

In addition to selecting which patients should undergo functional testing after successful intervention, a second major dilemma involves which is the optimal type of functional test to use. Calcium channel antagonists are frequently prescribed for the weeks following angioplasty to prevent coronary vasoconstriction or spasm. These agents are often inadvertently continued for months; they should be discontinued before follow-up functional testing.

Exercise Electrocardiography

The advantage of exercise treadmill testing is its wide availability and low cost. During the initial development of coronary angioplasty, exercise electrocardiography (ECG) appeared to have adequate predictive value for the determination of restenosis. In Gruentzig's early series of 169 patients,[85] 97% of whom had abnormal exercise ECGs before intervention, follow-up for a mean of 29 months indicated that coronary angioplasty improved peak exercise capacity significantly (from 74 ± 42 to 122 ± 47 beats/minute). These functional improvements were maintained with time; remarkably, only 10% of patients with successful dilatation in this original series had positive exercise stress tests 5 to 8 years later.[86] Scholl et al.[87] also noted improvements after angioplasty in ischemic endpoints in association with a significant increase in mean exercise time and augmentation of the rate pressure product; both of these parameters decreased when restenosis occured. An exercise-induced deterioration in regional wall motion or an abnormal (<5%) increase in left ventricular ejection fraction on a gated radionuclide ventriculogram was present in 75% of patients with restenosis after angioplasty.[88]

However, these data from the early angioplasty era include primarily patients with predominantly proximal, single-vessel disease. In the modern era, exercise ECG has only a limited role for the detection of restenosis for two predominant reasons. First, significant technologic improvements have occurred in coronary intervention, with the result that angioplasty is often used to treat patients with multivessel disease and those who are poor candidates for surgical revascularization. Fortunately, advances in functional testing have kept pace with advances in coronary intervention; for patients with multivessel disease, ECG combined with an imaging modality can provide higher levels of sensitivity and specificity, can assist in quantifying the amount of myocardium at risk, and can localize the ischemic terri-

Table 17-3. Sample of Data on the Sensitivity and Specificity of Exercise ECG in Identifying Restenosis After Coronary Angioplasty

	Timing of Test	Angiographic Follow-up (%)	Restenosis (%)	NPV (%)	PPV (%)
<8 Weeks after Angioplasty					
Scholl et al. (1982)[87]	1 month	83	12	27	40
O'Keefe et al. (1988)[120]	<1 month	100	13	73	29
Wijns et al.[23a]	3–8 weeks	89	40	52	60
Wijns et al.[43a]	3–7 weeks	74	35	65	50
el-Tamimi et al. (1990)[121]	1 month	100	45	94	100
8 Weeks or More After Angioplasty					
Rosing et al. (1984)[122]	8 months	100	34	76	47
Ernst et al. (1985)[90]	8 months	100	34	76	47
Honan et al. (1989)[123]	4–8 months	100	4	95	50
Scholl et al. (1982)[87]	6 months	88	58	64	57
Vlay et al. (1989)[25]	6 months	83	12	50	64
Honan et al. (1989)[123]	6 months	88	40	64	57
Kadel et al. (1989)[124]	4 months	100	33	75	66
el-Tamini et al. (1990)[121]	6 months	100	45	94	100

Abbreviations: NPV, negative predictive value; PPV, positive predictive value.

[a] In this study, the data for the positive and negative predictive values at 1 month are based on the angiographic follow-up at 6 months. (Modified from Califf et al.,[114] with permission.)

tory.[89] Second, exercise ECG has limited sensitivity for detecting restenosis, because many patients have uninterpretable ST segments (owing to baseline abnormalities) or cannot exercise maximally.

Table 17-3 summarizes the available data on the predictive value of exercise ECG in identifying restenosis after coronary angioplasty. Although these data are from nonrandomized, primarily retrospective series, we can conclude that exercise ECG has suboptimal predictive value, averaging 74%. With the exception of two studies that report negative predictive values of 84%[34] and 95%,[90] the negative predictive values cluster in the 50% to 70% range.

Thallium Scintigraphy and Radionuclide Ventriculography

The recommendations of the Subcommittee on Coronary Angioplasty of the ACC/AHA Task Force on the assessment of diagnostic and therapeutic cardiovascular procedures,[84] in its review of the appropriate use of coronary angioplasty and of the value of functional testing for the detection of restenosis in asymptomatic patients, recognized the incremental value of exercise thallium compared with ECG alone. In particular, the committee recognized the excellent negative predictive value of a normal stress perfusion study for the absence of restenosis.

The accuracy of thallium imaging in the post-angioplasty patient is discussed in Chapter 19. Table 17-4 summarizes available data on the accuracy of exercise thallium scintigraphy for the detection of restenosis in series that have high angiographic follow-up (55% to 100%). With respect to the diagnosis of angiographic restenosis, the positive predictive values have ranged from 37% to 100%, and the negative predictive values have ranged from 42% to 100%. As we have discussed, the percentage of patients undergoing angiographic follow-up affects the observed restenosis rate and thus the predictive accuracy of the noninvasive test. If we limit our analysis to those studies with a high rate of angiographic follow-up (>85%), the positive predictive value averages 66%, and the mean negative predictive value is 81%.

Tomographic imaging has been reported to be superior to planar imaging techniques for the detection of restenosis,[91] in part because tomographic imaging is able to identify the correct coronary territory in approximately 75% of scans. This advantage is

Table 17-4. Sample of Available Data on the Accuracy of Thallium Scintigraphy and Sestamibi Scintigraphy for Detection of Restenosis[a]

	No. of Patients	Timing of Test	Imaging Method	Angiographic Follow-up (%)	Restenosis (%)	NPV (%)	PPV (%)
Hardoff et al. (1990)[125]	90	12–24 hours	Atrial pacing	79	32	86	53
Jain et al. (1988)[126]	53	0–6 days	Oral dipyridamole SPECT thallium	55	14	88	79
Miller et al. (1987)[127]	50	2 weeks	Exercise thallium	76	39	94	76
Lam et al. (1987)[128]	43	2 weeks	Dipyridamole thallium	100	9	96	89
Wijns et al. (1985)[43]	91	5 weeks	Exercise thallium	74	35	83	74
Wijns et al. (1985)[23]	89	3–8 weeks	Exercise thallium	89	40	72	82
Scholl et al. (1982)[87]	54	1 month	Exercise thallium	83	12	42	56
Scholl et al. (1982)[87]	—	6 months	Exercise thallium	—	—	75	100
Renkin et al. (1990)[113]	111	6 months	Exercise thallium	83	31	74	75
Ernst et al. (1985)[90]	25	4–8 months	Exercise thallium	100	4	100	50
Rosing et al. (1984)[122]	66	8 months	Exercise thallium	100	21	83	37
Marie et al. (1993)[129]	62	6 months	Exercise SPECT Thallium	100	33	83	70
Schroeder et al. (1989)[130]	111	6 months	Exercise thallium	100	12[b]	98	63
Avery et al. (1993)[131]	21	4 months	Gated MIBI	76	25	100	57

[a] All studies included in this summary had an angiographic follow-up rate of at least 50%.
[b] For this single study angiographic restenosis was defined as the recurrence of a lesion ≥70%.
(Modified from Califf et al.,[114] with permission.)

particularly useful in assessing the patient before coronary intervention if there are several intermediate lesions in multiple coronary artery territories. In addition, much of the data regarding planar thallium is derived from the early days of coronary angioplasty; thus, studies share many of the inherent weaknesses already discussed under exercise ECG. These studies may underestimate slightly the predictive value of a positive thallium scintigram. Studies performed too soon (within 4 weeks) of coronary angioplasty may demonstrate flow heterogeneity resulting from abnormal microvascular function or ischemia that will continue to improve as the vessel continues to remodel favorably over the following 2 to 5 months (Fig. 17-2).

Several studies in the literature have evaluated the predictive accuracy of exercise-gated radionuclide ventriculography. With respect to the diagnosis of angiographic restenosis, the positive predictive values have ranged from 15% to 54%, and the negative predictive values have ranged from 50% to 100%. Again, limiting the analysis to those studies with a total of 178 patients with an angiographic follow-up rate of 80% or more gives mean positive and negative predictive values of 39% and 85%, respectively.

Thus, as with exercise testing for the initial diagnosis of coronary disease, currently available data suggests that thallium scintigraphy is superior to routine exercise ECG for the evaluation of restenosis.

Exercise Echocardiography

Exercise echocardiography detects provokable ischemia by comparing regional left ventricular wall motion and thickening before, during, and after exercise. Decreased endocardial movement and decreased myocardial thickening during and after exercise are interpreted as evidence of exercise-induced ischemia. In patients who have not undergone revascularization procedures, exercise echocardiography has a higher sensitivity and specificity than routine exercise ECG for the detection of coronary artery disease (CAD) and is also superior for localizing the anatomic distribution of critical steno-

Table 17-5. Data on the Accuracy of Exercise Echocardiography for Detection of Restenosis

	No. of Patients	Timing of Test (months)	Type of Echocardiography Test	Angiographic Follow up (%)	Restenosis (%)	Sensitivity	Specificity
Aboul-Enein et al. (1991)[132]	101	6 months	Treadmill	100	NR[b]	67	83
Mertes et al. (1993)[133]	86	6.5 months	Bicycle stress	100		83	85
Hecht et al. (1993)[134]	80	4–8 months	Bicycle stress	100	56	87	95

[a] Series with complete angiographic follow-up.
[b] Data were reported based on the number of diseased vessels at follow-up; data on restenosis of the index lesion were not reported separately.

ses and the extent of jeopardized myocardium.[92–96] In nonselected patients (i.e., those who may or may not have had previous coronary interventional procedures), the reported range of sensitivity has been from 66% to 100% and the range of specificity has been from 69% to 100%.

Table 17-5 summarizes the available data on the sensitivity and specificity of exercise echocardiography in identifying restenosis after coronary angioplasty. Unfortunately, there are few data regarding the sensitivity and specificity of exercise echocardiography derived specifically from patients after coronary intervention. Of course, in the 1 year after intervention a fraction of patients will experience restenosis and a smaller number will have progression of disease at other sites; for clinical purposes, the sensitivity and specificity of any functional test would apply to both disease recurrence and disease progression. Mertes et al.[96] used bicycle stress echocardiography in 86 patients who underwent single vessel coronary angioplasty at a mean of 6.5 ± 1.3 months previously. Importantly, these patients were not selected on the basis of recurrent chest pain or other anginal symptoms, and all patients underwent follow-up coronary angiography. After eliminating seven patients because of technically inadequate angiograms, exercise echocardiography had a sensitivity of 83% and a specificity of 85%. Of note, all patients with a false-negative result failed to reach their target heart rate at peak exercise.

In summary, although the available data on exercise echocardiography are somewhat limited, exercise echocardiography appears to be a reliable tool for evaluating the extent of ischemia after percutaneous coronary interventions. As discussed in the section on thallium scintigraphy, the limitations on the use of angiography as the gold standard for determining the accuracy of functional testing also apply to exercise echocardiography.

Other Adjunctive Imaging Modalities

Previous chapters have summarized the accuracy of positron emission tomography, dobutamine echocardiography, dipyridamole echocardiography and dipyridamole thallium scintigraphy in the initial diagnosis of CAD, but there are few data regarding these modalities for the detection of restenosis after coronary intervention. Dobutamine stress echocardiography has been used before and after coronary intervention to document improvement in regional wall motion abnormalities,[97,98] but the only study that has evaluated this technique for the detection of restenosis reported relatively low values for sensitivity and specificity.[99] Several limitations were acknowledged that may have led to these disappointing results, such as the large number of patients with single vessel disease and the continuation of antianginal medications in more than 90% of patients on the day of testing.

CLINICAL APPROACH TO FOLLOW-UP AFTER CORONARY ANGIOPLASTY

Investigation of the Post-PTCA Patient

Selection of the Best Functional Test

For patients with a recurrence of typical symptoms after angioplasty, many clinicians recommend repeat angiography, particularly if these symptoms are accelerating or occur with rest. If these symptoms are stable, a stress imaging test can still be very useful to identify the likely culprit vessel. *Patients who present with less typical or atypical symptoms* after coronary angioplasty should undergo functional testing. For *patients who were completely revascularized*, a positive functional test is moderately accurate in identifying patients with angiographic restenosis. A negative test provides an 80% to 90% level of certainty that angiographic restenosis is not present. In addition, regardless of the presence of an intermediate lesion on angiography, a negative thallium test suggests an excellent 5-year event-free survival; similar data are being collected that suggest that stress echocardiography also has similar predictive value. In *patients who were incompletely revascularized*, the accuracy of functional testing for predicting restenosis is less. Nevertheless, stress imaging tests may serve a vital function in these patients; if the functional test demonstrates a large amount of ischemia, additional therapy is often indicated, regardless of whether restenosis has occurred at a particular site. This is especially important in patients with impaired left ventricular systolic function.

In our practice, most patients with chronic angina will have had a functional test before their initial intervention. Although no data support this strategy, we often find it useful to employ the same imaging modality at follow-up. In our opinion, this allows more accurate comparison of one timepoint with another. However, the most important aspect of choosing a functional test is to choose that modality with which the hospital is most expert. As reported by Picano et al.,[100] in a particular hospital one or two types of studies are often performed with a greater degree of accuracy than others; this factor should far outweigh any theoretical or small differences reported in the literature from other centers.

Timing of Functional Testing

Most patients in whom functional testing is indicated should be tested at the time that restenosis is most likely to have occurred (i.e., within 6 months). Although some evidence suggests that coronary stents may delay the peak incidence of restenosis, this data does not yet warrant changing this recommendation. The ACC/AHA Committee classified postangioplasty functional testing as a class 1 indication ("a condition for which there is general agreement that exercise testing is justified"); we agree with this recommendation.

There are three potential indications for early functional testing (e.g., within 4 weeks of coronary angioplasty):

To Document Improvement in Perfusion for a "Suboptimal" Angiographic Result

Despite the advances in interventional technology, a suboptimal result on the postprocedure coronary arteriogram occurs in at least 5% to 10% of cases. Examples of such suboptimal results are tears, dissections, or an incomplete improvement in the percent diameter stenosis (for example, to 40% to 50%) despite attempts to obtain a better result. Another example of a suboptimal result that can be a potential indication for early functional testing is to assess the hazy postintervention angiogram. When a target vessel with any of these suboptimal results supplies a large area of myocardium, it can be important to confirm that perfusion has been adequately improved.

To Document Salvage After Primary Angioplasty

When primary (also called *direct* angioplasty) is performed as an alternative to thrombolytic therapy for the treatment of acute myocardial infarction, it can be important in particular cases to document myocardial salvage or to rule out residual ischemia, either in the territory of the infarct vessel or in other vessels with intermediate lesions.

Early Functional Testing to Predict Restenosis After Balloon Angioplasty?

In the 1980s and early 1990s, a series of publications reported on the ability of early functional testing in asymptomatic patients to predict the subsequent development of restenosis.[23,101] However, functional testing early after successful angioplasty is often unreliable in the early weeks following PTCA. Table 17-4 summarizes studies that have examined the predictive value of early perfusion imaging for restenosis. Taken together, these studies suggest that although the negative predictive value of a normal perfusion study is good, the positive predictive value of an abnormal study performed early varies considerably. For example, a study of rapid atrial pacing stress thallium 201 perfusion imaging in 90 patients demonstrated that 77% of reversible perfusion defects, found in 38% of patients at 12 to 24 hours after successful angioplasty, subsequently developed angiographic restenosis. In contrast, only 14% of patients with *normal* early thallium 201 studies developed restenosis. However, false positive reversible perfusion defects occurred early after angioplasty, probably related to abnormalities of vasomotor tone[102] or suboptimal early vessel remodeling. Thus, although the negative predictive value of early pacing stress thallium 201 imaging in these patients was good, the positive predictive value of an abnormal scan was low. False positive thallium 201 redistribution defects early after angioplasty that are not associated with later restenosis are also common in other reports.[103]

If much of the restenotic process takes place during a period of several months, why should a functional test performed within days or weeks of an intervention have *any* predictive value for restenosis? This phenomenon may reflect one of the limitations of angiography, namely, the tendency for angiography to overestimate lumen dimension after percutaneous interventions, particularly balloon angioplasty. Numerous studies have documented that in many patients, despite the appearance of angiographic success, there is actually a less dramatic improvement in the postprocedural lumen area. Therefore, in these patients, the postprocedural angiogram may be misleading with respect to the actual improvement in lumen area after intervention. In addition, recoil and thrombus deposition may occur soon after the procedure (i.e., between the final angiogram and the performance of the functional test).

Data from intravascular ultrasound studies that have only recently become available suggest that some coronary sites treated with angioplasty may actually demonstrate luminal enlargement in the 6 months after the procedure.[104] Remarkably, several investigators in the field of nuclear cardiology speculated about the mechanism of improvement in flow as early as the mid 1980s. Manyari et al.[105] assessed thallium results after various intervals before and after successful angioplasty. Within 1 to 3 weeks after angioplasty, myocardial perfusion improved in most patients; however, in approximately one third of patients thallium results reverted to normal 1 month or more after angioplasty. The authors speculated that this delay in thallium reperfusion may depend upon progressive improvements and coronary flow with continued arterial filling. Other studies confirm that a myocardial continuum of mildly to severely ischemic (but viable tissues) exist distal to angioplasty sites, in which marked differences in thallium 201 clearance create the appearance of a fixed three- to four-hour poststress defect that slowly improves after angioplasty reestablishes blood flow.

In conclusion, the optimal time to perform a functional test is at the time when the restenotic process is most likely to be complete (within 3 to 6 months). In certain situations, however, early testing is appropriate. These include patients with a suboptimal outcome (dissection, poor antegrade flow, or a suboptimal angiographic result) who are stable after an angiographically successful percutaneous intervention—who should be considered for study before hospital discharge. In an early perfusion test (within 1 month after angioplasty), the presence of a persistent defect may not indicate that the procedure was unsuccessful. If a perfusion test is performed within 1 month and is normal, the probability of restenosis is lower than average but is still at least 10% to 15% or more. Thus, in patients with very high-risk lesions (e.g., subtotal proximal or ostial stenosis of the left anterior descending), a negative perfusion test at 1 month may not obviate the need to repeat functional testing again at 6 months, to avoid missing asymptomatic restenosis.

Although the incidence of complications from exercise testing soon after coronary intervention is probably low, the literature contains several case reports of acute coronary occlusion in this setting. In addition, anecdotal reports suggest that this risk may be slightly higher for coronary stents treated without coumadin (Columbo A, personal communication.)

Psychological and Work-Related Issues

There are some patients who benefit significantly from the reassurance provided by a negative functional study after coronary intervention. For example, the clinician encounters a patient who is reluctant to resume sexual intercourse or a regular exercise program, perhaps because the first symptoms of angina pectoris occurred during these activities. Similarly, patients whose occupations require physical exertion (e.g., construction workers, policemen) or whose occupations involve psychological stress or public safety (e.g., pilots or other transportation personnel) may also derive reassurance from a negative maximal exercise test. This indication is one of the most important applications of exercise testing after coronary intervention because a negative result can have a significant favorable effect on the patient's quality of life.

Repeat Angiography in Lieu of Functional Testing

Some groups warrant *repeat angiography* rather than (or in addition to) repeat functional testing. Those with extremely high-risk anatomy, such as patients who undergo angioplasty of a vessel supplying a very large amount of myocardium (such as proximal left anterior descending lesions), those undergoing angioplasty of a vessel supplying the only remaining viable myocardium, and those undergoing angioplasty of the only remaining coronary vessel or vein graft (who presumably are not candidates for surgery because of concomitant illnesses or other contraindications) are at inherently higher risk and in some cases are best reevaluated with repeat angiography rather than functional testing (Fig. 17-6).

In addition, in patients with typical angina who have excellent symptom relief from their angioplasty but who develop typical angina within 6 months, the probability of restenosis is so high that angiography may be indicated even in the event that the functional test is negative. In this circumstance, some clinicians forego functional testing and proceed directly to angiography.

Issues Related to Patient Management

It must be emphasized that treatment decisions after a positive functional test must be individualized. The following represent an approach to the most common scenarios, but this should be modified, depending on other clinical considerations.

Extensive Ischemia on Functional Testing

If ischemia is documented and the amount of myocardium at risk is large, repeat angiography is usually warranted. According to the ACC/AHA Committee, objective evidence of myocardial ischemia (exercise-induced ST depression, large reversible thallium defects, or overt left ventricular dysfunction) is a class I indication for angioplasty in both symptomatic and asymptomatic patients; ischemia in a moderate-sized distribution is a class II indication. The presence or absence of symptoms has little effect—repeat intervention is probably justified in the asymptomatic patient who has a moderate or large area of myocardial ischemia on functional study. Deligonul et al.[106] have suggested that after angioplasty, patients who develop restenosis and asymptomatic ischemia documented by functional testing have the same prognosis as patients with symptomatic ischemia. The preliminary ACIP data suggest that the prognosis of these patients may be improved by elimination of the ischemia, but there is no prospective data on the precise role of repeat angioplasty in these patients.

In stable patients, angiography can be scheduled electively; in the interim, patients should be maintained on aspirin. Many interventional cardiologists will resume a calcium channel antagonist in anticipation of repeat angioplasty; for some patients, a β-blocker is more appropriate therapy. Restenosis usually presents with stable exertional angina; for the minority who develop rest angina or other unstable symptoms, admission and prompt angiography are indicated. Repeat angioplasty usually has a success rate at least as high and a lower complication rate than the initial procedure.[74,75] In general, restenotic lesions are somewhat easier to treat with percutaneous techniques than are de novo lesions with otherwise similar angiographic features. In addition, the restenosis rate after a second angioplasty is similar to that after the initial procedure.[74,76] In other patients, rather than repeat angioplasty, coronary artery bypass grafting may be warranted for the first episode of restenosis. Examples of such patients include those whose restenotic lesions are more complex (such as those that now involve an ostium or a side branch) or those with multiple restenoses at multiple sites.

Limited Ischemia on Functional Testing

If the amount of myocardium at risk is small, repeat angiography and angioplasty may be unnecessary. Not all patients with positive functional tests should undergo repeat angiography. Even the ACC/AHA Committee recommended that "in the absence of symptoms, a *modest* reversible defect on stress perfusions scintigraphy may not justify repeat angioplasty" or repeat coronary angiography. When the area of ischemia is small, the committee classified the indication for angioplasty as class III.

A difficult clinical dilemma is a positive functional study in the presence of only an intermediate lesion angiographically. As we have discussed, in these patients a new modality, such as intravascular ultrasound, coronary Doppler, or fractional flow reserve, may reveal that the *angiogram* is falsely negative and that repeat intervention is indeed justified.

No Ischemia on Functional Testing

In those patients in whom the functional test is negative or the subsequent angiogram does not reveal a significant stenosis, "annual testing may be appropriate," as recommended by the ACC/AHA Committee.

Not infrequently, clinicians are presented with patients who have a high-quality, negative functional test (with an adjunctive imaging modality) despite the presence of angiographic restenosis. In this situation, conventional criteria would label the functional study as "falsely negative," and clinicians faced with such a situation face a dilemma: Since both angiography and thallium studies have prognostic value, should one act on the basis of the angiogram, or defer repeat intervention on the basis of the thallium? It is our opinion that in the absence of symptoms, repeat intervention in patients with an intermediate lesion solely on the basis of the angiogram is empiric; for the majority of such patients, the small but definite risks of intervention warrant against its use. Many studies have documented the excellent clinical outcome of patients with negative thallium studies, as documented in a recent review[107] and in Chapter 27. When thallium imaging is performed after coronary angioplasty, a normal scan is associated with a very low incidence of subsequent cardiac events.[23,43] This observation can be extended to patients with multivessel disease who undergo intervention of only one target vessel: if ischemia is not provokable in the other myocardial segments, "incomplete" revascularization does not affect 1-year prognosis.[108]

PROGRESS IN INTERVENTIONAL CARDIOLOGY

As we have discussed, the probability of restenosis has a significant effect on the indications, timing, and method of follow-up. Several new developments in interventional cardiology may reduce the incidence or change the time course of restenosis; if so, they will also affect the indications or optimal timing of follow-up functional testing.

Platelet Glycoprotein IIb/IIIa Receptor Antagonists

In addition to demonstrating a reduction in acute ischemic events after high-risk angioplasty, the Evaluation of c7E3 to Prevent Ischemic Complications (EPIC) investigators have recently reported that specific glycoprotein IIb/IIIa inhibition with this chimeric antibody reduced clinical restenosis.[109] Although the EPIC trial did not include systematic angiographic follow-up as part of the study, among patients who did not have an acute ischemic complication, those who received the c7E3 as bolus-plus-infusion regimen had 26% fewer adverse events at 6-month follow-up, primarily a reduction in the need for repeat revascularization. Glycoprotein IIb/IIIa inhibition may reduce restenosis by inhibiting secretion of platelet-derived growth factor (PDGF) by interfering with the smooth muscle cell $a_v b_3$ receptor, or both of these mechanisms. Similarly, the Studio Trapidil versus Aspirin nella Restenosi Coronarica (STARC) investigators[110] reported a 37% reduction in angiographic restenosis among patients given trapidil (an antiplatelet agent that inhibits thromboxane A2 and competitively blocks the PDGF receptor) compared with aspirin. Ongoing trials are comparing the angiographic restenosis rates of patients who are randomized to glycoprotein IIb/IIIa inhibition versus standard therapy.

Intracoronary Stents

Restenosis frequently involves some component of plaque persistence and recoil; coronary stents attempt to reduce restenosis by addressing these components. Two recent randomized trials of intracoronary stents versus stand-alone balloon angioplasty in *de novo* native coronary lesions have recently reported a 10% reduction of restenosis compared with conventional balloon angioplasty. The Belgian-Netherlands Stent (BENESTENT) Trial[111] of 520 patients reported a restenosis rate of 22% in patients randomized to coronary stent deployment versus 32% in those randomized to balloon angioplasty. The Stent Restenosis Study (STRESS)[112] of 408 patients reported a restenosis rate of 32% in patients randomized to coronary stent deployment versus 42% in those randomized to balloon angioplasty. Both of these studies used the same binary definition of restenosis, a 50% or greater lumen diameter stenosis by quantitative angiography. In both studies, patients randomized to the stent had an improved event-free survival rate and required fewer repeat revascularization procedures during the 6- and 8-month follow-up periods.

Despite these impressive results, there is some concern that coronary stents may simply delay the time course of restenosis rather than provide a permanent solution. In both the BENESTENT and STRESS trials, patients who received a stent had a significantly greater "acute gain" in minimum lumen diameter, which was consumed by greater absolute "late loss." If the "late loss" process continues beyond 6 months, stented patients may demonstrate a "catch-up" phenomenon with respect to restenosis. Furthermore, there is concern that stents may not be equally beneficial in vessels of all sizes.

Intravascular Ultrasound and Doppler Flow Guidance

After percutaneous coronary intervention, intravascular ultrasound occasionally reveals that the actual gain in luminal dimension is less than the apparent gain by angiography. In addition, observational studies have suggested that the absolute amount of atheroma remaining at the target site is the strongest predictor of angiographic restenosis. These observations raise the possibility that an angiographic endpoint is insufficient for coronary interventions; improving the absolute gain in lumen area or minimizing the amount of residual atheroma with intraprocedural guidance may reduce conventional restenosis rates. Several trials examining this use of intravascular ultrasound and coronary Doppler flow are currently in progress. If the results of these trials are positive, they will significantly affect indications for functional testing after intervention.

SUMMARY AND RECOMMENDATIONS

In the past, the conventional indication for routine functional testing after coronary intervention was to diagnose angiographic restenosis. Failure of a functional test to demonstrate ischemia in a patient with proven angiographic restenosis was interpreted as inadequate sensitivity of the functional test. Recent insights from clinical, angiographic, and intravascular ultrasound studies have changed the restenosis paradigm in several ways that have critical interpretation for functional testing. The restenotic process is best conceptualized as a complex set of responses to the vascular injury induced by coronary intervention. Not all of the restenotic process is due to a hyperproliferative cellular response; a considerable amount is due to a large residual plaque burden and recoil and unfavorable vessel remodeling. All angiographic definitions of restenosis are to some extent arbitrary and have only a moderate correlation with clinical restenosis, whether the latter is defined by symptoms, the provocation of ischemia, or the need for repeat revascularization. Thus, when a high-quality functional test fails to indicate ischemia despite the presence of an apparent angiographic stenosis greater than 50% diameter, this may reflect an inadequate specificity of angiography rather than the inadequate sensitivity of the functional test.

These concepts suggest that a new paradigm for the assessment restenosis may be helpful in research trials and clinical practice. Ideally, in the future randomized trials of devices or drugs aimed at reducing restenosis will include endpoints of clinical restenosis, such as the probability of survival free from recurrent angina, provokable ischemia, myocardial infarction, and death. Although angiographic endpoints will remain valuable for comparison of the morphologic effects of different devices, clinical endpoints are more relevant to judge the relative benefit of coronary revascularization procedures. Unless a new device, drug, or a combination reduces the incidence of restenosis below that of recently reported trials, postprocedural functional testing will remain a vitally important component of coronary intervention. Furthermore, because restenosis can cause silent ischemia even in patients who were symptomatic before intervention, because ischemia (whether symptomatic or silent) worsens prognosis, routine functional testing can identify candidates for repeat revascularization (PTCA or surgery) or intensification of medical therapy.

REFERENCES

1. Forrester JS, Fishbein M, Helfant R et al: A paradigm for restenosis based on cell biology: clues for the development of new preventive therapies. J Am Coll Cardiol 17:758, 1991
2. Rensing BJ, Hermans WRM, Beatt KJ et al: Quantitative angiographic assessment of elastic recoil after percutaneous transluminal coronary angioplasty. Am J Cardiol 66:1039, 1990
3. Rensing BJ, Hermans WRM, Vos J et al: Angiographic risk factors of luminal narrowing after coronary balloon angioplasty using balloon measurements to re-

flect stretch and elastic recoil at the dilatation site. Am J Cardiol 69:584, 1992
4. Ardissino D, Barberis P, De Servi S et al: Abnormal coronary vasoconstriction as a predictor of restenosis after successful coronary angioplasty in patients with unstable angina pectoris. N Engl J Med 325:1053, 1991
5. Luo H, Nishioka T, Eigler N et al: Chronic vessel constriction is an important mechanism of restenosis after balloon angioplasty: an intravascular ultrasound analysis. Circulation 90:I, 1994
6. Mintz GS, Popma JJ, Pichard AD et al: Mechanism of arterial responses to transcatheter therapy: a serial quantitative angiographic and intravascular ultrasound study. Circulation 90:I, 1994
7. Arora R, Platko W, Bhadwar K et al: Role of intracoronary thrombus in acute complications during percutaneous transluminal coronary angioplasty. Cathet Cardiovasc Diag 16:226, 1989
8. Mabin T, Holmes D, Smith H et al: Intracoronary thrombus: role in coronary occlusion complicating percutaneous transluminal coronary angioplasty. J Am Coll Cardiol 5:198, 1985
9. Miller DD, Rivera FJ, Garcia OJ et al: Imaging of vascular injury with 99mTc-labeled monoclonal antiplatelet antibody S12. Preliminary experience in human percutaneous transluminal angioplasty. Circulation 85:1354, 1992
10. Miller DD, Boulet AJ, Tio FO et al: In vivo technetium-99m S12 antibody imaging of platelet alpha-granules in rabbit endothelial neointimal proliferation after angioplasty. Circulation 83:224, 1991
11. Ellis SG, Bates ER, Schaible T et al: Prospects for the use of antagonists to the platelet glycoprotein IIb/IIIa receptor to prevent postangioplasty restenosis and thrombosis. J Am Coll Cardiol 17:89B, 1991
12. den Heijer P, van Dijk R, Hillege H et al: Serial angioscopic and angiographic observations during the first hour after successful coronary angioplasty: a preamble to a multicenter trial addressing angioscopic markers for restenosis. Am Heart J 128:656, 1994
13. Schwartz RS, Holmes Jr D, Topol E: The restenosis paradigm revisited: an alternative proposal for cellular mechanisms. J Am Coll Cardiol 20:1284, 1992
14. Holmes DRJ, Vlietstra RE, Smith HC et al: Restenosis after percutaneous transluminal coronary angioplasty (PTCA): a report from the PTCA registry of the National Heart, Lung, and Blood Institute. Am J Cardiol 53:77C, 1984
15. Topol EJ, Leya F, Pinkerton CA et al: A comparison of directional atherectomy with coronary angioplasty in patients with coronary artery disease. The CAVEAT Study Group. N Engl J Med 329:221, 1993
16. Simonton C, Leon M, Kuntz R et al: Acute and late clinical and angiographic results of directional atherectomy in the optimal atherectomy restenosis study (OARS). Circulation 92:I, 1995
17. White C, Wright C, Doty D et al: Does visual interpretation of the coronary arteriogram predict the physiologic importance of a coronary stenosis? N Engl J Med 310:819, 1984
18. Galbraith J, Murphy M, Desoyza N: Coronary angiogram interpretation: interobserver variability. JAMA 240:2053, 1981
19. Zir L, Miller S, Dinsmore R et al: Interobserver variability in coronary angiography. Circulation 53:627, 1976
20. Bottner RK, Green CE, Ewels CJ et al: Recurrent ischemia more than 1 year after successful percutaneous transluminal coronary angioplasty. An analysis of the extent and anatomic pattern of coronary disease. Circulation 80:1580, 1989
21. The Epic Investigators: Use of a monoclonal antibody directed against the platelet glycoprotein IIb/IIIa receptor in high-risk coronary angioplasty. N Engl J Med 330:956, 1994
22. Rosing D, Cannon R, Watson R et al: Three-year anatomic, functional, and clinical follow-up after successful percutaneous transluminal coronary angioplasty. J Am Coll Cardiol 9:1, 1987
23. Wijns W, Serruys PW, Reiber JH et al: Early detection of restenosis after successful percutaneous transluminal coronary angioplasty by exercise-redistribution thallium scintigraphy. Am J Cardiol 55:357, 1985
24. Stuckey T, Burwell L, Nygaard T et al: Quantitative exercise thallium-201 scintigraphy for predicting angina recurrence after percutaneous transluminal coronary angioplasty. Am J Cardiol 63:517, 1989
25. Vlay SC, Chernilas J, Lawson WE et al: Restenosis after angioplasty: don't rely on the exercise test. Am Heart J 117:980, 1989
26. Leimgruber P, Roubin G, Hollman J et al: Restenosis after successful coronary angioplasty in patients with single-vessel disease. Circulation 73:710, 1986
27. Laarman G, Luijten HE, van Zeyl LG et al: Assessment of "silent" restenosis and long-term follow-up after successful angioplasty in single vessel coronary artery disease: the value of quantitative exercise electrocardiography and quantitative coronary angiography. J Am Coll Cardiol 16:578, 1990
28. Breisblatt W, Weiland F, Spaccavento L: Stress thallium-201 imaging after coronary angioplasty predicts

28. restenosis and recurrent symptoms. J Am Coll Cardiol 12:1199, 1988
29. Hernandez RA, Macaya C, Iniguez A et al: Midterm outcome of patients with asymptomatic restenosis after coronary balloon angioplasty. J Am Coll Cardiol 19:1402, 1992
30. Califf R, Fortin D, Frid D et al: Restenosis after coronary angioplasty: an overview. J Am Coll Cardiol 17:2B, 1991
31. Joye J, Schulman D, Lasorda D et al: Intracoronary Doppler guidewire versus single-photon emission computer tomographic thallium-201 imaging in assessment of intermediate coronary stenoses. J Am Coll Cardiol 24:940, 1994
32. Donohue TJ, Kern MJ, Aguirre FV et al: Assessing the hemodynamic significance of coronary artery stenoses: analysis of translesional pressure-flow velocity relations in patients. J Am Coll Cardiol 22:449, 1993
33. de Bruyne B, Bartunek J, Sys S et al: Feasibility and hemodynamic dependency of invasive indexes of coronary stenosis. Circulation 92:I, 1995
34. Bengtson JR, Mark DB, Honan MB et al: Detection of restenosis after elective percutaneous transluminal coronary angioplasty using the exercise treadmill test. Am J Cardiol 65:28, 1990
35. Falcone C, DeSevi S, Porna E et al: Clinical significance of exercise induced silent myocardial ischemia in patients with coronary artery disease. J Am Coll Cardiol 9:295, 1987
36. Kent KM, Rosing DR, Ewels CJ et al: Prognosis of asymptomatic or mildly symptomatic patients with coronary artery disease. Am J Cardiol 49:1823, 1982
37. Weiner DA, Ryan TJ, McCabe CH et al: Risk of developing an acute myocardial infarction or sudden coronary death in patients with exercise-induced silent myocardial ischemia. A report from the Coronary Artery Surgery Study (CASS) registry. Am J Cardiol 62:1155, 1988
38. Heller L, Tresgallo M, Sciacca RR et al: Prognostic significance of silent myocardial ischemia on a thallium stress test. Am J Cardiol 65:718, 1990
39. Pepine C, Cohn P, Deedwania P et al: Effects of treatment on outcome in mildly symptomatic patients with ischemia during daily life: the atenolol silent ischemia study (ASIST). Circulation 90:762, 1994
40. Knatterud G, MG B, Pepine C et al: Effects of treatment strategies to suppress ischemia in patients with coronary artery disease: 12-week results of the asymptomatic cardiac ischemia pilot (ACIP) study. J Am Coll Cardiol 24:11, 1994
41. Hecht HS, Shaw RE, Chin HL et al: Silent ischemia after coronary angioplasty: evaluation of restenosis and extent of ischemia in asymptomatic patients by tomographic thallium-201 exercise imaging and comparison with symptomatic patients. J Am Coll Cardiol 17:670, 1991
42. Popma JJ, van den Berg EK, Dehmer GJ: Long-term outcome of patients with symptomatic restenosis after percutaneous transluminal coronary angioplasty. Am J Cardiol 62:1298, 1988
43. Wijns W, Serruys PW, Simoons ML et al: Predictive value of early maximal exercise test and thallium scintigraphy after successful percutaneous transluminal coronary angioplasty. Br Heart J 53:194, 1985
44. Friedrich S, Kuntz R, Gordon P et al: "Moderate" restenosis has a favorable natural history. J Am Coll Cardiol 21:321A, 1993
45. Pfisterer M, Rickenbacher P, Kiowski W et al: Silent ischemia after percutaneous transluminal coronary angioplasty: incidence and prognostic significance. J Am Coll Cardiol 22:1446, 1993
46. Moliterno DJ: Restenosis following percutaneous coronary intervention. In: Textbook of interventional cardiology. Update 17. WB Saunders, Philadelphia, 1995
47. Carrozza J, Kuntz R, Fishman R et al: Restenosis after arterial injury caused by coronary stenting in patients with diabetes mellitus. Ann Intern Med 118:344, 1993
48. Lambert M, Bonan R, Cote G et al: Multiple coronary angioplasty: a model to discriminate systemic and procedural factors related to restenosis. J Am Coll Cardiol 12:310, 1988
49. Myler RK, Shaw RE, Stertzer SH et al: Recurrence after coronary angioplasty. Cathet Cardiovasc Diagn 13:77, 1987
50. Rupprecht HJ, Brennecke R, Bernhard G et al: Analysis of risk factors for restenosis after PTCA. Cathet Cardiovasc Diagn 19:151, 1990
51. Leimgruber PP, Roubin GS, Hollman J et al: Restenosis after successful coronary angioplasty in patients with single-vessel disease. Circulation 73:710, 1986
52. Bourassa MG, Lesperance J, Eastwood C et al: Clinical, physiologic, anatomic, and procedural factors predictive of restenosis after percutaneous transluminal coronary angioplasty. J Am Coll Cardiol 18:368, 1991
53. Simonton C, Mark D, Hinohara T et al: Late restenosis after emergent coronary angioplasty for acute myocardial infarction: Comparison with elective coronary angioplasty. J Am Coll Cardiol 11:698, 1988
54. Arora RR, Konrad K, Badhwar K et al: Restenosis after transluminal coronary angioplasty: a risk factor analysis. Cathet Cardiovasc Diagn 19:17, 1990
55. Hearn JA, Donohue BC, Ba'albake H et al: Usefulness

of serum lipoprotein (a) as a predictor of restenosis after percutaneous transluminal coronary angioplasty. Am J Cardiol 69:736, 1992
56. Reis GJ, Kuntz RE, Silverman DI et al: Effects of serum lipid levels on restenosis after coronary angioplasty. Am J Cardiol 68:1431, 1991
57. Johansson S, Wiklund O, Emanuelsson H: Lack of correlation between the serum level of lipoprotein (a) and restenosis after coronary angioplasty. Coron Artery Dis 3:839, 1992
58. Rozenman Y, Gilon D, Welber S et al: Plasma lipoproteins are not related to restenosis after successful coronary angioplasty. Am J Cardiol 72:1206, 1993
59. Sahni R, Maniet AR, Voci G et al: Prevention of restenosis by lovastatin after successful coronary angioplasty. Am Heart J 121:1600, 1991
60. Lovastatin Study Trial Group: Lovastatin Restenosis Trial: results in patients with cholesterol over 200 mg/dl. J Am Coll Cardiol 23:470A, 1994
61. Serruys PW, Rutsch W, Heyndricks GR et al: Prevention of restenosis after percutaneous transluminal coronary angioplasty with thromboxane A2-receptor blockade—a randomized, double-blind, placebo-controlled trial. Circulation 84:1568, 1991
62. MERCATOR Study Group: Does the new angiotensin-converting enzyme inhibitor cilazapril prevent restenosis after percutaneous transluminal coronary angioplasty? Results of the MERCATOR study: a multicenter, randomized, double-blind, placebo-controlled trial. Circulation 86:100, 1992
63. Faxon D, on behalf of the MARCATOR study group: Effect of high dose angiotensin-converting enzyme inhibition on restenosis: final results of the MARCATOR study, a multicenter, double-blind, placebo-controlled trial of cilazapril. J Am Coll Cardiol 25:362, 1995
64. Ohishi M, Fujii K, Minamino T et al: A potent genetic risk factor for restenosis [letter]. Nature Genetics 5:324, 1993
65. Hirshfeld JWJ, Schwartz JS, Jugo R et al: Restenosis after coronary angioplasty: a multivariate statistical model to relate lesion and procedure variables to restenosis. J Am Coll Cardiol 18:647, 1991
66. Rensing BJ, Hermans WRM, Vos J et al: Luminal narrowing after percutaneous transluminal coronary angioplasty. Circulation 88:975, 1993
67. Piovaccari G, Fattori R, Marzocchi A et al: Percutaneous transluminal coronary angioplasty of the very proximal left anterior descending artery lesions: immediate results and follow-up. Int J Cardiol 30:151, 1991
68. Clark D, Wexman M, Murphy M et al: Factors predicting recurrence in patients who have had angioplasty of total occluded vessels. J Am Coll Cardiol 7:20A, 1986
69. DiSciascio G, Vetrovec G, Cowley M et al: Early and late outcome of percutaneous transluminal coronary angioplasty for subacute and chronic total coronary occlusion. Am Heart J 111:833, 1986
70. Melchior J, Meier B, Urban P et al: Percutaneous transluminal coronary angioplasty for chronic total coronary arterial occlusion. Am J Cardiol 59:535, 1987
71. Meier B, King III SB, Gruentzig AR et al: Repeat coronary angioplasty. J Am Coll Cardiol 4:463, 1984
72. Rapold HJ, David PR, Val PG et al: Restenosis and its determinants in first and repeat coronary angioplasty. Eur Heart J 8:575, 1987
73. Bauters C, McFadden E, Lablanche J et al: Restenosis rate after multiple percutaneous transluminal coronary angioplasty procedures at the same site. A quantitative angiographic study in consecutive patients undergoing a third angioplasty procedure for a second restenosis. Circulation 88:969, 1993
74. Dimas AP, Grigera F, Arora RR et al: Repeat coronary angioplasty as treatment for restenosis. J Am Coll Cardiol 19:1310, 1992
75. Glazier JJ, Varricchione TR, Ryan TJ et al: Outcome in patients with recurrent restenosis after percutaneous transluminal balloon angioplasty. Br Heart J 61:485, 1989
76. Teirstein PS, Hoover CA, Ligon RW et al: Repeat coronary angioplasty: efficacy of a third angioplasty for a second restenosis. J Am Coll Cardiol 13:291, 1989
77. Weintraub W, Brown C, Liberman H et al: Effect of restenosis at one previously dilated coronary site on the probability of restenosis at another previously dilated coronary site. Am J Cardiol 72:1107, 1993
78. Berger PB, Bell MR, Holmes DR et al: Effect of restenosis after an earlier angioplasty at another coronary site on the frequency of restenosis after a subsequent coronary angioplasty. Am J Cardiol 69:1086, 1992
79. Bresee SJ, Jacobs AK, Gareber GR et al: Prior restenosis predicts restenosis after coronary angioplasty of a new significant narrowing. Am J Cardiol 68:1158, 1991
80. Gibson CM, Kuntz RE, Nobuyoshi M et al: Lesion-to-lesion independence of restenosis after treatment by conventional angioplasty, stenting, or directional atherectomy. Validation of lesion-based restenosis analysis. Circulation 87:1123, 1993
81. Adelman A, Cohen E, Kimball B et al: A comparison of directional atherectomy with balloon angioplasty

for lesions of the left anterior descending artery. N Engl J Med 329:228, 1993
82. Kuntz R, Gibson C, Nobuyoshi M et al: Generalized model of restenosis after conventional balloon angioplasty, stenting and directional atherectomy. J Am Coll Cardiol 21:15, 1993
83. Bourassa MG, Holubkov R, Yeh W et al: Strategy of complete revascularization in patients with multivessel coronary artery disease (a report from the 1985–1986 NHLBI PTCA Registry). Am J Cardiol 70:174, 1992
84. Ryan T, Bauman W, Kennedy J et al: The American College of Cardiology/American Heart Association Task Force on Assessment of Diagnostic and Therapeutic Cardiovascular Procedures. Subcommittee on Percutaneous Transluminal Coronary Angioplasty: Guidelines for percutaneous transluminal coronary angioplasty. J Am Coll Cardiol 22:2033, 1993
85. Meier B, Gruentzig A, Siegenthaler W et al: Long-term exercise performance after percutaneous transluminal coronary angioplasty and coronary artery bypass grafting. Circulation 68:796, 1983
86. Gruentzig AR, King SB, Schlumpf M et al: Long-term follow-up after percutaneous transluminal coronary angioplasty. The early Zurich experience. N Engl J Med 316:1127, 1987
87. Scholl J, Chaitman B, David P et al: Exercise electrocardiography and myocardial scintigraphy in the serial evaluation of the results of percutaneous transluminal coronary angioplasty. Circulation 66:380, 1982
88. DePuey G, Leatherman L, Leachman R et al: Restenosis after transluminal coronary angioplasty detected with exercise-gated radionuclide ventriculography. J Am Coll Cardiol 4:1103, 1984
89. Miller D: Evaluation of the patient with stable angina following coronary artery bypass surgery. p. 137. In Waters D, Bourassa M (eds): Care of the Patient with Previous Coronary Bypass Surgery. FA Davis, Philadelphia, 1991
90. Ernst SM, Hillebrand FA, Klein B et al: The value of exercise tests in the follow-up of patients who underwent transluminal coronary angioplasty. Int J Cardiol 7:267, 1985
91. Lefkowitz C, Ross B, Schwartz L et al: Superiority of tomographic thallium imaging for the detection of restenosis after percutaneous transluminal coronary angioplasty. J Am Coll Cardiol 13:161A, 1988
92. Limacher M, Quinones M, Poliner L et al: Detection of coronary artery disease with exercise two-dimensional echocardiography: description of a clinically applicable method and comparison with radionuclide ventriculography. Circulation 67:1211, 1983
93. Maurer G, Nanda N: Two-dimensional echocardiographic evaluation of exercise-induced left and right ventricular asynergy: correlation with thallium scanning. Am J Cardiol 48:720, 1981
94. Ginzton L: Stress echocardiography and myocardial contrast echocardiography. Cardiol Clin 7:494, 1989
95. Sawada S, Ryan T, Fineberg N et al: Exercise echocardiographic detection of coronary artery disease in women. J Am Coll Cardiol 14:1440, 1989
96. Mertes H, Erbel R, Nixdorff U et al: Stress echocardiography: a sensitive method for the detection of coronary artery disease. Herz 16:355, 1991
97. Akosah PO, Porter TR, Simon R et al: Ischemia-induced regional wall motion abnormality is improved after coronary angioplasty: demonstration by dobutamine stress echocardiography. J Am Coll Cardiol 21:584, 1993
98. McNeill AJ, Fioretti PM, El-Said EM et al: Dobutamine stress echocardiography before and after coronary angioplasty. Am J Cardiol 69:740, 1992
99. Heinle SK, Lieberman EB, Ancukiewicz M et al: Usefulness of dobutamine echocardiography for detecting restenosis after percutaneous transluminal coronary angioplasty. Am J Cardiol 72:1220, 1993
100. Picano E, Lattanzi F, Orlandini A et al: Stress echocardiography and the human factor: the importance of being expert. J Am Coll Cardiol 17:666, 1991
101. Hirzel H, Nuesch K, Gruentzig A et al: Short- and long-term changes in myocardial perfusion after PTCA assessed by thallium-201 exercise scintigraphy. Circulation 63:1001, 1981
102. Bates ER, McGillem MJ, Beals TF et al: Effect of angioplasty-induced endothelial denudation compared with medial injury on regional coronary blood flow. Circulation 76:710, 1987
103. Powelson S, DePuey E, Roubin G et al: Discordance of coronary angiography and 201-thallium tomography early after transluminal coronary angioplasty (abstract). J Nucl Med 27:900, 1986
104. Mitsuo K, Degawa T, Nakamura K et al: Serial intravascular ultrasound evaluation of the mechanism of restenosis after directional coronary atherectomy. Circulation 92:I, 1995
105. Manyari D, Knudtson M, Kloiber R et al: Sequential thallium-201 myocardial perfusion studies after successful percutaneous transluminal coronary artery angioplasty: delayed resolution of exercise-induced scintigraphic abnormalities. Circulation 77:86, 1988
106. Deligonul U, Vandormael MG, Younis LT et al: Prognostic significance of silent myocardial ischemia detected by early treadmill exercise after coronary angioplasty. Am J Cardiol 64:1, 1989

107. Brown K: Prognostic value of thallium-201 myocardial perfusion imaging: a diagnostic tool comes of age. Circulation 83:363, 1991
108. Breisblatt WM, Barnes JV, Weiland F et al: Incomplete revascularization in multivessel percutaneous transluminal coronary angioplasty: the role for stress thallium-201 imaging. J Am Coll Cardiol 11:1183, 1988
109. Topol E, Califf R, Weisman H et al: Randomised trial of coronary intervention with antibody against platelet IIb/IIIa integrin for the reduction of clinical restenosis: results at six months. Lancet 343:881, 1994
110. Maresta A, Balducelli M, Cantini A et al: Trapadil (triazolopyrimidine), a platelet-derived growth factor antagonist, reduces restenosis after percutaneous transluminal coronary angioplasty. Results of the randomized, double-blind STARC study. Circulation 90:2710, 1994
111. Serruys P, de Jaegere P, Kiemeniej F et al: A comparison of balloon-expandable-stent implantation with balloon angioplasty in patients with coronary artery disease. N Engl J Med 331:489, 1994
112. Fischman D, Leon M, Baim D et al: A randomized comparison of coronary-stent placement and balloon angioplasty in the treatment of coronary artery disease. N Engl J Med 331:496, 1994
113. Renkin J, Melin J, Robert A et al: Detection of restenosis after successful coronary angioplasty: improved clinical decision making with use of a logistic model combining procedural and follow-up variables. J Am Coll Cardiol 16:1333, 1990
114. Califf R, Ohram E, Frid D et al: Restenosis: the clinical issues. p. 363. In Topol E (Ed): Textbook of Interventional Cardiology. WB Saunders, Philadelphia, 1990
115. Zaidi A, Hollman J, Galan K et al: Predictive value of chest discomfort for restenosis following successful coronary angioplasty. Circulation, suppl. III, 72:456, 1985
116. Mabin T, Holmes DJ, Smith H et al: Follow-up clinical results in patients undergoing percutaneous transluminal coronary angioplasty. Circulation 71:754, 1985
117. Levine S, Ewels C, Rosing D et al: Coronary angioplasty: clinical and angiographic follow-up. Am J Cardiol 55:673, 1985
118. Jutzy K, Berte L, Alderman E et al: Coronary restenosis rates in consecutive patient series one-year post-successful angioplasty (abstract). Circulation, suppl. II, 66:331, 1982
119. Roth A, Miller HI, Keren G et al: Detection of restenosis following percutaneous coronary angioplasty in single-vessel coronary artery disease: the value of clinical assessment and exercise tolerance testing. Cardiology 84:106, 1994
120. O'Keefe J, Lapeyre A, Holmes D et al: Usefulness of early radionuclide angiography for identifying low-risk patients for late restenosis after percutaneous transluminal coronary angioplasty. Am J Cardiol 61:51, 1988
121. el-Tamimi H, Davies GJ, Hackett D et al: Very early prediction of restenosis after successful coronary angioplasty: anatomic and functional assessment. J Am Coll Cardiol 15:259, 1990
122. Rosing D, Van Raden J, Mincemoyer R et al: Exercise electrocardiographic and functional responses after percutaneous transluminal coronary angioplasty. Am J Cardiol 53:36C, 1984
123. Honan MB, Bengtson JR, Pryor DB et al: Exercise treadmill testing is a poor predictor of anatomic restenosis after angioplasty for acute myocardial infarction. Circulation 80:1585, 1989
124. Kadel C, Strecker T, Kaltenbach M et al: Recognition of restenosis: can patients be defined in whom the exercise-ECG result makes angiographic restudy unnecessary? Eur Heart J 10:22, 1989
125. Hardoff R, Shefer A, Gips S et al: Predicting late restenosis after coronary angioplasty by very early (12 to 24 h) thallium-201 scintigraphy: implications with regard to mechanisms of late coronary restenosis. J Am Coll Cardiol 15:1486, 1990
126. Jain A, Mahmarian J, Borges-Neto S et al: Clinical significance of perfusion defects by thallium-201 single photon emission tomography following oral dipyridamole early after coronary angioplasty. J Am Coll Cardiol 11:970, 1988
127. Miller DD, Liu P, Strauss HW et al: Prognostic value of computer-quantitated exercise thallium imaging early after percutaneous transluminal coronary angioplasty. J Am Coll Cardiol 10:275, 1987
128. Lam J, Chaitman B, Byers S et al: Can dipyridamole thallium imaging predict restenosis after coronary angioplasty? Circulation, suppl. IV, 76:373, 1987
129. Marie PY, Danchin N, Karcher G et al: Usefulness of exercise SPECT-thallium to detect asymptomatic restenosis in patients who had angina before coronary angioplasty. Am Heart J 126:571, 1993
130. Schroeder E, Marchandise B, De Coster P et al: Detection of restenosis after coronary angioplasty for single-vessel disease: how reliable are exercise electrocardiography and scintigraphy in asymptomatic patients? Eur Heart J 10:18, 1989
131. Avery PG, Hudson NM, Hubner PJ: Assessment of myocardial perfusion and function using gated methoxy-isobutyl-isonitrile scintigraphy to detect reste-

nosis after coronary angioplasty. Coron Artery Dis 4: 1097, 1993
132. Aboul-Enein H, Bengston JR, Adams DB et al: Effect of the degree of effort on exercise echocardiography for the detection of restenosis after coronary artery angioplasty. Am Heart J 122:430, 1991
133. Mertes H, Erbel R, Nixdorff U et al: Exercise echocardiography for the evaluation of patients after nonsurgical coronary artery revascularization. J Am Coll Cardiol 21:1087, 1993
134. Hecht HS, DeBord L, Shaw R et al: Usefulness of supine bicycle stress echocardiography for detection of restenosis after percutaneous transluminal coronary angioplasty. Am J Cardiol 71:293, 1993
135. Duerr RL, Lefkovits J, Pieper K, et al: The relationship between angiographic indices and clinical outcomes following percutaneous coronary revascularization. Submitted for publication, 1996
136. De Franco AC, Tuzcu EM, Abdelmeguid A et al: Intravascular ultrasound assessment of PTCA results: Insights into the mechanisms of balloon angioplasty, abstracted. J Am Coll Cardiol 21:485, 1993
137. Topol EJ, Nissen SE. Our preoccupation with coronary luminology. Circulation 92:2333, 1995

Chapter 18

Stress Echocardiography Before and After Interventional Therapy

Rainer Hoffmann

With the expansion of coronary interventions over the last two decades, decision making regarding both the selection and follow-up of patients undergoing interventional therapy has grown into a significant problem. Generally, myocardial revascularization is recommended for the treatment of severe symptoms or for prognostic reasons in the setting of substantial ischemia.[1-3] Functional testing may be used to identify the presence of "prognostically important" disease, indicating myocardium at risk, severe multivessel disease, and left main stenosis, as discussed previously.

Several ongoing studies are comparing angioplasty with surgery, in respect of patient selection, indications, and outcome. Angioplasty may be preferable to bypass surgery in patients with one-vessel and two-vessel disease, whereas coronary artery bypass grafting seems to be more adequate in patients with multivessel disease and left ventricular dysfunction. Nonetheless, the relative indications for these effective techniques for coronary revascularization are ill-defined, particularly with the increasing application of coronary angioplasty in situations traditionally reserved for bypass surgery. The ability of functional testing to identify the "culprit vessel" and then assess the adequacy of revascularization may be of value in assisting the selection between coronary angioplasty and coronary bypass grafting.

Stress echocardiography has been proven to be an accurate method for the evaluation of myocardial ischemia, one of the main criteria to assess the need for interventional therapy as well as its success. Thus, this chapter will focus on the utility of stress echocardiography for two purposes: (1) the functional evaluation of angiographically documented coronary lesions in patients considered for coronary interventions, and (2) the assessment of patients who have already undergone interventional procedures including angioplasty or bypass surgery (Table 18-1).

USE OF STRESS ECHOCARDIOGRAPHY IN DECISION MAKING PRIOR TO INTERVENTION

Prior to interventional therapy stress echocardiography can be used (1) to identify the functional significance of a coronary stenosis, (2) to determine the "culprit" vessel in multivessel disease, and (3) to determine myocardial viability in patients with impaired left ventricular function.

Assessment of the Functional Significance of a Coronary Stenosis

Evidence of the functional significance of an angiographically proven coronary stenosis is a critical factor in determining the need for coronary revascu-

Table 18-1. Indications for Stress Echocardiography Related to Interventional Therapy

Assessment of the functional signficance of an angiographically proven coronary stenosis
Determination of the culprit vessel prior to PTCA in multivessel disease
Assessment of myocardial viability in patients with impaired left ventricular function
Assessment of improved stress tolerence after intervention
Diagnosis of restenosis or bypass occlusion

---

larization. For both, angioplasty and bypass surgery recommendations concerning the indications of therapy have been made by the American College of Cardiology/American Heart Association ACC/AHA Task Force.[2,3] Three classes have been defined to classify the degree of consensus on patient management: class I, a condition for which there is general agreement that coronary angioplasty/bypass surgery is justified; class II, conditions for which there is divergence of opinion with respect to the justification of coronary angioplasty/bypass grafting; and class III, conditions for which there is general agreement that neither coronary angioplasty nor bypass grafting is ordinarily indicated. As left main stenosis or severe three-vessel disease is the commonest class I indication for bypass surgery, functional evidence of ischemia may be a less important factor influencing the indication for surgery. In contrast, patients undergoing coronary angioplasty more frequently have one- or two-vessel disease, so that evidence of myocardial ischemia during a stress test is the essential factor that will qualify a patient for a class I indication.

As discussed in Chapter 3, stress echocardiography is an accurate means of identifying inducible ischemia. In patients with normal left ventricular function stress echocardiography can evaluate the size of myocardium at risk due to a stenotic coronary artery, it can define the stress level at which myocardial ischemia occurs, and it can demonstrate the distribution of ischemic regions (and hence impute the presence of single- or multivessel disease). Thus, stress echocardiography may help in classifying patients according to the classes of treatment necessity defined by the ACC/AHA Task Force Reports.

Assessment of the "Culprit" Vessel in Multivessel Disease

Patients undergoing angioplasty currently include an increasing proportion with multivessel disease. Multivessel angioplasty has been shown to be a safe procedure, having success and complication rates comparable with those of single-vessel angioplasty. In managing multivessel disease by angioplasty, a decision has to be made whether multivessel angioplasty should be performed to provide the patient with complete revascularization, or incomplete revascularization should be considered, in which only the functionally most significant coronary stenosis is dilated. Although the argument for multivessel angioplasty is to provide the patient with complete coronary revascularization, it has not been proven consistently that complete revascularization is associated with improved outcome with respect to death, myocardial infarction, or need for late revascularization.[4] On the other hand, it has been shown that partial revascularization in patients with multivessel disease is already associated with important symptomatic relief.[5]

If incomplete revascularization is considered, it is important to determine which stenosis should be dilated. In contrast to the exercise electrocardiogram (ECG), with its poor correlation of the site of ST-segment change and the location of the diseased coronary ("culprit") vessel, the close correlation of regional wall motion abnormalities and the vessel responsible for ischemia allows an accurate prediction of the most significant stenosis by means of echocardiography. Once angioplasty of the culprit lesion has been performed, stress echocardiography allows separation of patients without inducible wall motion abnormalities and those with persistent positivity due to a territory fed by a less-stenotic coronary vessel. Thus, correction of the "culprit" lesion might unmask a stenosis to be functionally significant that had initially been thought to be less important.

Myocardial Viability

The highest priority of the cell is to feed those basic aspects of cell metabolism devoted to repairing itself. As discussed in subsequent chapters on myocardial viability, an important consideration in the revascularization of hypokinetic or akinetic myocardial areas is whether they represent viable myocardium with critically endangered local supply–demand balance (ischemia, hibernation, stunning) or whether these areas represent irreversibly damaged necrotic scar tissue.[6] Coronary revascularization is useful only if viability of dyssynergic segments can be demonstrated. Thus, the identification of hibernating myocardium is important for selection of patients who will profit from coronary revascularization. Pharmacological stress echocardiography has been used for detection of both stunned as well as hibernating myocardium to predict patients who will have spontaneous recovery of left ventricular function and those who might profit from revascularization therapy. Moreover, as discussed in Chapter 28, documentation of myocardial viability has prognostic as well as therapeutic implications.[7]

Dobutamine and dipyridamole stress echocardiography have been found useful in several studies for the assessment of myocardial viability early after an acute myocardial infarction.[8–13] A high level of concordance between dobutamine stress echocardiography and positron emission tomography in the identification of viable myocardial segments has been reported.[9] Similarly, both tests appear to identify viable tissue in patients with chronic left ventricular dysfunction,[15,16] this situation perhaps being more important with respect to coronary interventions.

Enoximone, a phosphodiesterase inhibitor independent of the β-adrenoceptor, has recently been claimed to be a useful alternative in combination with echocardiography for the detection of viable myocardium.[17] In comparison to dobutamine stimulation, enoximone offers the advantages of being independent of possible β-blockade and stimulation occurs without changes in hemodynamics.

ASSESSMENT WITH STRESS ECHOCARDIOGRAPHY AFTER INTERVENTIONAL THERAPY

Use of Stress Echocardiography to Assess the Effects of Angioplasty

Percutaneous transluminal coronary angioplasty and other interventional procedures for nonsurgical revascularization have been established as standard therapy in the treatment of patients with coronary artery disease. It is now reasonable to expect an overall initial success rate for single lesion dilations of greater than 90% by angiographic criteria (>20% change in luminal diameter, with the final-diameter stenosis being less than 50%).[18]

Stress Testing after Angioplasty

However, it has been difficult to accurately assess the physiologic and functional benefits of revascularization after angioplasty for a given angiographic result. The physiologic importance of residual stenosis is not reliably predicted by angiography. Exercise ECG is of limited value as it does not reach a high sensitivity for the diagnosis of significant coronary stenosis. This holds true especially in patients with one-vessel disease, in whom test results are often negative already prior to angioplasty. Perfusion scintigraphy has a greater diagnostic accuracy, however, it may reveal persistent reversible defects in the myocardial distribution of the dilated vessel for several weeks. In nearly one-third of patients persistently abnormal regional thallium uptake 4 to 18 days after successful angioplasty has been found by Manyari et al.[19] Hibernation and stunning have been suggested as possible reasons, although the exact mechanism remains unclear. The persistently abnormal thallium uptake limits the utility of thallium stress imaging for assessment of immediate improvements of left ventricular perfusion after angioplasty. While thallium uptake is determined by perfusion and metabolic integrity, stress echocardiography is dependent on the development of systolic dysfunction as an indicator of true myocardial ischemia.

Stress Two-Dimensional Echocardiography after Angioplasty

Several reports in the literature support the use of stress echocardiography for assessment of improved regional function after angioplasty (Table 18-2). The initial reports used exercise stress echocardiography to evaluate the effect of successful angioplasty on left ventricular function. Labovitz et al.[20] found that using exercise echocardiography, 12 of 17 patients demonstrated inducible ischemia prior to angioplasty compared to no patients postangioplasty. However, Broderick et al.[21] demonstrated that a significant number of patients still had inducible wall motion abnormalities after angioplasty. In a group of 36 patients examined before and after coronary

Table 18-2. Effect of Angioplasty Assessed by Stress Echocardiography

Author (Year) (Patient No.)	Positive Echo Prior to PTCA	Positive Post PTCA	Time Interval from PTCA to Echo	Stress Mode
Labovitz et al. (1989)[20] ($n=17$)	71%	0%	up to 14 days	Exercise
Broderick et al. (1990)[21] ($n=36$)	69%	39%	28 ± 26 days	Exercise
Hoffman et al. (1994)[37] ($n=47$)	90%	30%	13 ± 6 days	Exercise
McNeill et al. (1992)[23] ($n=23$)	61%	11%	28 days	Exercise
Akosah et al. (1993)[22] ($n=35$)	89%	28 patients improvement	up to 28 h	Dobutamine
McNeill et al. (1992)[23] ($n=28$)	71%	14%	up to 72 h	Dobutamine
Picano et al. (1989)[24] ($n=63$)	92%	25%	up to 72 h	Dipyridamole

Abbreviations: PTCA, percutaneous transluminal angioplasty; echo, echocardiography.

angioplasty, 69% had inducible wall motion abnormalities prior to angioplasty compared to 39% after angioplasty. However, the majority of patients still showing ischemia had less severe wall motion abnormalities, with an overall improvement in 81% of patients. One drawback of this study was that patients were reevaluated an average of 28 ± 26 days after angioplasty, at which time restenosis may have occurred in some patients.

Early reassessment of patients after angioplasty using exercise echocardiography may lead to the occurrence of bleeding complications at the puncture site. In situations in which immediate reassessment is desired, pharmacological stress testing may avoid these problems, as well as having the advantage that patients unable to perform a sufficient stress load due to peripheral artery disease or joint disease may be examined adequately. Akosah et al.[22] used dobutamine stress echocardiography to study 35 patients 24 hours before and 24 to 48 hours after angiographically successful coronary angioplasty. In the 31 patients with inducible wall motion abnormalities before angioplasty, 28 showed immediate significant improvement in regional wall motion. In a similar study performed by McNeill et al.[23] 28 patients were evaluated using dobutamine followed by atropine 1 day before and up to 3 days after elective coronary angioplasty. The frequency of dobutamine-induced new wall motion abnormalities decreased from 71% to 14% after angioplasty.

Dipyridamole echocardiography has been used to assess the functional benefit of angiographically successful angioplasty and the prognostic value of post-angioplasty echocardiography in a larger patient group.[24] Of 63 patients with successful angioplasty, 58 demonstrated a positive dipyridamole echocardiogram before angioplasty as compared to only 16 patients 1 to 3 days after the procedure. This latter group of patients was at high risk for recurrence of symptoms. Patients having a positive dipyridamole echocardiogram after angioplasty developed recurrent angina in a significant number of cases (11 of 16; 69%) after a follow-up time of 11 ± 6 months compared to those having a negative dipyridamole echocardiogram after angioplasty (8 of 47; 17%, $p < 0.01$).

It may be concluded that stress echocardiography enables the assessment of procedural efficacy. Clinical success may be assessed by objective demonstration of less myocardial ischemia, this being independent of subjective definitions based on symptom classes.

Stress Doppler Echocardiography after Angioplasty

Stress echocardiography normally assesses only systolic wall motion abnormalities. However, it is believed from the "ischemic cascade" that systolic wall motion abnormalities as a result of myocardial ischemia occur later than diastolic function abnormalities. Doppler echocardiography has been used in different disease entities for the assessment of diastolic function and has also proven to be a sensitive means for the detection of myocardial ischemia and stress-induced myocardial ischemia.

To evaluate the effect of angioplasty on diastolic function El Said et al.[25] studied Doppler parameters at rest and under dobutamine stress before and after angioplasty. Left ventricular filling parameters at rest were found to be comparable before and after angioplasty. However, during dobutamine stress a decreased peak early filling velocity identified patients with significant coronary artery disease. Successful angioplasty resulted in normalization of Doppler flows in response to dobutamine stress. Thus, in selected patients, Doppler indices during dobutamine stress were useful in identifying improvements in diastolic function postangioplasty.

Detection of Restenosis after Angioplasty

Pathophysiology

Restenosis after initially successful angioplasty remains one of the most important unresolved problems associated with this procedure. Traditionally, restenosis has been reported as a late phenomenon, occurring in between 20% and 40% of patients.[26] However, studies using quantitative angiography have shown that a reduction in luminal diameter occurs to some degree in practically all lesions treated by angioplasty. Rather then being a dichotomy of late success and failure, restenosis constitutes a spectrum,[27] characterized by a "Gaussian," bell-shaped, unimodal distribution with angiographic outcome being a continuous variable. This should be kept in mind while evaluating the diagnostic accuracy of noninvasive tests for restenosis after angioplasty. However, further factors such as collateralization and the length of stenoses may further modulate the influence of morphology on functional evidence of ischemia.

The increasing application of angioplasty and the higher rate of multivessel angioplasty with higher rates of restenosis have established the need for an accurate diagnostic tool for evaluating restenosis. Thus, any noninvasive approach that reliably identifies patients with hemodynamically significant restenosis has important clinical value. Exercise-induced chest pain is a very insensitive marker for restenosis. Some 12% to 20% of asymptomatic patients will have significant restenosis 6 months after angioplasty and the incidence of angina pectoris has been only 34% to 40% in patients with restenosis.[28] Exercise ECG is also quite insensitive in the detection of restenosis—probably reflecting the prevalence of relatively moderate single vessel stenoses—with studies reporting a sensitivity of exercise ECG in the range of 24% to 64%.[28-30] Rensing et al.[31] reported a sensitivity and specificity of 41% and 74% for bicycle ergometry after single-vessel angioplasty. In contrast, perfusion scintigraphy permits demonstration of ischemia in patients with restenosis with high diagnostic accuracy, allowing also the localization of ischemia.[30] Hecht et al.[30] reported a sensitivity and specificity of 93% and 77%, respectively, using thallium-201 scintigraphy.

Detection of Restenosis Using Exercise Echocardiography

Several reports have confirmed the utility of stress echocardiography for detection of restenosis after nonsurgical coronary interventions, including reports by Aboul-Enein et al.,[32] Hecht et al.[33] and Mertes et al.[34] Exercise echocardiography, pharmacological stress testing, and atrial pacing have all been used as stress modalities for this purpose (Table 18-3). The main advantage of stress echocardiography compared with exercise ECG is its greater diagnostic accuracy, which is comparable to that of perfusion scintigraphy. However, this technique is much cheaper, the examination is easily repeatable, and the necessary equipment is more widely available.

In a study of 101 patients examined at routine follow-up 6 months after coronary angioplasty, Aboul-Enein et al.[32] reported the sensitivity and specificity of exercise echocardiography for the detection of significant coronary obstruction to be 67% and 83%, respectively. This contrasted with respective values of 34% and 85% using the exercise ECG. Hecht et al.[33] evaluated 80 patients 6.1 ± 2.9 months after angioplasty, using supine bicycle echocardiography, and reported a somewhat higher sensitivity and specificity (87% and 95%, respectively). For specific coronary arteries sensitivity, specificity, and accuracy were 91%, 93%, and 92% for left anterior descending coronary artery (LAD), 77%, 94%, and 85% for the right coronary artery (RCA), and 76%, 96%, and 88% for the left circumflex coronary artery (LCx). However, the latter study was attended by a considerable referral bias, with studies being performed in 81% of patients for the evaluation of recurrent chest pain (with a high suspicion of having coronary restenosis), or because of unusually complex angioplasty or positive exercise ECG studies in the remaining patients. In the study by Mertes et al.[34] 86 patients underwent exercise echocardiography for the purpose of routine follow-up 6.5 ± 1.3

Table 18-3. Diagnostic Accuracy of Stress Echocardiography for Detection of Restenosis

Author (Year) (Patient No.)	Sensitivity	Specifity	Stress
Aboul-Enein et al. (1991)[32] (n = 101)	67%	83%	Exercise
Hecht et al. (1993)[33] (N = 80)	87%	95%	Exercise
Mertes et al. (1993)[34] (N = 86)	83%	85%	Exercise
Takeuchi et al. (1994)[35] (N = 45)	77%	84%	Dobutamine
Pirelli et al. (1993)[36] (N = 50)	75%	90%	Dipyridamole
Hoffmann et al. (1994)[37] (N = 60)	84%	85%	Pacing

months after a revascularization procedure. A sensitivity of 83% and a specificity of 85% were reported. In 50 patients with prior myocardial infarction, the sensitivity for the detection of a significant coronary artery disease was slightly higher (88%) than in those without prior myocardial infarction (75%).

Detection of Restenosis Using Nonexercise Techniques

Takeuchi et al.[35] and Pirelli et al.[36] reported on the use of pharmacological stress testing for the detection of restenosis. Takeuchi et al.[34] evaluated dobutamine echocardiography in a study on 45 patients referred for the evaluation of possible restenosis. They reported a sensitivity of 77% and a specificity of 84% for the detection of restenosis, these results being comparable to those of perfusion scintigraphy performed at the same time in this study. A somewhat different study was performed by Pirelli et al.[36] comparing dipyridamole echocardiography with exercise thallium scintigraphy for detection of restenosis. They studied 50 asymptomatic patients 3 months after successful coronary angioplasty, among whom restenosis occurred in 12 patients. Dipyridamole echocardiography had a sensitivity of 75% and a specificity of 90% for the detection of restenosis, again similar to the results of exercise thallium scintigraphy. Moreover, dipyridamole echocardiography and perfusion scintigraphy were highly concordant concerning the localization of an abnormal segment. The authors concluded that it appears reasonable for routine clinical practice to defer repeat angiography after angioplasty, unless the patient develops evidence of recurrent spontaneous or stress-induced ischemia. These findings suggest that pharmacological stress testing may be an adequate alternative to exercise stress tests, especially in patients with proven coronary artery disease and other medical problems that limit exercise capacity.

The combination of transesophageal echocardiography with pacing stress has been used by Hoffmann et al.[37] for the noninvasive diagnosis of restenosis. This technique had been established in prior studies[38] to result in a high image quality in nearly all patients and to be independent of the patients ability to perform a sufficient work load. However, as discussed in Chapter 13, its disadvantages include the invasiveness and discomfort of the technique, the less physiologic nature of the stress, and the restricted number of echo views, if a monoplane (or even biplane) transesophageal echocardiographic probe is used. The protocol used in the study by Hoffmann et al.[37] required a transesophageal short-axis view of the left ventricle at the level of the papillary muscle (Fig. 18-1). Square wave pulses obtained from a transesophageal cardiac stimulator were delivered to the left atrium; after baseline recording,

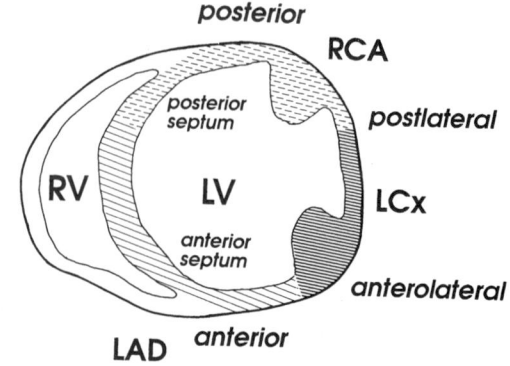

Fig. 18-1. Schematic diagram illustrating the relation of the two-dimensional transgastric echocardiographic short-axis view and coronary artery perfusion areas.

atrial pacing was started at 80 pulses/min and increased stepwise every 2 minutes by 20 pulses/min up to 85% of the age-predicted maximum heart rate. The development of stress-induced wall motion abnormalities using this technique Figs. 18-2 and 18-3; plate 18-1 was shown to have a sensitivity of 84% and a specificity of 85% for the detection of restenosis[37] among 60 patients presenting for routine follow-up angiography at an average of 5.4 months after angioplasty regardless of clinical status. These

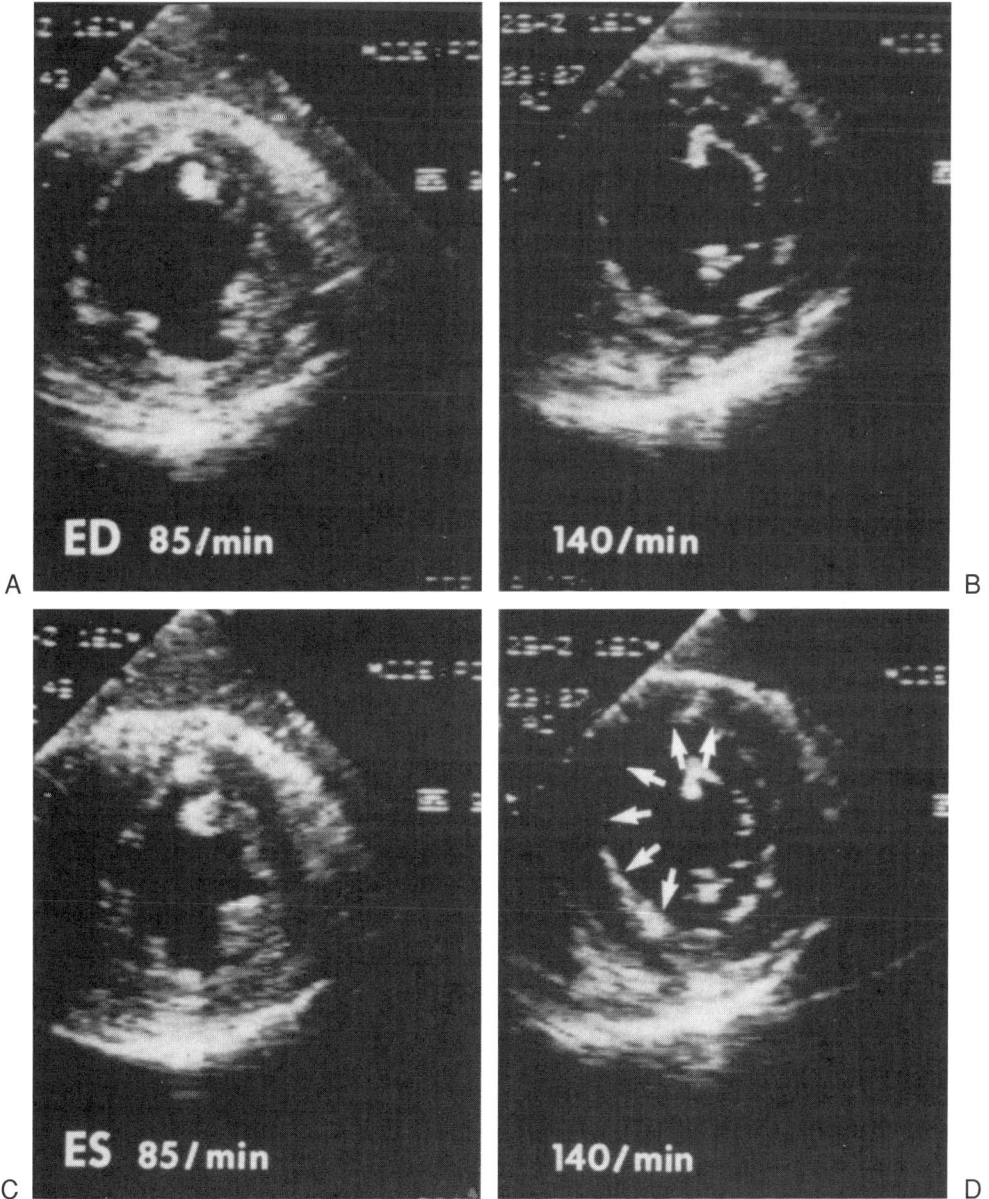

Fig. 18-2. Transesophageal pacing echocardiogram in the short axis view at midpapillary level of a patient with a predominant left anterior descending coronary artery stenosis. (**A&B**) End diastolic (ED) images; (**C&D**) end systolic images. (**A&C**) No wall motion abnormality is seen at baseline. (**B&D**) During rapid atrial pacing marked wall motion abnormalities occur in the septum indicated by arrows.

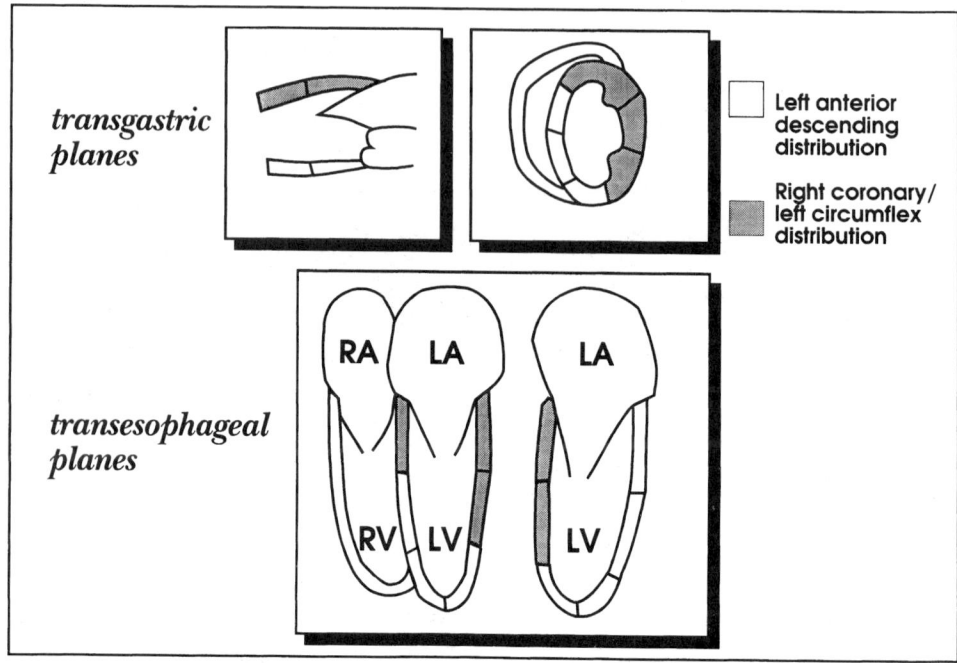

Fig. 18-3. Schematic representations of transgastric short-axis and long-axis as well as transesophageal four- and two-chamber views of the left ventricle.

results were comparable to those of perfusion scintigraphy performed at the same time, which demonstrated a sensitivity and specificity of 86% and 84%, respectively.

Sequential Stress Testing

Paired stress tests have been proposed for studies on angioplasty outcome to increase the interpretability of stress tests.[39] This enables the comparison of resting and postexercise images at different points in time. The aim is to document an ischemic response before angioplasty, to identify improvement after successful dilatation in a second study, and then document late functional state (persistent improvement or deterioration to baseline) in a third study. Thus, "worsening" of test results from early to late after angioplasty would be counted as a positive sign of restenosis.

Hoffmann et al.[40] investigated the incidence of inducible wall motion abnormalities before and early (2 weeks) after angioplasty as well as 4 months later, to evaluate the prognostic value of exercise echocardiography performed 2 weeks after angioplasty concerning the development of restenosis and to determine whether serial exercise tests increase the accuracy for detection of angiographically relevant restenosis. Exercise echocardiography performed 2 weeks after angioplasty had an overall accuracy for prediction of restenosis of 70%, with a positive predictive value of 50%, and a negative predictive value of 79%. Deterioration of exercise echocardiograms from 2 weeks to 4 months after angioplasty had a very high specificity of 94% for the diagnosis of restenosis, however, sensitivity was only 36%. Hoffmann et al.[40] concluded that improvement in regional function after angioplasty can be demonstrated by exercise echocardiography; nevertheless, a significant proportion of patients continues to have a positive stress echocardiogram 2 weeks after successful angioplasty due to delayed recovery, restenosis, or discrepancy between angiographic and functional outcome. Stress echocardiography performed early after angioplasty has only a moderate predictive value for restenosis. Deterioration between stress echocardiograms performed soon after angioplasty and those performed later is highly specific for restenosis.

Stress Echocardiography Early after Coronary Bypass Surgery

The detection of residual myocardial ischemia after bypass surgery has particular implications regarding further therapy. While complete revascularization is known to improve prognosis, incomplete revascularization is indicative of an increased future event rate. As exercise testing for the detection of residual ischemia is not feasible in the immediate postoperative period, if stress testing is required at this time, pharmacologic stress is preferable. Both Biagini et al.[41] and Bongo et al.[42] used dipyridamole stress echocardiography to assess the coronary reserve early after coronary bypass surgery. Biagini et al.[41] examined 11 patients, of whom all were found to have a positive stress test prior to surgery. As early as 2 hours after surgery, only 2 patients still showed inducible wall motion abnormalities using the transesophageal approach. One of these patients developed a perioperative myocardial infarction, while the second patient developed low-level effort angina in the follow-up period. This study, therefore, reported early dipyridamole echocardiographic stress testing was found to be useful in the assessment of completeness of revascularization early after bypass surgery. Bongo et al.[42] confirmed these results, showing that dipyridamole echocardiography was positive in 14 of 18 patients prior to surgery compared with only 4 patients after surgery. Although dipyridamole time increased in those 4 patients with a persistent positive test result, all of them showed obstructed grafts or native vessels obstructed distal to bypass graft insertion on coronary angiography. Thus, dipyridamole echo testing again proved to be useful in the evaluation of bypass graft patency early after surgery with a sensitivity of 80% and a specificity of 100%.

These results compare favorably to those of exercise ECG and perfusion scintigraphy. Greenberg et al.[43] reported a lower diagnostic accuracy for exercise ECG (sensitivity 60%, specificity 86%) and a comparable accuracy for perfusion scintigraphy (sensitivity 77%, specificity 100%) in patients after bypass surgery. The major limitation of dipyridamole stress echocardiography for this situation was reported to be abnormal ventricular septal motion early after surgery, which was observed in 61% of patients and restricted the ability to assess the ventricular septal motion and thus the patency of the LAD artery grafts.

Use of Stress Echocardiography to Assess Late Bypass Patency

Although coronary artery bypass grafting is an effective treatment in patients with coronary artery disease, progression of the underlying disease in native vessels as well as the obstruction or occlusion of bypass grafts are frequent events. Occlusion rates of venous bypass grafts at 10 years have been reported to approach 50%, while even patent grafts had significant disease in about 75%.[44] Thus, an accurate noninvasive method for the detection of recurrent ischemia in patients after coronary bypass surgery would be desirable.

The accuracy of chest pain and the exercise ECG in patients after coronary bypass surgery is often compromised by previous myocardial infarction, medication, or insufficient physical stress capability.[45] Reported sensitivities and specificities of exercise ECG for the detection of recurrent ischemia (graft disease or new native vessel disease) are in the range of 35% to 60% and 67% to 100%, respectively.[43,46,47]

The accuracy of stress echocardiography for the assessment of coronary artery bypass patency is summarized in Table 18-4. Sawada et al.[46] as well as Crouse et al.[47] investigated patients at a mean of 6.3 and 7 years, respectively, after coronary artery bypass grafting, using exercise echocardiography. Sawada et al.[46] examined 42 patients, among whom the detection of a stress-induced wall motion abnormality (Fig. 18-4) had a sensitivity of 94% for the identification of ischemia; the specificity was 83%. In addition to accurately detecting the presence of ischemia, the technique was also found to be reliable for its localization. Crouse et al.[47] examined 125 patients. Exercise echocardiography was again found to have a high sensitivity (98%) and specificity (92%) for the detection of compromised or uncompromised vascular supply, significantly higher than for stress ECGs. Thus, diagnostic accuracy is definitely higher than for exercise ECG and comparable to perfusion scintigraphy, for which a sensitivity of 77% to 80% and a specificity of 88% to 100% has been reported.[43,48] In some patients, however, excessive

Table 18-4. Diagnostic Accuracy of Stress Echocardiography for Assessment of Bypass Graft Patency

Author (Year) (Patient No.)	Sensitivity	Specificity	Stress	Echo Mode
Sawada et al. (1989)[40] (N=42)	94%	83%	exercise	TTE
Crouse et al. (1992)[47] (N = 125)	98%	92%	exercise	TTE
Hoffman et al. (1996)[50] (N=60)	93%	93%	dobutamine	TEE
	78%	86%	dobutamine	TTE

Abbreviations: Echo, echocardiographic; TTE, transthoracic echocardiogram; TEE, tranesophageal echocardiogram.

cardiac motion, displacement of the heart, and impaired echocardiographic penetration of the chest may pose problems in acquisition and interpretation of images after coronary artery bypass grafting.[49]

For this reason Hoffmann et al.[50] performed transthoracic as well as biplane transesophageal dobutamine stress echocardiography—with its proven high image quality—in 60 patients after coronary artery bypass grafting. The transthoracic dobutamine stress test reached a diagnostic accuracy of 80% with a sensitivity of 78% and a specificity of 86%. However, in patients with low image quality, not ena-

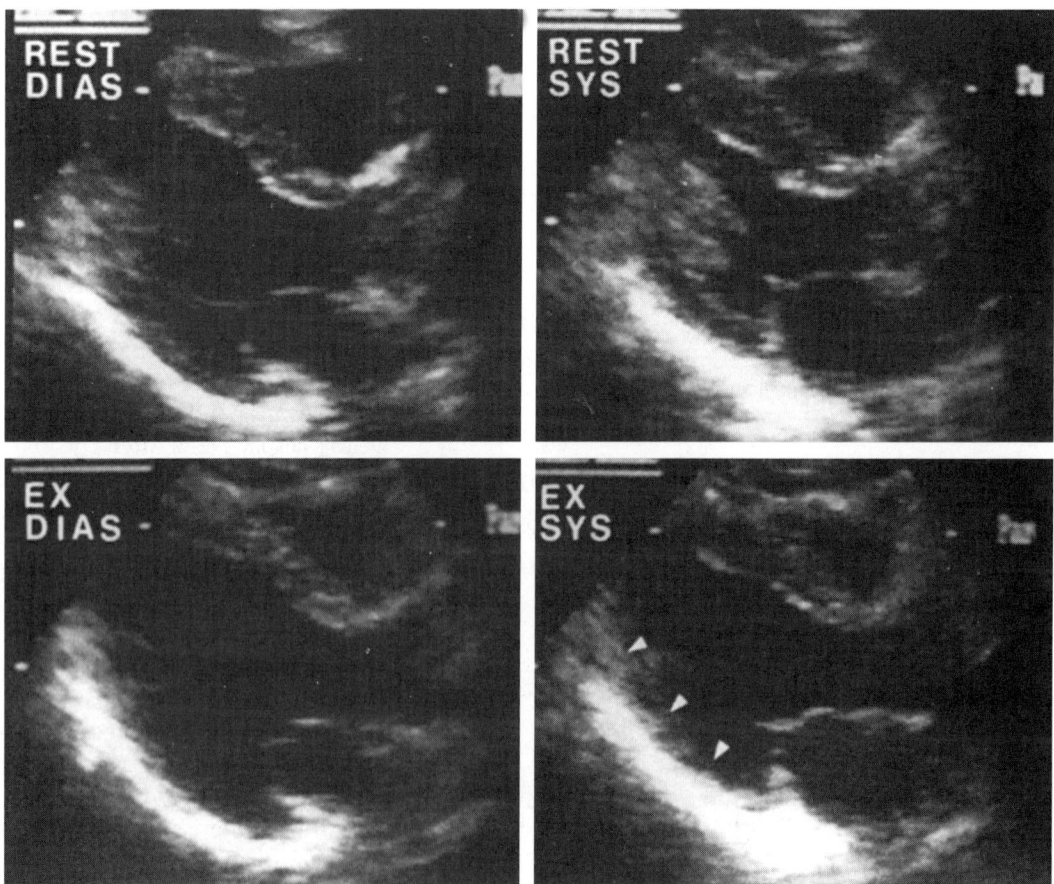

Fig. 18-4. Long-axis echocardiograms demonstrating left ventricular dilation and posterior wall akinesis (arrowheads) with exercise in a woman after coronary artery bypass grafting who had incomplete revascularization of all three major coronary arteries. (From Sawada et al.,[46] with permission.)

bling the visualization of a complete coronary territory, transesophageal dobutamine stress echocardiography reached a higher diagnostic accuracy. Most patients detected additionally by biplane transesophageal echocardiography as having vascular insufficiency had poor transthoracic image quality. Overall, biplane transesophageal dobutamine stress echocardiography had a sensitivity of 93%, a specificity of 93% and an accuracy of 93%. The overall higher diagnostic accuracy of biplane transesophageal echocardiography may be explained by the greater image quality in a larger number of patients. The authors concluded that in patients with impaired transthoracic echocardiographic windows, it may be reasonable to use biplane transesophageal dobutamine stress echocardiography, although this is limited by the disadvantages of being semi-invasive and thus more unpleasant to the patient.

CONCLUSIONS

Limitations of Stress Echocardiography after Intervention

Although both transthoracic and transesophageal echocardiography have proven useful in several studies for the detection and localization of inducible ischemia after coronary intervention, these techniques have their limitations. To date, most studies of stress echocardiography in relation to interventions have involved only small patient numbers, and should be validated in larger studies. These studies have shown variations in the pretest likelihood of disease, which should reflect clinical practice.

The utility of stress echocardiography for studying patients in relation to coronary angioplasty is colored by the extent of disease and the presence of prior infarction. Many patients treated with coronary angioplasty have only single-vessel disease, and the sensitivity of stress echocardiography for mild disease may be suboptimal. Furthermore, patients undergoing interventions have often had prior myocardial infarction, and the detection of additional ischemic regions may be difficult in patients with extensive resting wall motion abnormalities.[51]

After cardiac surgery, septal motion abnormalities may complicate the identification of left anterior descending artery disease. These may subside after weeks to months. In the interim, wall thickening rather than inward endocardial motion should be used to assess systolic function in these cases. Image quality may be impaired after surgery, and finding a good acoustic window may be difficult. Although Crouse et al.[47] and Sawada et al.[46] did not report problems using the transthoracic approach in this subset of patients, Hoffmann et al.[50] showed the benefit of the transesophageal approach in situations of poor image quality. However, this technique is semi-invasive and may be unpleasant for the patient.

Potential Future Directions

Interventional procedures using coronary angioplasty and bypass surgery are both effective in the reduction of morbidity and mortality in patients with coronary artery disease. However, both techniques involve high personal and financial burdens, and as medicine becomes more cost conscious, the need for an interventional procedure will have to be proven by demonstration that stenoses are functionally significant. Stress echocardiography has proven to be accurate for the diagnosis of functionally significant coronary artery disease, restenosis, and bypass patency. Several studies have demonstrated the equivalence of this technique to perfusion scintigraphy for diagnostic purposes, at a lower cost. Stress echocardiography may become the technique of choice for both documenting the need for intervention, as well as for follow-up.

REFERENCES

1. Wong JB, Sonnenberg FA, Salem DN, Pauker SG: Myocardial revascularization for chronic stable angina: analysis of the role of percutaneous transluminal coronary angioplasty based on data available in 1989. Ann Intern Med 113:852, 1990
2. Ryan TJ, Bauman WB, Kennedy JW et al.: Guidelines of percutaneous tranluminal coronary angioplasty. A report of the American College of Cardiology/ American Heart Association. J Am Coll Cardiol 22:2033, 1993
3. Kirklin JW, Akins CW, Blackstone EH et al.: Guidelines and indications for coronary artery bypass graft surgery. J Am Coll Cardiol 17:543, 1991
4. O'Keefe JH, Rutherford BD, McConahay DR et al.: Multivessel coronary angioplasty from 1980 to 1989: Procedural results and long-term outcome. J Am Coll Cardiol 16:1097, 1990

5. Vandormael MG, Chaitman BR, Ischinger T et al.: Immediate and short term benefit of multivessel coronary angioplasty: influence of degree of revascularization. J Am Coll Cardiol 6:983, 1985
6. Rahimtoola SH: A perspective on the three large multicenter randomized clinical trials of coronary bypass surgery for chronic stable angina. Circulation, suppl. Five, 72: V-123, 1985
7. Yoshida K, Gould KL: Quantitative relation of myocardial infarct size and myocardial viability by positron emission tomography to left ventricular ejection fraction and 3-year mortality with and without revascularization. J Am Coll Cardiol 22:984, 1993
8. Previtali M, Poli A, Lanzarini L et al.: Dobutamine stress echocardiography for assessment of myocardial viability and ischemia in acute myocardial infarction treated with thrombolysis. Am J Cardiol 72:124G, 1993
9. Pierard LA, De Lansheere CM, Berthe C et al.: Identification of viable myocardium by echocardiography during dobutamine infusion in patients with myocardial infarction after thrombolytic therapy: comparison with positron emission tomography. J Am Coll Cardiol 15:1021, 1990
10. Smart SC, Sawada S, Ryan T et al.: Low-dose dobutamine echocardiography detects reversible dysfunction after thrombolytic therapy of acute myocardial infarction. Circulation 88:405, 1993
11. Salustri A, Elhendy A, Garyfallydis P et al.: Prediction of improvement of ventricular function after first acute myocardial infarction using low-dose dobutamine stress echocardiography. Am J Cardiol 74:853, 1994
12. Barilla F, Gheorghiade M, Alam M et al.: Low-dose dobutamine in patients with acute myocardial infarction identifies viable but not contractile myocardium and predicts the magnitude of improvement in wall motion abnormalities in response to coronary revascularization. Am Heart J 122:1522, 1991
13. Picano E, Marzullo P, Gigli G et al.: Identification of viable myocardium by dipyridamole-induced improvement in regional left ventricular function assessed by echocardiography in myocardial infarction and comparison with thallium scintigraphy at rest. Am J Cardiol 70:703, 1992
14. Gould KL: Myocardial viability. What does it mean and how do we measure it? Circulation 83:333, 1991
15. La Canna G, Alfieri O, Giubbini R et al.: Echocardiography during infusion of dobutamine for identification of reversible dysfunction in patients with chronic coronary artery disease. J Am Coll Cardiol 23:617, 1994
16. Cigarroa CG, deFilippi CR, Brickner E et al.: Dobutamine stress echocardiography identifies hibernating myocardium and predicts recovery of left ventricular function after coronary revascularization. Circulation 88:430, 1993
17. Baumgart D, Buck T, Leischik R et al.: Enoximone echocardiography. Herz 19:227, 1994
18. King III SB: Percutaneous transluminal coronary angioplasty: The second decade. Am J Cardiol 62:2K, 1988
19. Manyari DE, Knudtson M, Kloiber R, Roth D: Sequential thallium 201 myocardial perfusion studies after successful percutaneous transluminal coronary angioplasty: delayed resolution of exercise induced scintigraphic abnormalities. Circulation 77:86, 1988
20. Labovitz AJ, Lewen M, Kern MJ et al.: The effect of successful PTCA on left ventricular function: assessment by exercise echocardiography. Am Heart J 117: 1003, 1989
21. Broderick T, Sawada S, Armstrong WF et al.: Improvement in rest and exercise-induced wall motion abnormalities after coronary angioplasty: an exercise echocardiographic study. J Am Coll Cardiol 15:591, 1990
22. Akosah KO, Porter TR, Simon R et al.: Ischemia-induced regional wall motion abnormality is improved after coronary angioplasty: demonstration by dobutamine stress echocardiography. J Am Coll Cardiol 21: 584, 1993
23. McNeill AJ, Fioretti PM, El-Said ELM et al.: Dobutamine stress echocardiography before and after coronary angioplasty. Am J Cardiol 69:740, 1992
24. Picano E, Pirelli S, Marzilli M et al.: Usefulness of high-dose dipyridamole echocardiography test in coronary angioplasty. Circulation 80:807, 1989
25. El-Said ESM, Fioretti PM, Roelandt RTC et al.: Dobutamine stress-Doppler echocardiography before and after coronary angioplasty. Eur Heart J 14:1011, 1993
26. Serruys PW, Luijten HE, Beatt KJ et al.: Incidence of restenosis after successful coronary angioplasty: a time-related phenomenon. Circulation 77:361, 1988
27. Rensing BJ, Hermans WRM, Deckers JW et al.: Lumen narrowing after percutaneous transluminal coronary balloon angioplasty follows a near Gaussian distribution: a quantitative angiographic study in 1445 successfully dilated lesions. J Am Coll Cardiol 19:939, 1992
28. Honan MB, Bengston JR, Pryor DB et al.: Exercise treadmill testing is a poor predictor of anatomic restenosis after angioplasty for acute myocardial infarction. Circulation 80:1585, 1989
29. Bengston JR, Mark DB, Honan MB et al.: Detection of restenosis after elective percutaneous transluminal coronary angioplasty using the exercise treadmill test. Am J Cardiol 65:28, 1990
30. Hecht HS, Shaw RE, Bruce TR et al.: Usefulness of

tomographic thallium-201 imaging for detection of restenosis after percutaneous transluminal coronary angioplasty. Am J Cardiol 66:1314, 1990
31. Rensing BJ, Hermans EWRM, Deckers JW et al.: Which angiographic variable best describes functional status 6 months after successful single-vessel coronary balloon angioplasty? J Am Coll Cardiol 21:317, 1993
32. Aboul-Enein H, Bengtson JR, Adams DB et al.: Effect of the degree of effort on exercise echocardiography for the detection of restenosis after coronary artery angioplasty. Am Heart J 122:430, 1991
33. Hecht HS, DeBord L, Shaw R et al.: Usefulness of supine bicycle stress echocardiography for detection of restenosis after percutaneous transluminal coronary angioplasty. Am J Cardiol 71:293, 1993
34. Mertes H, Erbel R, Nixdorff U et al.: Exercise echocardiography for the evaluation of patients after nonsurgical coronary artery revascularization. J Am Coll Cardiol 21:1087, 1993
35. Takeuchi M, Nandate H, Miura Y et al.: The usefulness of dobutamine stress echocardiography for detecting restenosis after PTCA. J Am Coll Cardiol, suppl. 23: 142, 1994
36. Pirelli S, Danzi GB, Massa D et al.: Exercise thallium scintigraphy versus high-dose dipyridamole echocardiography testing for detection of asymptomatic restenosis in patients with positive exercise tests after coronary angioplasty. Am J Cardiol 71:1052, 1993
37. Hoffmann R, Kleinhans E, Lambertz H et al.: Transesophageal pacing echocardiography for detection of restenosis after percutaneous transluminal coronary angioplasty. Eur Heart J 15:823, 1994
38. Lambertz H, Kreis A, Trümper H, Hanrath P: Simultaneous transesophageal atrial pacing and transesophageal two-dimensional echocardiography: a new method of stress echocardiography. J Am Coll Cardiol 16:1143, 1990
39. Popma JJ, Califf RM, Topol EJ: Clinical trails of restenosis after coronary angioplasty. Circulation 84:1426, 1991
40. Hoffmann R, Lethen H. Flachskampf FA, Hanrath P: Exercise echocardiography performed early and late after percutaneous transluminal coronary angioplasty for prediction of restenosis. Eur Heart J 16:1872, 1995
41. Biagini A, Maffei S, Baroni M et al.: Early assessment of coronary reserve after bypass surgery by dipyridamole transesophageal echocardiographic stress test. Am Heart J 120:1097, 1990
42. Bongo AS, Bolognese L, Sarasso G et al.: Early assessment of coronary artery bypass graft patency by high-dose dipyridamole echocardiography. Am J Cardiol 67:133, 1991
43. Greenberg BH, Hart R, Botvinick EH et al.: Thallium-201 myocardial perfusion scintigraphy to evaluate patients after coronary bypass surgery. Am J Cardiol 42:167, 1978
44. Fitzgibbon GM, Leach AJ, Kafka HP, Keon WJ: Coronary bypass graft fate: long-term angiographic study. J Am Coll Cardiol 17:1075, 1991
45. Gohlke H, Gohlke-Bärwolf C, Samek L et al.: Serial exercise testing up to 6 years after coronary bypass surgery: behavior of exercise parameters in groups with different degrees of revascularization determined by postoperative angiography. Am J Cardiol 51:1301, 1983
46. Sawada SG, Judson WE, Ryan T et al.: Upright bicycle exercise echocardiography after coronary artery bypass grafting. Am J Cardiol 64:1123, 1989
47. Crouse LJ, Vacek JL, Beauchamp GD et al.: Exercise echocardiography after coronary artery bypass grafting. Am J Cardiol 70:572, 1992
48. Pfisterer M, Emmenegger H, Schmitt HE et al.: Accuracy of serial myocardial perfusion scintigraphy with thallium-201 for prediction of graft patency early and late after coronary artery bypass surgery. Circulation 66:1017, 1982
49. Mann DL, Gillam LD, Weyman AE: Cross-sectional echocardiographic assessment of regional left ventricular performance and myocardial perfusion. Prog Cardiovasc Dis 29:1, 1986
50. Hoffmann R, Lethen H, Falter F et al.: Dobutamine stress echocardiography after coronary artery bypass grafting: transthoracic versus biplane transesophageal imaging. Eur Heart J 17:222, 1996.
51. Forster T, McNeill AJ, Salustri A et al.: Simultaneous dobutamine stress echocardiography and technetium-99m isonitrile single-photon emission computed tomography in patients with suspected coronary artery disease. J Am Coll Cardiol 21:1591, 1993

Perfusion Markers after Coronary Interventions

Oberdan Parodi and Gianmario Sambuceti

PATHOPHYSIOLOGY AND RELATED CLINICAL PROBLEMS AFTER REVASCULARIZATION

Coronary revascularization relieves the hydraulic effects of the focal obstructions in epicardial coronary arteries. The rationale for this procedure reflects the recognition of coronary stenosis as one of the major determinants of the clinical presentation of anginal patients.[1] Since a close relationship exists between the degree of epicardial obstruction and its impact on flow regulation in experimental animals,[2] it has been assumed that in patients with coronary artery disease (CAD), more severe stenoses are associated with larger reductions in maximal flow capacity, leading to more frequent occurrence of ischemic episodes. Indeed, a large literature has confirmed this assumption in numerous groups of patients.[1] Nevertheless, previous chapters have discussed the influence of factors other than the focal obstruction of an epicardial artery on the regulation of coronary blood flow, and their effect on the results of diagnostic testing in the evaluation of patients submitted to revascularization procedures.

We will briefly reconsider blood flow regulation in CAD, with particular attention to the role of coronary microcirculation. This subject is of particular relevance in the evaluation of revascularized patients.

Coronary Microcirculation

The degree and distribution of coronary resistance are modulated by a number of mechanisms able to provide a fine regulation of flow and pressure. The need for flow regulation is obvious considering the variability of metabolic demand; however, the need for regulation of capillary pressure (which is related to the number of open capillaries) is at least as important, since this influences the exchange of water and solutes between plasma and tissue and abrupt increases in endoluminal pressure might irreversibly damage the capillary wall. A number of mechanisms such as adenosine receptors,[3] myogenic response,[4] and endothelial control[5] operate together in an integrated fashion to maintain an adequate oxygen supply without deleterious gross changes in capillary pressure. Among these mechanisms, the endothelium plays a crucial role in modulating the conductance of large vessels in response to phenomena such as adenosine vasodilation, which involve the more distal microvascular compartment.[6]

It has recently been demonstrated that atherosclerosis can affect the microvascular endothelium, causing an increased microvascular sensitivity to vasoconstrictor stimuli[7] and a reduced sensitivity to the action of several endothelium-mediated vasodilators such as acetylcholine or bradykinin.[8] Theoretically, this alteration might also lead to a reduced response even to direct vasodilators such as adenosine. In fact, in the absence of the endothelial feedback on the upstream vasculature, the increase in flow should be associated with a marked reduction in pressure at the inlet of the capillary bed, leading, in turn, to a reduced overall flow response.[9]

In agreement with this concept, positron emission tomographic measurements of myocardial blood flow using either $H_2^{15}O$[10] or $^{13}NH_3$[11] showed that in patients with CAD, myocardial regions subtended by stenotic vessels had largest flow impairment; however, abnormal flow and coronary reserve values were also observed in contralateral regions supplied by normal vessels in a significant number of patients with single-vessel disease. Moreover, a recent study[12] in a similar patient population demonstrated that, besides the reduction in coronary reserve, the myocardial regions supplied by angiographically normal coronary arteries also showed a reduced perfusion response to atrial pacing tachycardia (Fig. 19-1), in contrast to the increment of flow in proportion to rate pressure product in normal subjects. If this finding is considered together with the reduced flow of these "control" areas, it may be concluded that this microvascular dysfunction might be associated with a myocardial metabolic alteration leading to a lower oxygen consumption for similar cardiac work.

Interventions used in the treatment of coronary artery disease palliate the hydrodynamic effects of epicardial stenoses. However, these microvascular changes, which are caused by the atherosclerotic "mileau," might be expected to persist, and may influence the results of functional testing.

Relation between Stenosis and Coronary Reserve

Animal Models

In the animal models of *external constriction* of an epicardial coronary artery, a close relationship exists between the degree of lumen obstruction and the severity of blood flow impairment in the downstream arterial bed.[13] Stenoses of intermediate severity are not associated with reductions in baseline myocardial perfusion, mainly because of an adaptive autoregulatory vasodilation in the downstream microvasculature. In fact, the arterial obstruction causes a pressure drop in the distal bed, that, in turn, induces an autoregulatory vasodilation in the downstream microvasculature, leading to the restoration of a nor-

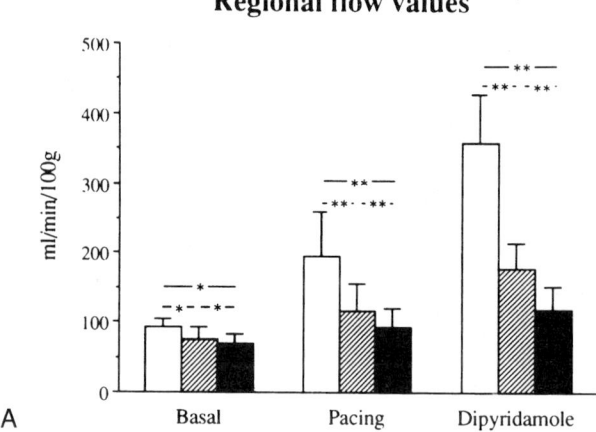

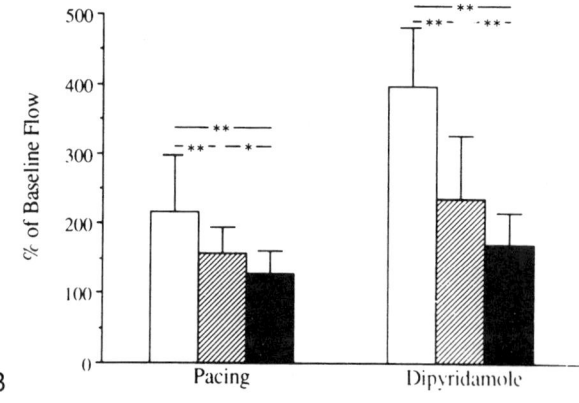

Fig. 19-1. (**A**) Average flow values at baseline (basal), during pacing tachycardia, and after dipyridamole in normal subjects (white columns), in regions supplied by nonstenotic (dashed columns) and stenotic (black columns) vessels of patients with single vessel coronary artery disease. (**B**) Percent increases in flow during pacing and after dipyridamole are shown. Both values observed in patients were lower than those observed in normal subjects.

mal overall baseline resistance. Nevertheless, the maximal flow capacity is reduced in this model; in fact, during maximal vasodilation (caused by a marked increase in metabolic demand, or by administration of potent vasodilator drugs), microvascular autoregulation is abolished, so the resistance offered by the stenosis cannot be counterbalanced, and hence reductions in flow can be observed.

In the presence of very severe stenoses, microvascular adaptation cannot counterbalance the resistance offered by the epicardial obstruction, despite maximal vasodilation; in this setting, a reduction in baseline flow can be observed.[14] While resting perfusion defects have been frequently considered as markers of maximal vasodilation, recent experimental[15] and clinical studies[12,16] have shown that residual vasomotor tone and vasodilator reserve can be observed even in myocardial regions with severe resting hypoperfusion. The mechanisms underlying this paradox have not been fully elucidated. Several authors have demonstrated an active downregulation of myocardial oxygen demand: during sustained moderate ischemia, anaerobic metabolism subsides[17] and energy stores of creatine phosphate[18] return to normal despite the persistence of a reduced contractility. These phenomena can be reversed by inotropic stimulation, with which induction of a moderate increase in function is associated with the reappearance of the metabolic markers of ischemia. Hence, various authors[19] have hypothesized that the myocardium can restore perfusion contraction matching, by actively reducing its own metabolic demand below the actual flow availability, thus restoring the balance between flow and demand. On the other hand, Chilian and Layne[20] demonstrated a paradoxic vasoconstriction of coronary microvessels exposed to marked reduction in perfusion pressure, and hypothesized that this mechanism might prevent an adequate adaptation to the effects of a severe stenosis. Whatever the mechanism, these findings suggest that despite the observed correlation between the degree of coronary reserve and the severity of epicardial stenosis in animals, this relationship may be more complex in humans.

Clinical Studies

In humans with CAD, stenosis is associated with disease of the endocardium rather than epicardial constriction. In fact, the documentation of microvascular abnormalities in hypercholesterolemic animals[7,8] and in nonstenotic vascular beds[10-12] of patients with CAD justifies the suspicion that this disorder might hamper the adaptation to the presence of the epicardial stenosis, thus influencing the pathogenesis of myocardial ischemia.[21]

Coronary reserve shows a particularly poor correlation with the angiographic severity of stenosis in patients with multivessel disease.[22] This finding has been ascribed to problems in defining the degree of coronary obstruction in patients with advanced CAD and diffuse atherosclerosis. In patients with single vessel CAD, the reduction in vasodilating capability (measured as the ratio of maximal to rest blood flow velocity) has been found to correlate better with the angiographic estimate of epicardial stenosis.[23] Nonetheless, even in patients with limited CAD, myocardial perfusion (measured by positron emission tomography) and stenosis severity have been found to correlate less than expected.[10-12] Among the number of reasons that might explain these differences, several studies have emphasized the importance of the microcirculatory adaptation to a severe epicardial stenosis, demonstrating the role of this compartment in the precipitation of myocardial ischemia in patients with angina on effort[21] or with unstable angina undergoing coronary angioplasty.[24] Similarly, in patients with angina on effort and isolated occlusion of one coronary branch, we observed a significant correlation between the degree of reduction in vasodilating capability of regions supplied by the nonstenotic arteries and that of collateral-dependent myocardium. This suggests that the global microvascular alteration might affect the vasodilating capability even in regions downstream from a severely stenotic (or occluded) vessel.[25]

Implications for Myocardial Perfusion Imaging

The impact of minor coronary disease on vasodilator capacity has important implications for conventional perfusion imaging. These methods do not provide quantitative measurements of blood flow, so that identification of coronary stenoses is based on the recognition of differences between myocardial regions supplied by nonstenotic vessels (supposed to be truly "control" regions) and those supplied by obstructed arteries (Fig. 19-2). The presence of a global microvascular dysfunction might obscure perfusion differences between jeopardized and "control" regions, thus masking a perfusion defect despite the presence of a significant coronary stenosis.[26] This phenomenon might explain an approximately 30% incidence of false-negative results

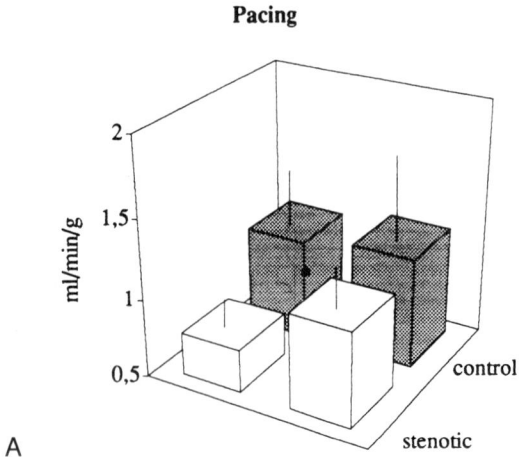

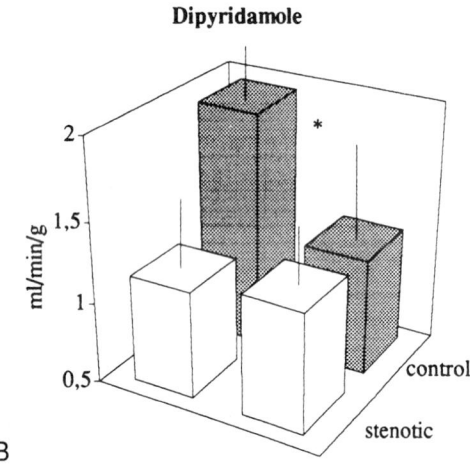

Fig. 19-2. Average flow values during pacing (**A**) and following dipyridamole (**B**) in stenotic regions (front, white columns) and in contralateral areas (back, dotted columns). During pacing, patients with perfusion defects (left columns) showed a larger reduction in flow to stenotic regions than patients with homogeneous perfusion (right columns). By contrast, after dipyridamole, patients with perfusion defects (left columns) showed similar flow values in stenotic regions but higher values in control areas (*$p < .005$) than patients with homogeneous distribution of blood flow (right columns).

in patients with native single-vessel disease evaluated with myocardial scintigraphy.[27]

A more complex relationship between epicardial coronary artery and blood flow regulation has been reported in patients submitted to revascularization. As noted above, relief of a stenosis by coronary angioplasty may not be associated with *normalization* of coronary reserve, even though an *improvement* in vasodilating capability can be observed in the majority of patients.[23] Interestingly, the residual vasodilating capability is unrelated to the severity of epicardial obstruction at the initial evaluation.[23] The mechanisms underlying this phenomenon have not been clearly identified; Uren and co-workers[28] hypothesized the presence of a global microvascular disturbance of unknown origin that might revert in a period of months. Other investigators[29] suggested the presence of vasoconstriction in the vascular bed distal to the site of dilation because of the abrupt increase in endoluminal pressure caused by the removal of obstruction. Whatever the mechanism, these data should indicate that the interpretation of a single measurement of coronary reserve might be an unreliable marker of the presence of restenosis or graft occlusion.

In the majority of perfusion studies, the results obtained in revascularized regions or vessels have been compared with findings in nonstenotic vessels. Gould and co-workers[30] suggested that this index ("relative flow reserve") has advantages over the measurement of the ratio between maximal and resting blood flow in a given myocardial region ("absolute flow reserve") by avoiding extrinsic influences such as arterial pressure and heart rate.[31] Unfortunately, relative flow reserve may instead be influenced by microvascular changes in the control segments. In fact, in comparison with a normal population,[32] coronary reserve, measured by digital subtraction angiography, was lower than normal in patients who underwent revascularization, despite significant improvement in symptoms and, mostly, despite the documentation of graft patency. Thus, although stress-induced ischemia identified in the early evaluation of asymptomatic patients following revascularization are considered an accurate marker of epicardial vessel disease (and hence restenosis or graft failure),[33] disturbances of flow reserve may limit sensitivity (because the control segment is abnormal) or specificity (because flow reserve changes are heterogeneous).

Revascularization of Dysfunctional Myocardium
Preoperative Evaluation

As discussed in other chapters on myocardial viability, the identification of reversible dysfunction should be required before considering revascularization in patients with depressed left ventricular function.[34,35] Unfortunately, myocardial perfusion is not a reliable marker of residual viability in patients with chronic left ventricular dysfunction, as baseline perfusion defects, downstream from a severely stenotic coronary artery, have been observed in a significant fraction of patients with CAD, in the absence of myocardial necrosis[36,37] despite the presence of residual vascular tone and vasodilator reserve even in those myocardial regions with concomitant reductions in resting blood flow and contractility.[12,16,25] Trying to understand whether this paradox is caused by an incomplete vascular response or by a primary metabolic downregulation, Testa and co-workers[38] evaluated regional perfusion and wall motion before and after coronary angioplasty (Fig. 19-3). Before revascularization, hypoperfused, dyssynergic segments still retained a significant vasodilator response to papaverine. Following coronary angioplasty, these territories showed an improved perfusion, despite ongoing impairment in wall motion, likely caused by superimposed myocardial stunning. If baseline hypoperfusion is caused only by a metabolic downregulation, flow should not increase after coronary angioplasty, especially in the presence of decreased contractility. Thus, the immediate beneficial effect of revascularization suggests the existence, below a severe stenosis, of an excessive coronary tone, which might hamper the adaptation to the hydraulic effects of the stenosis.[39]

These findings have generated some reservations about selecting patients for revascularization, based only on the evaluation of resting myocardial perfusion. Although very severe reductions in resting myocardial perfusion (i.e., below 0.25 ml/min/g) are often associated with the presence of necrotic tissue (and hence irreversible dysfunction) as suggested by Gewirtz and co-workers,[40] other studies[41,42] reported a large overlap in resting perfusion between dysfunctioning viable and necrotic segments. However, the identification of a residual coronary reserve might provide further information about residual viability. In patients with recent myocardial infarction, Marzullo and co-workers[42] observed that although viable segments (defined by [^{18}F]fluorodeoxyglucose uptake) had resting blood flow values similar to those observed in necrotic areas, only viable segments maintained a residual vasodilator reserve in response to dipyridamole.[42] At present, this goal can be achieved only by using methods able to provide quantitative measurements of regional perfusion; it is not feasible with conventional myocardial scintigraphy.

Postoperative Evaluation

Although the preoperative use of perfusion imaging may have limitations with respect to the prediction of viable myocardium, this technique may be of use postoperatively. Myocardial blood flow should improve immediately after revascularization; hence, perfusion scintigraphy might provide important insight in the evaluation of patients without functional recovery. Failure to normalize perfusion might indicate unsuccessful revascularization, while normaliza-

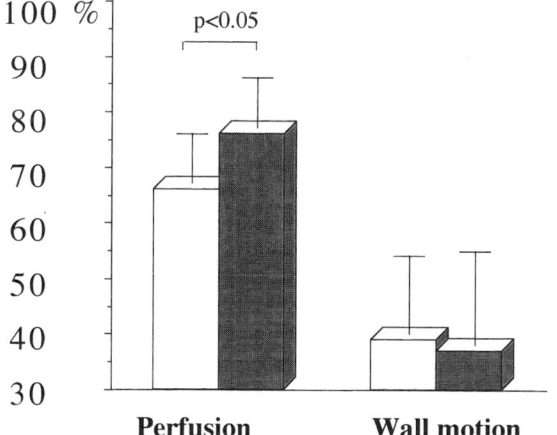

Fig. 19-3. Effect of coronary angioplasty (PTCA) on blood flow (left) and wall motion (right) of hypoperfused, dysfunctioning myocardial segments, in a selected population of patients with isolated severe stenosis of the left anterior descending coronary artery. Regional perfusion (expressed as percent of the maximum) was impaired before PTCA (white column) and significantly increased following revascularization (gray column). This behavior was not associated with an improvement of wall motion.

tion of blood flow distribution, despite persistence of wall motion abnormality, might be associated with later improvement in wall motion.[43] The practical value of this approach is unexplored, because of the limited number of patients undergoing follow-up studies on both flow distribution and regional function.

Timing of Postprocedural Evaluation of Myocardial Perfusion

Coronary reserve does not normalize immediately after revascularization in a significant proportion of patients, in whom persistent microvascular dysfunction has been observed up to several weeks following coronary angioplasty.[28,44] This phenomenon might lead to an abnormal perfusion scan, even in the absence of recurrent stenosis of the epicardial conductance vessels, particularly in the early months following revascularization. This phenomenon has little relationship to the occurrence of restenosis; in fact, in a significant fraction of patients, coronary reserve improves over time.[23] In patients submitted to successful coronary angioplasty and with no restenosis, Manyari et al.[44] demonstrated that an abnormal exercise thallium-201 scan can be observed in a significant number of patients (Fig. 19-4). The prevalence of these "false-positive" results decreases to a minimum of 30%, 6 months following the procedure. These studies suggest caution in interpreting results of perfusion scans observed early after these procedures, mainly in patients without angina who might show a high prevalence of false-positive results.

Nevertheless, an early evaluation may be needed, particularly in patients with impaired left ventricular function, in whom the actual benefit of the procedure must be carefully evaluated. The improvement of wall motion in this situation is heterogeneous, with reports of both immediate[45] and delayed recovery.[43] Since even in segments with a delayed recovery, myocardial perfusion shows early improvement,[38] persistent dysfunction in a region with normalized perfusion might suggest a potential for late recovery. In conclusion, the ideal time for patients to undergo imaging after coronary angioplasty is controversial, but 4 to 6 weeks after the procedure seems to be a good time to assess the functional results of angioplasty.

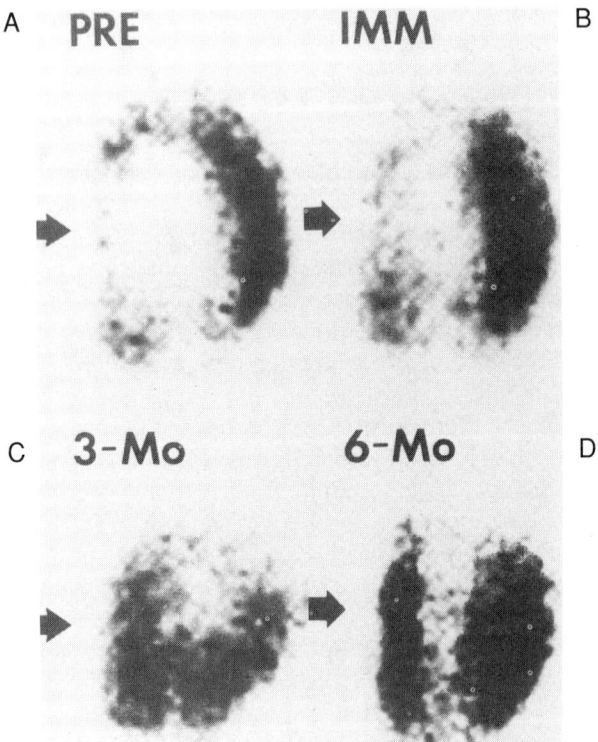

Fig. 19-4. (A–D) Sequential perfusion scans (40 degree left anterior oblique) in a patient with single-vessel disease treated with successful coronary angioplasty. Exercise myocardial perfusion did not normalize immediately after revascularization (IMM, **B**) despite the angiographic effectiveness of the procedure. A progressive normalization was observed up to 6 months [(3 Mo to 6 Mo): **C, D**] after restoration of vessel patency.

INDICATIONS FOR PERFUSION IMAGING IN PATIENTS AFTER MYOCARDIAL REVASCULARIZATION

Evaluation Early in the Postrevascularization Period

Patients with recent revascularization may warrant reevaluation for ischemia for a number of reasons, including diagnosis of perioperative ischemic complications, verification of benefit of the procedure on myocardial perfusion and function, and identification of residual ischemic tissue.

The recognition of adverse events is of great clinical relevance since it may determine the subsequent approach in patients who underwent bypass surgery. In this setting, the recognition of intraoperative myocardial damage may be difficult because of the limited accuracy of electrocardiogram or enzymes in the diagnosis of myocardial infarction. Similarly, the evaluation of regional wall motion is hampered by a number of artifacts (such as postsurgical septal asynergy). In these patients, the application of perfusion imaging with nuclear methods may be useful, particularly when a comparison with prerevascularization scans can be performed.

This issue is particularly relevant when patients with poor left ventricular function are submitted to aortocoronary bypass surgery. In these patients, a reliable evaluation of the benefit on left ventricular perfusion may predict subsequent functional outcome, as discussed in the previous section.[35] Failure of perfusion to recover might be ascribed to an incorrect preintervention characterization as well as to an incomplete revascularization procedure.

Patients with severe angina and multivessel disease may not be submitted to complete revascularization by aortocoronary bypass surgery, instead undergoing angioplasty to the "culprit lesion" identified by exercise perfusion scintigraphy. In this situation, a repeat stress perfusion study may be used to identify other areas of ischemia. This situation may occur in up to 44% of patients who underwent successful dilation of the "culprit lesion" in the presence of a multivessel disease (Plate 19-1).[46] In contrast, only 13% of patients with no evidence of ischemia on repeated testing required dilatation of a second vessel at 1 year follow-up.

In patients submitted to coronary angioplasty, the recurrence of atypical chest pain is relatively frequent, despite a successful procedure as evaluated by angiographic criteria. In these patients the characterization of myocardial perfusion with exercise thallium-201 scan has proved to be highly reliable. Although the persistence of a residual reversible perfusion defect does not identify the presence of restenosis, a normal perfusion scan at high heart rate or work-load during exercise should exclude the presence of a significant restenosis.

Evaluation at Follow-up

Symptomatic Patients

The evaluation of myocardial perfusion by means of scintigraphic methods may be particularly useful in patients who develop atypical angina[47] after successful coronary angioplasty. Symptoms may be referred either to extracardiac diseases or angina at rest, perhaps related to vasospasm.[48] In this situation, a normal perfusion scan at high workload effectively excludes the presence of significant restenosis.

In symptomatic patients after aortocoronary bypass surgery, identification of the site of ischemia (and thus the "culprit lesion") is particularly relevant. Although the occurrence of a positive exercise stress test at low work-load in such anginal patients indicates the need for coronary angiography, this technique does not provide accurate identification of the "culprit lesion," because of the presence of diffuse undetected atherosclerosis.[22] Considering the high risk of repeated surgical intervention, myocardial perfusion scintigraphy might be considered as a rational test to be performed in this subset of patients. This technique might localize the site of ischemia during exercise, thus providing complementary information to coronary angiography, which may be used in planning a catheter-based strategy for reintervention.

Myocardial perfusion scintigraphy is unquestionably of value for the investigation of symptomatic patients after revascularization. A more difficult issue is whether a systematic evaluation of patients submitted to revascularization should be performed or if only patients who develop typical or atypical angina after the procedure should be evaluated.

Identification of Restenosis or Graft Occlusion in Asymptomatic Patients

The cost-effectiveness of routinely performed myocardial perfusion scintigraphy in asymptomatic patients submitted to either coronary angioplasty or surgery has not been conclusively defined. Nonetheless, systematic study of asymptomatic patients submitted to coronary angioplasty is attractive because of the problems of incomplete revascularization and restenosis, which may occur in 40% of asymptomatic patients.[49]

Prediction of Restenosis

Although the accuracy of a reversible perfusion defect at thallium-201 scintigraphy performed early after revascularization has not been conclusively demonstrated,[23, 28,44, 50] several studies have indicated a favorable prognostic capability of thallium-

201 scintigraphy in the prediction of restenosis. Breisblatt et al.[51] evaluated the accuracy of myocardial perfusion scan in 104 asymptomatic patients at 4 to 6 weeks after angioplasty, 26 (25%) of whom had thallium-201 redistribution. Evidence of restenosis was present at 6 months in 22 (85%) and at 1 year in 25 (96%) of the latter group. Quantitative exercise thallium-201 scintigraphy was performed approximately 2 weeks after coronary angioplasty in 68 asymptomatic patients studied by Stuckey and coworkers.[52] At 10 months follow-up, 23 (34%) developed recurrent angina; multivariate analysis of a number of clinical, angiographic, and exercise test variables revealed that thallium-201 redistribution, any thallium-201 scan abnormality, the presence of distal stenosis, and treadmill time were the only significant predictors of recurrent angina. Only 9% of patients who remained asymptomatic throughout the follow-up period demonstrated thallium-201 redistribution at the initial study. However, despite the prognostic value of thallium imaging, only 9 of 23 patients with recurrent angina (39%) had thallium-201 redistribution at 2 weeks.

Wijns et al.[53] performed planar imaging 1 month following successful angioplasty in 89 patients, who then underwent angiographic follow-up at 6 months (earlier if symptoms recurred). The presence of an exercise-induced defect was predictive of the recurrence of angina in 66% of patients, and of restenosis in 74%. The predictive value of abnormal scan for restenosis was 74%, and the negative predictive value was 83%. By contrast, exercise electrocardiography was predictive of neither recurrent angina nor restenosis. In conclusion, while some studies indicate exercise thallium-201 imaging to have a relatively high sensitivity for the prediction of restenosis or recurrence of angina 4 to 6 weeks after coronary angioplasty, others in which thallium-201 imaging was performed earlier after dilation have demonstrated a lower sensitivity in predicting restenosis.

Dipyridamole may be a promising substitute of exercise for myocardial perfusion studies performed early after coronary angiography. In contrast to exercise, which may be associated with coronary vasoconstriction at the site of fixed lesions, dipyridamole exerts a generalized coronary vasodilation. Jain et al.[54] reported the use of thallium-201 single-photon emission computed tomography imaging in conjunction with orally administered dipyridamole in 53 patients studied 2.9 ± 2.7 days after coronary angioplasty, and followed clinically for a mean of 21.7 months. Of 14 patients with scan defects after coronary angioplasty, 10 (71%) developed restenosis. By contrast, of 27 patients with no ischemic abnormalities in the distribution of the dilated vessel, only 3 (11.5%) showed restenosis. These results, demonstrating that abnormalities in coronary flow reserve early after coronary angioplasty may not be so marked during dipyridamole test as during exercise, are promising but should be substantiated by other investigations involving direct comparison.

Identification of Bypass Graft Disease

The results obtained in the evaluation of patients submitted to aortocoronary bypass grafting are similar. Using the Doppler technique and papaverine infusion, Wilson et al.[55] demonstrated that surgical myocardial revascularization restored the normal maximal flow reserve capacity to the perfusion field of the graft, in the presence of a nonstenotic arterial segment downstream from the distal anastomosis supplying a normal myocardium. This effect on flow reserve suggests that perfusion imaging should be effective in the identification of ischemia after bypass surgery.

Iskandrian and co-workers[56] evaluated 30 consecutive patients with recurrent chest pain at a mean of approximately 20 months following revascularization. These authors observed a high specificity of thallium-201 scan in predicting graft failure or disease of the nongrafted vessels. However, normal images were observed in 35% of patients with incomplete revascularization, mainly in those who had graft or native vessel disease of the right coronary artery or the secondary branches of the left system.

In addition to this limited sensitivity, myocardial perfusion scintigraphy is hampered by further limitations in the evaluation of graft patency in asymptomatic patients. Sbarbaro and co-workers[57] demonstrated that in 15 asymptomatic patients evaluated prospectively before and after surgery, a postoperative increase of perfusion was an accurate marker of graft patency. A typical example of improved perfusion in the regions supplied by a patent graft is shown in Figure 19-5. However, regional graft occlusion was difficult to predict by analysis of post-treat-

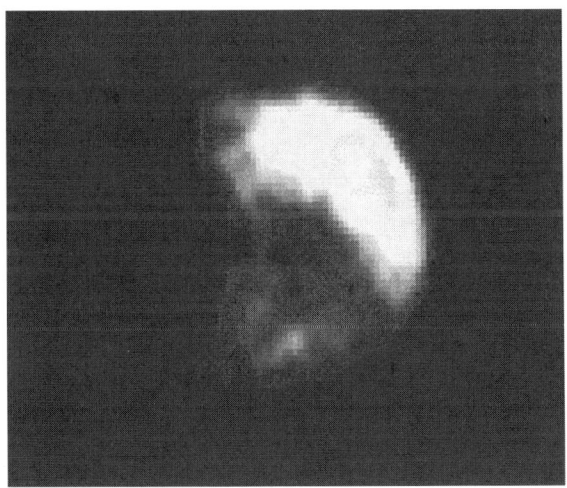 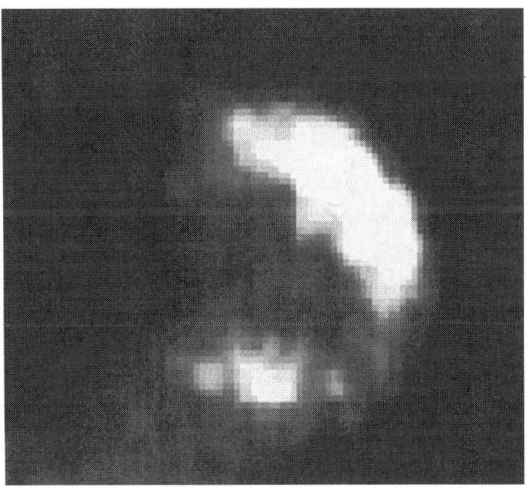

Fig. 19-5. Exercise ^{99m}Tc-Sestamibi perfusion scans before (**A**) and after (**B**) coronary artery bypass grafting. An improved perfusion, during exercise, can be observed in the inferior wall. This patient had an occluded right coronary artery and an open graft to the posterior descending branch.

ment scans, especially in the presence of irreversible perfusion defects, which may infer a failing graft or the presence of scar tissue within the revascularized region. It is worth noting that the majority of these studies have been performed by using the stress-redistribution protocol. To our knowledge, the usefulness of reinjection in identifying residual viability in dysfunctioning areas has not yet been evaluated in the clinical setting of patients with persistent defects following revascularization.

The identification of graft or progressive native-vessel disease may be facilitated by interpretation of the scans together with clinical and exercise data. The usual analysis of pretest probability is inappropriate in this group, as in patients submitted to revascularization procedures, the pretest probability of CAD is obviously 100%. Nevertheless, some idea of the pretest probability of *ischemia* may be gathered from the symptom status of the patient. Unfortunately, chest pain is often caused by mechanisms different from angina, especially in the postsurgical period. Likewise, while electrocardiographic changes with exercise are of help in defining the meaning of a perfusion defect, many patients in this group demonstrate abnormal ST- and T-wave segments at rest, or equivocal electrocardiographic findings during exercise stress testing.

Despite continuous improvement in techniques and results of myocardial revascularization, a substantial proportion of patients may have recurrent angina after bypass surgery. In these patients, a second surgical intervention represents a higher risk procedure,[58] and angioplasty is an attractive alternative. However, identification of the "culprit lesion" might be useful before cardiac catheterization, since it may allow a target vessel angioplasty during catheterization, a goal that is more difficult to obtain with the evaluation of angiography picture alone because of the presence of diffuse atherosclerosis.[22] In these patients, the exercise stress electrocardiogram does not provide any insight about the site of ischemia. In a study by Hirzel and co-workers,[59] 81% of patients showing normal postoperative regional perfusion had patent grafts at angiography, while the presence of a reversible perfusion defects at exercise myocardial scintigraphy was highly predictive of recurrent angina due to graft disease or occlusion. These data suggest that myocardial perfusion scintigraphy can provide information complementary to coronary angiography that could better address therapeutic choices in patients with graft failure.

In summary, these findings suggest that a normal perfusion scan should indicate the presence of normally functioning grafts. The detection of reversible perfusion defects at exercise myocardial perfusion scintigraphy performed late after revascularization

(> 4 to 6 weeks) should be considered as a marker of restenosis or graft failure.[60] Patients with early negative postoperative stress test results, which later become positive, usually have progressive ischemia caused either by progression of coronary atherosclerosis or graft failure. Myocardial perfusion imaging can help in determining the location, the extension, and the severity of the ischemic process.[61] The meaning of perfusion defects should be more cautiously interpreted in asymptomatic revascularized patients. Fixed defects are best interpreted by comparison of images obtained before and after revascularization.

Follow-up of Patients with Dysfunctioning Myocardium

In recent years, an increasing number of patients with left ventricular dysfunction have been submitted to coronary revascularization. This has been justified by the observations that patients submitted to successful revascularization show a greater life span than those treated with medical therapy alone,[62] and that patients with reduced left ventricular ejection fraction and CAD show the greatest prognostic benefit when treated surgically.[35] As discussed by Di Carli in Chapter 28, the presence of hibernating myocardium in patients with severe left ventricular dysfunction identifies a population with a poorer prognosis if not treated surgically.[35,63,64] Two possible mechanisms may contribute to this: first, revascularization may prevent the recurrence of infarction and worsening of myocardial dysfunction, and second, restoration of a normal perfusion in these areas might improve the left ventricular function and reduce the risk of death.

Early evaluation of myocardial perfusion or metabolism may be of value for risk stratification in patients who do not show a functional improvement after revascularization. Lack in contractile recovery may be due to several pathogenetic mechanisms. First, although the majority of hypocontracting segments show an immediate functional improvement after revascularization,[45] about 23% to 30% of segments improve function late in the follow-up.[43] Second, the revascularization procedure might be incomplete or unsuccessful, or early graft failure might have been developed. Finally, this unsuccessful result might have been caused by an incorrect presurgical characterization.

Follow-up Using Myocardial Perfusion Imaging

The evaluation of myocardial perfusion may be useful in patients with persistent dysfunction postoperatively, since incomplete revascularization should be easily picked up by the detection of perfusion defects in the dysfunctional segments. In a classic study of Berger and co-workers,[65] transient perfusion defects following rest injection of thallium-201 were observed in a significant number of patients with left ventricular dysfunction who were candidates for aortocoronary bypass surgery. Successful revascularization was associated with a normalization of early baseline perfusion scan, thus indicating a normalization of resting perfusion.

Nevertheless, although the restoration of a normal blood flow and homogeneous myocardial perfusion should indicate a successful procedure, the meaning of persistent perfusion defects has not been clearly elucidated. Iskandrian and co-workers[61] studied 95 patients divided into two groups based on left ventricular function before surgery. In both groups, a normal postrevascularization myocardial perfusion was associated with a higher left ventricular ejection fraction. However, in the 69 patients with ejection fraction greater than 50%, 28 still had abnormal resting perfusion, thus indicating that an improvement in global myocardial function can be also associated with the persistence of an abnormal perfusion scan.

Follow-up with Metabolic Imaging

Several studies have pointed out the persistence of abnormal metabolism in some hibernating segments, even after functional recovery. Tamaki et al.[66] identified persistent [^{18}F]fluorodeoxyglucose uptake at 5 to 7 weeks after revascularization. Using a dog model of 3 hour occlusion and reperfusion, Schwaiger et al.[67] showed a slow functional recovery over 4 weeks matched by continuing metabolic abnormalities, including increased [^{18}F]fluorodeoxyglucose uptake. In humans, a longitudinal follow-up 2 days and 2 months after angioplasty has been performed by Nienaber et al.[68] demonstrating early resolution of perfusion defects but delay in functional and metabolic recovery until later studies. Similarly, data obtained by Marwick and co-workers[69] demonstrated the persistence of increased uptake of [^{18}F]fluorodeoxyglucose after revascularization in

10 of 35 hibernating segments, with the more extensive impairment in presurgery perfusion and metabolism.

From a practical point of view, these data suggest that the normalization of myocardial perfusion in a previously hibernating segment can be considered as a marker of successful reperfusion. This finding should be associated with a normalization (early or late) of left ventricular function in those segments accurately evaluated before the procedure. The persistence of a perfusion defect in previously hibernating myocardium could be caused by a number of mechanisms and should be cautiously interpreted; however, if this behavior is associated with a lack of contractile improvement, it should indicate the need for a more accurate evaluation of graft patency.

Incomplete Revascularization

In patients with severe angina on effort and multivessel disease, a complete revascularization procedure by aortocoronary bypass grafting may not be possible because of the anatomy of coronary arterial tree. In these patients, important symptom relief may be achieved with partial revascularization by either coronary angioplasty or bypass surgery.[70-72] Data from the National Heart, Lung and Blood Institute Registry relative to 286 angioplasty patients with 26 months follow-up show that there were no differences in respect to death, myocardial infarction, and need for late surgery between patients with complete and incomplete revascularization.[70] Thus, revascularization by coronary angioplasty of the "culprit lesion" is being increasingly viewed as a rational approach in those patients with multivessel disease not suitable for complete revascularization.

While the frequency of "hard events" appears to be low in incompletely revascularized postangioplasty patients, the prognostic implications of this situation are unclear with respect to "soft" events. Identification of functional evidence of ongoing ischemia might be important in this context, and the sensitivity of myocardial scintigraphy is greater than that provided by exercise electrocardiography. Moreover, clinical or electrocardiographic criteria cannot reliably differentiate myocardial ischemia caused by the nontreated stenoses from that resulting from restenosis of the dilated vessel. Postangioplasty perfusion imaging is the most accurate technique in the evaluation and management of patients with multivessel disease submitted to incomplete myocardial revascularization. Using thallium-201 single-photon emission computed tomography imaging in 85 patients studied after angioplasty for multivessel disease, Breisblatt and co-workers[46] reported that ischemia was evident in a second vascular distribution territory in 38 of 85 (44%) patients. Over a 1-year follow-up period, 79% of these patients required repeated angioplasty compared to only 10% of patients with negative exercise perfusion scan.[46]

ADVANTAGES AND LIMITATIONS OF NUCLEAR IMAGING VERSUS ALTERNATIVE TECHNIQUES

Stress Electrocardiography

When compared with perfusion imaging, exercise electrocardiography offers obvious advantages in terms of costs and repeatability. However, in the setting of patients submitted to revascularization procedures, stress electrocardiography shows major limitations such as unreliability in the localization of ischemia, the possibility of equivocal findings in the presence of an abnormal resting electrocardiogram, and a limited accuracy in the prediction of restenosis. Accordingly, exercise electrocardiography can be considered as a method able to monitor the follow-up of patients to identify the presence of restenosis or graft failure in revascularized patients, more than a method to identify high-risk patients.

When performed early after coronary angioplasty, exercise electrocardiography shows limited accuracy in predicting the recurrence of both restenosis and angina. When incomplete revascularization has been performed by dilation of the culprit lesion in patients with multivessel disease, an early perfusion scan is able to adequately identify those patients at high risk for the recurrence of angina or need for a repeated angioplasty, a task that cannot be accomplished with electrocardiography alone. Similarly, if symptoms recur after bypass surgery, the importance of identifying the site of ischemia and thus the culprit vessel suggests that myocardial perfusion imaging is a more appropriate option than stress electrocardiography.

Stress Echocardiography

In comparison with nuclear imaging of myocardial perfusion, stress echocardiography offers significant advantages in terms of cost and repeatability, without a large reduction in diagnostic power. Indeed, the presence of left ventricular asynergy during stress is a more specific marker of myocardial ischemia than electrocardiographic or perfusion abnormalities. The accuracy of stress echocardiography in previously revascularized patients is discussed in Chapter 18.

To date, however, a direct comparison of these two techniques has not been obtained in a selected population of patients submitted to coronary revascularization. Since the accuracy of perfusion scintigraphy significantly increases when the postrevascularization results are directly compared with those obtained before the intervention,[57] this approach might be preferred in patients with a positive perfusion scan before revascularization, while stress echocardiography might be the first choice in those patients not evaluated by radioisotopic techniques before the procedure. In the absence of a conclusive demonstration of the relative advantages and disadvantages of these two techniques in the setting of revascularized patients, the choice of perfusion scintigraphy or stress echocardiography still remains highly subjective. Thus, the roles for perfusion imaging in the remainder of this chapter might be filled by stress echocardiography.

CLINICAL DECISION MAKING AFTER REVASCULARIZATION

Patients with Normal Left Ventricular Function

The evaluation of patients with normal left ventricular function after revascularization is most often focused on two major aims: (1) the early recognition of restenosis in case of coronary angioplasty, and (2) the documentation of benefit induced by revascularization. Normalization of left ventricular ejection fraction in patients with reversible left ventricular dysfunction can be observed early in patients submitted to successful coronary angioplasty,[73] while in patients undergoing coronary artery bypass surgery it can take longer because of the superimposition of myocardial stunning after a cardioplegic procedure.

Coronary angioplasty is frequently performed in patients with single-vessel disease, while aortocoronary bypass surgery is usually indicated in patients with multivessel disease. This may imply a different "threshold" of recognition of location and extent of ischemia following the two revascularization procedures.

Coronary Angioplasty

Patients with normal left ventricular function after successful coronary angioplasty represent a low-risk population, especially if the procedure was performed because of the presence of *single-vessel* CAD. In these patients the first step in evaluation is usually performed by electrocardiography. Patients with normal function before revascularization usually do not need a systematic assessment of left ventricular ejection fraction by echocardiography or gated blood pool imaging in the absence of complications.

In contrast, the recognition of a normalized function may be important in those patients with *stress-induced dysfunction* before the procedure. Exercise electrocardiography is often utilized as a first step in these patients[53] because of its repeatability and low cost, despite its limited accuracy. The need for a perfusion study can be evident in the presence of equivocal findings at exercise electrocardiography or when symptoms reappear. Myocardial imaging may thus verify the ischemic nature of the symptoms and ascertain whether ischemia is caused by restenosis or progression of disease in nonrelated vessels. The use of a viability imaging with either thallium-201 reinjection or [^{18}F]fluorodeoxyglucose and positron emission tomography should be applied to address specific diagnostic concerns.

A different approach should be considered in patients with *multivessel* disease who have had an incomplete revascularization due to angioplasty of the "culprit lesion."[46,70] In these patients, perfusion imaging can be the approach of first choice since normal perfusion during exercise can identify those patients with a low probability of recurrence of angina.

The best timing for evaluation after coronary angioplasty is still controversial. However, the reliability of myocardial perfusion scan seems to be higher at least 4 weeks after the procedure. Single-photon emission computed tomography should be preferred to planar scintigraphy, since it provides greater accuracy in the identification of left circumflex disease and a more accurate evaluation of the extent of ischemia; moreover, in these patients, the indexes of left ventricular function derived by planar scans (such as increased lung uptake, or transient dilation of the left ventricular chamber) are less important. Positron emission tomography can also be used, although its high cost and limited availability prevent its wide application. Moreover, the advantages of this method over single-photon emission computed tomography with conventional gamma emitters are not yet fully ascertained.

Coronary Artery Bypass Surgery

A systematic evaluation of patients submitted to surgical revascularization is not usually needed, but it is strongly indicated if symptoms recur. Patients with single-vessel disease seldom undergo surgical revascularization; in general, patients submitted to aortocoronary bypass surgery have diffuse atherosclerosis and a complete revascularization is attempted in all vascular territories, for treatment of severe angina. Exercise electrocardiography after surgical revascularization is often uninterpretable due to ST- and T-wave changes, and symptom responses are not easily interpreted because of the consequences of thoracotomy. Moreover, it does not provide data relating to the site of the ischemic process. Accordingly, myocardial imaging may be useful in these patients. This information is of crucial relevance; patients with normal ventricular function, after revascularization, have a good prognosis and a new surgical intervention represents a high risk procedure that may be avoided if relief of symptoms would be achievable by coronary angioplasty. Recognition of the site of stress-induced perfusion abnormalities may provide the rationale for selective coronary angioplasty more accurately than that achieved by the evaluation of the severity of epicardial stenosis at angiography.[22]

Patients with Dysfunctioning Myocardium

Persistent myocardial dysfunction or new onset of signs of heart failure may develop in patients who have undergone coronary revascularization. In these circumstances, there are two pertinent questions: (1) Is the depressed contractile performance secondary to persistent ischemia? and (2) Does dysfunctional myocardium retain the capacity for functional recovery? Confounding effects of interventions that may cause stunning of the revascularized territories (e.g., prolonged balloon inflation times at coronary angioplasty, effects of cardioplegia, or perioperative ischemia) may further complicate interpretation of the dysfunction. Active diagnostic approaches appear justified in this set of patients, on the basis of higher risk of adverse events in those with dysfunctioning, viable myocardium[35] and of the costs needed for subsequent interventions.

These patients may exhibit equivocal electrocardiographic findings during stress, as a result of previous myocardial infarction in the revascularized territories and ambiguous clinical symptoms. These reasons justify (1) a search for markers of ischemia, (2) tests that are able to evaluate myocardial viability, and (3) the use of advanced imaging technology such as positron emission tomography.

Coronary Angioplasty

Failure to improve contraction after coronary angioplasty may be caused by (1) ineffective procedure (i.e., persistence of a hemodynamically significant stenosis), (2) incomplete revascularization, or (3) subsequent restenosis. Worsening of previous dysfunction or occurrence of new myocardial dysfunction may occur following a complicated or emergency procedure. Myocardial perfusion imaging is particularly suited to the investigation of dysfunctional territories with reversible perfusion defects before coronary angioplasty, because improvement or normalization of perfusion precedes recovery of contraction abnormalities after a successful procedure. Improvement of perfusion in the dysfunctional area may indicate either stunning postcoronary angioplasty or delayed recovery of myocardial function. Persistence of perfusion defects may indicate that revascularization was ineffective. Whether thallium-201 reinjection or metabolic studies with [^{18}F]fluorodeoxyglucose, [^{11}C]acetate,[74] or $H_2{}^{15}O$ are indicated to assess viability in fixed defects at stress-redistribution imaging after revascularization remains to be determined.

Coronary Artery Bypass Surgery

The major problem with the use of perfusion imaging to evaluate revascularization after bypass surgery in patients with preoperative myocardial dysfunction is perioperative infarction. Perioperative infarction may further impair regional and global function; however, it may relieve anginal symptoms and resolve ischemia. Furthermore, stunning is more frequent and prolonged after aortocoronary bypass surgery than after coronary angioplasty, raising the question of whether depressed function after surgery is a result of extensive irreversible damage, stunning, or hibernation of nonrevascularized segments.

REFERENCES

1. Chaitman BR, Bourassa MG, Davis K et al.: Angiographic prevalence of high risk coronary artery disease in patients subsets (CASS). Circulation 64:360, 1981
2. Rubio R, Berne RM: Regulation of coronary blood flow. Prog Cardiovasc Dis 18:105, 1975
3. Kanatsuka H, Lamping KG, Eastham CL, Dellsperer KC, Marcus ML: Comparison of the effects of increased oxygen consumption and adenosine on the coronary microvascular resistance. Circ Res 65:1296, 1989
4. Kuo L, Chilian WM, Davis MJ: Interaction of pressure and flow-induced responses in porcine coronary resistance vessels. Am J Physiol 261:H1706, 1991
5. Jones CJH, Kuo L, Davis MJ et al.: Role of nitric oxide in the coronary microvascular responses to adenosine and increased metabolic demand. Circulation 91:1807, 1995
6. Cox AD, Vita JA, Treasure CB et al.: Atherosclerosis impairs flow-mediated dilation of coronary arteries in humans. Circulation 80:458, 1989
7. Heistad DD, Armstrong ML, Marcus ML et al.: Augmented responses to vasoconstrictor stimuli in hypercholesterolemic and atherosclerotic monkeys. Circ Res 54:711, 1984
8. Chilian WM, Dellsperger KG, Layne SM et al.: Effect of atherosclerosis on the coronary microcirculation. Am J Physiol 258:H529, 1990
9. Chilian WM: Small vessel phenomena in the coronary microcirculation: phasic intramyocardial perfusion and coronary microvascular dynamics. Prog Cardiovasc Dis 31:17, 1988
10. Uren NG, Marraccini P, Gistri R et al.: Altered coronary vasodilator reserve and metabolism in myocardium subtended by normal arteries in patients with coronary artery disease elsewhere. J Am Coll Cardiol 22:650, 1993
11. Sambuceti GM, Parodi O, Marcassa C et al.: Alteration in regulation of myocardial blood flow in single vessel coronary artery disease determined by positron emission tomography. Am J Cardiol 72:538, 1993
12. Sambuceti G, Marzullo P, Giorgetti A et al.: Global alteration in perfusion response to increasing oxygen consumption in patients with single vessel coronary artery disease. Circulation 90:1696, 1995
13. Gould KL, Lipscomb K, Hamilton GW: Physiologic basis for assessing critical coronary stenosis. Instantaneous flow response and regional distribution during coronary hyperemia as measures of coronary flow reserve. Am J Cardiol 33:87, 1974
14. Shipley RE, Gregg DE: The effect of external constriction of a blood flow. Am J Physiol 141:289, 1974
15. Pantely GA, Bristow JD, Swenson LJ et al.: Incomplete coronary vasodilation during myocardial ischemia in swine. Am J Physiol 249:H638, 1985
16. Parodi O, Sambuceti G, Roghi A et al.: Residual coronary reserve despite decreased resting blood flow in patients with critical coronary lesions. A study by technetium-99m human albumin microsphere myocardial scintigraphy. Circulation 87:330, 1993
17. Fedele FA, Gewirtz H, Capone RJ et al.: Metabolic response to prolonged reductions of myocardial blood flow distal to a severe coronary stenosis. Circulation 78:729, 1988
18. Pantely GA, Malone SA, Rhen WS et al.: Regeneration of myocardial phosphocreatine in pigs despite continued moderate ischemia. Circ Res 67:1481, 1990
19. Bristow JD, Arai AE, Anselone CG, Pantely GA: Response to myocardial ischemia as a regulated process. Circulation 84:2580, 1991
20. Chilian WM, Layne SM: Coronary microvascular responses to reductions in perfusion pressure: Evidence for persistent arteriolar vasomotor tone during coronary hypoperfusion. Circ Res 66:1227, 1990
21. Pupita G, Maseri A, Kaski JC et al.: Myocardial ischemia caused by distal coronary artery constriction in stable angina pectoris. N Engl J Med 323:514, 1990
22. White CW, Wright CB, Doy DB et al.: Does visual interpretation of the coronary arteriogram predict the physiologic significance of a coronary stenosis? N Engl J Med 310:819, 1984
23. Wilson RF, Johnson MR, Marcus ML et al.: The effect of coronary angioplasty on coronary flow reserve. Circulation 77:873, 1988
24. Wilson RF, Lesser JF, Laxon DD, White CW: Intense microvascular constriction after angioplasty of acute thrombotic arterial lesions. Lancet 1:807, 1989
25. Sambuceti G, Parodi O, Giorgetti A et al.: Microvascular dysfunction in collateral dependent myocardium. J Am Coll Cardiol 26:615, 1995
26. Sambuceti G, Parodi O: Role of coronary microvascu-

lar abnormalities in coronary artery disease: implications for perfusion imaging. J Nucl Cardiol 2:78, 1995
27. Beller GA, Gibson RS: Sensitivity, specificity, and prognostic significance of noninvasive testing for occult or known coronary disease. Prog Cardiovasc Dis 29:241, 1987
28. Uren NG, Crake T, Lefroy DC, et al.: Delayed recovery of coronary resistive vessel function after coronary angioplasty. J Am Coll Cardiol 21:612, 1993
29. Fishell TA, Bausback KN, McDonald TV: Evidence for altered epicardial coronary artery autoregulation as a cause of distal coronary vasoconstriction after successful percutaneous transluminal angioplasty. J Clin Invest 86:575, 1990
30. Gould KL, Kirkeeide RL, Buchi M: Coronary flow reserve as a physiologic measure of stenosis severity. J Am Coll Cardiol 15:459, 1990
31. Uren NG, Melin JA, De Bruyne B et al.: Relation between myocardial blood flow and the severity of coronary artery stenosis. N Engl J Med 330:1782, 1994
32. Bates ER, Aueron FM, Legrand V et al.: Comparative long-term effects of coronary artery bypass graft surgery and percutaneous transluminal coronary angioplasty on regional flow reserve. Circulation 72:833, 1985
33. Pirelli S, Massa D, Faletra F et al.: Exercise electrocardiography vs dipyridamole echocardiography testing in coronary angioplasty: early functional evaluation and prediction of angina recurrence. Circulation, suppl. III:III38, 1991
34. Tillisch J, Brunken R, Marshall R et al.: Reversibility of cardiac wall motion abnormalities predicted by positron emission tomography. N Engl J Med 314:884, 1986
35. Eitzman D, Al Aouar Z, Kanter HL et al.: Clinical outcome of patients with advanced coronary artery disease after viability studies with positron emission tomography. J Am Coll Cardiol 20:559, 1992
36. Rocco TP, Dilsizian V, Strauss HW, Boucher CA: Technetium-99m isonitrile myocardial uptake at rest. II. Relation to clinical markers of potential viability. J Am Coll Cardiol 14:1678, 1989
37. Parodi O, Marcassa C, Casucci R et al.: Accuracy and safety of technetium-99m hexakis 2-methoxy-2-isobutyl isonitrile (Sestamibi) myocardial scintigraphy with high dose dipyridamole test in patients with effort angina pectoris: a multicenter study. J Am Coll Cardiol 18:1439, 1991
38. Testa R, Sambuceti G, Roghi A et al.: Breakdown in perfusion contraction matching following successful coronary angioplasty, abstracted. Eur Heart J 14:474, 1993
39. Maseri A, Crea F, Cianflone D: Myocardial ischemia caused by distal vasoconstriction. Am J Cardiol 70:1602, 1992
40. Gewirtz H, Fischman AJ, Abraham S et al.: Positron emission tomographic measurements of absolute regional myocardial blood flow permit identification of nonviable myocardium in patients with chronic myocardial infarction. J Am Coll Cardiol 23:851, 1994
41. Czernin J, Porenta G, Brunken R et al.: Regional blood flow, oxidative metabolism and glucose utilization in patients with recent myocardial infarction. Circulation 88:884, 1993
42. Marzullo P, Parodi O, Sambuceti G et al.: Residual coronary reserve identifies segmental viability in patients with wall motion abnormalities. J Am Coll Cardiol 26:342, 1995
43. Mintz LY, Ingels HB, Daughters GI et al.: Sequential studies of left ventricular function and wall motion after coronary bypass surgery. Am J Cardiol 45:210, 1980
44. Manyari DE, Knudtson M, Roth D: Sequential thallium-201 myocardial perfusion studies after successful percutaneous transluminal coronary angioplasty: delayed resolution of exercise-induced scintigraphic abnormalities. Circulation 77:86, 1988
45. Topol EJ, Weiss JL, Guzman PA et al.: Immediate improvement of dysfunctional myocardial segments after coronary revascularization: detection by intraoperative transesophageal echocardiography. J Am Coll Cardiol 4:1123, 1984
46. Breisblatt WM, Barnes JV, Weiland F, Spaccavento LJ: Incomplete revascularization in multivessel percutaneous transluminal coronary angioplasty: The role for stress thallium-201 imaging. J Am Coll Cardiol 11:1183, 1988
47. Diamond GA: A clinically relevant classification of chest discomfort. J Am Coll Cardiol 1:578, 1983
48. Parodi O, Uthurralt N, Severi S et al.: Transient reduction of regional myocardial perfusion during angina at rest with ST-segment depression or normalization of negative T waves. Circulation 63:1238, 1981
49. Nobuyoshi M, Kimura T, Nosak H et al.: Restenosis after successful percutaneous coronary angioplasty: serial angiographic follow-up of 229 patients. J Am Coll Cardiol. 12:616, 1988
50. Zjilstra F, Den Boer A, Reiber JHC et al.: Assessment of immediate and long term functional results of percutaneous transluminal coronary angioplasty. Circulation 78:15, 1988
51. Breisblatt WM, Weiland F, Spaccavento LJ: Stress thallium-201 imaging after coronary angioplasty predicts

restenosis and recurrent symptoms. J Am Coll Cardiol 12:1199, 1988
52. Stuckey TD, Burrwell LR, Nygaard TW et al.: Value of quantitative exercise thallium-201 scintigraphy for predicting angina recurrence after percutaneous transluminal coronary angioplasty. Am J Cardiol 65:517, 1989
53. Wijns W, Serruys PW, Reiber JHC et al.: Early detection of restenosis after successful percutaneous transluminal angioplasty by exercise-redistribution thallium scintigraphy. Br Heart J 55:357, 1985
54. Jain A, Mahmarian JJ, Borges-Neto S et al.: Clinical significance of perfusion defects by thallium-201 single photon emission tomography following oral dipyridamole early after coronary angioplasty. J Am Coll Cardiol 11:970, 1988
55. Wilson RF, White CW: Does coronary artery bypass surgery restore a normal maximal coronary flow reserve? Circulation 76:563, 1987
56. Iskandrian AS, Haaz W, Segal BL, Kane SA: Exercise thallium 201 scintigraphy in evaluating aortocoronary bypass surgery. Chest 80:11, 1981
57. Sbarbaro JA, Karunaratne H, Cantez S et al.: Thallium-201 imaging in assessment of aortocoronary artery bypass graft patency. Br Heart J 42:553, 1979
58. Hochberg MS, Parsonnet V, Gielchinski I, Hussain SM: Coronary artery bypass grafting in patients with ejection fraction below forty percent. J Thorac Cardiovasc Surg 86:519, 1983
59. Hirzel HO, Nuesch K, Sialer G et al.: Thallium-201 exercise myocardial imaging to evaluate myocardial perfusion after coronary artery bypass surgery. Br Heart J 43:426, 1980
60. DePuey GE: Myocardial perfusion imaging with thallium-201 to evaluate patients before and after percutaneous transluminal coronary angioplasty. Circulation suppl I: I-59, 1991
61. McConahay DR, Valdes M, McAllister BD et al.: Accuracy of treadmill testing in assessment of direct myocardial revascularization. Circulation 56:548, 1977
62. Kron IL, Flanagan TL, Blackbourne LH et al.: Myocardial revascularization rather than cardiac transplantation for chronic ischemic cardiomyopathy. Ann Surg 210:348, 1989
63. DiCarli M, Davidson M, Little R et al.: Value of metabolic imaging with positron emission tomography for evaluating prognosis in patients with coronary artery disease and left ventricular dysfunction. Am J Cardiol 73:527, 1994
64. Lee KS, Marwick TH, Cook SA et al.: Prognosis of patients with left ventricular dysfunction, with and without viable myocardium after myocardial infarction. Circulation 90:2687, 1994
65. Berger BC, Watson DD, Burwell LR et al.: Redistribution of thallium at rest in patients with stable and unstable angina and the effects of coronary bypass surgery. Circulation 60:114, 1979
66. Tamaki N, Yonekura Y, Yamashita Y et al.: Positron emission tomography using F-18 deoxyglucose in evaluation of coronary artery bypass grafting. Am J Cardiol 64:860, 1989
67. Schwaiger M, Schelbert H, Ellison D et al.: Sustained regional abnormalities in cardiac metabolism after transient ischemia in the chronic dog model. J Am Coll Cardiol 6:336, 1985
68. Nienaber CA, Brunken RC, Sherman CT et al.: Recovery of myocardial metabolism precedes functional improvement following relief of chronic ischemia by PTCA, abstracted. J Nucl Med 30:838, 1989
69. Marwick TM, McIntyre WJ, Lafont A et al.: Metabolic response of hibernating and infarcted myocardium to revascularization: a follow up study of perfusion, function and metabolism. Circulation 85:1347, 1992
70. Reeder GS, Holmes DR, Detre K et al.: Degree of revascularization in patients with multivessel coronary disease: a report from the National Heart, Lung and Blood Institute Percutaneous Transluminal Coronary Angioplasty Registry. Circulation 77:638, 1988
71. Dorros G, Sterzer SM, Cowley MJ, Myler RK: Complex coronary angioplasty: multiple coronary dilations. Am J Cardiol 53:126, 1984
72. Vandormael MG, Chaitman BR, Ischinger T et al.: Immediate and short-term benefit of multilesion coronary angioplasty. Influence of the degree of revascularization. J Am Coll Cardiol 6:983, 1985
73. Renkin J, Wijns W, Ladha Z, Col J: Reversal of segmental hypokinesis by coronary angioplasty in patients with unstable angina, persistent T wave inversion, and left anterior descending coronary artery stenosis. Circulation 82:913, 1990

Chapter 20

Optimal SPECT Technique for Assessing Myocardial Viability

Philippe R. Franken and
Frank W. De Geeter

GENERAL CONSIDERATIONS

Clinical Importance of Assessing Myocardial Viability

In the clinical management of patients with coronary artery disease (CAD) and poor left ventricular function, the available treatment choices are medical therapy, cardiac transplantation, and myocardial revascularization. Myocardial revascularization is an attractive alternative because medical therapy is associated with a high mortality and cardiac transplantation is expensive and often impractical, due to the shortage of donor hearts. Myocardial revascularization is known to improve heart failure symptoms and survival in patients with severe CAD and depressed ventricular function, even if symptoms are minimal or absent. In the absence of symptoms of significant angina pectoris, however, myocardial revascularization should be recommended only in those patients in whom the procedure is very likely to reverse ventricular dysfunction since the surgery itself is associated with 5% to 37% mortality.[1] In addition, recent studies have shown that residual viable myocardium is an unstable substrate after myocardial infarction and is likely to lead to ischemic events if left unrevascularized.[2,3]

It should be emphasized that a clinical decision to revascularize cannot be made solely on the grounds of a viability study. Moreover, in some patients coronary revascularization may not improve regional or global left ventricular function, even though viable myocardium is present. Indeed improvement following coronary revascularization represents a complex interaction between compensatory mechanisms, coronary anatomy, surgical outcome, and patient selection.[4]

Definition of Myocardial Viability

Relation to Functional Recovery

Viable myocardium is identified by the presence of myocardial dysfunction that is reversible either spontaneously or after coronary revascularization, whereas nonviable myocardium can be defined as myocardial dysfunction that is irreversible after coronary revascularization. Irreversible dysfunction results from myocardial necrosis and scar, whereas reversible contractile dysfunction may be caused by stunning or hibernation. Stunning differs basically from hibernation in that recovery of function can occur without revascularization, since by definition it represents a transient dysfunction following an episode of ischemia. In contrast, the dysfunction due to hibernation is a chronic process associated with conditions of severely reduced coronary blood flow. In many clinical situations, however, a combination of normal, scar, hibernating, and stunned myocardium may coexist in different proportions not only in various parts of the myocardium, but even as overlapping strata within the thickness of individual segments. Therefore, a definite distinction between viable and nonviable myocardium is best made by comparison of prerevascularization and postrevascularization studies of regional and global left ventricular function.[5]

Myocardial Stunning

Myocardial stunning may result when severe acute ischemia is followed by reperfusion, and the regional ventricular dysfunction associated with stunning represents the combined results of ischemic injury and reperfusion injury.[6] The commonest clinical settings in which stunned myocardium is observed are thrombolytic therapy or acute revascularization therapy for acute myocardial infarction. Myocardial stunning also occurs in various settings in which the myocardium is exposed to transient ischemia including unstable angina, open-heart surgery, cardiac transplantation, and possibly exercise-induced angina.[7] By definition, myocardial dysfunction associated with stunning is completely reversible, but may persist for several days or weeks after reperfusion before resolving. Although the mechanisms for myocardial stunning have not be fully determined, this is a well-demonstrated and reproducible phenomenon with excellent animal models.

Hibernating Myocardium

Hibernating myocardium refers to the presence of persistent myocardial dysfunction at rest, associated with conditions of severely reduced coronary blood flow.[8] There are no adequate long-term animal models of hibernation, and there are no serial studies in patients that show whether hibernating myocardium is truly a chronic condition. It has been speculated that the process of hibernation maintains myocardial viability by reducing the metabolic demand to match the decreased supply for as long as myocardial perfusion is inadequate. The chronic impairment of contractile function in this setting is thus considered to represent a protective mechanism, minimizing the energy requirements and preventing the appearance of irreversible tissue damage.

This concept has been recently challenged by Vanoverschelde and colleagues.[9] In patients with noninfarcted but dysfunctional collateral-dependent myocardium, they found that absolute myocardial blood flow and oxygen consumption were nearly normal at rest, but that coronary flow reserve was extremely limited. The authors concluded that repetitive episodes of ischemia with a persistent stunning effect, rather than a chronic low-flow state of perfusion-contraction coupling, was responsible for chronic myocardial dysfunction in this circumstance. However, because the dysfunctional segments showed pronounced structural abnormalities (loss in myofibrillar content and excessive accumulation of glycogen), the tissue also differs from models of acute stunning, in which structural changes are mild. These findings strongly suggest that demand-induced ischemia and consequent postischemic dysfunction (rather than hibernation) are likely to play an important role in chronic left ventricular dysfunction and that recovery of dysfunctional segments after revascularization is likely to be delayed frequently by the ultrastructural changes that have occurred.

Assessing Myocardial Viability with SPECT

Among the available invasive and noninvasive modalities, nuclear cardiology techniques utilizing single-photon emission computerized tomography (SPECT) have achieved a preeminent position for the assessment of myocardial viability. This arises from the rather unique potential of scintigraphic methods to assess myocardial perfusion, cell membrane integrity, and metabolic activity, thereby providing greater diagnostic precision regarding viability than can be achieved by assessment of regional anatomy or function alone. In particular, thallium-201 scintigraphy has evolved over the past two decades as an imaging modality that may be used not only in diagnosing CAD but also in assessing myocardial viability in patients with proven CAD. The limitations of imaging thallium-201, however, are also well established, related primarily to its low-energy photons, which are readily scattered and attenuated, and to dosimetric considerations. These limitations have lead to considerable interest in the use of technetium-99m-based myocardial perfusion agents, particularly sestamibi, to predict residual viability. On the other hand, iodine-123 free fatty acid analogs represent unique metabolic probes for correlation of energy substrate metabolism with regional myocardial viability using SPECT. More recently, the feasibility of assessing regional myocardial uptake of the positron emitter fluorine-18 deoxyglucose (FDG) using SPECT has been demonstrated. Finally, the simultaneous imaging of a flow tracer and an infarct avid tracer (antimyosin) that demarcates regions of necrosis may help identify the viable segments.

FLOW TRACERS
Basic Principles

To be used as an agent for the detection of myocardial viability, a tracer needs to fulfill two basic requirements. First, its cellular accumulation should depend on active cellular metabolism, so that it will be retained in viable cells but not in necrotic ones. Second, its accumulation should not be limited by flow, so that it would be taken up in all cells that are viable, including those in low-flow areas. Thallium-201 and technetium-99m sestamibi are myocardial flow tracers showing biological properties that also reflect tissue viability.

Thallium-201: A Marker of Cellular Membrane Integrity

Relationship Between Net Thallium Uptake and Cellular Metabolism

Thallium is a cationic element with biological properties similar to those of potassium. Following intravenous administration, its initial distribution depends on regional blood flow and on extraction fraction into the myocardial myocyte, which is approximately 85% at normal flow rates. Extraction fraction increases at low flow rates but is not appreciably affected by acidosis, hypoxemia, or transient ischemia unless irreversible membrane injury is present.[10-12] Approximately 40% to 60% of the transport of thallium across the sarcolemmal membrane involves sodium–potassium adenosine triphosphatase (ATPase) and hence is dependent on metabolism to provide the adenosine triphosphate (ATP) necessary to drive the pump system.

Uptake in Low-Flow Areas: Importance of Tracer Redistribution

Following the initial distribution of thallium within the myocardium, a continuous exchange of the tracer over the sarcolemmal membrane takes place, resulting in a progressive redistribution of the tracer over time and leading to images that reflect the intracellular myocardial potassium pool. Pohost et al.[13] observed that some early thallium defects may fill in when delayed imaging is performed. Gewirtz and colleagues[14] first reported the occurrence of thallium defects on resting images in patients with severe CAD but without acute ischemic processes or previous myocardial infarction. They also recognized that many of these defects demonstrated redistribution over the next 2 to 4 hours, especially in regions with normal or hypokinetic wall motion. Thus, redistribution is not only active after changing the physiologic conditions from stress to rest, but may also come into play after rest injection in territories subserved by severely stenosed coronary arteries.

Further experimental studies showed that redistribution is due to an absolute reduction in thallium concentration in normal segments along with an absolute increase in thallium concentration in ischemic segments. The determinants of redistribution, however, are complex. Washout of thallium is slowed down when perfusion pressure falls or as the severity of the coronary stenosis increases; therefore, ischemic segments retain the tracer longer than normal segments. However, a continued accumulation of the tracer into the ischemic segments takes place concurrently, depending on the available blood levels of the tracer. If circulating levels of tracer between the time of initial and delayed imaging are low, delivery of tracer to low-flow areas may remain insufficient to cause detectable redistribution.

Eating, fasting, and ribose infusion may affect thallium clearance and, hence, may decrease or enhance the detection of defect reversibility. Eating or infusion of glucose–potassium–insulin impairs detection of reversibility by decreasing blood thallium concentration.[15] Ribose infusion, on the other hand, appears to enhance the detection of reversibility. The exact mechanism is unknown but has been suggested to be metabolic.[16]

Technetium-99m Sestamibi: A Marker of Mitochondrial Activity

Relationship between Net Sestamibi Uptake and Cellular Metabolism

Technetium hexaxis(2-methoxy)isobutyl isonitrile (sestamibi) is a lipophilic cationic complex. Like thallium, the initial distribution of sestamibi following intravenous injection is proportional to regional blood flow. Its uptake and retention in the myocardial myocyte, however, differ fundamentally from that of thallium. The uptake mechanism involves passive distribution across sarcolemmal and mitochondrial membranes due to its high lipophilicity. At equilibrium, sestamibi is predominantly (84%) concentrated and sequestered within the mitochondria by their large negative transmembrane potentials.[17] Depolarization of the plasma membrane potentials by changes in the extracellular potassium content reduces net accumulation of sestamibi. Additional depolarization of the mitochondria or incubation with a mitochondrial uncoupler rapidly and nearly completely depletes cellular sestamibi to levels comparable to that found in nonviable preparations. In contrast, hyperpolarizing the mitochondrial membrane with an ATP synthase inhibitor increases net uptake and retention of sestamibi.[17] Mitochondrial calcium overload, which is known to be the "point of no return" in the process of cellular ischemia and cell death, was found to release sestamibi from the mitochondria.[18] Consequently, uptake of sestamibi depends on cellular metabolism because metabolism is ultimately responsible for the maintenance of sarcolemmal and mitochondrial transmembrane electric gradients.

Necrotic myocardium does not retain sestamibi.[19-22] In a dog model studied by Sinusas et al.,[19] sestamibi was injected after 90 minutes of reperfusion following 3 hours of left anterior descending artery occlusion. The defect area defined by sestamibi autoradiography correlated very closely with the postmortem infarct area. On the other hand, the myocardial defect was significantly less than that measured with microspheres at the time of reperfusion, reflecting myocardial viability more than the degree of reperfusion flow in both necrotic and perinecrotic regions.

Myocardial Uptake in Low-Flow Areas

When sestamibi was introduced into clinical practice, it was emphasized that absence of redistribution would relieve the necessity of immediate imaging linked to the use of a redistributing tracer. Further experiments, however, showed some redistribution of sestamibi over time under conditions of occlusion and reperfusion and after resting injection in the presence of a critical stenosis.[23,24] Redistribution of sestamibi is much slower than that of thallium, a finding that is consistent with its faster blood clearance and the fact that sestamibi is compartmentalized into the mitochondria.[25]

Whether sestamibi redistributes to a clinically important level remains the subject of considerable debate. As an example, Taillefer et al.[26] demonstrated a decrease in planar ischemic-to-normal activity ratios between 1 and 3 hours after stress injection. On the other hand, Villanueva-Meyer et al.[27] reported no change in defect size between 1 and 4 hours after sestamibi stress injection, using serial quantitative SPECT imaging. Nevertheless, because sestamibi redistributes under conditions of sustained low flow,[24] imaging should be delayed after the resting injection of sestamibi when assessing myocardial viability in the presence of critical stenosis.

Comparison Between Thallium and Sestamibi as Markers of Cellular Viability

Cultured Cardiac Myocyte Model

Differences in the ways thallium and sestamibi react to metabolic insults have been highlighted in a key experiment by Piwnica-Worms and co-workers.[28] In cultured chick cardiac myocytes, these authors have simulated various depths of ischemic injury by applying, for various lengths of time, a blocker of glycolysis combined with an inhibitor of respiratory chain electron transport. These substances provide a complete metabolic inhibition and bring about a quick decline in cellular ATP levels. As shown on Figure 20-1, severe injury completely depletes sestamibi cell content while thallium uptake persists at around 40% of the reference value, corresponding to the part of uptake that is not mediated by the sodium–potassium ATPase. Moderate injury already depresses thallium uptake while sestamibi uptake is transiently enhanced, reflecting hyperpolarization of the cell. On the basis of this evidence, it appears that thallium uptake is more sensitive than sestamibi uptake to brief episodes of ischemia. However, in severe ischemic injury, sestamibi uptake is decreased more than thallium. The lesser uptake of sestamibi than thallium in necrotic cells has been confirmed in other experimental models.[12] Based on these results in non-flow-dependent experiments, sestamibi

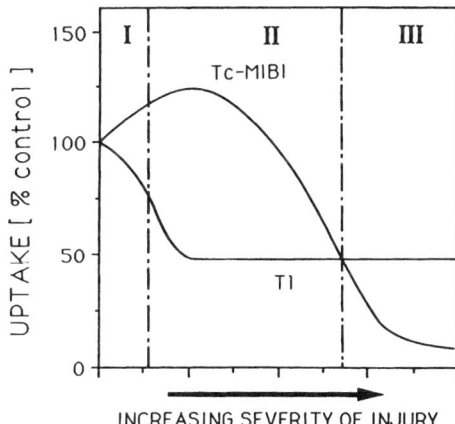

Fig. 20-1. Effect of the severity of injury on initial uptake rates of technetium-99m sestamibi and thallium-201 into cardiac myocytes. Zones I, II, and III represent mild, moderate, and severe myocellular injury, respectively. (From Piwnica-Worms et al.,[28] with permission.)

could better distinguish reversible from irreversible injury than could thallium.

Low Coronary Flow and Postischemic Dysfunction Dog Model

The myocardial uptake of thallium and sestamibi was correlated with microsphere flow in an open chest canine model of low coronary flow ("hibernating" myocardium) and postischemic dysfunction ("stunned" myocardium) by Sinusas and co-workers.[19] Regional dysfunction was documented by quantitative two-dimensional echocardiography. When the tracers were administered 40 minutes after partial left anterior descending artery occlusion producing left ventricular dysfunction without necrosis, thallium and sestamibi activities were comparable, respectively, for endocardial, midwall, and epicardial segments, and increased proportionally with flow. There was a good linear correlation between flow and both thallium and sestamibi activities (Fig. 20-2). Thallium and sestamibi activities were also comparable in asynergic myocardium in dogs undergoing 15 minutes of coronary occlusion followed by reperfusion. This transient occlusion resulted in severe postischemic dysfunction, which is characteristic of stunned myocardium.

These studies demonstrate that myocardial uptake of sestamibi closely parallels that of thallium under conditions of low coronary flow and during the period of postischemic regional myocardial dysfunction. In both pathophysiologic conditions, uptake of both tracers was directly proportional to flow.

Conclusion

In summary, it would appear that both thallium and sestamibi comply with the requirements for viability tracers. Their uptake is severely (thallium) or almost totally (sestamibi) depressed in nonviable cells. In low-flow myocardial areas, redistribution allows for incremental uptake of these tracers with the passage of time, although this phenomenon is quantitatively more important with thallium than with sestamibi.

Clinical Assessment of Myocardial Viability with Thallium-201

On basis of the favorable physiological characteristics demonstrated by animal experiments, the ability of thallium to delineate viable myocardium has been extensively studied in clinical practice and its advantages and disadvantages have now been well established. Although rest–redistribution thallium imaging may be adequate to assess myocardial viability, many clinical situations require the simultaneous assessment of both myocardial viability and exercise-induced ischemia, necessitating stress studies.

Stress–Early Redistribution Thallium Imaging

At first, two separate injections of thallium were given to study myocardial blood flow at peak exercise and at rest. After the initial report on redistribution of thallium by Pohost et al.,[13] however, stress and 3 to 4 hour redistribution imaging became the accepted standard. Redistribution of thallium, even in asynergic regions, was shown to predict improvement of regional contraction after revascularization, consistent with the presence of myocardial viability.

However, the *absence* of redistribution does not necessarily indicate myocardial scar because severely ischemic but viable myocardium as well as admixture of scar and viable myocardium may also produce an irreversible thallium defect. Blood et al.[29] and Ritchie et al.[30] found discordant results between conventional redistribution images (in which defects were present in 56%) and images acquired soon after resting injection (defects present in 32%). Moreover, Gibson et al.,[31] using quantitative planar imaging,

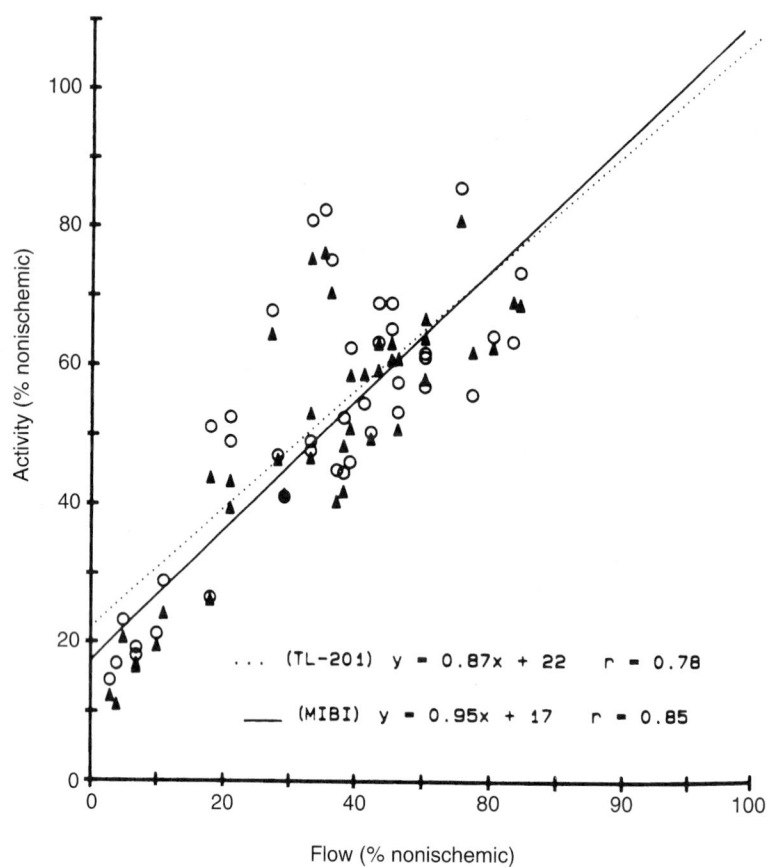

Fig. 20-2. Correlation of thallium-201 (open circles) and technetium-99m sestamibi (closed triangles) activity and stenotic flow among endocardial segments in which stenotic flow was reduced to 60% of preocclusion flow. (From Sinusas et al.,[19] with permission.)

showed that 45% of segments designated as irreversible on conventional redistribution images improved thallium uptake after coronary artery bypass grafting. Of note, segments that were likely to improve had greater than 50% of the thallium activity of normal regions (Fig. 20-3). In patients subjected to percutaneous transluminal coronary angioplasty, Liu et al.[32] and Manyari et al.[33] found 75% to 83% of segments with irreversible or only partially reversible thallium defects to have qualitatively normal thallium activity after successful intervention. Underestimation of myocardial viability with 3 to 4 hour redistribution imaging was further corroborated by metabolic studies using positron emission tomography (PET) and FDG as tracer. In small numbers of patients, 38% to 58% of myocardial regions with irreversible thallium defects were found to represent metabolically viable myocardium.[34–36]

These data suggest that 3 to 4 hour redistribution following stress injection frequently underestimates the presence of viable myocardium, and, therefore, the potential for recovery following revascularization. Recognizing these limitations, investigators have pursued two separate approaches to improve the accuracy of thallium imaging to identify myocardial viability: late redistribution imaging and reinjection imaging.

Stress–Late Redistribution Thallium Imaging

The first approach to overcome the low sensitivity of 3 to 4 hour thallium redistribution is to allow a longer time for redistribution to occur by repeating

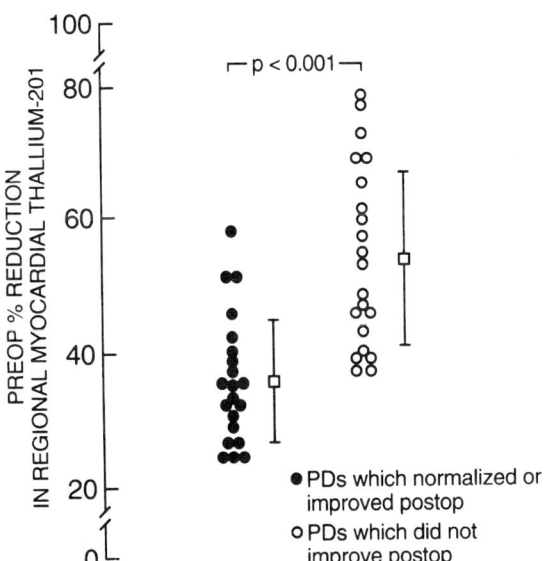

Fig. 20-3. Relationship between preoperative redistribution thallium activity (expressed in percent reduction) in segments with persistent defects (PD) 4 hours after stress injection and the postrevascularization perfusion pattern. Only 3 segments showing more than 50% reduction in thallium activity demonstrated improvement after surgery. (From Gibson et al.,[31] with permission.)

imaging at 8 to 24 hours after the stress imaging. In this protocol, three sets of images are acquired: early, 4-hour delayed, and late (8 to 24 hours). Gutman et al.,[37] using planar imaging, found that 21% of segments with irreversible defects on 3 to 4 hour images showed redistribution on images taken at 18 to 24 hours after injection. These segments were typically subserved by severely stenosed but patent coronary arteries. Cloninger et al.,[38] using SPECT, found further redistribution at 24 hour in 46% of patients with prior Q-wave infarction and in 92% of patients without previous infarction. In that study, none of the segments showing late reversibility was completely irreversible at 3 to 4 hours after injection. Kiat and colleagues,[39] however, found similar results in completely irreversible thallium defects: 61% of such irreversible segments on 3 to 4 hour images demonstrated redistribution at 18 to 72 hours. Since late imaging may have been performed preferentially in patients with anginal symptoms or exercise-induced electrocardiographic abnormalities, the high frequency of late reversibility might have been explained in part by selection bias. Therefore, the same group determined the frequency of late redistribution in a nonselected population consisting of 118 consecutive patients with CAD and irreversible defects at 4 hours.[40] Late redistribution occurred in 22% of segments (in 53% of the patients) with defects that were irreversible at 4 hour.

Late redistribution occurs because the initial uptake of thallium during exercise may be sufficiently reduced that the defect remains even after 3 or 4 hours. The passage of greater time until redistribution imaging allows for continued perfusion of the defect with thallium and resolution of the lower level of activity compared with a normal zone (viable regions from myocardial scar). On the other hand, the rate of thallium delivery may be reduced during the redistribution period in regions supplied by critically stenosed coronary arteries. Thus, late redistribution, when present, is an accurate indicator of viable myocardium. In the study by Kiat et al.,[39] 95% of segments with late redistribution showed improved function after revascularization. However, 37% of segments that remained irreversible after 4 and 24 hours also improved after revascularization, indicating limited negative predictive value of this protocol. These data indicate that although late thallium imaging improves the identification of viable myocardium, it continues to overstimate the frequency and severity of myocardial fibrosis.

Reinjection Thallium Imaging

Thallium reinjection, as described by Dilsizian and colleagues at the National Institutes of Health,[41] may demonstrate additional defect reversibility following a small dose of thallium reinjected immediately after the 3 to 4 hour redistribution image (Fig. 20-4). As previously pointed out, thallium redistribution depends not only on the severity of the initial defect but also on the continuing delivery of thallium over the subsequent 3 to 4 hours. If the blood thallium concentration decreases during this interval, the delivery of thallium may be insufficient and the thallium defect may remain irreversible despite underlying viable myocardium, even after 24 hours, unless the serum thallium concentration is augmented. Indeed, Kayden et al.[42] found that 39% of segments (in 44% of patients) that were irreversible after 4

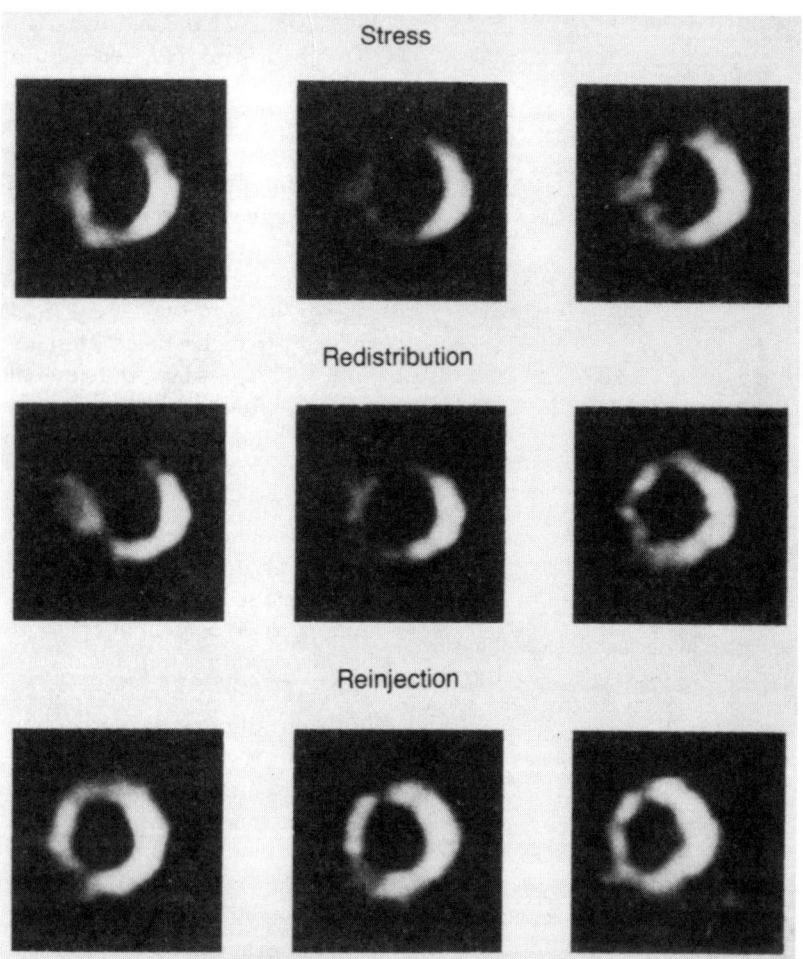

Fig. 20-4. Short axis thallium tomograms at stress, redistribution, and reinjection imaging in a patient with coronary artery disease. Extensive thallium abnormalities in the anterior and septal regions during stress persist on the 3 to 4 hour redistribution images but improved markedly on reinjection images. (From Dilsizian et al.,[41] with permission.)

and after 24 hours improved thallium uptake after reinjection.

The use of a postreinjection image offers information on segmental blood flow at rest relative to that during stress. Reinjection enhances thallium activity in 31% to 49% of regions with irreversible defects on the 3 to 4 hour redistribution images.[41,43-45] After revascularization, 80% to 87% of such regions showed increased thallium uptake during exercise or improved resting regional wall motion, indicating viability.[41,45] In contrast, regions that remained irreversible after reinjection showed improved regional function after revascularization in only 0% to 18% (Table 20-1). The stress–redistribution–reinjection protocol has also been compared to metabolic imaging with positron emission tomography, using FDG as a tracer. By means of thallium reinjection, Tamaki et al.[46] identified viable myocardium in 42% of regions that were irreversible at 3 to 4 hours after injection; in their study the concordance with PET was 85%. All regions that were reversible on reinjection were confirmed to be metabolically viable by PET, but 25% of irreversible segments also showed viability by PET. A study of 16 patients who underwent

Table 20-1. Predictive Accuracy for Functional Improvement Using Various Thallium Imaging Protocols

Reference	Method	Segments (Patients)	Predictive Accuracy (%)		
			Positive	Negative	Overall
Kiat et al. (1988)[39]	Stress–late redistribution (SPECT)	201 (21)	90	63	83
Dilsizian et al. (1990)[41]	Stress–redistribution–reinjection (SPECT)	23 (20)	87	100	91
Ohtani et al. (1990)[45]	Stress–redistribution–reinjection (SPECT	61 (24)	89	50	74
Tamaki et al. (1991)[46]	Stress–redistribution–reinjection (SPECT)	56 (11)	79	75	79
Mori et al. (1991)[54]	Rest–redistribution (planar imaging)	51 (17)	79	62	67
Marzullo et al. (1993)[62]	Rest–redistribution (planar imaging)	75 (14)	95	77	88
Ragosta et al. (1993)[55]	Rest–redistribution (planar imaging)	176 (21)	57	77	61
Udelson et al. (1994)[63]	Rest–redistribution (SPECT)	45 (18)	75	92	85
Total		689 (146)	78.4	71.0	76.1

Abbreviations: SPECT, single-photon emission computed tomography.

both PET and thallium reinjection[47] has emphasized the importance of quantitative analysis of thallium activity. In irreversible defects with only mild-to-moderate reduction in thallium activity (defined as 50% to 85% of peak activity), metabolic activity was present in 88%. In irreversible defects with severe reduction in thallium activity (<50% of peak activity), PET as well as thallium reinjection indicated viability in 51% of segments. In this study, PET and reinjection thallium were concordant regarding the presence of viable or nonviable myocardium in 88% of segments. Other studies have confirmed that the level of regional thallium activity in reinjection images is significantly related to the mass of preserved viable myocytes. Zimmermann et al.[48] found a significant correlation between relative thallium activity and the amount of interstitial fibrosis on transmural biopsies obtained during coronary artery bypass grafting in 37 patients.

Dilsizian and co-workers[49] found that little is to be gained from an additional acquisition at 24 hours after reinjection. In 50 patients with stable CAD, they found that only 11% of segments (in only 6% of patients) that remained irreversible after both 3 to 4 hour redistribution and reinjection showed late redistribution. However, there *is* a need for at least one redistribution study in the thallium imaging protocol.[50] In 50 patients, the same group acquired stress, 3 to 4 hour redistribution, reinjection, and late (24-hour) redistribution images. Among perfusion defects that redistributed at 3 to 4 hours, 25% appeared irreversible when only stress and reinjection images were compared. However, 24-hour images obtained after reinjection demonstrated further redistribution in these regions resulting in relative thallium activities indistinguishable from those on the 3 to 4 hour images (Fig. 20-5). Hence, elimination of the 3 to 4 hour redistribution images or the late redistribution images would incorrectly assign 25% of reversible thallium defects as irreversible and scarred. The apparent washout of such defects after reinjection results from smaller increases of thallium activity within the ischemic regions than in normal regions (presumably a consequence of low flow to the ischemic region).

To alleviate the logistic strains of acquiring three different sets of images, it has been suggested that thallium be reinjected immediately after acquisition of the stress images, thus saving the performance of one set of images. This way, both the stress and early reinjected thallium doses would be allowed to redistribute over the next 3 to 4 hours. The image subsequently obtained would combine the information of the 3 to 4 hour redistribution and reinjection studies. However, with one study in favor,[51] and another with unfavorable results,[52] this protocol remains controversial.

Rest–Redistribution Thallium Imaging

When the clinical question pertains only to the viability of a myocardial region, and not to the presence of inducible ischemia, stressing the heart is not really

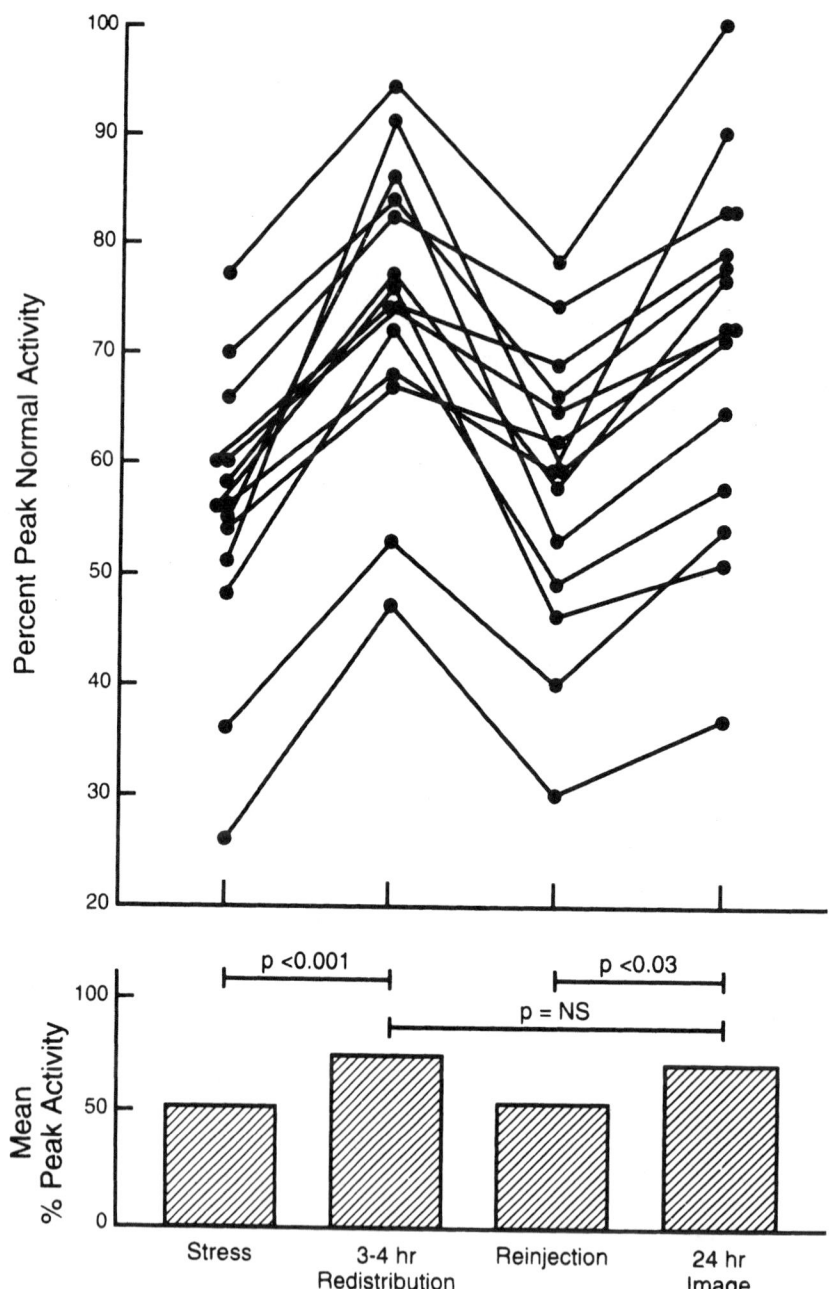

Fig. 20-5. Plot of regional thallium activity in regions demonstrating the phenomenon of apparent thallium washout caused by low differential uptake. If the 3 to 4 hour redistribution images were eliminated and the reinjection images were acquired alone, these regions would be incorrectly assigned to be irreversible. On the 24-hour images, redistribution is again apparent, indicating reversibility of the defect, and the relative thallium activity is similar to that observed on the 3 to 4 hour redistribution studies. (From Dilsizian et al.[50] with permission.)

necessary and rest–redistribution thallium imaging may be the procedure of choice.

Iskandrian et al.[53] examined the value of rest–redistribution thallium imaging in predicting improvement in left ventricular ejection fraction (LVEF) after coronary bypass surgery (Plate 20-1). Of 14 patients with left ventricular dysfunction at rest and normal thallium studies or reversible thallium abnormalities, 12 patients (86%) improved left ventricular function after surgery. In contrast, only 2 of the 9 patients (22%) with left ventricular dysfunction and irreversible thallium defects improved function after surgery. In the study by Mori et al.,[54] 79% of asynergic regions with thallium rest–redistribution improved wall motion after revascularization, but 38% of asynergic regions without thallium redistribution before surgery also showed improved wall motion after surgery. However, the severity of the irreversible thallium defect was not quantified in that study.

Improved results have been obtained with quantitative analysis in which the severity of reduction in thallium activity is considered within irreversible rest–redistribution thallium defects. In a recent study by Ragosta et al.,[55] 21 patients with severe left ventricular dysfunction underwent rest–redistribution planar thallium imaging and regional wall motion analysis prior to and 2 months after coronary bypass surgery. In that study the following criteria for viability were used: (1) normal initial thallium uptake, (2) initial defect of any magnitude showing delayed redistribution, and (3) mild (>50% of maximum) fixed defect. Severe reduction in viability was defined as a persistent defect with thallium activity less than 50% of maximal activity. Among severely asynergic regions showing normal flow, 62% improved ventricular function 2 months after coronary artery bypass grafting. In contrast, 54% of those with mildly reduced viability and only 23% of segments with a pattern of severely reduced viability improved function (Fig. 20-6). When only adequately revascularized segments were considered, the predictive

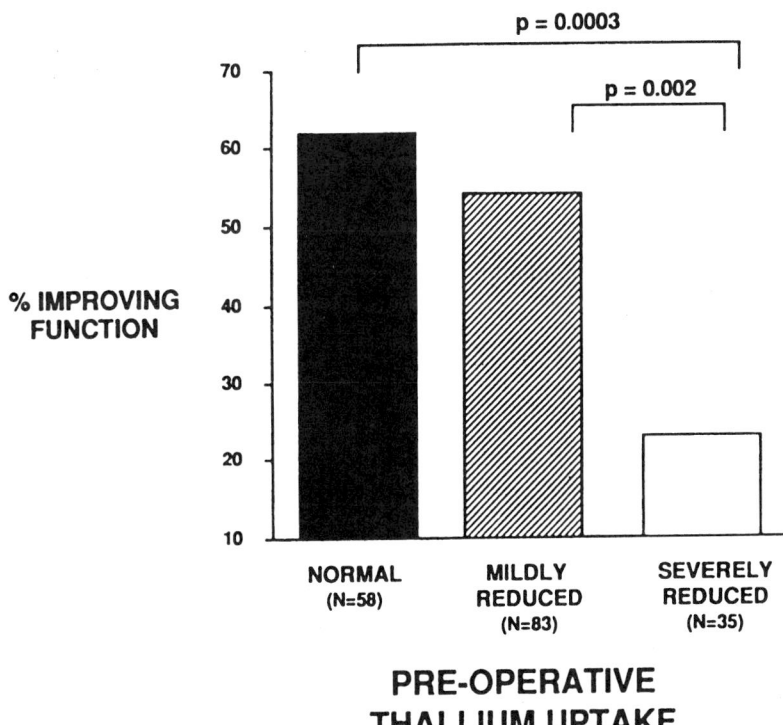

Fig. 20-6. Relationship between improvement in regional function after coronary artery bypass surgery and preoperative thallium uptake in segments with severe asynergy. (From Ragosta et al.,[55] with permission.)

value of a positive preoperative viability scan for segmental functional improvement was 73%. The greater the number of viable segments, the greater the improvement in global left ventricular function after operation. In patients with more than 7 viable, asynergic segments, mean LVEF rose by more than 12% after operation, whereas in patients with 7 or less such segments, no significant changes in LVEF were observed.

Dilsizian and co-workers[56] compared stress–redistribution–reinjection with rest–redistribution in 41 patients. In defects that were irreversible on conventional 4-hour redistribution images, concordant data on myocardial viability were obtained by these two methods in 79% of defects. Twenty patients also underwent PET with oxygen-15 water and FDG. In these patients stress–redistribution–reinjection and rest–redistribution provided concordant results in 72% of all segments. When thallium defects with mild to moderate reduction in activity (51% to 85%) were regrouped as viable, concordance improved to 94%. These data indicate that stress–redistribution–reinjection and rest–redistribution protocols are equivalent for the detection of viable myocardium.

Additional Protocols to Improve Detection of Myocardial Viability with Thallium

Other protocols have been proposed to enhance the detection of myocardial viability with thallium. Infusion of ribose, an adenine nucleotide precursor that possibly stimulates sodium–potassium ATPase, has been shown to result in faster thallium redistribution after transient ischemia in a swine model.[57] In a pilot study on 17 patients with CAD, Perlmutter et al.[58] identified nearly twice as many reversible thallium defects at both 1 and 4 hours postexercise when patients received intravenous ribose infusion during the redistribution period, compared to saline infusion.

The use of nitrates along with reinjection has been shown to improve thallium uptake in ischemic myocardium, and hence the detection of myocardial viability. In a study by He et al.,[59] 20 patients underwent two exercise and 4-hour redistribution thallium SPECT protocols, one with reinjection alone and the other with reinjection and 20 mg isosorbide dinitrate given immediately after postexercise imaging. Fifteen patients had reversible defects with reinjection alone, and three additional patients were defined as ischemic with the nitrate reinjection protocol.

Summary: Assessing Myocardial Viability with Thallium-201

The studies discussed above have outlined criteria to assess myocardial viability with thallium imaging. The criteria for viability reflect regional tracer tissue kinetics. The initial tracer uptake reflects regional myocardial blood flow. For delayed imaging, time is allowed for tracer equilibration between myocardium and blood pool; late images reflect the intracellular myocardial potassium pool. This must be distinguished from the reinjection approach, which is used often in conjunction with stress imaging protocols and where the postreinjection images provide information on the regional blood flow at rest relative to that during stress.

The presence of viable myocardium is associated with normal tracer uptake, completely or partially reversible defects, and fixed defects that are mild or moderate. Pooled data from 8 clinical studies encompassing a total of 689 segments in 146 patients (Table 20-1) show a positive predictive value of 78% and a negative predictive value of 71%, for an overall accuracy of 76% for functional improvement following coronary revascularization.

The optimal protocol to assess myocardial viability with thallium imaging depends on the clinical question to be addressed. If the question is one of myocardial viability alone in a patients with poor left ventricular function, it seems logical not to use a stress imaging protocol, but directly to inject the tracer at rest. Stress testing, however, provides a more comprehensive assessment of the extent and severity of CAD by demonstrating both reversible myocardial ischemia and viability. In this setting, two imaging options provide comparable information for identifying most of the ischemic but viable myocardium: stress–early redistribution–reinjection or stress–reinjection–late redistribution imaging. Not all patients require each of the three sets of studies, however, and the sequence can be stopped as soon as one of the criteria for viability is met.

Clinical Assessment of Myocardial Viability with Technetium-99m Sestamibi

In spite of data from relevant animal models of low-flow ischemia demonstrating that regional thallium activity and sestamibi activity are comparable at multiple time points after resting injection, the first human studies on the use of sestamibi for delineation of viable myocardium seemed rather disappointing. Rocco et al.[60] found by qualitative visual analysis on planar images that more than 25% of segments with markedly reduced sestamibi activity after resting injection exhibited preserved wall motion. However, analogous to the concept that quantitative analysis of thallium content within irreversible defects accurately discriminates viable from nonviable myocardium, quantitative uptake of sestamibi in territories with markedly reduced uptake was significantly higher in normal or hypokinetic segments (62 ± 15%) than in akinetic segments (39 ± 16%). Cuocolo et al.[61] compared a 2-day stress–rest sestamibi protocol with thallium stress–redistribution–reinjection in 20 patients with previous myocardial infarction and severe left ventricular dysfunction. Analysis of planar images was qualitative, by a five-point grading system. Among the 122 myocardial segments with irreversible defects on standard 4-hour redistribution images, 47% demonstrated increased (by at least one grade) thallium uptake after reinjection, whereas only 18% were reversible on the rest sestamibi study. These data suggest that myocardial regions with *severe* reduction of sestamibi uptake both on stress and rest images may contain viable myocardium. Unfortunately, this study had important shortcomings; first, the absence of quantification of tracer uptake, and second, the absence of functional data and follow-up, enhanced uptake of thallium after reinjection being arbitrarily chosen as a golden standard.

Prediction for Functional Recovery after Revascularization

Studies examining the prediction of viable myocardium using sestamibi are summarized in Table 20-2. Marzullo et al.[62] investigated 14 patients with left ventricular dysfunction at rest due to previous myocardial infarction. Planar rest–redistribution thallium images were quantitatively compared with planar sestamibi images at rest. All patients underwent revascularization and functional outcome was assessed by echocardiography before and after intervention. The average percent activity of delayed thallium and sestamibi in viable and nonviable segments was similar for the two tracers: 67 ± 9% versus 67 ± 13% and 46 ± 6% versus 48 ± 10%, respectively. The sensitivity and specificity to predict functional recovery after revascularization were 86% and 92% for delayed thallium imaging, and 75% and 84% for sestamibi, respectively.

Udelson et al.[63] performed quantitative comparisons of rest and redistribution thallium activity and sestamibi activity 1 hour after rest injection on short-axis tomograms obtained in 31 patients with CAD and left ventricular dysfunction. Quantitative analysis for all segments showed significant correlation between regional thallium redistribution activity and sestamibi activity in individual segments. Eighteen of these patients were revascularized. Segments exhibiting significant regional ventricular dysfunction before revascularization were classified as having reversible or irreversible dysfunction, based on the comparison of wall motion and thickening at preoperative and postoperative two-demensional echocardiography. Thallium and sestamibi regional activities were similar in those segments with reversible (72 ± 11% vs. 75 ± 9%, respectively) as well as irreversible ventricular dysfunction (51 ± 11% vs. 50 ± 8%) (Fig. 20-7). The probability of a scintigraphic segment representing viable myocardium was related to the magnitude of regional activity (Fig. 20-8). Using a 60% threshold cutoff point, the sensitivity (88% for thallium vs. 94% for sestamibi) and specific-

Table 20-2. Predictive Accuracy for Functional Improvement Using Various Sestamibi Imaging Protocols

Reference	Method	Segments (Patients)	Predictive accuracy (%)		
			Positive	Negative	Overall
Marzullo et al. (1993)[62]	Rest (planar imaging)	75 (14)	90	65	79
Udelson et al. (1994)[63]	Rest (SPECT)	45 (18)	84	96	91
Bisi et al. (1994)[67]	Rest–nitrates (SPECT)	45 (19)	91	88	89
Total		166 (51)	88.7	82.1	84.9

Abbreviations: SPECT, single-photon emission computed tomography.

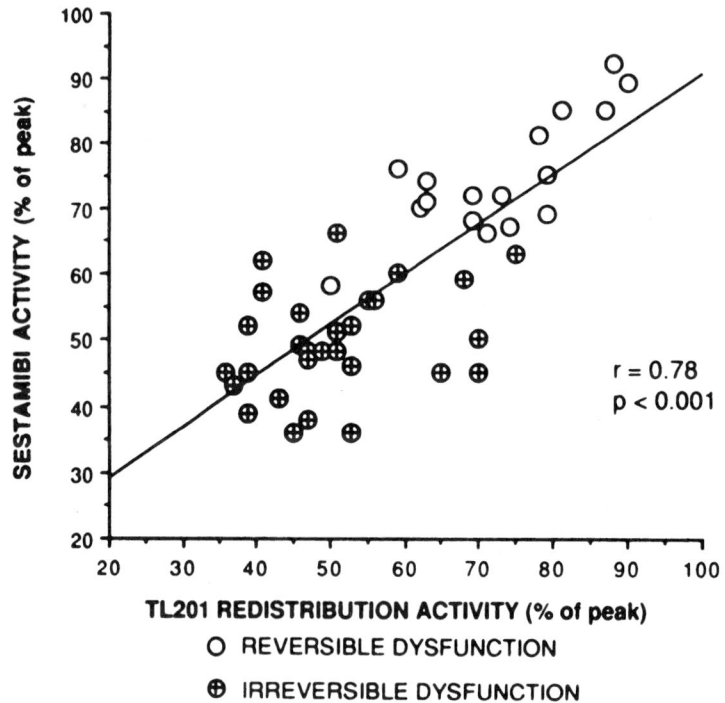

Fig. 20-7. Correlation of quantitative regional activities of thallium (at redistribution imaging) and regional activities of sestamibi among segments with significant regional dysfunction in patients undergoing revascularization. Open circles, reversible dysfunction, circles with plus, irreversible dysfunction. (From Udelson et al.,[63] with permission.)

ity (83% vs. 86%, respectively) for predicting recovery of regional ventricular dysfunction after revascularization were similar for the two agents.

These two studies demonstrate that quantitative analysis of regional activities of both thallium and sestamibi after resting injection can differentiate viable from nonviable myocardium. The two agents predict reversibility of significant regional wall motion abnormalities after revascularization in such patients with a similar level of accuracy.

Correlation of Sestamibi Results with Metabolic Activity at PET

Two studies have compared the results of sestamibi with PET imaging for the prediction of viable myocardium. Sawada et al.[64] studied a rather heterogeneous group of 20 patients who were from 3 weeks to more than 6 months postmyocardial infarction, including 6 patients with previous coronary artery grafts, and 3 others with previous coronary angioplasty. Patients underwent rest sestamibi imaging and PET using FDG as tracer. For the purpose of this study, regional FDG uptake greater than 60% peak activity was defined as metabolic evidence for tissue viability. Fifty-three percent of segments with moderate sestamibi defects (activity 50% to 59% of peak) and 47% of segments with severe sestamibi defects (activity < 50% of peak) had metabolic evidence for tissue viability. Evidence of viability was still present in 50% of segments with sestamibi activity less than 40%. Within the group of segments with severe defects, there was no significant difference in the mean sestamibi activity in segments with or without metabolic evidence for tissue viability. Although these data clearly indicate *underestimation* of metabolic viability by sestamibi, the authors emphasized that in the majority of patients, viability was underestimated in only one or two segments. Failure to detect small areas of viable myocardium would not affect appreciably clinical decision making in these patients.

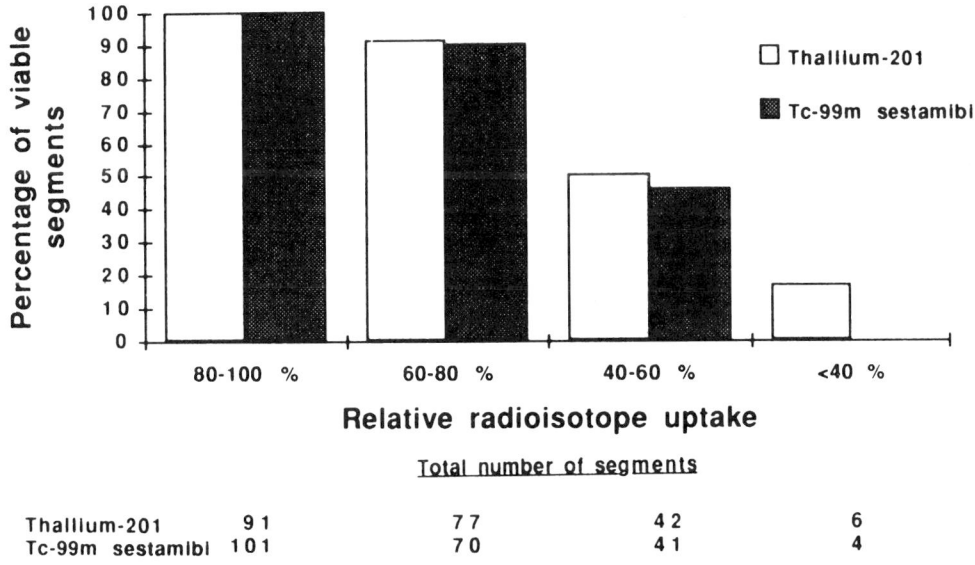

Fig. 20-8. Relationship between the probability that a scintigraphic segment represent viable myocardium (defined by either preserved wall motion or improved wall motion after revascularization) and the magnitude of regional activity for either thallium or sestamibi. (From Udelson et al.,[63] with permission.)

Altehoefer et al.[65] reported a more extensive comparison of rest sestamibi with FDG in 111 patients with stable CAD. Here, the PET study was obtained within 3 days of the sestamibi SPECT. Sestamibi and FDG uptake were normalized to the same reference region, which was the one with maximum sestamibi uptake in the patient. PET separated segments into viable segments (FDG uptake > 70% of peak), nonviable segments (FDG uptake < 50%), and intermediate segments with intermediate uptake values. The repartition of segments into viable and nonviable categories according to the uptake of sestamibi is shown in Figure 20-9. These results concur with those obtained by Udelson et al.,[63] in that prediction of viability is probabilistic rather than deterministic: the probability of viability increases with increasing sestamibi uptake; it is very small in segments with sestamibi less than 40% of peak, and very high in segments with sestamibi more than 70% of peak. This, however, leaves an important gray zone in the middle of the spectrum, in which additional studies are required to assess viability.

Dilsizian et al.[66] investigated 54 patients with chronic stable CAD and left ventricular dysfunction presenting with at least one irreversible perfusion defect on standard stress–redistribution thallium imaging. They underwent stress–redistribution–reinjection thallium imaging and one day rest–stress sestamibi imaging using the same exercise protocol. Segments with abnormal thallium activity at rest were classified as either normal or reversible, or as irreversible by both tracers. Results were concordant in 75% of segments; 23% of segments were discordantly irreversible with sestamibi, and only 2% were discordantly irreversible with thallium. A subgroup of 25 patients also underwent PET metabolic studies with FDG as tracer. Concordancy (70%) and discordancy (30%) in these patients were similar to the overall group. Segments were then divided into those with severe irreversible defects defined as less than 50% peak activity, and those with either reversible or mild to moderate defects. Regrouping the segments this way increased the concordance between thallium and sestamibi studies to 93%. Out of 26 segments that were incorrectly predicted as nonviable on the basis of irreversible sestamibi defects, only 7 had severe sestamibi defects (Fig. 20-10). Again, this study indicates that taking into account the severity of reduction in sestamibi activity enhances the detection of viability.

400 Cardiac Stress Testing and Imaging

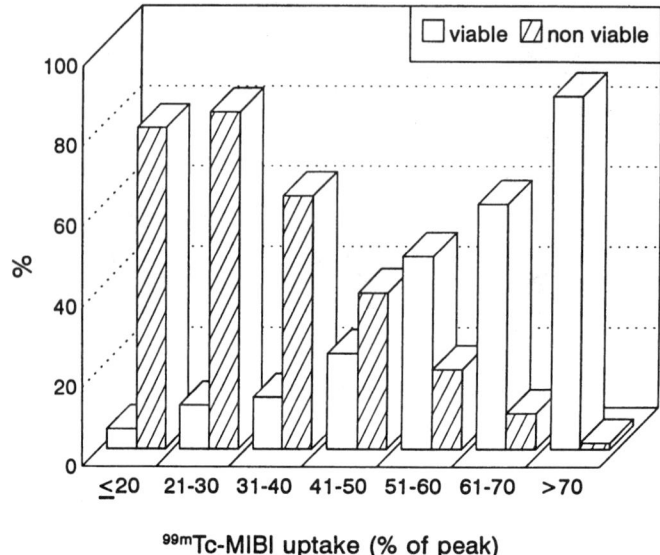

Fig. 20-9. Percentage of viable and nonviable segments according to metabolic positron emission tomography criteria in relation to sestamibi defect severity. (From Altehoefer et al.,[65] with permission.)

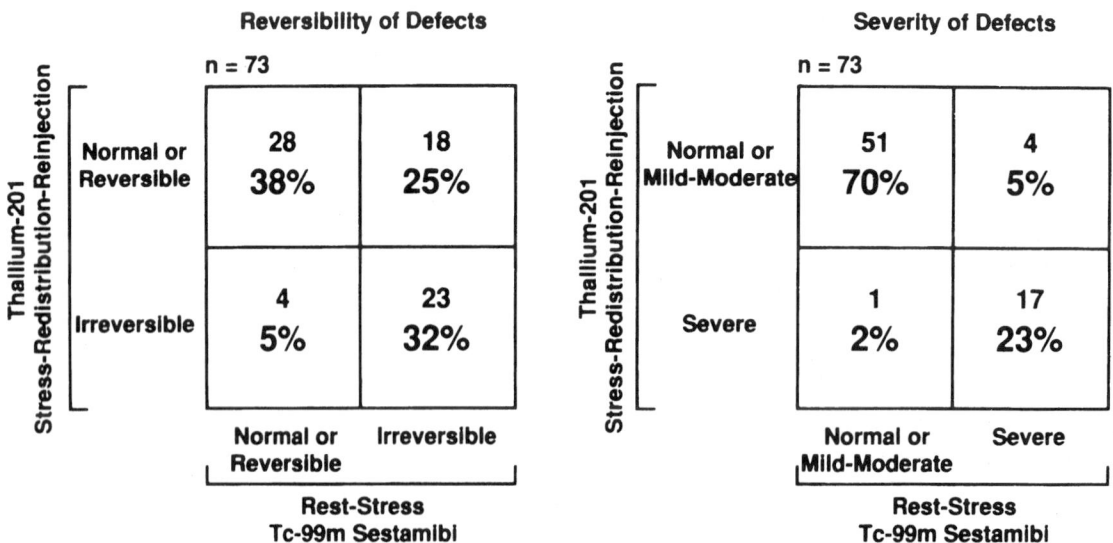

Fig. 20-10. Concordance and discordance between thallium stress–redistribution–reinjection and sestamibi rest–stress images. Reversibility of defects (normal or reversible vs. irreversible) is shown on the left, and severity of defects (normal or mild-to-moderate vs. severe) is shown on the right. (From Dilsizian et al.[66] with permission.)

Additional Protocols to Improve Detection of Myocardial Viability with Sestamibi

The value of redistribution of sestamibi after injection at rest for the prediction of myocardial viability has been addressed by Dilsizian et al.[66] In 18 patients with coronary artery disease and left ventricular dysfunction, a 4-hour sestamibi redistribution image was acquired after injection at rest. Using these redistribution images, concordance with stress–redistribution–reinjection thallium imaging was increased from 71% to 82%; 6 of 16 segments with normal or improving thallium activity but irreversible sestamibi defects on standard 1-hour sestamibi images showed reversibility after 4 hours.

A further method to enhance detection of viable myocardium has recently been proposed by Bisi et al.[67] They performed quantitative sestamibi SPECT at baseline and during isosorbide dinitrate infusion in 19 patients with a previous myocardial infarction and left ventricular dysfunction. In patients who recovered regional function after revascularization, nitrate infusion induced a reduction ($-37.4\% \pm 21.6\%$) in the extent of the global uptake defect. In contrast, in patients without functional recovery after revascularization, no change or a slight increase ($+5.8\% \pm 8.4\%$) was observed. The nitrate-induced changes in the extent of the uptake defect correlated with postrevascularization changes in ejection fraction. The uptake of sestamibi improved after nitrate administration in all 10 viable territories, but only in 4 of 34 territories considered as nonviable.

Summary: Assessing Myocardial Viability with Sestamibi

As of now, it would appear that sestamibi is a challenging alternative to thallium for viability delineation in patients with CAD and left ventricular dysfunction, provided that quantitation is performed, that redistribution images are acquired after rest injection, or that tracer administration takes place after nitrate administration. Pooled data from three clinical studies (Table 20-2) show a positive predictive value of 89%, negative predictive value of 82%, and overall accuracy of 85% for functional improvement following revascularization. These values compare favorably with the corresponding figures for thallium. However, the reader should be aware that the accuracy of sestamibi as a marker of viability has only been tested in a limited number of segments in an equally limited number of patients: functional follow-up has been reported in only 51 patients to date.

Conclusion: Assessment of Myocardial Viability with Flow Tracers

In the 197 patients in whom functional follow-up has been obtained after initial viability studies with either thallium-201 or technetium-99m sestamibi (Tables 20-1 and 20-2), an overall accuracy of 78% was obtained with a positive predictive value of 80% and a negative predictive value of 74%. Caution is warranted on the use of these values, however. First, the majority of studies have included *segments with normal function* along with dysfunctional segments. This enhances the predictive value for recovery of function. The clinical issue of viability is important only in asynergic areas, however, and hence, it would be more practical to define predictive values exclusively in such segments. Second, emphasis has been placed on recovery of segmental function, and it remains difficult to know how the use of flow tracers in viability studies would affect management on a patient basis. This is important as the extent of viable tissue is an important consideration in the decision to perform revascularization.

Three key points have emerged from recent publications on myocardial viability using flow tracers. First, quantitative analysis of defect severity dramatically enhances predictive accuracies. Second, sufficient amounts of tracer must be present and a sufficiently long time span has to be allowed, in order for the tracer to be able to reach all viable myocardial cells, even those in low-flow areas. Third, data presented have supported the concept of the probabilistic, rather than deterministic, character of the prediction of viability. In the continuum of probabilities of viability, a large group of intermediate values exists in between the extremely low and the extremely high values. In segments with such intermediate probabilities of viability based on flow tracer studies, the question arises whether metabolic imaging may not discriminate more precisely between viable myocardium and scar tissue.

In this context, looking into the ability of flow tracer studies to predict the outcome of metabolic PET studies, may shed some light on the potential

Table 20-3. Predictive Accuracy for Preserved Metabolic Activity on PET Using Thallium Imaging

Reference	Method	Segments (Patients)	Predictive Accuracy (%)		
			Positive	Negative	Overall
Tamaki (1991)[46]	Stress–redistribution–reinjection (SPECT)	95 (18)	100	75	93
Bonow et al. (1991)[47]	Stress–redistribution–reinjection (SPECT)	166 (16)	88	49	72
Dilsizian et al. (1994)[66]	Stress–redistribution–reinjection (SPECT)	73 (20)	93	56	79
Total		334 (54)	92.9	56.1	79.3

Abbreviations: PET, position emission tomography; SPECT, single-photon emission computed tomography.

of metabolic imaging to provide additional information on myocardial viability (Tables 20-3 and 20-4). Pooled data show rather adequate positive predictive values of 93% for thallium-201 and 83% for sestamibi, but deceivingly low negative predictive values of 56% and 53%, respectively. The low negative predictive values indicate that about one out of two segments categorized by flow tracers as low probability of viability, nevertheless, show metabolic activity with PET.

METABOLIC TRACERS

Basic Principles

The primary substrates for energy metabolism in the myocardium are long-chain fatty acids and glucose. The selection of these depends on energy demand, substrate supply, and oxygen availability for oxidative phosphorylation. Under fasting conditions, 60% to 70% of the metabolic needs of the myocytes are met by β-oxidation of fatty acids. Following their uptake into the cell, probably by active transport rather than passive diffusion, fatty acids are first activated by binding to coenzyme A. This energy-dependent process is irreversible. Fatty acids are then either utilized for the synthesis of various lipids and stored into the intracellular lipid pool, or are tranported via the carnitine shuttle into the mitochondria where they are rapidly catabolized.

The global effect of cardiac ischemia on myocardial fatty acid turnover is a reduction of uptake that is due to the conjunction of reduced perfusion, reduced transport capability due to release of fatty acid binding proteins from the cell during ischemia, and a temporary inhibition of oxidation resulting from limited oxygen supply. Concomitant changes are an increase in back-diffusion of fatty acids, an increase of storage in tissue lipids, mainly triglycerides, and an increase in glucose utilization.

Although technetium-99m is most widely used for scintigraphic work with the gamma camera in practice, it is unfortunately not well suited for metabolic imaging, since it does not covalently bind to carbon, nitrogen, or oxygen in organic molecules. The radionuclide iodine-123 at present appears to be the preferred choice for labeling metabolic substrates.

Iodine-123 Free Fatty Acids

Interest in the clinical use of iodine-123-labeled fatty acids is currently primarily focused on 15-(p-iodophenyl)pentadecanoic acid (IPPA) and "modified" fatty acid analogs such as 15-(p-iodophenyl)-3R,S-

Table 20-4. Predictive Accuracy for Preserved Metabolic Activity on PET Using Sestamibi Imaging

Reference	Method	Segments (Patients)	Predictive Accuracy (%)		
			Positive	Negative	Overall
Sawada et al. (1994)[64]	Sestamibi rest (SPECT)	153 (20)	73	53	69
Altehoefer et al. (1994)[65]	Sestamibi rest (SPECT)	713 (111)	86	53	72
Total		866 (131)	83.1	53.2	71.7

Abbreviations: PET, position emission tomography; SPECT, single-photon emission computed tomography.

methylpentadecanoic acid (BMIPP). Although the physiological basis is not completely understood, differences between regional fatty acid uptake and flow tracer distribution may reflect alterations in important parameters of metabolism that can be useful for patient management or planning therapy. These tracers may also represent unique metabolic probes for correlation of energy substrate metabolism with regional myocardial viability using SPECT.

Iodophenylpentadecanoic Acid

Until the last decade, studies had focused on the use of iodine-123-labeled straight-chain fatty acids, such as 17-iodoheptadecanoic acid (IHA), most of which are rapidly metabolized, requiring the use of sequential planar imaging to generate time-activity curves of regions of interest. Because of the rapid appearance of free [^{123}I]-iodine in the blood released from metabolism of the IHA tracer, special correction procedures involving the intravenous administration of [^{123}I]-sodium iodide were required to differentiate the myocardium from free blood activity. Because of inability to perform SPECT, the number of clinical studies with IHA has been limited.[68]

To stabilize the iodine-123 attached to the fatty acid to overcome the rapid loss of free iodide, ω-phenyl-substituted straight-chain fatty acids analogs were developed by Machulla and co-workers[69] as an alternative for myocardial metabolic studies with SPECT. The analog that has received the most attention is IPPA, in which the iodine radiolabel is attached to the *para* position of the terminal phenyl ring (Fig. 20-11). The amount of free iodide in the blood pool and soft tissue by metabolism of IPPA is very limited.

Myocardial Uptake and Metabolism of IPPA

Studies using Langendorf perfused rat hearts have demonstrated that IPPA behaves similarly to the physiological substrate palmitic acid (Fig. 20-12).[70] The uptake of IPPA is linearly correlated with blood flow over a wide spectrum (from very low flow to five times normal).[71] The metabolism of IPPA is linked to myocardial oxygen supply and consumption. The catabolism of IPPA follows the normal biochemical pathways for fatty acids, including activation by coenzyme A, transfer by carnitine into the mitochondria, and rapid β-oxidation with a half-time of 11

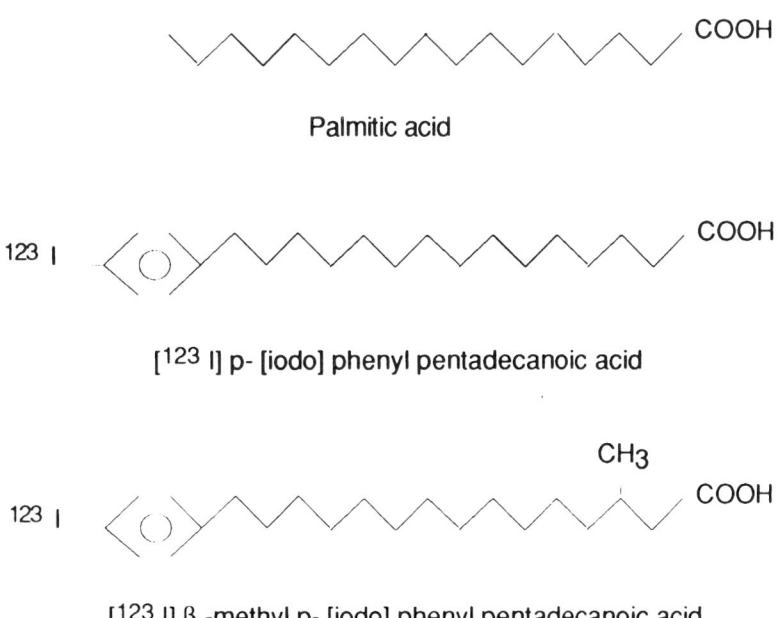

Fig. 20-11. Structure of palmitic acid and fatty acid analogs iodophenylpentadecanoic acid (IPPA) and β-methyliodophenylpentadecanoic acid (BMIPP) used for myocardial imaging.

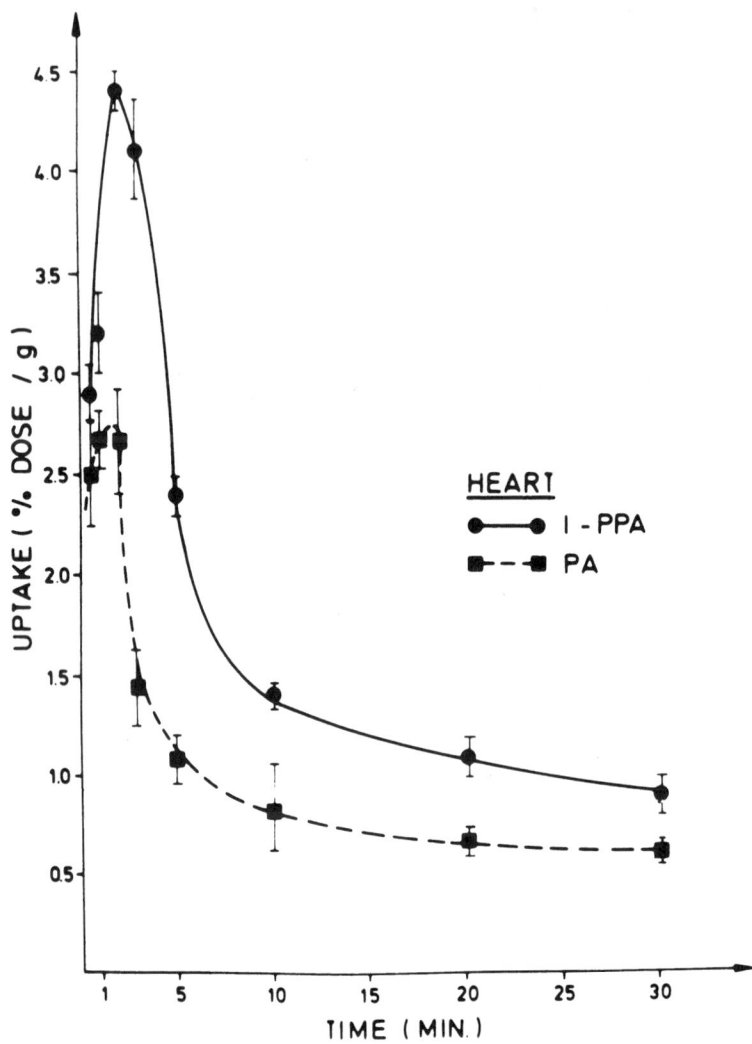

Fig. 20-12. Cardiac uptake of 15-(p-iodophenyl) pentadecanoic acid (IPPA) compared to the physiological substrate palmitic acid (PA) in an animal model. (From Reske et al.,[70] with permission.)

minutes to iodobenzoic acid. Iodobenzoic acid is then rapidly released from tissue into blood and is subsequently excreted rapidly via the kidneys in the form of hippuric acid so that catabolite recirculation becomes minimal and does not interfere with external measurement of myocardial lipid turnover. A portion of IPPA is metabolized more slowly with a half-time of 76 minutes, reflecting the fraction of IPPA that is incorporated into phospholipid and triglyceride pools and is subsequently also metabolized.

Assessment of Myocardial Viability with IPPA

The rationale of using IPPA imaging in the assessment of myocardial viability depends on the assumption that the uptake and washout of IPPA reflect myocardial blood flow and oxidation metabolism. IPPA uptake and oxidation are both reduced during myocardial ischemia. IPPA clearance in infarcted areas is significantly prolonged when compared to normal myocardium.[72] The differential washout from normal, ischemic, and infarcted myocardium has been exploited to characterize the myocardium, first in animal experiments, and later also in patients. Rellas and co-workers[73] were able to differentiate reversible and irreversible tissue damage by means of sequential IPPA-SPECT imaging of dogs with acute ischemia and reperfusion. Similar findings were reported by Reske et al.,[74] who found in an occlusion–reperfusion swine heart model that IPPA uptake was preserved in reversible ischemic viable tissue but severely reduced in irreversibly damaged myocardium.

Only a few studies have been published regarding the efficacy of IPPA for the identification of viable myocardium in patients. In an early study by Hansen et al.[75] comparing IPPA-SPECT with thallium SPECT for the detection of CAD, both approaches provided comparable sensitivities for the diagnosis of CAD. IPPA-SPECT was superior to thallium SPECT, however, for detecting reversible defects indicative of myocardial ischemia or potential viability. Kuikka et al.[76] evaluated 31 patients with CAD (25 patients with previous myocardial infarction) and at least one fixed perfusion defect on the rest–stress sestamibi study. Of the 57 segments showing persistent perfusion defects with sestamibi, 14 segments (25%) had a normal IPPA uptake and 22 segments (39%) showed a partial IPPA uptake indicating residual metabolically active myocardium. The remaining 21 segments (36%) showed no IPPA uptake. Unfortunately, no follow-up studies after revascularization were available in these studies.

More recently, Murray et al.[77] investigated 15 patients with CAD and severe left ventricular dysfunction (ejection fraction < 35%) who underwent resting metabolic cardiac imaging utilizing low-dose IPPA intravenously and a multicrystal gamma camera. Parametric images of regional rates of IPPA clearance and accumulation were generated. Forty-two vascular territories (22 infarcted) were evaluated by metabolic imaging as well as by transmural biopsies. Despite resting akinesis or dyskinesis in 20 of 22 infarcted territories, 73% of these territories were metabolically viable. Transmyocardial biopsies during coronary bypass surgery confirmed IPPA results in 91% of cases. When compared to biopsy, IPPA scintigraphy had a 92% sensitivity and a 86% specificity for viability. Eighty percent of bypassed, infarcted but IPPA viable segments demonstrated improved systolic wall motion postoperatively. Furthermore, when compared to the reinjection of thallium, concordance occurred in 77% of cases. When disagreement occurred, in each case, IPPA showed viability when thallium did not.[78]

Dynamic IPPA-SPECT imaging is a promising new technique now undergoing phase III clinical trial in the United States and Canada to assess myocardial viability. Sequential SPECT studies (8 minutes each) are obtained at 4, 12, 20, 28, and 36 minutes after rest injection using a multidetector gamma camera. The protocol is based on the pattern of differential washout between normal and ischemic myocardium: defects seen on first tomograms will appear reversible on late tomograms in ischemic but viable myocardium because the slower washout of IPPA compared to normal myocardium. In contrast, nonviable myocardium will demonstrate markedly reduced initial uptake of IPPA and no significant metabolism over time (Plate 20-2 and Fig. 20-13). In a pilot study of 18 patients with left ventricular dysfunction, the uptake of IPPA was compared to that of rest–redistribution thallium images.[79] In 10 patients the thallium images showed evidence of fixed defects and, in 8 patients, both reversible and fixed defects. On the other hand, with IPPA imaging, 2 patients had fixed defects, and 16 patients had reversible defects or both fixed and reversible defects. More reversible defects were detected by IPPA than by thallium imaging. In 12 patients, the LVEF was repeated after coronary revascularization and improved by greater than 5% in 6 of the 12 patients. The patients with improved ejection fraction had more reversible IPPA segments per patient than patients who did not show improvement.

Summary

In summary, the metabolism of IPPA is well understood and its unique properties for tracing perfusion and fatty acid turnover by the myocardial myocytes in one single investigation would make it an ideal tracer for detection of myocardial viability. Preliminary studies have shown that reversible defects following rest injection are predictive of recovery of left ventricular function after coronary revascularization. However, its rapid metabolism may result in poor quality SPECT images.

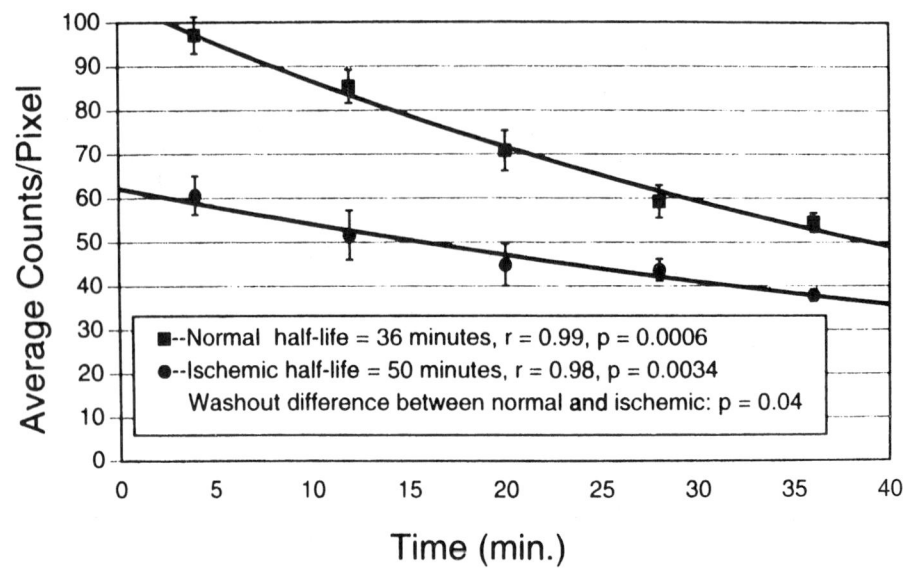

Fig. 20-13. Dynamic 15-(p-iodophenyl) pentadecanoic acid (IPPA)-SPECT imaging. Relative activity versus time in regions identified on the bull's-eye plot as ischemic (red) and normal (green) (see Plate 20-2). The nonischemic region is plotted as squares and the ischemic regions as circles. (From Hansen et al.,[99] with permission.)

β-Methyliodophenylpentadecanoic Acid (BMIPP)

Since straight-chain fatty acids are rapidly catabolized by β-oxidation, a variety of structural modifications have been introduced into fatty acid analogs to inhibit their oxidation. In particular, methyl-branched fatty acids such as BMIPP have been widely investigated. BMIPP is the 3-methyl-branched fatty acid analogue of IPPA (Fig. 20-11). The inhibitory effect of the methyl group on β-oxidation results in longer myocardial retention, which has been demonstrated in laboratory animal studies and, more recently, in humans.

Myocardial Uptake and Metabolism of BMIPP

BMIPP follows the same initial biochemical pathways of uptake and transport as do native fatty acids within the myocardial cells.[80,81] BMIPP undergoes irreversible enzymatic activation to acyl-coenzyme A (CoA) (Fig. 20-14), and its accumulation is positively correlated with the intracellular concentration of ATP, which is required in this activation process.[82] The BMIPP-CoA thus produced is hydrophilic (facilitating its intracellular retention) and cannot be catabolized directly via β-oxidation because the methyl group precludes the formation of the keto-acyl intermediate. Instead, BMIPP-CoA is esterified to triglycerides and stored into the cytosolic lipid pool.[80] The impediment caused by the methyl group can be removed by initial α-oxidation, and the resulting α-methyl catabolite can then serve as a substrate for the usual β-oxidative pathway.[83]

The accumulation of BMIPP therefore reflects the initial, energy-dependent metabolic sequestration and retention of fatty acids, rather than their β-oxidation.

Comparative Distribution of BMIPP and Flow Tracers

Discrepancies between BMIPP and regional myocardial blood flow have been reported in patients with myocardial infarction. In their preliminary clinical study, Saito et al.[84] found mismatching between BMIPP and thallium distribution in four of six patients investigated after an acute myocardial infarction. More reduced fatty acid uptake was found in the three patients who had successful reperfusion. In a larger series including 28 patients with myocardial infarction, Tamaki et al.[85] found that BMIPP uptake was decreased compared to thallium in 17 patients (61%) and in 49 of 196 myocardial segments (25%).

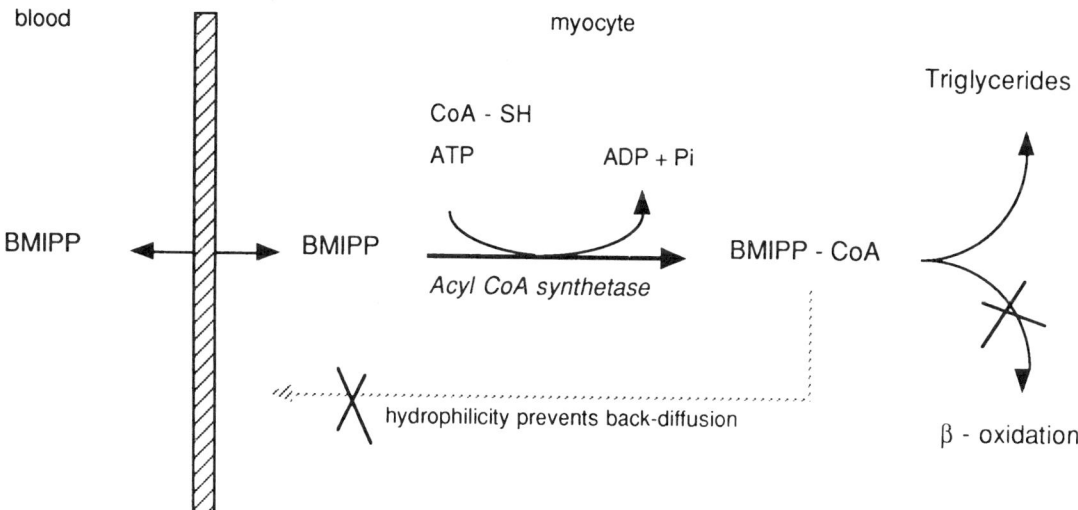

Fig. 20-14. Mechanism of uptake and retention of BMIPP. (Adapted from Fujibayashi et al.,[82] with permission.)

Such discordant BMIPP uptake was observed more often in areas of acute, as opposed to chronic, myocardial infarction, and more often in reperfused, as opposed to nonreperfused, areas. In addition, a discordant decrease in BMIPP was frequently seen in areas showing a regional wall motion abnormality with relatively preserved perfusion. Thus, the discordant decrease in BMIPP uptake may indicate a persistent metabolic abnormality associated with the failure of functional recovery after revascularization, particularly in patients with acute myocardial infarction. Nishimura et al.[86] investigated 25 patients with myocardial infarction, in whom BMIPP and thallium were administered simultaneously. Myocardial SPECT was carried out 15 to 30 minutes later. A dissociation between thallium and BMIPP defects was more frequently observed in successful reperfusion than in those with no reperfusion and chronic myocardial infarction. More importantly, the severity score for BMIPP uptake determined by SPECT correlated well with ventricular function, determined by measurement of ejection fraction.

Similar findings were observed by De Geeter et al.[87] using sestamibi as flow tracer. In this study, 26 patients were investigated within 2 weeks of an acute myocardial infarction. Ten patients had a history of previous infarction. BMIPP and sestamibi SPECT were performed after rest injection within 4 days of one another. Forty segments were defined on apical, midventricular and basal slices. Of the 477 abnormal segments for at least one tracer, 47% showed defects of similar intensity, 42% showed more reduced BMIPP than sestamibi uptake, and 11% showed a relative excess of BMIPP. Coronary arteriography and contrast ventriculography were obtained for each patient. Ninety-five percent of the defects occurred either in the infarct related coronary artery (77%) or in territories subserved by significant coronary stenoses (18%). Regions with relatively decreased BMIPP uptake occurred significantly more frequently in patients who had undergone thrombolysis and/or percutaneous transluminal angioplasty (PTCA) in the early phase of infarction, and appeared more often in areas supplied by patent, as opposed to occluded, coronary arteries. Areas with relative excess of BMIPP were observed at the periphery of previous infarction and severe regional wall motion abnormalities, presumably reflecting the higher metabolic needs of myocardium, which undergoes passive systolic wall stretch.

Prediction of Myocardial Viability in Subacute Myocardial Infarction

To determine whether BMIPP uptake can be used to differentiate viable myocardium from scar tissue soon after myocardial infarction, Franken et al.[88]

compared the relative uptake of BMIPP and sestamibi to regional wall motion and to contractile reserve assessed by two-dimensional echocardiography and low-dose dobutamine stimulation. Twenty-two patients with a first acute myocardial infarction were investigated 4 to 10 days after coronary thrombolysis. BMIPP was injected intravenously under resting conditions after an overnight fast. SPECT images were obtained 20 minutes after injection. Three segmental patterns were identified in the infarct-related coronary artery territory: normal uptake of both tracers, mismatched defects with more reduced BMIPP uptake than sestamibi uptake (Plate 20-3), and matched defects. All segments with both *normal BMIPP and sestamibi uptake* showed normal wall motion. Evidence of residual viability was found in 72% of the segments showing a *mismatch pattern*, i.e., wall motion was either normal at rest or demonstrated inotropic reserve during low-dose dobutamine stimulation. In segments with dysfunction, mismatching was significantly associated with inotropic reserve. All segments that improved function during dobutamine stimulation showed a mismatched uptake. In contrast, segments with *matched defects* always showed abnormal wall motion and none demonstrated inotropic reserve, regardless of the severity of the sestamibi defect. It was concluded from the study that mismatching is indicative of jeopardized but viable myocardium and that matched defects are associated with scar tissue.

The accuracy of combined BMIPP and sestamibi for prediction of functional outcome after acute myocardial infarction has been recently evaluated.[89] Rest BMIPP, rest sestamibi, and dobutamine echocardiography were obtained in 18 patients with echocardiographic wall motion abnormalities 1 week after acute myocardial infarction. Patients received appropriate treatment according to standard indications (including PTCA in 7 patients and coronary artery bypass grafting [CABG] in 6 patients), and all patients underwent a second echocardiographic study to assess functional outcome, 6 months after infarction. Wall motion improved in at least 50% of the dysfunctional segments in 9 patients and was unchanged in the 9 other patients. Baseline clinical data, findings on coronary arteriography before hospital discharge, and occurrence and type of revascularization procedure were similar in patients who improved function and in patients who did not. On the other hand, a highly significant association was found between the functional outcome and the relative uptake of BMIPP and sestamibi. Wall motion improved in 27 of the 33 segments (82%) showing a mismatch pattern and was unchanged in 19 of the 21 segments (90%) with matched defects. The overall accuracy of combined BMIPP and sestamibi in predicting segmental functional outcome was 85%. These values are similar to those obtained with metabolic studies using PET and FDG for differentiating viable from nonviable myocardium. The study shows that the probability of observing functional improvement in a patient was related to the extent of mismatch. The sensitivity, specificity, and predictive accuracy of combined BMIPP and sestamibi scintigraphy for patient functional improvement were 100%, 89%, and 94%, respectively.

The incremental value of combined BMIPP and sestamibi to predict segmental functional outcome over that provided by either sestamibi uptake alone or by low-dose dobutamine echocardiography was also evaluated in this study. Using an arbitrary cutoff of 50% of the maximal activity as the criterion for myocardial viability, sestamibi uptake alone had a positive predictive value of 84% and a negative predictive value of 72%. These values improved to 95% and 89%, respectively, when considering in addition the relative uptake of BMIPP (mismatched vs. matched defects). Improvement in wall thickening during low-dose dobutamine stimulation had a positive predictive value of 80% and a negative predictive value of 62%. These values increased to 94% and 94%, respectively, when considering the relative uptake of BMIPP and sestamibi.

Summary

In summary, the comparison of BMIPP uptake with flow tracer (thallium or sestamibi) allows for the characterization of the complete spectrum of postischemic myocardium, that is, from complete functional recovery (when the uptake of both tracers is normal) to complete transmural necrosis without residual viability (when the uptake of both tracers is severely and similarly reduced). A mismatch pattern (more severely depressed fatty acid metabolism than expected on the basis of flow) is indicative of jeopardized but viable myocardium and is predictive for long-term functional recovery following acute myocardial infarction. Matched defects are associated with scar. The additional information provided by BMIPP substantially increases the accuracy of flow tracer uptake alone or dobutamine echocardiography alone to predict functional outcome early after acute myocardial infarction.

Fluorine-18 Fluorodeoxyglucose

The positron emitter fluorine 18 FDG is an analog of glucose that crosses the capillary and sarcolemmal membranes at a rate proportional to that of glucose. Following myocardial uptake, FDG is phosphorylated to FDG-6-phosphate and is then trapped in the myocardium because, unlike glucose 6-phosphate, FDG-6-phosphate is a poor substrate for both glycogen synthesis and glycolysis. Regional myocardial uptake of FDG therefore reflects the regional rates of exogenous glucose utilization. Although fatty acids are the preferred substrate for ATP production in the nonischemic myocardium under fasting conditions, there is a shift from fatty acid oxidation to glucose utilization in ischemic myocardial regions. Imaging with FDG has been used to identify viable myocardium with PET. As will be discussed in Chapter 21, most clinical studies have shown that a pattern of enhanced FDG uptake (with normal or reduced perfusion) is associated with recovery of contractile function after revascularization in 75% to 85% of segments. Regions with concordantly diminished flow and FDG uptake do not improve after revascularization in 80% to 90% of cases. The clinical use of FDG-PET to assess viability, however, is still limited due to the limited availability and high costs of PET.

Recently, special high-energy collimators for detecting positron emitters with a standard gamma camera have been developed.[90–95] Preliminary results have demonstrated the feasibility of assessing regional myocardial uptake of FDG with planar,[92] and more recently with SPECT imaging.[93–95] Williams et al.[92] performed planar FDG imaging in patients after myocardial infarction who were evaluated before and after revascularization. Of the 46-stress–24-hour redistribution fixed thallium defects preoperatively, 30 demonstrated improvement in regional exercise thallium uptake or in regional systolic function after revascularization. Enhanced FDG activity relative to thallium was present in 83% of these regions.

Bax et al.[96] compared the myocardial distribution of thallium and FDG activity, both measured with SPECT, in nine healthy individuals. Mean profiles of midventricular short axis slices showed no significant difference between thallium and FDG activity, suggesting that no separate thallium and FDG reference values are needed for comparison in patient studies with SPECT. In another study, Bax et al.[93] studied nine patients with wall motion abnormalities. All patients underwent FDG-SPECT and resting thallium-SPECT as well as echocardiography. Of the 14 segments with thallium defects, 8 showed concordantly decreased FDG uptake (indicating myocardial scar), whereas the remaining 6 segments demonstrated a relatively increased FDG uptake suggesting viable myocardium. Contractility was preserved in 4 of the 6 segments with increased FDG uptake. In contrast, 7 of the 8 regions with a matching defect were akinetic. In the study by Stoll et al.[94] FDG was used together with sestamibi in dual-isotope acquisition.

More recently, Burt et al.[95] investigated 20 consecutive patients for myocardial viability using rest thallium-SPECT, FDG-PET, and FDG-SPECT imaging. FDG images obtained with the PET tomograph were aesthetically superior to the FDG-SPECT images (Plate 20-4). FDG-PET images were characterized by sharper myocardial wall margins and more accurate depiction of wall thickness than FDG-SPECT images. However, the authors found that the differences between the instruments were of little clinical relevance for the detection of segments with FDG uptake. Of the 60 segments with fixed thallium defects, 13 were shown probably viable by FDG-SPECT (8 of 20 patients), and 14 segments by FDG-PET (7 of 20 patients).

In summary, only limited data are currently available on the use of FDG-SPECT for the delineation of myocardial viability. This awaits further study in more extended patient groups. Issues to be addressed are the cost–benefit relationship (taking into account the elevated costs for the tracer as well as the equipment), and the relative position of this technique compared to other metabolic studies, particularly with fatty acids.

ANTIMYOSIN

Antimyosin is the Fab fragment of a murine monoclonal antibody directed against human heavy chain myocardial myosin. Antimyosin is bound via the chelator diethylenetriamine penta-acetic acid (DTPA) to indium-111, a gamma emitter suited for SPECT imaging. After intravenous injection in normal subjects, antimyosin is unable to bind its antigen, because the myosin is contained within the intact cell membrane. Dead myocardial cells, however, are characterized by ruptured cell membranes, which allow the circulating antibodies to reach, and bind to, the myosin. This way, antimyosin serves as an in vivo marker of myocardial necrosis, and, indirectly, of as a marker of viability. Apart from its use as an infarct-avid tracer, other useful applications for this tracer have been described in myocarditis, cardiomyopathy, and transplant rejection.

The combined use of antimyosin with flow tracers permits further characterization of the myocardium in patients with recent myocardial infarction. Several patterns of relative distribution of the flow tracer and the antimyosin may be observed.[97,98] In the "matched pattern," the defects on the flow study are filled in with antimyosin. These regions correspond with areas of transmural infarction. The "mismatched pattern" is characterized by the presence of areas that contain neither the flow tracer not antimyosin. The correlates of this pattern may be diverse: old scar, viable myocardium with reduced blood flow due to decreased supply, or stunned myocardium. In the latter case, the relatively decreased uptake of flow tracer in the stunned myocardium is explained by the compensatory hyperkinesis and the attending increase of flow in the normal myocardium. Finally, the "overlap pattern" shows segments that contain both tracers. This pattern represents nontransmural necrosis.

Several papers have addressed the prognostic implications of these patterns after myocardial infarction, in terms of ischemic in-hospital events (sudden death, arrhythmia, infarct extension, recurrent angina) or positive exercise tests. Johnson et al.[97] found evidence for continued ischemia in 70% of patients with the mismatched pattern, but no such evidence in any of the patients with the matched pattern. Schoeder et al.[98] observed exercise-induced ischemia in 53% of patients with overlap pattern, 14% with match pattern, and 0% with mismatch pattern. When ischemic risk was defined as either a positive stress test or the advent of major in-hospital complications, however, its incidence was not different among the three patterns.

Although combined flow tracer and antimyosin studies are potentially helpful in risk stratification early after myocardial infarction, at a clinical stage when stress tests are not usually performed, it seems that the evidence is as yet insufficient to endorse their routine use. The method may be further marred by the occurrence of false-negative antimyosin scans, especially in patients with inferoposterior infarctions. Moreover, it remains unclear whether patency of the infarct-related artery is a prerequisite for uptake of antimyosin in the infarction, at least in the absence of adequate collaterals.

CONCLUSION

The preceding sections describe a multiplicity of SPECT protocols that may be used for the identification of viable myocardium. In this last section, the relative merits of these techniques will be discussed and recommendations will be given on their use in patients with myocardial dysfunction, in whom the question of viability arises.

A logical way to approach the problem is to start with a study of myocardial perfusion, either at rest or following stress, since this provides an assessment of the status of the CAD. The use of various thallium protocols for viability determination is supported by a large body of literature. However, dosimetric and physical characteristics may give rise to suboptimal images in a number of patients. The technetium-99m-labeled tracer sestamibi does not suffer from such drawbacks, but fewer data are available to buttress its use in this indication, particularly since redistribution of this tracer into viable areas with severely compromised flow has been shown to be much less than that observed with thallium. However, a number of recent papers indicate that the use of sestamibi for viability delineation is warranted, provided that quantitation is performed, that late images are acquired after rest injection, or that the tracer is administered after nitrate administration.

Quantitative studies have shown that the prediction of myocardial viability with flow tracers is probabilistic. A continuum of segments exists between those with extremely low uptake of flow tracers, in which the probability of viability is very low, and those with high uptake values, which have high likelihood of being viable. Between those extremes, additional studies with metabolic tracers may be useful to obtain more precise data on viability.

Several tracers are available for metabolic imaging with SPECT, and the existing data have been encouraging for the use of these tracers in the subgroup of segments with intermediate probability of viability on flow imaging. IPPA has the advantage of measuring both uptake and β-oxidation of free fatty acids, but imaging may be hampered by its short biological half-life. On the other hand, BMIPP shows longer retention in the myocardium, allowing for excellent quality SPECT imaging, but only reflects the initial phases of fatty acid uptake and activation. Image interpretation with these two tracers is fundamentally different. With IPPA, early images reflect flow, while late images reflect viability because of differential washout from ischemic, as compared to normal areas. With BMIPP, jeopardized areas show up as segments with relatively decreased BMIPP uptake compared to flow tracer activity (mismatches). Flow and metabolism mismatches are also observed with FDG but, in this case, tracer uptake is enhanced relative to flow in jeopardized areas. Recently, the acquisition of images of FDG distribution has been shown to be feasible on a SPECT camera equipped with special collimators. No comparative data exist as yet to define the relative merits of these three tracers.

Hence, SPECT imaging provides an answer to the question of viability in the majority of cases. Flow studies may place the patient into either high or low probability categories. Patients with intermediate probability of viability may be further investigated by metabolic SPECT imaging.

REFERENCES

1. Louie HW, Laks H, Milgalter E et al.: Ischemic cardiomyopathy: criteria for coronary revascularization and cardiac transplantation. Circulation 84:III-290, 1991
2. Di Carli M, Davidson M, Little R et al.: Value of metabolic imaging with positron emission tomography for evaluating prognosis in patients with coronary artery disease and left ventricular dysfunction. Am J Cardiol 73:527, 1994
3. Lee KS, Marwick TH, Cook SA et al.: Prognosis of patients with left ventricular dysfunction, with and without viable myocardium after myocardial infarction. Circulation 90:2687, 1994
4. Iskandrian AS, Heo J, Stanberry C: When is myocardial viability an important clinical issue? J Nucl Med 35: 4S, 1994
5. Iskandrian AS, Van der Wall EE: Myocardial viability: summary and perspectives. p. 179. In: Iskandrian AS, Van der Wall EE (Eds): Myocardial Viability. Kluwer Academic Publishers, Dordrecht, The Netherlands, 1994
6. Braunwald E, Kloner RA: The stunned myocardium: prolonged, postischemic ventricular dysfunction. Circulation 66:1146, 1982
7. Bolli R: Myocardial 'stunning' in man. Circulation 86: 1671, 1992
8. Rahimtoola SH: The hibernating myocardium. Am Heart J 117:211, 1989
9. Vanoverschelde JL, Wijns W, Deprè C et al.: Mechanisms of chronic regional postischemic dysfunction in humans. Circulation 87:1513, 1993
10. McCall D, Zimmer LJ, Katz AM: Kinetics of thallium exchange in cultured rat heart cells. Circ Res 56:370, 1985
11. Meerdink DJ, Leppo JA: Comparison of hypoxia and ouabain effects on the myocardial uptake kinetics of technetium-99m hexakis 2-methoxyisobutyl isonitrile and thallium-201. J Nucl Med 30:1500, 1989
12. Maublant JC, Moins N, Gachon P et al.: Uptake of technetium-99m-teboroxime in cultured myocardial cells: comparison with thallium-201 and technetium-99m-sestamibi. J Nucl Med 34:255, 1993
13. Pohost GM, Zir L, Moore RH et al.: Differentiation of transiently ischemic from infarcted myocardium by serial imaging after a single dose of thallium-201. Circulation 55:294, 1977
14. Gewirtz H, Beller GA, Strauss HW et al.: Transient defects of resting thallium scans in patients with coronary artery disease. Circulation 59:707, 1979
15. Angello DA, Wilson RA, Gee D et al.: Effect of eating on thallium-201 redistribution postischemia. Am J Cardiol 60:528, 1987
16. Hegewald MG, Palac RT, Angello DA et al.: Ribose infusion accelerates thallium redistribution with early imaging compared with late 24-hour imaging without ribose. J Am Coll Cardiol 18:1671, 1991
17. Piwnica-Worms D, Kronauge JF, Chiu ML: Uptake and retention of hexakis (2-methoxyisobutyl isonitrile) technetium (I) in cultured chick myocardial cells: mito-

chondrial and plasma membrane potential dependence. Circulation 82:1826, 1990
18. Crane P, Laliberte R, Heminway S et al.: Effect of mitochondrial viability and metabolism on technetium-99m-sestamibi myocardial retention. Eur J Nucl Med 20:20, 1993
19. Sinusas AJ, Watson DD, Cannon JM, Beller GA: Effect of ischemia and postischemic dysfunction on myocardial uptake of technetium-99m-labeled methoxyisobutyl isonitrile and thallium-201. J Am Coll Cardiol 14:1785, 1989
20. Canby RC, Silber S, Pohost GM: Relations of the myocardial imaging agents Tc-99m MIBI and Tl-201 to myocardial blood flow in a canine model of myocardial ischemic insult. Circulation 81:289, 1990
21. Freeman I, Grunwald AM, Hoory S, Bodenheimer MM: Effect of coronary occlusion and myocardial viability on myocardial activity of technetium-99m-sestamibi. J Nucl Med 32:292, 1991
22. Beller GA, Glover DK, Edwards NC et al.: Tc-99m sestamibi uptake and retention during myocardial ischemia and reperfusion. Circulation 87:2033, 1993
23. Okada RD, Glover D, Gaffney T, Williams S: Myocardial kinetics of technetium-99m hexakis-2-methoxy-2-methylpropyl-isonitrile. Circulation 77:491, 1988
24. Sinusas AJ, Bergin JD, Edwards NC et al.: Redistribution of Tc-99m sestamibi and Tl-201 in the presence of a severe coronary artery stenosis. Circulation 89:2332, 1994
25. Li Q-S, Solot G, Frank TL et al.: Myocardial redistribution of Tc-99m-methoxyisobutyl isonitrile (sestamibi). J Nucl Med 31:1069, 1990
26. Taillefer R, Primeau M, Costi P, Lambert R et al.: Technetium-99m-sestamibi myocardial perfusion imaging in detection of coronary artery disease: comparison between initial (1-hour) and delayed (3-hour) postexercise images. J Nucl Med 32:1961, 1991
27. Villanueva-Meyer J, Mena I, Diggles L, Narahara KA: Assessment of myocardial perfusion defect size after early and delayed SPECT imaging with technetium-99m-hexakis 2-methoxyisobutyl isonitrile after stress. J Nucl Med 34:187, 1993
28. Piwnica-Worms D, Chiu ML, Kronauge JF: Divergent kinetics of thallium-201 and Tc99m-sestamibi in cultured chick ventricular myocytes during ATP depletion. Circulation 85:1531, 1992
29. Blood DK, McCarthy DM, Sciacca RR, Cannon PJ: Comparison of single-dose and double-dose thallium 201 myocardial perfusion scintigraphy for the detection of coronary artery disease and prior myocardial infarction. Circulation 58:777, 1978
30. Ritchie JL, Albro PC, Caldwell JH et al.: Thallium-201 myocardial imaging: a comparison of the redistribution and rest images. J Nucl Med 20:477, 1979
31. Gibson RS, Watson DD, Taylor GJ et al.: Prospective assessment of regional myocardial perfusion before and after coronary revascularization surgery by quantitative thallium-201 scintigraphy. J Am Coll Cardiol 1:804, 1983
32. Liu P, Kiess MC, Okada RD et al.: The persistent defect on exercise thallium imaging and its fate after myocardial revascularization: does it represent scar or ischemia? Am Heart J 110:996, 1985
33. Manyari DE, Knudtson M, Kloiber R, Roth D: Sequential thallium-201 myocardial perfusion studies after successful percutaneous transluminal coronary artery angioplasty: delayed resolution of exercise-induced scintigraphic abnormalities. Circulation 77:86, 1988
34. Tillisch J, Brunken R, Marshall R et al.: Reversibility of cardiac wall motion abnormalities predicted by positron tomography. N Engl J Med 314:884, 1986
35. Brunken R, Schwaiger M, Grover McKay et al.: Positron emission tomography detects tissue metabolic activity in myocardial segments with persistent thallium perfusion defects. J Am Coll Cardiol 10:557, 1987
36. Tamaki N, Yonekura Y, Yamashita K et al.: Relation of left ventricular perfusion and wall motion with metabolic activity in persistent defects on thallium-201 tomography in healed myocardial infarction. Am J Cardiol 62:202, 1988
37. Gutman J, Berman DS, Freeman M et al.: Time to completed redistribution of thallium-201 in exercise myocardial scintigraphy: relationship to the degree of coronary artery stenosis. Am Heart J 106:989, 1983
38. Cloninger KG, DePuey EG, Garcia EV et al.: Incomplete redistribution in delayed thallium-201 single photon emission computed tomographic images: an overestimation of myocardial scarring. J Am Coll Cardiol 12:955, 1987
39. Kiat H, Berman DS, Maddahi J et al.: Late reversibility of tomographic myocardial thallium-201 defects: an accurate marker of myocardial viability. J Am Coll Cardiol 12:1456, 1988
40. Yang LD, Berman DS, Kiat H et al.: The frequency of late reversibility in SPECT thallium-201 stress-redistribution studies. J Am Coll Cardiol 15:334, 1989
41. Dilsizian V, Rocco TP, Freedman NM et al.: Enhanced detection of ischemic but viable myocardium by the reinjection of thallium after stress-redistribution imaging. N Engl J Med 323:141, 1990
42. Kayden DS, Sigal S, Soufer R et al.: Thallium-201 for assessment of myocardial viability: quantitative comparison of 24-hour redistribution imaging with imag-

ing after reinjection at rest. J Am Coll Cardiol 18:1480, 1991
43. Rocco TP, Dilsizian V, McKusick KA et al.: Comparison of thallium redistribution with rest 'reinjection' imaging for the detection of viable myocardium. Am J Cardiol 66:158, 1990
44. Tamaki N, Ohtani H, Yonekura Y et al.: Significance of fill-in after thallium-201 reinjection following delayed imaging: comparison with regional wall motion and angiographic findings. J Nucl Med 31:1617, 1990
45. Ohtani H, Tamaki N, Yonekura Y et al.: Value of thallium-201 reinjection after delayed SPECT imaging for predicting reversible ischemia after coronary artery bypass grafting. Am J Cardiol 66:394, 1990
46. Tamaki N, Ohtani H, Yamashita K et al.: Metabolic activity in the areas of new fill-in after thallium-201 reinjection: comparison with positron emission tomography using fluorine-18-deoxyglucose. J Nucl Med 32:673, 1991
47. Bonow RO, Dilsizian V, Cuocolo A, Bacharach SL: Identification of viable myocardium in patients with coronary artery disease and left ventricular dysfunction: comparison of thallium scintigraphy with reinjection and PET imaging with 18F-fluorodeoxyglucose. Circulation 83:26, 1991
48. Zimmermann R, Mall G, Rauch B et al.: Residual thallium-201 activity in irreversible defects as a marker of myocardial viability. Circulation 91:1016, 1995
49. Dilsizian V, Smeltzer WR, Freedman NM et al.: Thallium reinjection after stress-redistribution imaging: does 24-hour delayed imaging following reinjection enhance detection of viable myocardium? Circulation 83:1247, 1991
50. Dilsizian V, Bonow RO: Differential uptake and apparent thallium-201 washout after thallium reinjection: options regarding early redistribution imaging before reinjection or late redistribution imaging after reinjection. Circulation 85:1032, 1992
51. van Eck-Smit B, van der Wall EE, Kujiper AFM et al.: Immediate thallium-201 reinjection following stress imaging: a time-saving approach for detection of myocardial viability. J Nucl Med 34:737, 1993
52. Kiat H, Friedman JD, Wang FP et al.: Frequency of late reversibility in stress-redistribution thallium-201 SPECT using early reinjection protocol. Am Heart J 122:613, 1991
53. Iskandrian AS, Hakki A, Kane SA et al.: Rest and redistribution thallium-201 myocardial scintigraphy to predict improvement in left ventricular function after coronary artery bypass grafting. Am J Cardiol 51:1312, 1983
54. Mori T, Minamiji K, Kurogane H et al.: Rest-injected thallium-201 imaging for assessing viability of severe asynergic regions. J Nucl Med 32:1718, 1991
55. Ragosta M, Beller GA, Watson DD et al.: Quantitative planar rest-redistribution thallium-201 imaging in detection of myocardial viability and prediction of improvement in left ventricular function after coronary bypass surgery in patients with severely depressed left ventricular function. Circulation 87:1630, 1993
56. Dilsizian V, Perrone-Filardi P, Arrighi JA et al.: Concordance and discordance between stress-redistribution-reinjection and rest-redistribution thallium imaging for assessing viable myocardium: comparison with metabolic activity by positron emission tomography. Circulation 88:941, 1993
57. Angello DA, Wilson RA, Gee D: Effect of ribose on postischemic thallium-201 kinetics. J Nucl Med 29:1943, 1988
58. Perlmutter NS, Wilson RA, Angello DA et al.: Ribose facilitates thallium-201 redistribution in patients with coronary artery disease. J Nucl Med 32:193, 1991
59. He ZX, Darcourt J, Guignier A et al.: Nitrates improve detection of ischemic but viable myocardium by thallium-201 reinjection SPECT. J Nucl Med 34:1472, 1993
60. Rocco TP, Dilsizian V, Strauss HW, Boucher CA: Technetium-99m isonitrile myocardial uptake at rest. II. Relation to clinical markers of potential viability. J Am Coll Cardiol 14:1678, 1989
61. Cuocolo A, Pace L, Ricciardelli B et al.: Identification of viable myocardium in patients with chronic coronary artery disease: comparison of thallium-201 scintigraphy with reinjection and technetium-99m-methoxyisobutyl isonitrile. J Nucl Med 33:505, 1992
62. Marzullo P, Parodi O, Reisenhofer B et al.: Value of rest thallium-201/technetium-99m sestamibi scans and dobutamine echocardiography for detecting myocardial viability. Am J Cardiol 71:166, 1993
63. Udelson JE, Coleman PS, Metherall J et al.: Predicting recovery of severe regional ventricular dysfunction: comparison of resting scintigraphy with 201Tl and 99m-Tc-sestamibi. Circulation 89:2552, 1994
64. Sawada SG, Allman KC, Muzik O et al.: Positron emission tomography detects evidence of viability in rest technetium-99m sestamibi defects. J Am Coll Cardiol 23:92, 1994
65. Altehoefer C, vom Dahl J, Biedermann M et al.: Significance of defect severity in technetium-99m-MIBI SPECT at rest to assess myocardial viability: comparison with fluorine-18-FDG PET. J Nucl Med 35:569, 1994
66. Dilsizian V, Arrighi JA, Diodati JG et al.: Myocardial viability in patients with chronic coronary artery dis-

ease: comparison of Tc99m-sestamibi with thallium reinjection and [F-18]fluorodeoxyglucose. Circulation 89:578, 1994
67. Bisi G, Sciagrà R, Santoro GM, Fazzini PF: Rest technetium-99m sestamibi tomography in combination with short-term administration of nitrates: feasibility and reliability for prediction of postrevascularization outcome of asynergic territories. J Am Coll Cardiol 24:1282, 1994
68. Dudczack R, Kletter K, Frichauf H et al.: The use of I-123-labeled heptadecanoic acid as a metabolic tracer. Eur J Nucl Med 9:81, 1984
69. Machulla HJ, Marsmann M, Dutschka KP: Biochemical concept and synthesis of a radioiodinated pheny fatty acid for in vivo metabolic studies of the myocardium. Eur J Nucl Med 5:171, 1980
70. Reske SN, Sauer W, Machulla HJ, Winckler C: 15-(p-[I-123] phenyl) pentadecanoic acid as tracer for lipid metabolism. Comparison with 1-C-14 palmitic acid in murine tissues. J Nucl Med 25:1335, 1984
71. Caldwell JH, Martin GV, Link JM et al.: Iodophenylpentadecanoic acid-myocardial blood flow relationship during maximal exercise with coronary occlusion. J Nucl Med 31:99, 1990
72. Reske SN, Knapp FF, Winkler C: Experimental basis of metabolic imaging of the myocardium with radioiodinated aromatic free fatty acids. Am J Physiol Imag 1:214, 1986
73. Rellas JS, Corbett JR, Kulkarni P et al.: Iodine-123-phenylpentadecanoic acid: detection of acute myocardial infarction and injury in dogs using an iodinated fatty acid and single-photon emission tomography. Am J Cardiol 52:1326, 1983
74. Reske SN, Knapp FF, Nitsche J et al.: Preserved I-123 phenyl-pentadecanoic acid uptake in the reperfused myocardium [abstr]. J Nucl Med 29:842, 1988
75. Hansen CL, Corbett JR, Pippin JJ et al.: Iodine-123-phenylpentadecanoic acid and single photon emission computed tomography in identifying LV regional metabolic abnormalities in patients with coronary artery disease: comparison with thallium-201 myocardial tomography. J Am Coll Cardiol 12:78, 1988
76. Kuikka JT, Musalo H, Hietakorpi S et al.: Evaluation of myocardial viability with technetium-99m hexaxis-2-methoxyisobutyl isonitrile and iodine-123 phenyl pentadecanoic acid and single photon emission tomography. Eur J Nucl Med 19:882, 1992
77. Murray G, Schad N, Ladd W et al.: Metabolic cardiac imaging in severe coronary artery disease: assessment of viability with iodine-123-iodophenylpentadecanoic acid and multicrystal gamma camera, and correlation with biopsy. J Nucl Med 33:1269, 1992
78. Murray G, Schad N, Magill L, Vander Zwagg R: Myocardial viability assessment with dynamic low-dose iodine-123-iodophenylpentadecanoic acid metabolic imaging: comparison with myocardial biopsy and reinjection SPECT thallium after myocardial infarction. J Nucl Med, suppl. 35:43S, 1994
79. Wolmer I, Powers J, Sung KK et al.: Detection of myocardial viability using dynamic SPECT I-123-IPPA imaging [abstr]. Circulation, suppl. I4, 88:I 200, 1993
80. Knapp FF Jr, Ambrose KR, Goodman MM: New radioiodinated methyl-branched fatty acid for cardiac studies. Eur J Nucl Med 12:S39, 1986
81. Ambrose KR, Owen BA, Goodman MM, Knapp FF Jr: Evaluation of the metabolism in rat hearts of two new radioiodinated 3-methyl-branched fatty acid myocardial imaging agents. Eur J Nucl Med 12:486, 1987
82. Fujibayashi Y, Yonekura Y, Takemura Y et al.: Myocardial accumulation of iodinated beta-methyl-branched fatty acid analogue, iodine-125-15-(p-iodo-phenyl)-3-(R,S) methylpentadecanoic acid (BMIPP), in relation to ATP concentration. J Nucl Med 31:1818, 1990
83. Yamamichi Y, Hideo BS, Kusuoka H et al.: Metabolism of I-123 labeled 15-(p-iodophenyl)-3-(R,S)-methyl-pentadecanoic acid (BMIPP) in perfused rat hearts: The evidence for initial alpha-oxidation and subsequent cycles of beta-oxidation, and dependency of substrates. J Nucl Med 36:1043, 1995
84. Saito S, Yasuda T, Gold HK et al.: Differentiation of regional perfusion and fatty acid uptake in zones of myocardial injury. Nucl Med Commun 12:663, 1991
85. Tamaki N, Kawamoto M, Yonekura Y et al.: Regional metabolic abnormality in relation to perfusion and wall motion in patients with myocardial infarction: assessment with emission tomography using an iodinated branched fatty acid analog. J Nucl Med 33:659, 1992
86. Nishimura T, Uehara T, Shimonagata T et al.: Clinical results with beta-methyl-p-iodophenylpentadecanoic acid, single-photon emission computed tomography in cardiac disease. J Nucl Cardiol 1:S65, 1994
87. De Geeter F, Franken PR, Knapp FF Jr, Bossuyt A: Relationship between blood flow and fatty acid metabolism in subacute myocardial infarction: a study by means of Tc-99m MIBI and I-123 beta-methyl iodophenyl pentadecanoic acid. Eur J Nucl Med 21:283, 1994
88. Franken PR, De Geeter F, Dendale P et al.: Abnormal free fatty acid uptake in subacute myocardial infarction after coronary thrombolysis: correlation with wall motion and inotropic reserve. J Nucl Med 35:1758, 1994
89. Franken PR, Demoor D, De Sadeleer C et al.: Free fatty acid uptake in myocardium with postischemic dysfunction: comparison with dobutamine echocardiogra-

phy to predict long term functional recovery. J Nucl Med 35:50P, 1994
90. Hoeflin F, Ledermann H, Noelpp U et al.: Routine 18F-deoxy-2-fluoro-d-glucose myocardial tomography using a normal large field of view gamma camera. Angiology 140:1058, 1989
91. van Lingen A, Huijgens PC, Visser FC et al.: Performance characteristics of a 511 keV collimator for imaging positron emitters with a standard gamma camera. Eur J Nucl Med 19:315, 1992
92. Williams KA, Taillon LA, Stark VJ: Quantitative planar imaging of glucose metabolic activity in myocardial segments with exercise thallium-201 perfusion defects in patients with myocardial infarction: comparison with late (24-hour) redistribution thallium imaging for detection of reversible ischemia. Am Heart J 124:294, 1992
93. Bax JJ, Visser FC, van Lingen A et al.: Feasibility of assessing regional myocardial uptake of 18F-fluorodeoxyglucose using single photon emission computed tomography. Eur Heart J 14:1675, 1993
94. Stoll HP, Hellwig N, Alexander C et al.: Myocardial metabolic imaging by means of fluorine-18 deoxyglucose/technetium-99m sestamibi dual-isotope single-photon emission tomography. Eur J Nucl Med 21:1085, 1994
95. Burt RW, Perkins OW, Oppenheim BE et al.: Direct comparison of fluorine-18-FDG SPECT, fluorine-18-FDG PET and rest thallium-201 SPECT for detection of myocardial viability. J Nucl Med 36:176, 1995
96. Bax JJ, Visser FC, van Lingen A et al.: Relation between myocardial uptake of thallium-201 chloride and fluorine-18 fluorodeoxyglucose imaged with single photon emission tomography in normal individuals. Eur J Nucl Med 22:56, 1995
97. Johnson LL, Seldin DW, Keller AM et al.: Dual isotope thallium and indium antimyosin SPECT imaging to identify acute infarct patients at further ischemic risk. Circulation 81:37, 1990
98. Schoeder H, Topp H, Friedrich M et al.: Thallium and antimyosin dual-isotope single-photon emission tomography in acute myocardial infarction to identify patients at further ischaemic risk. Eur J Nucl Med 21:415, 1994
99. Hansen CL: Preliminary report of an ongoing phase 1/11 dose range, safety and efficacy study of iodine-123-phenylpentadecanoic acid for the identification of viable myocardium, suppl. 4, 35:38S, 1994

Chapter 21

Assessment of Myocardial Viability Using Positron Emission Tomography

Richard C. Brunken

Positron emission tomography (PET) has evolved over the last 15 years from an exciting research tool into an affordable and clinically useful cardiac imaging technique. Observations made with cardiac PET imaging have substantially advanced our understanding of the interrelationships among myocardial perfusion, metabolism, and contractile function in acute and chronic ischemic heart disease. This new information has already had a substantial direct impact on patient care. The emergence of cardiac PET into the clinical arena has been paralleled by advances in imaging instrumentation and by the synthesis of new radioactive tracers for myocardial imaging. Current PET tomographs permit visualization of the entire heart with spatial and temporal resolutions that are far superior to those of early instruments; a variety of radiolabeled tracers that depict metabolism and perfusion have been synthesized, validated in animal experiments, and employed for imaging studies of human myocardium.

As the number of PET imaging centers continues to increase in the United States and around the world, physicians are finding that it is increasingly feasible to refer coronary heart disease patients with left ventricular dysfunction for myocardial viability studies. Prior experimental and clinical studies have yielded several alternative PET imaging methods for the determination of myocardial viability, and each of these methods has its own advantages and disadvantages. Because the results of these PET imaging studies directly affect the clinical decision-making process, it is important that physicians have an understanding of the fundamentals of cardiac PET imaging as well as a knowledge of the relative merits and limitations of each of the various imaging options for the determination of myocardial viability. This chapter provides a brief overview of the fundamentals of cardiac positron emission tomography, which supplements the observations of Schwaiger and co-authors, followed by a discussion of the PET imaging options available to clinicians to assess myocardial viability in patients with chronic coronary artery disease and left ventricular dysfunction.

METHODOLOGY OF CARDIAC PET
Fundamentals of PET

PET, a noninvasive nuclear medicine imaging technique, uses radioactive tracers labeled with positron-emitting atoms to characterize tissue processes in vivo.[1-3] The particular radioactive tracer used for imaging, along with its tissue distribution and disposition, determine the specific nature of the information provided by the PET imaging study. Carbon, oxygen, and nitrogen have short-lived radionuclide species that decay by positron emission; these iso-

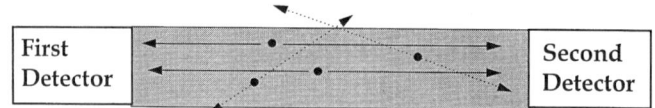

Fig. 21-1. Two 511 keV photons are created when an emitted positron encounters an electron and the two mutually annihilate. The photons depart from the annihilation site in opposite directions. When two detectors opposite each other simultaneously detect a scintillation event (*solid lines*), the site of the annihilation is localized to the volume between the two detectors. If only one photon is detected (*broken lines*) the requirement for coincidence detection is not satisfied and the scintillation event is not incorporated into that detector pair's contribution to the myocardial image. ●, site of β^+, β^- annihilation.

topes can readily be incorporated into biologically active molecules that depict naturally occurring cellular processes. In addition, an isotope of fluorine, fluorine-18, has chemical properties similar to the hydroxyl group (OH) and can be used to label a variety of biologically active molecules that are useful for myocardial imaging.

Each of the radioactive tracers employed in PET imaging decays by emitting a positron (or β^+ particle) from a proton-rich nucleus. This positron interacts with atoms in the surrounding medium, producing excitations and ionizations that slow the positron and decrease its kinetic energy. As the positron slows it comes into close proximity with one of the many electrons in the surrounding medium, at which point both the electron and the positron mutually annihilate. The energy liberated from this interaction results in the release of two 511 keV *annihilation photons*, which depart from the annihilation site about 180° apart.

Current PET tomographs use circular rings of individual detectors connected by sophisticated electronic circuitry to identify paired scintillation events occurring 180° apart (*annihilation coincidence detection*). If two detectors opposite each other simultaneously (within 10 to 20 nanoseconds) register photons in coincidence, then the annihilation event must have occurred somewhere in the volume between the two detectors (Fig. 21-1). If only one photon is detected, the requirement for coincidence detection is not satisfied and the scintillation event is not incorporated into the myocardial image.

The net *attenuation* (backscatter and/or absorption) of emitted annihilation photons in a cross-sectional slice of uniform medium is independent of the location of the annihilation event relative to the detectors.[1,2] In clinical practice, individualized attenuation correction factors are determined for each patient's images on a pixel by pixel basis. To determine the attenuation correction factors, a scan is first performed using a ring source of a positron-emitting substance placed about the edge of the field of view of the tomograph (*the blank scan*). The scan is then repeated with the patient in the field of view (*the transmission scan*). A matrix of attenuation correction factors is generated by dividing the blank scan by the transmission scan. The numerical factors thus calculated are then applied to the patient's emission scan count data to correct for photon attenuation by the structures of the chest.

The sensitivity for the detection of annihilation photons and the spatial resolution of current PET instruments reflect mainly the geometry and the size of the tomograph's detectors and photomultiplier tubes and are relatively insensitive to the depth of the annihilation event. Because an annihilation event can occur anywhere in the sensitive space between two detectors, coincidence detection effectively localizes scintillation events to the line defined by the two detectors (one dimension). To define the two-dimensional spatial distribution of the tracer, activity measurements are made from many different directions, using a ring of detectors. Because a given detector can be in coincidence with multiple detectors on the opposite side of the ring, the sensitive region for that detector is a fanlike area within the plane. A set of activity profiles is generated for each of the detectors in the ring. These profiles depend upon the angle about the ring (i.e., the particular detector) and each point in a detector's activity profile represents the sum of activity on a line between it and one of the opposite detectors. If the number of counts in each profile is adequate and a sufficiently high angular sampling frequency is employed, it is possible to solve for all unknown variables (somewhat analogous to solving n linear equations for an equal number of unknowns). Using standard back-projection and Fourier reconstruction techniques, it is then possible to reconstruct a two-dimensional image of the tracer distribution within the plane.

To define the three-dimensional spatial distribution of a labeled tracer, most PET tomographs use multiple rings of detectors adjacent to each other. In some PET tomographs, lead shielding is interposed between individual detector rings to reduce photon scatter. Despite the shielding, a detector in one plane can be in the "line of sight" of some of the opposite detectors in adjacent planes. By using interplane coincidences, current instruments provide an additional set of interpolated images midway between the direct planes defined by the detector rings. Current state-of-the-art tomographs can simultaneously acquire as many as 64 cross-sectional images over axial distances of 10 to 15 cm, at 4 to 7 mm spacing with effective slice thicknesses of 5 to 8 mm.

Clinical PET Imaging

When individuals with advanced coronary artery disease (CAD) undergo cardiac PET imaging, a knowledgeable physician is present to assist in monitoring the patient's condition and to treat promptly any complications that arise during the course of the study. The patient's cardiac rhythm is monitored continuously and cuff blood pressure measurements are obtained periodically. Measurements of peripheral oxygen saturation can also be monitored noninvasively using a pulse oximeter. Individuals with pronounced left ventricular dysfunction may experience orthopnea or an exacerbation of their cardiac arrhythmias if left in a supine position for prolonged periods. Some patients may therefore benefit from the use of supplemental oxygen during the imaging procedure.

Clinical PET imaging begins with careful positioning of the subject within the tomograph. Care is taken to make the patient as comfortable as possible to reduce movement during the imaging session. The precise location of the heart within the thorax is first determined. In some laboratories, this is accomplished using fluoroscopy or a supine chest radiograph. More frequently, rectilinear scans or short transmission scans are obtained using an external positron-emitting ring source. Once the position of the heart is determined, a 10- to 20-minute transmission scan is performed. The transmission scan is used to correct all subsequent emission images for attenuation of activity by the thorax. It is therefore important to assure that the patient does not move between transmission and emission image acquisition to prevent the introduction of artifacts into the emission images.[4] Although sometimes the emission images can be corrected for patient movement,[5] it is much easier to prevent the problem by ensuring that the patient is comfortable before the study begins.

Emission images are obtained after the administration of a radioactive tracer to the patient. The radioactive tracer can be administered intravenously or a radioactive gas can be administered by inhalation. Emission images are frequently acquired at the time of peak myocardial uptake of the tracer relative to background (*static image acquisition*). Alternatively, a whole series of images may be sequentially acquired (*dynamic image acquisition*). These images depict the changes in myocardial tracer concentrations as a function of time. A dynamic image-acquisition sequence is required to assess the kinetic behavior of the radioactive tracer within the myocardium and to quantitatively measure absolute rates of blood flow and metabolic processes. Images gated to the patient's electrocardiogram (ECG) may also be obtained, either as part of a static image-acquisition protocol or after a dynamic image-acquisition sequence. Gated images permit measurements of segmental wall motion and thickening, ventricular volumes, and ejection fractions[6-10] and may also reduce the inhomogeneities in the PET images that result from anatomic variations in regional wall thicknesses.[11]

Since all positron-emitting tracers liberate 511 keV photons, myocardial counts must decline to near background levels by physical decay or biologic clearance before a second set of images can be acquired. When tracers with different half-lives are used, imaging with the tracer with the shortest half-life is usually performed first, followed by the tracer with the next longest half-life, etc. The time required for the imaging procedure ranges from 1 to 4 hours, depending on the complexity of the imaging se-

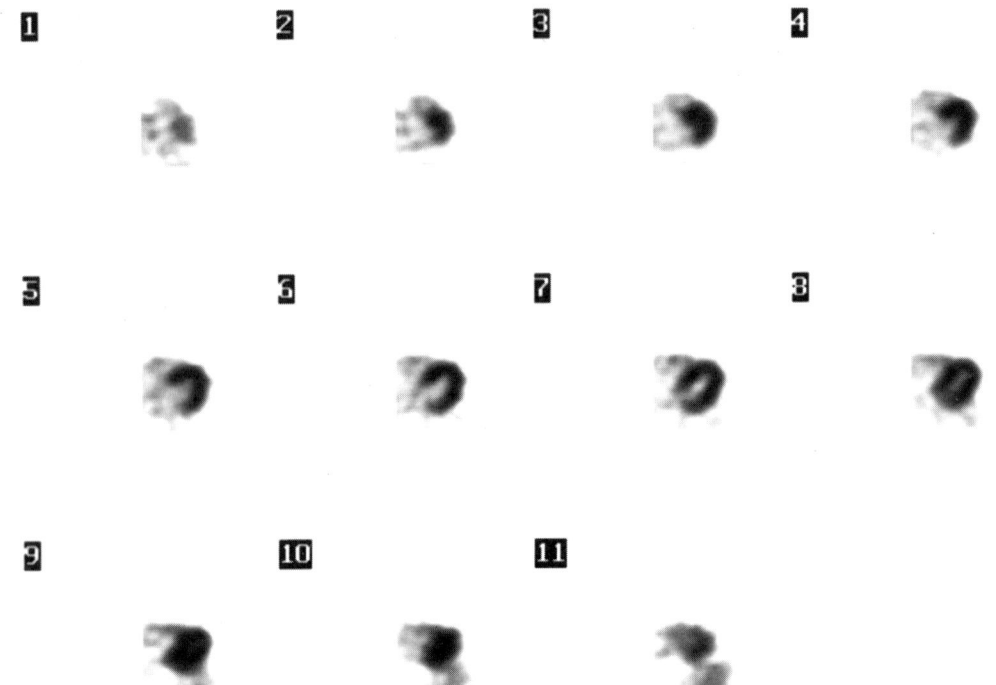

Fig. 21-2. The initial transverse images obtained during positron emission tomographic imaging are orthogonal to the body. Image 1 is the most cranial, while image 11 is most caudad. In this image display, the left ventricle points to the upper right. On the more inferior images, the horseshoe-shaped myocardial image changes into an eccentric ring and then into a solid confluence of activity as the image plane dips beneath the mitral valve.

quences employed and the number of radioactive tracers used in the imaging study.

The images acquired by the PET scanner, the *transaxial images*, are orthogonal to the body (Fig. 21-2). Because it may be difficult to visualize the inferior wall of the heart on these images, they are usually "resliced" into short-axis and vertical and horizontal long-axis images.[12–16] Semiquantitative analysis of realigned PET images can be achieved using methods analogous to those employed in single photon emission computed tomographic (SPECT) thallium-201 (^{201}Tl) scintigraphy,[17–19] in which relative myocardial tracer concentrations defined by automated edge-detection algorithms on short-axis images are referenced to normal databases and displayed as polar maps.[14–16,20–22]

Quantitation of Myocardial Tracer Concentrations

Absolute measurements of myocardial blood flows and metabolic rates require an analysis of the manner in which tissue and vascular radioactive tracer concentrations change over time. Tissue tracer concentrations are derived by drawing myocardial regions of interest on the images obtained in a dynamic PET imaging study. By knowing the framing rate used for image acquisition, counts within a region of interest can be graphed as a function of time (Fig. 21-3). Vascular tracer concentrations can be measured directly using arterial blood samples or determined noninvasively from regions of interest placed over the center of the left ventricular cavity or the left atrium. The count data are displayed as *time-activity curves*. Time-activity curves can be fit using appropriate mathematical models that describe the biologic behavior of the radioactive label. By fitting the data, the mathematical equations can be solved for the physiologic parameter of interest. If a dynamic image acquisition sequence is employed, it is also feasible in conjunction with the appropriate tracer kinetic models (below) to generate parametric myocardial images and polar maps that

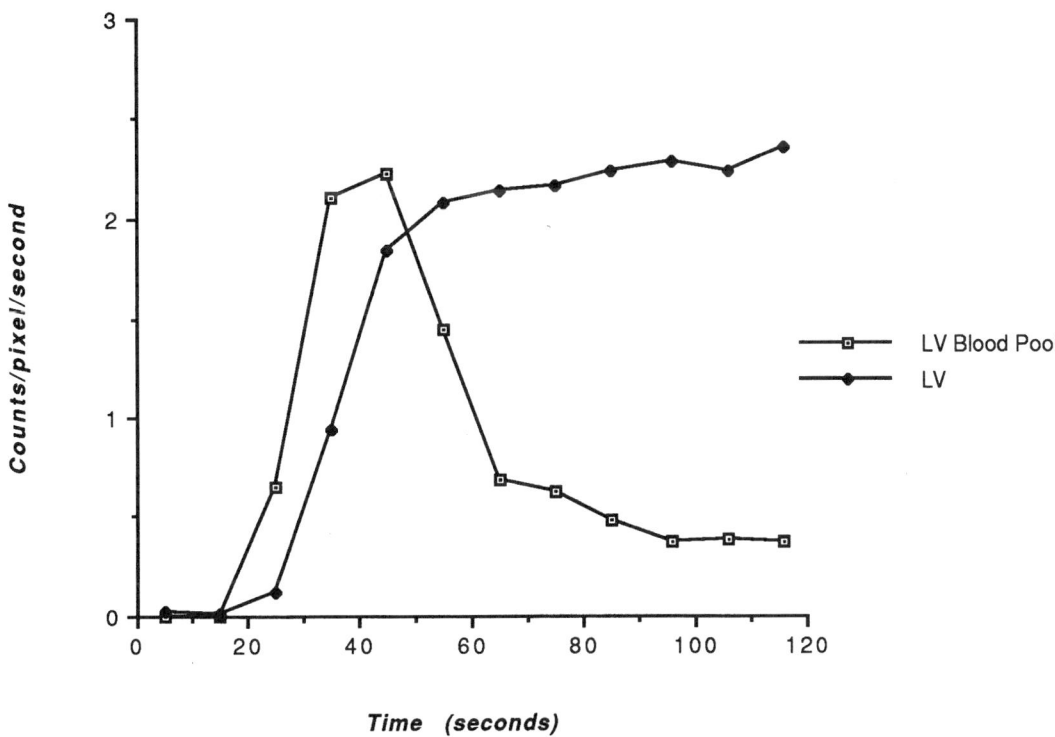

Fig. 21-3. Left ventricular myocardial and arterial time–activity curves derived from rapidly acquired nitrogen 13 ammonia positron emission tomographic cardiac images. Count data for the tissue curve were obtained by placing a region of interest over the free wall of the left ventricle on resliced short axis images, while data for the arterial (left ventricular blood pool) curve were obtained by placing a region of interest over the center of the left ventricular cavity.

depict absolute values of blood flow (in milliliters of blood flow per minute per gram of tissue) and tissue metabolic rates (in micromoles of substrate per minute per gram of tissue) on a pixel by pixel basis.[23-28]

Because correction for attenuation of myocardial activity by extracardiac structures is routinely performed during clinical cardiac PET imaging, the counts displayed on myocardial PET images reflect actual tissue tracer concentrations. As noted, the capability to accurately measure rapidly changing tissue tracer concentrations forms the basis for the measurements of absolute rates of flow and metabolism made with cardiac PET imaging. Two other physical factors also affect the myocardial tracer concentrations depicted on PET images: the *partial volume effect* and *spillover of activity*. The partial volume effect refers to the fact that radioactivity occupying a space less than the smallest volume element resolvable by the PET tomograph will be distributed over the entire resolvable volume element. For example, suppose that a point source of activity with 10,000 counts/s occupies an actual volume of 10 mm^3. The true activity concentration is 10,000/10 = 1,000 counts/s/mm^3. If the same point source is placed in a tomograph with a minimal resolvable volume of 1000 mm^3, the activity concentration observed with the PET camera will be about 10,000/1000 = 10 counts/s/mm^3.

From phantom studies, it can be shown that myocardial counts on PET images accurately reflect true tissue concentrations if the regional myocardial wall thickness is equal to or greater than twice the spatial resolution of the PET tomograph.[1,29] As wall thickness decreases, there is a nonlinear decrease in observed PET tissue tracer concentrations. Parodi[30] and his colleagues demonstrated that the loss of systolic thickening (as might be observed in patients with resting regional wall-motion abnormalities) will further reduce observed tracer concentrations, because of a decrease in the time-averaged ventricular wall thickness. The *recovery coefficient* (RC) reflects the relative amount of the true activity concentration observed with the PET tomograph; it is nonlinearly related to object size. The RC is determined by the performance characteristics of the tomograph and is measured for each type of instrument. If the regional myocardial wall thickness is known, then the true myocardial tissue tracer concentration C_m (in counts/s/ml) can be calculated. Measurements of regional wall thickness can be obtained from echocardiography, computed tomography, magnetic resonance imaging, or from gated PET images themselves.[10]

Spillover of activity refers to the inability of the PET camera to distinguish activity from two different sources that are physically close to each other. Activity within a region of interest reflects both intrinsic activity as well as "contaminating" counts from adjacent structures with activity. Early after the intravenous administration of a radioactive tracer, when vascular concentrations are high and myocardial concentrations are low, activity "spills" from blood within the left ventricular cavity into adjacent myocardium. Furthermore, since about 10% of the volume of the myocardium is composed of blood vessels, activity within this vascular space also "spills" over into tissue. Once tracer concentrations decline in blood, the opposite effect can be observed, that is, activity retained within tissue can "spill" into measured blood activities. Corrections for spillover of activity are feasible, based upon measurements of the size of the left ventricular cavity, the thickness of the myocardium, and the performance characteristics of the tomograph, or by incorporating a term reflecting spillover into the differential equations used to model the kinetic behavior of the tracer.[29,31]

Assessment of Myocardial Perfusion

Regional myocardial blood flow is usually assessed with either nitrogen 13 (^{13}N) ammonia, rubidium 82, or oxygen 15 (^{15}O) water. Each of these perfusion tracers has unique advantages and disadvantages that have been discussed in the previous chapter. Both ^{13}N ammonia (half-life, 9.96 minutes) and ^{15}O water (half-life, 2.07 minutes) require an on-site cyclotron for their production, while rubidium 82 (half-life, 1.26 minutes) is eluted at the bedside from a commercially available strontium 82 generator.[32,33]

Nitrogen 13 Ammonia

Nitrogen 13 (^{13}N) ammonia is a partially extractable tracer of myocardial perfusion.[34–37] Following the intravenous administration of the radioactive tracer, about 95% to 100% of the substance within the vascular space crosses the capillary membrane in the resting state, but as myocardial blood flow increases, an increasing proportion of the tracer diffuses back into the vascular space. The fraction of ^{13}N activity retained in the myocardium is thus inversely and nonlinearly related to flow, because the increase in the net tissue extraction of ^{13}N ammonia becomes progressively smaller for each increment in blood flow.[38–41] Once in the extracellular space, ^{13}N ammonia is trapped within the cell via the glutamic acid–glutamine reaction, in which the ^{13}N label is transferred to glutamine.[36,42,43]

For clinical imaging, 10 to 20 mCi of ^{13}N ammonia are administered as an intravenous bolus. Clearance of ^{13}N activity from blood pool and lungs is rapid in most individuals, so that static cardiac images may be acquired 4 to 7 minutes after tracer injection. In patients with markedly impaired left ventricular function or in those who are chronic smokers, pulmonary uptake of ^{13}N ammonia may be prominent. ^{13}N ammonia is also taken up by the liver, and hepatic ^{13}N activity occasionally impinges upon the inferior margin of the heart. Acquisition times for ^{13}N ammonia perfusion images range from 5 to 20 minutes, depending on the administered dose.

On static myocardial images, the distribution of ^{13}N activity may be heterogeneous, with a modest reduction in relative tracer activity in the posterolateral region of the ventricle.[44,45] The reason for this reduction is not understood, but it does not appear to be a technical artifact. It is not observed on static images obtained using other perfusion tracers or when absolute measurements of myocardial blood flow are made with ^{13}N ammonia.[45] Possibly a small amount of "redistribution" of ^{13}N ammonia metabolites occurs in this ventricular region. The reduction in posterolateral ^{13}N activity does not adversely affect the clinical interpretation of the PET perfusion images in most patients. However, in some individuals it may be necessary to use semiquantitative techniques such as circumferential profile analysis or polar mapping to compare the observed tracer distribution to that of a normal database.

Rubidium 82

Rubidium is a positively charged metallic ion whose biologic behavior is similar to potassium. Its myocardial uptake depends on blood flow. Several radioactive isotopes of this element have been explored as tracers of myocardial perfusion.[46-52] Rubidium 82 has several advantages for clinical perfusion imaging. First, its short half-life (1.26 minutes) permits performance of sequential perfusion studies in the same patient in a brief period, so full rest and pharmacologic stress perfusion studies can generally be acquired in less than 45 minutes. Second, it may be eluted directly from a strontium 82/rubidium 82 generator,[52] which permits performance of perfusion imaging at any time.

Rubidium 82 is actively transported across the cell membrane by the sodium–potassium adenosine triphosphate (ATP) dependent transmembranous ion-exchange system. Rate constants for the tissue uptake of rubidium 82 exhibit little variation from anatomic segment to segment in normal myocardium.[53] Net myocardial concentrations of rubidium 82 ultimately reflect two competing processes: cellular transport across the sarcolemma and back-diffusion into the vascular space. Back-diffusion of rubidium 82 depends upon blood flow; as a diffusable tracer the net tissue extraction of rubidium 82 declines nonlinearly with increasing blood flows.[54-57]

For clinical imaging, 30 to 60 mCi of rubidium 82 are administered intravenously over 30 to 60 seconds. Static cardiac images are acquired after blood pool activity has declined to acceptable levels, typically 1 to 3 minutes after tracer injection. Acquisition times for static rubidium 82 perfusion images are 5 to 8 minutes, depending on the dose administered. Rubidium 82 perfusion images are generally of good quality, demonstrating relatively homogeneous tracer activity,[44] but may be limited in some patients by relatively low counts resulting from the rapid decay of the tracer.

Oxygen 15 Water

Water labeled with ^{15}O (half-life, 2.07 minutes) is a freely diffusable tracer, which is nearly completely extracted on its initial pass through the coronary microcirculation, irrespective of alterations in blood flow or changes in tissue metabolic state.[58-63] Unfortunately, several technical factors render this tracer less than optimal for clinical imaging. First, blood pool activity in lungs and the vasculature contribute significantly to the ^{15}O water images, and image substraction using inhaled carbon dioxide (see below) may be compromised by patient movement. Second, counts on the final myocardial images may be relatively low, owing to substraction of vascular activity as well as to the relatively rapid decay of ^{15}O. Finally, it is time consuming and technically demanding.

For clinical imaging, 15 to 25 mCi of ^{15}O-labeled water are administered by either a bolus intravenous infusion or a slow intravenous infusion. Images are typically acquired over the subsequent 2 to 3 minutes. Alternatively, ^{15}O-labeled CO_2 may be administered by continuous inhalation for about 3 to 4 minutes.[64,65] In this technique, labeled CO_2 is rapidly converted to ^{15}O water by carbonic anhydrase within the lungs and vascular space. Images are acquired during and for 3 to 4 minutes after the inhalation of the gas. This method of tracer administration helps to obviate the high count rates that sometimes accompany the intravenous administration of ^{15}O water, thereby assuring that they do not exceed the capabilities of the PET instrument. Correction for vascular ^{15}O activity has been attained by subtraction of myocardial blood pool activity from the original image.[66,67] However, this is usually accomplished by obtaining a second set of images following inhalation of 40 to 50 mCi of ^{15}O-labeled carbon monoxide. Labeled carbon monoxide binds to hemoglobin in red blood cells to form ^{15}O carboxyhemoglobin and irreversibly label the vascular space. The blood pool images are normalized to the initial ^{15}O images and then subtracted from them to derive true myocardial ^{15}O activity.

Other Tracers of Myocardial Perfusion

Other positron-emitting tracers of myocardial perfusion have been studied but not extensively used for clinical imaging. These include potassium 38,[68-72] sestamibi labeled with technetium 94m,[73] and lipophilic complexes of gallium 68[74-76] and copper 62.[77-82] Potassium 38 (physical half-life, 7.6 minutes) and technetium-94m (half-life, 53 minutes) sestamibi require a cyclotron for their production while gallium 68 (half-life, 68.1 minutes) and copper 62 (half-life, 9.74 minutes) are eluted from commercially available generators.

Microspheres labeled with positron-emitting radionuclides have also been employed for myocardial perfusion imaging. Long considered the "gold standard" for laboratory measurements of myocardial blood flow,[83] radiolabeled microspheres must be administered into the systemic circulation (usually via an injection in the left ventricular cavity) to prevent trapping of the particles within the pulmonary capillaries. Biodegradable human serum albumin microspheres (15 to 20 μ) labeled with either gallium 68 or ^{11}C (^{11}C half-life, 20.4 minutes) have been used for qualitative and quantitative determinations of regional blood flows with PET.[59,84-87] Although the administration of labeled macroaggregated albumin by left ventricular injection appears to be well tolerated in CAD patients with regional dysfunction,[87] this imaging technique is infrequently used in the clinical setting because of the need to inject the radiolabeled microspheres directly into the systemic circulation.

Summary—Options for PET Perfusion Imaging

Each of the PET perfusion tracers has unique advantages and disadvantages for clinical cardiac imaging. An on-site cyclotron is required for imaging with either ^{13}N ammonia or ^{15}O water. In contrast, rubidium 82 can be used for perfusion imaging any time during the life of the strontium 92 generator. The short half-half of rubidium 82 permits performance of sequential studies (e.g., rest and pharmacologic stress) relatively rapidly. Off-setting the advantages of rubidium 82 as a perfusion tracer are its relatively energetic positrons, the cost of the strontium 82/rubidium 82 generator (about $30,000 per generator) and the fact that the elution volume for a given amount of radioactivity increases as generator strontium 82 activity decays with time. Although ^{15}O water also has a short physical half-life and biologic properties that make it the ideal blood flow tracer, relatively high background activity and the necessity to correct for blood pool activity may make it less than optimal for imaging in a busy clinical center. Because of the relatively rapid decay of both rubidium 82 and ^{15}O, images obtained with either of these agents may suffer from relatively low count density. ^{13}N ammonia, as the tracer with the longest half-life, permits imaging for longer periods and better image count density. Since some normal individuals may exhibit a relative reduction in ^{13}N activity in the posterolateral wall, visual interpretation of ^{13}N ammonia images may be somewhat difficult in some patients. Because all three perfusion tracers provide comparable diagnostic information about regional myocardial perfusion, the tracer best suited for clinical imaging will depend on the local needs and economics of each PET imaging center.

Quantitative Perfusion Measurements

Conventional planar or SPECT perfusion images, as well as static PET perfusion images, depict proportionate tissue tracer concentrations, and, therefore, only relative myocardial perfusion. Perfusion defect severity, for example, is often expressed as the reduction in activity relative to peak myocardial activity. This normalization process assumes that the highest tissue counts do indeed reflect normal myocardium; it does not account for the deficient recovery of counts in hypoperfused regions with impaired wall motion resulting from the partial volume effect. In patients with "balanced" coronary artery disease or homogeneous myocardial pathophysiology (e.g., nonischemic cardiomyopathies, heart transplant rejection, chest pain with normal coronary arteries), conventional imaging techniques may provide little additional useful information because there are no regional disparities in the disease process. Cardiac PET, however, can accurately measure rapidly changing blood pool and regional tissue tracer concentrations with a high temporal resolution immediately following the administration of the radioactive agent. This makes it possible to determine absolute rates of myocardial perfusion (in milliliters of blood flow per minute per gram of tissue) from the dynamic PET images.

The myocardial concentration of a perfusion tracer at time t after the injection of the tracer, or Q_t, is given by the formula:

$$Q_t = E \cdot F \cdot \int_0^t C_a(t)dt$$

where E is the first-pass unidirectional extraction fraction, $C_a(t)$ is the concentration of the tracer in arterial blood (the arterial input function), and F is myocardial blood flow.[3] The true myocardial concentration of the tracer, Q_f, can be determined from count data on the cardiac PET images if the instrument is appropriately calibrated using a reference standard with a known radioactivity concentration. $C_a(t)$, or the arterial input function, can be obtained directly by counting arterial blood samples or, alternatively, from count data obtained from a region of interest placed over the left ventricular cavity or the left atrium on the PET images.[88-90]

If radiolabeled microspheres are used for perfusion imaging, the extraction fraction, E, is equal to one because the tracer is completely trapped on the first pass through the coronary microcirculation. If arterial blood is continuously withdrawn at a constant rate, F_a, from an indwelling peripheral arterial catheter, then myocardial blood flow is readily calculated using the formula:

$$F = \frac{F_a \cdot Q_T}{C_T}$$

where Q_T is the regional myocardial tracer activity determined from the PET images, and C_T is the integral of the arterial input function from the time of injection to time T.[83]

Measurement of absolute myocardial blood flows with either freely diffusable (^{15}O water) or partially extractable perfusion tracers (rubidium 82, ^{13}N ammonia) is accomplished by careful analysis of the temporal changes in tissue and blood pool radioactivity concentrations on dynamic PET perfusion images. Myocardial and blood pool time-activity curves are obtained from regions of interest defined on the PET images. These data are then fit using operational mathematical equations based upon tracer kinetic models, which quantitatively describe the time-dependent behavior of the tracer within functional pools (or compartments) within the heart.[91,92] The fit of the experimental data to the operational differential equations describing the behavior of the tracer provides a quantitative estimate of absolute myocardial blood flow, in milliliters per minute per gram of tissue.

A single compartment tracer kinetic model is usually used to derive blood flow measurements from ^{15}O water studies (59, 63-66). It is assumed that ^{15}O water rapidly and fully equilibrates between plasma and tissue, that the uptake of the tracer is flow dependent and not limited by diffusion, that there are no arteriovenous shunts, and that blood flow is constant and homogeneous during the period of imaging. Tracer kinetic models that incorporate corrections for activity spillover, the partial volume effect, and the arterial blood volume of the tissue into the operational differential equations have been developed and validated in both experimental and clinical studies.

Quantification of myocardial blood flows with partially extractable tracers of perfusion such as ^{13}N ammonia or rubidium 82 is usually performed using a tracer kinetic model with two functional compartments.[38-40,57,93-97] The *fast exchangeable compartment* corresponds to the rapid exchange of tracer across the capillary membrane and back diffusion. Activity within this compartment represents activity within the vascular and interstitial spaces. The slow exchangeable compartment represents that portion of tracer activity retained within tissue. In the two-compartment model, myocardial blood flow (F) is considered constant over the period of image acquisition. Time-activity curves generated from myocardial regions of interest drawn on the early dynamic PET images are fit to estimate the parameters of the operational equations describing the two-compartment model. In some models, the operational equations include terms accounting for activity spillover and partial volume effects. Myocardial blood flow is then obtained as one of the desired parameters estimated by the curve-fitting process.

Quantitative blood flow measurements derived from dynamic ^{15}O water, rubidium 82 and ^{13}N ammonia PET images correlate well with microsphere blood flow measurements in animal experiments.[38,40,59,60,94,95-97] In human studies, noninvasive measurements of myocardial blood flow with dynamic ^{13}N ammonia PET images have been shown to have relatively small interobserver and interstudy variabilities.[98] Ratios of hyperemic-to-rest myocardial blood flows measured with PET are linearly related to ratios of hyperemic-to-rest coronary flow velocities measured directly with intracoronary Doppler flow probes in patients with coronary heart disease and in individuals with chest pain and angiographically normal coronary arteries.[99,100] Thus, reliable measurements of absolute myocardial blood flows can be simultaneously obtained in all regions of the heart in vivo using dynamic PET imaging and state of the art instruments.

Assessment of Myocardial Metabolism

To generate the vital energy used to sustain contraction, maintain membrane ion gradients, and support other critical cellular functions, the mammalian heart metabolizes a wide variety of substrates including free fatty acids, glucose, lactate, pyruvate, ketone bodies, and amino acids.[101–109] Myocardial substrate utilization is highly influenced by arterial substrate concentrations, regional blood flow, and oxidative capacity of myocardium, and the neurohormonal milieu. In the fasting state myocardial glucose utilization is suppressed by high free fatty acid levels in the plasma. Under these conditions about 60% of myocardial oxygen consumption is used to oxidize free fatty acids, 30% is used for oxidation of glucose, and the remaining oxygen consumption is accounted for by triglycerides, lactate, ketones, and pyruvate.[108] In contrast, a postprandial increase in plasma insulin and glucose levels results in an increase in myocardial glucose utilization. Following a carbohydrate-rich meal, about 70% of myocardial oxygen consumption is used for oxidative metabolism of glucose, and nearly all of the oxygen consumption of the heart can be attributed to the oxidation of carbohydrate, either as glucose, lactate, or pyruvate.[108] Qualitative and quantitative measurements of tissue metabolic processes made in vivo with PET must therefore be interpreted in light of the factors known to influence myocardial substrate selection.

Although a variety of positron-emitting tracers of myocardial metabolism have been synthesized, only three have had extensive clinical use: Carbon 11 (^{11}C) palmitate, ^{11}C acetate, and fluorine-18 2-fluoro-2-deoxyglucose (FDG). ^{11}C palmitate is a 16-carbon, naturally occurring, fatty acid labeled on the carboxyl (C-1) end with ^{11}C (half-life, 20.4 minutes).[110] Dynamic PET images depicting the myocardial uptake and clearance of ^{11}C palmitate provide quantitative information about regional fatty acid metabolism. ^{11}C acetate is a two-carbon molecule of intermediate metabolism that is labeled on the first carbon atom.[111] Dynamic ^{11}C acetate PET images depicting the myocardial uptake and clearance of this tracer provide information on the rate of substrate flux through the mitochondrial tricarboxylic acid cycle. This provides an indirect, quantitative measure of regional myocardial oxygen consumption that is largely independent of the patient's dietary state.[112–118] Myocardial glucose metabolism is assessed with FDG (half-life, 109.8 min), a glucose analog labeled on the second carbon atom with fluorine 18.[119] Rates of myocardial FDG uptake are proportional to the tissue consumption of exogenous glucose. If a dynamic FDG PET study is performed, absolute regional rates of myocardial glucose consumption, in micromoles of glucose per minute per gram of tissue, can be determined.

Carbon 11 Palmitate

^{11}C palmitate was one of the first tracers used in conjunction with PET imaging to assess myocardial metabolism in vivo in coronary heart disease patients.[120–122] These pioneering studies established that regional disturbances in myocardial metabolism could be characterized and quantified with noninvasive PET imaging and helped to inaugurate the use of metabolic imaging in clinical cardiology.

The initial myocardial uptake of ^{11}C palmitate reflects both regional blood flow and first pass extraction fraction. The first pass extraction fraction is inversely related to blood flow and directly related to the fatty acid concentration gradient between the plasma and the cytosol of the myocyte. This gradient depends upon plasma fatty acid concentrations and the rate of intracellular palmitate utilization through the thioesterification of ^{11}C palmitate, which sequesters the tracer within the cell.[123,124] Following activation to ^{11}C palmitoyl-coenzyme A (CoA), the acyl-CoA moiety can enter various biochemical pathways (e.g., mitochondrial oxidation, incorporation into triglyceride and phospholipid), the selection of which is incompletely understood. In the mitochondria, fatty acids are sequentially cleaved by β-oxidation into two-carbon fragments, which are then oxidized to carbon dioxide and water via the tricarboxylic acid (TCA) cycle. Each cycle produces reduced forms of the adenine dinucleotides, which generate ATP by reoxidation by the transfer of electrons to molecular oxygen by way of the electron transport chain.

For clinical imaging, 15 to 20 mCi of ^{11}C palmitate suspended in 6% albumin are administered by intravenous bolus infusion. Activity within the central circulation is present on early ^{11}C palmitate PET images and then declines over the next several minutes as the tracer accumulates within the myocardium. Myocardial uptake and regional distribution of ^{11}C palmitate can be evaluated on static images acquired after blood activity decreases, about 3 to 7 minutes after injection. Dynamic PET imaging may be performed for 40 to 60 minutes after tracer administration; peak myocardial ^{11}C palmitate uptake typically occurs 3 to 5 minutes after tracer injection. Following peak tracer accumulation, ^{11}C activity is gradually released from the tissue, and there is a progressive loss of counts from the cardiac image.

^{11}C palmitate images are quantitatively analyzed by assigning regions of interest to the myocardium and constructing tissue time-activity curves that depict regional ^{11}C activity as a function of time. Myocardial time-activity curves typically reveal a biexponential clearance of ^{11}C activity from tissue. The first component represents the initial rapid clearance phase of the tracer, caused by oxidation of ^{11}C palmitate. The relative size of this component and its rate constant, k_1, are proportional to cardiac work, rates of oxygen consumption, and ^{11}C-labeled CO_2 production.[125–130] The latter component of the curve, or that portion representing the slow clearance phase of tracer activity, is described by a second rate constant, k_2. This latter, slower phase of the tissue time-activity curve reflects incorporation of the radioactive label into the intracellular lipid pool, primarily as triglycerides and phospholipids.

As the clinical expression of biochemical processes occurring within living tissue, myocardial ^{11}C palmitate time-activity curves are significantly altered by the physiologic and pathophysiologic factors that affect cellular fatty acid metabolism. For example, increases in plasma glucose, acetoacetate, 3-hydroxybutyrate, or lactate levels suppress myocardial fatty acid utilization. This shift in tissue substrate utilization decreases the relative size and the slope of the early rapid clearance phase of the myocardial ^{11}C time-activity curve,[131–133] and increases the late slow phase of the curve, indicating that the proportion of the fatty acid stored in the endogenous lipid pool increases in response to the shift in substrate utilization.

Acute ischemia limits myocardial oxygen delivery relative to tissue needs and impairs mitochondrial fatty acid oxidation,[104,134,135] cellular uptake, cytosolic activation, and transmitochondrial transport.[104] In PET imaging studies with ^{11}C palmitate, acute ischemia and hypoxia have been shown to prolong the half-life of the early rapid clearance phase of this tracer and to decrease the relative size of this component of the ^{11}C time-activity curve,[136,137] reflecting the impaired oxidation of the fatty acid. The relative contribution of the second slow portion of the time-activity curve increases, indicating that the relative amount of the labeled fatty acid that enters the endogenous lipid pool increases as myocardial ischemia becomes more pronounced. These observations are consistent with histopathologic studies demonstrating an increase in intracellular lipid content in acutely ischemic myocardium.[138–141]

As tissue oxygen delivery becomes more impaired, the *back-diffusion* of ^{11}C palmitate (i.e., the egress of unaltered tracer from the myocyte back into capillary blood) increases.[142,143] Back-diffusion of the tracer also affects the myocardial ^{11}C time activity curves obtained from serial PET images because it is another means of clearing activity from tissue. Rosamond et al.[143] reported that 44% of unmetabolized tracer diffused back into the vascular space in ischemic myocardium compared with 16% in normal tissue. Back-diffusion therefore limits the value of the rapid clearance phase of the ^{11}C time-activity curve as a quantitative measure of fatty acid oxidation under ischemic or hypoxic conditions. Thus, assessment of myocardial oxidative metabolism with ^{11}C palmitate is complicated by the dependence of rates of fatty acid oxidation on plasma substrate levels and by the back-diffusion of unmetabolized label under ischemic or hypoxic conditions.

^{11}C Acetate

Myocardial oxidative metabolism can be assessed more directly using dynamic PET imaging with ^{11}C acetate, a labeled two-carbon molecule that traces substrate flux through the TCA cycle. Following the initial myocardial uptake of ^{11}C acetate from the vascular space, the initial rapid phase of clearance of the ^{11}C label from the tissue is linearly related to myocardial oxygen consumption under a variety of metabolic and hemodynamic conditions.

Under aerobic conditions nearly all the major substrates of the heart, including glucose, fatty acids, ketone bodies, lactate, and pyruvate, are catabolized by conversion to acetyl-CoA and oxidation via the TCA cycle to carbon dioxide and water. Since reduced forms of the adenine dinucleotides generated by the TCA cycle are major determinants of rates of oxidative phosphorylation,[144] TCA cycle substrate flux is linked to myocardial oxygen consumption. Dietary state, and therefore the particular substrate used by the myocardium, has only a minor effect on the relationship between TCA cycle flux and myocardial oxygen consumption. For example, if glucose, lactate, or palmitate are exclusively metabolized by the heart, the myocardium will consume 3.0, 3.0, and 2.9 moles of oxygen for each mole of acetate, respectively.[145]

Following intravenous administration, first-pass extraction fractions of ^{11}C acetate average 64% at myocardial blood flows of about 1.0 ml/min/g and decline only modestly to 47% as blood flows further increase to 5.0 ml/min/g.[146] Clearance of the ^{11}C label from the vascular space is rapid, and blood pool activity falls to about 10% of peak counts by 3 to 4 minutes after tracer injection.[147,148] Because of the high first-pass extraction fraction and the rapid clearance of the ^{11}C label from blood, images acquired early after tracer administration can also be used to semi-quantitatively and quantitatively assess regional myocardial perfusion.[149–151] ^{11}C acetate therefore has the advantage of permitting evaluation of both regional perfusion and oxidative metabolism with a single isotope injection, thereby reducing both the radiation dose to the patient and the acquisition time for the PET study.

Transport of ^{11}C acetate across sarcolemmal and mitochondrial membranes is believed to be carrier mediated but not energy dependent. Once inside mitochondria, ^{11}C acetate is activated to ^{11}C acetyl-CoA, so that ^{11}C activity rapidly appears in the intermediates of the TCA cycle as well as glutamate and aspartate.[152] Incorporation of the ^{11}C label to glutamate and aspartate probably results from transamination of α-ketoglutarate and oxaloacetate, two major TCA cycle intermediates. Macroscopically observed rates of clearance of the myocardial label therefore reflects ^{11}C activity flux through a pool that includes TCA cycle intermediates, glutamate, and aspartate. Although ischemia increases the size of the pool containing the TCA intermediates, it decreases the size of glutamate and aspartate pools to about the same extent. Thus, the aggregate size of the combined TCA and amino acid pools would appear to be relatively constant under most imaging conditions, providing the rationale for the assessment of regional oxidative metabolism with this tracer.[152] Ultimately, nearly all ^{11}C activity is released as $^{11}CO_2$.

In the clinical setting, dynamic PET imaging is performed after the intravenous administration of 10 to 20 mCi of ^{11}C acetate. On the early PET images, radioactivity can be identified within the vascular space (Plate 21-1). Sequential images then demonstrate prompt myocardial uptake of ^{11}C activity and a decline in blood pool activity, resulting in high tissue-to-background activity ratios 4 to 8 minutes following tracer injection. ^{11}C activity then clears from the myocardium over time, and ratios of myocardial-to-background activity gradually decline.

The myocardial clearance of ^{11}C activity after the administration of labeled acetate is best described mathematically as a biexponential function (Plate 21-2). Unlike ^{11}C palmitate, early rates of ^{11}C clearance following ^{11}C acetate administration are virtually independent of dietary state.[147,153,154] In animal and human studies, the rate constant k_1 of the initial rapid portion of the time–activity curve has been shown to be directly proportional to myocardial oxygen consumption (or its indirect index, rate pressure product), to measurements of wall stress, and to the appearance of $^{11}CO_2$ in coronary sinus effluent.[146,147,153–158] Furthermore, human ^{11}C acetate clearance rates increase with increasing myocardial workloads incited by inotropic stimulation.[151,157] Mathematical modeling[159] is probably not necessary for the interpretation of most ^{11}C acetate PET studies in routine clinical practice. The second slow clearance phase of the time–activity curve (described by the second exponential rate constant k_2) probably reflects the conversion of labeled glutamate to labeled glutamine[152] and is not related to myocardial oxygen consumption.

Under conditions of low myocardial oxygen consumption, clearance half-times for the first phase of the ^{11}C clearance curve may be prolonged and impinge on the late, slowly changing portion of myocardial time–activity curve. In these circumstances, the initial portion of the time–activity curve may be fit using a single monoexponential function. The derived clearance constant, k_{mono}, is less sensitive to errors resulting from low count rates and random noise. Although k_{mono} slightly underestimates k_1, this parameter can be ascertained using a shorter image acquisition protocol than that necessary for the determination of k_1. In addition, regional variability in k_{mono} may be less than that of k_1, because of minimization of statistical noise. k_{mono} measurements are also linearly related to myocardial oxygen consumption.[146,147]

Ischemia impairs oxidative substrate metabolism. This is manifest in the myocardial ^{11}C acetate time–activity curve as a reduction in initial uptake of tracer (paralleling the degree of blood flow reduction) and by a prolongation of the initial phase of activity clearance from tissue.[146,152] In hypoxic laboratory preparations, ^{11}C clearance rate constants parallel myocardial oxygen consumption and are not appreciably influenced by changes in myocardial blood flows.[152] Back-diffusion of tracer does not significantly impair the clinical assessment of regional oxidative substrate metabolism with ^{11}C acetate.[146]

Fluorine 18 2-fluoro-2-deoxglucose

FDG is the metabolic tracer employed most frequently in clinical PET imaging. After intravenous administration, FDG undergoes facilitated transport from the vascular space into the cardiac myocyte in proportion to the rate of glucose transport. Once inside the cell, FDG competes with unlabeled glucose for hexokinase, an enzyme capable of phosphorylating both moieties at the six-carbon position. FDG-6-phosphate, however, is not an effective substrate for either glycogen synthesis or glycolysis, and the phosphorylated radioactive tracer undergoes little further metabolism. FDG metabolic images thus reflect the myocardial utilization of glucose delivered by nutrient perfusion and do not provide direct information regarding the subsequent intracellular metabolism of this sugar.

Because FDG-6-phosphate is relatively impermeable to the sarcolemmal membrane, the radioactive tracer is effectively trapped within the myocyte. The tissue concentration of the tracer increases over time while vascular concentrations of FDG are declining owing to renal excretion and uptake by other organs. Thus, in contrast to ^{11}C palmitate or ^{11}C acetate, myocardial-to-background ratios, and hence image quality continue to improve over time until limited by the physical decay of fluorine 18 (Plate 21-3). This property can be used to advantage in clinical imaging: if initial FDG images demonstrate relatively low myocardial uptake and persistence of blood pool activity, delayed imaging may improve image quality.

Myocardial glucose utilization depends highly upon plasma substrate levels and the prevailing neurohormonal milieu. This variability in substrate selection is directly reflected in the PET FDG metabolic images.[160] In the fasting state, plasma free-fatty-acid levels are high, favoring preferential metabolism of free fatty acids, while insulin and glucose levels are low, inhibiting glycolysis; hence, relatively little myocardial uptake of FDG is observed on PET images obtained in the fasting state. Conversely, plasma insulin and glucose levels rise in the postprandial state, and the heart significantly increases its consumption of glucose. In normal volunteers, quantitative measurements of myocardial glucose utilization obtained after oral dextrose administration are almost three times higher than those in the fasting state.[161] FDG images obtained in the glucose-loaded state therefore exhibit higher counts, less heterogeneity in count activity, higher myocardial-to-background ratios, and higher absolute rates of glucose utilization,[161] with a visibly detectable improvement in image quality.

Insulin is also required for effective myocardial utilization of glucose. Insulin deficiency in diabetic patients is associated with lower rates of myocardial glucose utilization than in normal volunteers; supplementation with intravenous insulin during imaging increases glucose utilization rates and improves FDG image quality.[162,163] FDG image quality is also improved by reducing plasma levels of free fatty acids (e.g., by treatment with acipimox, a nicotinic acid derivative that inhibits lipolysis in peripheral

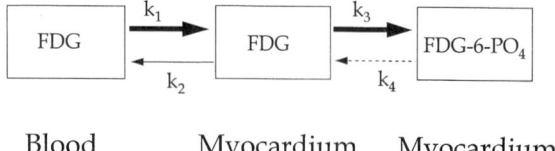

Fig. 21-4. Schematic of the three-compartment model used in conjunction with fluorine 18 2-fluoro-2-deoxyglucose (FDG) positron emission tomographic imaging to obtain absolute rates of myocardial glucose utilization in micromoles per minute per gram of tissue. FDG is extracted by the myocardial cell and then phosphorylated. The forward steps (*dark arrows*) and the rate constants k_1 and k_3, predominate. The reverse steps, described by rate constants k_2 and k_4, are much slower. For most clinical imaging protocols, the contribution of k_4 is negligible.

tissue[164,165]. As free-fatty-acid levels decline there is less inhibition of glycolysis; in addition, acipimox may separately stimulate glycogen synthase. Both factors enhance myocardial uptake of glucose, and therefore increase FDG uptake.

As originally described by Sokoloff and colleagues,[166] the biologic behavior of radiolabeled deoxyglucose is best described by a three compartment model (Fig. 21-4). Tracer within the vascular space (first compartment) undergoes facilitated transport into tissue (second compartment), where the FDG is phosphorylated by intracellular hexokinase to FDG-6-phosphate (third compartment). In this tracer kinetic model, each transition from one compartment to the next is described by a first order rate constant. k_1 and k_3 are the unidirectional rate constants for the forward steps, while k_2 and k_4 are the respective unidirectional rate constants for the reverse transitions. By using a least squares fitting curve fitting routine, data obtained from regional myocardial time activity curves can be analyzed to derive each of the unidirectional rate constants.[167,168] The rate of myocardial glucose utilization, MRGlc (in μmoles of glucose per minute per gram of tissue) is then given by

$$\text{MRGlc} = \frac{C_p}{\text{LC}} \cdot \frac{k_1 \cdot k_3}{k_2 + k_3}$$

where C_p is the plasma concentration of glucose and LC is a constant term, usually taken as 0.67, which relates the uptake of FDG to that of glucose[168]. Alternatively, instead of curve fitting to solve for each of the rate constants, rates of myocardial glucose consumption can be determined using a graphic approach originally proposed by Patlak and colleagues.[23,169–171] In this approach, values of the myocardial activity concentration at time t divided by plasma activity at time t are plotted against the integral of the plasma activity concentration to time t divided by the instantaneous plasma concentration at time t. The slope of the line is the ratio of the rate constants in the above equation. Multiplying the slope of the line by the plasma glucose concentration and dividing by the constant LC yields the myocardial metabolic rate for glucose in μmoles of glucose per minute per gram of tissue.

Clinical PET imaging with FDG is usually performed after the intravenous bolus administration of 5 to 10 mCi of the tracer. Either a static or dynamic image acquisition protocol can be used. Static images are usually acquired about 50 to 60 minutes following tracer administration, while dynamic images may be obtained over the subsequent 90 minutes. A dynamic imaging sequence is needed to measure absolute rates of myocardial glucose utilization, in μmoles/min/g of tissue, and the longer imaging times are employed to estimate more accurately the rate constants from the myocardial time–activity curves (Plate 21-4). For the assessment of myocardial viability, however, most centers rely on static images only. If only static images are obtained, the patient's chest can be marked with indelible ink and he or she can be taken off the scanner during the period of myocardial uptake. Metabolic images can then be obtained later by using the chest marks to reposition the patient in the scanner. This allows a second patient to be imaged during the period of FDG uptake for the first patient, increasing the number of imaging studies that can be performed in the PET imaging center.

Most PET imaging centers perform FDG metabolic imaging in the glucose loaded state to enhance myocardial uptake of the tracer and improve image quality. The standard oral glucose load consists of 50 to 100 of a dextrose-containing solution given 30 to 60 minutes before the injection of FDG. Alternatively, the patient's glucose levels may be maintained relatively constant by using an hyperinsulinemic euglycemic clamp.[165] This technique has found particular application in research studies, in which it is desirable to maintain steady-state conditions during clinical imaging. It is helpful to monitor blood glucose levels before and during imaging with FDG. If plasma glucose levels are low despite glucose loading, additional oral dextrose may be given. Much more frequently, plasma glucose levels are high (above 120 mg/dl), and supplementation with insulin (3 to 6 units IV) may be necessary to obtain FDG images of diagnostic quality.

PET imaging with the glucose analog FDG is attractive for the clinical assessment of tissue viability in coronary heart disease patients because of the effects of myocardial ischemia on substrate selection. Ischemia impairs mitochondrial oxidative metabolism and is associated with enhanced glycogenolysis and anaerobic glycolysis.[104,107,109,135,172–175] Glucose consumption is increased in ischemic human myocardium, reflecting an increase in the myocardial extraction of glucose from blood.[176] Intravenous infusion of low-dose glucose during atrial pacing lengthens the time to the onset of angina and reduces the severity of associated electrocardiographic ST-segment changes.[177] The increase in glucose consumption associated with ischemia is readily demonstrable on noninvasive PET imaging with FDG and, in conjunction with assessment of myocardial perfusion, provides important information regarding the metabolic integrity of dysfunctional cardiac tissue in coronary heart disease patients.

ASSESSING MYOCARDIAL VIABILITY
Perfusion Imaging

Several approaches, including quantitation of defect severity, determination of the relative amount of viable tissue within the myocardial wall using the water-perfusable index, and analysis of rubidium 82 washout rates, have been used to distinguish viable from nonviable tissue using PET perfusion imaging. This section discusses the relative merits of these approaches.

Perfusion Defect Severity
Rationale

The myocardium requires a steady supply of energy-rich substrates and molecular oxygen to sustain myocyte life, and complete cessation of nutrient perfusion rapidly precipitates cellular death. However, some hypoperfused dysfunctional regions, areas with "hibernating myocardium," exhibit improved wall motion following coronary revascularization, indicating that important tissue viability can be maintained in some situations in which resting myocardial blood flow is diminished but not completely absent.[178–181] One approach to the assessment of myocardial viability thus uses the severity of a perfusion defect to identify reversibly dysfunctional tissue. It is assumed that there is a certain minimum level of perfusion which is required to sustain myocardial life. If perfusion is less than this value then the myocardial region is considered nonviable and unlikely to exhibit improved contractility if coronary revascularization is performed. Dysfunctional regions with relative or absolute perfusion values above the minimum threshold are considered viable and therefore likely to benefit from revascularization.

Value of PET

Accurate measurements of perfusion defect severity are necessary if the presence or absence of viable tissue is to be inferred by this method, and PET imaging affords the clinician several advantages relative to SPECT. First, accurate correction for photon attenuation with PET means that relative myocardial activities accurately reflect true tissue tracer concentrations, whereas with SPECT perfusion images, a reduction in observed myocardial counts may be due either to a true perfusion defect or to a diminution of myocardial activity as a result of interposed soft tissue. Second, the spatial resolution of PET tomographs is better than that of SPECT gamma cameras, meaning that there is better ability to separate and distinguish counts from different sources that are close to each other. Thus, the activity observed within a defect using a higher resolution device is less likely to reflect spillover from adjacent normal myocardium. This is particularly problematic at the edges of perfusion defects, and less so for extensive defects (the activity in the center of large defects is further from normal tissue and less subject to spillover). Defect severity determinations may also be influenced by spillover of activity from abdominal organs and lungs, which can vary significantly from patient to patient and from stress to rest images. Myocardium with pronounced perfusion defects is most affected by spillover activity, because of the relatively low number of counts intrinsic to the tissue itself. The spatial resolution of PET renders spillover of background activity less problematic than SPECT.

In myocardial areas that are thinned as a result of prior infarction or in areas with impaired systolic thickening, the partial volume effect causes a nonlinear underestimation of true tissue tracer concentrations,[30] because the time-averaged myocardial thickness is small and the camera is inefficient at recovering myocardial counts. The greater the reduction in wall thickness and regional thickening, the greater the diminution in observed tracer activity within the corresponding perfusion defect. The partial volume effect is less problematic for PET than SPECT because PET tomographs are more efficient at recovering counts in thinner structures.

Clinical Efficacy of Relative Perfusion Criteria for Viability

Despite the difficulties inherent in accurately measuring relative perfusion defect severity, several clinical studies using single photon tracers have indicated that this is helpful in identifying tissue viability in dysfunctional myocardial regions.[182,183] For example, in a study of 37 patients undergoing coronary artery bypass surgery, Zimmermann and co-workers[184] reported that relative ^{201}Tl concentrations in myocardial areas with persistent perfusion defects on preoperative reinjection planar images were inversely related to the percent interstitial fibrosis noted in biopsy specimens obtained during the operation. This suggests that ^{201}Tl concentrations in myocardial areas with persistent perfusion defects on preoperative reinjection planar images were inversely related to the percent interstitial fibrosis noted in biopsy specimens obtained during the operation. This suggests that ^{201}Tl concentrations on the planar images paralleled the amount of viable tissue within affected myocardial regions.

To examine the utility of PET perfusion imaging for identifying viable tissue, Go and co-workers[185] performed rest and dipyridamole stress rubidium 82 perfusion imaging along with FDG metabolic imaging in 145 patients with chronic myocardial infarction. Normal myocardial segments were defined by relative rubidium 82 concentrations greater than or equal to 80% of peak activity. Persistent perfusion defects were defined by a change in relative rubidium 82 activity of less than 15% between the rest and dipyridamole stress perfusion images. The presence of preserved tissue glucose metabolism on FDG images was used to define myocardial viability. Metabolic tissue viability was identified in 381 (30%) of 1252 segments with persistent rubidium 82 perfusion defects, whereas concordant reductions in metabolic activity consistent with scar formation were noted in the remaining 871 segments. When perfusion defects with rubidium 82 concentrations of less than 70% of normal were examined, the relative proportion of myocardial perfusion defects with preserved metabolic activity was fairly constant, ranging from 23% for rubidium 82 concentrations of 30% to 35% of peak activity up to 35% of defects for rubidium 82 concentrations of 40% to 45% of peak activity. Thus, Go and his colleagues found no correlation between the severity of a persistent myocardial perfusion defect and residual tissue viability as defined by PET metabolic imaging with FDG.

Tamaki and his colleagues[186] studied 43 patients with prior myocardial infarction (mean left ventricular ejection fraction [LVEF], 41%) using rest and stress ^{13}N ammonia PET perfusion imaging along with FDG metabolic imaging in the fasting state. Viability was identified in 51 segments by an improvement of regional function on biplane contrast ventriculograms taken before and after surgery. As relative ^{13}N activity on the resting perfusion images in the asynergic segments decreased, the likelihood that the regions would improve functionally after revascularization also declined (Fig. 21-5). The single region with a relative ^{13}N concentration greater than 80% of peak normal improved functionally, and about half the regions with ^{13}N activity between 60% and 80% of peak normal activity improved. Fifteen of 38 (39%) regions with relative tracer concentrations between 50% and 60% improved after revascularization, as did 4 of 21 (19%) regions with ^{13}N tracer concentrations between 40% and 50%. None of the regions with relative ^{13}N concentrations below 40% of normal had postoperative improvement in

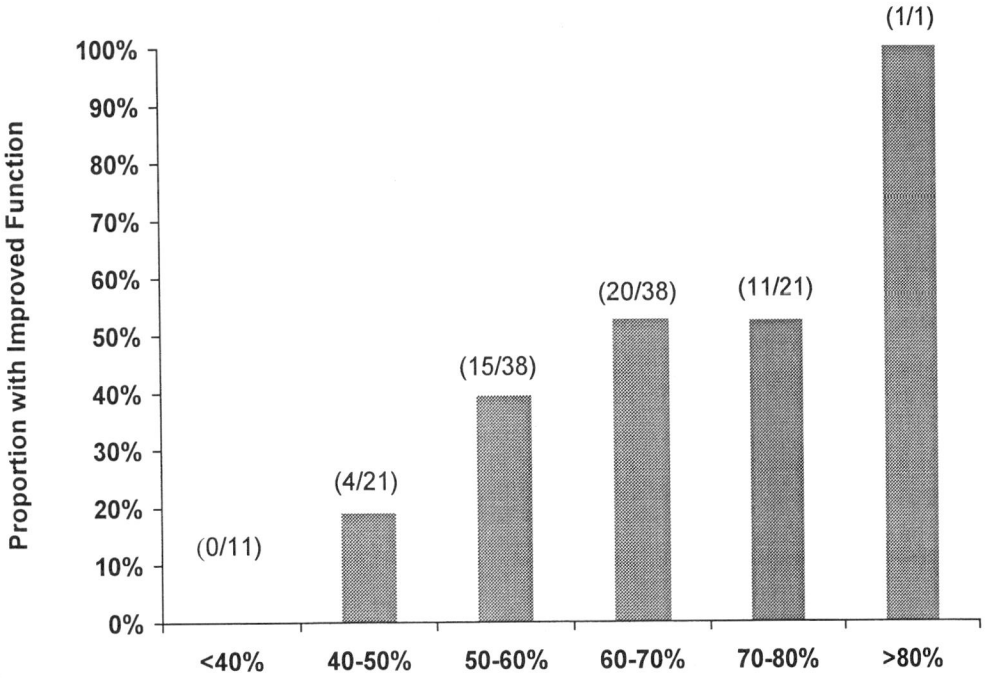

Fig. 21-5. Relationship between nitrogen 13 ammonia perfusion defect severity on preoperative positron emission tomographic images and the probability of improved wall motion following successful coronary revascularization. As the severity of a resting perfusion defect becomes less pronounced, the probability of functional improvement increases.[136]

function. The positive predictive value for a relative ^{13}N concentration greater than 50% for predicting improvement in function following revascularization was 48%, while the negative predictive value for a tracer concentration less than 50% was 87.5%. Stress-induced perfusion defects were identified in 68 of the 130 asynergic regions. Of these 68 regions, 43 (63%) improved after revascularization; 54 (87%) of the 62 regions without reversible defects had no improvement in wall motion. Identification of defect reversibility thus increased the positive predictive accuracy of the perfusion studies from 48% to 63% and did not have a significant effect on the observed negative predictive accuracy. On the FDG images, preserved glucose metabolism was identified in 59 of the 130 asynergic regions. Forty-five (76%) of the regions with metabolic viability improved functionally after revascularization while only 6 (8%) of the 71 regions without metabolic activity improved. PET metabolic imaging thus had a better overall diagnostic accuracy (85%, 110 of 130 regions) for predicting improvement in function than either the resting perfusion studies (75 of 130 regions, 58%) or the rest-stress studies (97 of 130 regions, 75%, $p < 0.05$ versus rest or versus metabolic imaging).

In a subsequent study Duvernoy and her coinvestigators[187] also related relative ^{13}N ammonia tracer concentrations on resting PET perfusion images to improvement in wall motion after coronary revascularization in 25 patients with chronic ischemic heart disease (mean LVEF 35%). An improvement in function was defined by an increase in visual wall motion score of 0.5 or more on gated radionuclide ventriculography. Of 107 segments with resting wall motion abnormalities, 45 (42%) had improved function after revascularization. Twenty-two (63%) of 35 segments with ^{13}N uptake of greater than 80% of normal improved, while only one (14%) of 7 segments with ^{13}N uptake less than 40% of normal improved. Of the 52 segments with ^{13}N tracer concentrations greater than 60%, 16 (31%) improved whereas 6 (46%) of 13 segments with ^{13}N activities greater than 40% improved. These investigators reasoned that resting ^{13}N ammonia perfusion defect severity was helpful in identifying myocardial viability, noting that segments with relative tracer concentrations of 80% or more tended to improve after revascularization whereas those with less than 40% relative activity usually derived no functional benefit from restoration of blood flow. For the perfusion defects of intermediate severity, there was no apparent relationship between relative ^{13}N ammonia tracer concentrations and functional improvement after revascularization. The authors thus concluded that FDG metabolic imaging would provide additional clinical benefit for identifying viable tissue with resting perfusion defects of intermediate severity.

Clinical Efficacy of Absolute Perfusion Criteria for Viability

To examine the clinical utility of absolute perfusion measurements for discriminating between viable and nonviable myocardium (defined by FDG metabolic imaging), Gewirtz and co-workers[188] quantitated resting regional blood flows in 26 patients with prior myocardial infarction using dynamic PET imaging with ^{13}N ammonia. Measured blood flows were compared with relative FDG concentrations and with regional wall motion as indicators of myocardial viability. Normal segments were defined by resting blood flows greater than or equal to 75% of peak values, while infarct zones were defined by blood flows less than 50% of maximum. Border zones around the infarct areas were defined by blood flow measurements between 50% and 75% of maximum.

Myocardial blood flows averaged 0.81 ± 0.32 ml/min/g in 40 normal areas, 0.59 ± 0.29 ml/min/g in 16 border zones ($p < 0.02$ versus normal regions), and 0.27 ± 0.17 ml/min/g in 22 infarct regions ($p < 0.001$ versus both border zones and normal regions). Metabolic viability was not identified on the FDG images in any myocardial area with less than 0.24 ml/min/g blood flow, a value that corresponded to 35% of peak perfusion tracer activity. Enhanced FDG uptake relative to perfusion was noted most frequently in areas with blood flows ranging from 40% to 70% of normal but was also observed in some areas with blood flows of 90% or more of normal, providing evidence for an abnormality in regional metabolism despite relatively well preserved perfusion.

Dyskinetic segments (n = 5) on contrast ventriculography had blood flows less than 0.25 ml/min/g, and none exhibited metabolic viability. Six of 28 segments (21%) with severe hypokinesis or akinesis had blood flows less than 0.25 ml/min/g and the mean blood flow for all severely hypokinetic/akinetic regions was 0.42 ± 0.21 ml/min/g. Four segments (three with akinesia, one with severe hypokinesia) had evidence of metabolic viability on the FDG images. Of the 45 regions with normal wall motion or mild hypokinesia, 43 (94%) had resting blood flows greater than or equal to 0.39 ml/min/g, and enhanced uptake of FDG was present in five of these regions. Thus, although severe myocardial blood flow reductions were associated with pronounced regional dysfunction, considerable variation in the blood flow measurements was noted when regions were grouped according to the severity of wall motion abnormality. Myocardial viability is unlikely to be present in regions with resting blood flows less than 0.25 ml/min/g. However, a prospective study is needed to determine the positive predictive accuracy for blood flows exceeding this value for identifying myocardial segments that will demonstrate functional improvement following coronary revascularization.

Marzullo and his colleagues[189] postulated that quantitative measurements of coronary flow reserve made with PET imaging could distinguish between myocardial regions with and without residual metabolic viability (defined by FDG imaging) in 14 patients with chronic Q-wave infarction. In 119 normal segments, resting myocardial blood flows averaged 1.00 ± 0.24 ml/min/g, and the mean coronary flow reserve was 2.76 ± 0.72. In 60 segments with mild dysfunction on echocardiography, resting blood flows averaged 0.69 ± 0.14 ml/min/g, and the mean flow reserve was 2.5 ± 1.6. More pronounced echocardiographic wall motion abnormalities were present in 73 segments with resting hypoperfusion; 25 were considered viable and 48 nonviable on metabolic imaging with FDG. In the metabolically viable hypoperfused segments, resting blood flows averaged 0.42 ± 0.12 ml/min/g, and the mean flow reserve was 2.6 ± 1.3. Resting blood flows in the nonviable hypoperfused segments were similar at 0.39 ± 0.27 ml/min/g, but the mean coronary flow reserve was significantly lower at 1.3 ± 0.5 ($p < 0.01$). A coronary flow reserve of 1.65 best discriminated between segments with and without metabolic viability. This study thus suggests that resting perfusion measurements alone do not reliably distinguish between viable and nonviable regions and that quantitative measurements of coronary flow reserve can provide further additional information about tissue viability.

The concept that perfusion defect severity can be used to identify viable tissue assumes that observed blood flow reductions generally parallel the extent of irreversible injury in dysfunctional myocardial regions. For example, if perfusion defect activity averages 60% of normal, then the assumption would be that about 40% of the tissue had been replaced by scar. However, a histopathologic study by Parodi and his coworkers[190] does not support that assumption. These investigators compared microsphere blood flow measurements[83] with the percent tissue fibrosis in myocardial specimens obtained in four patients with ischemic cardiomyopathy undergoing cardiac transplantation. Mean transmural myocardial blood flows averaged 0.38 ± 0.15 ml/min/g in the four patients with ischemic cardiomyopathy; the mean percent fibrosis was 25 ± 28%. There was no correlation between microsphere blood flow measurements and the amount of fibrosis as determined either by histologic measurements or by biochemical analysis of the exercised tissue (Fig. 21-6). Furthermore, there was no relationship between relative tracer concentrations on the scintigraphic images and the histologic amount of fibrosis. The authors concluded that the amount of myocardial fibrosis is not a primary determinant of blood flow in patients with end-stage ventricular dysfunction and suggested that inferences regarding the amount of residual tissue viability based upon the severity of a perfusion abnormality would be unreliable in patients with end-stage ischemic cardiomyopathy.

The Water Perfusable Index
Rationale
A second approach to the determination of myocardial viability using perfusion imaging involves measurement of the water perfusable index. The *water perfusable index* (measured as grams of perfusable tissue/grams of total anatomic tissue) is the relative amount of the anatomic myocardial wall capable of rapidly exchanging ^{15}O water.[191] Viable myocytes can rapidly exchange ^{15}O labeled water, while scar tissue is not capable of rapid exchange of this radioactive tracer. Calculation of the water perfusable index provides information about the mass of viable myocytes within the ventricular wall and permits normalization of relative and absolute perfusion measurements to the amount of viable tissue, as compared with total left ventricular anatomic mass.

Clinical Application
Yamamoto and his colleagues[191] used PET transmission images along with ^{15}O-labeled carbon monoxide, ^{15}O water, and FDG emission images to examine the clinical utility of the water perfusable index in 8 normal volunteers, 15 patients with chronic myocardial infarction, and 11 patients with acute myocardial infarction who had successful thrombolysis of the infarct-related vessel. Echocardiography was performed in the patients with acute infarction 2 to 4 days after the clinical event and at 4 months follow-up examination. A blood volume image was first generated by dividing counts on the ^{15}O carbon monoxide blood pool images by the product of the density of whole blood (1.06 g/ml) and the number of counts/sec/g measured in a venous whole blood sample. Images of extravascular tissue density were then obtained by subtracting images of blood density (the blood volume image multiplied by 1.06) from transmission images that had been converted to images of tissue density. This allowed the investigators to calculate the number of grams of anatomic tissue per milliliter in regions of interest of known volume. Using time–activity curves obtained from the dynamic ^{15}O water images, the authors were able to derive myocardial blood flows, in milliliters per minute per gram of perfusable tissue, as well as the number of grams of anatomic tissue per milliliter in the region of interest.[64,192] The water perfusable tissue index was then calculated by dividing the grams of perfusable tissue per milliliter by the grams of total anatomical tissue per milliliter. To identify areas of metabolic viability, uptake of FDG in asynergic zones was normalized to peak fluorine-18 counts and divided by blood flow measurements normalized to

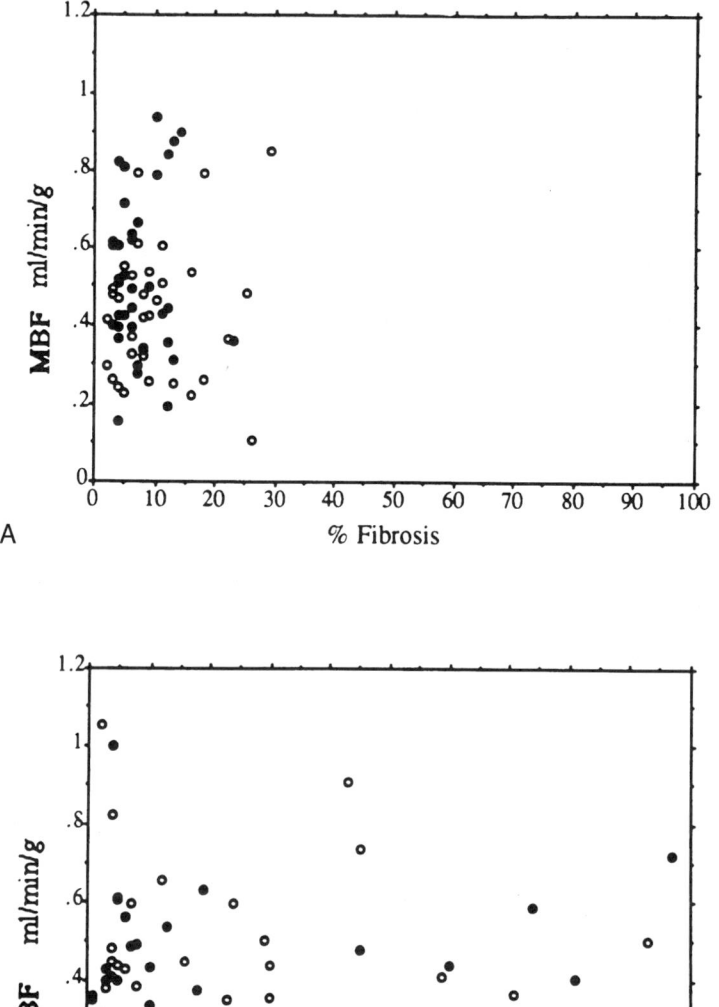

Fig. 21-6. Relationship between myocardial blood flow measurements and the percent tissue fibrosis assessed by biochemical analysis in patients with **(A)** idiopathic dilated cardiomyopathy (IDC) and **(B)** ischemic heart disease (IHD) undergoing cardiac transplantation. The closed and open circles represent endocardial and epicardial samples, respectively. There is no relationship between the relative amount of tissue fibrosis and myocardial blood flow. (From Parodi et al.,[190] with permission.)

peak blood flow determinations. Metabolically viable regions were defined by a metabolism to perfusion ratio greater than 1.2.

In the normal volunteers the water perfusable index was near unity, 1.08 ± 0.07 grams of perfusable tissue per grams of total anatomic tissue, while myocardial blood flows averaged 1.03 ± 0.18 ml/min/g of total anatomic tissue and 0.95 ml/min/g of water perfusable tissue. Six patients with chronic Q-wave myocardial infarction had perfusion defects without preserved metabolism, or completed infarctions, in the clinical infarct zone. In these areas of chronic infarction, blood flows averaged 0.33 ± 0.11 ml/min/g of anatomic tissue and 0.64 ± 0.23 ml/min/g of water perfusable tissue, while the corresponding values for remote normal myocardium were 0.98 ± 0.25 ml/min/g of anatomic tissue and 0.97 ± 0.25 ml/min/g of water perfusable tissue, respectively. Nine patients with chronic myocardial infarction had perfusion defects with preserved glucose metabolism. Blood flows in these infarct zones averaged 0.40 ± 0.17 ml/min/g of anatomic tissue and 0.51 ml/min/g of water perfusable tissue, respectively, while the values for remote normal myocardium were 1.10 ± 0.23 ml/min/g of anatomic tissue and 1.09 ± 0.23 ml/min/g of water perfusable tissue respectively. Neither blood flow per gram of total anatomic tissue nor blood flow per gram of water perfusable tissue reliably distinguished between myocardial infarct zones with and without preserved glucose metabolism on FDG PET images. However, the mean perfusable tissue index was significantly higher in the infarct areas with preserved tissue metabolism (0.75 ± 0.14 versus 0.53 ± 12 grams of perfusable tissue per grams of total anatomical tissue, $p < 0.01$), suggesting that the mass of viable tissue in the perfusion defects with preserved metabolism exceeded that in the areas with completed infarctions.

In the acute myocardial infarction patients, 12 regions had severely impaired systolic wall thickening after thrombolytic therapy. On follow-up echocardiography at 4 months, seven regions demonstrated improvement in systolic wall thickening while five had no functional recovery. In regions with improved function, blood flows averaged 0.61 ± 0.33 ml/min/g of anatomic tissue and 0.68 ± 0.32 ml/min/g of water perfusable tissue and did not differ statistically from the 0.33 ± 0.15 ml/min/g of anatomic tissue and 0.60 ± 0.18 ml/min/g of water perfusable tissue noted in the regions without recovery. Thus, measurements of absolute blood flow, whether normalized to total anatomic tissue or to the amount of water perfusable tissue, did not reliably discriminate between regions with and without functional recovery.

In contrast, the water perfusable tissue index was significantly higher in the regions with delayed functional improvement (0.88 ± 0.10 versus 0.53 ± 0.11 grams of perfusable tissue per grams of total anatomic tissue, $p < 0.02$). In the small number of patients with acute infarction who were studied, only those with a water perfusable index greater than 0.7 grams of perfusable tissue per grams of total anatomic tissue exhibited functional improvement, leading the authors to conclude that at least 70% of the tissue present in clinical infarct regions must be viable for the area to recover function after thrombolysis.

To explore the utility of the water perfusable tissue index for predicting functional improvement after coronary revascularization in individuals with chronic myocardial infarction, de Silva and coworkers[193] performed PET with ^{15}O carbon monoxide and ^{15}O water before revascularization in 12 patients with chronic coronary artery disease. Segmental ventricular function was assessed on echocardiography before and 3 to 5 months after elective coronary revascularization. Of 33 segments with preoperative resting wall motion abnormalities, 26 improved functionally after surgery while 7 segments did not.

Myocardial blood flows in the 26 segments with improved wall motion averaged 0.73 ± 0.18 ml/min/g perfusable tissue, significantly higher than the mean value of 0.45 ± 0.11 ml/min/g perfusable tissue in the 7 segments without improvement ($p < 0.02$). However, there was considerable overlap in the measured blood flows for the two groups. In 26 control segments, myocardial blood flows averaged 0.97 ± 0.22 ml/min/g perfusable tissue, significantly higher than blood flows in either group of asynergic segments ($p < 0.001$ for both). In the seven segments without functional improvement, water perfusable tissue indices averaged 0.62 ± 0.06 g perfusable tissue per gram of anatomic tissue and were consistently less than 0.7 g perfusable tissue per gram of anatomic tissue. In the 26 segments with improved wall motion the water perfusable index averaged 0.99 ± 0.15 gram perfusable tissue per gram of anatomic tissue ($p < 0.02$), and each segment that improved had a water perfusable tissue index greater than or equal to 0.70 gram perfusable tissue per gram of anatomic tissue. Furthermore, the water perfusable tissue index appeared to differentiate more clearly between hypoperfused segments with and without functional recovery than the measurements of absolute blood flow. The mean water perfusable tissue index in the control segments was 1.10 ± 0.15 gram perfusable tissue per gram of anatomic tissue; significantly greater than the corresponding values in either group of asynergic segments ($p < 0.02$ for both). These observations led the authors to conclude that 70% or more of the tissue mass in a dysfunctional myocardial segment must be viable, as determined by permeability to labeled water, for revascularization to benefit contractile function. However, this study could not discern whether interpatient differences in the transmural distribution of viable tissue might affect the degree of functional recovery after coronary revascularization.

Rubidium 82 Tissue Kinetic Analysis
Rationale
Finally, a third approach to the assessment of viability with myocardial perfusion images relies upon the fact that tissue uptake and retention of cations such as rubidium 82 requires energy and depends on maintenance of ionic gradients across cellular membranes. Following the administration of rubidium 82, the radioactive label is actively transported across cellular membranes. Rubidium 82 activity that is sequestered within viable myocytes will be slower to wash out than activity in scar tissue, owing to the inability of fibrous tissue to trap the cation effectively. Analysis of the rates of myocardial clearance of rubidium 82 might therefore be used to distinguish viable tissue from scar.

Reasoning that cellular membrane integrity would be important for the trapping of potassium analogues such as rubidium, Goldstein[194] examined the tissue kinetics of rubidium 82 in canine myocardium subjected to acute ischemic injury. Viable tissue in the risk zone retained or accumulated rubidium 82 over the first 150 seconds following tracer administration, while nonviable tissue leaked rubidium 82 following the initial uptake of the tracer. In contrast, Herrero and colleagues[195] reported that the backward rate transfer constant for rubidium 82 (the constant associated with leakage of rubidium 82 from tissue) was inversely related to the percent blood flow reduction in experiments in which intact dogs were subjected to ischemia and reperfusion, or both. Myocardial regions with severe ischemia (less than 35% of control myocardium) had significantly larger backward rate transfer constants than normal myocardium. In contrast, this kinetic parameter did not differ significantly from normal in reperfused areas or in areas with only mild ischemia.

Clinical Application
The clinical utility of rubidium 82 kinetic analysis technique for identifying myocardial viability was examined by Gould and his colleagues.[196] In 43 patients with prior clinical myocardial infarction, rubidium 82 images were acquired early (15 to 110 seconds) and late (120 to 360 seconds) following intravenous tracer administration and compared with FDG images as an indicator of tissue viability. Infarct size and location, derived from ratios of late to early rubidium 82 concentrations, correlated well with infarct size and location on the FDG metabolic images.

More recently, vom Dahl and colleagues[197] correlated the findings on dynamic rubidium 82 perfusion images with the results of metabolic imaging with FDG in 27 patients with coronary artery disease. In five normal subjects, rubidium 82 tissue clearance half-times were homogeneous throughout the left ventricle and averaged 90 ± 11 seconds. In 27 normally perfused regions in the patients with CAD, rubidium 82 clearance half-times averaged 95 ± 10 seconds and were significantly longer than the 57 ± 15 seconds noted in 17 regions with myocardial scar ($p < 0.0001$). In 21 regions with ischemically compromised tissue with preserved glucose metabolism, rubidium 82 half-times averaged 75 ± 9 seconds and differed significantly from the values observed in the normal and scarred regions ($p < 0.0001$ for both comparisons). In these patients, a tissue half-time for rubidium 82 greater than 76 seconds seemed to provide the best discrimination between viable and nonviable myocardium as defined by metabolic imaging with FDG. When myocardial regions were characterized as viable or scarred, rubidium 82 kinetic analysis and metabolic imaging with FDG yielded concordant results in 86% of the regions. While the analysis of rubidium 82 tissue kinetics appears to offer promise for identifying viable tissue in patients with CAD, further studies are needed to determine the reliability of this technique for identifying reversible asynergy in patients with chronic CAD.

Summary—Assessment of Viability Using Perfusion Tracers

Technical factors may limit the accuracy of measurements of relative perfusion defect severity in dysfunctional myocardial regions. PET perfusion images are less subject to these limitations than SPECT images, because of the higher spatial resolution of PET tomographs and correction for photon attenuation. Dysfunctional myocardial areas with pronounced perfusion defects are less likely to harbor viable tissue and are therefore less likely to derive benefit from coronary revascularization than areas with less pronounced perfusion defects. Between these extremes, Tamaki et al.[186] have shown that about one of every five segments with relative tracer concentrations of 40% to 50% of normal will derive functional benefit from coronary revascularization, while the study of Duvernoy et al.[187] indicates that about one in every two dysfunctional segments with relative tracer activities between 40% to 60% of normal will improve following restoration of blood flow. Thus, reliance upon the relative severity of a perfusion defect alone for the determination of clinically important tissue viability would not appear to be prudent.

Absolute perfusion measurements, obtained at rest and during pharmacologic stress, may provide additional information about the state of myocardial viability. Human myocardium is unlikely to harbor significant viability if resting blood flows are less than 0.25 ml/min/g of anatomic tissue,[188] but absolute resting blood flow greater than 0.25 ml/min/g cannot be assumed to denote the presence of clinically important viability. The report by Marzullo and his colleagues[189] suggests that myocardial regions with coronary flow reserves above 1.65 are likely to be viable, but further clinical studies are necessary to confirm these findings.

The water perfusable index, as an indicator of the amount of viable tissue mass within the myocardial wall, provides an additional means of identifying reversibly dysfunctional tissue,[191,193] although confirmation of these findings is needed. Derivation of the water perfusable index from ^{15}O water and ^{15}O carbon monoxide PET images is technically demanding and time consuming, rendering this method of viability determination less attractive for use in a busy nuclear cardiology practice. Similarly, relatively few patient studies have examined the utility of rubidium 82 tissue kinetic analysis for ascertaining myocardial viability; more studies are needed for validation of this approach before it can be implemented in clinical practice.

Metabolic Imaging

FDG Imaging

Early investigations of acute infarction and reperfusion in experimental preparations indicated that characterization of myocardium at risk with PET metabolic imaging shortly after an ischemic injury helped in predicting recovery of regional function.[198–201] Although initial patient studies employing PET metabolic imaging with FDG clearly indicated that preserved tissue glucose metabolism could be identified in hypoperfused human myocardium,[202] the clinical implications of these observations were uncertain.

To ascertain whether the scintigraphic identification of myocardial glucose metabolism in hypoperfused ventricular regions indicates significant tissue viability, Tillisch and colleagues[203] performed PET imaging with ^{13}N ammonia and FDG in 17 patients with resting wall motion abnormalities before elective coronary bypass surgery (Table 21-1). Segments with improved wall motion were considered viable and segments without functional improvement, nonviable. Of 67 segments with preoperative resting wall motion abnormalities that were revascularized, 41 had a metabolism–perfusion mismatch (Plate 21-5) and 26 showed a match pattern (Plate 21-6). Of the 41 metabolically viable segments, 35 (85%) improved wall motion postoperatively. In 11 individuals with preserved glucose metabolism in three or more asynergic segments, a significant increase in mean LVEF, from 30 ± 11% to 45 ± 14%, was noted after coronary revascularization. The patients with

Table 21-1. PET Metabolic Imaging For Recovery of Left Ventricular Function After Revascularization

Patients	Number of Segments	Tracer of Perfusion	Segments with Improved WM		LVEF		Reference
			With FDG uptake (%)	No FDG uptake (%)	Before	After	
17	67	$^{13}NH_3$	35/41 (85)	2/26 (8)	32 ± 14%	41 ± 15%	Tillisch et al. (1986)[203]
22	46	$^{13}NH_3$	18/23 (78)[a]	5/23 (22)	NR	NR	Tamaki et al. (1989)[204]
11	56	$^{13}NH_3$	40/50 (80)[a]	0/6 (0)	NR	NR	Tamaki et al. (1991)[205]
16	85	^{82}Rb	25/37 (68)[a]	10/48 (21)	NR	NR	Marwick et al. (1992)[206]
14	54	MIBI	37/39 (95)[a]	3/15 (20)	38 ± 5%	48 ± 4%	Lucignani et al. (1992)[207]
21	23	^{82}Rb	16/19 (84)	1/4 (25)	34 ± 14%	52 ± 11%	Carrel et al. (1992)[208]
34	116	$H_2^{15}O$, ^{11}C-acetate	38/73 (52)	8/43 (19)	NR	NR	Gropler et al. (1992, 1993)[209]
48	90	MIBI, ^{201}Tl	23/27 (85)	10/63 (16)	53 ± 11%	NR	Knuuti et al. (1994)
37	110	$^{13}NH_3$	24/59 (41)[b]	7/51 (14)[b]	34 ± 10%	36 ± 10%	vom Dahl et al. (1994)[212]
43	130	$^{13}NH_3$	45/59 (76)[a]	6/71 (8)	41%	NR	Tamaki et al. (1995)
12[c]	12	$^{13}NH_3$	12/12 (100)	—	55 ± 7%	65 ± 8%	Vanoverschelde et al. (1993)[216]
20[c]	20	$^{13}NH_3$	8/12 (67)	2/8 (25)	49 ± 9%	56 ± 9%	Maes et al. (1994)[217]
25	25	$^{13}NH_3$	16/19 (84)[d]	1/6 (17)	49 ± 11%	57 ± 15	Grandin et al. (1995)[213]
24[c]		$^{13}NH_3$	7/9 (78)	9/15 (60)	39 ± 15%	42 ± 19	Depre et al. (1995)[218]
Total 344	858		344/479 (72)	64/379 (17)	40%	47%	

[a] Metabolic imaging performed in the fasting state.
[b] Segments with moderate hypokinesis or worse function.
[c] Histopathologic correlation performed.
[d] FDG metabolic imaging results were incorporated into a discriminant model that also included absolute measurements of myocardial blood flow.

Abbreviations: FDG, fluorine 18 2-fluoro-2-deoxyglucose; $H_2^{15}O$, oxygen 15 water; LVEF, left ventricular ejection fraction; MIBI, technetium-99m sestamibi; $^{13}NH_3$, nitrogen 13 ammonia; NR, not reported; ^{11}C, carbon 11; PET, positron emission tomography; ^{201}Tl, thallium 201; WM, wall motion.

the largest amounts of dysfunctional tissue with preserved metabolism thus derived the greatest benefit from revascularization. In contrast, 24 of the 26 (92%) dysfunctional segments with concordant reductions in perfusion and metabolism on PET imaging had no improvement or further deterioration in wall motion after revascularization. Thus, this study indicated that metabolic imaging with FDG was clinically used for identifying viable but functionally compromised tissue that would benefit from restoration of blood flow.

Independent confirmation of the clinical utility of FDG metabolic imaging for identifying tissue viability in dysfunctional myocardial regions was provided by Tamaki et al.[204] They performed PET imaging with ^{13}N ammonia and FDG in the fasting state in 22 patients before elective coronary artery revascularization. Wall motion was abnormal in 46 segments in 20 of the 22 patients. On PET imaging, matching reductions in perfusion and glucose metabolism were present in 23 of 46 segments with abnormal wall motion, while FDG uptake was normal or increased in the other 23 segments. On follow-up 5 to 7 weeks after surgery, wall motion had improved in 18 (78%) of the 23 segments with metabolic evidence of viability, but only in five (22%) of the 23 segments with matching perfusion and metabolic defects on preoperative imaging (Table 21-1). The positive and negative predictive accuracies of metabolic imaging for predicting improvement in segmental function were 78% and 78%, respectively.

In a later study, these investigators[205] related changes in regional wall motion after coronary revascularization in 11 CAD patients with the findings on ^{201}Tl reinjection scintigraphy and PET-FDG metabolic imaging (Table 21-1). Improvement in segmental wall motion was present in 40 of the 56 segments with preoperative wall motion abnormalities. Forty (80%) of the 50 segments with preserved uptake of FDG on PET imaging improved function, while none of the six segments with matching perfusion and metabolic defects improved wall motion after surgery. The positive and negative predictive accuracies of PET metabolic imaging for predicting improvement in segmental wall motion were therefore 80% and 100%, respectively. In contrast, 11 of 17 (65%) segments with fill-in and two of eight segments without fill-in on ^{201}Tl reinjection improved function after revascularization, for positive and negative predictive accuracies of 65% and 75%, respectively.

Marwick and his colleagues[206] examined the effects of coronary revascularization on segmental function, perfusion, and metabolism in 16 patients with prior myocardial infarction. Two-dimensional echocardiograms, along with rest and dipyridamole rubidium 82 perfusion and fasting, post-exercise FDG PET images were obtained before and after coronary revascularization. Myocardial viability was defined by an improvement in echocardiographic wall motion score of one or more grades after revascularization. Of 85 segments with fixed perfusion defects and resting wall-motion abnormalities on the preoperative studies, 35 had improved function after revascularization and were considered viable, while 50 failed to improve and were considered to have completed infarction. On metabolic imaging with FDG, 25 (71%) of the 35 segments with reversible dysfunction were considered viable; 38 (76) of the 50 segments without improvement had matching perfusion and metabolic defects and were considered nonviable. The positive and negative accuracies for FDG metabolic imaging for predicting functional improvement after revascularization were 68% and 79%, respectively (Table 21-1). The relatively low positive predictive accuracy may reflect both that metabolic imaging was performed in the fasting state and also that the metabolic images were obtained after exercise. Increases in plasma lactate levels with exercise may have suppressed glucose utilization by normal myocardium in some patients, leading to an overestimation of FDG activity and hence viability in the hypoperfused ventricular areas.

As the information in these patient studies began to accumulate, it became apparent that PET metabolic imaging with FDG did provide useful information regarding the amount of salvageable tissue in dysfunctional myocardial regions. However, this imaging procedure was initially performed only in a limited number of centers. Because the half-life of FDG is just under 2 hours, it is feasible to compound this radiopharmaceutical at regional centers and to distribute it to community imaging facilities. To establish whether an imaging protocol incorporating SPECT perfusion imaging in conjunction with PET FDG imaging could also identify myocardial viability, Lucignani and co-workers[207] studied 14 patients with coronary artery disease before elective coronary revascularization. Myocardial perfusion was assessed using resting technetium 99m sestamibi SPECT images while myocardial metabolism was assessed on FDG-PET images in each of 54 segments with abnormal function. After surgery, function improved in 37 (95%) of 39 segments with preserved glucose metabolism and 3 (20%) of 15 segments without metabolic viability. The positive and negative predictive accuracies for this dual imaging technique were 95% and 80%, respectively (Table 21-1). The mean LVEF increased from 38 ± 4.9% to 47.9 ± 4.1% after coronary revascularization. Thus, FDG-PET metabolic imaging used in conjunction with conventional SPECT perfusion imaging also could be used to identify reversible asynergy in patients with coronary artery disease and left ventricular dysfunction.

Carrel and colleagues[208] performed PET imaging with rubidium 82 and FDG in 23 patients before coronary artery bypass surgery. In 21 patients with patent bypass grafts on postoperative angiography, revascularization resulted in a significant improvement in both the resting LVEF (34 ± 14% to 52 ± 11%, $p < 0.01$) and the exercise LVEF (31% ± 14% to 58 ± 13%, $p < 0.01$). Improvement in segmental function was noted in 16 (84%) of 19 hypoperfused segments with preserved FDG uptake, including 4 of 7 akinetic segments and 2 of 5 dyskinetic segments (Table 21-1). Only one (25%) of the four segments with concordant rubidium 82 and FDG defects had an improvement in segmental function after surgery.

PET Assessment of Oxidative Metabolism

To determine if characterization of oxidative substrate metabolism is helpful for identifying reversible asynergy, Gropler and his colleagues[209] performed PET imaging with ^{15}O water, ^{11}C acetate, and FDG in 16 patients with chronic coronary artery disease before revascularization. Viable myocardium was defined by an improvement in segmental function after revascularization. Of the 53 asynergic segments examined, 24 exhibited postoperative improvement in function and were considered viable, 29 had no functional improvement and were considered nonviable. Both groups had comparable resting wall motion abnormalities and relative reductions in segmental perfusion before surgery.

^{11}C acetate clearance constants (k_1 values) in the viable segments were significantly larger than those in the nonviable segments (0.061 ± 0.014 min^{-1} versus 0.042 ± 0.013 min^{-1}, $p < 0.003$) and were similar to values observed in normal segments (0.064 ± 0.015 min^{-1}). Relative rates of glucose utilization, normalized to relative myocardial perfusion, averaged 1.24 ± 0.41 in viable segments, and were 19% higher than in normal segments (1.04 ± 0.24, $p < 0.01$). The corresponding ratios for the nonviable segments (1.33 ± 0.85) did not differ statistically from those in normal or viable segments. Nineteen (79%) of 24 segments with enhanced uptake of FDG relative to perfusion had improved function after revascularization; 24 (83%) of 29 segments with matching FDG and perfusion defects had no functional improvement. This study thus confirmed the utility of PET imaging with FDG for identifying salvageable myocardium and further indicated that characterization of regional oxidative substrate metabolism with dynamic ^{11}C acetate PET imaging was also helpful for identifying individuals likely to benefit from coronary revascularization. However, a threshold for viability, as defined by a specific or relative value for ^{11}C acetate clearance constants, was not established.

In a subsequent investigation,[210] the same investigators compared the relative merits of metabolic imaging with ^{11}C acetate to that of FDG for identifying reversibly dysfunctional myocardium. The study population consisted of the 16 patients previously reported[209] and 18 additional subjects imaged with ^{11}C acetate and FDG. On the dynamic ^{11}C acetate images, myocardial areas were considered viable if the rate constants for tracer clearance were within two standard deviations of normal segmental values obtained in 10 healthy volunteers. In the normal volunteers, average ^{11}C acetate clearance constants ranged from 0.052 ± 0.007 min^{-1} in the apical area to 0.057 ± 0.006 min^{-1} in the inferior wall. Seventy of the 116 segments examined had no improvement in function after revascularization and were considered nonviable; 46 segments improved functionally and were considered viable. On the ^{11}C acetate images, 40 (67%) of the 60 segments with scintigraphic criteria for viability exhibited improved wall motion after revascularization, while 50 (89%) of the 56 segments considered nonviable by scintigraphic criteria did not improve in function. Thus, the positive and negative predictive accuracies for metabolic imaging with ^{11}C acetate were 67% and 89%, respectively. On the FDG images, myocardial viability was defined by a relative ^{18}F concentration that was within two standard deviations of the normal mean value, or by a ratio of relative ^{18}F activity/relative perfusion activity greater than two standard deviations from the mean. Importantly, ^{18}F counts were normalized to peak ^{18}F activities, rather than to ^{18}F activity in normally perfused myocardium. The authors reported that 38 (52%) of the 73 segments considered viable on the FDG studies exhibited improved function after revascularization, while 35 (81%) of the 43 segments considered nonviable had no improvement in wall motion after intervention ($p < 0.01$ for both positive and negative predictive accuracies versus corresponding values for ^{11}C acetate). Analysis of receiver operating characteristic curves indicated that ^{11}C acetate clearance constants were more robust for predicting functional recovery than the scintigraphic criteria used for viability assessment on the FDG images.

Although this investigation suggests that ^{11}C acetate imaging is more robust than metabolic imaging with FDG for identifying reversibly dysfunctional myocardium in patients with chronic CAD, several aspects of this report deserve further consideration. While the observed negative predictive accuracy for FDG imaging is similar to that of other clinical studies, the reported positive predictive accuracy is significantly smaller. This may reflect that tissue ^{18}F counts were referenced to the highest ^{18}F concentrations on the metabolic images for the circumferential profile analysis. Because ^{18}F concentrations in ischemically compromised myocardium can sometimes exceed those in normal tissue, it is probably better to reference ^{18}F activities to peak activities in the best perfused area of the heart. Variations in dietary and hormonal state are minimized using this latter approach.

Secondly, ^{11}C acetate clearance constants were considered normal or abnormal based on the results obtained in normal volunteers. Because ^{11}C acetate clearance constants indirectly reflect myocardial oxygen consumption, increases or decreases in cardiac workload (rate-pressure product) in the healthy subjects would also serve to increase or decrease the normal k_1 values. Rate–pressure products may be higher in patients with CAD and comparison of patient k_1 values to those of normal volunteers therefore assumes comparable rate–pressure products in both groups. Further studies comparing metabolic imaging with ^{11}C acetate to imaging with FDG for identifying clinically important myocardial viability would appear indicated.

Quantitative Techniques for Assessment of Myocardial Viability

Knuuti and co-workers[211] postulated that relative tissue concentrations of FDG could be used to identify viable myocardium. They performed FDG-PET imaging with rest SPECT perfusion imaging (^{201}Tl in 25 individuals, technetium-99m sestamibi in 18 patients) in 48 patients with prior myocardial infarction. On circumferential profile analysis, FDG concentrations were normalized to those in the myocardial segment with the highest tracer uptake on the perfusion images, or (in the five patients without perfusion images) to myocardial areas that were without clinical infarction and supplied by a normal coronary artery. Of 90 asynergic segments that were revascularized, 27 segments exhibited functional improvement after revascularization, while 63 segments had no change or deterioration in function. These investigators reported that a relative FDG concentration of 85% to 90% of peak provided a positive predictive accuracy of 85% and a negative predictive accuracy of 84%, respectively (Table 21-1) for improvement in segmental function following revascularization. This study illustrates the importance of appropriate normalization of FDG activity to healthy reference myocardium for determination of myocardial viability.

Vom Dahl[212] correlated the findings on preoperative PET imaging with ^{13}N ammonia and FDG with changes in segmental function in 37 patients with CAD undergoing elective coronary revascularization. Ventricular function was assessed on gated radionuclide ventriculography before and after coronary revascularization. Relative segmental tracer activity on the PET images was visually assessed according to the following scale: 1 = normal, 2 = slight reduction, 3 = severe reduction, 4 = tracer uptake comparable to background activity. Segments that appeared normal or that had incomplete matching defects of modest severity, or perfusion–metabolism mismatches were considered viable. Segments with more pronounced (scores greater than 2) matching perfusion and metabolic defects were considered nonviable. Of 191 segments with resting wall-motion abnormalities, 50 were considered normal on PET imaging, 43 were considered to have incomplete matching defects (viable without mismatch), 36 were considered viable with perfusion–metabolism mismatches, and 62 were considered nonviable.

On follow-up radionuclide ventriculography, mean wall motion scores improved significantly in the normal segments and in the segments with perfusion–metabolism mismatches. No significant improvement in mean wall motion scores was noted in either the segments with incomplete matching defects or in the nonviable segments. The negative predictive accuracy of FDG metabolic imaging for functional improvement was 86%. However, using the authors definition of viability (segments that appeared normal, had incomplete matches, or perfusion–metabolism mismatched), the positive predictive accuracy of PET imaging for identifying reversible left ventricular dysfunction was quite variable, ranging from 21% to 86%, and highly dependent on the severity of the associated wall-motion abnormality and the scintigraphic pattern. For segments with moderate hypokinesis or worse function, the overall positive predictive accuracy was only 41%. Segments that had incomplete matching perfusion and metabolic defects and that were considered viable without mismatch on PET imaging had positive predictive accuracies ranging from 21% to 31%, with the best predictive accuracy noted for segments that were akinetic or dyskinetic. Segments exhibiting the pattern of an incomplete matching defect were therefore not likely to exhibit improved wall motion following restoration of blood flow, suggesting nontransmural myocardial infarction. For segments considered normal, the positive predictive accuracies ranged from 53% to 75%, again improving as the severity of the associated wall-motion abnormality worsened. Segments with perfusion–metabolism mismatches tended to have the highest positive predictive accuracies, ranging from 48% for segments with mild hypokinesis to 86% for segments with akinesis or dyskinesis.

This study demonstrates that metabolic imaging with FDG is of particular clinical benefit for the characterization of myocardial regions with moderately severe resting perfusion defects. Hypoperfused ventricular regions that have matching reductions in glucose metabolism, the areas with incomplete matching defects, respond much differently to coronary revascularization than hypoperfused ventricular regions in which glucose metabolism is increased relative to blood flow (perfusion–metabolism mismatch). When blood flow and metabolism are concordantly reduced moderately, this likely represents a situation in which there is subendocardial fibrosis with essentially normal (adequately perfused) tissue in the midcardial and epicardial levels. If so, then the segmental dysfunction might reflect the inability of these regions to compensate for the loss of contractility in the subendocardial layer. Under these circumstances, segmental function would be unlikely to benefit from revascularization because the subendocardial scar will still continue to dominate transmural function. The distinction between normal, viable without mismatch, and nonviable on PET images will then reflect the severity of the reduction in tracer concentration on the perfusion and metabolic images.

In contrast is the myocardial region with a perfusion–metabolism mismatch, in which glucose consumption is truly increased relative to substrate delivery (perfusion). The myocardial extraction of glucose, in μmoles per milliliter of blood flow to the tissue, has increased in response to the reduction in tissue oxygen delivery. Viable tissue compensates for ischemia by increasing its consumption of exogenous glucose and by ceasing all noncritical energy-requiring functions. In areas of perfusion–metabolism mismatches, substantial amounts of viable myocardium may have down-regulated contractile function to compensate for the reduced tissue oxygen delivery. Restoration of blood flow to these areas would be expected to be of great clinical benefit since the wall motion abnormality primarily results from compensatory dysfunction of viable tissue.

It is also not surprising that the positive predictive accuracy for segments with relatively preserved function and perfusion–metabolism mismatches was lower than that for segments with more profound wall-motion abnormalities. Since assessment of wall motion was performed using visual analysis only, it may have been more difficult to identify accurately additional improvement in function in segments with mild wall-motion abnormalities. For the segments with more pronounced dysfunction, the observed positive and negative predictive accuracies of 86% and 100% agree quite well with the positive predictive accuracy of 85% and the negative predictive accuracy of 92% originally reported by Tillisch and his colleagues.[203] Thus, the study of vom Dahl and co-workers[212] does not contradict the previously reported observations indicating a high positive and negative predictive accuracy for identifying viable myocardium with PET metabolic imaging with FDG.

Prediction of Left Ventricular Function Recovery after Revascularization

Grandin and associates[213] used a multivariate discriminant model to identify the best predictors of improvement in ventricular function after revascularization, reasoning that recovery of ventricular function after restoration of myocardial blood flow was a complex phenomenon. Dynamic PET imaging with ^{13}N ammonia and FDG was performed before revascularization in 25 patients with chronic CAD and anterior wall dysfunction (coronary artery bypass graft in 7 patients, percutaneous transluminal coronary angioplasty in 18 patients). Two observers visually assessed changes in regional wall motion before and after surgery on contrast ventriculograms. Dysfunctional myocardial areas on the baseline study were considered to harbor viable tissue if the wall motion score improved at least one grade and if end-systolic volume decreased on the postoperative studies. Dysfunctional myocardial areas were considered nonviable if regional wall motion did not improve or if end-systolic volume increased after revascularization. The PET variables that were examined were absolute and normalized myocardial blood flows, absolute and normalized myocardial glucose uptake, absolute and normalized glucose extraction, relative ^{13}N ammonia and FDG uptake, and ratios of normalized FDG activities to normalized ^{13}N activities.

On follow-up assessment of ventricular function at 6 to 9 months after revascularization, 17 patients had improved regional wall motion and smaller end-systolic ventricular volumes and were considered to have viable myocardium. Eight patients had increases in end-systolic ventricular volumes and a variable change in anterior wall motion score (three had no change, two had an improvement of one grade, and three had deterioration) and were considered to have nonviable myocardium. Before revascularization, the severity of the anterior wall motion abnormality, left ventricular volume, LVEF, and coronary anatomy were similar in both groups of patients.

On step-wise linear discriminant analysis, absolute myocardial blood flow ($F = 12.21, p < 0.01$) and normalized glucose extraction ($F = 6.36, p < 0.05$) were independent predictors of the presence of viable myocardium, as defined by an improvement in both ventricular end-systolic volume and in regional wall motion score. An absolute myocardial blood flow of 0.64 ml/min/g alone identified 12 (70%) of 17 patients with viable myocardium and 7 (88%) of 8 patients with nonviable myocardium. Using the discriminant function f = 0.10* absolute blood flow + 0.0274* normalized glucose extraction − 9.57, a value greater than 0.69 correctly identified 14 (82%) of 17 patients with viable myocardium while a value less than this identified 7 (88%) of 8 patients without viable myocardium. Similar results were observed if myocardial viability was defined solely by an improvement in regional wall motion score. Absolute myocardial blood flow ($F = 8.90, p < 0.01$) and relative FDG uptake ($F = 5.29, p < 0.05$) were independent predictors of improved regional wall motion on stepwise linear discriminant analysis. Using both of these parameters, 16 (84%) of 19 patients with improved regional wall motion and 5 (83%) of 6 patients without improvement in regional wall motion were correctly identified. The results of this investigation thus confirm that metabolic imaging with FDG provides independent information, on and beyond that provided by assessment of myocardial perfusion alone, which is helpful for identifying clinically important tissue viability.

Histopathologic Correlation

Although most clinical studies have relied upon improved wall motion following coronary revascularization as indirect evidence of the presence of viable tissue in dysfunctional myocardium, several investigators have directly related the results of PET metabolic imaging to histopathologic findings in diseased human hearts. These clinicopathologic studies have provided direct evidence of the ability of PET metabolic imaging to identify viable tissue in patients with chronic CAD and left ventricular dysfunction.

Berry[214] reported the results of PET imaging with ^{13}N ammonia and FDG in nine patients before orthotopic cardiac transplantation; four had ischemic cardiomyopathy, and five had nonischemic cardiomyopathy. The mean LVEF in both groups was 13%. Planimetric measurements of the relative amount of viable tissue in each 10-degree sector of a midventricular transaxial slice from each explanted heart were compared with ^{13}N and ^{18}F circumferential profiles derived from PET images. In patients with nonischemic cardiomyopathy there was interstitial and perivascular fibrosis but no discrete areas of myocardial infarction. Relative ^{13}N and ^{18}F counts were highly correlated in these individuals, indicating a close coupling between perfusion and glucose metabolism. In the hearts with ischemic cardiomyopathy, there were extensive areas of myocardial infarction with varying degrees of transmural involvement. Histologically the regions of infarction exhibited large areas of confluent fibrosis and myocardial thinning. Circumferential profile analysis revealed a close correlation between the histologic determinations of the amount of viable myocardium and relative ^{13}N and ^{18}F tracer concentrations on the PET images. Relative tracer concentrations paralleled the percent of viable myocardium in most myocardial sectors. This study thus indicated that areas of matching perfusion and metabolic defects on PET images correspond closely in extent and severity to the amount of irreversible tissue damage identified pathologically in ischemic human cardiomyopathy. In a similar study involving 11 patients with end-stage ischemic cardiomyopathy, Delbeke[215] demonstrated that measurements of left ventricular infarct mass and infarct size derived from ^{13}N ammonia PET images acquired before cardiac transplantation were highly correlated with actual infarct mass and size in the explanted hearts.

Vanoverschelde and his colleagues[216] correlated the results of PET perfusion and metabolic imaging with the histopathologic findings on transmural myocardial biopsies obtained at the time of coronary bypass surgery in 26 patients without prior clinical infarction who had chronic occlusion of a major coronary artery. Nine of the patients had normal wall motion in the affected coronary distribution while 15 patients had resting regional wall-motion abnormalities. Global and regional wall motion at baseline ($n = 26$) and 5 to 8 months after coronary revascularization ($n = 12$) were evaluated using contrast ventriculography. In seven patients, transmural myocardial biopsies were obtained from collateral dependent myocardium at the time of coronary bypass surgery and examined with light and electron microscopy. Light microscopy was performed to quantitate the percent of connective tissue present in the biopsy specimens and to estimate the relative number of myocytes with and without structural alterations. Electron microscopy was used to define the ultrastructural abnormalities in affected myocardial areas.

In the patients with normal wall motion in the affected coronary territory, resting myocardial blood flows averaged 0.85 ± 0.14 ml/min/g and did not differ statistically from those in areas with a wall-motion abnormality, 0.77 ± 0.25 ml/min/g. Relative ^{13}N ammonia concentrations were $83 \pm 10\%$ in collateral dependent myocardium with normal function and $65 \pm 17\%$ in collateral dependent myocardium with abnormal function ($p < 0.001$). Ratios of relative FDG uptake to ^{13}N ammonia uptake averaged 1.2 ± 0.2 in normally contracting regions and 1.9 ± 1.6 in dysfunctional regions ($p < 0.05$), meaning that perfusion–metabolism mismatches tended to be associated with the resting wall-motion abnormalities. Absolute rates of glucose utilization were 0.38 ± 0.16 μmol/min/g in dysfunctional myocardium and 0.33 ± 0.11 μmol/min/g in normally functioning myocardium. Derived rates of glucose extraction (absolute glucose consumption/absolute myocardial blood flow) were therefore significantly higher in dysfunctional myocardium than in normally functioning myocardium (0.60 ± 0.27 versus 0.42 ± 0.16 μmol/ml, $p < 0.004$), indicating an alteration in regional myocardial glucose metabolism. Rates of acetate clearance, or k_{mono} in dysfunctional collateralized myocardium paralleled the relative reductions in myocardial blood flows and were not significantly different from those in collateralized myocardium with normal function (0.049 ± 0.015 versus 0.054 ± 0.010 min^{-1}, $p = $ NS). Thus, in collateral dependent myocardium with regional contractile dysfunction, modest relative reductions in blood flow and oxidative substrate metabolism were identified along with enhanced glucose consumption per unit of myocardial blood flow.

Dipyridamole stress perfusion imaging was performed in 11 patients with occlusion of the left anterior descending artery. In the affected areas with normal function, coronary flow reserves averaged 3.0 ± 0.6 as compared with 1.4 ± 0.6 in the areas with abnormal function ($p < 0.001$). An inverse relationship was noted between anterior wall motion scores and the coronary flow reserve measurements in the collateral-dependent segments ($r = 0.85$, $p < 0.001$). These data suggest that the most severe wall motion abnormalities are associated with the greatest impairment in coronary flow reserve.

Myocardial biopsies were obtained at the time of coronary revascularization in four patients with resting wall motion abnormalities and in three patients with normal function. On histologic examination, little fibrosis was noted in six of the seven patients. One patient had 50% fibrosis in the subendocardium, while the others had from 1% to 11% fibrosis in the subendocardium and 1% to 8% transmural fibrosis. However, a large proportion of the myocytes appeared abnormal. The relative number of abnormal cells ranged from 5% to 90% in the subendocardium and from 4% to 59% of cells across the entire myocardial wall. Biopsies from the patients with wall motion abnormalities revealed a greater number of abnormal cells than those from patients with normal function. The abnormal cells were characterized by a severe reduction in contractile filaments, by glycogen accumulation, by a reduction in the sarcoplasmic reticulum, and by the presence of numerous small mitochondria.

Supporting evidence of cellular viability was provided by follow-up assessment of regional wall motion in 12 patients with abnormal preoperative function. Mean regional wall motion scores improved significantly, and end-systolic volume decreased from 47 ± 10 to 34 ± 11 ml/m2, ($p < 0.005$). In addition, the global LVEF improved from $55 \pm 7\%$ to $65 \pm 8\%$ ($p < 0.005$). These investigators suggested that repeated episodes of ischemia, as opposed to chronic hypoperfusion and myocardial hibernation, were responsible for the observed impairment in wall motion, glucose metabolism, and cellular ultrastructural abnormalities. The investigation indicates that reversibly dysfunctional human myocardium is characterized histologically by abnormal but viable myocytes and by metabolic abnormalities that can characterized noninvasively with PET imaging.

Maes et al.[217] performed PET imaging with ^{13}N ammonia and FDG in 33 patients with chronic CAD before coronary revascularization. The presence of a perfusion–metabolism mismatch (defined as a relative metabolism/flow ratio >1.2) was correlated with the results of two transmural biopsies obtained at the time of surgery and with recovery of regional wall motion following revascularization. The amount of connective tissue was determined using a morphometric technique. Myocytes were planimetrically scored for the degree of myolysis (sarcomere loss), using a minimum of 100 cells per epicardial or endocardial segment; cells with greater than 10% loss of sarcomeres were considered affected cells. Electron microscopy was also performed to delineate the ultrastructural changes in areas of interest identified with light microscopy.

On the biopsies from 10 patients with normal function, the histologic appearance was relatively normal (Fig. 21-7). Quantitatively, the amount of fibrosis within the biopsy specimens averaged 8 ± 4 vol%, and 12 ± 8% of the myocytes exhibited an increase in cellular glycogen content (below). Of 23 patients with anterior wall motion abnormalities, 9 had matching perfusion and metabolic defects on PET imaging and 14 had perfusion–metabolism mismatches. Neither absolute nor relative blood flows distinguished between dysfunctional myocardial regions with or without enhanced glucose metabolism. Rates of glucose utilization in the myocardial regions with matching perfusion and metabolic defects averaged 0.37 ± 11 μmol/min/g, compared with 0.55 ± 0.10 μmol/min/g in reference segments. In contrast, rates of glucose utilization in the dysfunctional regions with perfusion–metabolism mismatches were similar to reference myocardium, 0.62 ± 0.15 μmol/min/g versus 0.60 ± 0.17 μmol/min/g. Relative to blood flow, therefore, absolute rates of glucose utilization were increased in the dysfunctional myocardial regions with perfusion–metabolism mismatches.

In the patients with perfusion–metabolism mismatches, most of the cardiac myocytes appeared normal histologically. However, on light microscopy some cells exhibited a loss of contractile material (sarcomeres), with preservation of cellular volume (Fig. 21-8). In these cells, the contractile proteins appeared to be replaced by glycogen. A slight increase in connective tissue was noted, but no necrotic myocytes were identified. On electron microscopy, the depletion of sarcomeres in affected cells appeared to be most prominent in the perinuclear area. Small mitochondria with normal-appearing cristae were noted in the glycogen-rich perinuclear zones with the sarcomere depletion. The nuclear contour appeared tortuous, and the sarcoplasmic reticulum was virtually absent. The sarcolemma did not project protrusions (T tubules) into the cytosol. However, cytoplasmic vacuolization, cytosolic edema, mitochondrial swelling, membrane disruption, and accumulation of secondary lysosomes and lipid droplets were virtually absent. On quantitative analysis, the amount of fibrosis in the biopsy specimens averaged 11 ± 6 vol% and the relative number of myocytes with reduced contractile material and increased glycogen content averaged 25 ± 13%. In the regions with matching perfusion and metabolic defects, the relative number of myocytes with sarcomere depletion and enhanced glycogen content was similar to the areas with perfusion–metabolism mismatches, at 24 ± 15%. However, extensive fibrosis averaging 35 ± 25% vol% was also identified (Fig. 21-9).

Assessment of ventricular function was performed in 29 patients after coronary revascularization. In nine individuals with normal preoperative wall motion, global LVEF and regional ejection fractions were unchanged. Similarly, no improvement was noted in global or regional ejection fractions in the eight patients with matching perfusion and metabolic defects. In contrast, in the 12 patients with perfusion–metabolism mismatches with regional wall-motion abnormalities, there was a 29% improvement in regional ejection fraction, from 42 ± 11% to 54 ± 13%, and an 18% improvement in global LVEF, from 51 ± 11% to 60 ± 10% ($p < 0.05$ for both). Neither the severity of the perfusion defect

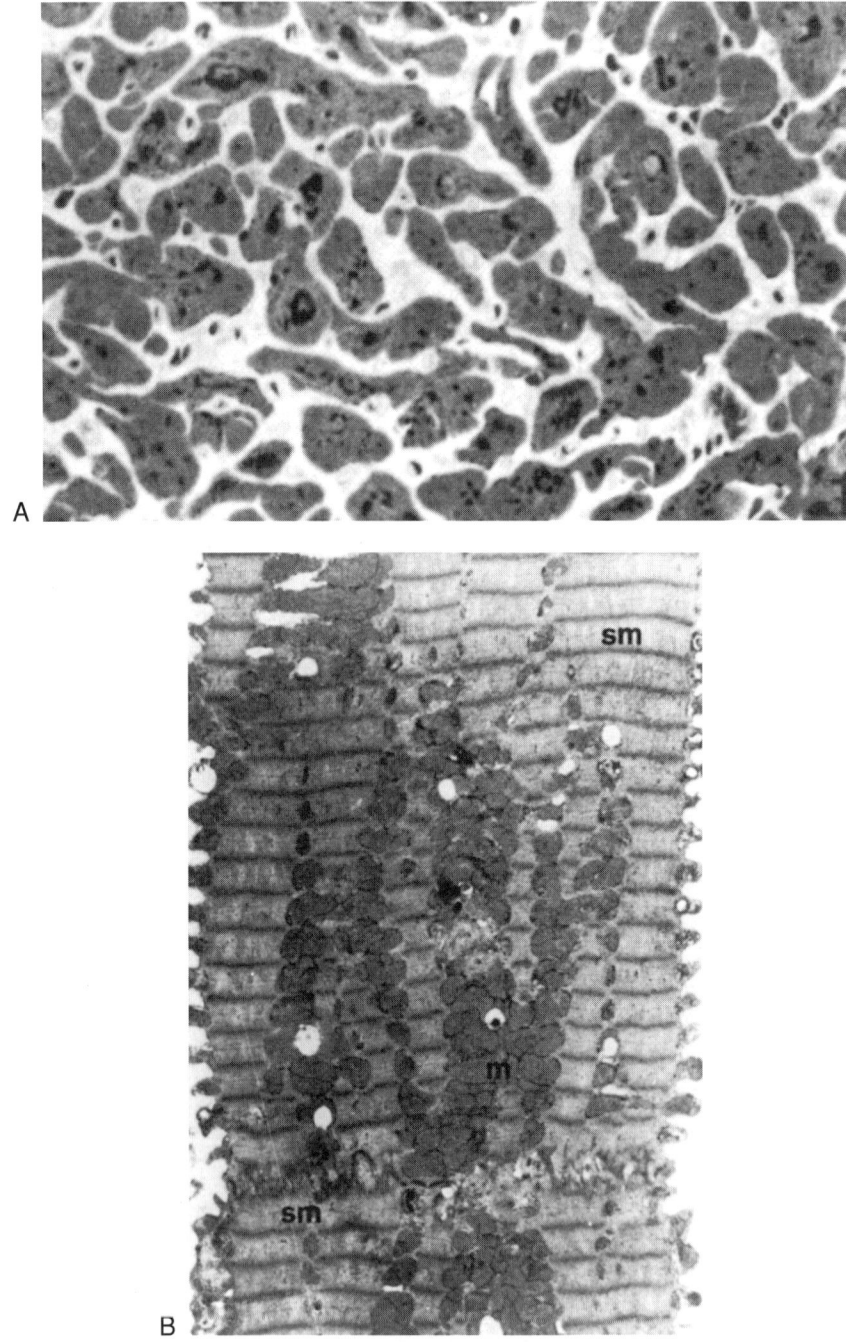

Fig. 21-7. Histopathologic findings in a coronary heart disease patient with normal regional function and normal nitrogen 13 ammonia perfusion and metabolic fluorine 18 2-fluoro-2-deoxyglucose images. On the light micrograph of the PAS-stained tissue **(A)**, a normal amount of glycogen is present. On the electron micrograph **(B)**, the cellular cytoplasm is filled with rows of sarcomeres (sm) and normal sized mitochondria (m). (From Maes et al.,[217] with permission.)

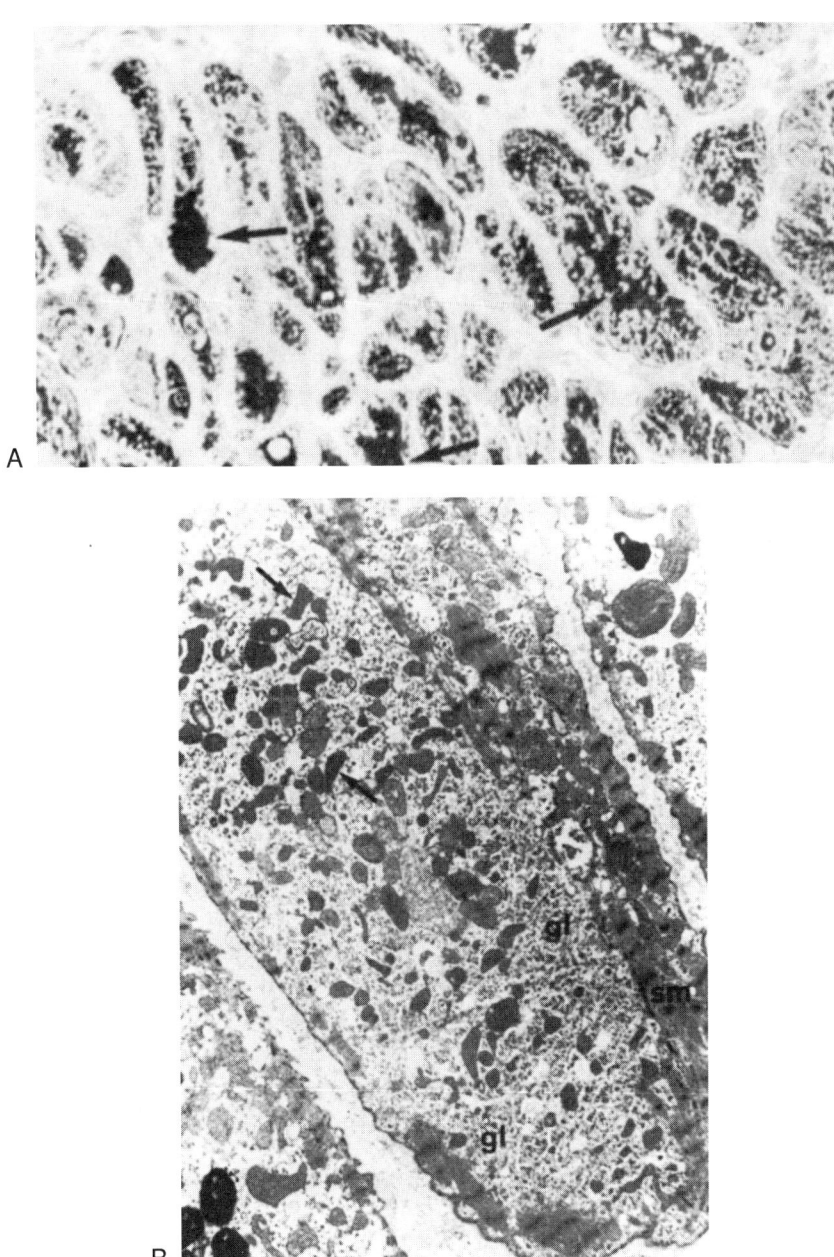

Fig. 21-8. Light **(A)** and electron microscopic **(B)** findings in a patient with anterior wall hypokinesis and a perfusion–metabolism mismatch on positron emission tomographic imaging. *Arrows* in panel 2a depict accumulation of glycogen in the PAS-stained specimen. On the electron micrograph, sarcomeres are absent from the center of the cell and are identified only at the periphery (sm). Cytosolic accumulation of glycogen is noted (gl) and small mitochondria are present (*arrows*). The regional ejection fraction in this area increased from 46% to 55% after coronary revascularization. (From Maes et al.,[217] with permission.)

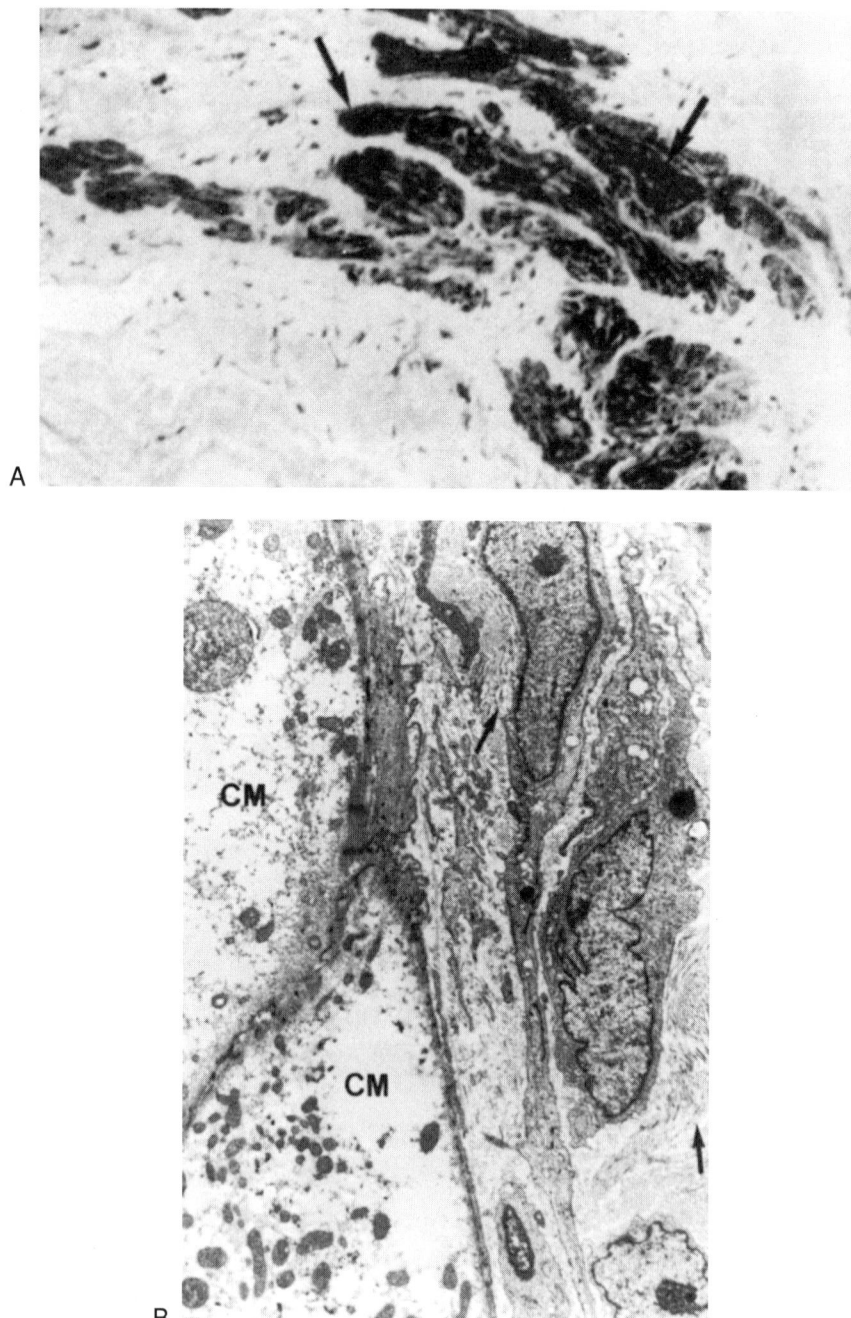

Fig. 21-9. Light **(A)** and electron microscopic **(B)** findings in a coronary artery disease patient with anterior wall hypokinesis and matching perfusion and metabolic defects on positron emission tomographic imaging. Extensive fibrosis is noted on the light micrograph, along with glycogen accumulating cells (*arrows*) on this PAS-stained specimen. On the electron micrograph, abundant collagen is noted (*arrows*) next to the cardiomyocytes (CM). Following revascularization, the regional ejection fraction decreased from 23% to 17%. (From Maes et al.,[217] with permission.)

nor the severity of the associated wall-motion abnormality predicted the improvement in regional ejection fraction after coronary revascularization. This investigation thus indicates that dysfunctional myocardial areas with matching perfusion and glucose metabolic defects on PET imaging contain extensive amounts of myocardial fibrosis, whereas dysfunctional myocardial areas with perfusion–metabolism mismatches contain a relatively high number of viable but abnormal myocytes with glycogen accumulation on histopathologic examination. The hypothesis that the abnormal myocytes identified in the areas with perfusion–metabolism mismatches are viable is supported further by the recovery of regional function after revascularization.

Depre and his colleagues[218] performed dynamic PET imaging with ^{13}N ammonia and FDG in 24 patients with CAD and anterior wall myocardial dysfunction before elective CABG. The scintigraphic findings were then correlated with the findings on transmural biopsies obtained at the time of surgery. Ventricular function improved after revascularization in 16 individuals, but there was no improvement in function in 8 patients. Compared with those in the patients without improvement in function, tissue biopsies in the individuals with functional recovery revealed significantly less transmural (24 ± 13 versus $49 \pm 20\%$, $p = 0.002$) and subendocardial (20 ± 13 versus $53 \pm 27\%$, $p = 0.008$) fibrosis. The authors noted that a value of 35% for the amount of transmural fibrosis best distinguished between regions with (12 of 16) and without (7 of 8) recovery of function after revascularization. Structurally altered myocytes were seen frequently in the specimens and were characterized by a loss of contractile material, small mitochondria, a virtual absence of sarcoplasmic reticulum and T tubules, and an increase in cellular glycogen content. The relative number of abnormal myocytes in the areas with reversible dysfunction was significantly greater than that in the areas with persistent dysfunction ($35 \pm 14\%$ versus $21 \pm 15\%$, $p < 0.05$) and the postoperative improvement in ventricular function was inversely related to the relative number of abnormal myocytes ($r = 0.48$, $p < 0.05$). This suggests that the greater the number of altered myocytes before surgery the greater the improvement in regional ventricular function after revascularization.

On the preoperative PET studies, relative ^{13}N ammonia uptake (74 ± 11 versus $58 \pm 12\%$, $p < 0.005$), absolute myocardial blood flow (0.88 ± 0.23 versus 0.61 ± 0.12 ml/min/g, $p = 0.005$), relative FDG uptake (88 ± 18 versus $66 \pm 26\%$, $p = 0.03$), and absolute glucose consumption (0.50 ± 0.21 versus 0.30 ± 0.13 μmoles/min/g, $p = 0.02$) were significantly higher in the areas exhibiting functional recovery than in the areas with no improvement in wall motion. In contrast to some other studies, relative FDG to ^{13}N ammonia ratios and absolute and normalized glucose extractions did not differ between the two groups. Interestingly, linear correlations were noted between the number of altered myocytes and relative FDG uptake, the amount of fibrosis and relative ^{13}N ammonia uptake, and the amount of fibrosis and absolute and normalized blood flows.

The authors constructed a multiple regression mathematical model to examine the factors that predicted improvement in segmental wall motion score that incorporated all flow, metabolic, and histologic data. On univariate analysis, improvement in wall motion score was significantly related to the severity of tissue fibrosis, absolute myocardial blood flow, the relative surface of the biopsy occupied by altered myocytes, left ventricular end-diastolic volume, and absolute myocardial glucose uptake. Step-wise multiple regression analysis selected severity of tissue fibrosis, left ventricular end-diastolic volume, and absolute myocardial blood flow as independent predictors of the improvement in regional function after revascularization. Depre et al. concluded that the recovery of contraction in their patients was related to the extent and severity of tissue fibrosis and to the residual relative amount of metabolically active, altered myocytes.

Summary

The clinical utility of PET metabolic imaging with FDG for identifying reversibly dysfunctional myocardium has been assessed in 344 patients with coronary artery disease in studies examining in excess of 800 myocardial segments (Table 21-1). These clinical investigations have involved major medical centers in Europe, the United States, and Japan. In the aggregate experience, the absence of FDG activity in hypoperfused myocardial segments has an 83% negative predictive value for identifying irreversible tissue injury. The positive predictive value, 72%, is somewhat less than that of initial reports, primarily because of the inclusion of studies performed in the fasting or postexercise state and in which visual (as opposed to circumferential profile) analysis of the PET images was performed. Thus, cumulative experience indicates that PET imaging with FDG is an accurate means of identifying reversibly dysfunctional myocardium in patients with chronic coronary artery disease.

CONCLUSION

Although the best method for identifying myocardial viability with PET in CAD patients with compromised ventricular function remains the subject of active investigation, the extensive accumulated experience with FDG imaging would seem to favor the use of this metabolic tracer for clinical viability determinations. As noted, FDG metabolic imaging is best performed in conjunction with a tracer of myocardial perfusion to distinguish regions with incomplete matching defects from areas with perfusion–metabolism mismatches, because the functional outcome of these two tissue types differs after revascularization. Future clinical investigations, in which the extent and severity of perfusion–metabolism mismatches along with other clinical descriptors, such as left ventricular volumes, absolute blood flows, and perfusable tissue indices, may well provide the means to predict not only whether ventricular function will improve but may also yield quantitative estimates of the magnitude of change in ventricular function that would reasonably be anticipated after coronary revascularization. This would afford the clinician a better estimate of the potential benefit of revascularization in the patient with coronary artery disease and pronounced left ventricular dysfunction and would assist in defining the optimal treatment approach for each specific individual, with the ultimate goal of reducing this disease's human morbidity and mortality.

REFERENCES

1. Hoffman EJ, Phelps ME: Positron emission tomography: principles and quantitation. p. 237. In Phelps ME, Mazziotta JC, Schelbert HR (eds): Positron Emission Tomography and Autoradiography. Principles and Applications for the Brain and Heart. Raven Press, New York, 1986
2. Bacharach SL: The physics of positron emission tomography. p. 13. In Bergmann SR, Sobel BE (eds): Positron Emission Tomography of the Heart. Futura Publishing, Mount Kisco, New York, 1992
3. Schelbert HR: Principles of positron emission tomography. p. 1140. In Marcus ML, Schelbert HR, Skorton DJ, Wolf GL (eds): Cardiac Imaging. A Companion to Braunwald's Heart Disease. WB Saunders, Philadelphia, 1991
4. McCord ME, Bacharach SL, Bonow RO et al: Misalignment between PET transmission and emission scans: its effect on myocardial imaging. J Nucl Med 33:1209, 1992
5. Andersson JLR, Vagnhammar BE, Schneider H: Accurate attenuation correction despite movement during PET imaging. J Nucl Med 36:670, 1995
6. Hoffman EJ, Phelps ME, Wisenberg G, Schelbert HR, Kuhl DE: Electrocardiographic gating in positron emission tomography. J Comput Assist Tomogr 3:733, 1979
7. Yamashita K, Tamaki N, Yonekura Y et al: Quantitative analysis of regional wall motion by gated myocardial positron emission tomography: validation and comparison with left ventriculography. J Nucl Med 30:1775, 1989
8. Yamashita K, Tamaki N, Yonekura Y et al: Regional wall thickening of left ventricle evaluated by gated positron emission tomography in relation to myocardial perfusion and glucose metabolism. J Nucl Med 32:679, 1991
9. Miller TR, Wallis JW, Landy BR, Gropler RJ, Sabharwal CL: Measurement of global and regional left ventricular function by cardiac PET. J Nucl Med 35:999, 1994
10. Porenta G, Kuhle W, Sinha S et al: Parameter estimation of cardiac geometry by ECG-gated PET imaging: validation using magnetic resonance imaging and echocardiography. J Nucl Med 36:1123, 1995
11. Bartlett ML, Bacharach SL, Voipio-Pulkki L, Dilsizian V: Artifactual inhomogeneities in myocardial PET and SPECT scans in normal subjects. J Nucl Med 36:188, 1995
12. Senda M, Yonekura Y, Tamaki N et al: Interpolating scan and oblique-angle tomograms in myocardial PET using N-13 ammonia. J Nucl Med 27:1830, 1986
13. Miller TR, Starren JB, Grothe RA: Three-dimensional display of positron emission tomography of the heart. J Nucl Med 29:530, 1988
14. Hicks K, Ganti G, Mullani N, Gould KL: Automated

quantitation of three-dimensional cardiac positron emission tomography for routine clinical use. J Nucl Med 30:1787, 1989
15. Miller TR, Wallis JW, Geltman EM, Bergmann SR: Three-dimensional functional images of myocardial oxygen consumption from positron tomography. J Nucl Med 31:2064, 1990
16. Kuhle WG, Porenta G, Huang SC, Phelps ME, Schelbert HR: Issues in the quantitation of reoriented PET images. J Nucl Med 33:1235, 1992
17. Garcia EV, Van Train K, Maddahi J et al: Quantification of rotational thallium-201 myocardial tomography. J Nucl Med 26:17, 1985
18. Klein JL, Garcia EV, DePuey EG et al: Reversibility of bull's-eye: a new polar bull's-eye map to quantify reversibility of stress-induced SPECT thallium-201 perfusion defects. J Nucl Med 31:1240, 1990
19. Garcia EV, DePuey EG, Sonnemaker RE et al: Quantification of the reversibility of stress-induced thallium-201 perfusion defects: A multicenter trial using bull's-eye polar maps and standard normal limits. J Nucl Med 31:1761, 1990
20. Ratib O, Bidaut L, Nienaber C et al: Semiautomatic software for quantitative analysis of cardiac positron tomography studies. SPIE 914:412, 1988
21. Porenta G, Kuhle WG, Czernin J et al: Semiquantitative assessment of myocardial blood flow and viability using polar map displays of cardiac PET images. J Nucl Med 33:1628, 1992
22. Sun KT, De Groof M, Yi J et al: Quantification of the extent and severity of perfusion defects in canine myocardium by PET polar mapping. J Nucl Med 35:2031, 1994
23. Choi Y, Hawkins RA, Huang SC et al: Parametric images of myocardial metabolic rate of glucose generated from dynamic cardiac PET and 2-[^{18}F]Fluoro-2-deoxy-d-glucose studies. J Nucl Med 32:733, 1991
24. Kotzerke J, Hicks RJ, Wolfe E et al: Three-dimensional assessment of myocardial oxidative metabolism: a new approach for regional determination of PET-derived carbon-11-acetate kinetics. J Nucl Med 31:1876, 1990
25. Muzik O, Beanlands R, Wolfe E, Hutchins GD, Schwaiger M: Automated region definition for cardiac nitrogen-13-ammonia PET imaging. J Nucl Med 34:336, 1993
26. Choi Y, Huang SC, Hawkins RA et al: A simplified method for quantification of myocardial blood flow using N-13-ammonia and dynamic PET. J Nucl Med 34:488, 1993
27. Blanksma PK, Willemsen ATM, Meeder JG et al: Quantitative myocardial mapping of perfusion and metabolism using parametric polar map displays in cardiac PET. J Nucl Med 36:153, 1995
28. Wu HM, Hoh CK, Buxton DB et al: Quantification of myocardial blood flow using dynamic nitrogen-13-ammonia PET studies and factor analysis of dynamic structures. J Nucl Med 36:2087, 1995
29. Henze E, Huang SC, Ratib O et al: Measurements of regional tissue and blood-pool radiotracer concentrations from serial tomographic images of the heart. J Nucl Med 24:987, 1983
30. Parodi P, Schelbert HR, Schwaiger M et al: Cardiac emission computed tomography: underestimation of regional tracer concentrations due to wall motion abnormalities. J Comput Assist Tomogr 8:1083, 1984
31. Bergmann SR: Quantification of myocardial perfusion with positron emisson tomography. p. 97. In Bergmann SR and Sobel BE: Positron Emission Tomography of the Heart. Futura Publishing, Mount Kisco, NY
32. Gennaro GP, Nierinckx RD, Bergner B et al: A radionuclide generator and infusion system for pharmaceutical quality Rb-82. p. 135. In Knapp FF, Butler TA (eds): Radionuclide Generators: New Systems for Nuclear Medicine Applications. ACS Symposium Series #241. American Chemical Society, Washington, D.C., 1984
33. Saha GB, Go RT, MacIntyre WJ et al: Use of the ^{82}Sr/^{82}Rb generator in clinical PET studies. International Journal of Radiation Applications and Instrumentation. Part B, Nuclear Medicine and Biology 17:763, 1990
34. Walsh WF, Harper PV, Resnekov L, Fill H: Noninvasive evaluation of regional myocardial perfusion in 112 patients using a mobile scintillation camera and intravenous nitrogen-13 labeled ammonia. Circulation 54:266, 1976
35. Schelbert HR, Phelps ME, Hoffman EJ et al: Regional myocardial perfusion assessed with N-13 labeled ammonia and positron emission computerized axial tomography. Am J Cardiol 43:209, 1979
36. Schelbert HR, Phelps ME, Huang SC et al: N-13 ammonia as an indicator of myocardial blood flow. Circulation 63:1259, 1981
37. Tamaki N, Senda M, Yonekura Y et al: Dynamic positron computed tomography of the heart with a high sensitivity positron camera and nitrogen-13 ammonia. J Nucl Med 26:567, 1985
38. Shah A, Schelbert HR, Schwaiger M et al: Measurement of regional myocardial blood flow with N-13 ammonia and positron emission tomography in intact dogs. J Am Coll Cardiol 5:92, 1985
39. Krivokapich J, Smith GT, Huang SC et al: ^{13}N ammo-

nia myocardial imaging at rest and with exercise in normal volunteers. Quantification of absolute myocardial perfusion with dynamic positron emission tomography. Circulation 80:1328, 1989
40. Bellina CR, Parodi O, Camici P et al: Simultaneous in vitro and in vivo validation of nirogen-13-ammonia for the assessment of regional myocardial blood flow. J Nucl Med 31:1335, 1990
41. Nienaber CA, Ratib O, Gambhir SS et al: A quantitative index of regional blood flow in canine myocardium derived noninvasively with N-13 ammonia and dynamic positron emission tomography. J Am Coll Cardiol 17:260, 1991
42. Krivokapich J, Huang SC, Phelps ME, MacDonald NS, Shine KI: Dependence of $^{13}NH_3$ myocardial extraction and clearance on flow and metabolism. Am J Physiol 242:H536, 1982
43. Krivokapich J, Barrio JR, Phelps ME et al: Kinetic characterization of $^{13}NH_3$ and [^{13}N]glutamine metabolism in rabbit heart. Am J Physiol 246:H267, 1984
44. Beanlands RSB, Muzik O, Hutchins GD, Wolfe ER, Schwaiger M: Heterogeneity of regional nitrogen-13-labeled ammonia tracer distribution in the normal human heart: comparison with rubidium-82 and copper-62-labeled PTSM. J Nucl Cardiol 1:225, 1994
45. de Jong RM, Blanksma PK, Willemsen ATM et al: Posterolateral defect of the normal human heart investigated with nitrogen-13-ammonia and dynamic PET. J Nucl Med 36:581, 1995
46. Love WD, Burch GE: Influence of the rate of coronary plasma flow on the extraction of Rb^{86} from coronary blood. Circ Res 7:24, 1959
47. Levy MN, de Olivera JM: Regional distribution of myocardial blood flow in the dog as determined by Rb-86. Circ Res 9:96, 1961
48. Cohen A, Zaleski EJ, Baberon H et al: Measurement of coronary blood flow using rubidium-84 and the coincidence counting method: a critical analysis. Am J Cardiol 19:556, 1967
49. Becker L, Ferreira R, Thomas M: Comparison of ^{86}Rb and microsphere estimates of left ventricular blood flow distribution. J Nucl Med 15:969, 1974
50. Berman DS, Salel AF, DeNardo GL, Mason DT: Noninvasive detection of regional myocardial ischemia using rubidium-81 and the scintillation camera. Circulation 52:619, 1975
51. Beller GA, Cochavi S, Smith TW, Brownell GL: Positron emission tomographic imaging of the myocardium with ^{81}Rb. J Comput Assist Tomogr 6:341, 1982
52. Gould KL, Goldstein RA, Mullani NA et al: Noninvasive assessment of coronary stenoses by myocardial perfusion imaging during pharmacologic coronary vasodilation. VIII. Clinical feasibility of positron cardiac imaging without a cyclotron using generator-produced rubidium-82. J Am Coll Cardiol 7:775, 1986
53. Coxson PG, Brennan KM, Huesman RH, Lim S, Budinger TF: Variability and reproducibility of rubidium-82 kinetic parameters in the myocardium of the anesthetized canine. J Nucl Med 36:287, 1995
54. Selwyn AP, Allan RM, L'Abbate A et al: Relation between regional myocardial uptake of rubidium-82 and perfusion: absolute reduction in cation uptake in ischemia. Am J Cardiol 50:112, 1982
55. Mullani NA, Goldstein RA, Gould KL et al: Myocardial perfusion with rubidium-82. I. Measurement of extraction fraction and flow with external detectors. J Nucl Med 24:898, 1983
56. Goldstein RA, Mullani NA, Marani SK et al: Myocardial perfusion with rubidium-82. II. Effects of metabolic and pharmacologic interventions. J Nucl Med 24:907, 1983
57. Huang SC, Williams BA, Krivokapich J et al: Rabbit myocardial ^{82}Rb kinetics and a compartmental model for blood flow estimation. Am J Physiol 256 (Heart Circ Physiol 25):H1156, 1989
58. Tripp MR, Meyer MW, Einzig S et al: Simultaneous regional myocardial blood flows by tritiated water and microspheres. Am J Physiol 232:H173, 1977
59. Bergmann SR, Fox KAA, Rand AL et al: Quantification of regional myocardial blood flow in vivo with $H_2^{15}O$. Circulation 70:724, 1984
60. Huang SC, Schwaiger M, Carson RE et al: Quantitative measurement of myocardial blood flow with oxygen-15 water and positron computed tomography: an assessment of potential and problems. J Nucl Med 26:616, 1985
61. Knabb RM, Fox KAA, Sobel BE, Bergmann SR: Characterization of the functional significance of subcritical coronary stenoses with $H_2^{15}O$ and positron-emission tomography. Circulation 71:1271, 1985
62. Walsh MN, Bergmann SR, Steele RL et al: Delineation of impaired regional myocardial perfusion by positron emission tomography with $H_2^{15}O$. Circulation 78:612, 1988
63. Bergmann SR, Herrero P, Markham J, Weinheimer CJ, Walsh MN: Noninvasive quantitation of myocardial blood flow in human subjects with oxygen-15-labeled water and positron emission tomography. J Am Coll Cardiol 14:639, 1989
64. Araujo LI, Lammertsma AA, Rhodes CG et al: Noninvasive quantification of regional myocardial blood flow in coronary artery disease with oxygen-15-labeled carbon dioxide inhalation and positron emission tomography. Circulation 83:875, 1991

65. Iida H, Takahashi A, Tamura Y, Ono Y, Lammertsma AA: Myocardial blood flow: comparison of oxygen-15-water bolus injection, slow infusion and oxygen-15-carbon dioxide slow inhalation. J Nucl Med 36:78, 1995
66. Lammertsma AA, De Silva R, Araujo LI, Jones T: Measurement of regional myocardial blood flow using $C^{15}O_2$ and positron emission tomography: comparison of tracer models. Clin Phys Physiol Meas 13:1, 1992
67. Bacharach SL, Cuocolo A, Bonow RO et al: PET myocardial blood flow by H_2O^{15} without a blood pool scan, abstracted. J Nucl Med 30:807, 1989
68. Tilbury RS, Myers WG, Chandra R, Dahl JR, LEE R: Production of 7.6-minute potassium-38 for medical use. J Nucl Med 21:867, 1980
69. Pierard LA, De Landsheere CM, Berthe C, Rigo P, Kulbertus HE: Identification of viable myocardium by echocardiography during dobutamine infusion in patients with myocardial infarction after thrombolytic therapy: comparison with positron emission tomography. J Am Coll Cardiol 15:1021, 1990
70. Duboc D, Kahan A, Maziere B et al: The effect of nifedipine on myocardial perfusion and metabolism in systemic sclerosis. Arthritis and Rheumatism 34:198, 1991
71. DeLandsheere C, Mannheimer C, Habets A et al: Effect of spinal cord stimulation on regional myocardial perfusion assessed by positron emission tomography. Am J Cardiol 69:1143, 1992
72. Melon PG, Brihaye C, Degueldre C et al: Myocardial kinetics of potassium-38 in humans and comparison with copper-62-PTSM. J Nucl Med 35:1116, 1994
73. Stone CK, Christian BT, Nickles RJ, Perlman SB: Technetium 94m-labeled methoxyisobutyl isonitrile: dosimetry and resting cardiac imaging with positron emission tomography. J Nucl Cardiol 1:425, 1994
74. Green MA, Welch MJ, Mathias CJ et al: Gallium-68, 1,1,1,-tris -(5-methoxysalicylaldiminomethyl) ethane: a potential tracer for evaluation of regional myocardial blood flow. J Nucl Med 26:170, 1985
75. Kung HF, Liu BL, Mankoff D et al: A new myocardial imaging agent: synthesis, characterization, and biodistribution of gallium-68-BAT-TECH. J Nucl Med 31:1635, 1990
76. Green MA, Mathias CJ, Neumann WL et al: Potential gallium-68 tracers for imaging the heart with PET: evaluation of four gallium complexes with functionalized tripodal tris(salicyladimine) ligands. J Nucl Med 34:228, 1993
77. Green MA, Klippenstein DL, Tennison JR: Copper (II) bis (thiosemicarbazone) complexes as potential tracers for evaluation of cerebral and myocardial blood flow with PET. J Nucl Med 29:1549, 1988
78. Shelton ME, Green MA, Mathhias CJ, Welch MJ, Bergmann SR: Kinetics of copper-PTSM in isolated hearts: a novel tracer for measuring blood flow with positron emission tomography. J Nucl Med 30:1843, 1989
79. Shelton ME, Green MA, Mathias CJ, Welch MJ, Bergmann SR: Assessment of regional myocardial and renal blood flow using copper-PTSM and positron emission tomography. Circulation 82:990, 1990
80. Green MA, Mathias CJ, Welch MJ et al: Copper-62-labeled pyruvaldehyde bis (N^4-methylthiosemicarbazonato) copper (II): synthesis and evaluation as a positron emission tomography tracer for cerebral and myocardial perfusion. J Nucl Med 31:1989, 1990
81. Beanlands RSB, Muzik O, Mintun M et al: The kinetics of copper-62-PTSM in the normal human heart. J Nucl Med 33:684, 1992
82. Herrero P, Markham J, Weinheimer CJ et al: Quantification of regional myocardial perfusion with generator-produced ^{62}Cu-PTSM and positron emission tomography. Circulation 87:173, 1993
83. Heymann MA, Payne BD, Hoffman JIE, Rudolph AM: Blood flow measurements with radonuclide-labeled particles. Prog Cardiovasc Dis 20:55, 1977
84. Beller GA, Alton WJ, Cochavi S, Hnatowich D, Brownell GL: Assessment of regional myocardial perfusion by positron emission tomography after intracoronary administration of Ga-68 labeled albumin microspheres. J Comput Assist Tomogr 3:447, 1979
85. Wisenberg G, Schelbert HR, Hoffman EJ et al: In vivo quantitation of regional myocardial blood flow by positron-emission computed tomography. Circulation 63:1248, 1981
86. Wilson RA, Shea MJ, De Landsheere CM et al: Validation of quantitation of regional myocardial blood flow in vivo with ^{11}C-labeled human albumin microspheres and positron emission tomography. Circulation 70:717, 1984
87. Selwyn AP, Shea MJ, Foale R et al: Regional myocardial and organ blood flow after myocardial infarction: application of the microsphere principle in man. Circulation 73:433, 1986
88. Weinberg IN, Huang SC, Hoffman EJ et al: Validation of PET-acquired input functions for cardiac studies. J Nucl Med 29:241, 1988
89. Iida H, Rhodes CG, de Silva R et al: Use of the left ventricular time-activity curve as a noninvasive input function in dynamic oxygen-15 water positron emission tomography. J Nucl Med 33:1669, 1992
90. Herrero P, Hartman JJ, Senneff MJ, Bergman SR:

Effects of time discrepancies between input and myocardial time-activity curves on estimates of regional myocardial perfusion with PET. J Nucl Med 35:558, 1994

91. Huang SC, Phelps ME: Principles of tracer kinetic modeling in positron emission tomography and autoradiography. p. 287. In Phelps ME, Mazziotta JC, Schelbert HR (eds): Positron Emission Tomography and Autoradiography. Principles and Applications for the Brain and Heart. Raven Press, New York, 1986

92. Carson RE: The development and application of mathematical models in nuclear medicine (editorial). J Nucl Med 32:2206, 1991

93. Hutchins GD, Schwaiger M, Rosenspire KC et al: Noninvasive quantification of regional blood flow in the human heart using N-13 ammonia and dynamic positron emission tomographic imaging. J Am Coll Cardiol 15:1032, 1990

94. Kuhle WG, Porenta G, Huang SC et al: Quantification of regional myocardial blood flow using ^{13}N-ammonia and reoriented dynamic positron emission tomographic imaging. Circulation 86:1004, 1992

95. Bol A, Melin JA, Vanoverschelde JL et al: Direct comparison of [^{13}N]ammonia and [^{15}O]water estimates of perfusion with quantification of regional myocardial blood flow by microspheres. Circulation 87:512, 1993

96. Herrero P, Markham J, Shelton ME, Weinheimer CJ, Bergmann SR: Noninvasive quantification of regional myocardial perfusion with rubidium-82 and positron emission tomography. Exploration of a mathematical model. Circulation 82:1377, 1990

97. Herrero P, Markham J, Shelton ME, Bergmann SR: Implementation and evaluation of a two-compartment model for quantification of myocardial perfusion with rubidium-82 and positron emission tomography. Circ Res 70:496, 1992

98. Sawada S, Muzik O, Beanlands RSB et al: Interobserver and interstudy variability of myocardial blood flow and flow-reserve measurements with nitrogen 13 ammonia-labeled positron emission tomography. J Nucl Cardiol 2:413, 1995

99. Shelton ME, Senneff MJ, Ludbrook PA, Sobel BE, Bergmann SR: Concordance of nutritive myocardial perfusion reserve and flow velocity reserve in conductance vessels in patients with chest pain with angiographically normal coronary arteries. J Nucl Med 34:717, 1993

100. Merlet P, Mazoyer B, Hittinger L et al: Assessment of coronary reserve in man: comparison between positron emission tomography with oxygen-15-labeled water and intracoronary doppler technique. J Nucl Med 34:1899, 1993

101. Bing RJ: Cardiac metabolism. Physiol Rev 45:171, 1965

102. Neely JR, Morgan HE: Relationship between carbohydrate and lipid metabolism and the energy balance of the heart muscle. Annu Rev Physiol 36:413, 1974

103. Randle PJ, Tubbs PK. Carbohydrate and fatty acid metabolism. p. 805. In Berne R, Sperelakis N (eds): Handbook of Physiology: Circulation. Section 2, The Cardiovascular System. Vol I. American Physiological Society. Williams & Wilkins, Baltimore 1979

104. Liedtke AJ: Alterations of carbohydrate and lipid metabolism in the acutely ischemic heart. Prog Cardiovasc Dis 23:321, 1981

105. Drake-Holland AJ: Substrate utilization. p. 195. In Drake-Holland AJ, Noble MIM (eds): Cardiac Metabolism. John Wiley & Sons, Chicester, 1983

106. Feigl EO, Neat GW, Huang AH: Interrelations between coronary artery pressure, myocardial metabolism and coronary blood flow. J Mol Cell Cardiol 22:375, 1990

107. Buxton D: Myocardial metabolism. p. 39. In Marcus ML, Skorton DJ, Schelbert HR, Wolf GL (eds): Cardiac Imaging. A Companion to Braunwald's Heart Disease. WB Saunders, Orlando, 1991

108. Opie LH. Fuels: carbohydrates and lipids. p. 208. In The Heart. Physiology and Metabolism (2nd ed.) Raven Press, New York, 1991

109. Stone CK, Liedtke AJ: Myocardial metabolism pertinent to cardiac positron tomography. p. 45. In Bergmann SR, Sobel BE: Positron Emisson Tomography of the Heart. Futura Publishing, Mount Kisco, NY, 1992

110. Schön HR, Schelbert HR, Robinson G et al: C-11 labeled palmitic acid for the noninvasive evaluation of regional myocardial fatty acid metabolism with positron-computed tomography. I. Kinetics of C-11 palmitic acid in normal myocardium. Am Heart J 103:532, 1982

111. Pike VW, Eakins MN, Allan RM, Selwyn AP: Preparation of [1-^{11}C]acetate—an agent for the study of myocardial metabolism by positron emission tomography. Int J Appl Radiat Isot 33:505, 1982

112. Brown M, Marshall DR, Sobel BE, Bergmann SR: Delineation of myocardial oxygen utilization with carbon-11-labeled acetate. Circulation 76:687, 1987

113. Buxton DB, Schwaiger M, Nguyen A, Phelps ME, Schelbert HR: Radiolabeled acetate as a tracer of myocardial tricarboxylic acid cycle flux. Circ Res 63:628, 1988

114. Brown MA, Myears DW, Bergmann SR: Noninvasive assessment of canine myocardial oxidative metabolism with carbon-11 labeled acetate and positron

emission tomography. J Am Coll Cardiol 12:1054, 1988

115. Brown MA, Myears DW, Bergmann SR: Validity of estimates of myocardial oxidative metabolism with carbon-11 acetate and positron emission tomography despite altered patterns of substrate utilization. J Nucl Med 30:187, 1989

116. Armbrecht JJ, Buxton DB, Schelbert HR: Validation of [1-^{11}C] acetate as a tracer for noninvasive assessment of oxidative metabolism with positron emission tomography in normal, ischemic and postischemic and hyperemic canine myocardium. Circulation 81:1594, 1990

117. Armbrecht JJ, Buxton DB, Brunken RC, Phelps ME, Schelbert HR: Regional myocardial oxygen consumption determined noninvasively in humans with [1-^{11}C] acetate and dynamic positron tomography. Circulation 80:863, 1989

118. Buck A, Wolpers HG, Hutchins GD et al: Effect of carbon-11-acetate recirculation on estimates of myocardial oxygen consumption by PET. J Nucl Med 32:1950, 1991

119. Gallagher BM, Fowler JS, Gutterson NI et al: Metabolic trapping as a principle of radiopharmaceutical design: some factors responsible for the biodistribution of [^{18}F] 2-deoxy-2-fluoro-D-glucose. J Nucl Med 19:1154, 1978

120. Sobel BE, Weiss ES, Welch MJ, Siegel BA, Ter-Pogossiam MM: Detection of remote myocardial infarction in patients with positron emission transaxial tomography and intravenous ^{11}C-palmitate. Circulation 55:853, 1977

121. Geltman EM, Biello D, Welch MJ et al: Characterization of nontransmural myocardial infarction by positron-emission tomography. Circulation 65:747, 1982

122. Billadello JJ, Smith JL, Ludbrook PA et al: Implications of "reciprocal" ST segment depression associated with acute myocardial infarction identified by positron tomography. J Am Coll Cardiol 2:616, 1983

123. Rose CP, Goresky CA: Constraints on the uptake of labeled palmitate by the heart. The barriers at the capillary and sarcolemmal surfaces and the control of intracellular sequestration. Circ Res 41:534, 1977

124. De Jong JW, Hulsmann WC: A comparative study of palmitoyl-CoA synthetase activity in rat-liver, heart and gut mitochondrial and microsomal preparations. Biochim Biophys Acta 197:127, 1970

125. Schön HR, Schelbert HR, Robinson G et al: C-11 labeled palmitic acid for the noninvasive evaluation of regional myocardial fatty acid metabolism with positron-computed tomography. I. Kinetics of C-11 palmitic acid in normal myocardium. Am Heart J 103:532, 1982

126. Vasdev SC, Kako KJ: Incorporation of fatty acids into rat heart lipids. In vivo and in vitro study. J Mol Cell Cardiol 9:617, 1977

127. Goldstein RA, Klein MS, Welch MJ, Sobel BE: External assessment of myocardial metabolism with C-11 palmitate in vivo. J Nucl Med 21:342, 1980

128. Klein MS, Goldstein RA, Welch MJ, Sobel BE: External assessment of myocardial metabolism with [^{11}C]palmitate in rabbit hearts. Am J Physiol 237 (Heart Circ Physiol 6):H51, 1979

129. Lerch RA, Ambos HD, Bergmann SR, Sobel BE, Ter-Pogossian MM: Kinetics of positron emitters in vivo characterized with a beta probe. Am J Physiol 242:H62, 1982

130. Weiss ES, Hoffman EJ, Phelps ME et al: External detection and visualization of myocardial ischemia with ^{11}C-substrates in vitro and in vivo. Circ Res 39:24, 1976

131. Schelbert HR, Henze E, Schon HR et al: C-11 palmitate for the noninvasive evaluation of regional myocardial fatty acid metabolism with positron computed tomography. III. In vivo demonstration of the effects of substrate availability on myocardial metabolism. Am Heart J 105:492, 1983

132. Schelbert HR, Henze E, Sochor H: Effects of substrate availability on myocardial C-11 palmitate kinetics by positron emission tomography in normal subjects and patients with left ventricular dysfunction. Am Heart J 111:1055, 1986

133. Vanoeverschelde JLJ, Wijns W, Kolanowski J et al: Competition between palmitate and ketone bodies as fuels for the heart: study with positron emission tomography. Am J Physiol 264 (Heart Circ Physiol 33):H701, 1993

134. Opie LH, Owen P, Riemersma RA: Relative rates of oxidation of glucose and free fatty acids by ischaemic and nonischaemic myocardium after coronary artery ligation in the dog. Eur J Clin Invest 3:419, 1973

135. Opie LH: Effects of regional ischemia on metabolism of glucose and fatty acids. Circ Res, Suppl. I, 38:I-52, 1976

136. Schon HR, Schelbert HR, Najafi A et al: C-11 labeled palmitic acid for the noninvasive evaluation of regional myocardial fatty acid metabolism with positron-computed tomography. II. Kinetics of C-11 palmitic acid in acutely ischemic myocardium. Am Heart J 103:548, 1982

137. Lerch RA, Bergmann SR, Ambos HD et al: Effect of flow-independent reduction of metabolism on re-

gional myocardial clearance of ^{11}C-palmitate. Circulation 65:731, 1982
138. Goldstein RA, Klein MS, Sobel BE: Distribution of exogenous labeled palmitate in ischemic myocardium: implications for positron emission tomography. p. 71. In Vogel JHK (ed): Advances in Cardiology. Vol. 27. S. Karger, Basel, 1980
139. Scheuer J, Brachfeld N: Myocardial uptake and fractional distribution of palmitate-1-C^{14} by the ischemic dog heart. Metabolism 15:945, 1966
140. Schwaiger M, Fishbein MC, Block M et al: Metabolic and ultrastructural abnormalities during ischemia in canine myocardium: noninvasive assessment by positron emission tomography. J Mol Cell Cardiol 19:259, 1987
141. Van der Vusse GJ, Roemen THM, Prinzen FW, Coumans WA, Reneman RS: Uptake and tissue content of fatty acids in dog myocardium under normoxic and ischemic conditions. Cir Res 50:538, 1982
142. Fox KAA, Abendschein, Ambos HD, Sobel BE, Bergmann SR: Efflux of metabolized and nonmetabolized fatty acid from canine myocardium. Implications for quantifying myocardial metabolism tomographically. Circ Res 57:232, 1985
143. Rosamond TL, Abendschein DR, Sobel BE, Bergmann SR, Fox KAA: Metabolic fate of radiolabeled palmitate in ischemic canine myocardium: implications for positron emission tomography. J Nucl Med 28:1332, 1987
144. Katz AM: p. 122. In: Physiology of the Heart. 2nd Ed. Raven Press, New York, 1992
145. Bergmann SR, Sobel BE: Quantification of regional myocardial oxidative utilization with positron emission tomography. p. 209. In Bergmann SR, Sobel BE: Positron Emission Tomography of the Heart. Futura Publishing, Mount Kisco, NY, 1992
146. Armbrecht JJ, Buxton DB, Schelbert HR: Validation of [1-^{11}C] acetate as a tracer for noninvasive assessment of oxidative metabolism with positron emission tomography in normal, ischemic, postischemic, and hyperemic canine myocardium. Circulation 81:1594, 1990
147. Buxton DB, Nienaber CA, Luxen A et al: Noninvasive quantification of regional myocardial oxygen consumption in vivo with [1-^{11}C] acetate and dynamic positron emission tomography. Circulation 79:134, 1989
148. Walsh MN, Geltman EM, Brown MA et al: Noninvasive estimation of regional myocardial oxygen consumption by positron emission tomography with carbon-11 acetate in patients with myocardial infarction. J Nucl Med 30:1798, 1989
149. Gropler RJ, Siegel BA, Geltman EM: Myocardial uptake of carbon-11 acetate as an indirect estimate of regional myocardial blood flow. J Nucl Med 32:245, 1991
150. Chan SY, Brunken RC, Phelps ME, Schelbert HR: Use of the metabolic tracer carbon-11-acetate for evaluation of regional myocardial perfusion. J Nucl Med 32:665, 1991
151. Krivokapich J, Huang SC, Schelbert HR: Assessment of the effects of dobutamine on myocardial blood flow and oxidative metabolism in normal human subjects using nitrogen-13 ammonia and carbon-11 acetate. Am J Cardiol 71:1351, 1993
152. Ng CK, Huang SC, Schelbert HR, Buxton DB: Validation of a model for [1-^{11}C] acetate as a tracer of cardiac oxidative metabolism. Am J Physiol 266(Heart Circ Physiol 35):H1304, 1994
153. Brown MA, Myears DW, Bergmann SR: Validity of estimates of myocardial oxidative metabolism with carbon-11 acetate and positron emission tomography despite altered patterns of substrate utilization. J Nucl Med 30:187, 1989
154. Armbrecht JJ, Buxton DB, Brunken RC, Phelps ME, Schelbert HR: Regional myocardial oxygen consumption determined noninvasively in humans with [1-^{11}C] acetate and dynamic positron tomography. Circulation 80:863, 1989
155. Brown MA, Myears DW, Bergmann SR: Noninvasive assessment of canine myocardial oxidative metabolism with carbon-11 labeled acetate and positron emission tomography. J Am Coll Cardiol 12:1054, 1988
156. Hicks RJ, Kalff V, Savas V, Starling MR, Schwaiger M: Assessment of right ventricular oxidative metabolism by positron emission tomography with C-11 acetate in aortic valve disease. Am J Cardiol 67:753, 1991
157. Henes CG, Bergmann SR, Walsh MN, Sobel BE, Geltman EM: Assessment of myocardial oxidative metabolic reserve with positron emission tomography and carbon-11 acetate. J Nucl Med 1489, 1989
158. Hicks RJ, Savas V, Currie PJ et al: Assessment of myocardial oxidative metabolism in aortic valve disease using positron emission tomography with C-11 acetate. Am Heart J 123:653, 1992
159. Buck A, Wolpers HG, Hutchins GD et al: Effect of carbon-11-acetate recirculation on estimates of myocardial oxygen consumption by PET. J Nucl Med 32:1950, 1991
160. Berry JJ, Baker JA, Pieper KS et al: The effect of metabolic milieu on cardiac PET imaging using fluorine-18-deoxyglucose and nitrogen-13 ammonia in normal volunteers. J Nucl Med 32:1518, 1991

161. Choi Y, Brunken RC, Hawkins RA et al: Factors affecting myocardial 2-[F-18]fluoro-2-deoxy-D-glucose uptake in positron emission tomography studies of normal humans. J Nucl Med 20:308, 1993
162. vom Dahl J, Herman WH, Hicks RJ et al: Myocardial glucose uptake in patients with insulin-dependent diabetes assessed quantitatively by dynamic positron emission tomography. Circulation 88:395, 1993
163. Ohtake T, Yokoyama I, Watanabe T et al: Myocardial glucose metabolism in noninsulin-dependent diabetes mellitus patients evaluated by FDG-PET. J Nucl Med 36:456, 1995
164. Knuuti MJ, Yki-Jarvinen H, Voipio-Pulkki LM et al: Enhancement of myocardial [fluorine-18] fluorodeoxyglucose uptake by a nicotinic acid derivative. J Nucl Med 35:989, 1994
165. Knuuti MJ, Nuutila P, Ruotsalainen U: Euglycemic hyperinsulinemic clamp and oral glucose load in stimulating myocardial glucose utilization during positron emission tomography. J Nucl Med 33:1255, 1992
166. Sokoloff L, Reivich M, Kennedy C et al: The [^{14}C]deoxyglucose method for the measurement of local cerebral glucose utilization: theory, procedure, and normal values in the conscious and anesthetized rat. J Neurochem 28:897, 1977
167. Krivokapich J, Huang SC, Phelps ME et al: Estimation of rabbit myocardial metabolic rate for glucose using fluorodeoxyglucose. Am J Physiol 243 (Heart Circ Physiol 12):H884, 1982
168. Ratib O, Phelps ME, Huang SC et al: Positron tomography with deoxyglucose for estimating local myocardial glucose metabolism. J Nucl Med 23:577, 1982
169. Patlak CS, Blasberg RG, Fenstermacher JD: Graphical evaluation of blood-to-brain transfer constants from multiple-time uptake data. J Cereb Blood Flow Metab 3:1, 1983
170. Patlak CS, Blasberg RG: Graphical evaluation of blood-to-brain transfer constants from multiple-time uptake data. Generalizations. J Cereb Blood Flow Metab 5:584, 1985
171. Gambhir SS, Schwaiger M, Huang SC et al: Simple noninvasive quantification method for measuring myocardial glucose utilization in humans employing positron emission tomography. J Nucl Med 30:359, 1989
172. Brachfeld N, Scheuer J: Metabolism of glucose by the ischemic dog heart. Am J Physiol 212:603, 1967
173. Marshall RC, Nash WW, Shine KI, Phelps ME, Ricchiuti N: Glucose metabolism during ischemia due to excessive oxygen demand or altered coronary flow in the isolated arterially perfused rabbit septum. Circ Res 49:640, 1981
174. Neely JR, Whitmer JT, Rovetto MJ: Effect of coronary blood flow on glycolytic flux and intracellular pH in isolated rat hearts. Circ Res 37:733, 1975
175. Vary TC, Reibel DK, Neely JR: Control of energy metabolism of heart muscle. Ann Rev Physiol 43:419, 1981
176. Most AS, Gorlin R, Soeldner JS: Glucose extraction by the human myocardium during pacing stress. Circulation 45:92, 1972
177. Thomassen A, Nielsen TT, Bagger JP, Henningsen P: Antianginal and cardiac metabolic effects of low-dose glucose infusion during pacing in patients with and without coronary artery disease. Am Heart J 118:25, 1989
178. Rahimtoola SH: A perspective on the three large multicenter randomized clinical trials of coronary bypass surgery for chronic stable angina. Circulation 72:V-123, 1985
179. Braunwald E, Rutherford JD: Reversible ischemic left ventricular dysfunction: evidence for the "hibernating myocardium" (editorial). J Am Coll Cardiol 8:1467, 1986
180. Rahimtoola SH: The hibernating myocardium. Am Heart J 117:211, 1989
181. Kloner RA, Przyklenk K, Patel B: Altered myocardial states: The stunned and hibernating myocardium. Am J Med, Suppl. 1A, 86:14, 1989
182. Ragosta M, Beller GA, Watson DD, Kaul S, Gimple LW: Quantitative planar rest-redistribution ^{201}Tl imaging in detection of myocardial viability and prediction of improvement in left ventricular function after coronary artery bypass surgery in patients with severely depressed left ventricular function. Circulation 87:1630, 1993
183. Mori T, Minamiji M, Kurogane H, Ogawa K, Yoshida Y: Rest-injected thallium-201 imaging for assessing viability of severe asynergic regions. J Nucl Med 32:1718, 1991
184. Zimmermann R, Mall G, Rauch B et al: Residual ^{201}Tl activity in irreversible defects as a marker of myocardial viability. Clinicopathological study. Circulation 91:1016, 1995
185. Go RT, MacIntyre WJ, Saha GB et al: Hibernating myocardium versus scar: severity of irreversible decreased myocardial perfusion in prediction of tissue viability. Radiology 194:151, 1995
186. Tamaki N, Kawamoto M, Tadamura E et al: Prediction of reversible ischemia after revascularization. Perfusion and metabolic studies with positron emission tomography. Circulation 91:1697, 1995
187. Duvernoy CS, vom Dahl J, Laubenbacher C, Schwaiger M: The role of nitrogen-13 ammonia posi-

188. Gewirtz H, Fischman AJ, Abraham S et al: Positron emission tomographic measurements of absolute regional myocardial blood flow permits identification of nonviable myocardium in patients with chronic myocardial infarction. J Am Coll Cardiol 23:851, 1994
189. Marzullo P, Parodi O, Sambuceti G et al: Residual coronary reserve identifies segmental viability in patients with wall motion abnormalities. J Am Coll Cardiol 26:342, 1995
190. Parodi O, De Maria R, Oltrona L et al: Myocardial blood flow distribution in patients with ischemic heart disease or dilated cardiomyopathy undergoing heart transplantation. Circulation 88:509, 1993
191. Yamamoto Y, de Silva R, Rhodes CG et al: A new strategy for the assessment of viable myocardium and regional myocardial blood flow using ^{15}O-water and dynamic positron emission tomography. Circulation 86:167, 1992
192. Iida H, Kanno I, Takahashi A et al: Measurement of absolute myocardial blood flow with $H_2^{15}O$ and dynamic positron emission tomography: strategy for quantification in relation to the partial volume effect. Circulation 78:104, 1988
193. de Silva R, Yamamoto Y, Rhodes CG et al: Preoperative prediction of the outcome of coronary revascularization using positron emission tomography. Circulation 86:1738, 1992
194. Goldstein RA: Rubidium-82 kinetics after coronary occlusion: temporal relation of net myocardial accumulation and viability in open-chested dogs. J Nucl Med 27:1456, 1986
195. Herrero P, Markham J, Shelton ME, Bergmann SR: Implementation and evaluation of a two-compartment model for quantification of myocardial perfusion with rubidium-82 and positron emission tomography. Circ Res 70:496, 1992
196. Gould KL, Yoshida K, Hess MJ et al: Myocardial metabolism of fluorodeoxyglucose compared to cell membrane integrity for the potassium analogue rubidium-82 for assessing infarct size in man by P.E.T. J Nucl Med 32:1, 1991
197. vom Dahl J, Muzik O, Wolfe ER et al: Myocardial rubidium-82 tissue kinetics assessed by dynamic positron emission tomography as a marker of cell membrane integrity and viability. Circulation 93:238, 1996
198. Bergmann SR, Lerch RA, Fox KAA et al: Temporal dependence of beneficial effects of coronary thrombolysis characterized by positron tomography. Am J Med 73:573, 1982
199. Schwaiger M, Schelbert HR, Keen R et al: Retention and clearance of C-11 palmitic acid in ischemic and reperfused canine myocardium. J Am Coll Cardiol 6:311, 1985
200. Knabb RM, Bergmann SR, Fox KA, Sobel BE: The temporal pattern of recovery of myocardial perfusion and metabolism delineated by positron emission tomography after coronary thrombolysis. J Nucl Med 28:1563, 1987
201. Schwaiger M, Schelbert HR, Ellison D et al: Sustained regional abnormalities in cardiac metabolism after transient ischemia in the chronic dog model. J Am Coll Cardiol 6:336, 1985
202. Marshall RC, Tillisch JH, Phelps ME et al: Identification and differentiation of resting myocardial ischemia and infarction in man with positron computed tomography, ^{18}F-labeled fluorodeoxyglucose and N-13 ammonia. Circulation 67:766, 1983
203. Tillisch J, Brunken R, Marshall R et al: Reversibility of cardiac wall motion abnormalities predicted by positron tomography. N Engl J Med 314:884, 1986
204. Tamaki N, Yonekura Y, Yamashita K et al: Positron emission tomography using fluorine-18 deoxyglucose in evaluation of coronary artery bypass grafting. Am J Cardiol 64:860, 1989
205. Tamaki N, Ohtani H, Yamashita K et al: Metabolic activity in the areas of new fill-in after thallium-201 reinjection: comparison with positron emission tomography using fluorine-18 deoxyglucose. J Nucl Med 32:673, 1991
206. Marwick TH, MacIntyre WJ, Lafont A, Nemec JJ, Salcedo EE: Metabolic responses of hibernating and infarcted myocardium to revascularization. A follow-up study of regional perfusion, function and metabolism. Circulation 85:1347, 1992
207. Lucignani G, Paolini G, Landoni C et al: Presurgical identification of hibernating myocardium by combined use of technetium-99m hexakis 2-methoxyisobutylisonitrile single photon emission tomography and fluorine-18 fluoro-2-deoxy-D-glucose positron emission tomography in patients with coronary artery disease. Eur J Nucl Med 19:874, 1992
208. Carrel T, Jenni R, Haubold-Reuter S et al: Improvement of severely reduced left ventricular function after surgical revascularization in patients with preoperative myocardial infarction. Eur J Cardiothorac Surg 6:479, 1992
209. Gropler RJ, Geltman EM, Sampathkumaran K et al: Functional recovery after coronary revascularization for chronic coronary artery disease is dependent on

maintenance of oxidative metabolism. J Am Coll Cardiol 20:569, 1992
210. Gropler RJ, Geltman EM, Sampathkumaran K et al: Comparison of carbon-11-acetate with fluorine-18-fluorodeoxyglucose for delineating viable myocardium by positron emission tomography. J Am Coll Cardiol 22:1587, 1993
211. Knuuti MJ, Saraste M, Nuutila P et al: Myocardial viability: fluorine-18-deoxyglucose positron emission tomography in prediction of wall motion recovery after revascularization. Am Heart J 127:785, 1994
212. vom Dahl J, Eitzman DT, Al-Aouar ZR et al: Relation of regional function, perfusion, and metabolism in patients with advanced coronary artery disease undergoing surgical revascularization. Circulation 90:2356, 1994
213. Grandin C, Wijns W, Melin JA et al: Delineation of myocardial viability with PET. J Nucl Med 36:1543, 1995
214. Berry JJ, Hoffman JM, Steenbergen C et al: Human pathologic correlation with PET in ischemic and non-ischemic cardiomyopathy. J Nucl Med 34:39, 1993
215. Delbeke D, Lorenz CH, Votaw JR et al: Estimation of left ventricular mass and infarct size from N-13-ammonia PET images based on pathological examination of explanted human hearts. J Nucl Med 34:826, 1993
216. Vanoverschelde JLJ, Wijns W, Depre C et al: Mechanisms of chronic regional postischemic dysfunction in humans. New insights from the study of noninfarcted collateral-dependent myocardium. Circulation 87:1513, 1993
217. Maes A, Flameng W, Nuyts J et al: Histologic alterations in chronically hypoperfused myocardium. Correlation with PET findings. Circulation 90:735, 1994
218. Depre C, Vanoverschelde JLJ, Melin J et al: Structural and metabolic correlates of the reversibility of chronic left ventricular ischemic dysfunction in humans. Am J Physiol 268(Heart Circ. Physiol 37):H1265, 1995

Chapter 22

Choice of Technique for the Assessment of Myocardial Viability

Jacques A. Melin, Bernhard Gerber, William Wijns, and Jean-Louis J. Vanoverschelde

CLINICAL ROLE OF ASSESSMENT OF MYOCARDIAL VIABILITY

Myocardial viability represents an impairment in contractile function that is potentially reversible if blood flow is adequately restored. Such impairment might result from different causes, such as acute myocardial ischemia, myocardial hibernation,[1-3] acute myocardial stunning,[4,5] or repetitive stunning.[6,7] The distinction between these latter pathophysiologic entities is probably not relevant for clinical decision making not only because these conditions often coexist but also because ultimately the proposed treatment will be complete revascularization.

The accurate diagnosis of viable but noncontracting myocardium in patients with ischemic heart disease and previous myocardial infarction permits treatment decisions to be made concerning heart failure symptoms and angina, as well as decisions regarding revascularization for prognosis. The latter is based on the rationale that while the severity of left ventricular dysfunction is a major determinant of prognosis, left ventricular dysfunction is not necessarily irreversible and may improve after myocardial revascularization procedures. Patients with severe left ventricular dysfunction are those who may benefit most from bypass surgery because they are the most vulnerable to further losses of contractile myocardium,[8] but they are also the most vulnerable to a higher operative mortality rate. The last few chapters have measured the benefit of revascularization in terms of improvement of regional function, but we should remember that this is also influenced by the adequacy of revascularization (including considerations relating to graft occlusion and restenosis) and the presence of coexisting myocardial disease (e.g., left ventricular hypertrophy, myopathic processes). Moreover, as physicians, we treat patients rather than segments of myocardium, and a new generation of studies are needed to consider global left ventricular function, exercise capacity, quality of life, and mortality as patient endpoints. Other considerations that will continue to remain important to defining a logical sequence of diagnostic tests will include their ease of application, local availability, and expertise of testers.

Several radionuclide approaches afford the noninvasive identification of viable myocardium.[9-11] The scintigraphic techniques follow three general strategies: estimates of myocardial perfusion, probes of the integrity of myocardial cell membranes, and the use of metabolic markers to study myocardial substrate retention as an indicator for maintained metabolism. The pathophysiologic basis of these measurements has been well documented in Chapters 20, 21, and 23. The aim of this chapter is to examine the relative merits and limitations of the radionuclide approaches for the assessment of myocardial viability and to examine whether a rational test ordering sequence could be followed in the context of chronic left ventricular dysfunction.

PERFUSION AND MEMBRANE INTEGRITY TRACERS

As discussed in Chapters 20 and 21, single photon emission computed tomography (SPECT) and positron emission tomography (PET) tracers for assessing perfusion and membrane integrity include thallium 201 (^{210}Tl), technetium 99m (^{99m}Tc) sestamibi (sestamibi), nitrogen 13 (^{13}N) ammonia, and oxygen 15 (^{15}O) water.

Thallium-201 Imaging

Experimental Basis

The uptake and redistribution kinetics of ^{201}Tl kinetics have been discussed in Chapter 20. Early myocardial uptake is proportional to regional blood flow and extraction fraction,[12–15] which is unaltered in experimental conditions, such as hypoxia[16] and stunning.[17] Interestingly, the initial trapping of ^{201}Tl by the myocardium appears to be proportional to flow without an independent influence of the viable or necrotic status of the myocardium.[18–21] Early after reperfusion, ^{201}Tl activity in necrotic samples does not significantly differ from that in the viable samples for a similar amount of myocardial blood flow.[22,23] The indirect estimate of flow by the initial trapping has already some potential relevance for viability assessment because a minimal level of myocardial blood flow is required to maintain cell membrane integrity and hence viability.[24–26]

Following the first-pass myocardial uptake phase after intravenous tracer injection, there is a constant exchange of ^{201}Tl between the myocardium and the extracellular compartments, with a clearance from normal myocardium and replacement by residual ^{201}Tl blood pool activity. This continuous exchange forms the basis of ^{201}Tl redistribution.[27] Redistribution or delayed defect resolution is observed when ^{201}Tl is injected during transient myocardial hypoperfusion[28] or with a chronic reduction in myocardial blood flow, which is referred to as rest redistribution.[29] The mechanism for rest redistribution during chronic ischemia is both a diminution in the initial ^{201}Tl uptake and a subsequent decrease in the tracer's intrinsic efflux rate.[28] ^{201}Tl washout over time from the stenotic region is substantially slower than the ^{201}Tl washout from nonischemic regions. When ^{201}Tl is given during coronary occlusion, ^{201}Tl gradients between normal and ischemic zones after reperfusion are significantly lower than the gradients measured during coronary occlusion and, thus, delayed redistribution of ^{201}Tl injected before reperfusion is an indication of viable myocardium.[29–31] If myocardial necrosis is present, no delayed ^{201}Tl redistribution is observed in the zone of irreversibly injured myocardial tissue.[20]

Rest-Redistribution Protocol

When the clinical question pertains only to the presence or absence of myocardial viability and not to the detection of inducible ischemia, rest-redistribution ^{201}Tl imaging (early and 4-hour delayed resting images) may be the procedure of choice. Patients suitable for such studies usually have severe left ventricular dysfunction and extensive resting perfusion defects—but in many circumstances, ischemia is an important consideration.

^{201}Tl defects may occur on resting images in patients with severe coronary artery disease (CAD). Gewirtz et al.[32] showed that a substantial number of defects that redistribute have normal or hypokinetic wall motion. Early studies by Berger et al.[33] and Iskandrian et al.[34] reported that patients showing initial resting defects with delayed rest redistribution preoperatively demonstrated an increase in regional and global function postoperatively. A number of recent studies[35–41] have reported on the accuracy of ^{201}Tl rest-redistribution imaging for prediction of the reversibility of wall motion abnormality following revascularization. Table 22-1 illustrates that the results of these studies have shown some heterogeneity, with generally high sensitivity but some reports of poor specificity. False positives are more likely when relative levels of ^{201}Tl uptake are used as criteria of viability; in these circumstances, areas of non-Q-wave infarction (admixed scar plus normal tissue)

Table 22-1. Sensitivity and Specificity of Resting Redistribution ^{201}Tl Imaging for Prediction of Reversible Segmental Dysfunction After Revascularization

Study	No. of Patients	Sensitivity (%) (No. of Segments)	Specificity (%) (No. of Segments)
Mori et al. (1991)[35]	17	44 (11/25)	88 (23/26)
Ragosta et al. (1993)[36]	21	93 (81/89)	31 (27/87)
Marzullo et al. (1993)[38]	14	86 (42/49)	92 (24/26)
Alfieri et al. (1993)[37]	13	93 (82/88)	44 (14/32)
Udelson et al. (1994)[40]	18	88 (15/17)	83 (24/29)
Marzullo et al. (1995)[39]	22	91 (50/55)	73 (36/50)
Total	105	87 (281/323)	59 (148/250)

may not be discriminated from "viable" myocardium, although the former is less likely to recover than the latter. If redistribution criteria are used, it is noteworthy that some of the regions without redistribution but with improved function after revascularization are characterized by a higher early ^{201}Tl uptake.

Only one study has compared quantitative rest-redistribution ^{201}Tl data with PET patterns of viability.[42] In this series, only 2% of the normal and 5% of the mismatch myocardial regions by PET had severe irreversible ^{201}Tl defects. However, 10 of the 59 myocardial regions (17%) with severely reduced F-18 2-fluorodeohyglucose (FDG) uptake by PET did *not* have severe (<50% of peak activity) irreversible ^{201}Tl defects. Thus, rest-redistribution approaches are sensitive but not necessarily specific. The three studies that used quantitative analysis and redistribution criteria for viability assessment had the best sensitivity and specificity figures.[38–40]

Stress-Redistribution-Reinjection Imaging

Clinical assessment and therapeutic management in many coronary patients with left ventricular dysfunction require evaluation of both inducible ischemia and viability. After stress and redistribution imaging are used as a first choice test for a comprehensive assessment of the extent and severity of myocardial ischemia, uptake of ^{201}Tl at redistribution or after reinjection of a small dose of ^{201}Tl would then indicate viable myocardium by analogy with the ^{201}Tl rest-redistribution protocol.

After exercise, an initial defect showing complete or partial delayed redistribution implies ischemia and viability. Defects that remain persistent from the initial to the delayed images indicate scar, although persistent ^{201}Tl defects may represent viable myocardium rather than scar if the redistribution ^{201}Tl defects are mild (i.e., ^{201}Tl uptake >50% of normal zone).[43] This phenomenon can be assessed by looking at the amount of ^{201}Tl activity on delayed ^{201}Tl imaging;[44,45] greater amounts of ^{201}Tl present in these images (rather than the presence or absence of redistribution) indicate larger amounts of viable myocardium. Severe persistent defects demonstrating less than 50% of normal ^{201}Tl counts may be further assessed for potential viability by late redistribution imaging at 18 to 24 hours,[46–48] although even late imaging may overestimate scar because one third of the segments irreversible at 18 to 72 hours show contractile recovery after revascularization.[47] The underestimation of viability on 24-hour ^{201}Tl imaging was also confirmed by the demonstration that the majority of myocardial regions with fixed ^{201}Tl defects on late images has preserved metabolic activity.[49] An additional limitation of the 24-hour imaging to detect late redistribution is the suboptimal count statistics.

An alternative to 24-hour delayed redistribution imaging, which circumvents these limitations, is to reinject ^{201}Tl at rest following acquisition of the 4-hour redistribution images[50] and re-image; late imaging after the reinjected dose is not necessary.[51] The predictive accuracy of stress-redistribution-reinjection ^{201}Tl imaging is summarized in Table 22-2.[49–55] Four-hour delayed redistribution imaging should not be omitted because some of the defects that demonstrate redistribution at 4 hours will revert to persistent defects after reinjection.[56] Attempts to avoid acquiring three sets of images have met with limited success; reinjection of ^{201}Tl immediately after the stress images with acquisition of a modified redistribution image 3 hours later (i.e., redistribution of both the stress and the reinjected ^{201}Tl doses) was associated with significantly fewer defects than those obtained using a standard 3-hour reinjection

Table 22-2. Sensitivity and Specificity of Stress-Redistribution-Reinjection ^{201}Tl Imaging for Prediction of Reversible Segmental Dysfunction After Revascularization

Study	No. of Patients	Sensitivity (%) (No. of Segments)	Specificity (%) (No. of Segments)
Dilsizian et al. (1992)[50]	20	100 (13/13)	80 (8/10)
Ohtani et al. (1990)[52]	24	89 (33/37)	50 (12/24)
Vanoverschelde et al. (1995)[55]	73	77 (129/167)	56 (155/277)
Haque et al. (1995)[53]	26	91 (30/33)	50 (5/10)
Arnese et al. (1995)[54]	22	89 (34/38)	48 (63/132)
Total	165	83 (239/288)	54 (243/453)

protocol.[57,58] Recent studies[53–55] have reported the postreinjection uptake of greater than 50% after stress as a sensitive, but not very specific, predictor of viability (defined by functional improvement after revascularization). Potential causes of "false positive" scans include detection of territories of jeopardized vital myocardial cells of inadequate size to influence left ventricular dysfunction despite successful revascularization; the presence of a subendocardial scar coexisting with the presence of viable myocardium in the subepicardial layers; and tethering by adjacent akinetic segments.

While the specificity of the ^{201}Tl reinjection method has been a source of some concern, comparison of this technique with PET (using the presence of metabolic activity as evidence for viability) has shown a high correlation between the tests.[59,60] The importance of quantifying residual ^{201}Tl activity after reinjection has been emphasized by a recent study showing that the level of regional ^{201}Tl activity after reinjection was significantly related to the mass of preserved viable myocytes.[61] This relation obtained on continuous values is important to note because the level of fibrosis is directly related to the absence of improvement of function after revascularization.[62]

In summary, the sequence of poststress, 4-hour redistribution and reinjection imaging is the most clinically appropriate protocol for the evaluation of inducible ischemia and detection of viability. The data relevant for predicting recovery of regional dysfunction can be provided by the quantitative analysis of ^{201}Tl content in the redistribution image as a first step[44,45] and in the reinjection image as a second step.[49]

Sestamibi Imaging

Experimental Basis

The use of sestamibi for the assessment of myocardial viability has been discussed in some detail in Chapter 20. In brief, this compound is retained only in viable myocytes,[63] and metabolic alterations consequent to ischemia or hypoxia (but not stunning) result in impaired sestamibi uptake independent of flow.[17,63,64] Sestamibi cannot be retained in myocardial regions that have been irreversibly injured by prolonged coronary occlusion followed by reperfusion.[65] The uptake of sestamibi and ^{201}Tl appear to be comparable in experimental settings of stenosis and infarction, although ^{201}Tl uptake exceeds sestamibi uptake during sustained low flow producing severe regional dysfunction.[66] Sestamibi redistribution has been observed under certain experimental conditions,[66–68] but the degree of redistribution is minimal.

Resting Studies

Early studies reported evidence of ^{201}Tl activity within sestamibi defects, either after resting ^{201}Tl injection with redistribution[69] or after reinjection after stress imaging.[70] Although these studies found that sestamibi underestimated regional viability compared with ^{201}Tl, we need to remember that specificity of ^{201}Tl uptake has not been shown to be optimal, and the differing resolution of ^{201}Tl and ^{99m}Tc could contribute to this discrepancy.[71] These data emphasize the need of independent standards of regional viability. The four studies[38–40,72] comparing resting sestamibi uptake with changes of regional wall motion after revascularization have shown the diagnostic accuracy of sestamibi to be comparable to that previously discussed with ^{201}Tl (Table 22-3). Clearly, larger studies of patients with left ventricular dysfunction directly comparing ^{201}Tl and sestamibi using quantitative techniques and independent gold standard are warranted.

Table 22-3. Sensitivity and Specificity of Resting Sestamibi Imaging for Prediction of Reversible Dysfunction after Revascularization

Study	No. of Patients	Sensitivity (%) (No. of Segments)	Specificity (%) (No. of Segments)
Marzullo et al. (1993)[38]	14	75 (37/49)	84 (22/26)
Udelson et al. (1994)[40]	18	94 (16/17)	86 (25/29)
Marzullo et al. (1995)[39]	22	73 (40/55)	55 (28/50)
Maublant et al. (1995)[72a]	27	100 (21/21)	67 (4/6)
Total	81	80 (114/142)	71 (79/111)

[a] patient analysis.

Exercise Studies

Similarly, exercise studies using sestamibi for prediction of viability have compared these results with either ^{201}Tl or PET, rather than independent parameters such as functional follow-up after revascularization.[70,73] These studies have been discussed at greater length in the Chapter 20; if only severe reduction in activity was considered as evidence for nonviability, then the overall concordance between ^{201}Tl and sestamibi studies was 93%.

Administration of nitrates before injection of sestamibi could enhance the detection of defect reversibility.[74] In this study, the changes in extent of perfusion defect induced by nitrate administration correlated well with the change in left ventricular ejection fraction after revascularization. However, the data are still too limited to draw firm conclusions.

Simultaneous Evaluation of Flow and Function

A unique feature of sestamibi imaging for viability evaluation is the capability to assess simultaneously regional perfusion and wall motion. Regional wall motion is assessed by gating either planar or SPECT perfusion images and viewing the end-systolic and end-diastolic images. Regions that show preserved sestamibi uptake despite abnormal systolic thickening would presumably be viable. New quantitation on gated images and regional normal values will have to be implemented before assessing the potential incremental value of this imaging modality for viability assessment.

PET Perfusion Tracers

The yield of PET perfusion tracers has to be examined separately because adequate myocardial perfusion is critical to tissue viability and because PET has intrinsic capabilities (i.e., spatial resolution, attenuation correction, and absolute quantification) instrumental in the accurate estimation transmural myocardial perfusion.

Resting Studies

As discussed in Chapter 21, a certain threshold of myocardial perfusion is required to maintain viability.[30,31] Using ^{13}N ammonia, relative perfusion at rest has been shown to correlate with regional glucose uptake[75] and predict recovery of regional function after revascularization.[76] Absolute measurements of myocardial perfusion have confirmed that myocardial viability is unlikely when basal regional myocardial blood flow is below a given threshold.[29,77,78]

Stress Perfusion Imaging

Using perfusion imaging with ^{13}N ammonia provides stress-induced flow defects that offer incremental predictive accuracy for viability beyond the resting data alone.[75] This may reflect the role of exercise-induced flow deficits as an integral part of the repetitive stunning phenomenon. Blood flow at rest may be well preserved or even normal in repetitively stunned myocardium, yet wall motion is reduced and flow reserve is blunted.[7] An increase in demand thus could produce ischemia followed by stunning. Revascularization eliminates the culprit and, consequently, wall motion would improve. Marzullo et al.[79] have also found a decreased maximal flow after dipyridamole in akinetic segments supposed to be viable by the persistence of metabolic activity.

PET METABOLIC TRACERS

Prediction of Recovery of Regional Function

Maintained or increased FDG has been shown to distinguish accurately reversible from irreversible injury.[9,10,22,27] The biochemical significance of FDG

Table 22-4. Sensitivity, Specificity of FDG/Flow PET Imaging for Prediction of Reversible Dysfunction After Revascularization

Study	Dietary Conditions	No. of Patients	Criteria for Positivity	Sensitivity (%) (No. of Segments)	Specificity (%) (No. of Segments)
Tillisch et al. (1986)[80]	Oral glucose load	17	Flow-metabolism mismatch	85 (35/41)	92 (24/26)
Tamaki et al. (1989)[81]	Fasted	22	Flow-metabolism mismatch	78 (18/23)	78 (18/23)
Marwick et al. (1992)[82]	After exercise	16	%FDG < 2SD	71 (25/35)	76 (38/50)
Carrel et al. (1992)[86]	Oral glucose load	23	Flow-metabolism mismatch	94 (16/17)	50 (3/3)
Gropler et al. (1993)[83]	Oral glucose load	34	%FDG < 2SD	83 (38/46)	50 (35/70)
Knuuti et al. (1994)[84]	Oral glucose load	48	%FDG < 2SD	100 (27/27)	63 (40/63)
Vom Dahl et al. (1994)[85]	Oral glucose load	37	Flow-metabolism mismatch	81 (50/62)	57 (82/143)
Tamaki et al. (1995)[76]	Fasted	61	%FDG < 2SD	88 (45/51)	82 (65/79)
Grandin et al. (1995)[77a]	IV glucose load	25	Flow-metabolism mismatch	89 (15/17)	50 (4/8)
Total		283		84 (269/319)	66 (309/465)

a Patient analysis.

uptake remains elusive; it may be observed during ongoing ischemia and postischemic stunning and in patients with chronic dysfunction or hibernating myocardium. While this engenders ambiguity regarding the mechanisms causing segmental dysfunction, all these conditions imply functional recovery after revascularization. However, FDG uptake may overestimate the amount of viable myocardium, because tracer uptake by inflammatory cells may lead necrotic myocardium to appear viable during the acute phase of reperfusing infarction, and because FDG uptake in chronic situations may occur in myocardium that shows profound structural alterations on pathologic examination.[7] The latter are characterized by significant loss of contractile material and may not return to normal function.

The sensitivity and specificity of FDG and flow PET imaging for prediction of reversible dysfunction following revascularization are summarized in Table 22-4.[75,77,80–87] Two major criteria have been evaluated: (1) flow-metabolism mismatch (the relative discordance between flow and metabolic activity profile), or (2) the FDG uptake expressed in absolute values or in normalized values relative to the remote myocardium. In the studies that compared separately the flow information to the FDG data,[75,77] the FDG information had always an incremental and independent value for the prediction of segmental recovery after revascularization. Additionally, some studies have employed a hybrid approach to derive a flow-metabolism comparison in which sestamibi SPECT imaging and PET-FDG were used respectively to evaluate flow and glucose utilization.[88] However, some caution needs to be applied to this approach; both modalities are influenced by the partial volume effect,[89] although this influence is different for the two modalities because different resolutions cause larger defect size and amplitude with SPECT than with PET.[90,91]

The kinetics of C-11 acetate have been shown to portend functional recovery, which clearly depends on the oxidative capacity of the myocardium.[83] In one study of 34 patients, predictive criteria of viability with C-11 acetate had better sensitivity (87%; 40/46) and specificity (71%; 50/70) than the criteria with FDG (sensitivity and specificity of 83 and 50%; see Table 22-4). This was shown for various criteria using an analysis by receiver-operating characteristic curves. Although very encouraging, these data need to be confirmed in larger series of patients with severe left ventricular dysfunction and with a comparison with FDG under other dietary conditions.

Prediction of Recovery of Global Function

As discussed at the beginning of the chapter, compared with the use of segmental improvement as an end-point, the important clinical question is whether revascularization will improve global left ventricular function and functional capacity and reduce mortality. The pioneering study by Tillisch et al.[80] suggested that if a substantial fraction of the left ventricular myocardium exhibited metabolic evidence of myocardial viability (flow-metabolism mismatch), the left ventricular ejection fraction was likely to improve after surgery (in their series, from 30 ± 11% to 45 ± 14%). Conversely, absence of metabolic evidence of viability or its presence in only a small portion of the left ventricular myocardium suggests that global left ventricular function will remain unchanged. Similar results have been reported by Depré et al.[59], vom Dahl et al.[85], and Maes et al.[87] Revascularization of patients with substantial amount of viable myocardium is followed by a marked improvement in symptoms related to congestive heart failure.[92,93] Finally, revascularization of patients with viable myocardium is associated with a lower incidence of ischemic events and improves survival. Four studies[92–95] in a total of 390 patients followed clinically for almost two years have addressed the long-term prognostic value of blood-flow–metabolism mismatches. Data from these studies point to greater cardiac-related mortality and morbidity rates in patients with blood-flow–metabolism mismatch when treated only medically.

SEQUENTIAL AND COMBINED APPROACHES

PET results and the ^{201}Tl or sestamibi approaches (Tables 21-1 to 22-4) must be compared cautiously because of differences in patient selection, study protocols, and viability criteria. Overall, the data suggest comparable predictive performances for SPECT and PET approaches, perhaps slightly favoring the sensitivity of PET. If FDG uptake expressed as a relative value from normal myocardium is effective for the prediction of functional recovery, this could support also the use of the FDG technique with SPECT.[96–99] Prospective studies are underway to test whether the predictive accuracy of this method will be influenced by the poorer resolution of the SPECT device.

Because clinical outcome in patients with left ventricular dysfunction and with signs of myocardial viability is better with revascularization than with conventional treatment,[92–95] tests for identification of potentially reversible dysfunction should be highly sensitive. As PET is more expensive and less available than SPECT, we recommend a sequential approach initially using SPECT, with PET as a secondary test in selected patients among whom ambiguity exists between the clinical situation and the presence or extent of viable myocardium. In a preliminary study,[100] 31 patients with low ejection fraction (33 ± 11%) had both ^{201}Tl SPECT stress-redistribution-reinjection and ^{13}N ammonia-FDG PET imaging. The predictive accuracy for recovery of function was tested for ^{201}Tl, PET, and a sequential testing strategy in which PET was performed only in patients with less than 50% ^{201}Tl uptake at reinjection. This latter strategy had a similar sensitivity ($^{16}/_{18}$; 89%) compared to the use of PET alone, using either the mismatch pattern or relative FDG uptake as the viability criterion. However, the advantage of this sequential strategy would be to avoid PET in 19 of 31 (61%) of the studied patients. The role of dobutamine echocardiography in relation to the nuclear techniques will be discussed in Chapter 23.

CONCLUSIONS

The available PET data suggest that patients with coronary artery disease and impaired left ventricular function may have a substantial improvement in outcome if identified and treated with myocardial revascularization. This would impact on the management of the whole group of patients with congestive heart failure in whom coronary disease is the leading cause. Although medical therapy improves outcome in these patients, the long-term results of medical management remain discouraging.[101–105] If patients with sufficient mass of viable myocardium to improve function can be identified accurately, these patients may be candidates for myocardial revascularization.

Which test modalities, criteria, and tracers should be selected? Because the decision making process in coronary patients with left ventricular dysfunction requires evaluation of both inducible ischemia and viability, stress SPECT imaging should be the first test. There are few situations (generally, unstable patients, in whom stress is not feasible) in which resting studies with ^{201}Tl or sestamibi could be performed as a first test, followed by FDG PET imaging only if tracer uptake in the corresponding dysfunctional area is lower than 50%. We use ^{201}Tl for stress-redistribution imaging, as this tracer has the largest experience in terms of comparative studies with independent gold standards of viability. Sestamibi may be a good alternative—but more studies are necessary. The stress-redistribution (or MIBI-rest) data will provide most of the clinically relevant information in a significant number of patients. The amplitude and extent of reversibility will indicate the amount of induced ischemia; the amplitude and extent of ^{201}Tl uptake and redistribution will indicate viability. After a review and a quantification of the stress-redistribution images, a decision can be made regarding the need for reinjection and reimaging. If after these data have been acquired, there is evidence of induced ischemia and significant amount of tracer uptake in the corresponding dysfunctional area, no other viability test would be necessary. If no or only a small area of induced ischemia is found and if tracer uptake is low in the dysfunctional area, an FDG study, preferably with PET and with myocardial glucose uptake maximized by glucose clamp or nicotinic acid, would be the next logical testing step; flow-metabolism mismatch and relative FDG uptake are the two best documented criteria of viability.

REFERENCES

1. Rahimtoola SH: The hibernating myocardium. Am Heart J 117:211, 1989
2. Braunwald E, Rutherford JD: Reversible ischaemic left ventricular dysfunction: evidence for "hibernating" myocardium. J Am Coll Cardiol 8:1467, 1986
3. Ross J Jr: Myocardial perfusion-contraction matching. Implications for coronary heart disease and hibernation. Circulation 83:1076, 1991
4. Braunwald E, Kloner RA: The stunned myocardium: prolonged postischemic dysfunction. Circulation 66:1146, 1982
5. Bolli R: Myocardial "stunning" in man. Circulation 86:1671, 1992
6. Vanoverschelde JL, Wijns W, Depré C et al: Mechanisms of chronic regional postischemic dysfunction in humans: new insights from the study of non-infarcted collateral dependent myocardium. Circulation 87:1513, 1993
7. Shen YT, Vatner SF: Mechanisms of impaired myocardial function during progressive coronary stenosis in conscious pigs. Hibernation versus stunning? Circ Res 76:479, 1995
8. Alderman EL, Fisher LD, Litwin P et al: Results of coronary artery bypass surgery in patients with poor left ventricular function (CASS). Circulation 68:785, 1983
9. Schelbert HR, Buxton D: Insights into coronary artery disease gained from metabolic imaging. Circulation 78:496, 1988
10. Schelbert HR: Metabolic imaging to assess myocardial viability. J Nucl Med 35(suppl.):8S, 1994
11. Dilsizian V, Bonow RO: Current diagnostic techniques of assessing myocardial viability in patients with hibernating and stunned myocardium. Circulation 87:1, 1993
12. Strauss HW, Harrison K, Langan JK, Lebowitz E, Pitt B: Thallium-201 for myocardial imaging. Relation of thallium-201 to regional myocardial perfusion. Circulation 51:641, 1975
13. Weich HP, Strauss HW, Pitt B: The extraction of thallium-201 by the myocardium. Circulation 56:188, 1977
14. Melin JA, Becker LC: Quantitative relationship between global left ventricular thallium uptake and blood flow: effects of propranolol, ouabain, dipyridamole and coronary artery occlusion. J Nucl Med 27:641, 1986
15. Sinusas AJ, Watson DD, Cannon JM Jr, Beller GA: Effect of ischemia and postischemic dysfunction on myocardial uptake of technetium-99m-labeled methoxyisobutyl isonitrile and thallium-201. J Am Coll Cardiol 14:1785, 1989
16. Leppo JA: Myocardial uptake of thallium and rubidium during alterations in perfusion and oxygenation in isolated rabbit hearts. J Nucl Med 28:878, 1987
17. Moore CA, Cannon J, Watson DD et al: Thallium 201 kinetics in stunned myocardium characterized by severe postischemic systolic dysfunction. Circulation 81:1622, 1990
18. Melin J, Becker L, Bulkley BH: Differences in thallium-201 uptake in reperfused and non-reperfused myocardial infarction. Circ Res 53:414, 1983
19. Chu A, Murdock RH, Cobb FR: Relation between regional distribution of thallium 201 and myocardial blood flow in normal, acutely ischemic and infarcted myocardium. Am J Cardiol 50:1141, 1982
20. Khaw Ban A, Strauss W, Pohost GM et al: Relation of immediate and delayed thallium-201 distribution to localization of iodine-125 antimyosin antibody in acute experimental myocardial infarction. Am J Cardiol 51:1428, 1983
21. Di Cola VC, Downing SE, Donabedian RK, Zaret BL: Pathophysiological correlates of thallium-201 myocardial uptake in experimental infarction. Cardiovasc Res 11:141, 1977
22. Sochor H, Schwaiger M, Schelbert HR et al: Relation-

ship between Tl-201, Tc-99m (Sn) pyrophosphate and F-18 2-deoxyglucose uptake in ischemically injured dog myocardium. Am Heart J 114:1066, 1987
23. Forman R, Kirk ES: Thallium-201 accumulation during reperfusion of ischemic myocardium: dependence on regional blood flow rather than viability. Am J Cardiol 54:659, 1984
24. Gewirtz H, Fischman AJ, Abraham S et al: Positron emission tomographic measurements of absolute regional myocardial blood flow permits identification of nonviable myocardium in patients with chronic myocardial infarction. J Am Coll Cardiol 23:851, 1994
25. Reimer KA, Jennings RB: The "wavefront phenomenon" of myocardial ischemic cell death. Transmural progression of necrosis within the framework of ischemic bed size (myocardium at risk) and collateral flow. Lab Invest 40:633, 1979
26. Jugdutt BI, Hutchins GM, Bulkley BM, Becker LC. Myocardial infarction in the conscious dog: three-dimensional mapping of infarct, collateral flow and region at risk. Circulation 60:1141, 1979
27. Pohost GL, Zir L, Moore RH et al: Differentiation of transiently ischemic from infarcted myocardium by serial imaging after a single dose of thallium-201. Circulation 55:294, 1977
28. Grunwald AM, Watson DD, Hozgrefe HH J, Irving JF, Beller GA: Myocardial thallium-201 kinetics in normal and ischemic myocardium. Circulation 64:610, 1981
29. Pohost GM, Okada RD, O'Keffe DD et al: Thallium redistribution in dogs with severe coronary artery stenosis of fixed caliber. Circ Res 48:439, 1981
30. Melin JA, Wijns W, Keyeux A et al: Assessment of thallium-201 redistribution versus glucose uptake as predictors of viability after coronary occlusion and reperfusion. Circulation 77:927, 1988
31. Granato JE, Watson DD, Flanagan TL et al: Myocardial thallium-201 kinetics and regional flow alterations with 3 hours of coronary occlusion and either rapid reperfusion through a totally patent vessel or slow reperfusion through a critical stenosis. J Am Coll Cardiol 1987;9:109–118.
32. Gewirtz H, Beller GA, Strauss HW et al: Transient defects of resting thallium scans in patients with coronary artery disease. Circulation 59:707, 1979
33. Berger BC, Watson DD, Burwell LR et al: Redistribution of thallium at rest in patients with stable and unstable angina and the effect of coronary artery bypass graft surgery. Circulation 60:1114, 1979
34. Iskandrian AS, Hakki aH, Kane SA et al: Rest and redistribution thallium-201 myocardial scintigraphy to predict improvement in left ventricular function after coronary artery bypass grafting. Am J Cardiol 51:1312, 1983
35. Mori T, Minamiji K, Kurogane H, Ogawa K, Yoshida Y: Rest-injected thallium-201 imaging for assessing viability of severe asynergic regions. J Nucl Med 32:1718, 1991
36. Ragosta M, Beller GA, Watson DD, Kaul S, Gimple L.: Quantitative planar rest-redistribution ^{201}Tl imaging in detection of myocardial viability and prediction of improvement in left ventricular function after coronary bypass surgery in patients with severely depressed left ventricular function. Circulation 87:1630, 1993
37. Alfieri O, La Canna G, Giubbini R et al: Recovery of myocardial infarction. The ultimate target of coronary revascularization. Eur J Cardiothorac Surg 7:325, 1993
38. Marzullo P, Parodi O, Reisenhofer B et al: Value of rest thallium-201/technetium-99^m sestamibi scans and dobutamine echocardiography for detecting myocardial viability. Am J Cardiol 71:166, 1993
39. Marzullo P, Sambuceti G, Parodi O et al: Regional concordance and discordance between rest thallium-201 and sestamibi imaging for assessing tissue viability: comparison with postrevascularization functional recovery. J Nucl Cardiol 2:309, 1995
40. Udelson JE, Coleman PS, Metherall J et al: Predicting recovery of severe regional ventricular dysfunction. Comparison of resting scintigraphy with ^{201}Tl and ^{99m}Tc-sestamibi. Circulation 89:2552, 1994
41. Lomboy CT, Schulman DS, Grill HP et al: Rest-redistribution thallium-201 scintigraphy to determine myocardial viability early after myocardial infarction. J Am Coll Cardiol 25:210, 1995
42. Dilsizian V, Perrone-Filardi P, Arrighi JA et al: Concordance and discordance between stress-redistribution and rest-redistribution thallium imaging for assessing viable myocardium. Comparison with metabolic activity by positron emission tomography. Circulation 88:941, 1993
43. Gibson RS, Watson DD, Taylor GJ et al: Prospective assessment of regional myocardial perfusion before and after coronary revascularization surgery by quantitative thallium-201 scintigraphy. J Am Coll Cardiol 1:804, 1983
44. Sabia PJ, Powers ER, Ragosta M et al: Role of quantitative planar thallium-201 imaging for determining viability in patients with acute myocardial infarction and a totally occluded infarct-related artery. J Nucl Med 34:728, 1993

45. Yamamoto K, Asada S, Masuyama T et al: Myocardial hibernation in the infarcted region cannot be assessed from the presence of stress-induced ischemia: usefulness of delayed image of exercise thallium-201 scintigraphy. Am Heart J 152:33, 1993
46. Cloninger KG, DePuey EG, Garcia EV et al: Incomplete redistribution in delayed thallium-201 single photon emission computed tomographic (SPECT) images: an overestimation of myocardial scarring. J Am Coll Cardiol 12:955, 1988
47. Kiat H, Berman DS, Maddahi J et al: Later reversibility of tomographic myocardial thallium-201 defects: an accurate marker of myocardial viability. J Am Coll Cardiol 12:1456, 1988
48. Yang LD, Berman DS, Kiat H et al: The frequency of late reversibility in SPECT thallium-201 stress-redistribution studies. J Am Coll Cardiol 15:334, 1990
49. Brunken RC, Modi FV, Hawkins RA et al: Positron emission tomography detects metabolic viability in myocardium with persistent 24-hour single photon emission computed tomography ^{201}Tl defects. Circulation 86:1357, 1992
50. Dilsizian V, Rocco TP, Freeman NMT, Leon MB, Bonow RO. Enhanced detection of ischemic but viable myocardium by the reinjection of thallium after stress-redistribution imaging. N Engl J Med 323:141, 1990
51. Dilsizian V, Smeitzer WR, Freedman NMT, Dextras R, Bonow RO. Thallium reinjection after stress-redistribution imaging: Does 24-hour delayed imaging following reinjection enhance detection of viable myocardium? Circulation 83:1247, 1991
52. Ohtani H, Tamaki N, Yonekura Y et al: Value of thallium-201 reinjection after delayed SPECT imaging for predicting reversible ischemia after coronary artery bypass grafting. Am J Cardiol 66:394, 1990
53. Haque T, Furukawa T, Takahashi M, Kinoshita M. Identification of hibernating myocardium by dobutamine stress echocardiography: Comparison with thallium-201 reinjection imaging. Am Heart J 130:553, 1995
54. Arnese M, Cornel JH, Salustri A et al: Prediction of improvement of regional left ventricular function after surgical revascularization. A comparison of low-dose dobutamine echocardiography with ^{201}Tl single photon emission computed tomography. Circulation 91:2748, 1995
55. Vanoverschelde JL, Gerber BL, Marwick T et al: Direct comparison of thallium SPECT with dobutamine echocardiography for delineation of myocardial viability. J Nucl Med 36:120, 1995
56. Dilsizian V, Bonow RO: Differential uptake and apparent thallium-201 "washout" after thallium reinjection: options regarding early redistribution imaging before reinjection or after redistribution imaging after reinjection. Circulation 85:1032, 1992
57. Kiat H, Friedman JD, Wang FP et al: Frequency of late reversibility in stress-redistribution thallium-201 SPECT using an early reinjection protocol. Am Heart J 122:613, 1991
58. Klingensmith WC III, Sutherland JD: Detection of jeopardized myocardium with ^{201}Tl myocardial perfusion imaging: comparison of early and late reinjection protocols. Clin Nucl Med 18:487, 1993
59. Tamaki N, Ohtani H, Yamshita K et al: Metabolic activity in the areas of new fill-in after thallium-201 reinjection: comparison with positron emission tomography using fluorine-18-deoxyglucose. J Nucl Med 32:673, 1991
60. Bonow RO, Dilsizian V, Cuocolo A, Bacharach SL: Identification of viable myocardium in patients with coronary artery disease and left ventricular dysfunction: comparison of thallium scintigraphy with reinjection and PET imaging with ^{18}F-fluorodeoxyglucose. Circulation 83:26, 1991
61. Zimmermann R, Mall G, Rauch B et al: ^{201}Tl activity in irreversible defects as a marker of myocardial viability. Clinicopathological study. Circulation 91:1016, 1995
62. Depré C, Vanoverschelde JL, Melin JA et al: Structural and metabolic correlates of the reversibility of chronic left ventricular ischemic dysfunction in humans. Am J Physiol 268:H1265, 1995
63. Piwnica-Worms D, Kronauge JF, Chiu ML: Uptake and retention of hexakis (2-methoxyisobutyl isonitrile) technetium(I) in cultured chick myocardial cells mitochondria and plasma membrane potential dependence. Circulation 82:1826, 1990
64. Beanlands RSB, Dawood F, Wen W-H et al: Are the kinetics of technetium-99m methoxyisobutyl isonitrile affected by cell metabolism and viability? Circulation 82:1802, 1990
65. Beller GA, Glover DK, Edwards NC et al: ^{99m}Tc-sestamibi uptake and retention during myocardial ischemia and reperfusion. Circulation 87:2033, 1993
66. Sansoy V, Glover DK, Watson DD et al: Comparison of thallium-201 resting redistribution with technetium-99m-sestamibi uptake and functional response to dobutamine for assessment of myocardial viability. Circulation 92:994, 1995
67. Li QS, Solot G, Frank TL, Wagner HN Jr, Becker LC. Myocardial redistribution of technetium-99m methoxyisobutyl isonitrile (sestamibi). J Nucl Med 31:1069, 1990
68. Sinusas AJ, Bergin JD, Edwards NC et al: Redistribu-

tion of ^{99m}Tc-sestamibi and ^{201}Tl in the presence of a severe coronary artery stenosis. Circulation 89:2332, 1994
69. Maurea S, Cuocolo A, Pace L et al: Left ventricular dysfunction in coronary artery disease: comparison between rest-redistribution thallium-201 and resting technetium-99m methoxyisobutyl isonitrile cardiac imaging. J Nucl Cardiol 1:65, 1994
70. Cuocolo A, Pace L, Ricciardelli B et al: Identification of viable myocardium in patients with chronic coronary artery disease: comparison of thallium-201 scintigraphy with reinjection and technetium-99m-methoxyisobutyl isonitrile. J Nucl Med 33:505, 1992
71. DePuey EG, Nichols K, Rozanski A et al: Defect reversibility with dual isotope SPECT: viability or just poorer contrast resolution with ^{201}Tl J Nucl Med 35:103, 1994
72. Maublant JC, Citron B, Lipiecki J et al: Rest technecium-99m-sestamibi tomoscintigraphy in hibernating myocardium. Am Heart J 129:306, 1995
73. Dilsizian V, Arrighi JAZ, Diodati JG et al: Myocardial viability in patients with chronic coronary artery disease. Comparison of ^{99m}Tc-sestamibi with thallium reinjection and [^{18}F]Fluorodeoxyglucose. Circulation 89:578, 1994
74. Bisi G, Sciagra R, Santoro GM, Fazzini PF. Rest technetium-99m sestamibi tomography in combination with short-term administration of nitrate: feasibility and reliability for prediction of postrevascularization outcome of asynergic territories. J Am Coll Cardiol 24:1282, 1994
75. Takahashi N, Tamaki N, Kawamoto M et al: Glucose metabolism in relation to perfusion in patients with ischaemic heart disease. Eur J Nucl Med 21:292, 1994
76. Tamaki N, Kawamoto M, Tadamura E et al: Prediction of reversible ischemia after revascularization. Perfusion and metabolic studies with positron emission tomography. Circulation 91:1697, 1995
77. Grandin C, Wijns W, Melin JA et al: Delineation of myocardial viability with PET. J Nucl Med 36:1543, 1995
78. Marinho NVS, Keogh BE, Costa DC et al: New insights into the pathophysiology of hibernating myocardium gained from the absolute measurement of myocardial blood flow and glucose utilization. Circulation (in press)
79. Marzullo P, Parodi O, Sambuceti G et al: Residual coronary reserve identifies segmental viability in patients with wall motion abnormalities. J Am Coll Cardiol 26:342, 1995
80. Tillisch J, Brunken R, Marshall R et al: Reversibility of cardiac wall motion abnormalities predicted by positron emission tomography. N Engl J Med 314:884, 1986
81. Tamaki N, Yonekura Y, Yamashita K et al: Positron emission tomography using fluorine-18 deoxyglucose in evaluation of coronary artery bypass grafting. Am J Cardiol 64:860, 1989
82. Marwick T, Nemec J, Lafont A, Salcedo E, MacIntyre W. Prediction by postexercise fluoro-18 deoxyglucose positron emission tomography of improvement in exercise capacity after revascularization. Am J Cardiol 69:854, 1992
83. Gropler RJ, Geltman EM, Sampathkumaran K et al: Comparison of carbon-11-acetate with fluorine-18-fluorodeoxyglucose for delineating viable myocardium by positron emission tomography. J Am Coll Cardiol 22:1587, 1993
84. Knuuti J, Saraste M, Nuutila P et al: Myocardial viability: fluorine-18-deoxyglucose positron emission tomography in prediction of wall motion recovery after revascularization. Am Heart J 127:785, 1994
85. Vom Dahl J, Eitzman D, Al-Aouar A et al: Relation of regional function, perfusion, and metabolism in patients with advanced coronary artery disease undergoing surgical revascularization. Circulation 90:2356, 1994
86. Carrel T, Jenni R, Haubold-Reuter S et al: Improvement of severely reduced left ventricular function after surgical revascularization in patients with preoperative myocardial infarction. Eur J Cardiothorac Surg 6:479, 1992
87. Maes A, Flameng W, Nuyts J et al: Histological alterations in chronically hypoperfused myocardium: correlation with PET findings. Circulation 90:735, 1994
88. Lucignani G, Paolini G, Landoni C et al: Presurgical identification of hibernating myocardium by combined use of technetium-99m hexakis 2-methoxyisobutylisonitrile single photon emission tomography and fluorine-18 fluoro-2-deoxy-D-glucose positron emission tomography in patients with coronary artery disease. Eur J Nucl Med 19:874, 1992
89. Parodi O et al: Cardiac emission computed tomography: underestimation of regional tracer concentrations due to wall motion abnormalities. J Comput Assist Tomog 8:1083, 1984
90. Baudhuin T, Coppens A, Bol A et al: Correlation of defect size and severity between ^{99m}Tc sestamibi SPECT and N-13 ammonia PET imaging. J Nucl Med 33:875, 1992
91. Baudhuin T, Coppens A, Bol A et al: Discrepancies in perfusion defect estimates between ^{99m}Tc MIBI SPECT and N-13 ammonia PET are not explained

by differences in tracer behavior. J Nucl Med 34:121, 1993
92. Di Carli M, Davidson M, Little R et al: Value of metabolic imaging with positron emission tomography for evaluating prognosis in patients with coronary artery disease and left ventricular dysfunction. Am J Cardiol 73:527, 1994
93. Eitzman D, Al-Aouar Z, Kanter H et al: Clinical outcome of patients with advanced coronary artery disease after viability studies with positron emission tomography. J Am Coll Cardiol 20:559, 1992
94. Tamaki N, Kawamoto M, Takahashi N et al: Prognostic value of an increase in fluorine-18 deoxyglucose uptake in patients with myocardial infarction: comparison with stress thallium imaging. J Am Coll Cardiol 22:1621, 1993
95. Lee K, Marwick T, Cook S et al: Prognosis of patients with left ventricular dysfunction, with and without viable myocardium after myocardial infarction. Circulation 90:2687, 1994
96. Bax JJ, Visser FC, van Lingen A et al: Feasibility of assessing regional myocardial uptake of 18F-fluorodeoxyglucose using single photon emission computed tomography. Eur Heart J 14:1675, 1993
97. Bax JJ, Visser FC, van Lingen A et al: Relation between myocardial uptake of thallium-201 chloride and fluorine-18 fluorodeoxyglucose imaged with single-photon emission tomography in normal individuals. Eur J Nucl Med 22:56, 1995
98. Burt RA, Perkins OW, Oppenheim BE et al. Direct comparison of fluorine-18-FDG SPECT, fluorine-18-FDG PET and rest thallium-201 SPECT for detection of myocardial viability. J Nucl Med 36:176, 1995
99. Sandler MP, Videlefsky S, Delbeke D et al: Evaluation of myocardial ischemia using a rest metabolism/stress perfusion protocol with fluorine-18 deoxyglucose/technetium-99m MIBI and dual-isotope simultaneous-acquisition single-photon emission computed tomography. J Am Coll Cardiol 26:870, 1995
100. Gerber B, Vanoverschelde JL, Bol A et al: Sequential use of ^{201}Tl SPECT and PET is better than single tests for identification of viable myocardium. J Nucl Med 36:143, 1995
101. The SOLVD Investigators: Effect of enalapril on survival in patients with reduced left ventricular ejection fractions and congestive heart failure. N Engl J Med 325:293, 1991
102. Cohn JN, Johnson G, Ziesche S et al: A comparison of enalapril with hyralazine-isosorbide dinitrate in the treatment of chronic congestive heart failure. N Engl J Med 325:303, 1991
103. The SOLVD Investigators: Effect of enalapril on mortality and development of heart failure in asymptomatic patients with reduced left ventricular ejection fractions. N Engl J Med 327:685, 1992
104. Swedberg K, Held P, Kjekshus J et al: Effects of the early administration of enalapril on morality in patients with acute myocardial infarction: results of the Cooperative New Scandinavian Enalapril Survival Study II (Consensus II). N Engl J Med 327:678, 1992
105. Pfeffer MA, Braunwald E, Move LA et al: Effect of captopril on mortality and morbidity in patients with left ventricular dysfunction after myocardial infarction: Results of the Survival and Ventricular Enlargement Trial. N Engl J Med 327:669, 1992

Chapter 23

Echocardiographic Techniques for Assessment of Myocardial Viability

Jean-Louis J. Vanoverschelde, Agneś Pasquet, and Jacques A. Melin

Over the past 50 years, ischemic heart disease has been a widespread cause of morbidity and the leading cause of mortality in the economically developed countries of the western world. Although the relative importance of coronary deaths has declined gradually during the last decade, "heart attacks" still account for approximately 25% of all deaths in the United States and in Europe. Mortality rates are higher in patients with severely depressed left ventricular LV function than in any other groups of patients, ranging from 15% to 60% per year.[1] Several studies have shown that surgical revascularization may improve survival and symptoms of heart failure in some of these patients.[2] The potential benefits of coronary revascularization should be balanced, however, with the higher surgical mortality in patients with LV dysfunction, which ranges from 5% to 37%.

Presumably, the beneficial effects of revascularization result from improving blood supply to dysfunctional but viable regions with subsequent improvement in regional and global LV function. This scenario is supported by the results of several studies in patients with severe LV dysfunction, showing that only patients with dysfunctional but "viable" myocardium are likely to benefit from coronary revascularization.[3-5] Although these studies were retrospective and nonrandomized, their results suggest that in addition to the evaluation of coronary anatomy, cardiac function, and myocardial perfusion, the selection of patients with severe LV dysfunction for coronary revascularization should also comprise a precise assessment of the presence of ischemically compromised but viable myocardium.

DEFINITION OF MYOCARDIAL VIABILITY

The successive emergence of coronary artery bypass surgery, percutaneous transluminal coronary angioplasty, and thrombolytic therapy has heightened our awareness of the diverse effects of perfusion on cardiac function and has drastically changed our way of thinking about coronary artery disease (CAD). Since the pioneering works of Tennant and Wiggers,[6] it has been known that total ischemia leads to a prompt cessation of contraction and eventually results in the appearance of cell damage and irreversible myocardial necrosis. Accordingly, the discovery of an abnormal regional contraction in a patient with coronary artery disease has long been equated with the presence of irreversible myocardial necrosis. With the advent of reperfusion therapy, however, evidence has accumulated that prolonged regional "ischemic" dysfunction did not always arise from irreversible tissue damage and, to some extent, could be reversed by restoration of blood flow. From laboratory and clinical investigations of reperfusion of ischemic myocardium, several associated phenomena were described, which have come to be known as myocardial "stunning"[7,8] and myocardial "hibernation."[9] The roles of these entities are discussed in Chapter 20, and will be reviewed briefly for the purpose of this discussion.

Myocardial stunning is a reversible form of contractile dysfunction that can occur after restoration of coronary blood flow following a relatively brief period of coronary occlusion. It was originally described in dogs by Heyndrickx et al.[7] and was subsequently shown to occur in humans as well,[8] where it is considered to participate in the prolonged contractile dysfunction seen after thrombolytic therapy or following attacks of unstable angina. Myocardial stunning is a form of reperfusion injury, whereby reintroduction of oxygen after a period of deprivation provokes a transient overload of calcium in cardiac myocytes and damages the contractile machinery. The ensuing contractile dysfunction typically lasts for hours or days, despite adequate restoration of myocardial blood flow and the lack of tissue necrosis. Nonetheless, in the absence of subsequent ischemic episodes, function always returns spontaneously and completely back to normal.

Myocardial hibernation is a term first used by Rahimtoola[9] for a postulated condition of chronic sustained abnormal contraction due to chronic underperfusion in patients with CAD, in whom revascularization or an improved oxygen supply–demand balance causes recovery of regional function. In his original description of the condition, Rahimtoola postulated that myocardial hibernation resulted from a "relatively uncommon response to reduced myocardial blood flow at rest whereby the heart downgrades its myocardial function to the extent that blood flow and function are once again in equilibrium, and as a result, neither myocardial necrosis or ischemic symptoms are present."[9] Although circumstantial evidence supports the existence of hibernation in humans, there is no experimental demonstration that it actually results from chronic underperfusion. Instead, there is increasing evidence that resting blood flow is normal in many patients with chronic but reversible ischemic dysfunction, whereas coronary vasodilatory reserve is severely altered.[10]

It is therefore possible that frequent, repeated, and incompletely resolutive episodes of ischemia followed by stunning could be the primary cause of reversible chronic dysfunction. In contrast to stunning, which does not usually result in significant structural changes, myocardial hibernation is characterized by marked structural alterations at both the myocyte and the extracellular matrix level, including the loss of myofibrillar content, the accumulation of glycogen, the lack of T-tubules and sarcoplasmic reticulum, and various phenotypic changes reminiscent of cellular dedifferentiation.[10–12]

While the existence of these altered myocardial states was receiving increasing recognition among basic and clinical cardiologists, ways to identify them in the clinical setting has become one of the most active areas of research in the field of ischemic heart diseases. Various approaches have been proposed to predict the reversibility of LV dysfunction after coronary revascularization. For the most part, these methods rely on assessing basic cellular mechanisms that are known to play a central role in the recovery of systolic function after coronary revascularization. These include sufficient resting perfusion to provide metabolic fuels and to allow washout of toxic metabolites, maintained membrane integrity (which includes the ability to generate transmembrane ionic gradients and to transport energy providing substrates), preserved metabolic machinery (to allow glucose, fatty acid, and oxygen consumption), and recruitable inotropic reserve. Several of these phenomena are identified using nuclear approaches and are discussed in other chapters. It is the purpose of this chapter to review some of the available echocardiographic modalities for assessment of the potential for recovery of contractile function following adequate restoration of coronary patency.

PREDICTION OF FUNCTIONAL RECOVERY WITH DOBUTAMINE ECHOCARDIOGRAPHY

Experimental and Early Clinical Observations

In experimental models of myocardial ischemic dysfunction, reversibly injured (including stunned,[13–15] short-term[16] and chronically hibernating[17]) myocardium has been shown to retain the ability to temporarily improve function upon stimulation with catecholamines or calcium, whereas infarcted myocardium usually remains unchanged. This diverging contractile response in dysfunctional but viable and infarcted myocardium may thus provide a basis for distinguishing between reversible and irreversible tissue injury in patients with CAD and LV ischemic dysfunction. Earlier investigators, attempting to predict the reversibility of LV ischemic dysfunction after revascularization, used the response of global left ventricular ejection fraction (LVEF) to an inotropic stimulus (epinephrine or postextrasystolic potentiation) at the time of cardiac catheterization as an index of myocardial viability. Nesto et al.[18] were among the first to use this approach. They showed that patients with an ejection fraction of less than 35% who demonstrated a greater than 10% increase in ejection fraction during inotropic stimulation improved global LV function after coronary revascularization. These patients also had better long-term survival than comparable patients lacking contractile reserve whether treated medically or surgically. Recent refinements in noninvasive functional imaging, particularly in digitized echocardiography, and the use of standardized dobutamine infusion protocols have allowed these concepts to be applied on a large scale in patients with severe LV ischemic dysfunction. Over the past decade, dobutamine stress echocardiography has received considerable attention as a safe, noninvasive means of diagnosing CAD. This technique uses progressively increasing doses of dobutamine, a synthetic catecholamine, to induce ischemic wall motion abnormalities by increasing oxygen demand in the setting of a coronary stenosis. However, low doses of dobutamine may elicit an improved contractile response from myocardial segments that are abnormal at rest, thus demonstrating contractile reserve (Fig. 23-1).

Prediction of Reversible Dysfunction Early after Myocardial Infarction

The use of dobutamine echocardiography for prediction of reversible dysfunction after myocardial infarction is summarized in Table 23-1. Piérard et al.[19] were the first to propose the use of low-dose dobutamine echocardiography to predict reversible dysfunction after acute reperfused myocardial infarction. These authors compared the accuracy of dobutamine echocardiography with that of positron emission tomography (PET) for detection of viable myocardium in 17 patients treated with thrombolytic therapy for a first acute anterior myocardial infarction. Their criteria for viable myocardium in the infarct zone were both an improved wall motion and evidence of viability by PET 9 ± 7 months after infarction. Dobutamine was infused at a rate of 10 μg/kg/min. As shown in Figure 23-2, in five patients with normal perfusion and fluorodeoxyglucose (FDG) uptake by PET (corresponding to myocardial stunning), dysfunctional myocardium at baseline improved contraction with dobutamine and subsequently normalized at follow-up. In six additional patients with reduced perfusion and maintained FDG uptake by PET (the so-called "flow-metabolism mismatch" pattern—corresponding to hibernation), dobutamine evoked a significant contractile response in three patients. Although not all of this group underwent revascularization, function subsequently improved in only one patient, whose dobutamine test was negative. In the last six patients, who showed a concordant decrease of flow and FDG uptake ("flow-metabolism match" pattern) by PET, no contractile response could be evoked by dobutamine and function did not improve at follow-up. Both techniques were concordant in 79% of the dysfunctional segments, with a slight, albeit nonsignificant advantage in favor of dobutamine echocardiography in terms of specificity and diagnostic accuracy.

Subsequently, in a selected group of 21 patients with incomplete infarction, Barilla et al.[20] observed that most dobutamine-responsive regions improved after revascularization. Nonrevascularized segments also responded to dobutamine, but showed less improvement at follow-up. Similar results were reported by Previtali et al.[21] and Watada et al.[22] Interestingly, in this last study, which included 21 patients with reperfused anterior myocardial infarction, the authors observed that the extent of improvement in wall motion during low-dose dobutamine (10 μg/kg/min) correlated closely ($r = 0.93$, $p < 0.0001$) with the extent of recovery of wall motion at follow-up (25 days after infarction).

The optimal dose of dobutamine for stimulating reversibly dysfunctional myocardium was studied by Smart et al.[23] in 51 patients treated with thrombolytic therapy for acute myocardial infarction. These authors investigated the contractile response of dys-

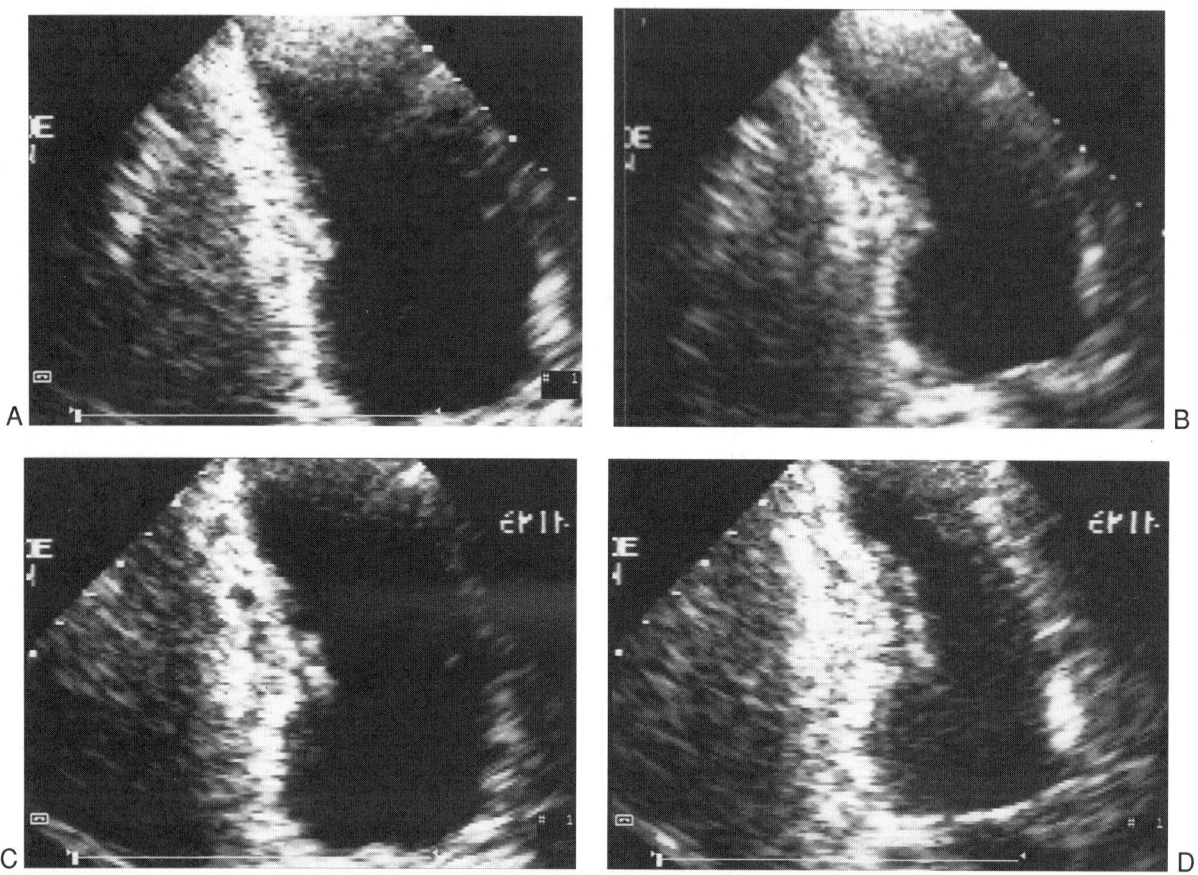

Fig. 23-1 Representative (**A** & **C**) end-diastolic and **B** & **D** end-systolic freeze frames in the apical two-chamber view, obtained at baseline (**A** & **B**) and after 10 μg/kg/min of dobutamine (**C** & **D**) in a patient with recent (3 weeks) anterior myocardial infarction. Note the significant improvement in anterior wall motion evidenced by reduction of left ventricular (LV) diameter.

Table 23-1. Sensitivity, Specificity, and Accuracy of Dobutamine Echocardiography for Prediction of Reversible Dysfunction following Acute Myocardial Infarction

Study	Number of Patients	Sensitivity	Specificity	Accuracy
Acute myocardial infarction				
Piérard et al. (1990)[19][a]	17	5/6 (83%)	8/11 (73%)	13/17 (76%)
Previtali et al. (1993)[21]	59	50/63 (79%)	109/158 (68%)	159/221 (72%)
Watada et al. (1995)[22]	21	55/66 (83%)	43/50 (86%)	98/116 (84%)
Smart et al. (1993)[23][a]	51	19/22 (86%)	26/29 (90%)	45/51 (88%)

[a] Patient-based analysis.

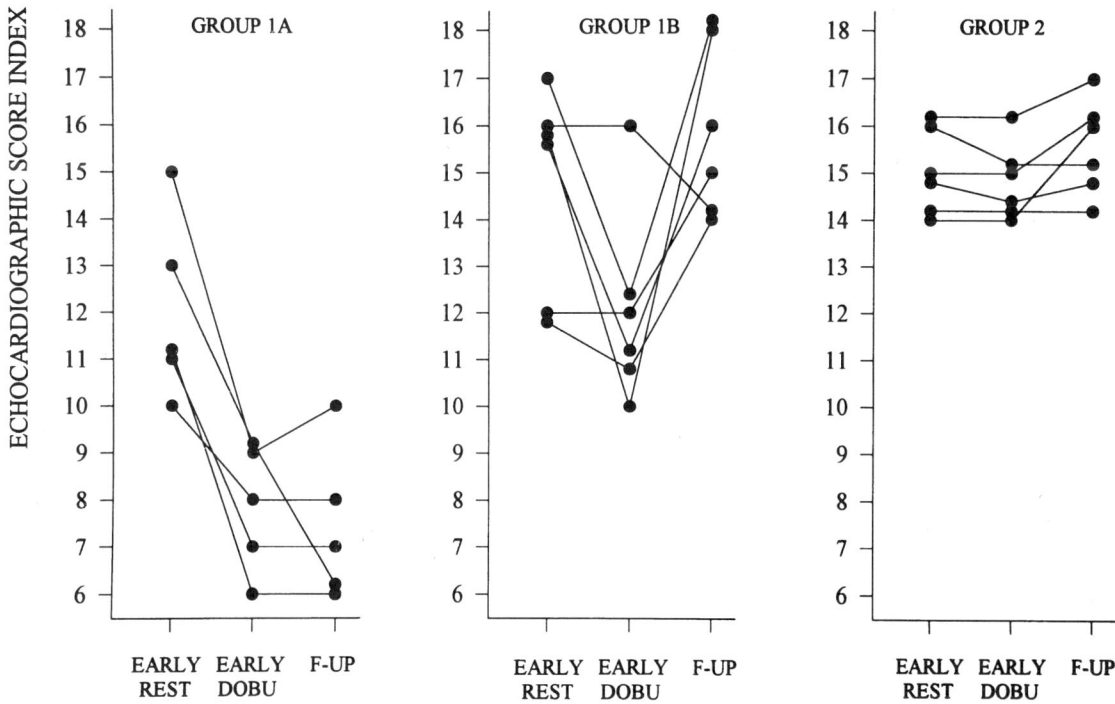

Fig. 23-2 Individual changes in the echocardiographic score index between the early study at rest and during dobutamine (DOBU) infusion and the follow-up (F-UP) study in 5 patients with normal perfusion (group 1A), 6 patients with a flow-metabolism mismatch pattern (group 1B) by positron tomography, and 6 patients with concordant decrease in flow and metabolism (group 2). (Adapted from Pierard et al.,[19] with permission.)

functional myocardium at three different doses of dobutamine (i.e., 4, 12, and 23 ± 10 μg/kg/min). While dobutamine-responsive wall motion was specific at all doses (90%, 93%, and 90%, respectively), sensitivity decreased in a dose-dependent manner, as the number of segments deteriorating increased (86%, 55%, and 35%, respectively). They also showed that dobutamine echocardiography was equally accurate in detecting reversible dysfunction in anterior, inferior, posterior, or lateral regions. Finally, like Watada et al.,[22] they found that the extent of wall motion improvement at follow-up correlated closely with that during low-dose dobutamine infusion, thus allowing prediction of the extent of recovery at follow-up.

Prediction of Reversible Dysfunction in Chronic LV Ischemic Dysfunction

Studies focused on the prediction of reversible dysfunction in chronic LV ischemic dysfunction are summarized in Table 23-2. While existing data suggest that augmentation of regional function in response to dobutamine reflects myocardial viability early after infarction, fewer data are available to support the efficacy of this technique in patients with chronic LV ischemic dysfunction, the so-called "chronic myocardial hibernation." In contrast to the early postinfarction period, where stunned myocardium is probably predominant, chronic myocardial hibernation likely involves both postischemic dysfunction and ongoing reduction of myocardial blood flow. It is known to be associated with marked ultrastructural alterations of the myocytes, including a loss of myofilaments and contractile material,[10-12] and with no or a very limited residual coronary flow reserve.[10] Thus, it would not be surprising if chronically dysfunctional but hibernating myocardium was less responsive to inotropic stimulation than purely stunned myocardium. However, on the contrary, there is increasing experimental and clinical evidence that chronically hibernating myocardium dis-

Table 23-2. Sensitivity, Specificity, and Accuracy of Dobutamine Echocardiography for Prediction of Reversible Dysfunction following Revascularization in Patients with Chronic Coronary Disease

Study	Number of Patients	Sensitivity	Specificity	Accuracy
Chronic coronary artery disease				
Marzullo et al. (1993)[24]	14	40/49 (82%)	24/26 (92%)	64/75 (85%)
Alfieri et al. (1993)[25]	14	85/93 (91%)	25/32 (78%)	110/125 (88%)
Cigarroa et al. (1993)[26] [a]	25	9/11 (82%)	12/14 (86%)	21/25 (84%)
La Canna et al. (1994)[27]	33	178/205 (87%)	89/109 (82%)	267/314 (85%)
Perrone-Filardi et al. (1995)[28]	18	42/48 (88%)	27/31 (87%)	69/81 (85%)
Afridi et al. (1995)[30]	20	28/38 (74%)	55/76 (73%)	83/114 (73%)
Arnese et al. (1995)[32]	38	24/33 (74%)	130/137 (95%)	154/170 (91%)
Vanoverschelde et al. (1996)[33]	73	123/167 (76%)	238/277 (86%)	361/444 (81%)

[a] Patient-based analysis.

plays recruitable inotropic reserve, and low-dose dobutamine echocardiography has permitted prediction of the reversibility of dysfunction in chronically hibernating myocardium as well.

In 25 patients undergoing coronary revascularization, Cigarroa et al.[26] showed that a greater than 20% improvement of the systolic wall thickening score during dobutamine had sensitivity of 82% and a specificity of 86% for recovery at follow-up. Similar results (87% sensitivity and 82% specificity) were recently reported by La Canna et al.[27] in 33 selected patients undergoing coronary artery bypass surgery. In 18 patients with chronic CAD undergoing revascularization, Perrone-Filardi et al.[28] showed that dobutamine echocardiography allowed prediction of functional outcome in more than 87% of dysfunctional myocardial segments with a reduced thallium uptake at rest (defined as < 80% maximal activity in two consecutive sectors).

We recently investigated the accuracy of this technique in 40 patients with an ejection fraction of less than 35% undergoing revascularization by either bypass surgery ($n = 33$) or angioplasty ($n = 7$).[29] Recovery of LV function was evaluated by echocardiography 5.3 ± 2.4 months after revascularization and patients were retrospectively categorized into groups with or without functional improvement defined by a greater than 5% increase in ejection fraction and greater than 10 ml decrease in end-systolic volume. Before revascularization, patients who improved LV function postoperatively had smaller end-diastolic volume and less wall motion abnormalities than patients with persistent postoperative dysfunction. They also showed greater improvement of wall motion score with dobutamine (6.1 ± 2.4 vs. 1.8 ± 4.2 grades, $p < 0.001$). Discriminant analysis selected the improvement in wall motion score with dobutamine and baseline end-diastolic volume as independent predictors of postoperative recovery. Consideration of both parameters allowed prediction of functional outcome in 84% of the patients with and 81% of those without postoperative improvement.

The optimal dose of dobutamine that stimulates chronically but reversibly dysfunctional myocardium was studied by Afridi et al.[30] in 27 patients with stable CAD and segmental dysfunction scheduled for coronary angioplasty. These authors investigated the contractile response of dysfunctional myocardium to incremental doses of dobutamine of 2.5, 5, 7.5, 10, 20, 30, and 40 μg/kg/min. Recovery of function occurred in 33% of initially dysfunctional segments that were revascularized. During dobutamine infusion, dysfunctional segments exhibited one of four responses: sustained improvement (from low to peak dose) in 18%, a biphasic response (improvement at low-dose with deterioration at high dose) in 28%, deterioration of wall motion in 15%, and no contractile response in 39%. In segments with a biphasic response, improvement always occurred within the 10 μg/kg/min dose, with the greatest prevalence at 7.5 μg/kg/min (Fig. 23-3). As the number of segments with deterioration increased in a dose-dependent manner, starting at 7.5 μg/kg/min with as much as 18% at 10 μg/kg/min and 54% at 20 μg/kg/min, they recommended that both the 5 and 10 μg/kg/

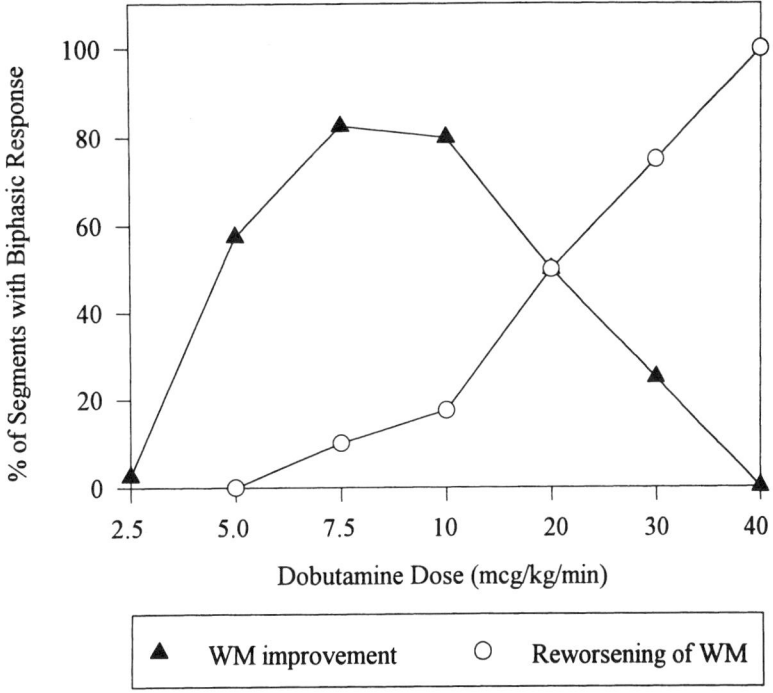

Fig. 23-3 Plot showing prevalence at various doses of dobutamine of maximal wall motion (WM) improvement and renewed worsening of wall motion in segments exhibiting a biphasic response. (Adapted from Afridi et al.,[30] with permission.)

min stages be recorded and analyzed to avoid missing a transitory improvement in wall motion, followed by rapid deterioration.

Comparison of Dobutamine Echocardiography with Other Techniques

Nuclear cardiology techniques are widely used to predict the reversal of LV dysfunction after revascularization. Because these methodologies are well established, the efficacy of dobutamine echocardiography as an adjunct or perhaps an alternative warrants particularly careful consideration. However, despite the favorable records of nuclear techniques, they have disadvantages in terms of cost (of imaging equipment, isotopes and disposable) and availability. Nevertheless, the dominant issue in the selection of one or the other technique must remain accuracy.

Few published studies offer a direct comparison between dobutamine echocardiography and nuclear medicine techniques for assessment of tissue viability. Because a number of variables may potentially influence the results of either tests, we have focused only on those studies in which both echocardiography and nuclear imaging were obtained in the same patients by observers who were equally expert in their respective field.

Dobutamine Echocardiography versus Thallium-201 Imaging

As discussed in Chapter 20, the uptake of thallium by the myocardium is dependent on the presence of an intact membrane Na^+–K^+-ATPase activity. Clinically, the absolute level of thallium uptake and the redistribution phenomenon are the most commonly used parameters for assessment of myocardial viability.

Panza et al.[31] recently reported the results of a direct comparison between rest–redistribution thallium single-photon emission computed tomography (SPECT) and low-dose dobutamine echocardiography in 30 patients with ischemic LV dysfunction. They observed that the number of dysfunctional segments with preserved thallium uptake significantly exceeded that of segments with residual inotropic reserve (54% vs. 30%). Likewise, Arnese et al.[32] reported that thallium SPECT indicated residual viability more frequently than dobutamine echocardiography (61% vs. 20%). At first glance, this could indicate that the myocardial processes necessary to maintain thallium uptake are less sensitive to the deleterious consequences of CAD than those responsible for the inotropic response to dobutamine. It is indeed likely that the maintenance of cell viability more critically depends on a preserved transmembrane pump activity than on a maintained inotropic reserve. Accordingly, Panza et al.[31] speculated that a spectrum of myocardial dysfunction actually existed in patients with coronary disease; a mild degree of myocyte dysfunction was characterized by both a preserved membrane integrity and the capacity to respond to an inotropic stimulus, whereas the more severe form of reversible dysfunction would lose the capacity to respond to inotropic stimuli, despite a persistently normal membrane function. Thus, the higher prevalence of viable segments detected by thallium SPECT as opposed to dobutamine echocardiography could indicate the greater capacity of thallium to predict potentially reversible dysfunction. It should be emphasized, however, that only the serial measurement of mechanical function following revascularization allows determination of the reversibility or irreversibility of injury. One should therefore be very cautious in interpreting the results of studies lacking an adequate gold standard (functional recovery) and, ideally, should focus only on those in which a direct comparison of the two approaches with the postoperative functional outcome is provided. So far, only two such studies are available.[32-33]

Arnese et al.[32] recently studied 38 patients with chronic LV ischemic dysfunction (ejection fraction < 40%) undergoing uncomplicated bypass surgery. Low-dose dobutamine echocardiography and exercise–redistribution–reinjection thallium SPECT were performed in every patient before revascularization and their respective accuracy was determined according to the return of regional function at follow-up. While both techniques were equally sensitive in predicting postoperative functional improvement (74% for dobutamine echocardiography, 89% for thallium), dobutamine echocardiography was significantly more specific than thallium SPECT for identification of persistent postoperative dysfunction (95% vs. 48% for thallium SPECT, $p < 0.001$). These results thus suggest that *although thallium may be valuable for identifying segments that are unlikely to recover after revascularization, it may significantly overestimate the amount of salvageable myocardium*, resulting in a low specificity and a low positive predictive accuracy.

We recently confirmed these observations in 73 consecutive patients with severe LV dysfunction (mean ejection fraction of 36%) undergoing revascularization.[33] As in the studies of Panza et al.[31] and Arnese et al.[32] more segments in our study were viable by thallium than by echocardiographic criteria (64% vs. 37%, Fig. 23-4). We also evaluated the ability of the two tests to predict the functional outcome 5.5 ± 2.5 months after revascularization. Criteria for presence of viable myocardium were a greater than 50% thallium uptake in the dysfunctional area at reinjection, with thallium SPECT, and a decrease in regional wall motion score of at least 1 grade from baseline to the 10 μg/kg/min dose, with dobutamine echocardiography. Prerevascularization thallium correctly predicted functional outcome in 77% of the segments that improved functionally following revascularization and in 56% of those that remained dysfunctional; the overall accuracy was 64%. Prerevascularization dobutamine echocardiography allowed correct prediction in 76% of the segments that improved after revascularization (p = ns vs. thallium) and in 86% of those that remained dysfunctional after revascularization ($p < 0.01$ vs. thallium). The diagnostic performance of both tests was also investigated on an *individual patient* basis. Forty-three patients improved LV ejection fraction by greater than 5% following revascularization, while 30 patients showed no significant changes. Before revascularization, patients who improved LV function postoperatively had higher thallium uptake in the dysfunctional area at reinjection (59 ± 10% vs. 48 ± 11%, $p < 0.001$), a larger proportion of dysfunctional segments with a greater than 50% thallium uptake at reinjection (71 ± 24% vs. 47 ± 32%, $p < 0.001$) and a greaer improvement of wall motion score with low-dose dobutamine (6.3 ± 3.0 vs. 1.1 ± 3.6 grades, $p < 0.001$). Empiric receiver operating curves were used to select the optimal SPECT and echocardiographic criteria for prediction of func-

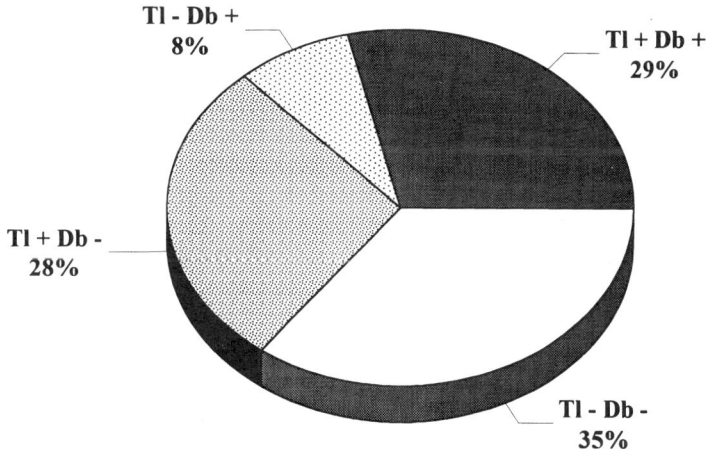

Fig. 23-4 Pie chart showing the distribution of akinetic segments according to preoperative thallium single-photon emission computed tomography (SPECT) and response to low-dose dobutamine infusion in 73 patients with coronary artery disease and chronic left ventricular ischemic dysfunction.

tional recovery after revascularization (Fig. 23-5). According to a mean thallium uptake of greater than 54% in the dysfunctional area at reinjection, thallium SPECT correctly identified 72% of the patients with and 73% of those without postoperative improvement in global ejection fraction. The overall accuracy of thallium SPECT was 73%. Similarly, according to an improvement in wall motion score of at least 3.5 grades during low-dose dobutamine, echocardiography correctly classified 88% of the pa-

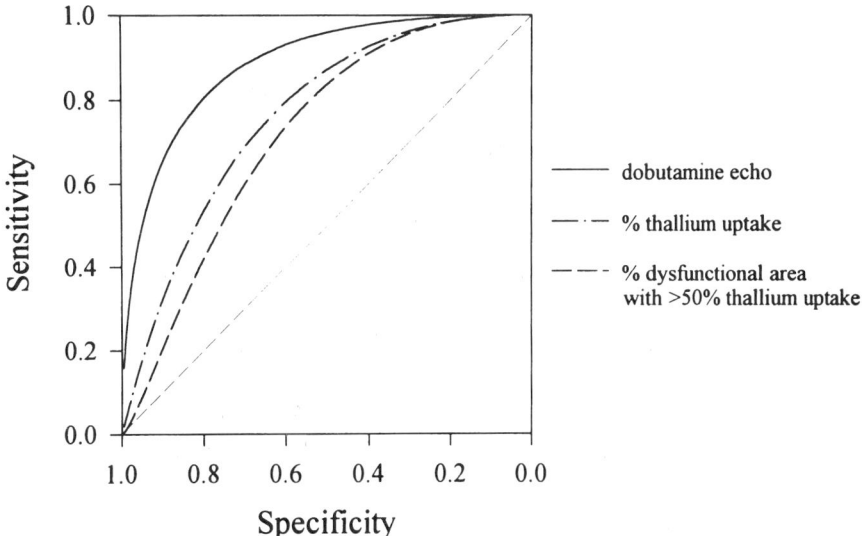

Fig. 23-5 Empiric receiver operating curves generated for selected thallium single-photon emission computed tomography (SPECT) and dobutamine echocardiographic criteria in the same 73 patients as in Figure 23-4. Criteria used to construct the curves were the mean thallium uptake at reinjection in the dysfunctional area, the proportion of the dysfunctional area with greater than 50% thallium uptake, and the degree of improvement in global wall motion score at 10 μg/kg/min dobutamine.

tients with and 77% of those without postoperative functional improvement. The overall accuracy of dobutamine echocardiography was 84% ($p = 0.054$ vs. thallium).

We also observed that with both methods, specificity was less in hypokinetic segments than in initially akinetic segments (68% by low-dose dobutamine test and 29% by thallium SPECT). There are several potential reasons for these poor specificity figures in hypokinetic segments. Segmental hypokinesis may reflect the presence of a subendocardial scar and be unaffected by revascularization. Nonetheless, if enough noninfarcted myocardium remains in mid and epicardial layers, such segments could still manifest improvement with dobutamine or exhibit near normal thallium uptake. Tethering by adjacent akinetic segments could also be an explanation. In this case, the segmental response to revascularization will largely depend on the recovery of the adjacent segments, while that to dobutamine will also reflect the changes in segmental contractility, cavity size, and afterload.

Dobutamine Echocardiography versus PET

Because regional contractile ischemic dysfunction reflects underlying alterations of myocardial perfusion and metabolism, much attention has focused on flow and metabolic imaging with PET. Positron imaging has a unique capacity to measure regional physiologic function by tracing the biological fate of compounds that have been tagged with positron-emitting radioisotopes. As discussed in Chapter 21, [^{18}F] FDG has been the preferred tracer for the assessment of myocardial viability. Results of studies using PET and FDG have shown that the persistence of residual glucose utilization in hypoperfused segments (a condition often referred to as "flow-metabolism mismatch") could identify the segments that will eventually resume function following revascularization. Using this approach, myocardial viability has been detected with sensitivity of 78% to 85% and specificity of 78% to 92%. Although several studies have demonstrated the merits of FDG and PET for the prediction of functional recovery after revascularization, very few have compared its accuracy with that of dobutamine echocardiography.

Piérard et al.[19] were the first to compare low-dose dobutamine echocardiography and PET for prediction of the reversibility of LV dysfunction after myocardial infarction. As mentioned previously, in a study of 17 patients with a first reperfused anterior myocardial infarction within 1 week of the acute event, they found both methods to be concordant in 79% of the patients, with a small, albeit nonsignificant advantage in favor of dobutamine echocardiography in terms of specificity and diagnostic accuracy. An 80% concordance of the FDG mismatch pattern with dobutamine echocardiography has also been reported by Williams et al.[33a] in 56 patients with chronic LV dysfunction (EF < 30%). In this series, FDG-PET was more sensitive than dobutamine echocardiography for the prediction of functional recovery at 8 weeks (85% vs. 69%, $p < 0.02$), but was less specific (50% vs. 79%, $p < 0.001$). The number of viable segments by dobutamine echocardiography correlated better with the degree of functional improvement than did the number of viable segments by PET. Similar levels of concordance were subsequently reported by Baer et al.[34] using dobutamine transesophageal echocardiography, although no follow-up data were presented in the latter series.

Combination of Dobutamine Echocardiography and Scintigraphy

It is obvious from the above that none of the techniques currently available for assessment of myocardial viability is clearly superior to the alternatives. We therefore reasoned that instead of opposing these techniques, one could perhaps use them sequentially and obtain better results than with any of the tests used separately. Thus, we recently investigated whether the sequential use of dobutamine echocardiography and PET could be a valuable option for delineation of viable myocardium.[35] We studied 47 patients with coronary disease and anterior wall dysfunction who underwent both dobutamine echocardiography and FDG-PET before coronary revascularization. Six months after revascularization, 29 patients had improved wall motion and global ejection fraction and were considered to have viable myocardium, while the remaining 18 were considered to have nonviable myocardium. Dobutamine echocardiography alone correctly identified 86% of the patients with and 78% of those without viable myocardium. We then evaluated the results of a sequential strategy in which dobutamine echocardiography would have been performed in all patients, as a first step (because it is less expensive and more widely available), and PET only in those patients ($n = 18$) showing no evidence of viability with dobutamine. This strategy would have identified all 29 patients with viable myocardium and had therefore the highest sensitivity (100%), while it retained a satisfactory specificity (67%). Such a sequential approach could thus obviate the performance of PET in about two-thirds of the patients.

Prognostic Value of Dobutamine Echocardiography

While there is little doubt that dobutamine echocardiography enables accurate prediction of reversible dysfunction after coronary revascularization, preliminary data are now emerging as to its prognostic implications in patients with LV dysfunction. In a series of 136 consecutive patients with moderate or severe LV dysfunction (ejection fraction 30 ± 5%) reported by Williams et al.[36] the presence of an ischemic or viable response was associated with a 46% event rate over the ensuing 16 ± 8 months, compared with a more stable pattern (8% event rate) associated with scar. Indeed, the presence of ischemic or viable tissue was the most important independent predictor of events (adjusted χ^2 5.7, $p = 0.02$).

We recently performed a 21-month (1 to 48 months) follow-up of 150 consecutive patients with coronary disease and depressed LVEF (36% ± 14%) who had undergone low-dose dobutamine echocardiography.[36a] Coronary revascularization was performed in 99 patients (77 by surgery, 22 by angioplasty), and the remaining 51 patients were treated medically. Four groups were retrospectively defined according to treatment strategy and the results of the pretreatment dobutamine echocardiographic study. Twenty-five patients (19%) died of cardiac causes during follow-up. As shown in Figure 23-6, analysis of Kaplan-Meier survival curves indicated that the 3-year survival rate was significantly better in the group of patients with echocardiographic evidence of myocardial viability who had been revascularized (61 of 63, 97%) than in any other groups of patients (23 of 31 [74%] in those with viable myocardium treated medically; 26 of 36 [72%] in those with nonviable myocardium undergoing revascularization, 15 of 20 [75%] in those with nonviable myocardium treated medically). These data suggest that among patients with LV ischemic dysfunction, only those with residual inotropic reserve invariably benefit from coronary revascularization in terms of survival. These data thus lend further support to the use of dobutamine echocardiography for assessment of myocardial viability, as this technique not only allows accurate identification of which patient will improve regional and global LV function after coronary revascularization, but also may indicate those most likely to benefit with respect to prognosis.

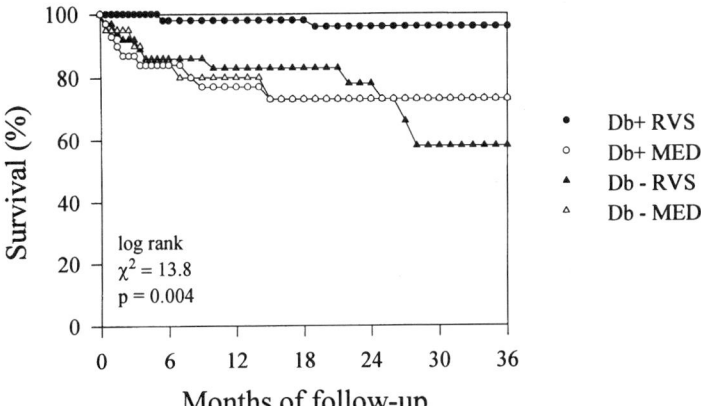

Fig. 23-6 Kaplan-Meier survival curves of cardiac death in 150 patients with left ventricular ischemic dysfunction categorized into those with (Db+) and without (Db−) residual inotropic reserve and undergoing either revascularization (RVS) or medical treatment (MED).

Potential Limitations of Dobutamine Echocardiography for Prediction of Myocardial Viability

Despite the very encouraging results of dobutamine echocardiography for delineation of myocardial viability, a few caveats are nonetheless appropriate. First, the changes in regional wall motion seen during low-dose dobutamine infusion are often quite subtle (hypokinetic tissue becoming more normal or akinetic tissue developing hypokinesis), requiring both sophisticated digital processing and highly expert interpretation. Most of the studies reported so far were performed by investigators who have been in the field of stress-echocardiography for many years and who have acquired an enormous experience in the analysis of digital echocardiographic loops. Despite this wealth of expertise, disagreement between experienced observers has been noted in as much as 10% of the readings. It is unlikely that the average echocardiographer will ever achieve such a high level of expertise, unless she or he has the discipline to ensure adequate interpretation of regional wall motion. Thus, the accuracy of the method is likely to decrease as it becomes more widely utilized by less experienced observers. Another difficulty with this technique is the extremely transient nature of the improvement in wall motion in some patients. That wall motion frequently and rapidly degrades after initial improvement makes the detection of the initial improvement all the more uncertain, especially with the semiquantitative categorical grading system used in most echocardiographic analysis. Finally, the difficulty of obtaining echocardiograms of diagnostic quality in every patient must be acknowledged. Although in experienced hands, the number of patients in whom the appropriate diagnostic information cannot be obtained is probably less than 5% to 10%, this number will likely be higher among technicians or echocardiographers with less experience.

PREDICTION OF FUNCTIONAL RECOVERY WITH MYOCARDIAL CONTRAST ECHOCARDIOGRAPHY

Recently, myocardial contrast echocardiography (MCE) has been investigated for prediction of functional recovery after myocardial infarction.[37] This technique, which is currently limited to the cardiac catherization laboratory, employs the intracoronary injection of air microbubbles and the imaging of their transmural distribution with two-dimensional echocardiography.[37] During acute coronary occlusion, MCE was shown experimentally to allow determination of residual collateral-dependent perfusion [30,38] and to provide excellent delineation of the area at risk.[39] Following reperfusion, the myocardial distribution of the echo-contrast may permit evaluation of spatial patterns of flow and hence the amount of salvaged myocardium, provided that sufficient time is allowed between reflow and the echo-contrast investigation.[39,40] The persistence of significant reactive hyperemia during the early hours of reperfusion may indeed lead to underestimation of infarct size by myocardial contrast echocardiography, particularly when the residual stenosis on the infarct-related vessel is not severe enough to attenuate the hyperemic response.[41] Twenty-four hours after reperfusion, however, when hyperemia is no longer present, MCE provides excellent estimation of infarct size.

MCE has also been used for the prediction of reversible dysfunction after myocardial infarction. Several experimental studies have demonstrated that in acute myocardial infarction, myocellular necrosis was often associated with the loss of microvascular integrity,[40,42] whereas the presence of residual microvascular perfusion within the risk area usually indicated the presence of viable myocardium.[40] Accordingly, several groups have investigated whether the persistence of residual myocardial perfusion, as determined by MCE, could be valuable in identifying patients whose LV function will recover after successful thrombolysis. Ito et al.[43] assessed the recovery of microvascular perfusion in 39 consecutive patients with a first anterior myocardial infarction. MCE was performed before and immediately upon restoration of coronary patency by intracoronary thrombolysis or direct angioplasty. They observed that despite successful recanalization of the infarct-related artery, more than a quarter of patients had severe persistent perfusion deficit by MCE and did not normalize myocardial function at follow-up. This contrasted with the situation in patients whose microvascular perfusion improved after recanalization who demonstrated an improved regional wall motion and global ejection fraction at follow-up. Along the same lines, Ragosta et al.[44] performed MCE in 105 patients undergoing cardiac catheterization within the first week of a first acute myocardial infarction. They calculated a contrast score index (combining the severity and extent of the perfusion defect by MCE) for each patient; this index was then correlated with the improvement of wall motion score after 1 month. Among the clinical, angiographic, and echocardiographic variables analyzed in this study, the contrast score index was the single most powerful independent correlate of the 1-month functional recovery ($r = -0.64$, $p < 0.001$). Agati et al.,[45] and more recently Camarano et al.,[46] confirmed these initial observations, thus supporting further the use of MCE for assessing microvascular perfusion and viability in patients with reperfused myocardial infarction.

Currently, MCE requires injection of the air mi-

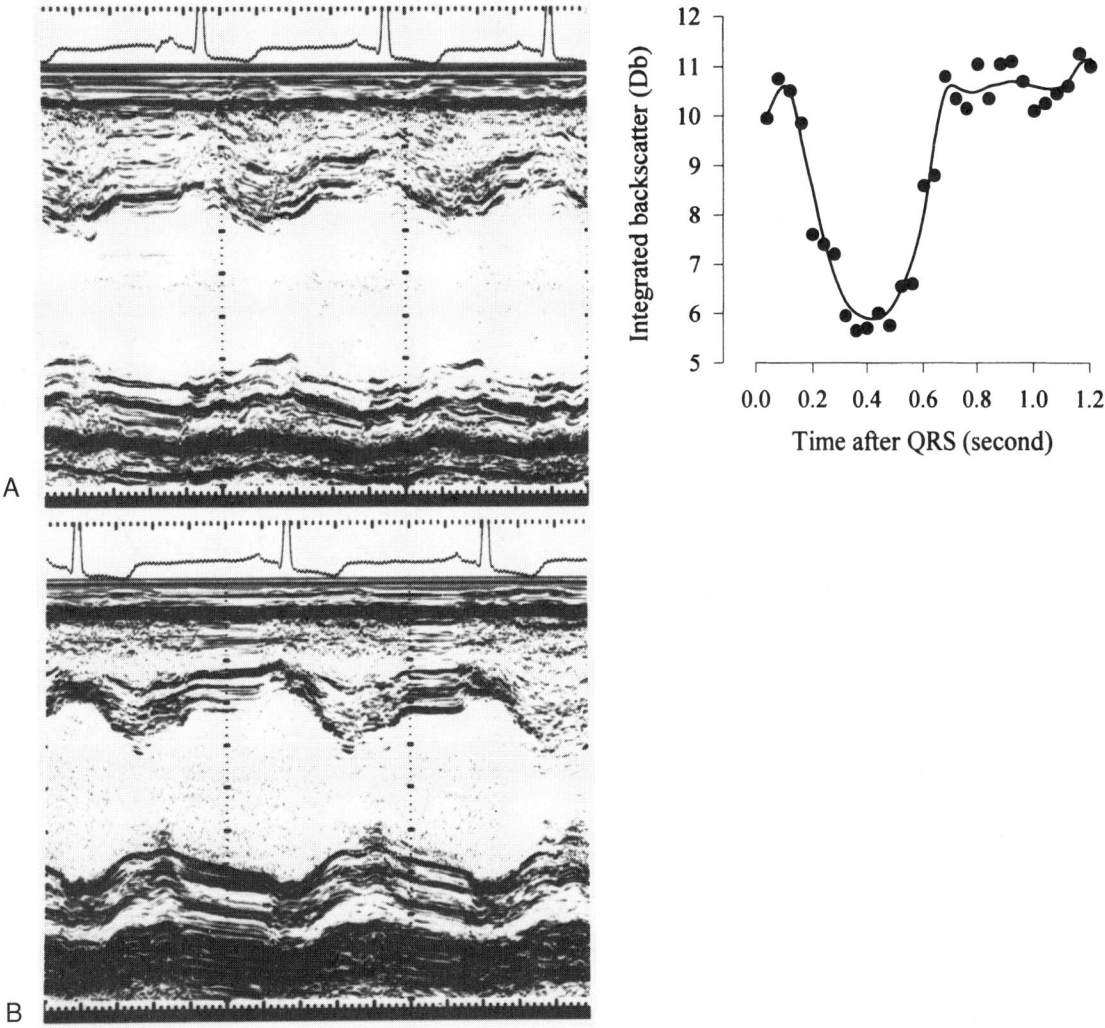

Fig. 23-7 Representative M-mode echocardiographic recordings of the left ventricular septum and anterior wall (**A**) before and (**B**) after revascularization are shown along with the amplitude of the time-dependent cyclic variations of integrated backscatter in the anterior wall before revascularization (**C**). Note that despite complete akinesis, significant cyclic variations of integrated backscatter are present in the anterior wall before revascularization, portending the improvement in systolic wall thickening after revascularization.

crobubbles directly in the aortic root via a pigtail catheter positioned in the ascending aorta, which limits its potential use to patients undergoing cardiac catheterization. The development of newer contrast agents that can cross the pulmonary capillary bed (and can therefore be injected intravenously) will probably improve the clinical applicability of this new and promising approach, possibly to include patients with chronic LV dysfunction.

ULTRASONIC TISSUE CHARACTERIZATION FOR PREDICTION OF FUNCTIONAL RECOVERY

Ultrasonic tissue characterization provides a novel approach for defining the physical state of myocardium that complements assessment of LV wall motion and chamber dimensions by two-dimension echocardiography. Recent studies have indicated that physiologic myocardial contraction and relaxation were paralleled by a cycle-dependent variation of integrated backscatter that reflects regional, intramural contractile performance and that cyclic variations of the backscatter signal were preserved in stunned as opposed to infarcted myocardium, despite similar severity of regional dysfunction.[47] This approach has been recently used in patients with reperfused myocardial infarction and was shown to allow accurate delineation of reversible (stunning) from irreversible (infarction) injury, thus providing a potentially useful adjunct for noninvasive evaluation of regional contractile function and for the detection of potentially reversible dysfunction (Fig. 23-7).[48] Its application to more chronic circumstances, however, awaits further study.

CONCLUSIONS

Echocardiography is the least expensive and most versatile cardiac imaging test, and has been found to be effective for the diagnosis of myocardial ischemia. Dobutamine echocardiography has recently emerged as a safe, noninvasive, and accurate means of identification of viable myocardium, as well. The clinically relevant data regarding the recovery of regional function are obtained by use of doses less than 10 μg/kg/min, while detection of inducible ischemia at a distance or within the dysfunctional area usually requires higher doses (up to 40 μg/kg/min). Several studies have now demonstrated that dobutamine echocardiography allows prediction of which patient is likely to improve LV function after coronary revascularization, as well as defining the prognosis of individual patients with CAD. The application of new echocardiographic features (contrast, backscatter) to this modality is likely to further strengthen its promise as a test for myocardial viability.

REFERENCES

1. Emond M, Mock MB, Davis KB et al.: Long-term survival of medically-treated patients in the Coronary Artery Surgery Study (CASS) registry. Circulation 90: 2645, 1994
2. Alderman EL, Fisher LD, Litwin P et al.: Results of coronary artery bypass surgery in patients with poor left ventricular function (CASS). Circulation 68:785, 1983
3. Eitzman D, Al-Aouar Z, Kanter HL et al.: Clinical outcome of patients with advanced coronary artery disease after viability studies with positron emission tomography. J Am Coll Cardiol 20:559, 1992
4. Lee KS, Marwick TH, Cook SA et al.: Prognosis of patients with left ventricular dysfunction, with and without viable myocardium after myocardial infarction. Relative efficacy of medical therapy and revascularization. Circulation 90:2687, 1994
5. Di Carli MF, Davidson M, Little R et al.: Value of metabolic imaging with positron emission tomography for evaluating prognosis in patients with coronary artery disease and left ventricular dysfunction. Am J Cardiol 73:527, 1994
6. Tennant R, Wiggers CJ: The effects of coronary occlusion on myocardial contraction. Am J Physiol 112:351, 1935
7. Heyndrickx GR, Millard RW, Mc Ritchie RJ et al.: Regional myocardial functional and electrophysiological alterations after brief coronary occlusions in conscious dogs. J Clin Invest 56:978, 1975
8. Bolli R: Myocardial "stunning" in man. Circulation 86: 1671, 1992
9. Rahimtoola SH: The hibernating myocardium. Am Heart J 117:211, 1989
10. Vanoverschelde JLJ, Wijns W, Deprè C et al.: Mechanisms of chronic regional postischemic dysfunction in humans: New insights from the study of non-infarcted collateral dependent myocardium. Circulation 87: 1513,1993

11. Depre, C, Vanoverschelde J-L, Melin JA et al.: Structural and metabolic correlates of the reversibility of chronic left ventricular ischemic dysfunction in humans. Am J Physiol 268:H1265, 1995
12. Borgers M, Thonè F, Wouters L et al.: Structural correlates of regional myocardial dysfunction in patients with critical coronary artery stenosis: Chronic hibernation? Cardiovasc Pathol 2:237, 1993
13. Becker LC, Levine JH, DiPaula AF et al.: Reversal of dysfunction in postischemic stunned myocardium by epinephrine and postextrasystolic potentiation. J Am Coll Cardiol 7:580, 1986
14. Ellis SG, Wynne J, Braunwald E et al.: Response of reperfusion-salvaged, stunned myocardium to inotropic stimulation. Am J Heart J 107:13, 1984
15. Sklenar J, Ismail S, Villanueva S, Goodman C et al.: Dobutamine echocardiography for determining the extent of myocardial salvage after reperfusion. An experimental evaluation. Circulation 90:1502, 1994
16. Chen C, Li L, Chen LL et al.: Incremental doses of dobutamine induce a biphasic response in dysfunctional left ventricular regions subtending coronary stenoses. Circulation 92:756, 1995
17. Gerber B, Laycock SK, Melin JA et al.: Perfusion-contraction matching, inotropic reserve and vasodilatory capacity in a canine model of dysfunctional collateral-dependent myocardium, abstracted. Circulation 92:I-314, 1995
18. Nesto RW, Cohn LH, Collins JJ et al.: Inotropic contractile reserve: a useful predictor of increased 5-year survival and improved postoperative left ventricular function in patients with coronary artery disease and reduced ejection fraction. Am J Cardiol 50:39, 1982
19. Piérard LA, De Landsheere CM, Berthe C et al.: Identification of viable myocardium by echocardiography during dobutamine infusion in patients with myocardial infarction after thrombolytic therapy: comparison with position emission tomography. J Am Coll Cardiol 15:1021, 1990
20. Barilla F, Gheorghiade M, Alam M et al.: Low-dose dobutamine in patients with acute myocardial infarction identifies viable but not contractile myocardium and predicts the magnitude of improvement in wall motion abnormalities in response to coronary revascularization. Am Heart J 122:1522, 1991
21. Previtali M, Poli A, Lanzarini L et al.: Dobutamine stress echocardiography for assessment of myocardial viability and ischemia in acute myocardial infarction treated with thrombolysis. Am J Cardiol 72:124G, 1993
22. Watada H, Ito H, Oh H et al.: Dobutamine stress echocardiography predicts reversible dysfunction and quantitates the extent of irreversible damaged myocardium after reperfusion of anterior myocardial infarction. J Am Coll Cardiol 24:624, 1995
23. Smart SC, Sawada S, Ryan T et al.: Low-dose dobutamine echocardiography detects reversible dysfunction after thrombolytic therapy of acute myocardial infarction. Circulation 88:405, 1993
24. Marzullo P, Parodi O, Reisenhofer B et al.: Value of rest thallium-201 / technetium-99m sestamibi scans and dobutamine echocardiography for detecting myocardial viability. Am J Cardiol 71:166, 1993
25. Alfieri O, La Canna G, Giubbini R et al.: Recovery of myocardial function: The ultimate target of coronary revascularization. Eur J Cardio-Thorax Surg 7:325, 1993
26. Cigarroa CG, deFilippi CR, Brickner E et al.: Dobutamine stress echocardiography identifies hibernating myocardium and predicts recovery of left ventricular function after coronary revascularization. Circulation 88:430, 1993
27. La Canna G, Alfieri O, Giubbini R et al.: Echocardiography during infusion of dobutamine for identification of reversible dysfunction in patients with coronary artery disease. J Am Coll Cardiol 23:617, 1994
28. Perrone-Filardi P, Pace L, Prastaro M et al.: Dobutamine echocardiography predicts improvement of hypoperfused dysfunctional myocardium after revascularization in patients with coronary artery disease. Circulation 91:2556, 1995
29. Vanoverschelde J-L, Gerber BL, D'Hondt A-M et al.: Preoperative selection of patients with severely impaired left ventricular function for coronary revascularization: Role of low-dose dobutamine echocardiography and exercise-redistribution-reinjection thallium SPECT. Circulation 92:II-37, 1995
30. Afridi I, Kleiman NS, Raizner AE et al.: Dobutamine echocardiography in myocardial hibernation. Optimal dose and accuracy in predicting recovery of ventricular function after coronary angioplasty. Circulation 91:663, 1995
31. Panza JA, Dilsizian V, Laurienzo JM et al.: Relation between thallium uptake and contractile response to dobutamine. Implications regarding myocardial viability in patients with chronic coronary artery disease and left ventricular dysfunction. Circulation 91:990, 1995
32. Arnese M, Cornel JH, Salustri A et al.: Prediction of improvement of regional left ventricular function after surgical revascularization. A comparison of low-dose dobutamine echocardiography with ^{201}Tl single photon emission computed tomography. Circulation 91:2748, 1995

33. Vanoverschelde J-L, D'Hondt A-M, Marwick TH et al: Head to head comparison of exercise-redistribution—reinjection thallium SPECT and low-dose dobutamine ecocardiography for prediction of the reversibility of chronic left ventricular ischemic dysfunction. J Am Coll Cardiol, in press, 1996
33a. Williams J, Odabashian J, Lytle B et al.: Prediction of viable myocardium in severe left ventricular dysfunction—Follow-up study of dobutamine echocardiography and positron emission tomography, abstracted. Circulation 92:I-266, 1995
34. Baer FM, Voth E, Deutsch HJ et al.: Assessment of viable myocardium by dobutamine transesophageal echocardiography and comparison with fluorine-18 fluorodeoxyglucose positron emission tomography. J Am Coll Cardiol 24:343, 1994
35. Gerber B, Vanoverschelde J-L, Bol A et al.: Sequential use of dobutamine echo and PET to identify viable myocardium. Circulation (abstract) (in press), 1995
36. Williams MJ, Odabashian J, Lauer MS et al.: Prognostic value of dobutamine echocardiography in patients with left ventricular dysfunction. J Am Coll Cardiol (in press), 1996
36a. Pasquet A, Gerber B, D'Hondt A-M et al.: Value of dobutamine echocardiography and FDG-PET in evaluating prognosis in patients with chronic left ventricular ischemic dysfunction, abstracted. Circulation 92:I–268, 1995
37. Kaul S: Assessment of coronary microcirculation with myocardial contrast echocardiography: current and future clinical applications. Br Heart J 71:490, 1995
38. Sabia PJ, Powers ER, Ragosta M et al.: An association between collateral blood flow and myocardial viability in patients with recent myocardial infarction. N Engl J Med 327:1825, 1992
39. Villanueva FS, Glasheen WP, Sklenar J et al.: Assessment of risk area during coronary occlusion and infarct size after reperfusion with myocardial contrast echocardiography using left and right atrial injections of contrast. Circulation 88:596, 1993
40. Villanueva FS, Glasheen WP, Sklenar J et al.: Characterization of spatial patterns of flow within reperfused myocardium using myocardial contrast echocardiography. Implications in determining the extent of myocardial salvage. Circulation 88:2596, 1993
41. Kaul S, Pandian NG, Guerrero JL et al.: The effects of selectively altering the collateral driving pressure on regional perfusion and function in the occluded coronary bed in the dog. Circ Res 61:77, 1987
42. Kloner RA, Ganote CE, Jennings RB: The "no-reflow" phenomenon after temporary coronary occlusion in the dog. J Clin Invest 54:1496, 1974
43. Ito H, Tommoka T, Sakai N et al.: Lack of myocardial perfusion after successful thrombolysis: a predictor of poor recovery of left ventricular function in anterior infarction. Circulation 85:1699, 1992
44. Ragosta M, Camarano G, Kaul S et al.: Microvascular integrity indicates myocellular viability in patients with recent myocardial infarction. New insights using myocardial contrast echocardiography. Circulation 89:2562, 1994
45. Agati L, Voci P, Bilotta F et al.: Influence of residual perfusion within the infarct zone on the natural history of left ventricular dysfunction after acute myocardial infarction. A contrast echocardiography study. J Am Coll Cardiol 24:336, 1994
46. Camarano G, Ragosta M, Grimple LW et al.: Identification of viable myocardium with myocardial contrast echocardiography in patients with poor left ventricular systolic function caused by recent or remote myocardial infarction. Am J Cardiol 75:215, 1995
47. Milunski MR, Mohr GA, Wear KA et al.: Early identification with ultrasonic integrated backscatter of viable but stunned myocardium in dogs. J Am Coll Cardiol 14:462, 1989
48. Milunski MR, Mohr GA, Pèrez JE et al.: Ultrasonic tissue characterization with integrated backscatter. Acute myocardial ischemia, reperfusion, and stunned myocardium in patients. Circulation 80:491, 1989

Chapter 24

Role of Functional Testing for Prognostic Evaluation

W. Wijns and Thomas H. Marwick

SCOPE OF THE PROBLEM

Clinical Decision-Making

In clinical medicine, decisions regarding therapeutic interventions should inevitably include an evaluation of the patient's prognosis, albeit implicitly. Most patients with coronary artery disease (CAD) have mild symptoms, which are easily controlled by medication and adaptation of the life-style. Revascularization procedures are prescribed to reduce the uncertainty about possible future events and prevent any reduction in life expectancy from sudden death or infarction. While the number of therapeutic options for patients with CAD has increased recently, many such options are a source of both potential complications and cost. Therefore, an accurate evaluation of prognosis has become mandatory. The ability to identify low-risk subjects in whom medical care will portend a very low long-term event rate is as important as the ability to identify patients at high risk for subsequent death or infarction. Identification of the latter will enable the selection of procedures that have a demonstrable impact on the natural history of the disease.

The art of clinical decision making is to select the path with the smallest risk (and cost) for any given patient. To this end, data on natural history and treatment effects need to be considered. Mortality and infarction are appropriate endpoints for these studies, while the need for revascularization is less desirable, as illustrated in recent trials on primary coronary stenting. In the Benestent[1] trial, for instance, the incidence of clinical events was significantly ($p = 0.017$) reduced in patients randomized to stent implantation (20.1%) versus balloon dilatation (29.6%). Yet, statistical significance was entirely accounted for by the reduced rate of repeat target lesion revascularization in the stent group while no difference in mortality or infarction rates was observed. Skeptics have argued that the need for repeat percutaneous transluminal coronary angioplasty (PTCA) or coronary artery bypass grafting (CABG) represents a soft end-point, which may be reached for reasons that are highly susceptible to patient and doctor prejudice.

Numerous useful prognosticators are readily available at little cost from the patient's history, physical examination, and resting electrocardiogram (ECG).[2] A number of reports have indicated that the use of stress imaging tests is of limited value in patients with normal resting ECGs. The question thus arises as to which patients with known or suspected CAD should undergo additional functional evaluation; this question will be addressed for different patient groups, according to the clinical presentation of the disease.

Unresolved issues

Much is known about the risk stratification of patients with CAD, but there remain important unresolved areas. For example, the diagnosis of CAD is more difficult in women than in men, because many tests are gender sensitive and yield a higher proportion of technically less adequate studies in women. An illustration of this would be the problem of breast attenuation with nuclear studies, which may affect their prognostic value as much as their diagnostic accuracy.[3] Together with the fact that the natural history of CAD is less well known in women than in men,[4] these problems suggest that the prognostic evaluation of women with CAD deserves more attention in future studies. Without these data, it will be difficult to evaluate the beneficial or detrimental impact of therapeutic interventions, considering also the possibility that treatment modalities such as PTCA or CABG may be associated with an increased procedural risk in women.[5-7]

PATIENTS WITH KNOWN OR SUSPECTED CORONARY ARTERY DISEASE

Relationship of Risk to Jeopardized Tissue

As will be outlined in Chapters 25 to 27, overwhelming evidence indicates that the various cardiac stress tests convey important prognostic information when applied to patients with suspected CAD. At each test, indices of left ventricular dysfunction and, particularly, the extent and severity of inducible ischemia (whether painful or not) relate directly to the likelihood of adverse outcome. A very low incidence of events may be anticipated when little or no ischemia can be demonstrated, irrespective of the results of coronary arteriography.[8,9] The performance of coronary angiography in low-risk cases consumes resources unnecessarily, without generating prognostic benefit. Unfortunately, the avoidance of angiography in these situations, while predicated by many, is practiced by few.

The benefits of functional testing over angiography reflect the fact that the accumulation of plaque within coronary arterial walls usually remains a well-tolerated and mild disease for many years. A number of adaptive mechanisms result in preservation of a normal myocardial perfusion and contraction under resting conditions, even despite the presence of sometimes severe disease by arteriography.[10] At the coronary level, these adaptive mechanisms include compensatory wall remodeling[11] as well as the recruitment and development of collateral channels.[12] Indeed, in patients with seemingly comparable disease, there may be marked differences in the extent of plaque accumulation that are undetected by angiography, the residual flow reserve distal to obstructions, and the efficacy of collateral blood supply, all of which will influence the functional response to stress testing. In other words, in the low-risk patient, a good response to stress reveals that the adaptive mechanisms acting both at the coronary and myocardial level still permit normal cardiac function despite the progressive accumulation of atherosclerotic plaque. Conversely, a positive stress result indicates the level of residual myocardial perfusion and/or contraction reserve, thereby identifying those parts of the myocardium that are potentially jeopardized and need to be protected by revascularization. Under those circumstances, bypass surgery (and presumably PTCA) will result in a lower incidence of subsequent cardiac events when compared with medical therapy.[13]

Life-threatening events such as unstable angina and myocardial infarction result from acute plaque rupture at sites with only moderate stenosis.[14-16] Abnormal responses to stress merely result from the presence of severe flow-limiting stenoses, and none of the noninvasive tests can detect mild coronary lesions that are prone to disruption. Thus, it might seem paradoxical that cardiac stress testing and imaging would have any predictive value at all—but yet, the powerful predictive value of each stress testing modality has been undoubtedly established. These findings may be reconciled if one considers that the predictive value of stress testing results from the integration of a number of variables that are important for the patient's outcome, *should* an acute plaque event and coronary occlusion occur.[17]

Clinical Implications

Given the influential role of the presence of jeopardized myocardium on prognosis and the poor correlation of symptom status with disease extent, we believe that all patients with suspected or known stable CAD should undergo some form of stress testing for

Table 24-1. Mortality Rates by Risk Groups Based on the VA Prognostic Score^a

	3-yr Mortality (%)	Patients %
Low Risk	< -2	2	77
Moderate Risk	-2 to $+2$	7	18
High Risk	$> +2$	15	6

^{a} The VA score incorporates signs of heart failure and exercise variables (ST segment depression, changes in blood pressure, exercise capacity).
(Adapted from Marcus et al.[19], with permission.)

prognostic evaluation. The selection of tests for prognostic purposes parallels that for diagnostic purposes; individuals with nondiagnostic stress ECG, or those unable to exercise maximally, require some form of stress-imaging study. Of those who are able to exercise and have a normal resting ECG—which infers normal resting ventricular function—little incremental benefit is obtained by performance of a stress imaging test.[18] Whichever test is used, its findings may be applied as a gatekeeper for diagnostic coronary angiography (Table 24-1).[19]

A difficult (and all too frequent) scenario arises when the results of coronary angiography are available in the absence of any functional evaluation. The performance of revascularization in low-risk patients is controversial, although when disease has been visualized, both the patient and the doctor are eager to have the problem fixed, for example by PTCA. Published guidelines require that only hemodynamically significant stenoses should undergo PTCA or related procedures, so that the demonstration of inducible ischemia, albeit painless, should be required before coronary interventions are applied.[20,21] However, a recently published survey has shown that evidence of demonstrable ischemia was present in only a minority of the PTCA cases that had been reviewed.[22] This problem relates to practical issues; ad hoc PTCA[23] is being performed more frequently, leaving no time for adequate functional testing, if these are unavailable before angiography. The advent of velocity and pressure monitoring guidewires that can be used during catheterization for the invasive measurement of velocity or fractional flow reserve certainly represents a unique opportunity to interrogate the physiologic significance of a given stenosis during the procedure.[24,25] The prognostic value of these studies has been recently demonstrated, particularly in patients who were denied intervention based on preserved flow velocity reserve,[26] and they may be used as a surrogate for the results of noninvasive stress tests.[27,28] A detailed discussion of these techniques is presented in Chapter 15.

PATIENTS WITH CHRONIC ISCHEMIC LEFT VENTRICULAR DYSFUNCTION

In the presence of a *moderately* depressed left ventricular function resulting from prior healed myocardial infarction, revascularized patients enjoy a survival benefit.[13] In this group of patients with permanently reduced functional reserve, the identification of jeopardized myocardium in vascular supply regions that are remote from the infarcted area has a strong independent value for the prediction of improved prognosis following revascularization.[29]

In patients with *severely* depressed left ventricular function, prognosis is poor. In a subset of patients with large areas of hibernating myocardium, functional improvement can be anticipated following revascularization.[30] However, revascularization usually requires CABG, as multivessel coronary disease is usually present, and the risk of surgery in this group is substantial.[31] The use of functional studies permits the detection of viable myocardium, which is associated with adverse outcome if left nonrevascularized.[32] These tests may thus alter surgical planning to the extent of referral of patients for heart transplantation or assist devices.

PATIENTS WITH ACUTE CORONARY SYNDROMES

The Acute Chest Pain Syndrome

Ruling out acute coronary insufficiency in patients presenting at the emergency room with chest pain syndromes is a daily task. The initial evaluation includes close clinical and ECG monitoring, repeated recording of 12-lead ECGs, and measurements of cardiac enzymes. In the absence of evidence of an ongoing ischemic insult, further evaluation is guided by the results of the noninvasive stress testing, most often using exercise, perhaps in combination with nuclear imaging procedures. Submission of all patients to diagnostic coronary arteriography will reveal apparently normal coronary arteries in a high proportion of cases.[33]

Unstable Angina Pectoris

In patients with documented unstable angina pectoris, prognostication can be readily achieved by using the Braunwald classification, which is based on the circumstances and the severity of anginal symptoms.[34] This clinical classification has been shown to be related to the angiographic evidence of instability (presence of complex lesions, intracoronary thrombus) and is predictive of further events.[35,36] The pattern of symmetric T-wave inversion in the anterior precordial leads is associated with proximal left anterior descending CAD and poor prognosis on medical treatment.[37] Continuous monitoring of the ST segment changes also permits the identification of a subgroup of patients in whom spontaneous changes in the severity of the unstable plaque and the ensuing episodes of flow reduction are associated with a poor outcome.[38,39] Thus, stress modalities have no place in the initial management of these patients.

From a physiopathologic point of view, plaque disruption is recognized as the initiating factor that precipitates acute coronary syndromes, although the majority of plaque events go unnoticed.[15,16] The outcome depends on the interplay between the importance of plaque rupture, the size of the intraluminal thrombus, the efficacy of the fibrinolytic system, local blood flow, and collateral perfusion to the distal myocardium. Repair processes involve proliferation of neo-intima and production of new connective tissue leading to plaque stability again, as shown on Plate 24-1.[40,41]

The major clinical dilemma is whether these reparative processes will be successful and can be given the time to operate without taking the chance of an acute infarction to occur. Therefore, useful indications to guide therapy in the individual patient are not likely to be obtainable from stress testing but rather from biological markers reflecting the interaction between plaque and its milieu.[42,43]

Subsequently, when symptoms eventually stabilize, protagonists of the invasive approach would recommend systematic angiography and revascularization. With the more conservative strategy, patients are first submitted to a functional study, the results of which determine the indication for coronary angiography and guide the decision for revascularization.[44] At present, there is no consensus on which of these approaches is preferable, nor on the ideal timing for performing the invasive study. Randomized data from the TIMI IIIB trial showed no difference in terms of mortality, infarction, and revascularization at 1 year between early, routine angiography versus initial conservative therapy with revascularization for recurrent ischemia.[45] Furthermore, the use of thrombolytic therapy was found to be of no benefit in patients with unstable angina.[46]

Acute Myocardial Infarction

The prognosis of patients suffering from an evolving myocardial infarction can be derived from history, clinical examination, and the ECG, and the performance of stress testing is appropriate only after stabilization of these patients. There is an ongoing controversy regarding the relative merits of the conservative approach (thrombolysis without any delay) versus the invasive approach (immediate revascularization).[47] A detailed discussion of all the issues is beyond the scope of this chapter, but a few points are relevant to the role of stress testing in this context.

The debate stems from the recognition that even aggressive thrombolysis does not result in optimal reperfusion (i.e., TIMI III grade flow) in most cases, one out of many factors being the incomplete patency of the epicardial vessel.[48,49] As a consequence, the degree of myocardial salvage is marginal, and both the residual viability of the distal myocardium and the potential for stress-inducible ischemia have to be considered when evaluating the need for subsequent revascularization. Although some argue that having a patent vessel subtending dead myocardium is of prognostic importance, none of the currently completed randomized trials supports the systematic use of percutaneous revascularization.[45,50] This is irrespective of the period following thrombolysis that was selected for performing the invasive study. Thus, the triage of patients into conservative or aggressive treatment strategies after thrombolysis should be based on the detection of both inotropic reserve and inducible ischemia within the infarcted zone. To this end, as discussed in Chapters 13 and 26, pharmacologic stress echocardiography, which can be performed safely early after infarction, appears currently to be the most appropriate and easily applicable technique.

CLINICAL APPLICATION OF PROGNOSTIC TESTING: A CRITICAL REVIEW

The Independent and Incremental Benefits of Functional Testing

Integrating the published data on the prognostic value of functional testing in the clinical decision process often appears difficult for several reasons. Results are frequently presented as group mortality rates or survival or event-free curves, none of which can be easily translated into probability figures applicable to an individual patient. Just as disease prevalence influences diagnostic accuracy, the predictive value of any test depends on the event rate in the population under study, being maximal when the event rate is highest (for example, around 50%). Since death or infarction are rather unlikely events in coronary patients in general, stress testing is more accurate in predicting good than poor outcome. Therefore many "statistically significant" results are the consequence of the inclusion of (nearly) normal subjects in whom prognosis is not an issue, as can be judged from simple interrogation. Thus, study populations should be representative of the patients in whom prognosis actually needs to be evaluated.

To be practically useful, one would require an estimate of the event rate expressed either as an odds ratio or as a probability figure, together with its confidence limits. More important than determining the univariate prognostic value of testing, its benefit must be shown to be incremental, beyond that of readily available clinical data.[51–53] The need for studies integrating all information available to the clinician is not different whether diagnosis or prognosis is to be evaluated.

The Place of Coronary Angiography

Coronary angiography has numerous limitations, particularly when it comes to prognosis.[54] As discussed above, the main reason for this is that life-threatening events result from acute plaque disruption, and vulnerable plaque prone to instability may not necessarily be severe in terms of diameter reduction on the coronary angiogram. In fact, while the probability of plaque rupture is much higher with increasing stenosis severity, the majority of events still occur at moderately stenosed sites because the number of mild lesions far outweighs the severe ones.[16,40] Many of these sites may not even be detectable at angiography because plaque mostly becomes visible only when the encroachment on the luminal area exceeds 40%. This dissociation between prognosis and coronary angiography forms the basis for criticizing the ongoing "preoccupation with coronary lumenology" and justifies the increasing interest for imaging techniques, such as intravascular ultrasound, which interrogate the coronary wall, rather than the lumen.

At the same time, it would be foolish to deny any prognostic value to the coronary arteriogram. Certain anatomic subsets (left-main and triple-vessel disease) are associated with poor outcome, and this simple finding is sufficient to trigger revascularization.[13,56] A more careful and detailed analysis of the morphology of coronary lesions permits the identification of sites that are prone to induce unstable symptoms or to increase in severity, at least in the short term.[57,58] Patient stratification on the basis of the crude distinction between single, double, and triple vessel disease has unfortunately gained wide clinical acceptance. However, a better description of the degree of plaque accumulation and the amount of myocardium at risk has been obtained by use of several coronary scores, taking into account the severity of the stenoses, their location, the collateral circulation, and the contraction pattern of the myocardium.[59] When applied to the large population of the Coronary Artery Surgery Study (CASS), several of these coronary scores were shown to convey powerful prognostic information, similar to the degree of prognostication achieved by the ventriculogram, as illustrated by Figure 24-1.

Clinical studies on prognosis should be oriented toward the patient (rather than technique). Quite often, prognostic information available to the physician is neglected while every effort is made to promote the use of a single technique. As mentioned earlier, the most meaningful studies integrate all available data and by multivariate analysis or other

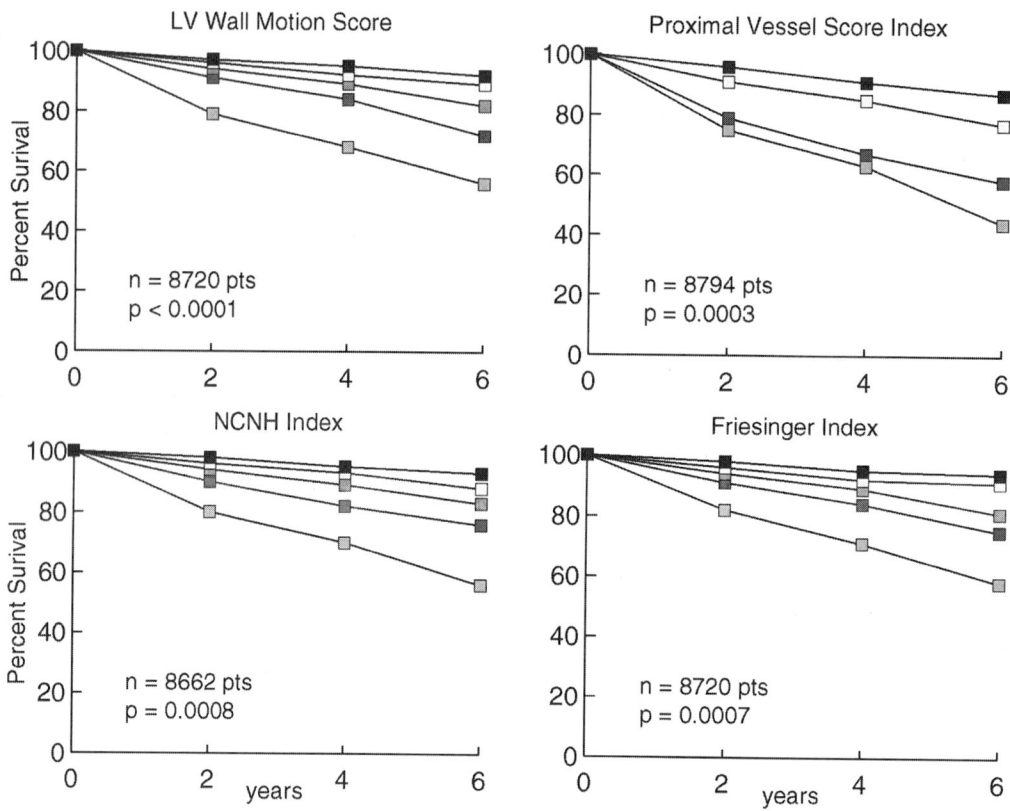

Fig. 24-1. Medical survival at 6 years for the left ventricular wall motion score ($p < 0.0001$) and for three coronary arteriographic indexes: the proximal vessel score index ($p = 0.0003$), the National Heart and Chest Hospital (NHCH) score ($p = 0.0008$) and the Friesinger index ($p = 0.0007$). The p values refer to the final p value in the stepwise Cox analysis of the prognostic value of nine angiographic indices of coronary artery disease. The coronary scores convey significant prognostic information that is independent from the ventricular function, while the number of diseased vessels do not. (Adapted from Ringqvist et al.,[59] with permission.)

statistically appropriate methods, allow the physician to select the combination of variables that will contribute to the most accurate prognostication in the individual patient.

REFERENCES

1. Serruys PW, De Jaegere P, Kiemeneij F et al: A comparison of balloon-expandable-stent implantation with balloon angioplasty in patients with coronary artery disease. N Engl J Med 331:489, 1994
2. Detre K, Peduzzi P, Murphy M et al: Effect of bypass surgery on survival in patients with low- and high-risk groups delineated by the use of simple clinical variables. Circulation 63:1329, 1981
3. Goodgold HM, Rehder JG, Samuels LD, Chaitman BR: Improved interpretation of exercise thallium-201 scintigraphy in women: characterization of breast attenuation artifacts. Radiology 165:361, 1987
4. Wenger NK, Speroff L, Packard B: Cardiovascular health and disease in women. N Engl J Med 329:247, 1993
5. Kelsey S, James M, Holubkov A et al: Results of percutaneous transluminal coronary angioplasty in women. 1985–1986 National Heart, Lung, and Blood Institute's Coronary Angioplasty registry. Circulation 87:720, 1993
6. Khan SS, Nessim S, Gray R et al: Increased mortality of women in coronary artery bypass surgery: evidence for referral bias. Ann Intern Med 112:561, 1990
7. Mickleborough LL, Takagi Y, Maruyama H et al: Is

sex a factor in determining operative risk for aortocoronary bypass graft surgery? Circulation 92:II-80, 1995
8. Gohlke H, Samek L, Betz P, Roskamm H: Exercise testing provides additional prognostic information in angiographically defined subgroups of patients with coronary artery disease. Circulation 68:979, 1983
9. Wijns W, Beauthier-Musschaert E, Van Domburg R et al: Prognostic value of symptom limited exercise testing in men with a high prevalence of coronary artery disease. Eur Heart J 6:939, 1985
10. Uren NG, Melin JA, de Bruyne B et al: Relation between myocardial blood flow and the severity of coronary artery stenosis. N Engl J Med 330:1782, 1994
11. Glagov S, Weisenberg E, Zarins CK et al: Compensatory enlargement of various human atherosclerotic coronary arteries. N Engl J Med 316:1371, 1987
12. Schaper W, Schaper J: Collateral Circulation. Heart, Brain, Kidney, Limbs. Kluwer Academic Publishers, Boston, 1993
13. Mark DB, Nelson CL, Califf RM et al: Continuing evolution of therapy for coronary artery disease. Initial results from the era of coronary angioplasty. Circulation 89:2015, 1995
14. Constantinides P: Plaque fissures in human coronary thrombosis. J Atheroscler Res 61:1, 1966
15. Davies MJ, Thomas AC: Plaque fissuring—the cause of acute myocardial infarction, sudden ischaemic death, and crescendo angina. Br Heart J 53:363, 1985
16. Falk E, Shah PK, Fuster V: Coronary plaque disruption. Circulation 92:657, 1995
17. Borges-Neto S, Puma J, Jones RH et al: Myocardial perfusion and ventricular function measurements during total coronary artery occlusion in humans: a comparison with rest and exercise radionuclide studies. Circulation 89:278, 1994
18. Christian TF, Miller TD, Bailey KR, Gibbons RJ: Exercise tomographic thallium-201 imaging in patients with severe coronary artery disease and normal electrocardiograms. Ann Intern Med 121:825, 1994
19. Marcus R, Lowe R III, Froelicher VF: The exercise test as gatekeeper. Limiting access or appropriately directing resources? Chest 107:1442, 1995
20. Ryan TJ, Faxon DP, Gunnar RM et al: Guidelines for percutaneous transluminal coronary angioplasty. A report of the American College of Cardiology/American Heart Association task force on assessment of diagnostic and therapeutic cardiovascular procedures (subcommittee on percutaneous transluminal coronary angioplasty). J Am Coll Cardiol 12:529, 1988. Circulation 78:486, 1988
21. Ryan TJ, Bauman WB, Kennedy JW et al: Guidelines for percutaneous transluminal coronary angioplasty. A report of the American Heart Association/American College of Cardiology task force on assessment of diagnostic and therapeutic cardiovascular procedures (committee on percutaneous transluminal coronary angioplasty). Circulation 88:2987, 1993. J Am Coll Cardiol 22:2033, 1993
22. Topol EJ, Ellis S, Cosgrove D et al: Analysis of coronary angiography practice in the United States with an insurance-claims data base. Circulation 87:1489, 1993
23. Meier B: Combining coronary angiography and angioplasty. Heart 75:8, 1996
24. Pijls NHJ, Van Son JAM, Kirkeeide RL et al: Experimental basis of determining maximum coronary, myocardial, and collateral blood flow by pressure measurements for assessing functional stenosis severity before and after percutaneous transluminal coronary angioplasty. Circulation 86:1354, 1993
25. Donohue TJ, Kern MJ, Aguirre FV et al: Assessing the hemodynamic significance of coronary artery stenoses: analysis of translesional pressure-flow velocity relationship in patients. J Am Coll Cardiol 22:449, 1993
26. Kern MJ, Donohue TJ, Aguirre FV et al: Clinical outcome of deferring angioplasty in patients with normal translesional pressure-flow velocity measurements. J Am Coll Cardiol 25:178, 1995
27. de Bruyne B, Bartunek J, Sys SU, Heyndrickx GR: Relation between myocardial fractional flow reserve calculated from coronary pressure measurements and exercise-induced myocardial ischemia. Circulation 92:39, 1995
28. Pijls NHJ, Van Gelder B, Van der Voort P et al: Fractional flow reserve. A useful index to evaluate the influence of an epicardial coronary stenosis on myocardial blood flow. Circulation 92:3183, 1995
29. Beller GA: Radionuclide assessment of prognosis. p. 137. In Zaret B, Beller GA (eds): Clinical Nuclear Cardiology. WB Saunders, Philadelphia, 1995
30. Braunwald E, Rutherford JD: Reversible ischemic left ventricular dysfunction: evidence for the hibernating myocardium. J Am Coll Cardiol 8:1467, 1986
31. Mickleborough LL, Maruyama H, Takagi Y et al: Results of revascularization in patients with severe left ventricular dysfunction. Circulation 92:II-73, 1995
32. Lee KS, Marwick TH, Cook SA et al: Prognosis of patients with left ventricular dysfunction, with and without viable myocardium after myocardial infarction. Relative efficacy of medical therapy and revascularization. Circulation 90:2687, 1994
33. Lee TH, Juarez G, Cook EF et al: Ruling out myocardial infarction—a prospective multicenter validation of a 12-hour strategy for patients at low risk. N Engl J Med 324:1239, 1991

34. Braunwald E: Unstable angina. A classification. Circulation 80:410, 1989
35. Ahmed WH, Bittl JA, Braunwald E: Relation between clinical presentation and angiographic findings in unstable angina pectoris, and comparison with that in stable angina. Am J Cardiol 72:544, 1993
36. Calvin JE, Klein LW, VandenBerg BJ et al: Risk stratification in unstable angina. Prospective validation of the Braunwald classification. JAMA 273:136, 1995
37. Haines DE, Raab DS, Gundel WD et al: Anatomic and prognostic significance of new T-wave inversion in unstable angina. Am J Cardiol 52:14, 1983
38. Gottlieb SO, Weisfeldt ML, Ouyang P et al: Silent ischemia as a marker for early unfavorable outcomes in patients with unstable angina. N Engl J Med 314:1214, 1986
39. Gottlieb SO, Weisfeldt ML, Ouyang P et al: Silent ischemia predicts infarction and death during 2-year follow-up of unstable angina. J Am Coll Card 10:756, 1987
40. Fuster V: Mechanisms leading to myocardial infarction: insights from studies of vascular biology. Circulation 90:2126, 1994
41. Davies MJ: Acute coronary thrombosis—the role of plaque disruption and its initiation and prevention. Eur Heart J 16:L-3, 1995
42. Liuzzo G, Biasucci LM, Gallimore JR et al: The prognostic value of C-reactive protein and serum amyloid A protein in severe unstable angina. N Engl J Med 331:417, 1994
43. Neri Serneri GG, Gensini GF, Poggesi L et al: The role of extraplatelet thromboxane A2 in unstable angina investigated with a dual thromboxane A2 inhibitor: importance of activated monocytes. Cor Art Dis 5:137, 1994
44. Butman SM, Olson HG, Gardin JM et al: Submaximal exercise testing after stabilization of unstable angina pectoris. J Am Coll Cardiol 4:667, 1984
45. The TIMI IIIB Investigators. Effects of tissue plasminogen activator and a comparison of early invasive and conservative strategies in unstable angina and non-Q wave myocardial infarction. Results of the TIMI IIIB trial. Circulation 89:1545, 1994
46. Topol EJ, Fuster V, Harrington RA et al: Recombinant hirudin for unstable angina pectoris. A multicenter, randomized angiographic trial. Circulation 89:1557, 1994
47. Michels KB, Yusuf S: Does PTCA in acute myocardial infarction affect mortality and reinfarction rates? A quantitative overview (meta-analysis) of the randomized clinical trials. Circulation 91:476, 1995
48. Simes RJ, Topol EJ, Holmes DR et al: Link between the angiographic substudy and mortality outcomes in a large randomized trial of myocardial reperfusion: the importance of early and complete infarct artery reperfusion. Circulation 91:1923, 1995
49. Lincoff MA, Topol EJ: Illusion of reperfusion. Does anyone achieve optimal reperfusion during acute myocardial infarction. Circulation 88:1361, 1993
50. Califf RM, Topol EJ, Gersh BJ: From myocardial salvage to patient salvage in acute myocardial infarction: the role of reperfusion therapy. J Am Coll Cardiol 14:1382, 1989
51. Lee KL, Pryor DB, Pieper KS et al: Prognostic value of radionuclide angiography in medically treated patients with coronary artery disease: a comparison with clinical and catheterization variables. Circulation 82:1705, 1990
52. Pollock SG, Abbott RD, Boucher CA et al: Independent and incremental prognostic value of tests performed in hierarchical order to evaluate patients with suspected coronary artery disease. Validation of models based on these tests. Circulation 85:237, 1992
53. Iskandrian AS, Heo J, Lemlek J et al: Identification of high-risk patients with left-main and three-vessel coronary artery disease using stepwise discriminant analysis of clinical, exercise and tomographic thallium data. Am Heart J 125:221, 1993
54. Little WC, Braden G, Applegate RJ: Angiographic evaluation of the extent and progression of coronary artery disease: limitations of "lumenology." Circulation 78:1157, 1988
55. Topol EJ, Nissen SE: Our preoccupation with coronary luminology. The dissociation between clinical and angiographic findings in ischemic heart disease. Circulation 92:2333, 1995
56. Campeau L, Corbara F, Crochet D et al: Left main coronary artery stenosis. The influence of aortocoronary bypass surgery on survival. Circulation 57:1111, 1978
57. Ambrose JA, Winters SL, Arora RR et al: Angiographic evolution of coronary artery morphology in unstable angina. J Am Coll Cardiol 7:472, 1986
58. Kaski JC, Chester MR, Chen L, Katritsis D: Rapid angiographic progression of coronary artery disease in patients with angina pectoris. The role of complex stenosis morphology. Circulation 92:2058, 1995
59. Ringqvist I, Fischer LD, Mock M et al: Prognostic value of angiographic indices of coronary artery disease from the Coronary Artery Surgery Study (CASS). J Clin Invest 71:1854, 1983

Chapter 25

Routine Exercise Electrocardiographic Testing for Prognostic Evaluation

Donald A. Weiner

The indications for performing exercise testing have evolved over the past 50 years.[1] Although initially used to assess functional capacity and heart rate and blood pressure responses to exercise, the test currently is also utilized to help confirm the presence and severity of coronary artery disease (CAD), to predict future coronary events among patients who have documented CAD or who have had a prior myocardial infarction, to screen asymptomatic individuals for silent myocardial ischemia, and to evaluate the effectiveness of medical or surgical therapy.[2] Despite all the recent technological advances in cardiac imaging techniques, standard exercise testing remains the most commonly ordered test for the assessment of patients with ischemic heart disease.

PROGNOSTIC VALUE OF EXERCISE TESTING

Assessment of the relative risk for subsequent cardiac events is an increasingly important aspect of the evaluation of patients with known CAD.[1,2] This risk is determined not only by the anatomic degree of coronary stenosis and by the degree of left ventricular dysfunction, but also by the physiological significance of the stenoses as determined by exercise testing with or without imaging techniques. Stratification of the risk for future coronary events can be made by analyzing multiple exercise test variables. Once higher risk patients are identified, they would be candidates for cardiac catheterization studies and coronary artery revascularization procedures.

Natural History of CAD

The prognostic value of exercise testing is best evaluated by analyzing several natural history studies of CAD.[3] Investigations performed 10 to 30 years ago evaluating the follow-up of patients with angina pectoris but without anatomic confirmation documented an overall annual mortality of 4 to 5%.[4–8] Other studies utilizing findings from cardiac catheterization showed that the annual mortality varied between 2% and 15%, according to the number of diseased coronary vessels and the left ventricular function.[9–12]

The more up-to-date survival data on medically treated patients with anatomically defined CAD emanate from three large multicenter clinical trials of coronary artery bypass graft (CABG) surgery.[13–15] These studies, which were started about 20 years ago and have follow-up data up to 15 years, revealed annual mortalities between 2.1% and 3.9%. The Coronary Artery Surgery Study (CASS) population, which excluded patients with left main CAD, disabling or unstable angina, and severe congestive heart failure, has shown an annual medical mortality of 2%.[15] The annual mortality may even be less today, given the wide proliferation of newer antianginal, antithrombotic, and antilipidemic medications. Identification of certain clinical factors such as a history of congestive heart failure and evidence of a prior myocardial infarction as well as baseline electrocardiographic (ECG) abnormalities were important predictors of higher risk.[16] For example, in the CASS trial, patients without heart failure had a 4-year survival rate of 90%, those with moderate heart failure had a survival of 62%, while those with severe heart failure had a very low survival rate of 18%.[17]

Stable Angina Pectoris

Risk stratification by exercise testing among patients with stable angina pectoris has been used to predict outcome and to identify patients who may have an improved survival following CABG surgery.[18] Four large studies[17,19–21] have correlated the results of exercise testing with outcome in patients with angina pectoris, as summarized in Table 25-1.

The Seattle Heart Watch study defined a high-risk group as patients with left ventricular dysfunction manifested by cardiomegaly, ability to exercise less than 3 minutes on the Bruce protocol, a peak systolic blood pressure of less than 130 mmHg during exercise testing, or a combination of these criteria.[19] The annual mortality rate of this high-risk group was 5.6%. By contrast, a low-risk group (no evidence of cardiomegaly, no exertional ischemia, and an absence of the nonischemic exercise parameters defined for the high-risk group) had an annual mortality rate of 1.2%. An intermediate-risk group (exertional myocardial ischemia alone) had an annual mortality rate of 2.2%. The study concluded that patients with preserved ventricular function and exercise tolerance, even with ischemia, have a good prognosis with medical therapy.

The Duke University Data Base study also identified a low-risk subgroup with a survival of 99% at 12 months and 93% at 48 months. This group was characterized by a negative exercise test result, an exercise duration greater than or equal to Stage IV of the Bruce protocol, a maximal heart rate of 160 or more beats/min, or any combination of these factors. By contrast, patients with a positive result in Stage I or II had a significantly greater risk for cardiac mortality, with a 12-month survival of 85% and a 48-month survival of 63%.[20] The average annual mortality rate for this high-risk group was 10%. These results indicated that the presence of ischemia at a low work load is associated with a poorer outcome.

A later study from Duke University evaluated the prognostic value of treadmill exercise test results in 2,842 consecutive patients with chest pain.[21] An exercise treadmill score based on total exercise duration, ST-segment deviation during exercise testing, and a treadmill angina index yielded 5-year survival rates varying from 72% to 97%. The exercise score added independent prognostic information to that provided by clinical data, coronary anatomy, and left ventricular function. Subset analysis revealed that among patients with three-vessel CAD, those patients with an abnormal exercise score had a 5-year survival rate of 67% compared with 93% for those with more normal exercise scores.

Data using exercise testing from 4,083 CASS registry patients, who underwent medical therapy and were prospectively followed, revealed that risk stratification could create subsets of patients with a fivefold difference in annual mortality rates.[17] A low-risk subgroup with an annual mortality rate of less than 1% consisted of patients without ischemia and a

Table 25-1. Prognostic Significance of Exercise Testing

Reference	Number of Patients	Follow-up (years)	% Annual Mortality		
			High	Moderate	Low Risk
Bruce et al. (1979)[19]	2,001	4.1	5.6	2.2	1.2
McNeer et al. (1979)[20]	1,472	4	10.0	—	2.0
Mark et al. (1987)[21]	2,842	5	5.6	1.8	0.6
Weiner et al. (1984)[17]	5,303	5	5.3	2.0	0.8

(From Weiner,[1] with permission.)

Table 25-2. Studies Evaluating Exhanced Survival after Coronary Artery Bypass Graft Surgery

| | Survival | | | |
Reference	Surgical (%)	Medical (%)	Duration (years)	ExT Markers of Improved Survival
Bruce et al (1979)[19]	94	67	5	Cardiomegaly, <stage 1, maximum systolic BP < 130 mmHg (2 of 3)
Varnauskas et al. (1988)[14]	75	62	10	>1.5 mm ST-segment depression
Peduzzi et al. (1986)[22]	67	31	11	>2 mm ST-segment depression, exercise PVCs, peak HR >140 at a low exercise level (2 of 3)
Weiner et al. (1986)[23]	82	72	7	>1 mm of ST-segment depression and <stage 1

Abbreviations: BP, blood pressure; HR, heart rate; PVCs, premature ventricular contractions.
(From Weiner,[1] with permission.)

moderate exercise duration (less than 1 mm ST depression and exercise capacity greater than stage 3 on a standard Bruce protocol). In contrast, patients with more severe ST depression and extremely limited exercise tolerance (≥1 mm ST depression and ability to complete stage 1 or less of the Bruce protocol) constituted a high-risk subgroup whose annual mortality was greater than 5%. Patients with preserved exercise tolerance but more significant ischemia (>1 mm of ST depression and final exercise stage >3) constituted an intermediate-risk subgroup, with an annual mortality of approximately 2%. These results indicate that patients with ischemia and poor exercise tolerance constitute a high-risk group.

An improved survival following CABG surgery has been shown in patients with abnormal exercise test results in four studies[14,19,22,23] (Table 25-2). Among patients with evidence of left ventricular dysfunction by chest x-ray or exercise testing, Bruce et al. found that the 5-year survival rate in the operated subset of these patients was 94%, compared with 67% for the subset without surgery.[19] By contrast, among patients with only exertional myocardial ischemia, the survival rates were not different with medical (91%) or surgical (92%) therapy. Peduzzi et al. found that the survival rate among patients with abnormal exercise test results was 69% with coronary bypass surgery versus 31% with medical management at 11 years.[22] Another study reported that patients who had at least 1.5 mm of ischemic ST-segment depression during exercise testing were found to have an improved survival after surgical therapy compared to medical therapy.[14] Results from the CASS trial revealed that among patients with early positive exercise test results, survival at 7 years was 82% after surgical therapy and 72% after medical therapy.[23] By contrast, survival was not different between surgical and medical therapy among patients without ischemic ST depression who could exercise into stage 3 or greater. The greatest difference in survival among patients with early positive exercise test results was found in the subset with three-vessel CAD, in whom the 7-year survival was 81% for the surgical group and 58% for the medical group.

Unstable Angina

The majority of patients who are admitted to the hospital with unstable angina pectoris undergo cardiac catheterization and coronary artery revascularization. Some patients, especially those whose pain quickly disappears during hospitalization, are treated solely with increasing antianginal and antithrombotic medications. These patients frequently undergo predischarge exercise testing. One study reported the results of exercise testing that was performed on patients who were admitted to the hospital for unstable angina but became pain-free after admission.[24] Exercise testing using a modified, low level protocol was performed on patients 3 days after their last episode of chest pain. The investigators found that the predictive value of a positive exercise test was higher than that of a negative test for adverse events during follow up (83% vs. 33%, respectively).[24]

Non-Q Wave Myocardial Infarction

Exercise testing has been used to determine higher risk subsets among patients with non-Q wave myocardial infarction. Early exercise testing was useful in predicting the extent and severity of CAD among survivors of non-Q wave myocardial infarction in an investigation reported by Sia and coinvestigators.[25] Another study divided patients with non-Q wave myocardial infarction into those with or without pulmonary congestion.[26] Exercise testing did not add any additional information among patients without pulmonary congestion. By contrast, ischemic ST-segment depression was a potent predictor of future events in patients with pulmonary congestion. The event rate was 71% for those with ST-segment depression versus 5% for those without this abnormality.

Q-Wave Myocardial Infarction

The role of exercise testing in evaluating patients after myocardial infarction has been well established.[27] The benefits of early exercise testing include assessment of functional capacity and of the patients' ability to perform tasks at home and work and an evaluation of the patients' current medical regimen. Exercise tests also are performed to assess the prognosis of the postinfarction patient.

Risk stratification of these patients can serve two purposes. It can identify certain patients ascertained to be at higher risk for a future coronary event who then could be given more intensive medical treatment, or be subject to revascularization procedures.[28] Conversely, it can be of help in determining which patients are considered at lower risk, so that they would not need more complicated studies and could have a more accelerated return to normal daily activities.[29]

Screening patients for suitability to undergo exercise testing early after myocardial infarction constitutes the initial step in risk assessment. Many studies have determined that patients who are deemed too ill to undergo exercise testing have an excessive mortality.[28] In a multicenter postinfarction study, the 1-year mortality was 17% in the group of 192 patients who did not undergo early exercise testing compared with 6% in the subset of 607 patients who were tested.[30]

The results of many earlier studies that analyzed the prognostic value of exercise testing soon after acute myocardial infarction showed that patients with ischemic ST depression were at increased risk for adverse outcomes. The annual mortality of such patients was as high as 20%.[31] Several selection processes are brought to bear on this analysis, however. Recent reports have suggested that patients referred to the exercise laboratory after myocardial infarction have a much better survival rate than previously reported, because they have been extensively screened and more aggressively treated. Similarly, many higher risk patients with complications are revascularized with coronary angioplasty or with bypass surgery early after infarction, and are not represented in the group undergoing exercise testing. Even patients without early complications leading to coronary revascularization frequently have been treated with thrombolytic therapy and with a variety of antiischemic and antithrombotic medications before exercise testing. These referral factors favor the survival of these patients after discharge.[32]

In contrast to the earlier reports of 1-year mortality of 10% to 15% after myocardial infarction, more recent trials have shown 1-year mortality rates of 2.0% to 3.3%.[33,34] This very low mortality rate has substantially reduced the predictive accuracy of early exercise test risk stratification. The mere occurrence of 1 mm of ST depression is not predictive of a significantly increased mortality. Among patients treated with thrombolytic therapy and referred for exercise testing in the Thrombolysis in Myocardial Infarction (TIMI) II trial, the 1-year mortality was actually lower in patients with, compared with those without exercise-induced ST-segment depression (0.6% vs. 2.4%, respectively).[35] Only a combination of high-risk exercise ECG variables (e.g., ST-segment depression occurring early in exercise) had any significant positive predictive value, but the sensitivity of combinations of exercise variables is very low.[36] Non-ECG variables, such as the inability to perform three to four metabolic equivalents (METs) or to achieve a peak systolic blood pressure greater than 110 mmHg, seem to have greater prognostic value. By contrast, the ability to perform at least five METs and to show a normal rise in the systolic blood pressure during exercise have great negative predictive value.[37]

Froelicher and colleagues, who did a metaanalysis

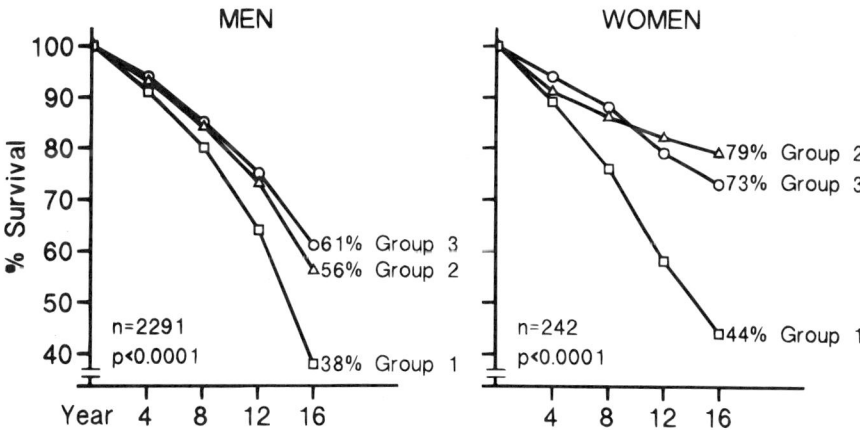

Fig. 25-1 Cumulative survival for men and women based on the results of exercise testing. Group 1 (high risk): >1 mm ST depression, final stage <1. Group 2 (intermediate risk): >1 mm ST depression, final stage >1, or no ST depression, final stage <2. Group 3 (low risk): no ST depression, final stage >3. (From Weiner et al.,[39] with permission.)

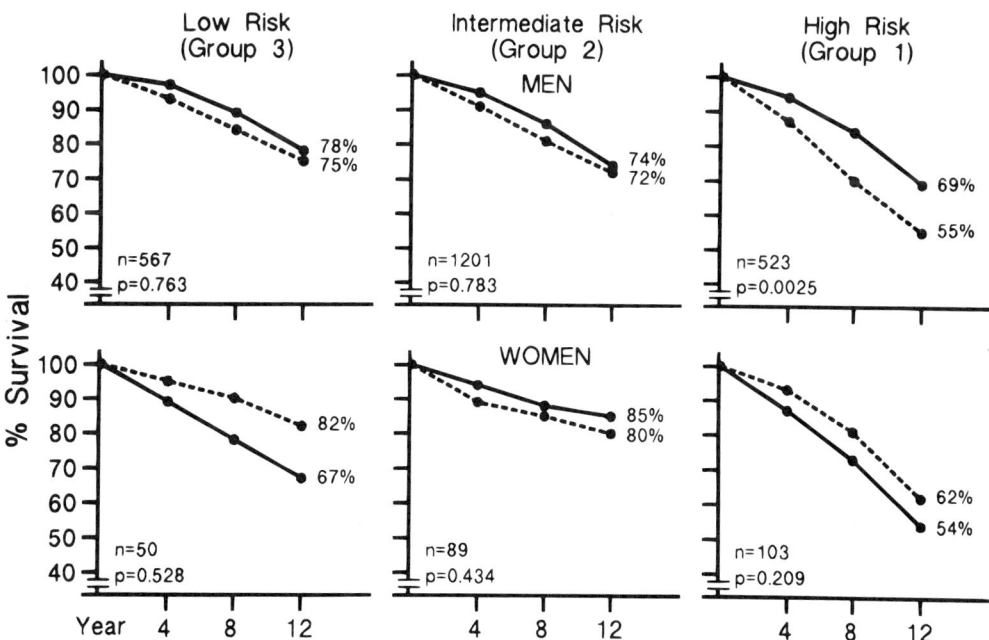

Fig. 25-2 Cumulative survival rates for the medically (dashed line) and surgically (solid line) treated men and women according to the exercise test risk classification. Coronary artery bypass surgery was associated with improved survival in group 1 men. (From Weiner et al.,[39] with permission.)

of 24 postinfarction studies, also confirmed the lack of prognostic value of 1 mm of ischemic ST-segment depression during exercise testing.[38] They suggested that interventions after myocardial infarction should be considered only for patients with at least 2 mm of ST-segment depression or for those with multiple abnormal exercise responses such as an abnormal blood pressure response combined with a poor exercise capacity.

Lower risk patients also can be identified by exer-

Table 25-3. American College of Cardiology/American Heart Association Guidelines for Indications of Exercise Testing

Class I   General consensus agreement that it is justified
Class II Frequently used but divergence of opinion regarding justification
Class III General agreement regarding little or no value, inappropriate or contraindications

A. Patients with signs/symptoms of CAD or with known CAD
   Class I   1. Diagnosis in male patients with atypical signs/symptoms of CAD
             2. Assess functional capacity
             3. Prognostication
             4. Evaluate patients with symptoms consistent with recurrent exercise-induced arrhythmias
   Class II 1. Diagnosis in women with chest pain
             2. Diagnosis with digoxin, right bundle branch block
             3. Evaluate functional capacity and response to therapy
             4. Evaluate variant angina
             5. To follow serially (1 year or longer) patients with CAD
   Class III 1. To evaluate patients with single PVCs
             2. To evaluate patients serially in rehabilitation
             3. To diagnose CAD in patients with Wolff-Parkinson-White syndrome or left bundle branch block
B. Screening of apparently healthy individuals
   Class I   None
   Class II To evaluate asymptomatic males over 40:
             1. In special occupations
             2. With 2 or more risk factors (cholesterol >240, HBP, cigarettes, DM, family history of CAD <55 yr)
             3. Who are sedentary and plan to enter a vigorous exercise program
   Class III To evaluate asymptomatic men or women:
             1. With no risk factors
             2. With chest discomfort not thought to be cardiac
C. Exercise testing soon after MI
   Class I   To evaluate prognosis and functional capacity in uncomplicated MIs
   Class II 1. Those with baseline ECGs or medical problems that effect responses
             2. Those with complicated MIs
   Class III 1. To evaluate acute ischemia
             2. Patients who are unstable or have complicating illnesses
D. Exercise testing after specific procedures
   Class I   To evaluate after CABS or PTCA
   Class II To follow yearly asymptomatic patients with CABS or PTCA
E. Exercise testing in patients with valvular heart disease
   Class I   Not used
   Class II To evaluate functional capacity
   Class III To evaluate symptomatic critical aortic stenosis or asymmetrical septal hypertrophy
F. Exercise testing in the management of patients with HPB or cardiac pacemakers
   Class I   Not used
   Class II To evaluate BP response in patients treated for HBP who do not plan to exercise, to evaluate pacemaker function

Abbreviations: CAD, coronary heart disease; PVC, premature ventricular contractions, HBP, high blood pressure; DM, diabetes mellitus; MI, myocardial infarction; ECG, electrocardiogram; CABS, coronary bypass surgery; PTCA, percutaneous transluminal coronary angioplasty.
(Modified from Subcommittee on Exercise Testing,[40] with permission.)

cise testing. Krone and co-workers identified a subset of 137 patients (from a total population of 298 patients) without pulmonary congestion who increased their exercise systolic blood pressure to at least 110 mmHg and who completed the 9-minute modified-exercise protocol.[30] There were no deaths in the year after the myocardial infarction in this subset of patients.

EXERCISE TESTING IN WOMEN

Exercise testing in women is used to evaluate the diagnostic accuracy of chest pain complaints and to predict the outcome of women with established heart disease. The influence of gender on the accuracy of exercise testing in women is discussed in Chapters 1 and 7.

The use of exercise testing in predicting the outcome of women with CAD has not been well studied. One recently published study analyzed the long-term prognostic value of exercise testing in 3,086 men and 747 women from the CASS registry.[39] The exercise test was classified as high-, intermediate-, and low-risk based on the degree of ST-segment depression and the final exercise stage achieved. Among men, 16-year survival varied from 74% with a low-risk exercise test to 48% with a high-risk test; similarly, among women, corresponding 16-year survival rates ranged from 91% to 58% (Fig. 25-1). Thus, the exercise test was useful in assessing the long-term survival for both men and women. The men and women in the three exercise test group classifications who were treated medically were then compared with those who underwent coronary artery bypass surgery (Fig. 25-2). Among men with a high-risk exercise test classification, surgery was associated with a survival advantage when compared with medical therapy (respective survivals 68% and 57%). The difference was especially true for men with three-vessel CAD. By contrast, among women, there was no subgroup based on exercise test results in which coronary bypass surgery was associated with increased survival. These results occurred even among women with three-vessel CAD.

SUMMARY

Approximately 10 years ago, a joint report from the American Heart Association and the American College of Cardiology Task Force on assessment of cardiovascular procedures listed guidelines regarding the indications for exercise testing (Table 25-3).[40] Class I (i.e., justified) indications include diagnosing CAD in male patients without known CAD, assessing the functional capacity and the prognosis of patients with known CAD, and evaluating patients after coronary artery revascularization procedures. The report emphasized the importance of considering the prevalence of CAD in the population under study when evaluating the predictive accuracy of diagnostic exercise testing.

The use of multivariate analysis of multiple exercise test variables becomes important when using the exercise test to evaluate the prognosis of patients with known CAD. Patients who demonstrate marked exercise test abnormalities (Table 25-4), such as substantial ST-segment depression at an early work load, would have much higher mortality risk. Once identified, such patients would be candidates for cardiac catheterization procedures and would likely

Table 25-4. Exercise Test Parameters Associated with Poor Prognosis and/or Increased Severity of CAD

1. Duration of symptom-limiting exercise
   a. Failure to complete State I of Bruce protocol or equivalent workload (i.e., <5 METs)
2. Exercise HR at onset of limiting symptoms
   a. Failure to attain HR>120/min (without medications)
3. Time of onset, magnitude, morphology, and postexercise duration of abnormal horizontal or downsloping ST-segment depression
   a. Onset at HR<120/min or <6.5 METs
   b. Magnitude >2.0 mm
   c. Postexercise duration >6 min
   d. Depression in multiple leads
   e. Downsloping configuration
4. Systolic BP response during or following progressive exercise
   a. Sustained decrease of >10 mmHg or flat BP response (<130 mmHg) during progressive exercise
5. Other potentially important determinants
   a. Exercise-induced ST-segment elevation in leads other than aVR
   b. Angina pectoris during exercise
   c. Exercise-induced ventricular tachycardia
   d. ST/HR slope <6 μV/beat/min

Abbreviations: CAD, coronary artery disease; METs, metabolic equivalent; HR, heart rate; BP, blood pressure.

benefit from coronary revascularization procedures if the coronary anatomic disease was suitable.

REFERENCES

1. Weiner DA: Risk stratification in angina pectoris. p. 39. In Abrams J (ed): Cardiology Clinics. Angina pectoris. Mechanisms, Diagnosis, and Therapy. W. B. Saunders Company, Philadelphia, 1991
2. Goldschlager N, Sox HC Jr: The diagnostic and prognostic value of the treadmill exercise test in the evaluation of chest pain, in patients with recent myocardial infarction, and in asymptomatic individuals. Am Heart J 116:523, 1988
3. Deering TF, Weiner DA: Prognosis of patients with coronary artery disease. J Cardiopulmon Rehab 5:325, 1985
4. Block W, Crumpacker E, Day T, Gage R: Prognosis of angina pectoris: observations in 6,882 cases. JAMA 150:239, 1952
5. Richard DW, Bland EF, White PD: A completed twenty-five year follow-up study of 456 patients with angina pectoris. J Chronic Dis 4:423, 1956
6. Frank CW, Weinblatt E, Shapiro S: Angina pectoris in men: Prognostic significance of selected medical factors. Circulation 47:509, 1973
7. Graham I, Mulcahy R, Hickey N, O'Neill W, Daly L: Natural history of coronary heart disease: A study of 586 men surviving an initial acute attack. Am Heart J 105:249, 1983
8. Kannel WB, Feinleib M: Natural history of angina pectoris in the Framingham study: prognosis and survival. Am J Cardiol 29:154, 1972
9. Moberg CH, Webster JS, Sones FM Jr: Natural history of severe proximal coronary artery disease as defined by cineangiography (200 patients, 7 year follow-up) (abstract). Am J Cardiol 29:282, 1972
10. Oberman A, Sones WB, Riley CH et al: Natural history of coronary artery disease. Bull NY Acad Med 48:1109, 1972
11. Burggraff GW, Parker JO: Prognosis in coronary artery disease: angiographic, hemodynamic, and clinical factors. Circulation 51:146, 1975
12. Proudfit WL, Bruschke AVG, Sones FM Jr: Natural history of obstructive coronary artery disease: ten-year study of 601 nonsurgical cases. Prog Cardiovasc Dis 21:53, 1978
13. The Veterans Administration Coronary Artery Bypass Surgery Study Group: Eleven-year survival in the Veterans Administration randomized trial of coronary bypass surgery for stable angina. N Engl J Med 311:1333, 1984
14. Varnauskas E, and the European Coronary Surgery Study Group: Twelve-year follow-up of survival in the randomized European coronary surgery study. N Engl J Med 319:332, 1988
15. Alderman EL, Bourassa MG, Cohen LS et al: Ten-year follow-up of survival and myocardial infarction in the randomized Coronary Artery Surgery Study. Circulation 82:1629, 1990
16. Harris PJ, Harrell FE Jr, Lee KL, Behar VS, Rosati RA: Survival in medical treated coronary artery disease. Circulation 60:1259, 1979
17. Weiner DA, Ryan TJ, McCabe CH, et al: Prognostic importance of a clinical profile and exercise test in medically treated patients with coronary artery disease. J Am Coll Cardiol 3:772, 1984
18. Weiner DA: Medical versus surgical management of the cardiac patient. p. 105. In Pollack ML, Schmidt DH (eds): Heart Disease and Rehabilitation. Human Kinetics, Champaign, Illinois, 1995
19. Bruce RA, DeRouen TA, Hammermeister KE: Noninvasive screening for enhanced 4-year survival after aortocoronary bypass surgery. Circulation 60:638, 1979
20. McNeer JF, Margolis JR, Lee KL et al: The role of the exercise test in the evaluation of patients for ischemic heart disease. Circulation 57:64, 1979
21. Mark DB, Hlatky MA, Harrell FE Jr et al: Exercise treadmill score for predicting prognosis in coronary artery disease. Ann Intern Med 106:793, 1987
22. Peduzzi F, Hultgren H, Thomsen J, Angell W: Prognostic value of baseline exercise tests. Prog Cardiovasc Dis 28:285, 1986
23. Weiner DA, Ryan TJ, McCabe CH et al: The role of exercise testing in identifying patients with improved survival after coronary artery bypass surgery. J Am Coll Cardiol 8:741, 1986
24. Butman SM, Olsen HG, Butman LK: Early exercise testing after stabilization of unstable angina: Correlation with coronary angiographic studies and subsequent cardiac events. Am Heart J 111:11, 1986
25. Sia T, MacDonald PS, Horowitz JD et al: Usefulness of early exercise testing after non-Q wave myocardial infarction in predicting prognosis. Am J Cardiol 57:738, 1986
26. Krone RJ, Duryer EM, Greenberg H et al: Risk stratification in patients with first non-Q wave infarction: Limited value of the early low level exercise test after uncomplicated infarcts. J Am Coll Cardiol 14:31, 1989
27. DeBusk FR: Specialized testing after recent myocardial infarction. Ann Intern Med 110:470, 1989
28. Weiner DA: Role of exercise testing after myocardial infarction. J Am Coll Cardiol 8:1020, 1986
29. DeBusk RF, Blomqvist CC, Kouchoukos NT et al: Identification and treatment of low-risk patients after acute

myocardial infarction and coronary artery bypass surgery. N Engl J Med 314:161, 1986
30. Krone RJ, Gillespie JA, Weld FM et al: Low-level exercise testing after myocardial infarction: Usefulness in enhancing clinical risks. Circulation 71:80, 1985
31. Weiner DA: Predischarge exercise testing after myocardial infarction: prognostic and therapeutic features. Cardiovasc Clin 15:95, 1985
32. Reeder GS, Gibbons RJ: Acute myocardial infarction: risk stratification in the thrombolytic era. Mayo Clin Proc 70:87, 1995
33. William DO, Braunwald E, Knatterud G et al: One-year results of the Thrombolysis in Myocardial Infarction (TIMI) phase II trial. Circulation 85:553, 1992
34. SWIFT (Should We Intervene Following Thrombolysis?) Trial Study Groups: SWIFT trial of delayed elective intervention v conservative treatment after thrombolysis with antistreplase in acute myocardial infarction. BMJ 302:555, 1991
35. Chaitman BR, McMahon RP, Terrin M et al: Impact of treatment strategy on predischarge exercise test in the Thrombolysis in Myocardial Infarction (TIMI) II trial. Am J Cardiol 71:131, 1993
36. Moss AJ, Goldstein RE, Hall J, for the Multicenter Myocardial Ischemia Research Group: Detection and significance of myocardial ischemia in stable patients after recovery from an acute coronary event. JAMA 269:2379, 1993
37. Piccalo G, Pirelli S, Massan D et al: Value of negative predischarge exercise testing in identifying patients at low risk after acute myocardial infarction treated by systemic thrombolysis. Am J Cardiol 70:31, 1992
38. Froelicher VF, Perdue S, Pewen W et al: Application of meta-analysis using an electronic spread sheet to exercise testing in patients after myocardial infarction. Am J Med 83:1045, 1987
39. Weiner DA, Ryan TJ, Parsons L et al: Long-term prognostic value of exercise testing in men and women from the Coronary Artery Surgery Study (CASS) registry. Am J Cardiol 75:865, 1995
40. Subcommittee on Exercise Testing. Guidelines for Exercise Testing: A report of the American College of Cardiology/American Heart Association Task Force on Assessment of Cardiovascular Procedures. J Am Coll Cardiol 8:725, 1986

Chapter 26

Implications of Stress-Induced LV Dysfunction on Risk Stratification

Janine Krivokapich

Stress testing is routinely used to diagnose the presence of coronary disease, to guide therapy, and to prognosticate future cardiac events. As discussed in Chapters 24 and 25, the nonimaging variables that provide the most useful prognostic information with exercise testing have been reduced exercise capacity, ischemic electrocardiographic changes, and angina. The addition of imaging to stress testing improves the sensitivity and specificity of diagnosing coronary artery disease (CAD). This chapter will review the additional prognostic information that is derived from assessment of regional myocardial function with either echocardiography or with radionuclide angiography in combination with various types of stress testing.

STRESS ECHOCARDIOGRAPHY

Stress echocardiography is used as an adjunct to stress ECG to improve the noninvasive detection of CAD. As detailed in previous chapters, the sensitivities and specificities of stress echocardiography for diagnosing the presence of significant CAD average over 80% with any of the commonly used stress modalities. Exercise is the most common stress utilized, with treadmill testing predominating over bicycle testing in the United States. Pharmacologic stress testing, usually with dobutamine or dipyridamole, is used when a patient is unable to exercise for any reason. As discussed in a Chapter 13, the mechanisms of action of these agents differ, with dobutamine simulating exercise by increasing both heart rate and blood pressure, and dipyridamole inducing a maldistribution of flow that is proportional to the degree of coronary artery narrowing.

The methodology of stress echocardiography has been discussed in detail in Chapters 3 and 13. Briefly, echocardiographic imaging of four views of the left ventricle is obtained at rest and immediately after treadmill stress testing or at peak stress, in the case of dipyridamole, dobutamine, or bicycle stress testing. The heart is divided into segments (usually 16), and the wall motion of each segment is graded at rest and with stress as hyperkinetic, normal, mildly hypokinetic, moderately to severely hypokinetic, or akinetic/dyskinetic. Rest and stress images are compared in a side-by-side format for each view, to determine if the wall motion has worsened; myocardial ischemia is detected as a decrease in segmental thickening following stress. If the wall motion in any segment deteriorates by one or more grades, the stress echocardiogram is considered to be positive for ischemia. In this contribution, a positive stress echocardiogram will always refer only to new and/or worsened wall motion abnormalities on the echocardiogram. References to the stress part of the test, whether it be ECG changes, duration of exercise, or angina, will be listed separately and not included in the designation "positive stress echocardiogram."

Known or Suspected CAD

A major goal of the noninvasive assessment of patients with known or suspected CAD is to predict prognosis. The prognosis of these patients is dependent on many variables, some of which may be the target of intervention (for example, ischemia), and others of which may not (for example, age). However, while the detection of significant ischemia by stress echocardiography may influence the subsequent management of patients, the results obtained when evaluating the usefulness of any test should be taken in the context of the patient population being studied. For example, in a patient population with a high pretest likelihood of CAD, it is more likely to have a positive stress echocardiogram result, as well as more cardiac events in the follow-up period. The results of several follow-up studies, which are summarized in Table 26-1, have varied depending on the patient population studied. However, in all populations studied, the presence of ischemia has been found to be an important variable in the prediction of future cardiac events.[1-9]

Exercise Echocardiography

Our laboratory examined the prognostic usefulness of positive and negative treadmill stress echocardiography for predicting cardiac events within 12 months of the test.[1] The results of exercise echocardiography and the cardiac event rate for 360 patients referred for evaluation of possible ischemia, who had 1 year of follow-up or a cardiac event within 1 year of follow-up, or both, were correlated. Only patients with a recent percutaneous transluminal angioplasty (PTCA) or with a cardiac transplant were excluded from the analysis. Cardiac events were defined as death, myocardial infarction (MI), coronary artery bypass grafting (CABG), or PTCA. Rest wall motion abnormalities were present in 60% of the patients. Forty-one percent of patients had a history of a prior MI or a revascularization procedure.

A positive stress echocardiogram was present in 18% of the patients, and one or more cardiac events occurred in 14% of the patients (Table 26-2). Multiple stepwise logistic regression using clinical and demographic variables was used to determine predictors of a cardiac event. The independent variables that were most predictive of a subsequent cardiac event by both univariate and multivariate analysis were exercising less than or equal to 6 minutes on a Bruce protocol, or the equivalent, a positive stress

Table 26-1. Prognostic Value of Stress Echocardiography in Patients with Known or Suspected CAD

Reference	Stress Test	Number of Patients Studied	Risk CAD	F/U (months)	Cardiac Events (%) + SE	Cardiac Events (%) − SE	Cardiac Events (%) Sensitivity[a]	Cardiac Events (%) Specificity[b]
Krivokapich et al. (1993)[1]	Treadmill	360	Medium	12	34	9	45	91
Mazeika et al. (1993)[3]	Dobutamine	51	High	24 ± 4	68	23	74	71
Afridi et al. (1994)[4]	Dobutamine	77	Medium	10	50	13		
Poldermans et al. (1994)[5]	Dobutamine	430	Medium	17 ± 5	26	13		
Picano et al. (1989)[6]	Dipyridamole	539	Medium	36	26 hd; 41 ld	6		
Amanullah et al. (1993)[8] and (1992)[9]	Bike	36	Unstable angina	30 ± 6	81	33	77	71

Abbreviations: CAD, coronary artery disease; F/U, average follow-up in months; hd, high dose; ld, low dose; SE, stress echocardiogram; +SE, stress echocardiogram positive; −SE, stress echocardiogram negative.
[a] Sensitivity of SE for predicting cardiac event.
[b] Specificity of SE in predicting cardiac event.

Table 26-2. Summary of Cardiac Events within First Year of Follow-up

	Patients		MI		PTCA		CABG		Death		Any Event	
	N	(%)	N	(%)	N	(%)	N	(%)	N	(%)	N	(%)
Total in category												
All patients	360		13	(4)	26	(7)	21	(6)	3	(1)	49	(14)
Subcategories												
Pts ≤6 min Bruce or equivalent	125		9	(7)	16	(13)	17	(14)	2	(2)	34	(27)
Pts >6 min Bruce or equivalent	235		4	(2)	10	(4)	4	(2)	1	(0.5)	15	(6)
SE positive												
All patients	65	(18)	6	(9)	9	(14)	13	(20)	1	(2)	22	(34)
Subcategories												
Pts ≤6 min Bruce or equivalent	31	(25)	5	(16)	6	(19)	11	(35)	1	(3)	17	(55)
Pts >6 min Bruce or equivalent	34	(14)	1	(3)	3	(9)	2	(6)	0	(0)	5	(15)
SE negative												
All patients	295	(82)	7	(2)	17	(6)	8	(3)	2	(1)	27	(9)
Subcategories												
Pts ≤6 min Bruce or equivalent	94	(75)	4	(4)	10	(11)	6	(6)	1	(1)	17	(18)
Pts >6 min Bruce or equivalent	201	(85)	3	(2)	7	(3)	2	(1)	1	(0.5)	10	(5)

Abbreviations: Any event, patients with one or more cardiac events during first 1 year of follow-up (some patients had more than one cardiac event); CABG, coronary artery bypass grafting; equivaluent, equivalent to Bruce protocol; MI, myocardial infarction; N, number of patients; PTCA, percutaneous transluminal coronary angioplasty after stress echocardiogram; SE, stress echocardiogram.
(From Krivokapich et al., reprinted with permission from The American Journal of Cardiology.[1])

echocardiogram, and a positive exercise ECG (Table 26-3). The change in left ventricular ejection fraction (LVEF) between rest and exercise was not a significant variable for discriminating between patients with and without a cardiac event. The cardiac event rates were 34% for patients with a positive stress echocardiography and 9% for patients with a negative stress echocardiography (Table 26-2), 28% and 7%, respectively, for patients with positive and negative exercise ECGs (Table 26-4, and 27% and 6%, respectively, for patients who exercised less than or equal to 6 minutes on the Bruce protocol (or its

Table 26-3. Significant Independent Variables for Prediction of a Cardiac Event (Stepwise Logistic Regression)

	Univariate Analysis		Multivariate Analysis	
Variable	Odds Ratio	95% CI	Odds Ratio	95% CI
≤ 6 min Bruce or equivalent	5.48	2.84–10.60	5.93	2.83–12.40
SE+	5.08	2.65–9.73	3.09	1.47–6.50
Male sex	2.57	1.20–5.51	3.16	1.31–7.59
ECG+	3.35	1.73–6.49	3.41	1.53–7.57
Baseline WMA	3.93	1.78–8.69	2.15	0.84–5.46

Abbreviations: Cardiac event, one or more cardiac events (some patients had more than one cardiac event); CI, confidence interval; ECG+, ischemic stress ECG; equivalent, equivalent to Bruce protocol; SE+, positive stress echocardiogram; WMA, wall motion abnormality.
(From Krivokapich et al., Reprinted with permission from The American Journal of Cardiology.[1])

Table 26-4. Correlation of Electrocardiogram Results with Cardiac Events and Stress Echocardiography during First Year of Follow-up

	Patients		MI		PTCA		CABG		Death		Any Event	
	N	(%)	N	(%)	N	(%)	N	(%)	N	(%)	N	(%)
All patients	360		13	(4)	26	(7)	21	(6)	3	(1)	49	(14)
ECG +	64	(18)	3	(5)	10	(16)	8	(12)	1	(2)	18	(28)
ECG ±	92	(25)	8	(9)	4	(4)	9	(10)	1	(1)	16	(17)
ECG −	204	(57)	2	(1)	12	(6)	4	(2)	1	(0.5)	15	(7)
All SE positive patients	65	(18)	6	(9)	9	(14)	13	(20)	1	(2)	22	(34)
ECG +	18	(5)	3	(17)	4	(22)	5	(28)	1	(6)	9	(50)
ECG ±	22	(6)	3	(14)	1	(5)	6	(27)	0	(0)	8	(36)
ECG −	25	(7)	0	(0)	4	(16)	2	(8)	0	(0)	5	(20)
All SE negative patients	295	(82)	7	(2)	17	(6)	8	(3)	2	(1)	27	(9)
ECG +	46	(13)	0	(0)	6	(13)	3	(6)	0	(0)	9	(20)
ECG ±	70	(19)	5	(7)	3	(4)	3	(4)	1	(1)	8	(11)
ECG −	179	(50)	2	(1)	8	(5)	2	(1)	1	(0.5)	10	(6)

Abbreviations: Any Event, one or more cardiac events (some patients had more than one cardiac event); CABG, coronary artery bypass graft surgery; MI, myocardial infarction; N, number of patients; PTCA, percutaneous transluminal coronary angioplasty; SE, stress echocardiogram; +, positive; −, negative; ±, equivocal.
(From Krivokapich et al., reprinted with permission from The American Journal of Cardiology.[1])

equivalent) and those who exercised greater than 6 minutes (Table 26-2). Of those patients with a cardiac event with a negative stress echocardiogram, the exercise capacity was diminished in 63% making it difficult to rule out ischemia. Therefore, it is important to take all three variables into account when assessing risk in patients. For example, a patient with both a positive stress echocardiogram and a positive ECG has a 50% chance of a cardiac event, compared to a 6% chance if both tests are negative. If the stress echocardiography is positive and the ECG is negative, or vice versa, the risk is 20% (Table 26-4). Thus, it is important to appreciate that both in relation to diagnosis or prognosis, the complete stress echocardiographic study provides a gradation of positivity, which reflects a gradation of risk, rather than a binary "positive or negative" answer.

Sawada et al.[2] reported a unique group of 148 patients who had both a normal resting and normal post-treadmill exercise echocardiogram. During a mean follow-up of 28 ± 8 months, only six patients, 4% of the total, had a cardiac event, which included two nonfatal MI and four revascularization procedures. All patients with an event exercised to a workload of less than 6 METs (equivalent to < 6 minutes on the Bruce protocol) or achieved less than 85% of their age-predicted maximal heart rate. Thus, patients with a good exercise capacity and a negative stress echocardiogram have an excellent prognosis.

Dobutamine Echocardiography

Mazeika et al.[3] evaluated 51 patients with a high pretest likelihood of having myocardial ischemia (Table 26-1). All patients were symptomatic and were awaiting coronary angiography. Dobutamine stress echocardiography was performed using 5 to 20 µg/kg/min in incremental doses. Patients were followed for an average of 24 ± 4 months (19 to 32 months) for the development of all cardiac events, including death, MI, unstable angina, CABG, and PTCA. A test was considered positive if a new or worsened wall motion abnormality appeared in greater than or equal to 1 segment. Forty-five percent of these patients had at least one cardiac event during follow-up, and 74% of these 23 patients had a positive stress echocardiogram. The 23 patients with events included 1 with MI, 9 with unstable angina, and 13 with revascularization (including 10 CABG, and 3 PTCA). Only 29% of patients without a cardiac event had a positive stress echocardiogram. The incidence of unstable angina or MI was eight times more frequent in patients with a positive versus a negative stress echocardiogram (32% vs. 8%). Another perspective of the same data is that 68% of patients with a positive stress echocardiogram had a cardiac event, whereas only 23% of patients with a negative stress echocardiogram had an event (Table 26-1). The baseline clinical variables including age, gender, symptoms, drug treatment, history of hypertension, abnormal baseline ECG, abnormal baseline echocardiogram, and baseline ejection fraction were not different between the patients with and without a cardiac event. In addition, the peak rate pressure product with dobutamine, time elapsed until the development of a wall motion abnormality, infusion duration, and incidence of ischemic ECG changes were not different between patients with and without a cardiac event. Moreover, the only dobutamine stress testing variable that was predictive of a future cardiac event was a positive stress echocardiogram, and evaluation of ejection fractions at rest and with dobutamine did not help discriminate between those patients with and without a cardiac event in the follow-up period.

A retrospective study of 77 patients with known or suspected CAD who underwent dobutamine stress echocardiography and were followed up for an average of 10 months was reported by Afridi et al.[4] Dobutamine was delivered up to a maximum dose of 40 µg/kg/min. Unlike the other studies, in this study, congestive heart failure was included as a cardiac event (and occurred in 7 patients), but revascularization was not considered as an event. One patient died and six had MI. Forty patients had normal wall motion at rest and with dobutamine; these patients had a 5% incidence of cardiac events. Patients who developed a new wall motion abnormality had a 50% incidence of cardiac events, whereas patients who had wall motion abnormalities at rest that did not change with dobutamine had a 26% event rate. If only MI or death were considered, the "hard" events occurred in 40% of patients with new wall motion abnormalities, in 7% with no change in resting wall motion abnormalities, and in 2.5% of patients with normal wall motion. Revascularization was performed in 5 of 6 patients who had new wall motion abnormalities but no event. Thus, 9 of 10 patients with a positive dobutamine stress echocardiogram, defined as new wall motion abnormalities, had revascularization, MI, or death. In addition to emphasizing that patients with a positive dobutamine stress echocardiogram have a much greater incidence of future cardiac events than do patients with a negative study, Afridi et al.[4] emphasize that patients with rest wall motion abnormalities that do not change are at an intermediate risk for future cardiac events. The most common event in these patients with a fixed wall motion abnormality was congestive heart failure. No other studies have addressed the incidence of congestive heart failure in this group with resting defects.

Poldermans et al.[5] used dobutamine–atropine stress echocardiography to evaluate 430 patients with chest pain who were unable to exercise adequately. This study is unique in the respect that the dobutamine study results were considered as research data, and the test results were not used in clinical management decisions. A bias toward more coronary angiography and subsequent revascularization in patients with positive studies may have been avoided. The follow-up was for at least 6 months (average 17 ± 5 months), over which time cardiac events occurred in 79 patients, comprising 11 deaths, 18 nonfatal MIs, and 50 revascularization procedures. Univariate and multivariate regression analysis was used to assess the prognostic value of the stress test in addition to the available clinical variables. When only cardiac death was considered, the two strongest univariate predictors were older than 70 years of age and a new wall motion abnormality with normal resting wall motion. If consideration was given to both cardiac death and myocardial infarction, a history of infarction, new wall motion abnormalities, rest wall motion abnormalities, and age over 70 years were all significant univariate predictors. Finally, when all cardiac events were combined, the best univariate predictors were new wall motion abnormalities and resting wall motion abnormalities. Multivariate regression analysis yielded similar correlations. New wall motion abnormalities induced by dobutamine provided prognostic information that was independent of clinical variables.

Dipyridamole Echocardiography

Dipyridamole echocardiography (DET) has been popularized by Picano et al.[6] As discussed previously, the "high dose" DET protocol involves initial delivery at a rate of 0.56 mg/kg over 4 minutes; if the test is negative after waiting 4 minutes, an additional 0.28 mg/kg is given over 2 minutes. The prognostic value of this test was assessed in 539 consecutive patients referred for evaluation of possible ischemia and followed for 3 years. Cardiac events (which included death, nonfatal myocardial infarction, PTCA, and CABG) occurred in 6% of patients with a normal DET, in 41% with a DET positive at low dose (0.56 mg/kg), and in 26% with a DET positive at high dose (0.84 mg/kg) (Table 26-1). Analysis of multiple clinical and test variables revealed that a positive DET, ischemic changes during DET, angina during DET, a previous MI, an abnormal basal echocardiogram, age, and an abnormal basal ECG were all univariate predictors of clinical events. However, a positive DET was by far the strongest predictor of all future cardiac events. In a subset of 341 patients who also had coronary arteriography, a positive DET was a stronger predictor of future cardiac events than was a pathologic coronary arteriogram.

Another large series of patients studied with both DET and exercise ECG was also reported more recently by the same group of investigators.[7] The study group consisted of 429 consecutive inpatients who were followed for 38 ± 14 months. Clinically, they were characterized by requiring coronary arteriography for the diagnosis of chest pain; they had no history of prior MI or evidence of significant wall motion abnormalities on baseline echocardiographic study. They had been off antianginal therapy for at least 2 days. Cardiac events, including 20 deaths, 13 nonfatal MI, and 126 revascularization procedures, occurred in 159 patients. The cumulative incidence rate for revascularization over the 5-year period was 36%. Exercise stress testing alone, DET alone, and angiography alone each provided good stratification of survival. Specifically, patients had an excellent survival if they had a negative exercise stress test or a negative DET or no evidence of CAD by angiography. In contrast, the 5-year survival rate was approximately 84% if a patient had a positive exercise test with a rate pressure product of less than 20,000 beats/min/mmHg, a positive DET at less than 8 minutes of dipyridamole infusion, or had multivessel CAD. The most powerful predictors of either future death or any event were the time to dipyridamole-induced ischemia, DET positivity, exercise ECG positivity coupled with low rate pressure product, and number of vessels narrowed to greater than or equal to 75%. In an effort to determine if the DET data provided prognostic information additional to that already provided by clinical information and exercise test results, a modified interactive stepwise procedure was used. Using this procedure, it was determined that the dipyridamole time provided independent and prognostic information additional to that available clinically, including the results of the exercise testing. The authors emphasize that all aspects of the test should be considered when evaluating prognosis—specifically, the time to onset of dipyridamole-induced ischemia, the severity of induced wall motion abnormalities, and the extent of induced wall motion abnormalities.

Unstable Angina

The outcomes in patients admitted to the hospital with unstable angina vary significantly. One of the clinical challenges in these patients is to select those most likely to require further intervention after medical stabilization. The greater sensitivity of stress echocardiography may make it more attractive than the currently used exercise ECG for this purpose.

Stress echocardiography using a bicycle ergometer was performed in 36 patients after medical stabilization for unstable angina.[8,9] Exercise echocardiography was positive in 22 of the patients and negative in 14 patients. Of those patients with a cardiac event, either a subsequent MI or a revascularization procedure, during a 30 ± 6 month follow-up, 81% had a positive exercise echocardiogram (Table 26-1). Only 33% of those without a cardiac event had a positive exercise echocardiogram. Stepwise logistic regression analysis identified both a positive exercise ECG and a positive exercise echocardiogram as significantly predictive of future events. These promising results suggest the need for further studies in this group.

Prognostication Post-Myocardial Infarction

The degree of left ventricular dysfunction and the presence of additional myocardium at risk are major factors influencing the prognosis of patients who have suffered an acute MI. Stress echocardiography may be used to address both of these issues with a single test (Table 26-5). Both exercise and pharmacologic approaches have been used for this purpose, although the prognostic importance of exercise capacity favors the use of exercise echocardiography

Table 26-5. Prognostic Value of Stress Echocardiography in Patients with Myocardial Infarction

Reference	Stress Test	Number of Patients Studied	F/U (months)	Cardiac Events (%)		Cardiac Events (%)	
				+ SE	− SE	Sensitivity[a]	Specificity[b]
Ryan et al. (1987)[10]	Treadmill	40	6–10	94	17	80	95
Applegate et al. (1987)[11]	Treadmill	67	11	50	13	63	80
Picano et al. (1993)[15]	Dipyridamole	925	14	50	18		
Camerieri et al. (1993)[16]	Dipyridamole	190	14 ± 10	52	17		
Chiarella et al. (1994)[17]	Dipyridamole	251	0.3	33	3	94	50
Iliceto et al. (1990)[18]	Pacing	83	14 ± 5	65	8	75	87

Abbreviations: F/U, average follow-up in months; SE, stress echocardiogram; + SE, stress echocardiogram positve; − SE, stress echocardiogram negative.
[a] Sensitivity of SE for predicting cardiac event.
[b] Specificity of SE in predicting cardiac event.

if the patient can exercise. On the other hand, pharmacologic stress may be more useful if risk stratification is required early after infarction or if questions arise regarding the presence and extent of viable myocardium.

Exercise Echocardiography

The prognostic value of exercise stress echocardiography in patients with a recent MI was first addressed in 1987.[10,11] In the study by Ryan et al.,[10] 40 patients recovering from an acute MI underwent exercise echocardiography 10 to 21 days after the infarction. Each was followed for at least 6 months or until the occurrence of a cardiac event, including death, recurrent MI, unstable angina, or CABG. Twenty patients did not have a cardiac event, and only 1 of these patients had a positive stress echocardiogram. In contrast, of the 20 patients with a cardiac event, 16 had a positive stress echocardiogram. The sensitivities and specificities for predicting a good versus a poor outcome were 80% and 95%, respectively, for the stress echocardiograms (Table 26-5), whereas they were only 55% and 65%, respectively, for the stress ECG data. Linear discriminant analysis of multiple clinical and test variables revealed that only a positive stress echocardiogram reached significance as a predictor of adverse outcome.

The usefulness of exercise stress echocardiography early post-MI was also addressed by Applegate et al.[11] A total of 67 patients were studied with exercise echocardiography and followed for an average of 11 months (3 to 24 months) for the occurrence of cardiac events including death, recurrent MI, and CABG. In addition to evaluation of wall motion abnormalities, rest and stress left ventricular ejection fractions were measured, and the difference between rest and stress ejection fraction was calculated. As in the study by Ryan et al.,[10] the sensitivity (63%) and specificity (80%) for stress echocardiography (Table 26-5) were greater than the respective values for stress ECG (38% and 76%). Univariate and multivariate analysis of risk both identified a positive stress echocardiogram as the most significant predictor of future cardiac events. A decrease in recovery ejection fraction greater than 10% below the rest value, angina during treadmill testing, and rest ejection fraction were three other significant predictive variables.

Dobutamine Echocardiography

Berthe et al.[12] introduced dobutamine stress echocardiography to the study of patients post-MI. They did not follow the patients over time but rather used the test in 30 patients with recent infarctions to identify multivessel CAD, a known risk factor for greater morbidity post-MI.[13] Dobutamine was well tolerated beginning at a dose of 5 μg/kg/min up to a maximum dose of 40 μg/kg/min. The dobutamine echocardiogram was considered positive for multivessel disease if a new wall motion abnormality developed in a region remote from the recent MI. The sensitivity and specificity of dobutamine stress echocardiography for detecting multivessel disease were 85% and 88%, respectively. Additional studies of dobutamine echocardiography focusing on the significance of both ischemia and viable myocardium to subsequent events are warranted.

Dipyridamole Echocardiography

DET has been evaluated in post-MI patients and found to be safe.[14] The sensitivity and specificity of dipyridamole stress echocardiography in detecting multivessel disease were 68% and 100%, respectively, in a series of 73 patients with a recent uncomplicated myocardial infarction.[14] As with dobutamine, a test was considered positive for multivessel disease if a new wall motion abnormality developed in a region remote from the recent MI.

The largest study to date evaluating the prognostic value of any type of stress echocardiography is that presented by Picano[15] for the EPIC Study Group (Echo Persantine Italian Cooperative Study Group). This multicenter trial included 925 patients who were evaluated with DET at a mean of 10 days after an uncomplicated acute MI,[15] and followed for an average of 14 ± 10 months. The endpoints selected for this study included class III or IV angina, as well as the more standard endpoints of reinfarction and death. The most important univariate predictor of any subsequent cardiac event was a positive DET. Age and a positive dipyridamole stress were the strongest predictors of death, which occurred in 7% of patients with a low-dose positive DET, in 4% with a high-dose positive DET, and in 2% with a negative DET. Although no randomization to treatment was performed, an important aspect of this study was that the value of revascularization was demonstrated by comparison of survival in the patients with positive DET findings who did and did not undergo revascularization. Those with revascularization had an 0.8% mortality versus a 7% mortality in those without revascularization. There were no significant differences in the rest or stress wall motion scores, nor the time to ischemia in these two populations to otherwise explain the difference in survival.

A subset analysis of the EPIC study was reported in 190 patients with an uncomplicated infarction who were considered elderly, defined as older than 65 years of age.[16] Cardiac events in the subsequent follow-up period, which averaged 14 ± 10 months, included death, nonfatal MI, class III or IV angina, or revascularization. Fifty-two percent of patients with a positive DET had a cardiac event, whereas only 17% with a negative DET had an event (Table 26-5). If only death or recurrent infarction were considered events, the event rate was 16% with a positive DET and 6% with a negative DET. The death rate was 13% with a positive DET and 3% with a negative DET. Thus, DET was very effective in risk stratifying this population of older patients. Moreover, the study revealed that unlike the larger study, which included younger patients, these older patients had less revascularization despite positive test results, which may have accounted for their significantly higher mortality rate in the presence of a positive DET. This suggests that revascularization might well have favorably improved the prognosis in this older population, as it did with the younger patients.

Many postinfarction complications occur early after admission, so there is an interest in risk-stratifying patients prior to discharge. Very early risk stratification, using DET 70 ± 6 hours after the acute MI, has been studied by Chiarella et al.[17] in a group of 251 patients. The test was well tolerated by patients and there were no significant complications or side-effects. Ischemia, defined by deterioration in the function of any wall segment, was present in 59% of patients. Cardiac events including death, reinfarction, or angina occurred in 52 patients during their hospital stay, which averaged 13 ± 3 days. DET was positive in 49 of the 52 patients with an event (94%). The event rate in hospital was 33% in those with a positive DET, and 3% in those with a negative DET. The negative predictive value exceeded 90%. Thus, very early testing using DET in patients with an acute myocardial infarction is useful in stratifying patients into high- and low-risk groups for future cardiac events. This study also emphasized the importance of considering the ECG findings along with the DET findings when assessing risk. For example, patients with a positive DET and an ECG positive for ischemia had a cardiac event rate of 42%, and those with a positive DET plus angina had a 49% event rate. No patient had a positive ECG without a positive DET. Multivariate logistic analysis revealed that DET positivity was the strongest independent predictor of cardiac events during the hospital stay after uncomplicated acute MI. Moreover, a low-dose positive DET was more predictive of future cardiac events than a high-dose positive DET.

Atrial Pacing

Transesophageal atrial pacing (TAP) is a nonexercise stress that offers the capacity to maximally stress the heart while maintaining complete control over the stress, including the ability to stop it abruptly. This technique has also been used to predict cardiac events (angina, heart failure, MI death, and CABG) after uncomplicated MI.[18] The stress echocardiogram in 83 patients followed for 14 ± 5 months was considered positive if wall motion abnormalities developed remote from the infarcted area. Cardiac events occurred in 15 of 23 patients (65%) with a positive stress echocardiogram, and in 5 of 60 (8%) with a negative stress echocardiogram (Table 26-5).

Summary

The ability of stress echocardiography to provide information about resting left ventricular function and stress-induced changes of regional wall motion makes this technique useful in the prognostic evaluation of patients. Regional left ventricular dysfunction may occur when global ejection fraction is not affected, and it is not surprising that several studies have shown that evaluation of wall motion abnormalities appears to prognosticate better than does evaluation of ejection fraction. The value of stress echocardiography for prognostic assessment appears to be independent of the circumstances in which it is used (chronic stable coronary disease, unstable angina, MI) as well as the type of stressor employed.

RADIONUCLIDE ANGIOGRAPHY

Radionuclide angiography (RNA) may be used to evaluate left and right ventricular ejection fraction, as well as the wall motion of the left ventricle.[19-24] The methodology of this test has been discussed previously. Briefly, the left ventricular cavity is labeled by intravenous injection of technetium-99m-labeled red blood cells, and the heart is imaged with a gamma camera. Equilibrium RNA (MUGA, referring to multigated acquisition) is performed by data acquisition over several minutes in multiple views (45° and 70° left anterior oblique, anterior, and left lateral or posterior oblique). Acquisition of data begins with the R-wave on the ECG; each cardiac cycle is divided into intervals; multiple cycles are added together to obtain adequate counts. Assuming that changes in radioactivity are proportional to volume changes, a comparison of the area-counts in the left ventricle in systole with those in diastole, after subtraction of background counts, allows calculation of the LVEF. In addition, the entire cycle of counts beginning at the R-wave can be presented in a cine format, which allows assessment of regional wall motion. It is possible to obtain right ventricular ejection fractions by equilibrium imaging,[25] but it is not felt to be as accurate as first pass imaging.

Exercise (usually bicycle stress) can be combined with RNA. However, as most patients cannot sustain peak exercise for more than a few minutes, exercise imaging is usually done only using one view of the heart (usually 45° left anterior oblique view) because of the limited acquisition time. If time allows, the anterior view may also be imaged during exercise. Rest and exercise ejection fractions and wall motion are then compared, in a manner similar to that employed with stress echocardiography. The normal response of LVEF to exercise has been evaluated by many investigators,[26-30] but there has not been uniform agreement as to what constitutes a normal response. Some investigators report an absolute change, whereas others evaluated a percentage change. The most common criterion used to define an abnormal response is a failure to increase the LVEF by at least 0.05 in absolute terms. A literature review of 259 patients with and 203 patients without significant coronary disease who had no prior MI revealed that the mean rest and exercise LVEF were 0.64 ± 0.09 and 0.74 ± 0.10 for patients with normal coronary arteriograms and 0.63 ± 0.09 and 0.58 ± 0.11 for patients with significant CAD.[30] The left ventricular response to exercise is influenced by the exercise protocol,[31] as well as the level of resting left ventricular function.[32] Rozanski et al.[30] emphasized the disadvantage of evaluating only the absolute change of LVEF with exercise rather than taking that change into consideration with the level of rest LVEF, as well as the wall motion assessment. These investigators developed a statistical algorithm, based on the pooled patients described above and then successfully applied prospectively to 854 patients, which incorporates this additional information. This algorithm explicitly identifies equivocal test responders, as opposed to designating a test as either abnormal or normal.

Not all reports of exercise nuclear ventriculography have been favorable, however. Gibbons et al.[33,34] published two studies examining the ejection fraction response to exercise in patients with chest pain.

Table 26-6. Prognostic Value of Radionuclide Angiography in Patients with Known or Suspected CAD

Reference	CAD	Number of Patients Studied	Rest LVEF	Best Predictor(s) of Subsequent Cardiac Events
Bonow et al. (1984)[35]	Known CAD	117	>0.40	Exercise LVEF Change in LVEF with exercise
Jones et al. (1983)[36]	Known CAD	278	>0.20–<0.55	Failure of LVEF to increase with exercise New or worsened WMAs Increase in ESV >20 ml
Pryor et al. (1984)[37]	Known CAD	386		Exercise LVEF
Lee et al. (1990)[38]	Known CAD	571[a]		Exercise LVEF
Taliercio et al. (1988)[39]	67% with CAD	424		Rest LVEF

Abbreviations: CAD, coronary artery disease; ESV, end-systolic volume; LEVF, left ventricular ejection fraction; WMA, wall motion abnormality.
[a] Includes 386 patients in study listed above.

In the first, 281 patients had CAD,[33] and in the other study of 60 patients, coronary arteriography was normal.[34] In both studies, there was a wide range of LVEF responses to exercise, with decreases of up to 36% and increases of up to 26%. Their analyses indicated that the ejection fraction response to exercise is very complex and influenced by many pathophysiologic variables, with or without the presence of coronary artery disease.[33,34]

Known or Suspected CAD

Bonow et al.[35] evaluated the prognostic value of RNA results in a cohort of 117 mildly symptomatic, medically treated patients with CAD who had an LVEF of greater than 0.40 (Table 26-6). Subsequent mortality was significantly associated with the absolute value of the exercise LVEF. The difference between rest and exercise LVEF was significantly associated with increased angina requiring coronary artery bypass surgery. No patient died within 4 years if the LVEF during exercise did not change or increased from rest, whereas the 4 year mortality rate was 7% if the LVEF decreased with exercise. If death or progressive symptoms requiring surgery are both considered as events, the event rate was 15% for patients with an increased or unchanged LVEF with exercise, compared to a 35% event rate in patients whose LVEF decreased with exercise.

Jones et al.[36] evaluated the prognostic value of positive and negative RNA in patients who had an LVEF between 0.20 and 0.55, and had known CAD documented by angiography (Table 26-6). The study consisted of 278 patients, 172 treated medically and 106 who underwent surgical revascularization, who were followed for up to 3 years. The decision regarding medical or surgical therapy was made individually by the patient's primary physician using all of the clinical data available including the results of RNA. An abnormal RNA exercise result was defined as a failure of the LVEF to increase, or the appearance of new or worsened wall motion abnormality, or an increase of end-systolic volume of greater than 20 ml. An abnormal exercise RNA response was identified in 192 (69%) of the patients: 113 were treated medically and 79 were treated with bypass surgery. Of the 86 patients with a negative exercise RNA response, 59 had medical therapy and 27 had surgical therapy. Patients treated medically had a significantly poorer survival (6% less at 1 year) if they had a positive RNA versus a negative RNA. Of patients with a positive RNA, those treated medically had a significantly poorer survival (8% less at 1 year) than those treated surgically. Patients with a negative RNA had similar survival rates with both medical and surgical therapy. Thus, a positive RNA was successful in identifying patients who were most likely to derive a survival benefit with surgery, as opposed to medical therapy. Moreover, a negative RNA identified a patient population unlikely to derive a survival benefit with surgery as opposed to medical treatment.

Duke investigators reported additional prognostic data on 386 symptomatic patients with known significant CAD who were treated only medically and followed for cardiovascular deaths and nonfatal MI over 4.5 years (Table 26-6).[37] Rest and exercise LVEF, wall motion abnormalities at rest or with exercise, and exercise time were univariate predictors of future events. However, using multivariate analyses, the exercise LVEF was the only independent variable that predicted future cardiac events. This variable was a better predictor of future cardiac events than the resting LVEF, cardiac anatomy, exercise ECG changes, or exercise time. An exercise LVEF of less than 0.35 was associated with an 82% survival rate at 1 year and a 56% survival rate at 3 years in contrast to a 100% survival at 1 year and 95% survival at 3 years for patients with an exercise LVEF greater than or equal to 0.50. Patients with reduced exercise LVEFs were also more likely to have nonfatal MIs. The event rates were correlated with the exercise LVEF, but not with the difference between rest and exercise LVEF.

More recently, Duke investigators[38] used their extensive database of patients to report on 571 stable patients with documented symptomatic CAD who were followed for a median of 5.4 years (Table 26-6). This is the largest patient series available, with the longest follow-up. It compared the prognostic value of RNA evaluation with that of clinical and catheterization data. This study included the 386 patients included in their previous report[37] with an extended follow-up. Each patient had upright rest and exercise first-pass RNA within 3 months of catheterization. All patients were initially treated medically for at least 3 months, but 149 (26%) of the patients eventually underwent either CABG or PTCA. Once again, the exercise ejection fraction was the single most important predictor of mortality, which was highest when the LVEF was the lowest. However, this relationship was not linear, and above an LVEF of 0.50, there was no further mortality gradient. The rest LVEF and the change in LVEF with exercise were not independent predictors of outcome, although the heart rate change from rest to exercise and the rest end-diastolic volume index did provide additional prognostic information. The RNA variables were equally predictive of mortality as the catheterization variables, which were also available. In fact, RNA contributed 84% of the information that was available from clinical and catheterization data, plus additional prognostic information. The prognostic value of RNA was similar but not as strong when cardiovascular events including both death and nonfatal MI were considered.

Mayo Clinic investigators have published prognostic data in 424 medically treated patients who had both RNA and coronary angiography, followed for a median of 21.7 months (Table 26-6).[39] Thirty-one percent of the patients did not have significant CAD by angiography, whereas patients from the Duke studies all had significant CAD.[36–38] The only variable from RNA that was independently associated with cardiac events, including death, nonfatal MI, or nonfatal cardiac arrest, was rest LVEF. Both rest and exercise LVEF were significant predictive variables of future cardiac events using univariate analysis. However, in contrast to the previous studies, no additional prognostic information was provided from exercise RNA beyond that available from resting RNA and angiographic data. However, the prognostic information available from RNA if the angiographic data were not known was not explicitly addressed.

Prognostic Assessment after Myocardial Infarction

Several investigators have found radionuclide ventriculography to be of prognostic value in patients with a recent MI. In fact, only one study has not shown the test to be of prognostic value. Borer et al.[40] evaluated LVEF by RNA at rest and during submaximal exercise in 45 patients studied 1 day prior to discharge after a MI (Table 26-7). The rest LVEF was 0.39 ± 0.05 and did not change significantly with exercise (0.37 ± 0.05). There was a normal increase of LVEF by greater than 0.05 in only 8 of 45 patients. All 4 of the 45 patients who died in the subsequent 1 year had a rest LVEF of less than 0.35. Determination of the absolute exercise LVEF or the change in LVEF with exercise did not add additional prognostic information to the rest LVEF in this population with significant dysfunction at rest.

The latter study, which may have been influenced by the failure of LVEF to change with exercise in all patients, is outweighed by more favorable results from six other studies. In an initial study by Corbett et al.,[41] submaximal exercise testing with RNA was performed prior to hospital discharge in 61 patients with a recent MI, having a mean resting LVEF of 0.55 (Table 26-7). The rest and exercise LVEF, wall

Table 26-7. Prognostic Value of Radionuclide Angiography in Patients with Myocardial Infarction

Reference	Number of Patients Studied	Rest LVEF	Best Predictor(s) of Subsequent Cardiac Events
Borer et al. (1980)[40]	45	0.39 ± 0.05	Rest LVEF
Corbett et al (1981)[41]	61	0.55	Exercise change in LVEF, ESV, or pressure/volume index
Corbett et al. (1983)[42]	117[a]		Exercise change in LVEF or ESV
Hung et al. (1984)[43]	117	0.49 ± 0.17	Fall in LVEF >0.05 with exercise
Kuchar et al. (1987)[44]	153	0.46 ± 0.12	Fall in LVEF >0.05 with exercise New/Worsened WMAs
Morris et al. (1985)[45]	106		Exercise and rest LVEF
Abraham et al. (1987)[46]	75	0.48 ± 0.15	Rest and exercise LVEF

Abbreviations: ESV, end-systolic volume; LVEF, left ventricular ejection fraction; WMA, wall motion abnormality.
[a] Includes 61 patients in study listed above.

motion score, end-diastolic volume, end-systolic volume, and ratio of systolic blood pressure to end-systolic volume were measured. All but one patient was followed for at least 6 months with a mean follow-up of 9.6 months. By the 6th month of follow-up, 37 of the patients had had a cardiac event—either major (death, recurrent MI, unstable or medically refractory angina) or minor (persistent congestive heart failure, or limiting angina). The most significant variables for predicting any event were the exercise change in LVEF, end-systolic volume, and pressure/volume index. A less than 0.05 increase in the exercise LVEF had a sensitivity and specificity of predicting cardiac events at 6 months of 95% and 96%, and a decrease in wall motion score with exercise had a sensitivity and specificity of 81% and 88%. In contrast, an ischemic ECG with exercise only had a sensitivity of 54% and a specificity of 58% in predicting events. This study demonstrated that RNA prior to hospital discharge was safe and revealed important clinical and prognostic information. Patients could be divided into two groups: one with a very low risk of subsequent events and a second group, with abnormal RNA results, that has a significant risk for subsequent cardiac events.

Corbett et al.[42] extended their study[41] to include 117 patients (Table 26-7). As in the initial study, the exercise change in LVEF and the exercise change in end-systolic volume were the best predictors of future cardiac events when considering all clinical, exercise, arteriographic, and scintigraphic variables for all patients. The predictive accuracy of a change in exercise LVEF was 93%. If only patients with an anterior transmural MI or patients with rest LVEF of less than 0.40 were considered, the peak submaximal LVEF was the best predictor of future cardiac events.

Hung et al.[43] also studied the prognostic value of rest and exercise RNA in 117 patients within 3 weeks of an uncomplicated MI, who were followed-up for a mean of 11.6 months (Table 26-7). Multivariate analysis revealed that a decrease in LVEF of 0.05 or more below the rest value during submaximal effort was most predictive of future cardiac events, including cardiac death, nonfatal ventricular fibrillation, or recurrent MI in this selected population without significant left ventricular dysfunction (rest LVEF 0.49 ± 0.17). In this study, neither rest nor exercise LVEF provided additional prognostic information.

In another RNA study including 153 patients[44] with a rest LVEF of 0.46 ± 0.12 after an acute MI, an abnormal response of LVEF to exercise (fall in LVEF by ≥ 0.05) or a new or worsened wall motion was predictive of future cardiac events (Table 26-7). Significant cardiac events occurred in 17% of patients with a positive RNA, and in only 6% without a positive test. The occurrence of death was significantly more likely with a rest LVEF of less than 40% (11% vs. 1% with an LVEF > 0.40), but the rest LVEF did not predict total cardiac events. Cardiac events were highly predicted by a peak exercise LVEF of less than 0.30.[44]

Morris et al.[45] reported on 106 patients post-MI who performed RNA (Table 26-7). Both rest and exercise LVEF were factors highly predictive of subsequent death by univariate analysis, with exercise LVEF having the higher χ^2 value. Both of these variables yielded significant independent prognostic information beyond that contained in the clinical data. Only the exercise LVEF remained significant in predicting events when a bivariate model was used. The exercise LVEF contained all the prognostic information contained within the rest LVEF. As the exercise LVEF fell less than 0.40, the mortality increased dramatically. The change in LVEF with exercise and the development of new or worsened wall motion abnormalities were not significant variables in predicting future events.

Finally, 75 patients were included in the post-MI study of Abraham et al.[46] (Table 26-7). In this group with relatively well-preserved left ventricular function (rest LVEF 0.48 ± 0.15 and exercise LVEF 0.49 ± 0.15), once again both rest and exercise LVEF were found to be predictive of future events. The change in LVEF from rest to exercise, however, did not help predict prognosis. Using a threshold of rest LVEF of greater than or equal to 0.50 yielded a 2-year cardiac event rate of 16% versus 46% with a rest LVEF of less than 0.50. Using this cutoff for exercise LVEF, event rates were 17% and 58%. In this study, a low rest LVEF predicted future complications, but the change of LVEF did not provide additional information in contrast to other studies cited above.

Use of Nuclear Ventriculography for Risk Assessment after PTCA

The use of nuclear techniques for post-PTCA risk assessment has been discussed fully in Chapter 19. Exercise RNA has been used to identify patients with and without restenosis after PTCA. O'Keefe et al.[47] report on 48 patients with successful PTCA, who underwent exercise RNA within 1 month of PTCA and cardiac catheterization a mean of 8 months after PTCA. A normal RNA was defined as no new wall motion abnormalities with exercise and a greater or equal to 0.05 increase in LVEF with exercise. Restenosis was detected in 13 (27%) of the 48 patients at angiography, and none of the 17 patients with a normal RNA had restenosis. All 13 patients with restenosis had an abnormal exercise RNA. Thus, the results of early, exercise RNA define a low-risk and a high-risk group of patients for subsequently developing restenosis.

Summary

The RNA studies detailed above do not agree as to what constitutes an abnormal response to exercise, and they do not all include the same cardiac events in their analysis of prognosis. However, they have demonstrated that data obtained from RNA can be very helpful in prognosticating future cardiac events in patients with recent MI. Although there is no uniform consensus as to the single best variable to predict future cardiac events, a combination of rest and exercise LVEF, as well as the change in LVEF with exercise, have been shown to add additional prognostic information. Since all are available to the clinician after routine RNA, it is not necessary for clinicians to restrict themselves to one variable. One of the major lessons learned from these studies is that although RNA adds additional prognostic information, it is most helpful to consider all of the information available for an individual patient when making a clinical decision regarding therapy.

CONCLUSION

Stress echocardiography and RNA have both been shown to be useful in the prediction of future cardiac events. Both techniques are routinely successful in providing reproducible rest and stress LVEFs. The induction of ischemia, however, is often not manifest as a change in global LVEF, but rather by a segmental wall motion abnormality. With stress echocardiography, evaluation of wall motion was superior to evaluation of LVEF in predicting future cardiac events. With RNA, the wall motion analysis was not as predictive as LVEF analysis.

No studies have been reported that directly compare the prognostic capabilities of each technique. However, it is likely that stress echocardiography has several advantages over exercise RNA. It provides complete assessment of the contraction of all walls as opposed to the one view usually imaged with exercise RNA. Instantaneous beat-to-beat analysis of LVEF and wall motion are possible with echocardiography in contrast to the summation of several minutes of data with RNA to obtain an average of LVEF and wall motion. Results are immediately available in contrast to requiring computer processing with RNA. Finally, stress echocardiography is completely noninvasive and usually less costly than RNA. Once further data are obtained to confirm the prognostic accuracy of stress echocardiography in larger groups of patients, it seems likely that stress echocardiography will be preferred over RNA for prognosticating future events in patients with known or suspected CAD.

REFERENCES

1. Krivokapich J, Child JS, Gerber RS et al.: Prognostic usefulness of positive or negative exercise stress echocardiography for predicting coronary events in ensuing twelve months. Am J Cardiol 71:646, 1993
2. Sawada SG, Ryan T, Conley JJ et al.: Prognostic value of a normal exercise echocardiogram. Am Heart J 120: 49, 1990
3. Mazeika PK, Nadazdin A, Oakley CM: Prognostic value of dobutamine echocardiography in patients with high pretest likelihood of coronary artery disease. Am J Cardiol 71:33, 1993
4. Afridi I, Quinones MA, Zoghbi WA, Cheirif J: Dobutamine stress echocardiography: Sensitivity, specificity, and predictive value for future cardiac events. Am Heart J 127:1510, 1994
5. Poldermans D, Fioretti PM, Boersma E et al.: Dobutamine-atropine stress echocardiography and clinical data for predicting late cardiac events in patients with suspected coronary artery disease. Am J Med 97:119, 1994
6. Picano E, Severi S, Michelassi C et al.: Prognostic importance of dipyridamole-echocardiography test in coronary artery disease. Circulation 80:450, 1989
7. Severi S, Picano E, Michelassi C et al.: Diagnostic and prognostic value of dipyridamole echocardiography in patients with suspected coronary artery disease: Comparison with exercise electrocardiography. Circulation 89:1160, 1994
8. Amanullah AM, Lindvall K, Bevegard S: Prognostic significance of exercise thallium-201 myocardial perfusion imaging compared to stress echocardiography and clinical variables in patients with unstable angina who respond to medical treatment. Int J Cardiol 39:71, 1993
9. Amanullah AM, Lindvall K, Bevegard S: Exercise echocardiography after stabilization of unstable angina: correlation with exercise thallium-201 single photon emission computed tomography. Clin Cardiol 15:585, 1992
10. Ryan T, Armstrong WF, O'Donnell JA, Feigenbaum H: Risk stratification after acute myocardial infarction by means of exercise two dimensional echocardiography. Am Heart J 114:1305, 1987
11. Applegate RJ, Dell'Italia LJ, Crawford MH: Usefulness of two-dimensional echocardiography during low-level exercise testing early after uncomplicated acute myocardial infarction. Am J Cardiol 60:10, 1987
12. Berthe C, Pierard LA, Hiernaux M et al.: Predicting the extent and location of coronary artery disease in acute myocardial infarction by echocardiography during dobutamine infusion. Am J Cardiol 58:1167, 1986
13. Taylor GJ, Humphries JO, Mellitis ED et al.: Predictors of clinical course, coronary anatomy and left ventricular function after recovery from acute myocardial infarction. Circulation 62:960, 1980
14. Bolognese L, Sarasso G, Aralda D et al.: High dose dipyridamole echocardiography early after uncomplicated acute myocardial infarction: Correlation with exercise testing and coronary angiography. J Am Coll Cardiol 14:357, 1989
15. Picano E, Landi P, Bolognese L et al.: Prognostic value of dipyridamole echocardiography early after uncomplicated myocardial infarction: A large-scale, multicenter trial. Am J Med 95:608, 1993
16. Camerieri A, Picano E, Landi P et al.: Prognostic value of dipyridamole echocardiography early after myocardial infarction in elderly patients. J Am Coll Cardiol 22:1809, 1993
17. Chiarella F, Domenicucci S, Bellotti P et al.: Dipyridamole echocardiographic test performed 3 days after an acute myocardial infarction: feasibility, tolerability, safety and in-hospital prognostic value. Eur Heart J 15:842, 1994
18. Iliceto S, Caiati C, Ricci A et al.: Prediction of cardiac events after uncomplicated myocardial infarction by cross-sectional echocardiography during transesophageal atrial pacing. Int J Cardiol 28:95, 1990
19. Strauss HW, Zaret BL, Hurley PJ et al.: A scinti-photographic method for measuring left ventricular ejection fraction in man without cardiac catheterization. Am J Cardiol 28:575, 1971
20. Alpert NM, McKusick KA, Pohost GM et al.: Noninvasive nuclear kinecardiography. J Nucl Med 15:1182, 1974
21. Green MV, Ostrow HG, Couglas MA et al.: High temporal resolution ECG-gated scintigraphic angiocardiography. J Nucl Med 16:95, 1975
22. Bacharach SL, Green MV, Borer JS et al.: A real-time system for multi-image gated cardiac studies. J Nucl Med 18:79, 1977
23. Steele P, Kirch D, LeFree M, Battock D: Measurement of right and left ventricular ejection fractions by radionuclide angiography in coronary artery disease. Chest 70:51, 1976
24. Burow RD, Strauss HW, Singleton R et al.: Analysis of left ventricular function from multiple-gated acquisition cardiac blood pool imaging: Comparison to contrast angiography. Circulation 56:1024, 1977
25. Maddahi J, Berman DS, Matsuoka DT et al.: A new

technique for assessing right ventricular ejection fraction using rapid multiple-gated equilibrium cardiac blood pool scintigraphy: description, validation and findings in chronic coronary artery disease. Circulation 60:581, 1979
26. Greenberg PS, Ellestad MH, Berge R et al.: Radionuclide angiographic correlation of the R wave, ejection fraction, and volume responses to upright bicycle exercise. Chest 80:459, 1981
27. Berger HJ, Reduto LA, Johnstone DE et al.: Global and regional left ventricular response to bicycle exercise in coronary artery disease: Assessment by quantitative radionuclide angiography. Am J Med 66:13, 1979
28. Jones RH, McEwan P, Newman GE et al.: Accuracy of diagnosis of coronary artery disease by radionuclide measurement of left ventricular function during rest and exercise. Circulation 64:586, 1981
29. Manyari DE, Kostuk WJ: Left and right ventricular function at rest and during bicycle exercise in the supine and sitting positions in normal subjects and patients with coronary artery disease: assessment by radionuclide ventriculography. Am J Cardiol 51:36, 1983
30. Rozanski A, Diamond GA, Jones R et al.: A format for integrating the interpretation of exercise ejection fraction and wall motion and its application in identifying equivocal responses. J Am Coll Cardiol 5:238, 1985
31. Foster C, Dymond DS, Anholm JD et al.: Effect of exercise protocol on the left ventricular response to exercise. Am J Cardiol 51:859, 1983
32. Port S, McEwan P, Cobb FR, Jones RH: Influence of resting left ventricular function on the left ventricular response to exercise in patients with coronary artery disease. Circulation 63:856, 1981
33. Gibbons RJ, Lee KL, Cobb FR et al.: Ejection fraction response to exercise in patients with chest pain, coronary artery disease and normal resting ventricular function. Circulation 66:643, 1982
34. Gibbons RJ, Lee KL, Cobb F, Jones RH: Ejection fraction response to exercise in patients with chest pain and normal coronary arteriograms. Circulation 64:952, 1981
35. Bonow RO, Kent KM, Rosing DR et al.: Exercise-induced ischemia in mildly symptomatic patients with coronary-artery disease and preserved left ventricular function. N Engl J Med 311:1339, 1984
36. Jones RH, Floyd RD, Austin EH, Sabiston DC: The role of radionuclide angiography in the preoperative prediction of pain relief and prolonged survival following coronary artery bypass grafting. Ann Surg 197:743, 1983
37. Pryor DB, Harrell FE, Lee KL et al.: Prognostic indicators from radionuclide angiography in medically treated patients with coronary artery disease. Am J Cardiol 53:18, 1984
38. Lee KL, Pryor DB, Pieper KS et al.: Prognostic value of radionuclide angiography in medically treated patients with coronary artery disease: a comparison with clinical and catheterization variables. Circulation 82:1705, 1990
39. Taliercio CP, Clements IP, Zinsmeister AR, Gibbons RJ: Prognostic value and limitations of exercise radionuclide angiography in medically treated coronary artery disease. Mayo Clin Proc 63:573, 1988
40. Borer JS, Rosing DR, Miller RH et al.: Natural history of left ventricular function during 1 year after acute myocardial infarction: comparison with clinical, electrocardiographic and biochemical determinations. Am J Cardiol 46:1, 1980
41. Corbett JR, Dehmer GJ, Lewis SE et al.: The prognostic value of submaximal exercise testing with radionuclide ventriculography before hospital discharge in patients with recent myocardial infarction. Circulation 64:535, 1981
42. Corbett JR, Nicod P, Lewis SE et al.: Prognostic value of submaximal exercise radionuclide ventriculography after myocardial infarction. Am J Cardiol 52:82A, 1983
43. Hung J, Goris ML, Nash E et al.: Comparative value of maximal treadmill testing, exercise thallium myocardial perfusion scintigraphy and exercise radionuclide ventriculography for distinguishing high-and low-risk patients soon after acute myocardial infarction. Am J Cardiol 53:1221, 1984
44. Kuchar DL, Freund J, Yeates M, Sammel N: Enhanced prediction of major cardiac events after myocardial infarction using exercise radionuclide ventriculography. Aust NZ J Med 17:228, 1987
45. Morris KG, Palmeri ST, Califf RM et al.: Value of radionuclide angiography for predicting specific cardiac events after acute myocardial infarction. Am J Cardiol 55:318, 1985
46. Abraham RD, Harris PJ, Roubin GS et al.: Usefulness of ejection fraction response to exercise one month after acute myocardial infarction in predicting coronary anatomy and prognosis. Am J Cardiol 60:225, 1987
47. O'Keefe JH, Lapeyre AC, Holmes DR, Gibbons RJ: Usefulness of early radionuclide angiography for identifying low-risk patients for late restenosis after percutaneous transluminal coronary angioplasty. Am J Cardiol 61:51, 1988
48. Krivokapich J: Diagnostic and prognostic application of stress echocardiography in coronary disease. Primary Cardiol 20:25, 1994

Chapter 27

Prognostic Evaluation of CAD Patients Using Perfusion Imaging

J. Machecourt, G. Vanzetto, and D. Fagret

BACKGROUND TO THE USE OF PERFUSION SCINTIGRAPHY FOR PROGNOSTIC ASSESSMENT

The "Stenosis at Risk" Hypothesis

A major aim of functional evaluation in patients with known coronary artery disease (CAD) whether they have symptoms or not, is to predict the occurrence of future coronary events liable to compromise survival. This evaluation is extremely important for several reasons:

1. The mortality rate due to chronic CAD is 0.3% per year; it is responsible for the deaths of 500,000 Americans and one million Europeans each year. The aim of recognizing patients at high risk is to submit these patients for myocardial revascularization to improve their prognosis.
2. In this era of cost rationalization, prognostic evaluation aims to define cost-efficient strategies for diagnosis and treatment. For example, in a patient with a low risk of coronary events, further investigation is not justifiable.

As most coronary catastrophes are due to atherosclerotic coronary lesions, the traditional parameters of prognostic evaluation are based on the proof of coronary stenosis, whether the patient has symptoms or not. This proof can be provided directly by coronary angiography, the justification of this tradional approach is based on the results of large-scale angiographic studies that date back to the 1980s. These studies clearly demonstrate the relationship first between presence and extent of coronary stenosis and prognosis, and second between impairment of left ventricular (LV) function and prognosis.[1,2] Indirect markers of myocardial ischemia, which express the consequences of coronary stenosis on myocardial perfusion (exercise stress test, myocardial perfusion scintigraphy, stress radionuclide angiography), have also been shown to have prognostic value.

The rationale of prognostic assessment based upon pre-existent coronary stenosis has been revisited, notably by Fuster.[3] Fully 65% of serious cardiac events occur due to the occlusion of a single coronary stenosis, initially reducing the arterial diameter by less than 50%. Inversely, tighter, more biologically evolved stenoses carry a lower risk of causing transmural necrosis when they become occluded (Fig. 27-1), even though they are liable to cause more ischemia than milder stenoses. These findings would seem to contradict the presence of relationship between the presence and extent of ischemia and the occurrence of a cardiac event. Moreover, this relationship is not present in all studies, or in all clinical situations, or even with all the different markers of ischemia. Thus, after a myocardial infarction, ST-

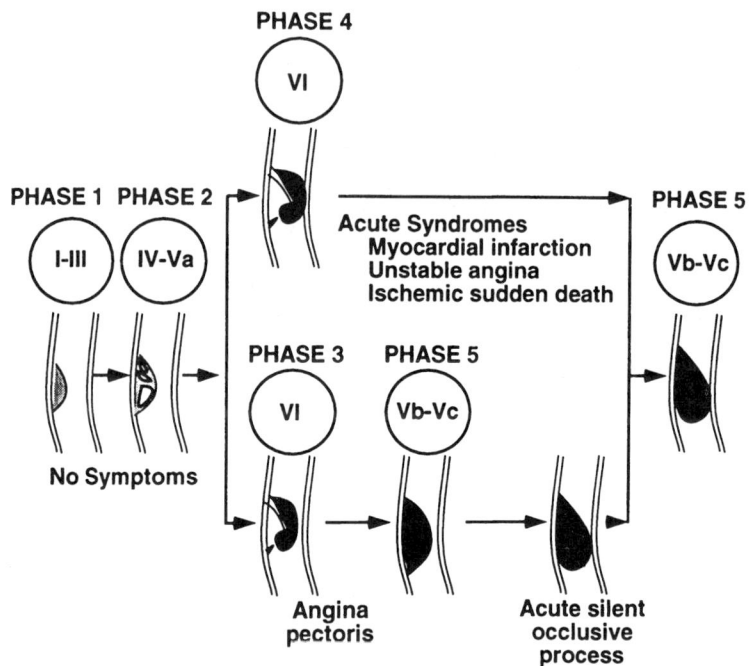

Fig. 27-1. Diagram of lesion morphology and phases of progression of coronary atherosclerosis according to clinical evaluation. Acute life-threatening syndromes (phase 4) develop more often from plaque rupture of a moderate stenosis (phase 2), whereas occlusion from a severe stenosis (phase 5) more often leads to a less severe clinical presentation (acute silent occlusive process, non-Q-wave myocardial infarction). (From Fuster,[3] with permission.)

segment depression, appearing during a test or during an ambulatory electrocardiogram (ECG) recording, has questionable value in the prediction of future cardiac accidents.[4] Identical findings have been reported in patients without prior myocardial infarction.[5] Certain teams even found an inverse relationship between the existence of postinfarction electrical ischemia and the occurrence of a severe coronary event in the following 5 years.[6] On the basis of these data, myocardial ischemia has been labeled "benign,"[7] and therefore this finding has been thought by some to be of little value prognostically.

Despite these findings, the recent definition of the concept of "stenosis at risk" does not threaten the prognostic value of ischemic markers on a conceptual level:

1. Over one-third (35%) of serious cardiac accidents *are* due to the rupture of lesions initially reducing the arterial diameter by more than 50% on the angiography. Therefore, these lesions are, in theory, detectable by perfusion markers.

2. The data on "stenosis at risk" are angiographic. As discussed in previous chapters, coronary angiography greatly underestimates the importance of coronary atheroma and its consequences on myocardial blood flow. This point becomes evident when an intravascular ultrasound is carried out in the face of a discordance between minimal angiographic stenosis severity and the observation of myocardial ischemia.[8]

3. In a patient suffering from CAD, lesions of various degrees and potentialities generally coexist. While the identification of the most threatening lesions requires the availability of high performance markers of myocardial ischemia, which are both sensitive (capable, in particular, of detecting "young," moderate coronary stenoses) and specific, the discovery of at least one significant steno-

sis inevitably signifies a high probability of having others, admittedly less occlusive, but carrying a higher risk of plaque rupture.

4. Lesions having a high risk of fracture cause more myocardial ischemia than do stable lesions. In a population of patients with mainly stable angina and single-vessel coronary disease studied by Picano et al.,[9] complex coronary lesions caused more ischemia (measured by stress echocardiography) than simple ones, even if the two were associated with equal degrees of stenosis (Fig. 27-2). The difference could be explained by the loss of endothelial integrity in high-risk lesions. While this degeneration alters the vasodilatory capabilities of the coronary artery when stimulated by effort or by dipyridamole, it may also facilitate the susceptibility to vasoconstrictor stimuli. Such complex lesions, which are very frequent after unstable angina or myocardial infarction, are also found in 20% to 30% of cases of stable angina, and are not easily recognized by quantitative angiography.[10,11] Thus, there probably *is* a link between the severity of myocardial ischemia and the risk of plaque rupture.

In light of these somewhat discordant data, this chapter will try to define the prognostic value of perfusion scintigraphy under various circumstances, including suspected disease, known disease, and after myocardial infarction. It is important to emphasize

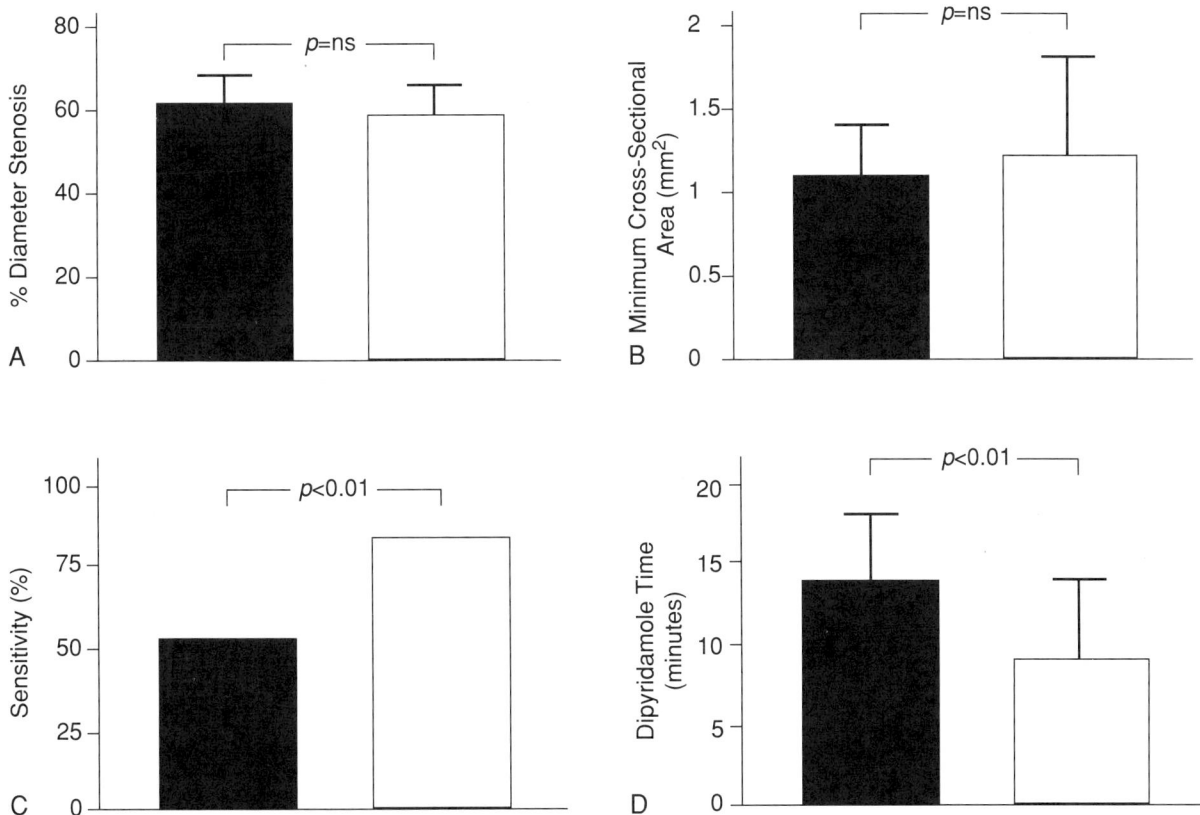

Fig. 27-2. Comparison of severity of myocardial ischemia (as assessed by stress echocardiography) in patients with simple (filled bar) and complex (open bar) coronary lesion morphologies. In spite of the same severity of coronary stenosis on quantitative coronary angiography percent diameter reduction (**A**) and minimum cross sectional area (**B**), complex type plaques exhibit higher prevalence of positivity (**C**) and shorter dipirydamole time (**D**). (From Lu et al.,[9] with permission.)

from the outset that these perfusion markers [thallium-201 and to a lesser extent technetium-99m (^{99m}Tc)-sestamibi] are markers of both myocardial ischemia (and therefore of territory at risk, keeping in mind the restrictions already mentioned), and also of previous irreversible LV damage. An attempt will be made to differentiate between the contribution of each of these aspects toward the prognostic value of perfusion agents. The prognostic value of perfusion imaging will be compared with other markers of CAD, including exercise stress testing, stress radionuclide angiography and stress echocardiography, and coronary stenosis detected by coronary angiography. In light of this review and cost considerations, we will propose decision trees concerning the need to refer the patient for coronary and myocardial revascularization.

Limitations of Nuclear Cardiology

Cost and Availability

Isotopic studies have several handicaps in comparison to other techniques (conventional stress testing, stress echocardiography, coronary angiography) used for prognostic assessment. The cost of the test is high, reflecting both capital and running expenses. The investigation is not performed by the referring cardiologist and sometimes is not directly interpreted by him, as specialized training and credentialing are needed. For these reasons, conventional exercise stress testing, the sensitivity and specificity of which are inferior to those of isotopic techniques, has the advantage of being immediately available. Stress echocardiography entails less financial investment and is more rapidly available, although this technique demands a long learning curve. Coronary angiography is the diagnostic "gold standard" due to its direct visualization of the vasculature, and the sensitivity and specificity of noninvasive techniques are calculated with respect to angiography. In extrapolation, sometimes rightly but often wrongly, the cardiologist tends to think that this examination is also the "gold standard" of prognostic evaluation. In fact, all these investigations are only adjuncts to history taking and clinical examination of the patient, which remain the first indispensable steps. All of these tests have meaning only if they provide significant incremental information with regard to the preceding steps.

In the domain of prognostic evaluation, myocardial perfusion scintigraphy possesses decisive advantages in terms of cost efficiency over other investigations, which justifies its present development in medicoeconomic terms.

Artifacts

Stringent quality control and a highly trained team are imperative for the performance of all invasive and noninvasive techniques, but this is particularly true of nuclear cardiology.[13] While artifacts may arise due to the intrinsic limitations of thallium as a perfusion marker, discussed in Chapter 2 by Schwaiger and co-workers, this problem may be overstated. While good quality data acquisition and image reconstruction are indispensable in the prevention of artifacts, the recognition of certain artifacts (e.g., interposition of the diaphragm in patients with short thoraxes, positional variations of the left ventricle, relative apical hypoperfusion, and, most of all, breast tissue attenuation in women) by the interpreting physician is critical. An experienced observer should recognize these artifacts and give unambiguous answers without altering the specificity of the investigation.[14] Greater uniformity in processing and presenting modalities of nuclear imaging would certainly promote more confidence in the results and hence the optimal performance of the tests used.

Perfusion scintigraphy is often wrongly held responsible for discrepancies caused by problems with the angiogram, such as underestimation of significant complex stenoses (which can now be recognized with intravascular ultrasound), or overestimation of the severity of short stenoses. It is often forgotten that there is only a loose relationship between the angiographic degree of a stenosis, its presumed anatomical territory, and its consequences on myocardial flow. The referring clinician will accept these apparent dissonances if he or she has confidence in the quality of the noninvasive data.

Interpretation

The reproducibility of interpretation is important in prognostic evaluation because the prognostic implications of perfusion defects depend on their extent and severity. The absence of standardization in image processing brings about poor agreement of interpretation from one center to another. In a multicentric study of planar scintigraphy at 24 centers,[15] interinstitutional variability was much less pronounced between two centers using equivalent techniques, although in other studies, a major disagreement was reported in 15% of these interpretations.[16] Quantitative planar thallium scintigraphy seems to increase the reproducibility of interpretation,[17] and the use of single-photon emission computed tomography (SPECT) improves it further. In a study of two observers of the same institution using visual and quantitative analysis of thallium-SPECT, Alazraki et al.[18] reported an agreement of 95% for the defect size and 100% for the location of the perfusion defect and the degree of redistribution. In the same study, the degree of reproducibility between two investigations performed within a short lapse of time was 94%. The level of effort attained on the size of the ischemic region plays an important role in the accuracy of perfusion imaging,[19,20] and probably also in the reproducibility between investigations.

Influence of Medical Therapy

The influence of β-blocker therapy on the prognostic significance of perfusion imaging is controversial.[21] In our experience,[22] as in that of Brown and Rowen,[23] β-blocker therapy does not significantly modify the prognostic value of scintigraphy. On the other hand, treatment with nitrates or calcium blockers may have an important effect if myocardial ischemia is related to a spastic component superimposed on a stenosis.

In practice, the performance of myocardial scintigraphy off anti-ischemic therapy is to be recommended. If, however, drugs cannot be withdrawn due to a supposed risk, we recommend that the administration of nitrate derivatives, β-blockers, and calcium blockers be interrupted for 24 hours. The prognostic examination can also be performed with dipyridamole stress.

PROGNOSTIC VALUE OF PERFUSION MYOCARDIAL SCINTIGRAPHY IN PATIENTS WITH SUSPECTED CAD

Diagnostic versus Prognostic Indications

In patients with suspected coronary disease, the first aim is to use a test that is sufficiently effective to allow us to confidently reassure the patient when it is negative. The second objective is to be able to discriminate between patients with a positive scan who are at moderate or high risk of a "major" event such as cardiac death or nonfatal myocardial infarction. Coronary angiography, with or without revascularization, is justified immediately in high-risk situations, whereas in patients at moderate risk, it will be carried out only if the patient continues to complain of symptoms on medical treatment. Thus, even in patients with suspected disease, the prognostic and diagnostic relevance of the investigation are directly linked. If the patient has extensive or occlusive coronary lesions, the risk of a serious coronary event is high, and coronary angiography followed by myocardial revascularization (if necessary) is appropriate. If the patient has either mild or no coronary lesions, the situation is prognostically benign, and escalation of diagnostic testing should be avoided. In this sense, perfusion imaging is the "gatekeeper" of an invasive strategy.

Factors Influencing Prognostic Value of Thallium Scintigraphy

Since the first work of Brown et al. in 1983,[24] a large body of literature has become available on this subject. An extensive review of these works has been carried out by Brown,[13] and, more recently, by Beller.[25] The principal results, including reanalysis of some of these studies,[26-33] are summarized in Table 27-1. Specific attention should be paid to the presence of defects, their extent, and whether the defects are fixed or reversible.

Prognostic Value of a Normal Perfusion Scintigraphy

The absence of scintigraphic abnormalities corresponds with an extremely low probability of coronary events. In Brown's review of the literature,[13] in more than 3,500 patients followed on average for 29 months after planar scintigraphy, the probability of the occurrence of myocardial infarction or of cardiovascular death was 0.9% per year. In the series of Pamelia et al.,[26] which used quantitative planar scintigraphy, the annual mortality rate of a population of patients investigated for angina and having a low to moderate pretest probability was 0.5% per year. This favorable prognostic implication of a normal scintigraphy seems to be maintained at late follow-up.[35] Our investigations[22] have shown the annual

Table 27-1. Predictive Value of Perfusion Imaging for Occurrence of Major Events[a]

Reference	Number of patients	Study	F/U (years)	Deaths (n)	Nonfatal MI (n)	Significant predictive variables	RR
Brown (1983)[13]	100	Planar exercise thallium	3.7	0	6	Presence of reversible defects Number of reversible defect	
Ladenheim et al. (1986)[30]	1689	Planar exercise thallium	1.0	12	20	Perfusion abnormalities Number of reversible defects Severity of detects	5.1
Gill et al. (1987)[40]	525	Planar exercise thallium	5.0	25	33	Increased lung/heart ratio Fixed defects	8.5 6.6
Stratmann et al. (1989)[38]	195	Planar atrial pacing thallium	1.6	12	6	Perfusion abnormalities Number of reversible defects Severity of defects	2.7
Hendel et al. (1990)[47]	504	Planar dipyridamole	1.8	23	43	Perfusion abnormalities Presence of reversible defects	3.8 2.1
Pollock et al. (1992)[82]	503	Planar stress thallium	4.4	61	30	Increased lung/heart ratio Presence of reversible defects Number of reversible defects	2.4 2.0
Iskandrian et al. (1993)[83]	316	SPECT exercise thallium	2.2	35	35	Extent perfusion abnormality >15% Number of reversible defects	5.0
Travin et al. (1993)[39]	261	Planar exercise thallium	2.1	12	12	For MI: ≥ 4 reversible defects For death: increased lung/heart ratio	5.6 3.7
Machecourt et al. (1994)[22]	1926	SPECT exercise thallium SPECT dipyridamole thallium	2.8	52	48	Extent perfusion abnormality Extent fixed defects Extent reversible defects	15.0 21.0 9.1
Lette et al. (1995)[42]	753	Planar dipyridamole thallium	1.3	53	32	Transient LV dilatation Presence of reversible defects Extent of reversible defects	23.0 7.7
Stratmann et al. (1994)[51]	210	SPECT stress-rest MIBI	1.1	13	11	Perfusion abnormalities Presence of reversible defects	13.8 3.2

Abbreviations: F/U, follow-up; MI, myocardial infarction; SPECT, single-photon emission computed tomography; LV, left ventricle.
[a] Major events include cardiovascular death or nonfatal myocardial infarction. The most predictive variables for each study are indicated, as well as the relative risk (RR) for events when this RR is noted in the paper or can be recalculated from the data of the study.

incidence of deaths of cardiovascular origin to be 0.10%, while the incidence of nonfatal infarction was 0.45%; these values are similar to those measured in the same country in an unselected population (1.2% of major coronary events, deaths, or nonfatal infarction). The predictive value of a normal thallium-SPECT on future freedom from coronary events seemed even greater in our population of patients than in those reported in the literature. This probably reflects the increased sensitivity of thallium-SPECT over planar imaging.[36]

It must be emphasized that the population studied in most of these papers was chosen because of suspected angina or stable ischemia, and that patients with unstable angina or evolving infarction were excluded. The conclusions drawn may not necessarily be applicable to these latter patients. While the inability of thallium imaging to identify nonstenosing coronary atheroma (which can sometimes rupture, leading to coronary thrombosis, myocardial infarction, and sudden death[3]) might be expected to lead to some false negatives, only a few patients who had normal imaging died. This suggests that the probability of evolution toward rupture is low in patients presenting with *only* such minor or mild plaques.

Prognostic Value of Perfusion Defect Extent

It is well known that the number of coronary stenoses determined by coronary angiography is an important prognostic indicator.[1,2] However, when thallium-SPECT detects a large ischemic region, it not only predicts the presence of coronary lesions (generally involving several vessels), but also demonstrates that these stenoses are enough to provoke ischemia. The literature suggests that the extent of the initial defect rather than the degree of hypoperfusion is the primary criterion for long-term prognosis (Fig. 27-3). This relationship between thallium perfusion defect extent and the occurrence of subsequent coronary events was initially described using planar imaging.[24–30]

The main advantage of SPECT over planar imaging is its ability to provide much finer segmental analysis, avoiding the problem of superimposition that occurs with planar imaging, as well a permitting a polar map display, which facilitates quantitation of the extent of ischemia (Plate 27-1). In our experience using SPECT,[22] the probability of cardiovascular mortality was 0.25% in patients without perfusion defects, 2% in patients in whom 16% of the myocardium showed an initial hypoperfusion, 5% in patients with defects in greater than 32% of the myocardium, and 17% in those with greater than 50% of the myocardium presenting an initial perfusion defect. The degree of hypoperfusion on initial SPECT is directly related to the extent of the myocardium either already destroyed by a previous infarct, or ischemic but viable. As destruction of more than 40% of the myocardium is incompatible with survival, it is not surprising that patients with hypoperfusion in greater than 40% of myocardial segments have a poor prognosis.

Prognostic Value of Reversible versus Fixed Defects

The presence of both reversible and fixed defects is predictive of coronary events. Early studies emphasized the prognostic importance of the presence of a reversible defect and established a link between the presence of ischemic territories at risk and the occurrence of a subsequent event.[24] In these studies,

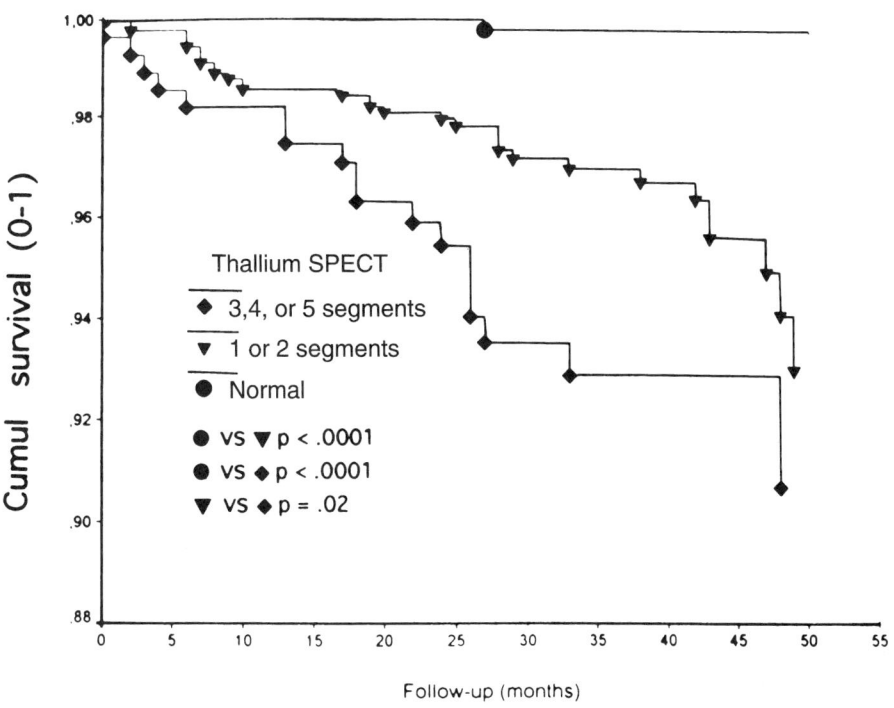

Fig. 27-3. Cumulative cardiovascular survival rate (cumul) according to the number of abnormal segments on initial thallium SPECT imaging. (From Machecourt et al.,[22] with permission.)

a limited fixed defect appeared to be a sign of good prognosis.[37] Later studies showed that extensive fixed defects, and even more so, mixed defects, were associated with an adverse prognosis.[29-31,33-38] In our experience, analysis according to the type of initial defect (transient, mixed, or permanent) demonstrated that these abnormalities were all predictive of cardiovascular events and mortality (the relative risk of annual cardiovascular death being respectively 9%, 18%, and 21%). Hence, in our study, as in that of Stratman et al.,[38] the frequency of cardiac events was even higher in the presence of fixed defects than in that of transient ones.

These discrepancies in the importance of ischemia and scar reflect several issues. First, fixed defects in a postinfarction patient usually (but not always) correspond to the presence of an irreversible myocardial scar, especially when they are extensive. The relationship between prognosis and the severity of ventricular dysfunction (itself related to the extent of scar) is well known. Second, the presence of transient defects may be associated with angina and this combination leads to coronary angiography and then myocardial revascularization. Unfortunately, patients revascularized in the 2 to 3 months following the test were generally excluded from these follow-up studies. Even among the patients revascularized more belatedly, surgery decreases the frequency of serious events. Hence, the presence of a reversible defect is predictive of "soft" coronary events (i.e., revascularization).

On review of the previous studies it appears that among major events, an extensive reversible defect is predictive of the occurrence of subsequent myocardial infarctions, whereas extensive fixed defects, or particularly increased lung activity, are predictive of future death. Hence, in the first study by Brown and Rowen,[23] the presence of a transient defect was predictive of infarction and not of death. In our own study, 52 patients died during follow-up, of which 58% had a fixed defect and 38% a transient defect; 45 patients underwent a nonfatal myocardial infarction, of which 44% had a fixed defect and 48% a transient defect. Mixed defects carried a particularly adverse prognosis. These findings were confirmed in the work of Travin et al.[39] Parameters of LV dysfunction (LV dilation, persistent defect, increased lung activity) indicate that the patient will not survive a new coronary thrombosis if it arises, whereas patients with pure ischemia have more chance of surviving a coronary thrombosis (by having a nonfatal myocardial infarction). This does not mean that myocardial ischemia is benign; however it is certainly better to have an ischemic but viable territory (whose probability of evolution toward necrosis is hypothetical) than an already necrosed territory.

In our opinion, it is the existence of extensive CAD (manifest as extensive or multiple myocardial defects—whether fixed, transient, or mixed), and not the presence of reversible ischemia, that is predictive of future coronary events. This is concordant with the "stenosis at risk" hypothesis, as the ischemic territory does not necessarily reflect the site of future events. The presence of extensive perfusion defects is an index of increased statistical risk of plaque rupture, and also identifies patients with limited reserve to tolerate such an episode, on the basis of LV dysfunction. A normal thallium-scintigram is associated with less plaque burden and hence less chance of a plaque rupture. However, whether this relationship holds true in younger patients (e.g., asymptomatic athletic patients) is unclear.

Prognostic Value of Other Thallium Parameters

Increased lung uptake of thallium-201 (^{201}Tl), as described in 1980 by Boucher et al.,[40] is a parameter which reflects both resting left ventricular dysfunction and the extent of coronary artery disease, as it corresponds with the presence of effort-induced acute pulmonary edema. This parameter is therefore rarely present in patients without CAD. It is most valuable when myocardial revascularization surgery is being discussed (Fig. 27-4). In this case it is most often associated with the presence of multiple or extensive defects on the scintigram.[39]

Transient LV dilatation is also a specific marker of severe coronary lesions.[41] The unfavorable prognostic association of this parameter persists even with dipyridamole-stress scintigraphy (Fig. 27-5).[42]

Choice of Perfusion Imaging Techniques for Prognostic Evaluation

Planar Scintigraphy versus SPECT?

This question is relevant only if the technical quality of SPECT is well controlled. Planar scintigraphy used with good methodology is infinitely better than imperfect SPECT.

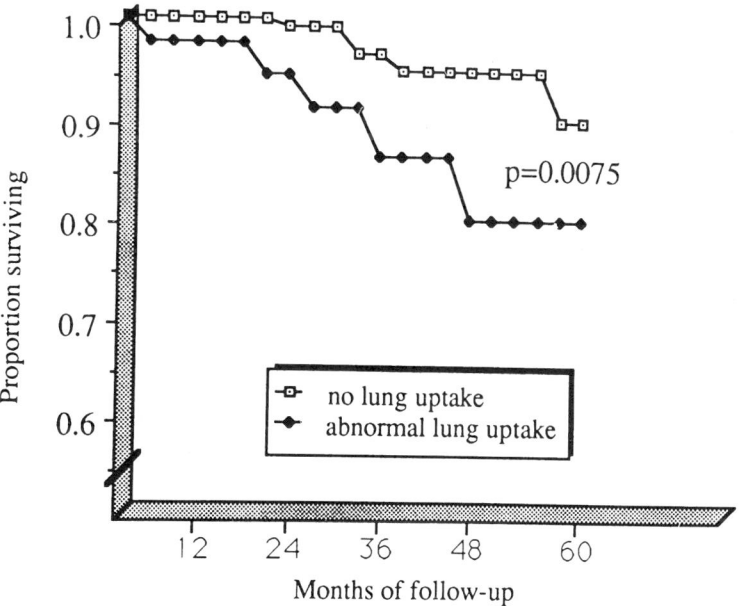

Fig. 27-4. Survival of patients whose thallium-201 showed abnormal lung uptake (i.e., lung–heart ratio > 0.5) compared with patients with normal lung uptake. (From Travin et al.,[39] with permission.)

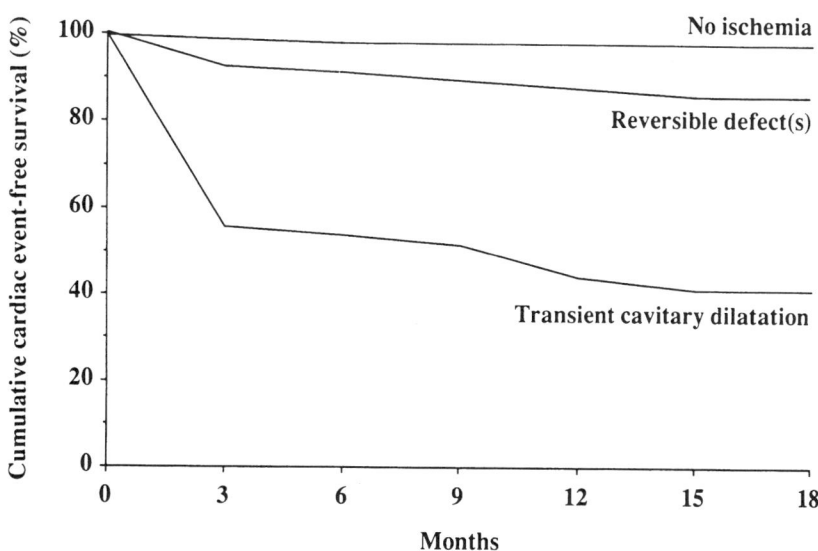

Fig. 27-5. Additive predictive value for prediction of cardiac events of presence of transient dipyridamole-induced left ventricular cavity dilatation, over the presence of only a reversible defect. (From Lette et al.,[42] with permission.)

Due to its greater complexity in the acquisition and processing of images, the true specificity of SPECT is probably inferior to that of planar scintigraphy. The normalcy rate of quantitative thallium-SPECT (the percentage of normal tests in a population that has a very low prevalence of CAD, avoiding posttest referral bias) is 82%, which is 1% to 6% less than that normalcy rate obtained by planar scintigraphy.[43] This slightly lower specificity of thallium-SPECT in comparison with planar scintigraphy is more than compensated, in prognostic studies, by the following advantages: greater sensitivity, higher reproducibility, and superior topographic value. These advantages also appear in Fintel's receiver operating characteristic (ROC) analysis.[36] It should be noted, however, that SPECT does not allow direct evaluation of pulmonary activity, therefore a planar image should be acquired at the beginning of the examination.

Exercise versus Pharmacological Agents?

In patients capable of performing both tests under favorable conditions, the sensitivity and specificity of exercise- and dipyridamole-stress scintigraphy for the detection of coronary artery disease are identical.[44,45] In patients unable to exercise properly, the performance of dipyridamole scintigraphy is superior to that with submaximal exercise. Moreover, the reproducibility of interpretation, in terms of the defect size, is related to the level of exercise attained and thus could be influenced by any anti-ischemic treatment. Dipyridamole-stress scintigraphy could, therefore, be more reproducible in patients on medical therapy over long-term follow-up. Published studies on the prognostic significance of myocardial scintigraphy with administration of dipyridamole demonstrate that, as for exercise stress, a normal dipyridamole scintigram corresponds to a favorable prognosis,[46] and that patients can be divided into low-, moderate-, and high-risk categories according to the extent of the perfusion defect observed.[47,48] The same conclusions may be drawn the study of ^{99m}Tc-sestamibi with dipyridamole[49] and adenosine.[50]

In summary, it seems preferable to use exercise stress thallium- or ^{99m}Tc-sestamibi scintigraphy whenever possible. The use of exercise recreates physiological conditions closer to those of everyday life and the exercise ECG provides additional diagnostic and prognostic information. In patients unable to exercise correctly for various reasons, dipyridamole stress appears to be an excellent alternative for prognostic evaluation.

Thallium-201 versus ^{99m}Tc-Sestamibi

Most of the experimental data published have been collected using either planar or SPECT thallium imaging, coupled with either exercise or dipyridamole. The introduction of ^{99m}Tc-sestamibi has been more recent, but some prognostic studies with this agent are emerging. Stratmann et al.[51] have shown that a normal rest-stress ^{99m}Tc-sestamibi SPECT imparts an excellent 1 year prognosis. The same conclusions were made by Brown et al.[49] using gated rest-stress planar ^{99m}Tc-sestamibi, coupled with exercise or dipyridamole stress. Moreover, the presence of a reversible defect, and, to a lesser extent, a fixed defect on either exercise[51] or dipyridamole[52] stress ^{99m}Tc-sestamibi SPECT identifies patients at high risk of severe events (Fig. 27-6).

The correlation between the extent of ^{99m}Tc-sestamibi perfusion defects and prognosis has not yet been clearly established. The above studies still comprise a limited number of patients with only a short-term follow-up, and often focus on composite endpoints (major events and other coronary events). However, as the diagnostic performance of ^{99m}Tc-sestamibi is similar to that of thallium in the evaluation of myocardial perfusion, we can presume that future studies will confirm a prognostic value comparable to that of thallium. While experimentally ^{99m}Tc-sestamibi[53] shows a greater underestimation of the flow disparity between stenotic and normal perfusion bed (compared with microspheres) than does thallium imaging, this marker is favored by its optimal physical properties. Thus, in obese patients or in women with breast attenuation, in which both the sensitivity and specificity of thallium-SPECT are decreased, the performance of ^{99m}Tc-sestamibi may be superior.

Prognostic Value of Perfusion Imaging versus Other Techniques

Nuclear Ventriculography

As discussed in Chapter 26, resting left ventricular ejection fraction is a major determinant of long-term prognosis. Only 57% of patients with an ejection

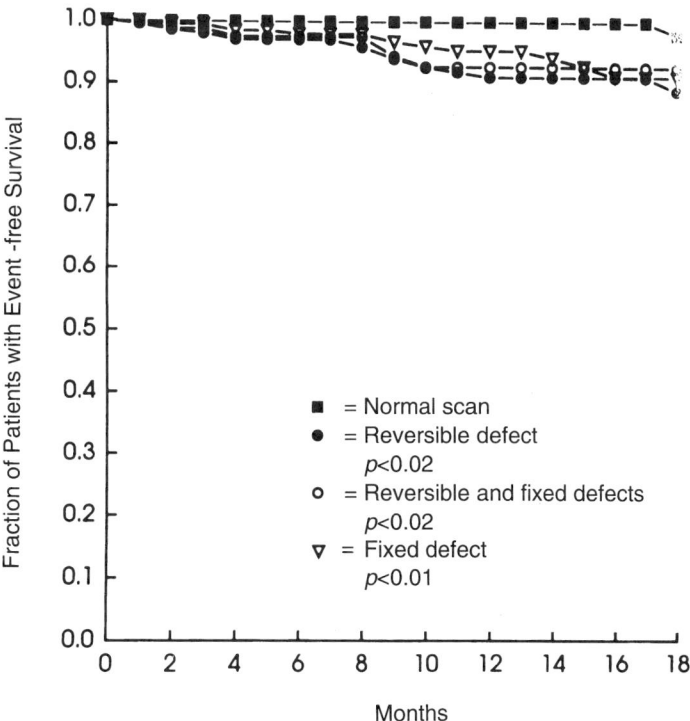

Fig. 27-6. Survival curves for major cardiac events in patients with normal, reversible defect, or fixed defect on sestamibi imaging. Patients with reversible, fixed, and mixed defects had significantly lower event-free survival rates than those with a normal scan. (From Stratmann et al.,[51] with permission.)

fraction less than 35% survive for 4 years, whereas the survival rate is 92% for those having normal ventricular function, whatever their degree of coronary artery disease.[1] Several studies have clearly demonstrated that exercise radionuclide angiography possesses additive prognostic value in such patients.[54–56] Decreased stress ejection fraction, and even more the observation of a peak ejection fraction less than 50%, are markers of poor prognosis. The additive prognostic value of stress-radionuclide angiography over coronary angiography appears well established in patients with basal LV dysfunction and three-vessel disease,[55] or one- or two-vessel disease.[57] In patients with preserved LV function, those with scans indicating inducible ischemia have a more unfavorable prognosis than nonischemic patients.[58] However, the incremental prognostic value of stress radionuclide angiography over the conventional exercise stress test remains controversial in patients with normal resting function[59] or less extensive coronary lesions.[5]

On a conceptual level, the difference between perfusion markers and markers of LV function is that the former are modified earlier in the ischemic cascade. A perfusion abnormality due to a significant stenosis precedes that appearance of myocardial ischemia. The development of ischemia (i.e., worsening of the perfusion abnormality to the extent that an imbalance develops between oxygen supply and myocardial needs) leads to diastolic and systolic LV dysfunction. Therefore, in theory, perfusional myocardial scintigraphy should be more sensitive than stress radionuclide ventriculography or stress echocardiography for evaluating ischemia. Moreover, radionuclide angiography is less specific than perfusional scintigraphy under certain circumstances, and it is rather more difficult to perform. Perfusion scintigraphy and first pass radionuclide angiography

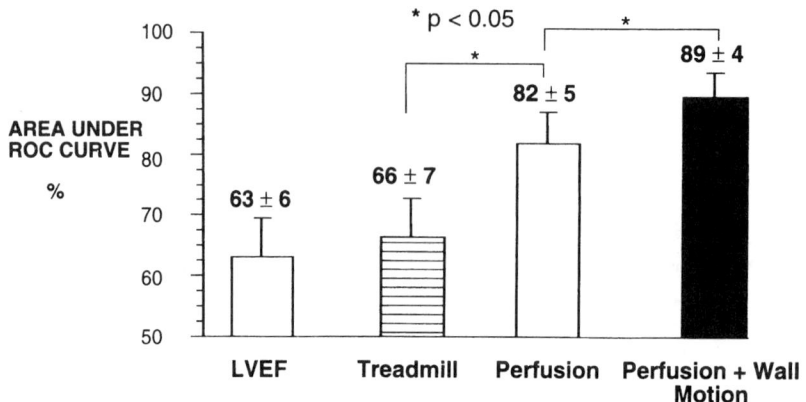

Fig. 27-7. Incremental value of simultaneous assessment of perfusion and left ventricular function with MIBI for prediction of multivessel disease. The perfusion study adds prognostic information over exercise test, and the perfusion plus wall motion study adds prognostic information over the perfusion study. (From Palmas et al.,[60] with permission.)

may be performed at the same time using ^{99m}Tc-sestamibi techniques. In a study of 70 patients, Berman et al.[64] has recently shown that this technique enhances the diagnostic value of perfusion scintigraphy over conventional stress tests, and that the joint analysis of first-pass-radionuclide angiography has incremental value over simple perfusion scintigraphy (Fig. 27-7).

Stress Echocardiography

Stress echocardiography represents an alternative to stress radionuclide angiography. Perfusion scintigraphy and stress echocardiography have been compared in Chapters 4 and 32. From the prognostic standpoint, comparitive prognostic data are not available. However, a recent review by O'Keefe et al.[61] identifies some features that might influence such a prognostic comparison. The sensitivity for detection of coronary artery disease is lower for stress echocardiography than for perfusion scintigraphy, but the specificity is higher. Pooling of these studies suggests that perfusion scintigraphy recognizes multivessel disease better than stress echocardiography (72% vs. 50%, p less than 0.0001). This might suggest that the predictive value of a negative test could be higher with perfusion imaging, but that the value of a positive test would be higher with stress echocardiography. Unfortunately, few large follow-up studies have been published using stress echocardiography; based on early studies, Brown[62] concluded that the cardiac event rate appeared to be three to six times higher among patients with negative stress echocardiography compared with negative myocardial perfusion imaging. These figures may not be true on the basis of more recent data utilizing newer digital equipment and maximal stress.

Prognostic Value of Thallium Scintigraphy in Comparison with Clinical Status

The pretest probability of CAD, which may be derived from age, gender, and clinical status,[63] has a major influence on both diagnostic and prognostic evaluation. From the standpoint of a purely diagnostic evaluation, perfusion scintigraphy should be performed mainly in patients with an intermediate pretest probability (20% to 80%) whereas patients with a high probability should directly undergo coronary angiography. Patients with low probability do not require further investigation. In clinical practice the situation is rather more complex. We must, at the same time, reconcile the imperatives of accurate diagnosis and prognostication of CAD, with cost requirements (to optimize the results of stress testing and to avoid redundant investigations). These issues must be addressed while honoring the patient's demand for an explanation of their symptoms (whether typical or not) and an exclusion of significant coronary disease.

The prognostic value of myocardial scintigraphy has been assessed in groups of patients having var-

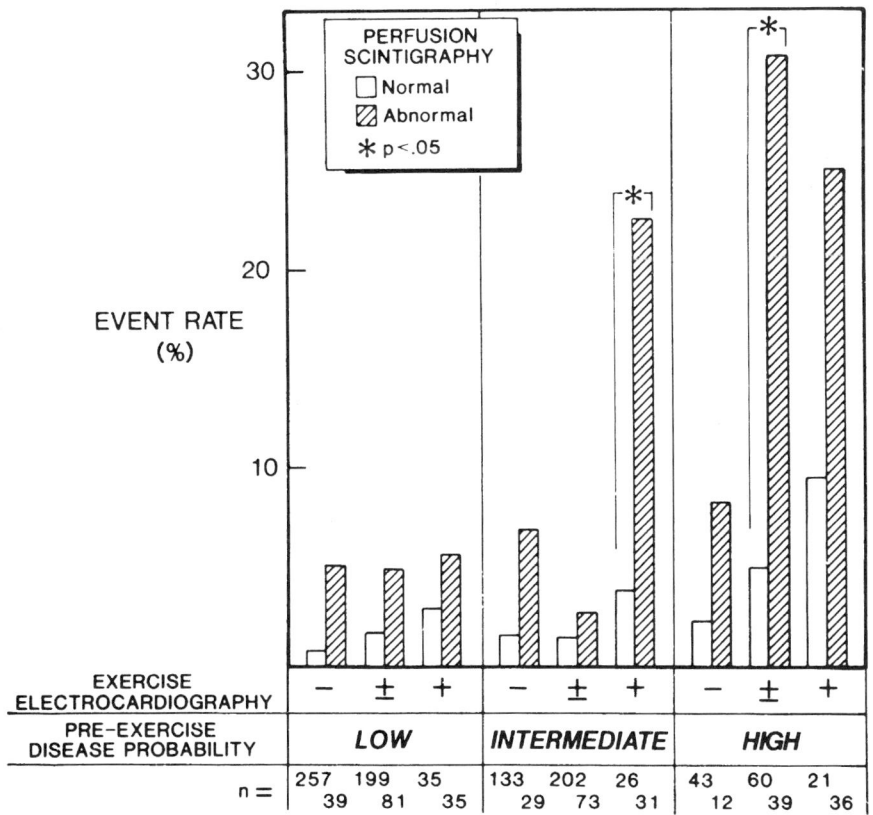

Fig. 27-8. Prognostic value of perfusion scintigraphy according to disease probability, and according to results of exercise electrocardiography. The highest incremental value of thallium is noticed in patients with intermediate or high prevalence of disease. (From Ladenheim et al.,[30] with permission.)

ious probabilities of CAD, determined by clinical data or by exercise stress-testing results. Ladenheim et al.[30] have shown that thallium myocardial scintigraphy has prognostic value in patients of low, intermediate, and high pretest probability, although this increment was higher in patients with a high probability of disease (Fig. 27-8). The same findings have been reported using ^{99m}Tc-sestamibi,[64] and it has been particularly emphasized that this investigation retains a high prognostic value in patients with a high pretest probability of disease.

The difficulties in diagnosing CAD in women are discussed in Chapter 9. From the diagnostic standpoint, several aspects are important. The positive predictive value of these tests is influenced by a lower prevalence of CAD in women under age 60, as well as a lower specificity of the stress ECG and thallium scintigraphy due to breast attenuation. The sensitivity of thallium-SPECT seems to be lower in women than in men.[65] In light of these findings, it might be feared that the prognostic value of perfusion scintigraphy would be compromised in women. In fact, preliminary studies published on this subject suggest that the prognostic value of thallium imaging is maintained. Pancholy et al.[66] reported that in a study of 212 women, the number of abnormal vascular territories was an independent predictor of events. Machecourt et al.[22] followed 623 female patients for on average 33 months and showed that the relative risk of cardiovascular death after a *normal* SPECT (0.10% per year) was as low in women as in men. The relative risk of coronary death following an *abnormal* scintigram was increased 12 times in women ($p < 0.003$); the positive predictive value of thallium-SPECT was, however, lower in women than in men. Hendel et al.[67] have also shown that the presence of a perfusion defect is predictive of coronary events at 1 year in middle-aged women presenting lower-limb arteriopathy.[67] These studies suggest that stress perfusion myocardial scintigraphy (with exercise or with pharmacologic agents) retains its prognostic relevance in women.

Prognostic Value of Thallium Scintigraphy versus Exercise Stress Testing

The features of conventional exercise stress testing that have prognostic significance (either for the existence of extensive coronary lesions, or a high probability of severe long-term cardiac events) have been discussed in Chapter 25. These include signs of a "strongly positive" test: decreased exercise capability, diminished peak maximum heart rate, and ST-segment depression of greater than 2 mm appearing at a low workload and persisting for more than 6 minutes after the end of exercise. The use of a treadmill score, taking into account these factors as a whole, provides additive prognostic data.[68] Some of these parameters reflect LV dysfunction, whereas others reflect the quantity of threatened ischemic myocardium. However, while these ECG parameters certainly have value in a homogeneous population of coronary patients, in a more heterogeneous population of patients investigated for suspected CAD, the lack of specificity of these signs alters their prognostic value. For example, inability to attain a high workload may be due to various extracardiac causes (physical, pharmacologic, or psychological) as well as due to severe CAD. Likewise, due to the suboptimal specificity of the exercise ECG, significant ST-segment depression is often due to nonischemic etiologies.

Thallium myocardial scintigraphy has been shown to offer prognostic information independent and incremental to the standard exercise stress test (Fig. 27-9). Machecourt et al.[22] have shown that a submaximal exercise ECG corresponds to a greater coronary risk than a negative or even a positive maximal exercise ECG. Among patients with submaximal tests, however, a normal thallium scan is associated with a substantially better prognosis that the observation of an abnormal one. These nondiagnostic exercise tests represent 20% to 30% of ergometric tests, and mainly occur because it is impossible to reach a sufficient heart rate during effort (85% of the maximal predicted heart rate), usually because of recent withdrawal of antianginal medication (primarily β-blockers). Although the prognostic value of thallium scintigraphy has been questioned in some studies when anti-ischemic drugs have not been stopped,[18,20,21] these treatments may have a lesser influence on the prognostic interpretation of the scintigraphy.[23] Thallium-SPECT also provides additional prognostic information in patients after a maximal exercise ECG. This is a population with a lower probability of events than patients with submaximal test. However, the incidence of major events was 10 times higher in our series after an abnormal thallium-SPECT than after a normal one ($p < 0.02$).

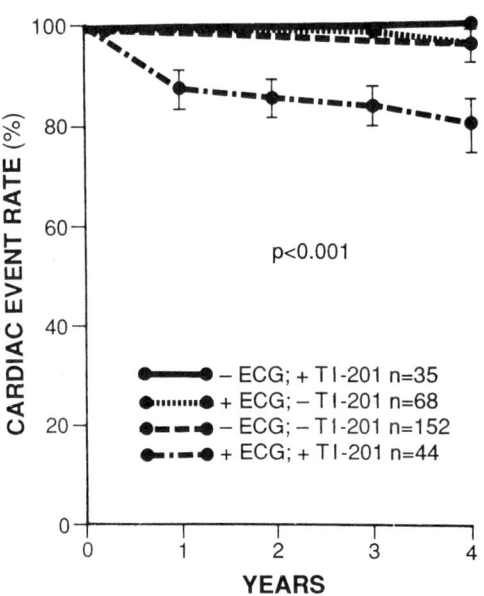

Fig. 27-9. Actuarial event-free survival curve according to combinations of exercise electrocardiographic and scintigraphic results in patients with maximal exercise test: in patients with moderate probability of disease, the rate of cardiac events was greatest in patients having both an abnormal exercise electrocardiogram and abnormal thallium scan. (From Fagan et al.,[72] with permission.)

By comparing patients with slightly positive and strongly positive exercise tests, Taylor et al.[71] recently demonstrated that the magnitude of ST-segment depression is poorly correlated with the ischemic mass measured by scintigraphy (Fig. 27-10). In patients with a positive exercise stress test, Krish-

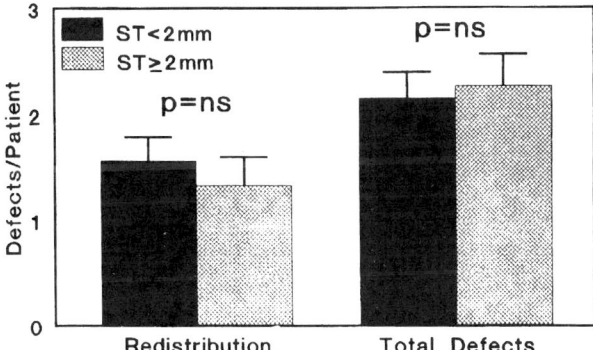

Fig. 27-10. In patients with unequivocal positive exercise stress test there is no correlation between the number of Tl redistribution defects, and total defects per patient, for patients with less than 2 mm (dark bars) and greater than 2 mm (hatched bars) of exercise induced ST depression. (From Taylor et al.,[71] with permission.)

nan et al.[69] also demonstrated that among those having a strongly positive exercise ECG, thallium scintigraphy identifies two groups having different prognosis: patients with normal or nearly normal scans had minimal coronary lesions and thus a much better prognosis under medical treatment than those presenting an abnormal scan.

In patients with a negative exercise test, perfusion imaging has the potential of offering additional prognostic stratification. In our series,[22] the event rate was 0.55% per year after a maximum negative exercise test and 0.10% per year following a normal SPECT. Among patients with a maximal negative exercise test, patients with a negative thallium scan had a major event rate (death or myocardial infarction) three times lower than patients with an abnormal scan. However for Krishnan et al.,[69] in patients with normal maximal exercise tests and low or moderate probability of disease, thallium scintigraphy did not provide additional prognostic information. These results are concordant with those of Schalet et al.[70]

In summary, myocardial scintigraphy has better predictive value than conventional exercise testing in the evaluation of extent of coronary lesions and the prediction of cardiovascular events. The superiority of perfusion scintigraphy over exercise ECG persists even when rest ECG is normal.[73] Hence, in clinical practice, myocardial scintigraphy has supplementary prognostic value when associated with a nondiagnostic exercise test, or after a strongly positive exercise stress test in patients having moderate or ambiguous chest pain. However, it is redundant in patients with high pretest probability of disease, as such patients can undergo coronary angiography immediately following a positive exercise test.

Prognostic Values of Perfusion Imaging versus Coronary Angiography

Patients without Significant Stenoses

The high predictive value of a normal coronary angiogram is well established, with up to 10 years of follow-up in some studies.[74,75] This incidence of cardiovascular events is comparable to that reported in the literature following normal thallium scintigraphy. Several recent studies of relatively small numbers of patients (75 and 93, respectively) reveal that the long-term cardiac event-rate is low (around 1% per year) in patients with a normal thallium scan despite abnormal coronary angiography, even among patients with multivessel disease.[76,77] The observation of normal perfusion in a territory supplied by a stenosed vessel may be explained by several phenomena: the stenosis is, in fact, less severe than it appears on visual or even quantitative angiographic analysis, the region situated downstream of the stenosis is too small for ischemia to be detected, or there exists a collateral circulation that protects this distal territory. In the last two instances, the prognosis following an eventual occlusion is benign.

Patients with Significant Disease

The relative prognostic significance of multivessel and single vessel disease is well established.[1,2] Nonetheless, even if single-vessel lesions have a good overall prognosis, adverse consequences do occur in some patients. Conversely, although the prognosis of patients with multivessel disease is globally more severe, this is not universally deleterious (50% of these patients are alive at 10-year follow-up).

Numerous studies have demonstrated that the presence of extensive perfusion defects, especially on SPECT,[78] and increased pulmonary activity[79] are reliable predictors of multivessel or left main disease as well as coronary events. Despite these observations, coronary lesions that appear identical may have very different cardiovascular prognoses, depending on whether they are responsible for a sizable ischemic region. Mahmarian et al.[80] have shown that proximal stenosis of the left anterior descending artery can lead to a perfusion defect of between 0% and 44% of the left ventricle. No relationship was found between the degree of stenosis and the extent of myocardial hypoperfusion in such patients.

Exercise planar thallium-201 scintigraphy is as powerful a prognostic determinant as coronary angiography,[81] and adds significantly to the data obtained by clinical and exercise ECG when viewed on an incremental basis.[82] Indeed, Kaul et al.[81] reported that coronary angiography provided little additional prognostic information to clinical, ECG, and thallium data. Iskandrian et al.[83] have shown that in patients with CAD, thallium-SPECT provides incremental prognostic information once catheterization data are available (Fig. 27-11). As in our series, the extent of the initial perfusion defect was found to be the most important prognostic factor with thallium scanning. We note that in these works, the angiographic ejection fraction was not always taken into account. Marie et al.[84] recently showed that in patients with high pretest probability, the ejection fraction and the extent of myocardial hypoperfusion using thallium are the two independent survival predictors. The number of coronary lesions defined by angiography has less value.

In summary, among patients with angiographically defined coronary disease, whether they have single-vessel or extensive lesions, the presence and extent of myocardial ischemia during myocardial perfusion scintigraphy allow us to better identify those having a high risk of complications. It is important to distinguish among these patients, as those at highest risk will benefit from myocardial revascularization. Conventional stress testing possesses additive prognostic value over coronary angiography, and perfusion scintigraphy adds further information. The extent of the ischemia reflects not only the size of the jeopardized myocardial territory, but perhaps also the risk of coronary thrombosis.[9]

Prognostic Evaluation in Patients with Silent Myocardial Ischemia

Increasing attention has been paid over the past few years to the diagnosis of silent myocardial ischemia. In patients without known CAD, this diagnosis is relevant only if it permits discrimination of those patients having a high probability of future coronary events, despite their lack of symptoms. As in symptomatic patients, it is the evaluation of pretest probability that allows good stratification and effective use of tests, in particular, of myocardial perfusion scintigraphy. Three prognostic groups may be identified:

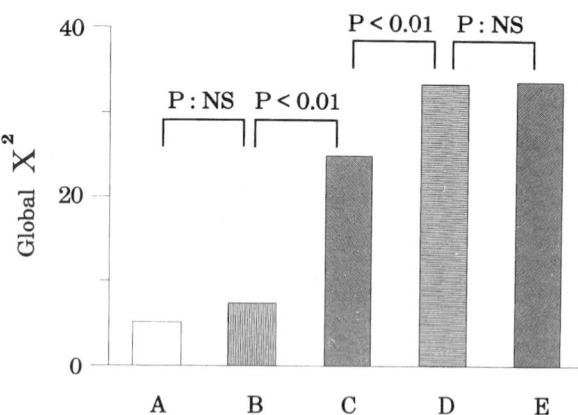

Fig. 27-11. Comparison of incremental prognostic power of clinical, exercise, catheterization, and single-photon emission computed tomography (SPECT) variables. Clinical + exercise + SPECT data, D, provide more prognostic information than clinical + exercise + catheterization data, C; A, gender; B, exercise metabolic equivalent as assessed on exercise; E, exercise + SPECT + catheterization data. (From Iskandrian et al.,[83] with permission.)

1. Asymptomatic patients having a low to moderate risk, but liable to make their first presentation of CAD with an inaugural cardiac event (type I silent myocardial ischemia according to Cohn). The coronary risk in athletic individuals falls into this category.
2. Asymptomatic patients having a statistically high long-term coronary risk: patients suffering from type I or II diabetes, chronic renal failure with microalbuminuria, or lower limb arteriopathy. These patients also belong to Cohn's group 1.
3. Patients with known coronary disease who no longer present symptoms, for example after an myocardial infarction or an episode of unstable

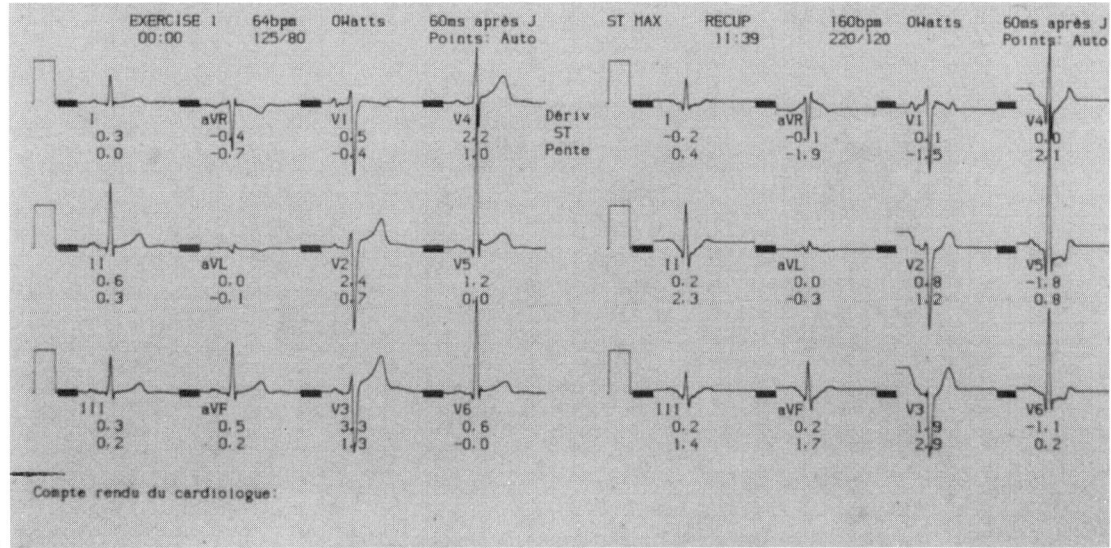

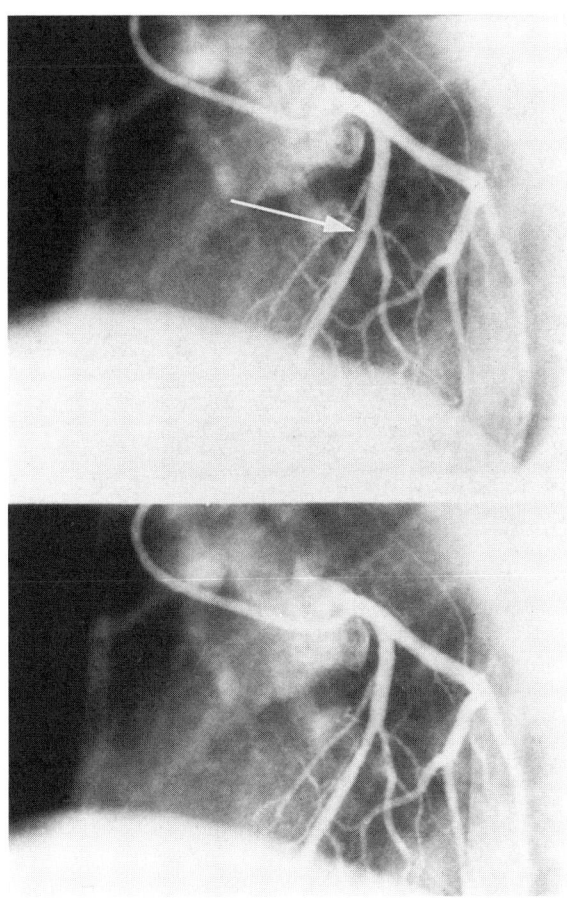

Fig. 27-12. (**A**) Detection of silent ischemia in an asymptomatic, 46-year-old athelete, studied because of hypercholesterolemia and a family history of coronary disease. Exercise ECG—1.8 mm ST-segment depression at 93% maximum predicted heart rate. (**B**) Coronary angiography (left anterior oblique [LAO] view)—apparently mild mid-left anterior descending coronary disease (approx 45% stenosis, minimal lumen diameter 1.5 mm). *(Figure continues.)*

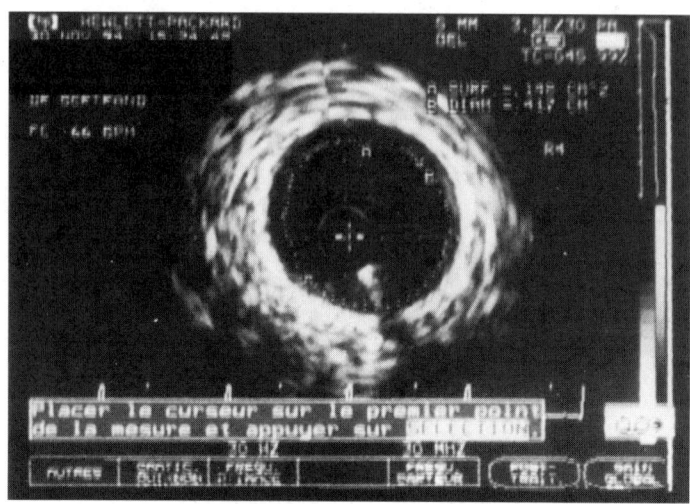
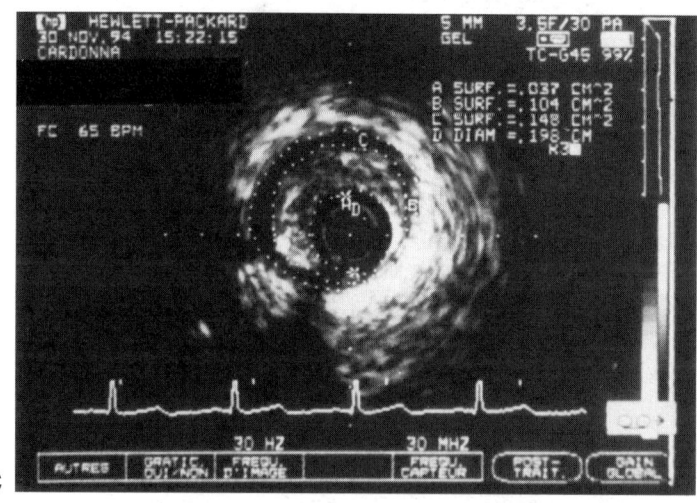

Fig. 27-12. *(Continued).* **(C)** Intravascular ultrasound—significant diffuse disease (56% stenosis, minimal lumen diameter 1.5 mm). The patient was treated with aspirin, β-blockade, and cholesterol-lowering therapy. (See Plate 27-2 for SPECT-Thallium.)

angina (silent myocardial ischemia type II). These will not be considered further.

Asymptomatic Patients with a Low Risk

The utility and advantage of using screening tests for the prognostication of such patients are controversial issues. Effectively, even if we know that ST-segment depression during stress test is a risk factor for future events, the positive predictive value of this sign is extremely low in patients with a low pretest probability of CAD.

The work of Fleg et al.[85] clearly shows the complimentary value, but also the limitations in the use of perfusion scintigraphy in such patients. This study involved 407 asymptomatic volunteers (mean age 60 years, range 40 to 94), with relatively few risk factors (3% diabetics, 10% to 14% current smokers or having dyslipidemia). It showed that the frequency of concordant positive results (positive stress test and scintigraphy), in favor of myocardial ischemia, drastically increased with age. In patients under 59, this frequency was 2%, whereas in patients over 70 it reached 12%; 48% of these patients with concordant positive results suffered a coronary event at an average follow-up of 4.6 years. However, of 40 recorded coronary events (of which 20 were deaths or infarcts), 23 (13 of which were deaths or infarcts) occurred in patients having double negative results in these tests, and only 11 (5 of which were deaths or infarcts) arose in patients having double concordant positive results. The yield of this search for asymptomatic myocardial ischemia (which increased with the patient's age) was therefore relatively limited even if, for a patient considered, the observation of a double positive result indicated a poor prognosis and provoked further investigations. Thus, in clinical practice, silent ischemia should be searched for only in populations at high coronary risk based upon age (> 40 for men, > 55 for women), family history of myocardial infarction or sudden juvenile death, and two or more other classical risk factors (smoking, dyslipidemia, high blood pressure, diabetes).

The detection of coronary risk (myocardial infarction or death) in athletic individuals or during sport poses problems of its own. Effectively, 4.4% of infarcts arise following heavy physical exertion, and this risk is related inversely to the level of fitness of the subject.[86] However, the occurrence of acute coronary accidents is not rare after strenuous physical exertion even in trained athletes. When an angiogram is immediately performed in such patients, there is nearly always a coronary occlusion or subtotal occlusion due to a ruptured plaque.[87] While few data are available concerning the previous state of their coronary arteries, the fact that most of these events occur in patients over 40, with at least one major risk factor, suggests that these patients had significant coronary lesions before the accident. In the absence of more precise published data, we limit the search for silent myocardial ischemia to high-risk athletes having a family history or major risk factors (Fig. 27-12 and Plate 27-2). However, for reasons of cost containment, this quest cannot be applied to athletes as a whole, and as pre-event lesion severity is probably moderate, it is likely that the majority of these events will remain unpredictable.

Asymptomatic Patients with an Intermediate or High Risk

This group includes patients with diabetes or chronic renal failure, who despite their asymptomatic status are at greater risk than the previous group of patients. Diabetics belong to a population of patients having an intermediate prevalence of coronary artery disease[88] with a high cardiovascular mortality rate, especially if other risk factors are present,[89] and even more so if renal damage is associated.[90] This has prompted attempts to screen for myocardial ischemia, either systematically or before surgery (especially kidney transplantation).

The works published on risk stratification in renal disease are based on a limited number of patients, and provide relatively contrasting findings. Each of these studies reveals a high number of false-positive defects in diabetics,[90,91] possibly because of the prevalence of small vessel CAD and LV hypertrophy. The low positive predictive value of thallium scintigraphy is also a consequence of the intermediate pretest probability in these asymptomatic patients. The value of a reversible thallium defect for detecting patients at risk of cardiac accidents, especially before renal transplantation,[92–96] is discussed in Chapter 11. A long-term prognostic study comprising a large number of patients with diabetic nephropathy is needed. At present, our practice follows the recommendations of Le et al.[97] and Eagle et al.,[98] and involves the performance of stress thallium imaging in patients presenting at least two classical clinical risk factors (age > 60, history of angina, arterial hypertension, peripheral vascular disease, abnormal ECG, microalbuminuria), followed by angiography in case of high-risk abnormalities and by myocardial revascularization if necessary.

Detection Strategy for Type I Silent Myocardial Ischemia

In accordance with the above definition, this involves assessment of high-risk asymptomatic patients (Fig. 27-13). The conventional exercise ECG should be the first step. If maximal and negative it imparts a low coronary risk, justifying a strategy of risk factor control, and simple surveillance. If positive or highly positive, a myocardial perfusion study is indicated: coronary angiography is necessary if the latter pro-

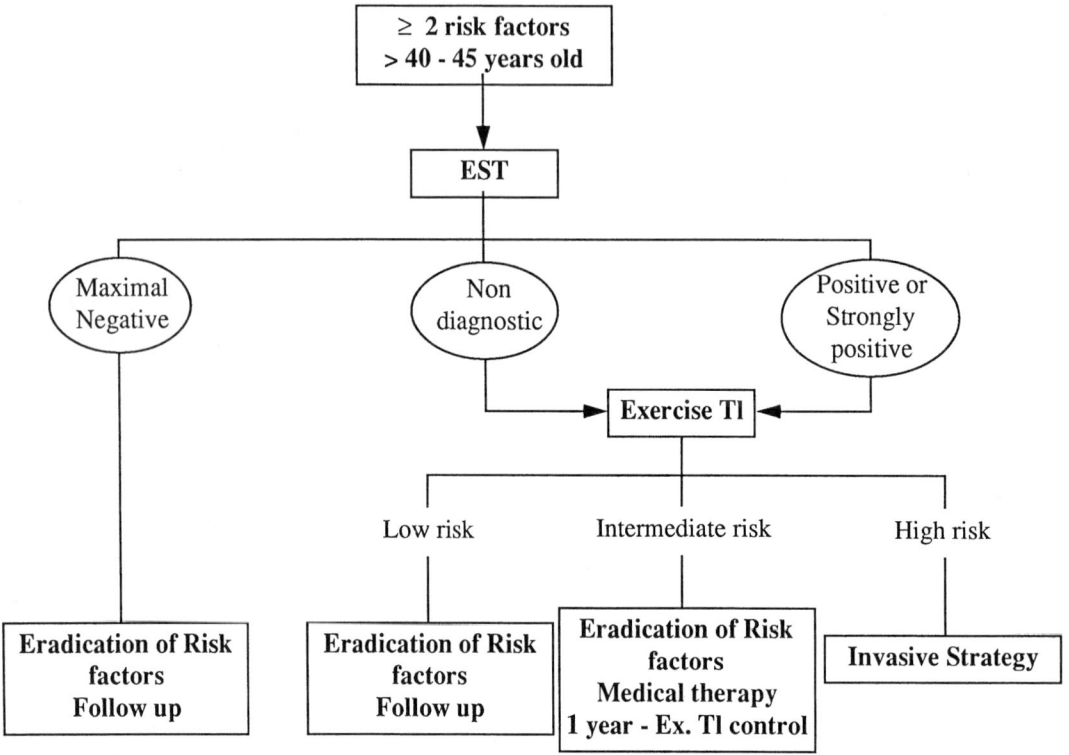

Fig. 27-13. Decision tree for risk stratification in patients with suspected silent myocardial ischemia (see text for explanations).

vides a concordant positive result, especially if the perfusion defect is extensive and associated with lung uptake or cavity dilatation. Whatever the result of the stress ECG, if the scintigram is negative, angiography should not be carried out. If the exercise ECG is nondiagnostic, we proceed to thallium imaging with maximal exercise, or pharmacologic stress thallium imaging. In such asymptomatic patients, an equivocal or slightly ischemic thallium scan (a single abnormal territory, with or without redistribution) does not justify the performance of angiography.

Proposed Decision Tree in Patients with Suspected Coronary Artery Disease (Fig. 27-14)

The following decision pathway is employed at our center, in light of the above data. In patients with low pretest probability (< 20%—group 1) or with high coronary probability (> 80%—group 3), myocardial perfusion imaging is not immediately justified; exercise ECG is the first line exploration of choice. If the exercise test in a group 1 patient is negative at greater than 85% of age-predicted maximal heart rate, this is very reassuring on both a diagnostic and prognostic level. If the exercise ECG is markedly ischemic in a group 3 patient, this justifies performance of coronary angiography. However, if the results of the stress ECG diverge from the clinical status (i.e., positive stress test in a group 1 patient or negative result in a group 3 patient), then these patients fall into a category of intermediate probability and therefore a scintigram should be carried out, either coupled with a second exercise test or with pharmacologic stress. The use of perfusion scintigraphy in group 1 and 3 patients is thus in series with clinical examination and exercise ECG, in a conditional manner. A group 1 patient with a positive exercise ECG, with a scintigram suggestive of extensive disease, should undergo coronary angiography and treatment. A normal or nearly normal scintigram in a group 3 patient having a negative stress ECG

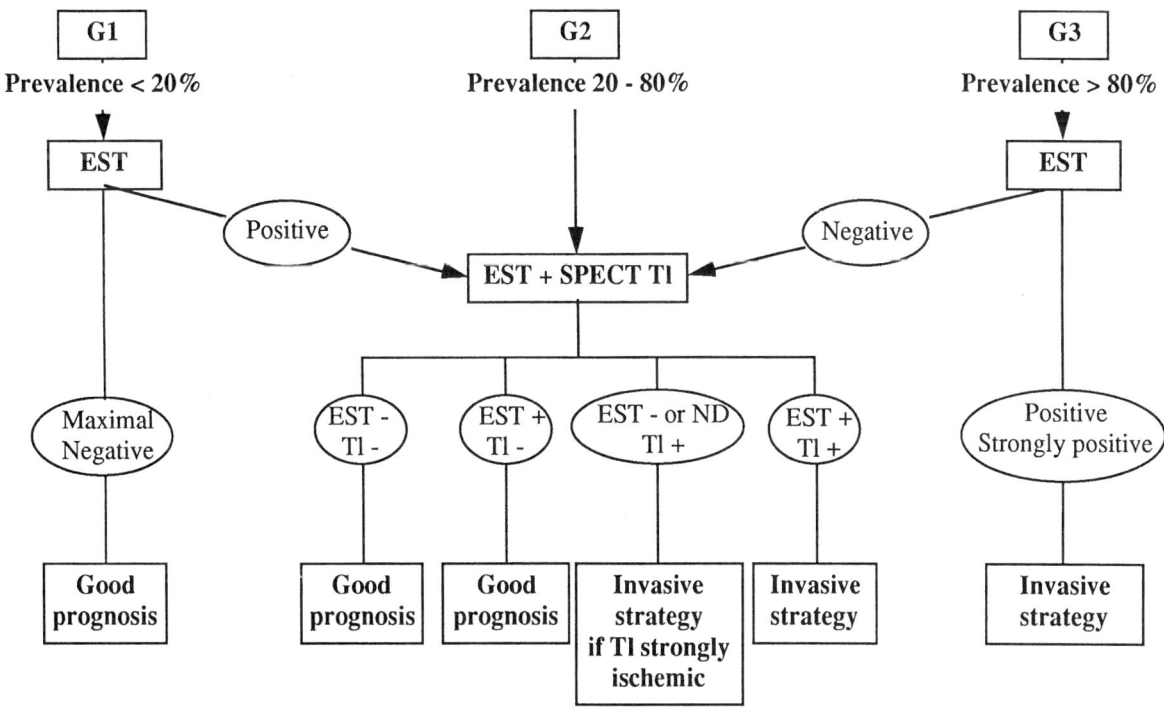

Fig. 27-14. Decision tree for risk stratification and prognostication in patients with suspected coronary artery disease (see text for explanations).

should not lead to an angiography, but to surveillance and, in the majority of cases, to medical treatment.

Patients of intermediate pretest probability may be so defined on the basis of classical clinical parameters (group 2) or with the help of diagnostic findings from the conventional exercise ECG (as we have already seen in groups 1 and 3). In these groups, myocardial perfusion scintigraphy should be carried out in parallel with the stress ECG. In such patients, a double positive test generally leads to coronary angiography (especially if the patient is symptomatic and/or the scintigram reveals a poor prognosis). The observation of a double negative test is reassuring, and leads us to abort all further investigations. If divergent results are observed, they should be considered case by case, with more emphasis on the scintigram, as a normal test corresponds with a good prognosis and a highly pathological scintigram generally justifies a coronary angiogram.

PROGNOSTIC RELEVANCE OF MYOCARDIAL PERFUSION SCINTIGRAPHY IN PATIENTS WITH KNOWN CAD

Prognostic Relevance in Patients with Stable CAD

In patients with known coronary disease, perfusion imaging may enhance decision making, the selection of myocardial revascularization (coronary artery bypass grafting or percutaneous transluminal coronary angioplasty), and medical treatment. Yusuf et al.[99] recently reported a meta-analysis of large-scale therapeutic trials, comparing results 10 years after surgical or medical treatment of stable angina. This work showed the most important indicators of a prognostic benefit with revascularization to be the extent of coronary lesions on angiography, the status of LV function, and the importance of myocardial ischemia. Demonstration of the benefit of surgical revascularization in patients with multivessel disease has required large populations, because of the heterogeneity of the group with multivessel disease.[1,2] Many of these patients have stenoses of intermediate severity, in which the anatomic interpretation of functional significance may be problematic. Perfusional scintigraphy may elucidate the functional character of stenosis in the patients with ambiguous coronary arteriograms, and thus aid in the decision of whether to carry out myocardial revascularization.

In most cases, the importance of myocardial ischemia is appreciated in a fairly simple way in these large trials: either by classing patients according to their ischemic score (based on the severity of the angina and on rest ECG modifications), or to the findings of conventional stress testing. Patients defined as being at high risk according to the degree of ischemia benefit from surgery in prognostic terms, whereas patients defined as being at low risk according to the degree of ischemia do not. Iskandrian et al.[100] have shown that myocardial scintigraphy allows a better stratification of patients' future risk than clinical findings or the results of exercise ECG. If for a given patient medical treatment is effective in improving symptoms and if the patient is classed as "low risk"—as previously defined—coronary an-

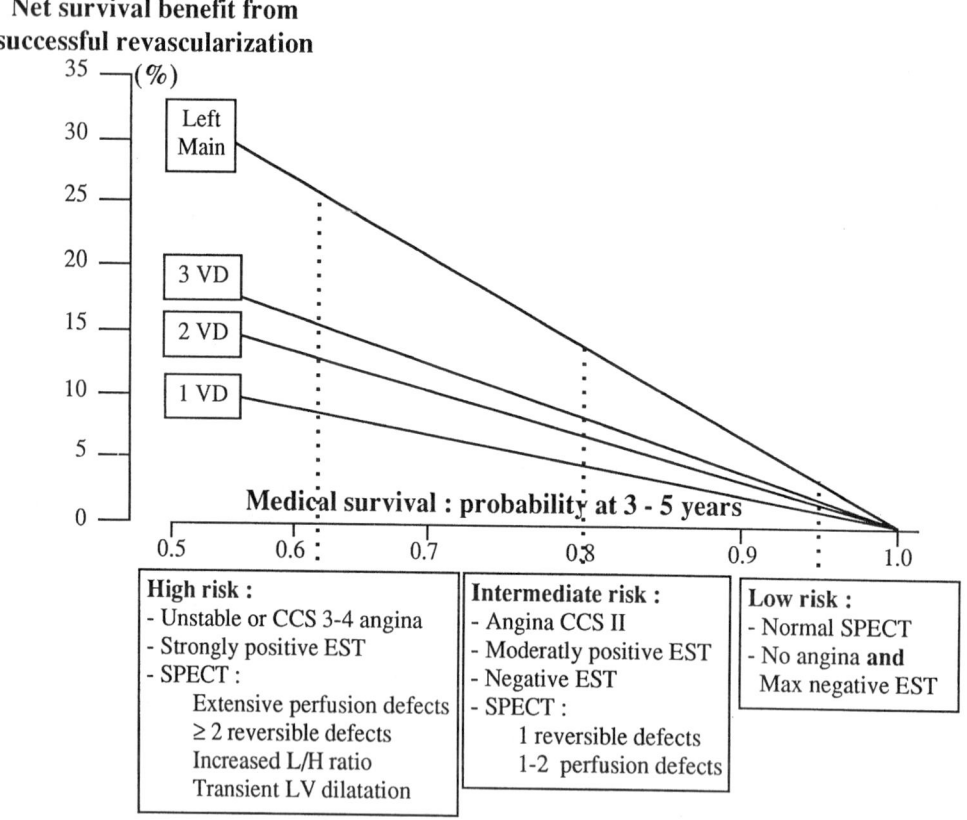

Fig. 27-15. Survival benefit that can be expected from successful revascularization, according to extent of coronary lesions and to prognostic variables obtained from functional tests (clinical variables, exercise electrocardiogram, perfusion imaging). On the x-axis the probability of survival at 3 to 5 years derived from the functional tests is plotted. For a given patient, a probability of occurrence of a serious cardiovascular event can be estimated. Afterward the net survival benefit from revascularization, according to the number and site of diseased vessels, can be anticipated. It should be remembered that functional tests, especially perfusion imaging, give additive and independent prognostic information to those provided by coronary angiography. Three different patients are described (a low-risk patient, an intermediate-risk patient, a high-risk patient). (Adapted from Califf et al.[101] and Yusuf et al.,[99] with permission)

giography should not generally be performed. A more systematic functional prognostic analysis in such patients would certainly avoid a number of "oculostenotic reflexes" responsable for unnecessary and costly myocardial revascularizations.

We utilize a strategy using clinical, stress ECG, and myocardial scintigraphy data to help in the decision-making process regarding myocardial revascularization. A functional prognostic score derived from these variables defines the pretest risk of events before obtaining the results of angiography, which themselves have further prognostic implications (Fig. 27-15). Adapting the diagram proposed by Califf et al.[101] permits definition of the probability of future cardiovascular death or myocardial infarction. In this way, very low-risk patients (essentially those with a normal thallium scan) can expect only minimal benefit from myocardial revascularization, whatever the state of their coronary arteries. Similarly, low-risk patients (essentially those with a maximum exercise test and a mildly abnormal or equivocal perfusion imaging) can expect to benefit only if they have stenosis of the left main artery. Moderate-risk patients (e.g., two abnormal territories in the scintigraphy) necessitate myocardial revascularization in the event of two- or three-vessel disease. Patients defined as being at high functional risk (extensive thallium abnormality, increased lung activity) should always undergo revascularization, even if they have single-vessel disease. Figure 27-15 also categorizes the prognostic risk according to the association of findings from exercise ECG and scintigraphy.

Prognostic Relevance in Patients with Unstable CAD

In the clinical situation of unstable angina (either new-onset type angina or progressive angina), myocardial scintigraphy is of limited interest because of the serious prognostic implications of these clinical entities.[102] After an attempt at medical stabilization, these patients are generally directed toward coronary angiography, followed more often than not by myocardial revascularization. There has been some experience with patients examined after a suspected or real episode of unstable angina and stabilized by medical treatment. Several studies have shown that patients presenting redistribution on the thallium scan have a high middle-term risk of serious coronary events.[104,105]

Sometimes the clinical scene is not as typical, and perfusion scintigraphy is therefore useful. The use of ^{99m}Tc-sestamibi can be proposed as, due to the near absence of redistribution of this isotope, it can be injected during chest pain with image acquisition 1 or 2 hours later. In 102 patients with an "atypical" presentation (unstable angina but dubious ECG), Hilton et al.[103] have shown that a normal scintigram (69% of scans) was associated with no coronary events during their hospital stay, although their long-term outlook is unknown. In this heterogeneous group, ^{99m}Tc-sestamibi investigation may exclude the diagnosis of unstable myocardial ischemia in patients with ambiguous symptoms, rather than differentiating among subgroups of patients with unstable angina.

To sum up, the place of myocardial perfusion scintigraphy in patients with unstable angina appears limited to the phase immediately after stabilization of the episode. We are in agreement with the conclusion of the ACC/AHA "Guidelines for Clinical uses of Cardiac Radionuclide Imaging" where the only class I application is the identification of the site of the culprit lesion.[106]

USE OF MYOCARDIAL PERFUSION SCINTIGRAPHY FOR RISK STRATIFICATION AFTER MYOCARDIAL INFARCTION

General Considerations

The aim of prognostic evaluation after myocardial infarction is similar to that sought in other coronary patients—to select a group at low risk (< 1% to 2% risk of severe coronary events per year). Such patients do not justify extensive investigations and are able to rapidly resume their normal physical activity. On the other hand, it is necessary to recognize patients at high risk of further events, who should be directed toward angiography and, if necessary, toward myocardial revascularization. Major complications (death, new myocardial infarction, unstable angina) following the acute phase are maximal in the first 3 months, especially the first month, and then decrease exponentially with time up to the third to fifth year. Thus, the performance of risk stratification is an urgent consideration after the acute phase.

The prognosis of myocardial infarction has changed enormously in the past decade, going from 10% to 20% of serious coronary accidents in the year following the myocardial infarction to figures eight times lower in certain circumstances. For example, in the GISSI 2 study,[4] a large cohort of patients underwent thrombolysis and was then followed medically. Despite a negligible rate of revascularization, the 1 year mortality rate was only 3.5%, which corresponds to a low or intermediate coronary risk. As many patients still do not receive thrombolytic therapy, this represents a "best case" scenario, but it does attest to the importance of subgroup analysis in this highly heterogeneous group.

Following a myocardial infarction, we distinguish three groups of patients on clinical grounds, having different levels of risk, in whom the additive prognostic value of the scintigraphy is different:

1. High risk—patients have a high clinical evolutive risk due to their initial clinical presentation and to the presence of factors clearly defined in numerous studies.[107] The principal factors corresponding to a high relative risk are an initial episode of left heart failure, multiple infarcts, electrical instability (especially late ventricular dysrhythmias), history of myocardial infarction, and age greater than 70. These patients should rapidly undergo coronary angiography. In this population, perfusion scintigraphy or other functional studies might be useful as an adjunctive test (*e.g.*, evaluating the possibility of myocardial recovery after revascularization in the event of severe LV dysfunction), but this group will not be discussed further.
2. Intermediate risk—patients whose initial course is uncomplicated. It is this group of patients that justifies supplementary investigations to evaluate their future risk.
3. Lowest risk—this corresponds to post-thrombolysis patients, with an initially uncomplicated course. These patients are often young without any associated pathology, having presented with their first myocardial infarction and with less extensive coronary lesions. While thrombolysis improves the prognosis by decreasing the size of the myocardial infarction (at least theoretically), it increases the ischemic potential within the reperfused zone. We will examine the value of myocardial scintigraphy in this third group.

Despite this theoretical model, myocardial infarction poses some specific problems. First, this major coronary event is often dramatic for the patient and family, and a relapse is often feared. Second, patients are often admitted to hospital, which facilitates access to coronary angiography without prolonging the duration of stay. Certain authors recommend the systematic performance of coronary angiography, but once performed, this often leads to myocardial revascularization, either of the infarct-related artery (according to the theory that it is better to have a patent artery than a severely stenosed or occluded one), or more complete surgical revascularization in patients with multivessel disease. However, the benefit of wide-scale secondary revascularization over more conservative attitudes has not been shown definitively.

Use of Perfusion Imaging in Low-Risk Patients without Thrombolytic Therapy

Prognostic Value of Conventional Exercise Stress Test

As discussed in Chapter 25, the conventional exercise ECG has prognostic value in these patients. By pooling the results of different prethrombolytic era studies, Beller[108] showed that 29% of postmyocardial infarction patients demonstrate ST-segment depression with stress and that the long-term mortality of these patients is 15.6% compared with 4.8% when the submaximal exercise test is normal. However, this test has important limitations: the specificity of ST depression in asymptomatic patients after an inferior wall myocardial infarction has been questioned, and the sensitivity in predicting myocardial ischemia is decreased after an anterior wall myocardial infarction. The manifestation of ST-segment elevation during exercise is of controversial significance, corresponding with a large irreversible dyskinetic scar for Haines et al.[109] or, on the contrary, with possible functional recovery for Margonato et al.[110] Moreover, symptom-limited exercise testing is not performed immediately after a myocardial infarction, when submaximal tests (which are less sensitive) are used. Even at subsequent follow-up, reduced exercise capacity is an adverse prognostic factor, but numerous extracardiac causes (physical, pharmacological) may also be responsible.

Advantages of Perfusion Imaging over Conventional Exercise Stress Test

Thallium perfusion imaging presents important theoretical advantages over exercise testing alone. It permits quantitation of the extent of both the infarcted and jeopardized myocardium, which represent two major prognostic factors. It is more sensitive than exercise ECG testing in the detection of ischemia and the use of SPECT permits accurate localization of the site of ischemia, permitting the discrimination of ischemia in the infarcted region from that remote from the infarct. Examination of pooled studies shows that the frequency of detected ischemia is doubled by the use of myocardial thallium imaging compared with conventional submaximal exercise testing (57% vs. 29%).[111] Furthermore, patients presenting the association of a negative stress test and a positive thallium scan have an unfavorable prognosis.[112] Most studies have noted the superior prognostic value of scintigraphy compared to conventional exercise testing.[111,113,114]

The scintigraphic parameters linked to prognosis are identical to those mentioned above for the general population of coronary patients: presence of redistribution, extent of redistribution, presence of a multivessel defect, increased lung activity, and stress-provoked LV dilation. Thus, in a series of 92 patients, one-third of whom had undergone thrombolysis, Mahmarian et al.[114] found that the conjunction of a perfusion defect of less than 20%, or of a reversible defect of less than 10% of the myocardium with an ejection fraction greater than 40%, defined a low-risk population. Conversely, all the patients in this study who died possessed a defect of greater than 30% of the myocardium. Similarly, Olona[113] proposed comparison of the information of a parameter studying myocardial ischemia (e.g., redistribution on the thallium scan) with a parameter evaluating LV kinetics (e.g., echocardiographic ejection fraction). The association of absence of ischemia on the thallium scan and ejection fraction greater than 40% defined a population with very good postmyocardial infarction prognosis. The extent of coronary lesions, assessed by coronary angiography, did not contribute any supplementary predictive information.

Prognostic Value of the Presence of a Reversible Defect after Myocardial Infarction

It is important to note that in these patients, the presence of reversible ischemia on the thallium scan has predictive value for events, unlike the presence of a fixed defect. *This finding differs from that observed in patients not having had a myocardial infarction, in whom reversible as well as irreversible defects are predictive of events*. Hence, in contrast to the situation in a patient without infarction, the criteria for defining reproducibility are important. Unfortunately, the scintigraphic definition of reversible ischemia using thallium varies somewhat from one study to the next. We define redistribution as being complete if the second image is either normalized or presents less than 25% activity decrease compared to the reference zone. Redistribution is incomplete if the later image reveals an improvement on the initial image but with a decrease in activity of greater than 25% compared to the reference zone or to normal. The quantification of this activity for defining the redistribution appears superior to simple visual analysis (decreased variability, increased reproducibility), provided that a strict methodology is observed.

Between 40% and 67% of patients demonstrate thallium redistribution after a myocardial infarction. The majority of transient defects are situated in the infarcted territory and the minority outside the infarct zone. According to Brown et al.,[115] thallium redistribution occurs in 50% of infarcted areas and in 27% of regions remote from the myocardial infarction. Using ^{99m}Tc-sestamibi, Travin et al.[116] reported an ischemic defect in 70% of patients, and in slightly more than a third of cases it exceeded the infarcted region.

It has been demonstrated that if redistribution is localized exclusively in the infarcted territory, this aspect has prognostic value. Thus in Gibson's series, 12 of the 13 single-vessel patients having a postinfarct coronary event demonstrated redistribution in this territory. Similarly, Wilson et al.[117] noted that the occurrence of coronary events after myocardial infarction was 42% within 39 months in patients with single-vessel disease and thallium redistribution. However, it should be noted that most of these events comprised recurrent unstable angina and not death or reinfarction. Other studies[114,118] confirmed that the positive predictive value of transient ischemia in the infarcted area is moderate (ranging from 33% to 36%).

This positive predictive value of a stress-induced perfusion defect is greater when the redistribution is situated outside the infarct zone, and more so if multiple transient defects are present. This pattern indicates the presence of occlusive multivessel coronary lesions.[111] Mahmarian et al.[114] note that the risk increases by 82% for each increase of 10% in the amount of ischemic myocardium and that, inversely, the risk is decreased by 32% for each improvement of 10% in ejection fraction. The probability of events is greatest when associated with increased pulmonary activity.

Prognostic Value of Fixed Defects after Myocardial Infarction

The existence of a fixed defect on the redistribution scan appears to have prognostic value only if it is extensive, multifocal, or associated with reversible ischemia. In contrast, a fixed defect in the infarct zone appears to be an element of good prognosis. By considering the results of a large multicentric study using evaluation by thallium redistribution imaging 1 to 6 months after a myocardial infarction, Bodenheimer et al.[119] noted that the observation of only a fixed defect corresponds with a good long-term prognosis, and that there is no relationship between the size of the defect and the occurrence of end points. Conversely, in this work, the greater the size of reversible defects, the greater the risk of death or of myocardial infarction. The relatively good prognosis of a fixed defect limited to the infarct site has been reported by other authors,[115,117] whereas the observation of a large *defect associated with LV dilation and/or with extensive perfusion defects* corresponds with an unfavorable prognosis.[120]

In summary, the observation of an isolated fixed defect, even an extensive one, has no adverse prognostic value. However, when associated with criteria of either significant LV dysfunction (LV dilation, increased lung activity), or of associated reversible myocardial ischemia, it is predictive of poor outcome.[114]

Prognostic Value of "Reverse-Redistribution" Defect after Myocardial Infarction

The presence of a "reverse" abnormality after a myocardial infarction (worsening of an initial hypofixation on the redistribution scan) should be considered to indicate the presence of a viable and ischemic area, generally downstream from a reperfused coronary stenosis.[121] This aspect is most frequent after an incomplete myocardial infarction or after a non-Q-wave myocardial infarction. The presence of reversible ischemia is particularly frequent in this situation. While no specific studies dealing with the prognostic implications of this finding have been published to our knowledge, the association with non-Q-wave infarction and ischemia suggests an adverse risk.

Relationship between Myocardial Viability, Ischemia, and Prognosis

The relationships between residual myocardial viability, residual ischemia, and prognosis are important. Myocardial viability is defined as reversible dysfunction characterized by the persistence of myocardial metabolism and may be expressed by residual thallium uptake. As discussed Chapters 20 to 22, certain infarct-related territories without redistribution remain metabolically active and liable to recuperate after revascularization (especially in the case of moderate fixed defects). Some of these redistribution-free, viable territories are detected by the technique of reinjection.[122] The problem of knowing if risk stratification could be appreciated better by thallium reinjection protocols than by thallium scan with redistribution imaging remains to be identified by subsequent studies. However, the fact that the prognosis is excellent in the presence of fixed defects on the redistribution scan seems to demonstrate that reinjection study is not necessary for prognostic evaluation. On the other hand, by comparing the prognostic value of stress thallium redistribution with that of FDG scintigraphy. Tamaki et al.[123] found more events in patients without thallium redistribution but with increased FDG uptake than in patients without either redistribution or increased FDG uptake. Due to the very limited number of patients, segments, and events and the large number of patients lost from follow-up in this retrospective study, this element remains to be clarified by subsequent studies. In the present state, stress-redistribution myocardial thallium scintigraphy appears to be the best validated method for postmyocardial infarction prognostic evaluation.

Use of Perfusion Scintigraphy in Post-thrombolysis Patients

Several studies have suggested that the prognostic value of scintigraphy in post-thrombolysis patients is inferior to its value in other postinfarction patients.[124–127] This population is at moderate or even low risk of hard events for the reasons explained earlier. As the pretest probability of an event is low in this group, the positive predictive value of an abnormal scintigram is even lower.

These patients frequently undergo catheterization—the rationale behind this being the persistent presence of the underlying stenosis after lytic therapy, as well as concerns regarding rethrombosis. However, this systematic invasive strategy is not rational. First, the group has a good spontaneous prognosis, second, the risk of rethrombosis exists but cannot be predicted by early angiography,[128] and third, large trials comparing medical treatment to systematic myocardial revascularization have shown no benefit for the latter.

Despite the unfavorable results to date, we believe that functional testing is appropriate in this group. Such an approach permits detection of viable and ischemic myocardium supplied by an artery remaining blocked despite thrombolysis. In such patients, secondary revascularization may be justified on a prognostic basis. Our approach is to use exercise or dipyridamole stress perfusion imaging in these patients: the absence of redistribution defines a population at very low risk, and the presence of redistribution (especially if extensive or present in multiple territories) justifies angiography and myocardial revascularization if necessary.

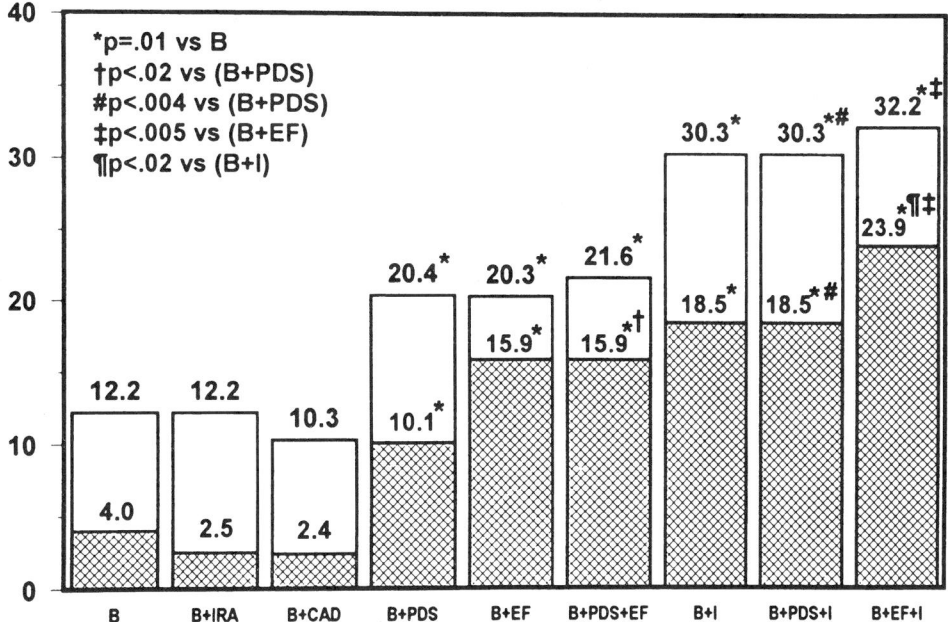

Fig. 27-16. Comparison of prognostic value of ejection fraction (EF), coronary angio variables (IRA, patency of the infarct related artery; CAD, extent of coronary artery disease), and scintigraphic variables (PDS, perfusion defect size; I, scintigraphic ischemia) after acute myocardial infarction. Coronary angiography adds no prognostic value from baseline clinical model (B). EF and/or PDS adds prognostic information from B. Extent of ischemia adds incremental prognostic information from both B, EF, and perfusion defect size. Patients were studied with adenosine thallium-201-SPECT. (From Mahmarian et al.,[114] with permission.)

Selection of Stress Perfusion Imaging Technique in Postinfarction Patients

Selection of Exercise or Pharmacologic Stress

As discussed, early risk stratification is favored after myocardial infarction, because coronary events are most common in the first days and weeks, and because this strategy reduces as much as possible the duration of inpatient hospital care and guides the choice of patients submitted for myocardial revascularization. For early stress testing, pharmacologic agents appear to be an excellent alternative to exercise, which is often submaximal, and the prognostic value of which is probably inferior to a symptom-limited stress test. Brown has shown that using vasodilatory agents, scintigraphy can be performed without risk as early as 36 hours after the acute phase of myocardial infarction.[115]

The predictive value of transient ischemia in dipyridamole-thallium scanning was initially documented in 1982.[118] Similar data have recently been presented using adenosine.[114] The latter study confirmed that adenosine-SPECT has additive value to classical clinical prognostic criteria, especially in the presence of dysfunction criteria or extensive reversible ischemia. Incidently, in this study, as in others, coronary angiography has a lower predictive value than perfusion scintigraphy (Fig. 27-16).

In practice, we recommend vasodilator-stress scintigraphy early after myocardial infarction if the patient is cared for in a center possessing nuclear imaging facilities. If this is not the case, this investigation is postponed until the exploration can be performed as an outpatient with exercise stress and after 24 hours of withdrawal of anti-ischemic drugs.

Selection of Thallium or ^{99m}Tc-sestamibi

Identical conclusions have been provided by the use of ^{99m}sestamibi.[116] Theoretically, in view of the differences in cellular uptake between thallium and ^{99m}sestamibi, and due to the absence of redistribu-

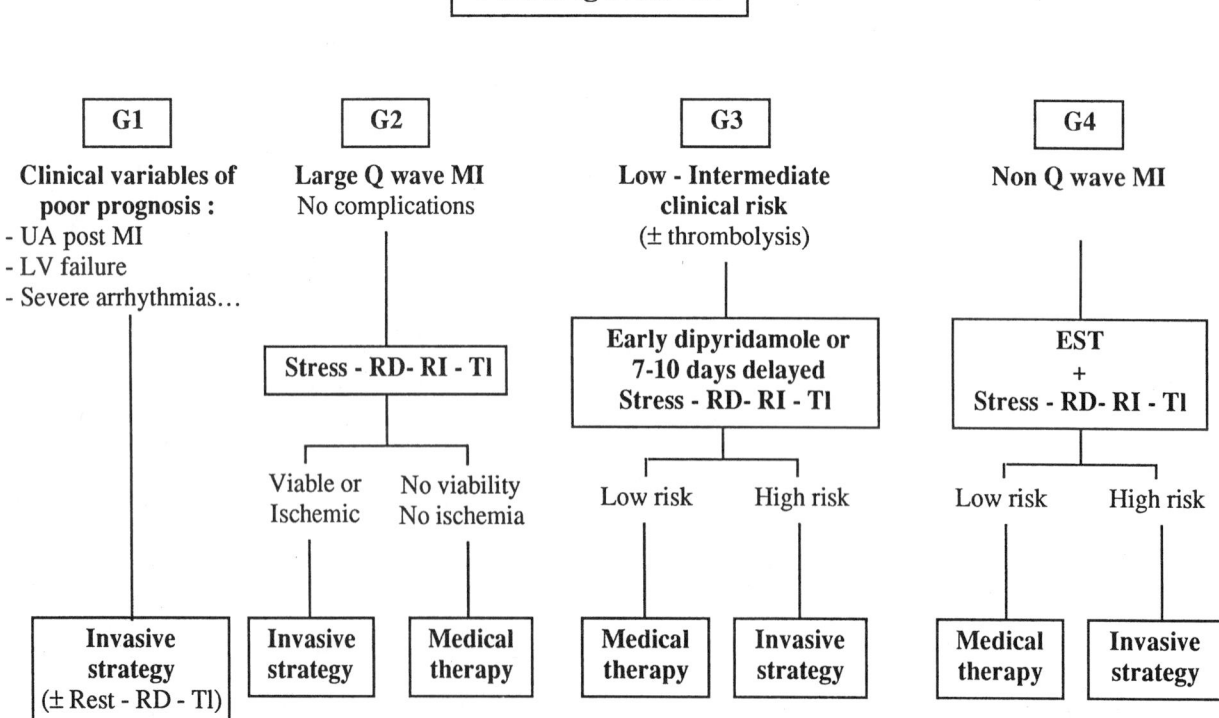

Fig. 27-17. Decision tree for risk stratification after acute myocardial infarction (for explanations see text).

tion with sestamibi, we could expect to detect less postmyocardial infarction ischemia with this agent than with thallium. In fact, using a stress-rest ^{99m}sestamibi protocol, Travin et al.[116] noted the presence of reversible ischemia in 70% of patients 1 week after a myocardial infarction. As with thallium, two-thirds of this ischemia was in the infarct zone. Similarly, the extent and number of reversible defects were directly linked to the long-term complication rate (death, myocardial infarction, unstable angina). The cardiac event rate (15% at 15 months) in nonrevascularized patients was very low, and only 4% died and 4% suffered reinfarction. The event rate was only 3.8% (with no deaths) in patients without multiple territory ^{99m}sestamibi defects, although it was nearly 50% in patients with multiple vascular territory defects. The low event rate in patients with milder disease reflects performance of thrombolysis in 40% of patients, and early revascularization in one in three patients, based upon scintigraphic findings.

Proposed Decision Tree for Prognostic Evaluation after Myocardial Infarction

Following a myocardial infarction, a general strategy can be schematized (Fig. 27-17). A systematic invasive strategy is justified only in group I (high clinical risk) patients. For patients of the other three groups, a functional noninvasive test is needed to act as "gatekeeper" for invasive strategy. Olona[113] estimates that angiography is justifiable in 50% to 70% of postinfarct patients, if the indications are based on a prognostic algorithm reflecting clinical data and noninvasive investigations (essentially exercise ECG and perfusional myocardial scintigraphy).

The systematic use of coronary angiography in the four clinical groups of patients after myocardial infarction risks the performance of intervention on the basis of the coronary anatomy rather than prognostic information. If "systematic" use of coronary angiography is used for group 3 and 4 patients, conventional stress testing should be the minimum requirement to supplement this angiography. If there is any doubt about this result (submaximal stress, nondiagnostic ECG or equivocal ST-segment changes) it should be complemented by perfusion scintigraphy. In groups 1 and 2, perfusion imaging should be performed before myocardial revascularization—if not, a number of revascularizations are liable to be performed without prognostic justification.

REFERENCES

1. CASS Principal Investigators and their associates: Coronary artery surgery study (CASS): A randomized trial of coronary artery bypass surgery survival data. Circulation 68:939, 1983
2. European Coronary Surgery Study Group: Long term results of prospective randomized study of coronary artery bypass surgery in stable angina pectoris. Lancet 2:1173, 1982
3. Fuster V: Mechanisms leading to myocardial infarction: insights from studies of vascular biology. Circulation 90:2126, 1994
4. Volpi A, De Vita C, Franzosi MG et al: Determinants of 6-month mortality in survivors of myocardial infarction after thrombolysis. Results of the GISSI-2 data base. Circulation 88:416, 1993
5. Chang J, Atwood JE, Froelicher V: Prognostic impact of myocardial ischemia. J Am Coll Cardiol 23:225, 1994
6. Mickley H, Nielsen JR, Berning J et al: Prognostic significance of transient myocardial ischemia after first acute myocardial infarction: five year follow up study. Br Heart J 73:320, 1995
7. Miller TD, Christian TF, Talierco CP et al: Severe exercise-induced ischemia does not identify high risk patients with normal left ventricular function and one- or two-vessel coronary artery disease. J Am Coll Cardiol 23:219, 1994
8. Yamagishi M, Miyatake K, Tamai J et al: Intravascular ultrasound detection of atherosclerosis at the site of focal vasospasm in angiographically normal or minimally narrowed coronary segments. J Am Coll Cardiol 23:352, 1994
9. Lu C, Picano E, Pingitore A et al: Complex coronary artery lesion morphology influences results of stress echocardiography. Circulation 91:1669, 1995
10. Ambrose JA, Tannenbaum MA, Alexopoulos D: Angiographic progression on coronary artery disease and the development of myocardial infarction. J Am Coll Cardiol 12:56, 1988
11. Taeymans Y, Théroux P, Lespérance J, Waters D: Quantitative angiographic morphology of the coronary artery lesions at risk of thrombotic occlusion. Circulation 85:78, 1992
12. Di Carli M, Czerni J, Hoh CK et al: Relation among stenosis severity, myocardial blood flow, and flow reserve in patients with coronary artery disease. Circulation 91:1944, 1995

13. Brown KA: Prognostic value of thallium 201 myocardial perfusion imaging. A diagnostic tool comes of age. Circulation 83:363, 1991
14. Desmarais R, Kaul S, Watson DD, Beller GA: Do false positive thallium-201 scans lead to unnecessary catheterization? Outcome of patients with perfusion defects on quantitative planar thallium 201 scintigraphy. J Am Coll Cardiol 21:1058, 1993
15. Wackers FJ Th, Bodenheimer M, Fleiss J et al.: Factors affecting uniformity in interpretation of planar thallium-201 imaging in a multicenter trial. J Am Coll Cardiol 21:1064, 1993
16. Trogaugh GB, Wackers FJ, Busemann-Sokole E et al.: Thallium-201 myocardial imaging: an interinstitutional study of observer variability. J Nucl Med 19:359, 1978
17. Sigal SL, Soufer R, Fetterman RC et al.: Reproducibility of quantitative planar thallium-201 scintigraphy: quantitative criteria for reversibility of myocardial perfusion defects. J Nucl Med 32:759, 1991
18. Alazraki NP, Krawczynska EG, DePuey EG et al.: Reproducibility of thallium-201 exercise SPECT studies. J Nucl Med 35:1237, 1994
19. Steele P, Sklar J, Kirsh D et al.: Thallium-201 myocardial imaging during maximal and submaximal exercise: comparison of submaximal exercise with propranolol. Am Heart J 106:1353, 1983
20. Iskandrian AS, Heo J, Kong B, Lyons E: Effect of exercise level on the ability of thallium-201 tomographic imaging in detecting coronary artery disease: analysis of 461 patients. J Am Coll Cardiol 14:1477, 1989
21. Burns RJ, Kruzyk GC, Armitage DL, Druck MN: Effect of antianginal medications on the prognostic value of exercise thallium scintigraphy. Can J Cardiol 5:29, 1989
22. Machecourt J, Longere Ph, Fagret D et al.: Prognostic value of thallium-201 single-photon emission computed tomographic myocardial perfusion imaging according to extent of myocardial defect. J Am Coll Cardiol 23:1096, 1994
23. Brown KA, Rowen M: Impact of antianginal medications, peak heart rate and stress level on the prognostic value of a normal exercise myocardial perfusion imaging study. J Nucl Med 34:1467, 1993
24. Brown KA, Boucher CA, Okada RD et al.: Prognostic value of exercise thallium-201 imaging in patients presenting for evaluation of chest pain. J Am Coll Cardiol 1:994, 1983
25. Beller GA: Radionuclide assessment of prognosis. p 137. In: Clinical Nuclear Cardiology. W.B. Saunders Company, Philadelphia, 1995
26. Pamelia FX, Gibson RS, Watson DD et al.: Prognosis with chest pain and normal thallium-201 exercise scintigrams. Am J Cardiol 55:920, 1985
27. Wackers FJTh, Russo DJ, Russo D, Clements JP: Prognostic significance of normal quantitative planar thallium-201 stress scintigraphy in patients with chest pain. J Am Coll Cardiol 6:27, 1985
28. Bairey CN, Rozanski A, Maddahi J et al.: Exercise thallium-201 scintigraphy and prognosis in typical angina pectoris and negative exercise electrocardiography. Am J Cardiol 64:282, 1989
29. Iskandrian AS, Hakki AH, Kane-Marsch S: Prognostic implications of exercise thallium-201 scintigraphy in patients with suspected or known coronary artery disease. Am Heart J 110:135, 1985
30. Ladenheim ML, Pollock BH, Rozanski A et al.: Extent and severity of myocardial hypoperfusion as predictors of prognosis in patients with suspected coronary artery disease. J Am Coll Cardiol 7:464, 1986
31. Staniloff HM, Forrester JS, Berman DS, Swan HJC: Prediction of death, myocardial infarction, and worsening chest pain using thallium scintigraphy and exercise electrocardiography. J Nucl Med 27:1842, 1986
32. Wahl JM, Hakki AH, Iskandrian AS: Prognostic implications of normal exercise thallium-201 images. Arch Intern Med 145:253, 1985
33. Koss JH, Kobren SM, Grunwald AM, Bodenheimer MM: Role of exercise thallium-201 myocardial perfusion scintigraphy in predicting prognosis in suspected coronary artery disease. Am J Cardiol 59:531, 1987
34. Iskandrian A, Chae S, Heo J et al.: Independent and incremental prognostic value of exercise in single photon emission tomography (SPECT) thallium imaging in coronary artery disease. J Am Coll Cardiol 22:665, 1993
35. Steinberg EH, Koss JH, Lee M et al.: Prognostic significance from 10-year follow-up of a qualitatively normal planar exercise thallium test in suspected coronary artery disease. Am J Cardiol 71:1271, 1993
36. Fintel DJ, Links JM, Brinker JA et al.: Improved diagnostic performance of exercise thallium-201 single photon emission computed tomography over planar imaging in the diagnosis of coronary artery disease: a receiver operating characteristic analysis. J Am Coll Cardiol 13:600, 1989
37. Brown KA, Rowen M, Altland E: Prognosis of patients with an isolated fixed thallium-201 defect and no prior myocardial infarction. Am J Cardiol 72:1199, 1993
38. Stratmann HG, Mark AL, Walter KE, Williams GA: Prognostic value of atrial pacing and thallium-201

scintigraphy in patients with stable chest pain. Am J Cardiol 64:985, 1989
39. Travin MI, Boucher CA, Newell JB et al.: Variables associated with a poor prognosis in patients with an ischemic thallium-201 exercise test. Am Heart J 125:335, 1993
40. Gill JB, Ruddy TD, Newell JB et al.: Prognostic importance of thallium uptake by lung during exercise in coronary artery disease. N Engl J Med 317:1485, 1987
41. Weis AT, Berman DS, Lew AS et al.: Transient ischemic dilation of the left ventricle on stress thallium-201 scintigraphy: a marker of severe and extensive coronary artery disease. J Am Coll Cardiol 9:752, 1987
42. Lette J, Bertrand C, Gossard D et al.: Long-term risk stratification with dipyridamole imaging. Am Heart J 129:880, 1995
43. Van Train KF, Maddahi J, Berman DS et al.: Quantitative analysis of tomographic stress thallium-201 myocardial scintigrams: a multicenter trial. J Nucl Med 31:1168, 1990
44. Albro PC, Gould KL, Wescott PJ et al.: Non invasive assessment of coronary stenoses by myocardial imaging during pharmacologic coronary vasodilatation. III. Clinical trial. Am J Cardiol 42:751, 1978
45. Machecourt J, Denis B, Wolf JE et al.: Sensibilité et spécificité respective de la scintigraphie myocardique réalisée après injection de 201Tl au cours de l'effort, après injection de dipyridamole et au repos. Comparaison chez 70 sujets coronarographiés. Arch Mal Cœur 2:147, 1981
46. Lette J, Waters D, Champagne P et al.: Prognostic implications of a negative dipyridamole-thallium scan: results in 360 patients. Am J Med 92:615, 1992
47. Hendel RC, Layden JJ, Leppo JA: Prognostic value of dipyridamole thallium scintigraphy for evaluation of ischemic heart disease. J Am Coll Cardiol 15:109, 1990
48. Leppo JA: Dipyridamole myocardial perfusion imaging. J Nucl Med 35:730, 1994
49. Brown KA, Altland E, Rowen M: Prognostic value of normal technetium-99m-sestamibi cardiac imaging. J Nucl Med 35:554, 1994
50. Mahmarian JJ, Mahmarian AC, Marks GF et al.: Role of adenosine thallium-201 tomography for defining long-term risk in patients after acute myocardial infarction. J Am Coll Cardiol 25:1333, 1995
51. Stratmann HG, Williams GA, Wittry MD et al.: Exercise technetium-99m sestamibi tomography for cardiac risk stratification of patients with stable chest pain. Circulation 89:615, 1994
52. Stratmann HG, Tamesis BR, Younis LT et al.: Prognostic value of dipyridamole technetium-99m sestamibi myocardial tomography in patients with stable chest pain who are unable to exercise. Am J Cardiol 73:647, 1994
53. Glover DK, Ruiz, M, Edwards NC et al.: Comparison between 201-thallium and 99mTc sestamibi uptake during adenosine-induced vasodilation as a function of coronary stenosis severity. Circulation 91:813, 1995
54. Bonow RO, Kent KM, Rosing DR et al.: Exercise-induced ischemia in mildly symptomatic patients with coronary artery disease and preserved left ventricular function: identification of subgroups at risk of death during medical therapy. N Engl J Med 311:1339, 1984
55. Lee KL, Pryor DB, Peiper KS et al.: Prognostic value of radionuclide angiography in medically treated patients with coronary artery disease: A comparison with clinical and catheterization variables. Circulation 82:1705, 1990
56. Iqbal A, Gibbons RJ, Zinsmeister AR et al.: Prognostic value of exercise radionuclide angiography in a population-based cohort of patients with known or suspected coronary artery disease. Am J Cardiol 74:119, 1994
57. Mazzotta G, Bonow RO, Pace L et al.: Relation between exertional ischemia and prognosis in mildly symptomatic patients with single or double vessel coronary artery disease and left ventricular dysfunction at rest. J Am Coll Cardiol 13:567, 1989
58. Gohlke H, Samek L, Betz P, Roskamm H: Exercise testing provides additional prognostic information in angiographically defined subgroups of patients with coronary artery disease. Circulation 68:979, 1983
59. Gibbons RJ, Fyke FE, Clements IP et al.: Non invasive identification of severe coronary artery disease using exercise radionuclide angiography. J Am Coll Cardiol 11:28, 1988
60. Palmas W, Friedman JD, Diamond GA et al.: Incremental value of simultaneous assessment of myocardial function and perfusion with technetium-99m sestamibi for prediction of extent of coronary artery disease. J Am Coll Cardiol 25:1024, 1995
61. O'Keefe JH, Barnhart CS, Bateman TM: Comparison of stress echocardiography and stress myocardial perfusion scintigraphy for diagnosing coronary artery disease and assessing its severity. Am J Cardiol 75:25D, 1995
62. Brown KA: Prognostic value of cardiac imaging in patients with known or suspected coronary artery disease: Comparison of myocardial perfusion imaging,

stress echocardiography and positron emission tomography. Am J Cardiol 75:35D, 1995
63. Diamond GA, Forrester JS: Analysis of probability as an aid in the clinical diagnosis of coronary artery disease. N Engl J Med 300:1350, 1979
64. Berman DS, Kiat H, Friedman JD, Diamond G: Clinical applications of exercise nuclear cardiology studies in the era of healthcare reform. Am J Cardiol 75:3D, 1995
65. Chae S, Heo J, Iskandrian A, Wasserleben V, Cave V: Identification of extensive coronary artery disease in women by single-photon emission computed tomographic (SPECT) thallium imaging. J Am Coll Cardiol 21:1305, 1993
66. Pancholy S, Fattah AA, Kamal AM et al.: Use of Exercise SPECT thallium imaging in risk assessment in women with coronary artery disease, abstracted. J Am Coll Cardiol 62A:716, 1994
67. Hendel RC, Chen MH, L'Italien GJ et al.: Sex differences in perioperative and long-term cardiac event-free survival in vascular surgery patients: an analysis of clinical and scintigraphic variables. Circulation 91:1044, 1995
68. Mark DB: An overview of risk assessment in coronary artery disease. Am J Cardiol 73:19B, 1994
69. Krishnan R, Lu J, Dae MW et al.: Does myocardial perfusion scintigraphy demonstrate clinical usefulness in patients with markedly positive exercise tests? An assessment of the method in a high-risk subset. Am Heart J 127:804, 1994
70. Schalet BD, Kegel JG, Heo J et al.: Prognostic implications of normal exercise SPECT thallium images in patients with strongly positive exercise electrocardiograms. Am J Cardiol 72:1201, 1993
71. Taylor AJ, Sackett MC, Beller GA: The degree of ST-segment depression on symptom-limited exercise testing: relation to the myocardial ischemic burden as determined by thallium-201 scintigraphy. Am J Cardiol 75:228, 1995
72. Fagan LF, Shaw L, Kong BA et al.: Prognostic value of exercise thallium scintigraphy in patients with good exercise tolerance and a normal or abnormal exercise electrocardiogram and suspected or confirmed coronary artery disease. Am J Cardiol 69:607, 1992
73. Nallamothu N, Ghods M, Heo J, Iskandrian AS: Comparison of thallium-201 single-photon emission computed tomography and electrocardiographic response during exercise in patients with normal rest electrocardiographic results. J Am Coll Cardiol 25:830, 1995
74. Proudfit WL, Bruschke AVG, Sones FM: Clinical course of patients with normal or slightly or moderately abnormal coronary arteriograms: 10 years follow-up of 521 patients. Circulation 62:712, 1980
75. Kemp HG, Kronmal RA, Vliestra RE, Frye RL, and participants in the Coronary Artery Surgery Study: Seven year survival of patients with normal or near normal coronary arteriograms: a CASS registry study. J Am Coll Cardiol 7:479, 1986
76. Brown KA, Rowen M: Prognostic value of a normal exercise myocardial perfusion imaging study in patients with angiographically significant coronary artery disease. Am J Cardiol 71:865, 1993
77. Fattah AA, Kamal AM, Pancholy S et al.: Prognostic implications of normal exercise tomographic thallium images in patients with angiographic evidence of significant coronary artery disease. Am J Cardiol 74:769, 1994
78. Iskandrian AS, Heo J, Lemlek J, Ogilby JD: Identification of high-risk patients with left main and three-vessel coronary artery disease using stepwise discriminant analysis of clinical, exercise, and tomographic thallium data. Am Heart J 125:221, 1993
79. Pollock SG, Abbott RD, Boucher CA et al.: A model to predict multivessel coronary artery disease from the exercise thallium-201 stress test. Am J Med 90:345, 1991
80. Mahmarian JJ, Pratt CM, Boyce TM, Verani MS: The variable extent of jeopardized myocardium in patients with single vessel coronary artery disease: quantification by thallium-201 single photon emission computed tomography. J Am Coll Cardiol 17:355, 1991
81. Kaul S, Lilly DR, Gasho JA et al.: Prognostic utility of the exercise thallium-201 test in ambulatory patients with chest pain: comparison with cardiac catheterization. Circulation 77:745, 1988
82. Pollock SG, Abott DA, Boucher CA et al.: Independent and incremental prognostic value of test performed in hierarchical order to evaluate patients with suspected coronary artery disease. Circulation 85:237, 1992
83. Iskandrian AS, Chae SC, Heo J et al.: Independent and incremental prognosis value of exercise single-photon emission computed tomographic (SPECT) thallium imaging in coronary artery disease. J Am Coll Cardiol 22:665, 1993
84. Marie PY, Danchin N, Durand JF et al.: Long term prediction of major ischemic events by exercise thallium 201 single photon emission computed tomography: incremental prognostic value compared with clinical, exercise testing, catheterization and radionuclide angiographic data. J Am Coll Cardiol 26:879, 1995

85. Fleg JL, Gerstenblith G, Zonderman AB et al.: Prevalence and prognostic significance of exercise-induced silent myocardial ischemia detected by thallium scintigraphy and electrocardiography in asymptomatic volunteers. Circulation 81:428, 1990
86. Mittleman MA, Maclure M, Tofler GH et al.: Triggering of acute myocardial infarction by heavy physical exertion. N Engl J Med 329:1677, 1993
87. Ciampricotti R, Taverne R, El Gamal M: Clinical and angiographic observations on resuscitated victims of exercise-related sudden ischemic death. Am J Cardiol 68:47, 1991
88. Koistinen MJ, Huikuri HY, Pirttiaho H et al.: Evaluation of exercise electrocardiography and thallium tomographic imaging in detecting asymptomatic coronary artery disease in diabetic patients. Br Heart J 63:7, 1990
89. Stamler J, Vaccaro O, Neaton JD et al.: Diabetes, other risk factors, and 12-yr cardiovascular mortality for men screened in the multiple risk factor intervention trial. Diabetes Care 16:434, 1993
90. Manskle CL: Coronary artery disease in diabetic patients with nephropathy. Am J Hypertens 6:3675, 1993
91. Holley JL, Fenton RA, Arthur RS: Thallium stress testing does not predict cardiovascular risk in diabetic patients with end-stage renal disease undergoing cadaveric renal transplantation. Am J Med 90:563, 1991
92. Brown KA, Rimmer J, Haisch C: Noninvasive cardiac risk stratification of diabetic and non diabetic uremic renal allograft candidates using dipyridamole-thallium-201 imaging and radionuclide ventriculography. Am J Cardiol 64:1017, 1989
93. Camp AD, Garvin PJ, Hoff J et al.: Prognostic value of intravenous dipyridamole thallium imaging in patients with diabetes mellitus considered for renal transplantation. Am J Cardiol 65:1459, 1990
94. Derfler K, Kletter K, Balcke P et al.: Predictive value of thallium-201-dipyridamole myocardial stress scintigraphy in chronic hemodialysis patients and transplant recipients. Clin Nephrol 36:192, 1991
95. Brown JH, Vites NP, Testa HJ et al.: Value of thallium myocardial imaging in the prediction of future cardiovascular events in patients with end-stage renal failure. Nephrol Dial Transplant 8:433, 1993
96. Marwick TH, Steinmuller DR, Underwood DA et al.: Ineffectiveness of dipyridamole SPECT thallium imaging as a screening technique for coronary artery disease in patients with end-stage renal failure. Transplantation 49:100, 1990
97. Le A, Wilson R, Douek K et al.: Prospective risk stratification in renal transplant candidates for cardiac death. Am J Kidney Dis 24:65, 1994
98. Eagle KA, Singer DE, Brewster DC et al.: Dipyridamole-thallium scanning in patients undergoing vascular surgery: optimizing pre-operative evaluation of cardiac risk. JAMA 257:2185, 1987
99. Yusuf S, Zucker D, Peduzzi P et al.: Effect of coronary artery bypass graft surgery on survival: overview of 10-year results from randomised trials by the Coronary Artery Bypass Graft Surgery Trialists Collaboration. Lancet 344:563, 1994
100. Iskandrian AS, Ghods M, Helfeld H et al.: The treadmill exercise score revisited: coronary arteriographic and thallium perfusion correlates. Am Heart J 124:1581, 1992
101. Califf RM, Harrell FE, Lee KL et al.: The evolution of medical and surgical therapy for coronary artery disease. A 15-years perspective. JAMA 261:2077, 1989
102. Calvin JE, Klein LW, Vanderberg BJ et al.: Risk stratification in unstable angina. Prospective validation of the Braunwald classification. JAMA 275:136, 1995
103. Hilton TC, Thompson RC, Williams HJ et al.: Technetium-99m sestamibi myocardial perfusion imaging in the emergency room evaluation of chest pain. J Am Coll Cardiol 23:1016, 1994
104. Freeman MR, Chisholm RJ, Armstrong PW: Usefulness of exercise electrocardiography and thallium scintigraphy in unstable angina pectoris in predicting the extent and severity of coronary artery disease. Am J Cardiol 62:1164, 1988
105. Brown KA: Prognostic value of thallium-201 myocardial perfusion imaging in patients with unstable angina who respond to medical treatment. J Am Coll Cardiol 17:1053, 1991
106. Guidelines for Clinical Use of Cardiac Radionuclide Imaging: Report of the American College of Cardiology/American Heart Association Task Force on assessment of diagnostic and therapeutic cardiovascular procedures (Committee on Radionuclide Imaging), developed in collaboration with the American Society of Nuclear Cardiology. J Am Coll Cardiol 25:521, 1995
107. Tavazzi L, Fresco C, Volpi A et al.: Prognostic stratification after acute myocardial infarction. J Cardiovasc Risk 1:287, 1994
108. Beller GA: Radionuclide imaging in acute myocardial infarction: noninvasive risk stratification using exercise stress and perfusion imaging. p 210. In: Clinical Nuclear Cardiology. W.B. Saunders Company, Philadelphia, 1995
109. Haines DE, Beller GA, Watson DD et al.: Exercise-

109. induced ST segment elevation 2 weeks after uncomplicated myocardial infarction: contributing factors and prognostic significance. J Am Coll Cardiol 9:996, 1987
110. Margonato A, Chierchia SL, Xuereb RG et al.: Specificity and sensitivity of exercise-induced ST segment elevation for detection of residual viability: comparison with fluorodeoxyglucose and positron emission tomography. J Am Coll Cardiol 25:1032, 1995
111. Gibson RS, Watson DD: Value of planar 201Tl imaging in risk stratification of patients recovering from acute myocardial infarction. Circulation 84:148, 1991
112. Gibson RS, Beller GA, Kaiser DL: Prevalence and clinical significance of painless ST segment depression during early postinfarction exercise testing. Circulation 75:36, 1987
113. Olona M, Candell-Riera J, Permanyer-Miralda G et al.: Strategies for prognostic assessment of uncomplicated first myocardial infarction: 5-year follow-up study. J Am Coll Cardiol 25:815, 1995
114. Mahmarian JJ, Mahmarian AC, Marks GF et al.: Role of adenosine thallium-201 tomography for defining long-term risk in patients after acute myocardial infarction. J Am Coll Cardiol 25:1333, 1995
115. Brown KA, Weiss RM, Clements JP, Wackers FJTh: Usefulness of residual ischemic myocardium within prior infarct zone for identifying patients at high risk late after acute myocardial infarction. Am J Cardiol 60:15, 1987
116. Travin MI, Dessouki A, Cameron T, Heller GV: Use of exercise technetium-99m sestamibi SPECT imaging to detect residual ischemia and for risk stratification after acute myocardial infarction. Am J Cardiol 75:665, 1995
117. Wilson WW, Gibson RS, Nygaard TW et al.: Acute myocardial infarction associated with single vessel coronary artery disease: an analysis of clinical outcome and the prognostic importance of vessel patency and residual ischemic myocardium. J Am Coll Cardiol 11:223, 1988
118. Leppo JA, Boucher CA, Okada RD et al.: Serial Tl-201 myocardial imaging after dipyridamole infusion: diagnostic utility in detecting coronary stenoses and relationship to regional wall motion. Circulation 66:649, 1982
119. Bodenheimer MM, Wackers FJTh, Schwartz RG et al.: Prognostic significance of a fixed thallium defect one to six months after onset of acute myocardial infarction or unstable angina. Am J Cardiol 74:1196, 1994
120. Krawczynska EG, Weintraub WS, Garcia EV et al.: Left ventricular dilatation and multivessel coronary artery disease on thallium-201 SPECT are important prognostic indicators in patients with large defects in the left anterior descending distribution. Am J Cardiol 74:1233, 1994
121. Weiss AT, Maddahi J, Lew AS et al.: Reverse redistribution of thallium-201: a sign of non transmural myocardial infarction with patency of the infarct related coronary artery. J Am Coll Cardiol 7:61, 1986
122. Bonow RO, Dilsizian V, Cuocolo A et al.: Identification of viable myocardium in patients with chronic coronary artery disease and left ventricular dysfunction. Comparison of thallium scintigraphy with reinjection and PET imaging with fluorine 18 deoxyglucose. Circulation 83:26, 1991
123. Tamaki N, Kawamoto M, Takahashi N et al.: Prognostic value of an increase in fluorine-18 deoxyglucose uptake in patients with myocardial infarction: comparison with stress thallium imaging. J Am Coll Cardiol 22:1621, 1993
124. Tilkemeier PL, Guiney TE, Laraia PJ, Boucher CA: Prognostic value of predischarge low-level exercise thallium testing after thrombolytic treatment of acute myocardial infarction. Am J Cardiol 121:1033, 1991
125. Sutton JM, Topol EJ: Significance of a negative exercise thallium test in the presence of a critical residual stenosis after thrombolysis for acute myocardial infarction. Circulation 83:1278, 1991
126. Moss AJ, Goldstein RE, Hall WJ et al., and the Multicenter Myocardial Ischemia Research Group. Detection and significance of myocardial ischemia in stable patients after recovery from an acute coronary event. JAMA 269:2397, 1993
127. Haber HL, Beller GA, Watson DD, Gimple LW: Exercise thallium-201 scintigraphy after thrombolytic therapy with or without angioplasty for acute myocardial infarction. Am J Cardiol 71:1257, 1993
128. Reiner JS, Lundergan CF, Van Den Brand M et al.: Early angiography cannot predict postthrombolytic coronary reocclusion: observations from the GUSTO angiographic study. J Am Coll Cardiol 24:1439, 1994

Chapter 28

Prognostic Evaluation of CAD Patients Using Positron Emission Tomography

Marcelo F. Di Carli

BACKGROUND

Prognostic Implications of Left Ventricular Dysfunction

Studies of the natural history of coronary artery disease (CAD) have demonstrated that patients with severely depressed left ventricular (LV) function have a poor prognosis when treated with medical therapy alone.[1] Coronary artery bypass surgery in selected patients improves survival and symptoms,[2-4] presumably by preventing further loss of ventricular function and, importantly, by recruiting viable but asynergic myocardium to improve LV function. However, because operative mortality remains considerable, cardiac surgeons are often reluctant to operate on these patients unless there is convincing evidence that revascularization will improve LV function, and, consequently, enhance exercise capacity and survival.[5,6]

In some patients with severely depressed LV function, myocardial asynergy results from myocardial infarction with attendant necrosis and scar formation. As discussed previously, recent studies suggest that in many patients such asynergy may be reversible with revascularization;[7] this is often referred to as hibernating myocardium.[8] The notion that chronic myocardial dysfunction in patients with CAD may be a reversible process has important clinical implications. Indeed, the presence of reversible asynergy in patients with low ejection fraction is not only a prognostic factor for improvement of ventricular function, but also correlates with long-term survival after surgical revascularization.[9] Therefore, identification of hibernating myocardium in CAD patients with depressed LV function may be critically important in selecting those who will benefit most from bypass surgery.

Viable tissue may be distinguished from infarcted myocardium using ^{18}F-labeled deoxyglucose positron emission tomography (PET), [10,11] or various thallium-201 protocols, as discussed in previous chapters. Recent evidence suggests that both PET and thallium-201 imaging approaches can effectively select patients with CAD and depressed ejection fraction in whom coronary revascularization may provide both significant symptomatic and prognostic benefit.[12-15]

Pathophysiology of LV Dysfunction in CAD

Chronic left ventricular contractile dysfunction may improve spontaneously or after revascularization,[16] depending on whether the myocardium is stunned[17] or hibernating.[8] Stunned myocardium has been documented in numerous clinical settings including unstable angina,[19] acute myocardial infarction with early reperfusion,[20] post-open-heart surgery[21] or cardiac transplantation,[22] and in patients with exercise-induced ischemia.[23] Although commonly regarded as an acute phenomenon, stunning may contribute to chronic LV dysfunction if myocardium is unable to recover fully between recurrent episodes of ischemia (symptomatic or asymptomatic). In contrast, hibernation is thought to represent a protective mechanism to reduce energy expenditure to ensure myocyte survival. Considerable clinical evidence supports the notion that contractile dysfunction due to hibernation may improve significantly if chronic ischemia is relieved by revascularization.[7,24–26]

All of these categories of dysfunctional myocardium (infarction, stunning, and hibernation) may commonly coexist in an individual patient. For example, a chronic reduction of function due to hibernation could be worsened further by acute and transient reductions of flow, followed by stunning. Moreover, asynergic myocardium may contain an admixture of subendocardial necrosis interspersed with areas of viable myocardium in which stunning and hibernation can both occur. The concept of reversible ventricular asynergy in patients with ischemic cardiomyopathy is supported by the fact that histologic examination of these hearts generally demonstrates only a modest amount of myocardial loss due to infarction.[27] Such potentially reversible asynergy has important functional and prognostic implications in patients with ischemic cardiomyopathy.[28–36] In such patients, severe heart failure may be attributed to severe, widespread hibernation (or stunning or both) rather than to necrosis of a critical mass of myocardium. Indeed, marked improvement in LV function following revascularization is frequently seen in patients with severely depressed ejection fraction in whom large areas of hibernating myocardium can be demonstrated before surgery.[7]

IDENTIFICATION OF HIBERNATING MYOCARDIUM IN PATIENTS WITH SEVERELY DEPRESSED LV FUNCTION

Clinical Parameters

In patients with LV dysfunction, the presence of angina has been traditionally accepted as evidence of reversible ischemia and, therefore, myocardial viability. Conversely, the lack of anginal symptoms in these patients was considered for many years a clinical marker of myocardial necrosis and a predictor of poor outcome following revascularization.[4] However, the occurrence or frequency of anginal chest pain is not a reliable marker of myocardial ischemia, as determined by exercise stress testing, Holter monitoring, or myocardial perfusion imaging.[37,38] Deanfield and co-workers[38] demonstrated in chronic CAD patients that only 24% of the episodes greater than 1 mm ST-segment depression were accompanied by chest pain. They also showed that angina occurred in only 37% of episodes greater than 3 mm ST-depression. Further, Hirzel and colleagues[39] demonstrated that silent myocardial ischemia during exercise stress testing was frequently associated with significant changes in cardiac hemodynamics and LV ejection fraction (EF).

It is now apparent that symptoms of cardiac dysfunction, such as dyspnea and heart failure or their hemodynamic correlates, may be the primary clinical manifestation of ischemic myocardium in patients with severely depressed LV function. Indeed, extensive areas of viable, yet dysfunctional, myocardium may be found in many patients with severe heart failure.[35,36] Finally, the presence of angina appears to be a poor predictor of improvement in LV function after revascularization.[35]

Hemodynamic Parameters

Clinical and hemodynamic parameters are unreliable for identifying hibernating myocardium in patients with CAD presenting with severe congestive heart failure. Observations by investigators at University of California, Los Angeles, UCLA School of Medicine[40] in 57 patients referred for evaluation for cardiac transplantation demonstrated that important clinical variables such as prior myocardial infarction, duration of heart failure, New York Heart Association (NYHA) heart failure class, and angina failed to discriminate between patients with and without hibernating myocardium as determined by PET. In addition, they reported that cardiac hemodynamics and echocardiographic indices of resting LV function such as ejection fraction and LV diameter were not useful markers of potentially reversible myocardial dysfunction.

Similarly, Ragosta and collaborators[35] demonstrated significant areas of hibernating myocardium, as assessed by preoperative rest–redistribution thallium scintigraphy, in 17 of 21 (81%) patients with ischemic cardiomyopathy presenting with advanced symptoms of congestive heart failure. These authors reported a lack of correlation between the presence of preoperative angina and improvement in LVEF after revascularization, suggesting that anginal symptoms are an indicator of exercise-induced ischemia rather than resting hibernation. Di Carli and colleagues[36] demonstrated significant areas of hibernating myocardium (ranging from 5% to 71% of the left ventricle) in 36 patients with ischemic cardiomyopathy and class III/IV heart failure. In this study, the presence of angina was neither associated with more extensive areas of hibernating myocardium, as determined by PET, nor predicted a change in heart failure class after surgical revascularization.[36]

In summary, these data suggest that clinically significant hibernating myocardium rather than massive myocardial necrosis may be found in many patients with CAD and severely depressed LV function. The lack of anginal symptoms in these patients does not necessarily reflect underlying myocardial fibrosis and, hence, this should not be interpreted as evidence of no reversible potential. Moreover, clinical symptoms of advanced heart failure or their hemodynamic correlates do not exclude the presence of extensive areas of hibernating myocardium. Thus, patients with poor LV function in whom surgical intervention (transplantation or myocardial revascularization) might be contemplated should undergo an imaging test, such as PET metabolic imaging, before rejecting the option of revascularization in a patient with ischemic cardiomyopathy, severe heart failure, and bypassable coronary arteries.

PET Imaging

While various protocols have been proposed to evaluate myocardial viability using PET,[7,28] the combined assessment of regional myocardial perfusion and glucose utilization is the most widely used in routine clinical practice.[10] Increased glucose uptake in dysfunctional segments with reduced blood flow at rest (*perfusion–metabolism mismatch*) indicates presence of metabolic activity and, hence, viable myocardium (Plate 28-1).[7,10] In contrast, a concordant reduction in regional blood flow and glucose uptake (*perfusion–metabolism match*) indicates reduced or absent metabolic activity as a result of myocardial necrosis and scar tissue formation (Plate 28-2).[7,10] The presence of a PET mismatch pattern has been shown to correlate with the presence of postinfarct angina, with electrocardiographic changes during ischemia, and with the presence of segmental wall motion abnormalities.[10] With the use of "mismatch" criteria, 78% to 85% of asynergic segments with a PET mismatch were correctly identified as reversible and 78% to 92% of myocardial segments with a PET match as nonreversible.[7,28-34]

DETERMINANTS OF PROGNOSIS IN PATIENTS WITH IMPAIRED LV FUNCTION

Left Ventricular Function and Provocable Ischemia

The prognosis of patients with CAD is dependent on the degree of LV dysfunction and the extent of CAD.[1] Myocardial ischemia may be the acute precipitating event for either ventricular arrhythmias or recurrent myocardial infarction, which are common underlying mechanisms of death in patients with low ejection fraction.[41] Myocardium involved in these processes must exhibit residual tissue viability and be supplied by a severely stenosed coronary artery.

As discussed in previous chapters, evidence of residual ischemia or exercise intolerance is associated with poor prognosis in postinfarction patients with low ejection fraction who are treated medically.[42] Further, exercise thallium-201 myocardial perfusion imaging has been shown to provide prognostic information independent of that derived by exercise parameters and/or electrocardiographic variables alone in postinfarction patients.[43] In patients who are unable to exercise, dipyridamole stress myocardial perfusion imaging has also been shown to be very effective for prediction of subsequent infarction and cardiac death.[44]

Although demonstrating reversible ischemia has important implications for selecting patients with LV dysfunction for revascularization, many patients may have a prognostic and functional benefit from revascularization even in the absence of significant clinical or scintigraphic evidence of exercise-induced ischemia.[12,14] In such patients, the beneficial effect of revascularization might be a result of improving blood flow to hibernating myocardium, thereby improving LV function, which ultimately results in improving exercise capacity and prognosis. Failure to recognize potentially reversible ventricular dysfunction may preclude these patients from undergoing revascularization, thereby missing an opportunity to improve LV function and prognosis.

Prognostic Significance of Hibernating Myocardium

Recent investigations have evaluated the prognostic significance of hibernating myocardium, as assessed by the perfusion–metabolism PET mismatch pattern, in patients with depressed LV function.[12–14] These studies examined the relative efficacy of medical therapy versus revascularization in patients with impaired LV function, with and without evidence of viable myocardium. It is important to note that these investigations were retrospective observations and not prospective randomized trials. Nevertheless, in the absence of randomized studies evaluating the outcomes of treatment decisions in patients with low ejection fraction on the basis of the presence or absence of viable myocardium, these observational studies provide useful information.

A summary of important clinical and angiographic information of the patients studied in these published series[12–14] is shown in Table 28-1. They included CAD patients with depressed LV function (average LVEF < 40%). Most of these patients had a history of myocardial infarction and multivessel CAD. Approximately one-third of the patients presented with angina and 20% to 68% of them had severe heart failure (NYHA class III-IV). In these studies, survival and recurrent ischemic events (myocardial infarction, unstable angina, and arrhythmia) were evaluated over an average of 12 to 17 months. In all three studies, the patients were grouped based on the presence (or absence) of a perfusion–metabolism PET mismatch, as evidence of viable myocardium (Fig. 28-1). Treatment decisions (i.e., revascularization or medical therapy) in patients with and without a PET mismatch were made on clinical grounds. However, no significant differences in relevant clinical and angiographic variables known to affect prognosis were found between these two groups.

The results of these studies showed a quite consistent trend with respect to several points (Fig. 28-2). In patients with a PET mismatch pattern, indicating hibernating myocardium, 1-year event-free survival was consistently poor with medical therapy, but 1-year event-free survival was significantly improved by prompt revascularization. In patients without

Table 28-1. Patient Populations from Three Observational Studies Evaluating the Efficacy of Medical Therapy and Revascularization in Patients with Coronary Artery Disease and Severe Left Ventricular Dysfunction

Variables	Eitzman et al. (1992)[13]	Di Carli et al. (1994)[12]	Lee et al. (1994)[14]
Number of patients	82	93	129
Age	59 ± 10	65 ± 10	62 ± 11
Male	88%	84%	79%
Previous MI	[a]	68%	100%
Severity of angina	1.9 ± 0.7 (CCS)	37%[b]	40%[b]
Heart failure class (NYHA)	1.8 ± 0.8	68%[c]	19%[c]
LVEF	34 ± 13%	25 ± 6%	38 ± 16%
Multivessel CAD	84%	82%	74%
Mean follow-up (months)	12	13	17
Observation period	1988–1990	1989–1991	1989–1991
End-point	Combined[d]	Cardiac mortality	Combined[d]

Abbreviations: MI, myocardial infarction; CCS, Canadian Cardiovascular Society; NYHA, New York Heart Association; CAD, coronary heart disease; LVEF, left ventricular ejection fraction.
[a] Not reported.
[b] Expressed as proportion of patients with class III-IV of the CCS.
[c] Denotes proportion of patients in NYHA class III-IV.
[d] Combined end-point of cardiac mortality, nonfatal MI, arrhythmia, unstable angina, and late revascularization.

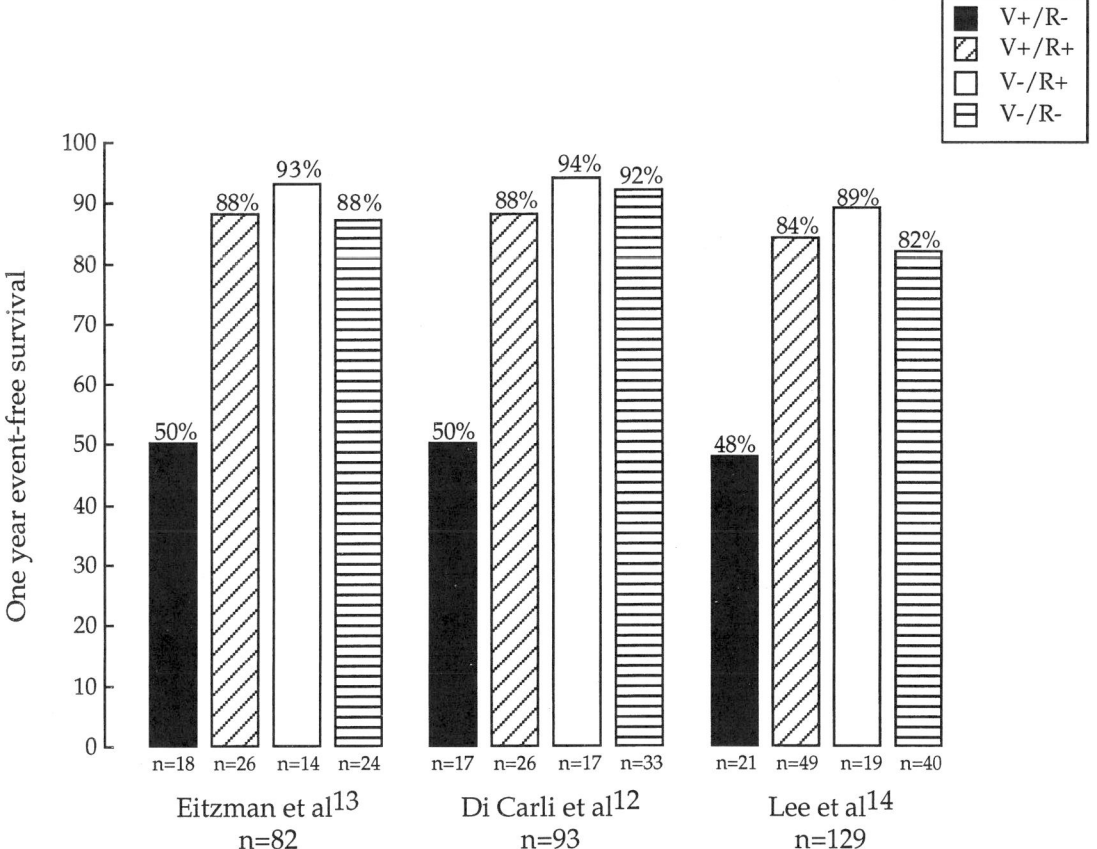

Fig. 28-1. One-year event-free survival of patients with depressed left ventricular function undergoing medical therapy or revascularization by presence or absence of viable myocardium on positron emission tomography (PET) imaging. V +, presence of a perfusion–metabolism PET mismatch; R +, revascularization.

hibernation, 1-year event-free survival was similar with either medical therapy or revascularization. Two of these studies also demonstrated that the presence of a PET mismatch pattern and the lack of revascularization were the most significant independent predictors of cardiac events in multivariate analysis.[12,14] In the study by Di Carli et al.[12] the relative risk (hazard) of cardiac death associated with a PET mismatch pattern in unrevascularized patients increased by 3.5% with each unit of increment in the percent extent of mismatch; the more extensive the perfusion–metabolism mismatch the higher the risk of dying during the follow-up period. In contrast, revascularization was associated with a positive effect on survival, decreasing the risk of cardiac death by 28%.

Other investigators have reported similar trends in patients with mild to moderate degrees of LV dysfunction (LVEF ≥ 40%) after myocardial infarction.[45,46] In a retrospective evaluation of 84 patients, Tamaki and colleagues[46] reported that the number of diseased vessels, a decreased LVEF, the presence of thallium redistribution, and the presence of a PET mismatch pattern were significant univariate predictors of ischemic events during a 2-year follow-up. However, only the presence of multivessel coronary disease and metabolically active tissue (PET mismatch) within the infarct zone were significant predictors of cardiac events on multivariate analysis. In this study, the presence of a PET mismatch was associated with a 39% event rate over 2 years, primarily unstable angina and revascularization procedures.

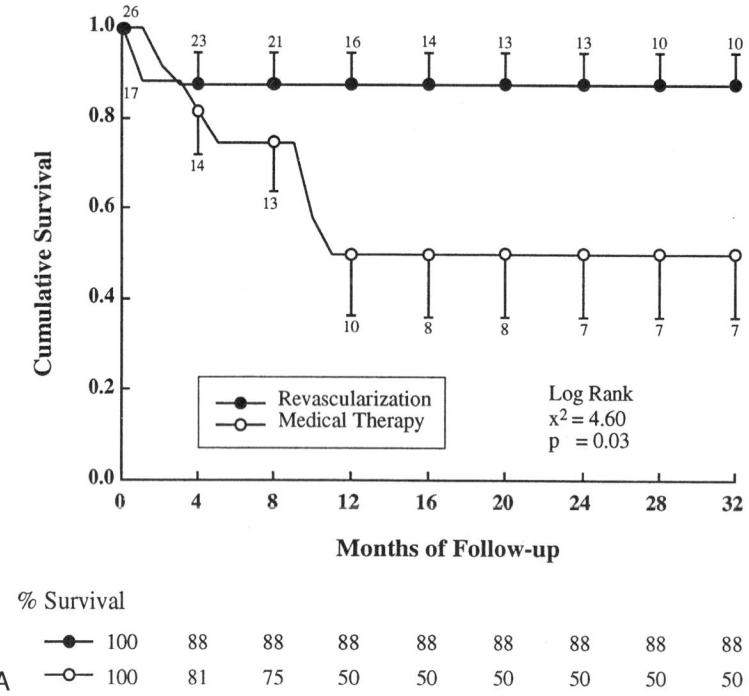

Fig. 28-2. Cumulative survival of patients, by (**A**) presence or (**B**) absence of a positron emission tomography mismatch and mode of treatment (i.e., medical therapy or revascularization). (From Di Carli et al.,[12] with permission.)

One study by Yoshida and Gould[46] did not show an increased event rate during a 3-year follow-up of patients with residual tissue viability in the infarct zone; however, this was a small group (only 5 of the 35 patients in the study). The low 3-year event rate (10%) in patients with viable myocardium undergoing revascularization was similar to that observed in patients with viable myocardium but severely depressed ejection fraction undergoing bypass surgery.

More recently, Gioia and colleagues[15] reported similar findings using rest–redistribution thallium-201 imaging for evaluating myocardial viability. This observational study included 85 coronary disease patients with LV dysfunction (LVEF < 50%). They evaluated the prognostic significance of the presence of thallium redistribution within myocardial regions with resting perfusion defects (the correlate of a perfusion–metabolism mismatch on PET imaging) over a 31-month follow-up. The degree of LV dysfunction, severity of clinical symptoms, and extent of CAD were comparable to those in the previous PET series. The results of this study are remarkably consistent with those presented in the previous PET reports: (1) in the medically treated group, the survival of patients with reversible defects was lower than that of those with fixed resting perfusion defects (55% vs. 74%), and (2) the survival of patients with reversible defects was better with revascularization than with medical treatment alone (94% vs. 55%).

The consistently lower event rate among those patients without evidence of viable myocardium by PET or thallium criteria may be explained by the lower risk of reinfarction or an unstable coronary syndrome

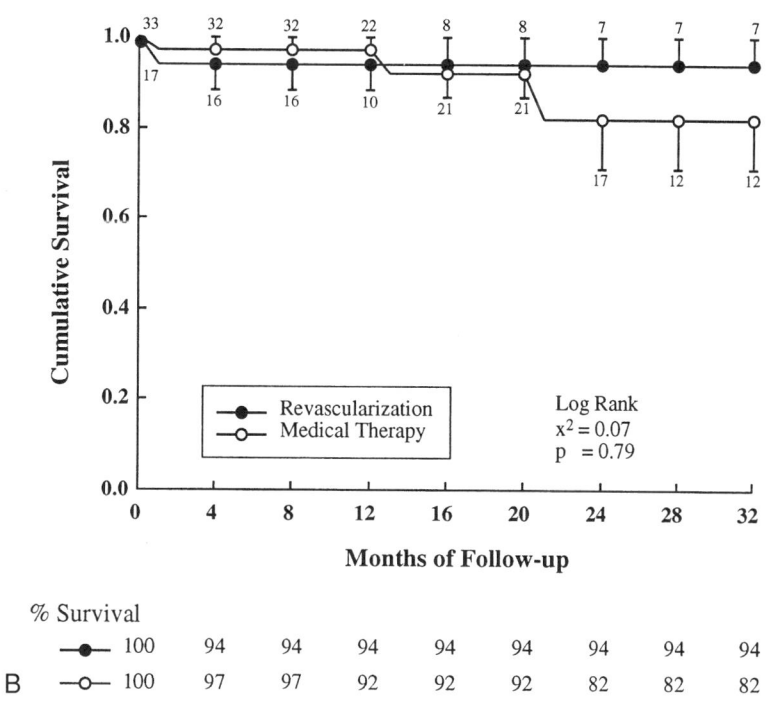

Fig. 28-2. (continued).

when a severely stenosed coronary artery supplies an area of infarcted rather than viable myocardium.

CLINICAL IMPLICATIONS

Optimization of Management Decisions by Integration of Clinical, Angiographic, and Scintigraphic Information

Patients with CAD and severely impaired LV function treated with medical therapy alone are exposed to frequent hospitalizations and early death.[1] In these patients, long-term survival with surgical revascularization is superior.[2-4] Indeed, it has been demonstrated that the patients most likely to benefit from bypass surgery are precisely those with the highest medical risk.[3,4] However, much controversy remains about the proper selection of patients with severe LV dysfunction for coronary revascularization. A rational approach to maximize the benefits from the operation would be to identify those patients in whom revascularization would likely improve LV function, symptoms, and survival. The presence of a perfusion–metabolism mismatch on PET imaging appears to effectively select patients with low ejection fraction in whom revascularization would likely improve exercise capacity and prognosis (Fig. 28-2).[12-14] Using this approach, the operative mortality rate ranges from 3% to 10%.[6,12,15] These numbers represent an improvement over the initial results in patients with severe LV dysfunction,[47] rendering revascularization a more acceptable treatment option in selected patients. However, these results may not apply to all patients with severe LV dysfunction. In patients who are primarily considered for cardiac transplantation, the operative risk and annual survival may also be affected by the LV size, hemodynamic condition, and previous bypass surgery.[6]

Predicting the Improvement of LV Function after Revascularization

The accuracy of PET for the prediction of regional improvements in LV function[7,28–34] has been summarized in Chapter 21. Similar data are also available for rest–redistribution thallium-201 imaging.[35,48,49]

The major question, however, is whether revascularization can provide a clinically meaningful improvement in LVEF in patients with severely depressed LV function, which may translate into improved exercise capacity and survival. Several studies in limited numbers of patients have addressed this issue.[7,35,50] In these reports, the improvement in global LV systolic function following revascularization was related to the preoperative presence of relatively large areas of viable myocardium. In the study by Tillisch et al.,[7] LVEF improved from 30 ± 11% to 45 ± 14% after bypass surgery only in patients with greater than 2 myocardial regions with a preoperative PET mismatch pattern.[7] Similarly, Ragosta et al.[35] reported a significant correlation between the number of asynergic but viable segments by thallium criteria and the improvement in LVEF after bypass surgery. In this study, the mean LV ejection increased significantly (29 ± 7% to 41 ± 11%) after revascularization in patients with more than 7 dysfunctional but viable myocardial regions, whereas it remained unchanged (27 ± 5% vs. 30 ± 8%) in those with less than 7 viable segments.

Predicting the Improvement of Functional Status after Revascularization

Another important question in patients with poor LV function under consideration for bypass surgery is whether revascularization of viable, asynergic myocardium will provide a significant alleviation of heart failure symptoms. Indeed, heart failure is often their primary functional limitation and in many patients it is the main reason to seek medical attention. Recent studies have focused on the relation between the preoperative detection of viable myocardium and the postoperative improvement in heart failure symptoms and exercise capacity in patients with poor cardiac function.

An early study by Marwick and colleagues[51] in patients post infarction, examined the efficacy of preoperative PET imaging for predicting improvement in LV function and exercise capacity after revascularization. In 23 postinfarction patients with LV dysfunction (LVEF 35 ± 14%) and impaired functional capacity (70% in NYHA class II-III), they demonstrated that the amount of viable myocardium before revascularization was predictive of a significant improvement in exercise parameters after revascularization. Peak rate–pressure product, maximal heart rate, and exercise capacity increased significantly after revascularization only in patients with multiple postexercise glucose-avid regions on preoperative PET imaging. In a more recent study, Di Carli and co-workers[36] demonstrated a significant linear correlation between the global extent of a preoperative perfusion–metabolism mismatch and the percent improvement in functional capacity after bypass surgery in 36 patients with ischemic cardiomyopathy (LVEF 28 ± 6%) (Fig. 28-3). The authors reported that a perfusion–metabolism PET mismatch involving greater than 18% of the LV on quantitative analysis was associated with a sensitivity of 76% and a specificity of 78% for predicting a significant improvement in heart failure class following bypass surgery. After revascularization, patients with large PET mismatches (> 18% of the LV), particularly in the left anterior descending coronary territory, had the greatest clinical benefit, improving their functional status by 107%, which was significantly greater than the 34% change observed in those with minimal or no PET mismatch (107% vs. 34%).

These data suggest that assessment of contractile reserve with PET or potentially with thallium scintigraphy before surgery can effectively select patients with CAD and severely depressed LV function likely to improve systolic function and symptoms after revascularization. Minimal or no evidence of anginal symptoms in these patients did not preclude them from undergoing bypass surgery and did not portend unsuccessful coronary revascularization.

CONCLUSIONS

The experimental and clinical data presented here indicate that preoperative PET imaging can effectively select patients with CAD and severely depressed ejection fraction who would most likely show an improvement in LV function, exercise capacity,

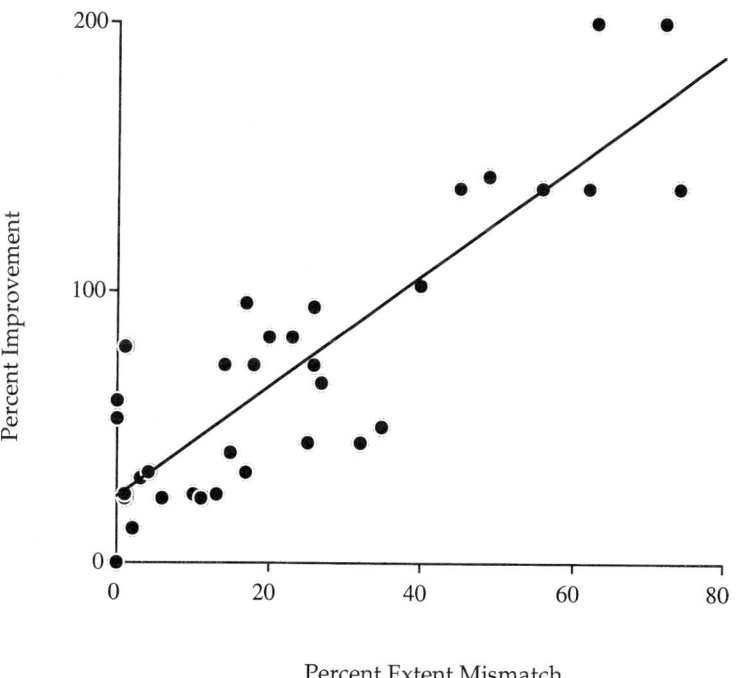

Fig. 28-3. Scatter plot showing the relation between the anatomic extent of perfusion–metabolism positron emission tomography mismatches, expressed as percent of the left ventricle, and the change in functional state post-coronary artery bypass grafting, expressed as percent improvement from baseline ($r = 0.87$, $p < 0.001$). (From Di Carli et al.,[36] with permission.)

and prognosis following coronary revascularization. Revascularization in patients with ischemic cardiomyopathy, bypassable coronary arteries, and relatively large areas of viable myocardium may be performed with acceptable operative mortality. Long-term survival after bypass surgery in these patients appears to be comparable to that achieved with cardiac transplantation.

Patients with markedly depressed ejection fraction ($< 30\%$) may have considerable amounts of hibernating myocardium even if presenting with severe heart failure and with no evidence of significant exercise-induced ischemia. Consideration of bypass surgery in a patient with poor cardiac function would be more attractive if there were objective evidence that such a patient has a high probability of improving LV function after revascularization. Demonstration of preserved metabolic activity in a myocardial region with reduced perfusion at rest (perfusion–metabolism mismatch) on PET imaging may provide such evidence. More importantly, the association of excess cardiac mortality and ischemic events with failure to revascularize viable myocardium, as demonstrated by a PET mismatch, further suggests that coronary revascularization in patients with depressed LV function may be justified on prognostic grounds. Because the cost of PET imaging is small in comparison to that of transplantation, we believe that its use is cost-effective in patients with severely depressed LV function due to CAD.

ACKNOWLEDGMENTS

The author is most grateful to Dr. Zoltan G. Turi for his excellent editorial comments, Barbara Fromm for her valuable suggestions, and Doris Robbins for her secretarial assistance.

REFERENCES

1. Emond M, Mock MB, Davis KB et al.: Long-term survival of medically treated patients in the Coronary Artery Surgery Study (CASS). Circulation 90:2645, 1993

2. Pigott JD, Kouchoukos NT, Oberman A: Late results of surgical and medical therapy for patients with coronary artery disease and depressed left ventricular function. J Am Coll Cardiol 5:1036, 1985
3. Bounous EP, Mark DB, Pollock BG et al.: Surgical survival benefits for coronary disease patients with left ventricular dysfunction. Circulation, suppl. I, 78: I - 151 1988
4. Alderman EL, Fisher LD, Litwin P et al.: Results of coronary artery surgery in patients with poor left ventricular function (CASS). Circulation 68:785, 1985
5. Kron IL, Flanagan TL, Blackbourne LH et al.: Myocardial revascularization rather than cardiac transplantation for chronic ischemic cardiomyopathy. Ann Surg 210:348, 1985
6. Louie HW, Laks H, Milgalter E et al.: Ischemic cardiomyopathy. Criteria for myocardial revascularization and cardiac transplantation. Circulation, suppl. III, 84: III-290, 1991
7. Tillisch J, Brunken R, Marshall RC et al.: Reversibility of cardiac wall motion abnormalities predicted by positron tomography. N Engl J Med 314:884, 1986
8. Rahimtoola SH: The hibernating myocardium. Am Heart J 117:211, 1989
9. Nesto RW, Cohn LH, Collins JJ Jr et al.: Inotropic contractile reserve: a useful predictor of increased 5-year survival and improved postoperative ventricular function in patients with coronary artery disease and reduced ejection fraction. Am J Cardiol 50:39, 1982
10. Marshall RC, Tillisch JH, Phelps ME et al.: Identification and differentiation of resting myocardial ischemia and infarction in man with positron computed tomography 18F-labeled fluorodeoxyglucose and N-13 ammonia. Circulation 64:766, 1981
11. Maddahi J, Schelbert H, Brunken R et al.: Role of thallium-201 and PET imaging in evaluation of myocardial viability and management of patients with coronary artery disease and left ventricular dysfunction. J Nucl Med 35:707, 1994
12. Di Carli MF, Davidson M, Little R et al.: Value of metabolic imaging with positron emission tomography for evaluating prognosis in patients with coronary artery disease and left ventricular dysfunction. Am J Cardiol 73:527, 1994
13. Eitzman D, Al-Aouar Z, Kanter HL et al.: Clinical outcome of patients with advanced coronary artery disease after viability studies with positron emission tomography. J Am Coll Cardiol; 20:559, 1992
14. Lee KS, Marwick TH, Cook SA et al.: Prognosis of patients with left ventricular dysfunction, with and without viable myocardium after myocardial infarction. Relative efficacy of medical therapy and revascularization. Circulation 90:2687, 1994
15. Gioia G, Powers J, Heo J, Iskandrian AS: Prognostic value of rest-redistribution tomographic thallium-201 imaging in ischemic cardiomyopathy. Am J Cardiol 75: 759, 1995
16. Kloner RA, Przyklenk K, Patel B: Altered myocardial states. The stunned and hibernating myocardium. Am J Med 86:14, 1989
17. Braunwald EB, Kloner RA: The stunned myocardium: prolonged, postischemic ventricular dysfunction. Circulation 66:1146, 1982
18. Bolli R: Mechanism of myocardial stunning. Circulation 82:723, 1990
19. Kolibask AJ, Goodenow JS, Busk CA: Improvement in myocardial perfusion and left ventricular function after coronary artery bypass grafting in patients with unstable angina. Circulation 59:66, 1979
20. Stack RS, Philips HR III, Grierson DS et al.: Functional improvement of jeopardized myocardium following intracoronary streptokinase infusion in acute myocardial infarction. J Clin Invest 72:84, 1983
21. Gray R, Maddahi J, Berman D et al.: Scintigraphic and hemodynamic demonstration of transient left ventricular dysfunction immediately after uncomplicated coronary artery bypass grafting. J Thorac Cardiovasc Surg 77:504, 1979
22. Wicomb WN, Cooper DKC, Novitzky D et al.: Cardiac transplantation following storage of the donor heart by a portable hypothermic perfusion system. Ann Thorac Surg 37:243, 1984
23. Kloner RA, Allen J, Cox Tae et al.: Stunned left ventricular myocardium after exercise treadmill testing in coronary artery disease. Am J Cardiol 68:329, 1991
24. Chaterjee K, Swan HJC, Parmley WW et al.: Depression of left ventricular function due to acute myocardial ischemia and its reversal after aortocoronary saphenous-vein bypass. N Engl J Med 286:117, 1972
25. Brundage BH, Massie BM, Botvinik EH: Improved regional ventricular function after successful surgical revascularization. J Am Coll Cardiol 3:902, 1984
26. Popio KA, Gorlin R, Bechtel D et al.: Postextrasystolic potentiation as a predictor of potential myocardial viability: preoperative analysis compared with studies after coronary artery bypass surgery. Am J Cardiol 39: 944, 1977
27. Schuster EH, Bulkley BH: Ischemic cardiomyopathy: a clinicopathologic study of fourteen patients. Am Heart J 100:506, 1980
28. Gropler RJ, Geltman EM, Sampathkumaran K et al.: Comparison of carbon-11-acetate with fluorine-18-fluorodeoxyglucose for delineating viable myocardium by positron emission tomography. J Am Coll Cardiol 22(6):1587, 1993

29. Tamaki N, Yonekura Y, Yamashita K et al.: Positron emission tomography using fluorine-18 deoxyglucose in evaluation of coronary artery bypass grafting. Am J Cardiol 64:860, 1989
30. Lucignani G, Paolini G, Landoni C et al.: Presurgical identification of hibernating myocardium by combined use of technetium-99m hexakis 2-methoxyisobutylisonitrile single photon emission tomography and fluorine-18 fluoro-2-deoxy-D-glucose positron emission tomography in patients with coronary artery disease. Eur J Nucl Med 19(10):874, 1992
31. Carrel T, Jenni R, Haubold-Reuter S et al.: Improvement of severely reduced left ventricular function after surgical revascularization in patients with preoperative myocardial infarction. Eur J Cardiothorac Surg 6:479, 1992
32. Tamaki N, Ohtani H, Yamashita K et al.: Metabolic activity in the areas of new fill-in after thallium-201 reinjection: comparison with positron emission tomography. J Nucl Med 32:673, 1991
33. Gropler RJ, Siegel BA, Sampathkumaran K et al.: Dependence of recovery of contractile function on maintenance of oxidative metabolism after myocardial infarction. J Am Coll Cardiol 19:989, 1992
34. Tamaki N, Kawamoto M, Tadamura E et al.: Prediction of reversible ischemia after revascularization. Perfusion and metabolic studies with positron emission tomography. Circulation 91:1697, 1995
35. Ragosta M, Beller GA, Watson DD et al.: Quantitative planar rest-redistribution Tl-201 imaging in detection of myocardial viability and prediction of improvement in left ventricular function after coronary artery bypass surgery in patients with severely depressed left ventricular function. Circulation 86:1630, 1993
36. Di Carli M, Asgarzadie F, Schelbert HR et al.: Quantitative relation between myocardial viability and improvement in heart failure symptoms after revascularization in patients with ischemic cardiomyopathy. Circulation 92:3436, 1995
37. Weiner DA, Ryan TJ, McCabe CH et al.: Exercise stress testing. Correlation among history of angina, ST segment response and prevalence of coronary artery disease in the Coronary Artery Surgery Study (CASS). N Engl J Med 301:230, 1979
38. Deanfield JE, Maseri A, Selwin AP et al.: Myocardial ischemia during daily life in patients with stable angina: Its relation to symptoms and heart rate changes. Lancet 2:753, 1983
39. Hirzel HO, Leutwyler R, Krayenbuehl HR: Silent myocardial ischemia: hemodynamic changes during dynamic exercise in patients with proven coronary artery disease despite absence of angina pectoris. J Am Coll Cardiol 6:275, 1985
40. Czernin J, Chan A, Müller P, et al.: Can hemodynamic and clinical parameters identify CHF patients with viable myocardium? (abstract) J Am Coll Cardiol 21:103A, 1993
41. Franciosa JA, Wilen M, Ziesche S et al.: Survival in men with severe chronic left ventricular failure due to either coronary heart disease or idiopathic dilated cardiomyopathy. Am J Cardiol 51:831, 1983
42. Weiner DA, Ryan TJ, McCabe CH et al.: Value of exercise testing in determining the risk classification and the response to coronary artery bypass grafting in three-vessel coronary artery disease: a report from the Coronary Artery Surgery Study (CASS) registry. Am J Cardiol 60:262, 1987
43. Gibson RS, Watson DD, Craddok GB et al.: Prediction of cardiac events after uncomplicated myocardial infarction: a prospective study comparing predischarge exercise thallium-201 scintigraphy and coronary angiography. Circulation 68:321, 1983
44. Leppo JA, O'Brian J, Rothendler JA et al.: Dipyridamole thallium-201 scintigraphy in the prediction of future cardiac events after acute myocardial infarction. N Engl J Med 310:1014, 1984
45. Tamaki N, Kawamoto M, Takahashi N et al.: Prognostic value of an increase in fluorine-18 deoxyglucose uptake in patients with myocardial infarction: comparison with stress thallium imaging. J Am Coll Cardiol 22:1621, 1993
46. Yoshida K, Gould KL: Quantitative relation of myocardial infarct size and myocardial viability by positron emission tomography to left ventricular ejection fraction and 3-year mortality with and without revascularization. J Am Coll Cardiol 22:984, 1993
47. Yatteau RF, Peter RH, Behar VS et al.: Ischemic Cardiomyopathy: The myopathy of coronary artery disease. Natural history and results of medical versus surgical treatment. Am J Cardiol 34:520, 1974
48. Mori T, Minamiji K, Kurongane H et al.: Rest-injected thallium-201 imaging for assessing viability of severe asynergic regions. J Nucl Med 23:1718, 1991
49. Alfieri O, La Canna G, Guibbini R et al.: Recovery of myocardial function. Eur J Cardiothorac Surg 7:325, 1993
50. Iskandrian AS, Hakki AH, Kane SA et al.: Rest and redistribution thallium-201 scintigraphy to predict improvement in left ventricular function after coronary artery bypass grafting. Am J Cardiol 51:1312, 1983
51. Marwick TH, Nemec JJ, Lafont A et al.: Prediction by postexercise fluoro-18 deoxyglucose positron emission tomography of improvement in exercise capacity after revascularization. Am J Cardiol 69:854, 1992

Chapter 29

Clinical Evaluation of Cardiac Risk Before Major Noncardiac Surgery

Alan K. Halperin and David L. Bronson

Perioperative cardiac events are the most common serious complication of noncardiac surgery. Each year, more than 25 million patients undergo noncardiac surgical procedures, of whom one million have known coronary artery disease (CAD), 2 to 3 million have multiple cardiac risk factors, and 4 million are older than 65 years. Eighty percent of the one million patients who suffer perioperative cardiac morbidity and mortality each year come from these groups.[1] This suggests that the patients at highest risk may be identified preoperatively, using clinical criteria and new noninvasive technology. Once high-risk patients are identified, interventions can be recommended with the goal of decreasing risk. This chapter will review the current literature on the physiologic stresses of surgery; risk stratification using the history, physical examination, electrocardiogram, and noninvasive technology (when necessary); and the approach to patients to reduce the risk of cardiac complications.

PHYSIOLOGIC STRESSES OF SURGERY

The physiologic stressors of surgery are related to the direct and indirect effects of anesthetic agents and the responses to surgical-induced hypotension, blood loss, anemia, and postoperative pain. During anesthesia induction, tachycardia and hypertension occur in response to anxiety and the mechanical effects of tracheal manipulation with intubation. Later, hypotension may occur due to vasodilation and myocardial depression associated with anesthetic agents, intermittent positive pressure ventilation, hemorrhage, or infection. Balanced anesthetic techniques using opiates, sedative hypnotics, neuromuscular blockers, and inhalational agents have enabled the anesthesiologist to provide anesthesia with less cardiovascular effects than with inhalational agents alone.[2] Newer inhalational agents such as isoflurane produce less myocardial depression than older agents.[2] In the early postoperative period, pain, hypertension, and increased catecholamines may increase cardiovascular stress by increasing myocardial oxygen demands and coronary vascular tone. In addition, enhanced platelet aggregation and hypercoagulability due to tissue injury may increase the risk of coronary occlusion. Limited cardiovascular reserve increases the risk of a cardiac event and predisposes to a poorer outcome.

The severity of the physiologic stress is proportional to the risk of the planned procedure. Procedures associated with higher levels of cardiac risk include craniotomies, cardiac procedures, large bowel surgery, thoracotomy, vascular surgery, major joint replacements, and exploratory laparotomies. Patients undergoing these higher levels of surgical trauma and physiologic stress are the subject of this chapter. Lower levels of risk are usually associated with plastic surgical procedures, tubal ligation, dilation and curettage (D&C), hysterectomy, eye and oral surgery, transurethral resection of the prostate, and herniorrhaphy. Low levels of surgical trauma and shorter duration of anesthesia are generally associated with lower levels of risk. Newer anesthetic agents and perioperative care techniques have substantially improved the outcomes of the surgical patients with medical problems.[2]

CLINICAL EVALUATION OF THE PREOPERATIVE PATIENT
General Considerations

The cardiologist or internist is commonly consulted to assess the cardiac risk of patients scheduled for surgery. The goal is to decrease perioperative cardiac complications, which include cardiac death, myocardial infarction (MI), transient myocardial ischemia, arrhythmias, and congestive heart failure.

The cornerstones of the preoperative evaluation are the history, physical examination, and resting electrocardiogram (ECG). Essential elements are a history of CAD, heart failure, valvular heart disease, and the presence of multiple risk factors. The physical examination should include a detailed cardiovascular exam. After the initial history and physical examination, patients with defined high-risk factors can be further stratified by placing them into high-, medium-, or low-risk groups (Table 29-1). At the end of the initial clinical assessment (history, physical examination, and ECG), patients should be categorized into one of four groups:

1. proceed with surgery without further evaluation,
2. proceed with surgery but take steps to further reduce perioperative risk by intensifying medical therapy,
3. proceed to further risk stratification before surgery, possibly culminating in myocardial revascularization prior to surgery, or
4. cancel surgery because of unacceptable risk.

Placing the patient in the latter category requires careful discussion with the surgical team to determine other alternatives for treatment.

Table 29-1. Goldman Multifactorial Index

Finding	Points
Myocardial infarction within 6 months	10
Age >70 years	5
S_3 gallop or jugular venous distention	11
Important aortic valve stenosis	3
Rhythm other than sinus, or sinus rhythm and atrial premature contractions on last preoperative electrocardiogram	7
Poor general medical status[a]	3
Intraperitoneal, intrathoracic or aortic operation	3
Emergency operation	4

Class	(Points)	Life-Threatening Complications (%)	Cardiac (%)
I	0–5	0.7	0.2
II	6–12	5	2
III	13–25	11	2
IV	≥26	22	56

[a] PaO_2 <60 mmHg, $PaCO_2$ >50 mmHg, serum potassium <3.0 mEq/L, serum bicarbonate <20 mEq/L, blood urea nitrogen >50 mg/dl, serum creatinine >3.0 mg/dl, abnormal asparate aminotransferase, signs of chronic liver disease, bedridden from noncardiac causes.
(From Goldman et al.,[14] with permission.)

Frequent Clinical Presentations
Patients without Known CAD

Patients with no clinical history or exam findings of CAD are low risk and can proceed with surgery without further evaluation. An ECG is frequently recommended for men older than 45 years of age and women older than 55 years of age to identify patients with abnormal rhythms and silent MI[3] (the use of an older age cutoff in women reflects the later development of CAD in women). The Framingham Study has demonstrated that approximately 25% of Q-wave MI may be silent,[4] and these patients have increased risk of cardiac complications in the long term.[5]

Patients with Known CAD

MI occurs perioperatively in 0.15% of patients without prior clinical evidence of heart disease and 3% to 18% of patients with a history of prior MI.[6] Patients with a prior history of CAD have a 25% to 50% higher mortality than those without disease,[7] although the absolute event rate is quite low. In the setting of emergency surgical procedures, this risk increases by four times compared to those without CAD. A 1993 study of consecutive noncardiac surgery procedures in 1487 men older than 40 years of age scheduled for major elective or urgent noncardiac surgery[8] classified patients clinically into four groups, based upon their cardiac history:

1. High-risk category—defined in patients with known CAD as shown by a history of MI, an old MI by ECG, typical angina, a history of coronary artery bypass grafting (CABG), or angiographic CAD with stenoses greater than 70%. These patients had a 4.1% risk of MI and a 2.3% risk of cardiac death.
2. Intermediate-risk category—defined as those patients with other vascular disease or atypical chest pain syndromes, but without known CAD. They experienced a 0.8% risk of MI and a 0.4% risk of cardiac death.
3. Low-risk category—patients with no known atherosclerosis, but older than 75 years of age or high risk by the Framingham criteria (> 15% risk of CAD in 6 years). They experienced no MIs and a 0.4% risk of cardiac death.
4. Negligible-risk group—patients with no atherosclerosis and low-risk profile. These experienced no cardiac deaths.

One can conclude from the above data that even with the presence of known CAD the risk of noncardiac surgery remains relatively low, as long as recent MI and unstable angina are absent.

Chronic stable angina can be managed safely without further intervention in many patients. A patient who can climb two flights without angina or significant dyspnea has adequate cardiopulmonary reserve, and additional preoperative testing is usually unnecessary. Perioperative administration of nitrates and β-blockers should be considered. Patients with unstable angina require further investigation prior to surgery. Those who have had previous myocardial revascularization and have no clinical symptoms of active ischemia are at low risk and do not require further investigation.[9]

Patients with Recent MI

MI within 6 months carries a significant risk of perioperative infarction, although modern anesthetic techniques emphasizing careful monitoring and hemodynamic intervention have lowered this risk. For elective surgical procedures, the perioperative reinfarction rate for patients who have had a MI within 3 months is 5.8%, between 3 and 6 months 2.3%, and after 6 months it falls to 1.3%.[10] Patients who have had a MI within 3 months carry a 16.7% rate of reinfarction or cardiac death when faced with urgent or emergent procedures.[11] Elective procedures should be delayed until 6 months after MI. If surgery is essential, preoperative perfusion imaging or stress ventriculographic assessment using radionuclide or echocardiographic techniques should be undertaken.[12,13] Patients at greatest risk are those with postinfarction angina, severe left ventricular LV dysfunction, or extensive inducible ischemia. For these subsets of early postinfarction patients, revascularization should be considered to minimize cardiovascular instability, depending on the balance between the risk of revascularization and that of surgery without prior intervention. Patients undergoing high-risk procedures with recent MI, ischemia on preoperative testing (without prior myocardial revascularization), or poor left ventricular function (ejection fraction < 30%) might be benefited by invasive monitoring during anesthesia.

Patients with Heart Failure

The presence of a third heart sound denotes a severity of left ventricular failure (LVF) indicating added risk for cardiac death or complications.[14] Echocardiographic assessment of active LVF can further define risk, and hemodynamic monitoring with aggressive management may lead to improved outcomes. Every effort to maximize LVF should be made prior to surgery. In all circumstances, the anesthesiologist needs to be aware of LVF to manage fluids, invasive monitoring, and anesthetic choice appropriately.

Patients with Aortic Stenosis

Valvular aortic stenosis increases the risk of cardiac events.[15] These patients are at a risk for endocarditis, embolization, and congestive heart failure. Severe aortic stenosis is a contraindication to most high-risk elective surgery, and evaluation for valvuloplasty or valve replacement should precede the elective procedure. When recognized and managed carefully, a Mayo Clinic series found a 10% incidence of intraoperative hypotension, but low risk of cardiac events (cardiac death or MI).[16] Hypotension responded promptly to standard treatments.

Patients with Hypertension

Patients with severe hypertension have increased morbidity and mortality compared with controlled hypertensives or normotensives. Patients with severe hypertension (diastolic blood pressure > 110 mmHg) have a larger absolute drop in systolic blood pressure BP, operative BP lability, more arrhythmias, myocardial ischemia and infarctions, neurologic complications, renal failure, congestive heart failure, and postoperative hypertension.[17] In contrast, patients with mild to moderate diastolic hypertension (90 to 109 mmHg) do not have increased operative mortality or complications. There are no differences between controlled and uncontrolled hypertensive patients with respect to their intraoperative BP, use of vasopressors or intravenous fluids during surgery, or incidence of postoperative hypertension. There are inadequate data to assess the risk of patients with isolated systolic hypertension.

Patients with Peripheral Vascular Disease

Because of the high prevalence of CAD in patients with peripheral vascular disease and increased risk of perioperative cardiac complications in patients undergoing vascular surgery, many recommend an aggressive evaluation for CAD including noninvasive testing and, if necessary, cardiac catheterization and revascularization prior to the elective vascular surgery.[5,9,10,14,17–21] Because of exercise limitations in these patients, pharmacologic stress tests are preferred. The value of an aggressive work-up in all patients has, however, been questioned, because 30% of patients will not have significant anatomic CAD, and even more have no perioperative events.

Eagle and colleagues[20] outlined a series of clinical predictors that identify vascular surgical patients at greatest risk for cardiac events. In 200 vascular surgery patients referred for dipyridamole-thallium stress testing prior to surgery, five clinical predictors were identified: age older than 70 years of age, a history of angina, significant Q-waves on ECG, congestive heart failure, and diabetes requiring treatment. Those patients with none of the predictors had a 3.1% rate of perioperative ischemic events, defined as unstable angina, ischemic pulmonary edema, MI, or cardiac death. Patients with one or two predictors had a 15.5% risk of events, while those with three or more had a 50% event risk. Clinical predictors alone correctly classified these patients into risk categories 71% of the time, compared to 69% for thallium imaging alone and 81% for combined thallium and clinical variables.

The role of testing in unselected patients remains uncertain, and recent studies by Mangano et al.[32] and Baron et al.[33] question the value of dipyridamole—thallium stress testing in these circumstances. Poldermans et al.[19] studied 430 patients undergoing major vascular surgery who had known or suspected CAD and correlated the results of the dobutamine-atropine stress echocardiography and clinical data in predicting cardiac events in patients undergoing major vascular surgery.[19] Patients without clinical risk factors (angina, diabetes, Q-waves on the ECG, symptomatic ventricular tacharrythmias, and age > 70 years) were at low risk. Patients with more than one clinical variable and a positive test defined a high-risk group with increased cardiac events. Clinical information also increased the predictive value of the dipyridamole-thallium test.[6,21] It is therefore recommended that all patients undergoing major vascular surgery with at least one of the above clinical variables and unable to exercise have a pharmacologic stress test. The choice of the test (dobutamine echocardiography or dipyridamole thallium) should depend on the local availability and expertise.

Quantification of Cardiac Risk Using Clinical Criteria

Goldman Index

The Goldman index of cardiac risk assessment remains the most useful instrument to assess cardiac risk in a multivariate model, primarily because of its ease of use and relative weighting of risk factors[14] (Table 29-1). Goldman studied 1001 patients older than 40 years of age to determine which preoperative risk factors predicted the development of cardiac complications in patients undergoing major noncardiac surgery. By multivariate analysis, nine independent correlates of fatal and nonfatal cardiac complications were identified and weighted:

Table 29-2. Rates of Death and Major Complications According to Goldman Multifactorial Cardiac Risk Index

Reference	Type of Patient	Class I			Class II			Class III			Class IV		
		Events	Pts	%	Events	Pts	%	Events	Pts	%	Events	Pts	%
Goldman et al. (1977)[5]	>40 years	5	537	1	21	316	7	18	130	14	14	18	78
Zeldin (1984)[22]	>40 years	4	590	1	13	453	3	11	74	15	7	23	30
Detsky et al. (1986)[15]	Preoperative consults	8	134	6	6	85	7	9	45	20	4	4	100
Pooled data		17	1261	1.3	40	854	4.7	38	249	15.3	25	45	56

1. a third heart sound or jugular venous distention,
2. MI in the preceding 6 months,
3. more than five premature ventricular contractions per minute documented any time before operation,
4. rhythm other than sinus or presence of premature atrial contractions on ECG,
5. emergency surgery,
6. age over 70 years,
7. intraperitoneal intrathoracic or aortic operation,
8. important valvular aortic stenosis, and
9. poor general medical condition.

The pooled performance of the index in three studies using modification of the Goldman index demonstrated death and major complication rate of 1.3% in Class I patients, 4.7% in Class II, 15.2% in Class III, and 56% in Class IV (Table 29-2).

However, the Goldman index has limitations. First, it was developed from a data set in the mid-1970s and, hence, does not reflect the modern practices of anesthesia, medicine, or surgery. Second, it may not fairly represent the pretest probabilities of events from other institutions, other surgical teams at the same institution, or specific surgical procedures. Third, the level of risk for patients in Class IV is higher than has been found at most institutions (for which a 30% complication rate is more representative[22]). Fourth, the data set included relatively few vascular surgical patients.[21] Finally, although this index is useful in predicting risk, its sensitivity is relatively low, and important CAD may be missed, especially in elderly patients. Nevertheless, the index is a measure that can be combined with other factors such as the nature of the surgical procedure, the extent to which risk factors reversible, and the benefits of the proposed surgery.

One of the most important roles of the Goldman index has been to alert physicians of the major risk factors for noncardiac surgery. This information has probably led to significant reductions in risk through identification of risk factors, aggressive interventions to correct them, and closer perioperative monitoring.

Detsky Score

Detsky et al.[15] found that the Goldman index did not perform as well in a validation set at another institution. In addition they modified the index by adding factors such as the Canadian Cardiovascular Society angina (Class III or IV), unstable angina, and the presence of recent or remote pulmonary edema. Table 29-2 displays the results compared to the Goldman score.

Eagle Score

The clinical criteria cited by Eagle et al.[20] are probably the most effective clinical tool for evaluation of cardiac risk in patients undergoing vascular surgery. This was previously discussed in the section on peripheral vascular disease.

NONINVASIVE TESTING FOR EVALUATION OF PERIOPERATIVE CARDIAC RISK

Exercise Testing

Exercise Electrocardiogram

The exercise ECG is widely used for the diagnosis of CAD and assessment of prognosis. The accuracy of the exercise ECG varies widely among studies, but pooled data demonstrate a sensitivity of 71% and a specificity of 73%.[23] The variation can be attributed to differences in disease severity, testing protocols, criteria for a positive test, and definitions of significant CAD. The exercise ECG is an acceptable test if the resting ECG (ST-T waves) is normal. Patients who are able to exercise less than 3 minutes should be considered to be at high risk.[24]

Myocardial Perfusion Imaging

The diagnostic and prognostic implications of exercise testing using thallium scintigraphy have been discussed in details in other chapters. It has a higher sensitivity and specificity than routine exercise ECG testing.[25] Thallium imaging is much more expensive than routine exercise ECG testing, but it is an important alternative in patients with resting ECG abnormalities and high-risk patients. Unfortunately, the sensitivity of both exercise techniques is highly dependent on the performance of adequate exercise.

Pharmacologic Stress Testing

Most patients with peripheral vascular disease or undergoing other major noncardiac surgery are unable to exercise maximally. Because the reliability of the exercise ECG with or without imaging is dependent on the performance of maximal exercise, patients who cannot exercise must have pharmacologic stressors such as dobutamine or dipyridamole.

Dipyridamole Thallium Perfusion Imaging

The results of dipyridamole-thallium perfusion imaging for the prediction of cardiac events is discussed in detail in Chapter 30 by Younis. In the pooled data of several prominent series,[26-33] dipyridamole-thallium has a positive predictive value of 22%, and a negative predictive value of 94%. The high predictive value of a negative stress perfusion imaging study is consistent with a high sensitivity for CAD. Not only reversible but also fixed thallium defects are associated with this increased risk, due to the difficulty of distinguishing severe ischemia from scar using standard thallium protocols.

The studies of Marwick and Underwood,[30] Mangano et al.,[32] and Baron et al.[33] appear to contradict these results, but these findings most likely reflect the importance of population selection on the predictive value of a test. According to Bayes' theorem, the posttest probability of an event pertains to both the accuracy of the results, and the pretest probability of an event. If a patient at high probability of disease is studied using perfusion imaging, and the test is negative, the patient continues to have a high probability of disease. It is important, therefore, that these studies are used on patients at intermediate probability of events, rather than in all patients presenting prior to surgery.

Some perioperative cardiac events are unpredictable, irrespective of the accuracy of the test performed. The most common source of cardiac events in the absence of preoperative ischemia is MI, which occurs due to formation of a thrombus on a ruptured plaque, and in many instances the stenosis severity due to the plaque rupture is only mild. Stenoses of less than 50% diameter do not significantly limit maximal hyperemic flow, and consequently do not produce perfusion defects even using the most accurate techniques such as positron emission tomography (PET). Indeed, the use of PET is predictive of outcome, but remains limited by the occurrence of MI in the absence of significant ischemia, presumably reflecting minor stenoses.[42]

The predictive value of a positive test is much lower than that of a negative test. This reflects both the lower specificity of perfusion imaging (due to the introduction of false positives due to artifacts), together with the fact that the identification of a positive scan may indicate the presence of mild coronary disease, which is generally prognostically benign. Consequently, not every patient with a positive perfusion imaging result, even if it truly reflects coronary disease, will suffer a cardiac event. These results may be improved by taking account of the nature of the perfusion defect, especially its size, as discussed in Chapter 30.

Dobutamine Stress Echocardiography

As discussed in Chapter 4, the accuracy of stress echocardiography (in experienced hands) for the identification of CAD has been shown to be comparable to that of myocardial perfusion imaging. For diagnostic purposes, the sensitivity of stress echocardiography is probably somewhat lower than that of perfusion imaging, with most of the discrepancies being due to patients with single-vessel coronary disease. On the other hand, the specificity of stress echocardiography is higher than that of perfusion imaging, because artifacts are less frequent.

At least theoretically, these findings should translate to a slightly lower predictive value of a negative test, but a somewhat higher predictive value for a positive test, both because of fewer false positives and (paradoxically) because of the lower sensitivity for prognostically benign single-vessel coronary disease. The results of the existing studies using stress echocardiography for risk stratification in patients undergoing vascular surgery is discussed in Chapter 31. When pooled, the data show a positive predictive value of 45% and a negative predictive value of 98% for pharmacologic stress echocardiography.[34–39] However, it should be noted that the pooling of data for both perfusion imaging and stress echocardiography has important limitations, because patients were treated differently and showed a range of results. Nonetheless, individual studies support the conclusion that abnormal results of pharmacologic stress echocardiography in vascular surgery patients signify increased risks of serious cardiac events.

Dobutamine stress echocardiography may have some advantages over dipyridamole-thallium testing.[34] First, it measures both LVF and the potential for ischemia, the major determinants of cardiac risk. Second, dobutamine more closely mimics the physiology of perioperative stress than dipyridamole. Additionally, it can detect unsuspected or underappreciated valvular disease. However, ischemic changes at stress echocardiography are less quantifiable and probably more dependent on operator interpretation and experience than are the changes seen at perfusion imaging. Few data are available to compare the predictive values of scintigraphy and stress echocardiography in the same patients, but on the basis of diagnostic comparisons, these choices should be made according to local experience and availability. A summary of available stress tests and costs is given in Table 29-3.

APPROACH TO PATIENTS WITH CAD

In the previous section of this chapter, we discussed individual and grouped clinical criteria that can be used to risk stratify patients prior to surgery. Once the risk is defined, the clinician must decide whether further investigation and/or interventions are indicated. To justify the expense and risk of interventions, there must be evidence that the risk is increased and that intervention (i.e., revascularization) substantially decreases the risk of an event. The presence of CAD alone does not necessarily increase risk or justify intervention. Clinical factors remain the most important part of risk stratification (Table 29-4).

A group of negligible to low-risk patients for adverse cardiac events can be identified by the history, physical examination, and ECG (the latter being of value in men > 45 years and women > 55 years). Low-risk patients have no history of previous CAD and no symptoms of angina. In these patients, the cardiac risk is low and no further investigation is indicated.

Another group of patients can be identified who have either CAD or high probability of CAD but in whom the probability of perioperative cardiac complications is low. While this group has a slightly higher risk than the low-risk patients, the absolute risk of cardiac events is extremely low. Patients undergoing nonvascular procedures with mild chronic stable angina,[5,9] ECG criteria of an old MI,[9] or history of previous coronary revascularization (CABG or percutaneous transluminal coronary angioplasty [PTCA]) with no current symptoms,[9] or

Table 29-3. Costs of Stress Tests

Test	Inducible Ischemia	Charges (in $)
Exercise test		
Treadmill	ST Depression	405
Stress thallium	Redistribution	2,105
Stress echocardiography	New wall motion abnormality	1,303
Pharmacologic stress tests		
Dipyridamole thallium	Redistribution	2,362
Dobutamine echocardiography	New wall motion abnormality	1,303

Table 29-4. Guidelines for Cardiac Testing Prior to Major Noncardiac Surgery

Category	Risk for Cardiac Complications	Guidelines
No known CAD		
Men <45 years, women <55 years	Negligible	No further testing
Men >45 years, women >55 years	Negligible	Resting ECG
Known CAD		
MI <6 months ago	High	Postpone surgery if possible; stress test; cardiac catheterization if positive
MI >6 months ago; now asymptomatic	Low	Resting ECG
Unstable angina	High	Postpone surgery if possible; cardiac catherization
Stable angina (moderate high exercise threshold)	Low	Resting ECG
History of revascularization (now asymptomatic)	Low	Resting ECG, stress test if patient has multiple risk factors
Vascular surgery patient		
No clinical variables[a]	Low	Resting ECG
>1 clinical variable	Medium/high	Stress test; cardiac catheterization if positive
Hypertension (BP >110 mgHg)	High	Lower BP prior to surgery
Multiple risk factors	High	Stress test—cardiac catheterization if positive

Abbreviations: CAD, coronary artery disease; ECG, electrocardiogram; MI, myocardial infarction; BP, blood pressure.
[a] Eagle criteria.

with peripheral vascular disease without Eagle criteria[20] (age > 70 years, angina, Q-waves, congestive heart failure, arrhythmias requiring treatment, diabetes requiring treatment) are included in this group. Although many of these patients have CAD, no further investigation may be needed because the cardiac event rate is still very low. Medical management of concurrent conditions such as angina, hypertension, and heart failure should be intensified prior to surgery.

The high-risk group includes patients with unstable angina, MI within 6 months, peripheral vascular disease with any of the clinical criteria listed above[10] and multiple risk factors. These patients have a high risk of perioperative cardiac complications and further evaluation is indicated.[9,16,29] The patient with unstable angina or a recent MI should probably be evaluated with coronary angiography prior to the planned intervention. If the multiple risk factor or vascular surgery patient can exercise and has an abnormal resting ECG, an exercise ECG with echocardiography or scintigraphy should be performed. If the patient cannot exercise, a pharmacologic stress should be performed using dobutamine (echocardiography or scintigraphy) or dipyridamole (preferably with scintigraphy). If the test is normal, the patient may proceed with surgery after medical therapy has been optimized. Those with inducible ischemia should be considered for coronary angiography, depending on its extent and cardiac workload at onset.

The risk and benefit of preoperative coronary angiography and coronary revascularization have recently been studied in vascular surgery patients with a positive dipyridamole-thallium scan prior to surgery.[40] In this decision analysis, proceeding directly to vascular surgery led to lower morbidity and cost, and only if inoperable CAD was found and the surgery was canceled did the strategy of preoperative coronary angiography lead to better outcomes. The reason for this surprising finding seems to be that exposing the patient to the risk of three procedures (coronary angiography, coronary revascularization, and vascular surgery) leads to event rates that are close to that of proceeding directly to vascular surgery, but with greater costs. An alternative approach might be to reduce postoperative event rates by intensification of medical therapy.[41]

While there may be grounds to question the efficacy of preoperative revascularization for risk reduction, it is important to remember that late cardiac events are highly prevalent in patients with vascular disease. In a group of patients followed after elective aortic aneurysmectomy, the cardiac event rate at 8 years was 61% among those with suspected or overt coronary disease preoperatively, compared with 15% in those without disease.[29] Similarly, Younis has shown that patients with preoperative evidence of ischemia on thallium imaging have an event rate of about 50% over 2 years after vascular surgery if they do not undergo myocardial revascularization. More research is needed to explore the optimal selection and timing of revascularization in these patients.

Although controversy exists, revascularization should be performed prior to surgery if it is deemed essential on its own merits. If the coronary anatomy is unsuitable for revascularization or if the surgery is deemed urgent, medical therapy should be intensified and hemodynamic monitoring during surgery should be considered. It should be kept in mind that most patients undergoing surgery will do well, even high-risk patients.

FUTURE DIRECTIONS

Cardiac risk stratification and intervention to reduce risk are important problems that continue to be actively investigated. Future advancements in reducing cardiac complications of major surgery are likely to focus on correlation of clinical variables with testing tools, the utility of revascularization, and perioperative monitoring during surgery and pharmacologic intervention.

Since resources are limited, it is not possible to evaluate every patient with further noninvasive testing. Future studies need to focus on new noninvasive technologies to assess and quantitate risk. Although it is clear that patients with vascular disease and other multiple risk factors are at high risk, the advisability of prophylactic revascularization before surgery remains controversial. There are now available methodologies to intensify medical treatment before surgery. These include perioperative monitoring with continuous ECG monitoring, transesophageal echocardiography, and pulmonary artery catheterization. In addition, prophylactic use of nitroglycerine, β-blockers, and calcium antagonists to intensify ischemic medical treatment needs further study. It is unclear whether using these modalities can lessen cardiac risk in high-risk patients. A randomized study comparing prophylactic revascularization and intensive medical therapy should be completed. Until then, clinicians need to continue to use their best judgment in evaluating and managing high-risk patients.

REFERENCES

1. Massie BM, Mangano DT: Risk stratification for noncardiac surgery; how (and why)? Circulation 87:1752, 1993
2. Higgins TL: The changing profile of anesthetic practice: an update for internists. Cleve Clin J Med 60(3):219, 1993
3. Jones T, Isaacson JH: Preoperative screening. Cleve Clin J Med 62:374, 1995
4. Kannel WB, Abbott RD: Incidence and prognosis of unrecognized myocardial infarction: an update in the Framingham Study. N Engl J Med 311:1144, 1984
5. Goldman L, Caldera DL, Nussbaum SR et al.: Multifactorial index of cardiac risk of noncardiac surgical procedures. N Engl J Med 297:845, 1977
6. Freeman WK, Gibbons RJ, Shub C: Preoperative evaluation of the cardiac patient undergoing non-cardiac surgery. Mayo Clin Proc 64:1105, 1989
7. Goldman L, Caldera DL, Southwick FS et al.: Cardiac risk factors and complications in non-cardiac surgery. Medicine 57:357, 1978
8. Ashton CM, Petersen NH, Wray NP et al.: The incidence of perioperative myocardial infarction in men undergoing non-cardiac surgery. Ann Intern Med 118:504, 1993
9. Foster E, Davis K, Carpenter J et al.: Risk of noncardiac operation in patients with defined coronary artery surgery study. (CASS) Registry Experience. Ann Thorac Surg 41:42, 1986
10. Rao TLK, Jacobs KH, El-Etr AA: Reinfarction following anesthesia in patients with myocardial infarction. Anesthesiology 59:499, 1983
11. Shah KB, Kleinman BS, Rao TK et al.: Angina and other risk factors in patients with cardiac diseases undergoing non-cardiac operations. Anesth Analg 70:240, 1990
12. Eagle KA, Singer DE, Brewster DC et al.: Dipyridamole-thallium scanning in patients undergoing vascular surgery. JAMA 257:185, 1987
13. Tischler MD, Lee TH, Hirsch AT et al.: Prediction of major cardiac events after peripheral vascular surgery using dipyridamole echocardiography. Am J Cardiol 68:593, 1991
14. Goldman L, Caldera DL, Nussbaum SR et al.: Multifac-

torial index of cardiac risk of non-cardiac surgical procedures. N Engl J Med 297:845, 1977
15. Detsky AS, Abrams HB, McLaughlin JR et al.: Predicting cardiac complication in patients undergoing noncardiac surgery. J Gen Intern Med 1:211, 1986
16. O'Keefe JH Jr, Shub C, Rettke SR: Risk of non-cardiac surgical procedures in patients with aortic stenosis. Mayo Clin Proc 64:400, 1989
17. Prys-Roberts C: Anesthesia and hypertension. Br J Anesth 56:711, 1984
18. Goldman L, Caldera DL: Risks of general anesthesia and elective operation in the hypertensive patient. Anesth 50:285, 1979
19. Poldermans D, Arnese M, Fioretti P et al.: Improved cardiac risk stratification in major vascular surgery dobutamine atropine stress echocardiography. J Am Coll Cardiol 26:648, 1995
20. Eagle KA, Coley CM, Newell JB et al.: Combining clinical and thallium data optimizes preoperative assessment of cardiac risk before major vascular surgery. Ann Intern Med (11):859, 1989
21. Jeffrey CC, Kunsman J, Cullen DJ, Brewster DC: A prospective evaluation of the cardiac risk index. Anesthesiology 58:462, 1983
22. Zeldin RA: Assessing cardiac risk in patients who undergo non-cardiac surgical procedures. Can J Surg 27:402, 1984
23. Detrano R, Froelicher VF: Exercise testing: uses and limitations considering recent studies. Prog Cardio Dis 31:173, 1988
24. Mark DB, Shaw L, Harrel FE Jr: Prognostic importance of a clinical profile and exercise test in medially treated patients with coronary artery disease. J Am Coll Cardiol 325:849, 1991
25. Landenheim ML, Kotler TS, Pollock BH et al.: Incremental prognostic power of clinical history, exercise electrocardiography and myocardial perfusion scintigraphy in suspected coronary artery disease. Am J Cardiol 59:270, 1987
26. Hendel RD, Whitfield SS, Villegas BJ et al.: Prediction of late cardiac events by dipyridamole thallium imaging in patients undergoing elective vascular surgery. Am J Cardiol 79(15):1243, 1992
27. Cambria RP, Brewster DC, Abbott WM et al.: The impact of selective use of dipyridamole thallium scans and surgical factors on the current morbidity of aortic surgery. J Vasc Surg 15(1):43, 1992
28. Andrews TC, Goldman L, Creager MA et al.: Identification and treatment of myocardial ischemia in patients undergoing peripheral vascular surgery. J Vas Med Bill 5:8, 1994
29. Roger VL, Ballard DJ, Hallett JW et al.: Influence of coronary artery disease on morbidity and mortality after abdominal aortic aneurysmectomy: a population based study, 1971–1987. J Am Coll Cardiol 14:1245, 1989
30. Marwick TH, Underwood DA: Dipyridamole thallium may not be a reliable screening test for coronary artery disease in patients undergoing vascular surgery. Clin Cardiol 13(1):14, 1990
31. Lette J, Waters D, LaPointe J et al.: Usefulness of the severity and extent of reversible perfusion defects during thallium dipyridamole imaging for cardiac risk assessment before noncardiac surgery. Am J Cardiol 64(5):276, 1989
32. Mangano DR, Siliciano D, Hollenberg M et al.: Postoperative myocardial ischemia: therapeutic trials using intensive analgesia following surgery. Anesthesiology 76:342, 1992
33. Baron J, Mundler O, Bertyrand M et al.: Dipyridamole thallium scintigraphy and gated radionuclide angiography to assess cardiac risk before abdominal aortic surgery. N Engl J Med 330:663, 1994
34. Poldermans MD, Paolo M, Fioretti MD et al.: Dobutamine stress echocardiography for assessment of perioperative cardiac risk in patients undergoing major vascular surgery. Circulation 87:1506, 1993
35. Marwick TM, Vincent M, D'Ondt AM: Predictions of perioperative events. Circulation 86:I-790, 1992
36. Lane RT, Sawada SG, Segar DS et al.: Dobutamine stress echocardiography for assessment of cardiac risk before noncardiac surgery. Am J Cardiol 68:976, 1991
37. Lalka SG, Sawada SG, Dalsing MC et al.: Dobutamine stress echocardiography as a predictor of cardiac events associated with aortic surgery. J Vasc Surg 15: 831; discussion 841, 1992
38. Davila-Roman VG, Waggoner AD, Sicard GA et al.: Dobutamine stress echocardiography predicts surgical outcome in patients with an aortic aneurysm and peripheral vascular disease. J Am Coll Cardiol 21:957, 1993
39. Langan EM, Youkey JR, Franklin DP et al.: Dobutamine stress echocardiography for cardiac risk assessment before aortic surgery. J Vasc Surg 18:905; discussion 912, 1993
40. Mason JJ, Owens DK, Haris RA et al.: The role of coronary angiography and coronary revascularization before noncardiac vascular surgery. JAMA 273:1919, 1995
41. Andrews TC, Goldman L, Creager MA et al.: Identification and treatment of myocardial ischemia in patients undergoing peripheral vascular surgery. J Vas Med Bill 5:8, 1994
42. Marwick TH, Shan K, Go RT et al.: Use of positron emission tomography for prediction of peri-operative and late cardiac events prior to vascular surgery. Am Heart J 1995 130:1196, 1995

Chapter 30

Myocardial Perfusion Imaging in the Preoperative Evaluation of Vascular Patients

Liwa T. Younis and Henry G. Stratmann

IMPORTANCE OF CAD IN PATIENTS WITH VASCULAR DISEASE

As discussed in previous chapters, patients undergoing vascular surgery (carotid, peripheral, or aortic) have a significant risk of perioperative cardiac complications.[1-3] The incidence of nonfatal myocardial infarction or cardiac death during the perioperative period ranges from 4% to 19%,[2-7] and about half of all deaths are cardiac in origin. This increased cardiac risk is related to the frequent presence of concomitant significant coronary artery disease (CAD) in these patients. While many of these patients will also have clinical evidence of coronary disease, it is often present in asymptomatic patients. In a consecutive series of 1,000 patients being considered for vascular surgery who had coronary angiography, significant coronary disease (one or more lesions > 70%) was seen in 78% of those with clinically suspected disease, but was also present in 37% of those in whom it was unsuspected.[8] The prevalence of significant CAD was 57%, 65%, and 59% in patients with peripheral vascular, abdominal aortic aneurysm, and carotid artery disease, respectively (Fig. 30-1).

Thus, patients being considered for vascular surgery require a through preoperative assessment of their cardiac risk. The goal of this evaluation is to identify those who are at higher than average perioperative and postoperative risk. These patients are likely to benefit from specific risk-reduction management strategies to enhance the postoperative outcome and reduce the mortality and morbidity associated with concomitant CAD. As discussed in Chapter 29, such strategies might include preoperative coronary angiography and coronary revascularization, use of anti-ischemic medical therapy or intraoperative hemodynamic monitoring, modification of anesthesia type, performance of a lower-risk vascular procedure, or, in patients at particularly high risk, even deferral of any kind of surgery.

ASSESSMENT OF CARDIAC RISK USING MYOCARDIAL PERFUSION IMAGING

Myocardial perfusion imaging using thallium-201 or newer radiotracers such as technetium-99m-sestamibi or teboroxime can be used in combination with exercise or pharmacological stress testing to diagnose the presence of CAD.[9-12] Using either planar or tomographic imaging, these methods have been found to provide prognostic information regarding the risk of subsequent cardiac events in various subgroups of patients with known or suspected coronary disease, including those being evaluated for vascular surgery.[22,25-27] The presence of a reversible

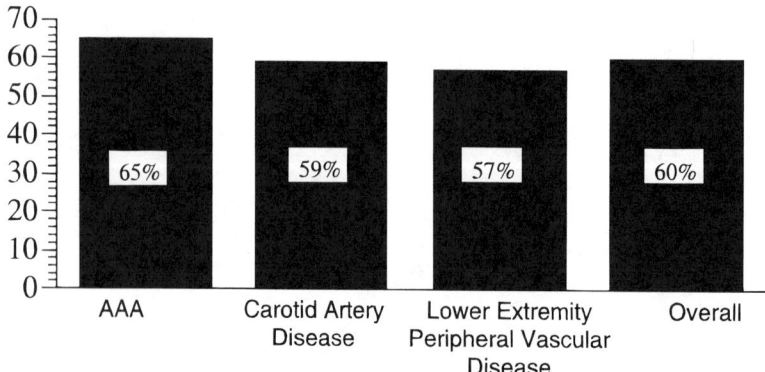

Fig. 30-1. Prevalence of significant coronary artery disease vascular patients. (From Hertzer et al.,[3] with permission.)

perfusion defect, consistent with the presence of myocardial ischemia, has generally been found to be an indicator of increased risk of postoperative cardiac mortality and morbidity.

Exercise Myocardial Perfusion Imaging

Little information is available concerning the combined use of exercise stress testing and myocardial perfusion imaging for preoperative assessment. McFalls et al.[7] studied 88 men with either treadmill or arm ergometry exercise and tomographic thallium-201 scintigraphy (stress and 3 to 4 hour delayed images) who subsequently underwent vascular surgery. An abnormal thallium-201 scan was seen in 75% of patients who had a perioperative cardiac event (nonfatal or fatal myocardial infarction), compared to 47% of those who had uneventful postoperative course ($p < 0.05$). However, in a multivariable analysis, the only independent predictors of complications were a history of angina pectoris and the presence of a fixed perfusion defect. A possible reason suggested for the latter finding was that some fixed perfusion defects may represent viable but severely ischemic myocardium rather than scar. This may be evident if thallium-201 reinjection techniques are used. The lack of increased risk associated with a reversible perfusion defect might reflect the low level of exercise achieved in these patients (average exercise time was only about 5 minutes), or possible changes in patient management by treating physicians based on knowledge of this result. Pending further studies using this method and confirmation of these findings, however, the value of exercise testing with thallium-201 for preoperative assessment prior to vascular surgery is uncertain.

Dipyridamole Stress Perfusion Imaging

A much larger number of studies (Table 30-1) have used myocardial perfusion imaging with intravenous or, rarely, oral dipyridamole testing for cardiac risk assessment prior to vascular surgery.[13-30] The imaging method and radioisotope most commonly employed in these studies has been planar thallium-201 scintigraphy. However, tomographic methods and other tracers, such as technetium-99m-sestamibi, have also been used.[23,24,31]

As discussed in the Chapter 13, intravenous infusion of low-dose dipyridamole usually produces little if any increase in myocardial oxygen demand, and its value for assessing the presence of CAD is based on its action as a potent coronary vasodilator. In patients with coronary artery lesions, dipyridamole causes a smaller increment in blood flow in vessels with mild to moderate stenosis than in those that are more normal; rarely, it may induce ischemia by a "steal" mechanism in an area of myocardium supplied by a vessel with a severe stenosis.[12] Ischemia is not necessary for the induction of a relative perfusion defect by dipyridamole.

Accuracy for Perioperative Risk Stratification

In one of the earliest reports using this method for preoperative cardiac risk assessment, Boucher et al.[16] described 48 patients tested with dipyrida-

Table 30-1. Prognostic Value of Dipyridamole Thallium-201 Myocardial Perfusion Imaging for Assessment of Perioperative Cardiac Risk

Reference	Patients (n)	Types of Surgery	Imaging Method	Cardiac Events	Significant Scintigraphic Predictors of Cardiac Events	Percent of Patients with Perioperative Cardiac Events	
						REV	No REV
McEnroe et al. (1990)[13]	95	AA	Planar	CD, MI, ISCH	REV, FIXED	26 (9/34)	11 (7/61)
Lette et al. (1991)[14]	125	AA, LE, C	Planar	CD, MI	REV	21 (13/62)	0 (0/63)
Eagle et al. (1989)[15]	200	AA, LE, C	Planar	CD, MI, UA, IPE	REV	30 (25/82)	4 (5/118)
Boucher et al. (1985)[16]	48	AA, LE	Planar	CD, MI UA	REV	50 (8/16)	0 (0/32)
Leppo et al. (1987)[17]	89	AA, LE	Planar	CD, MI	REV	33 (14/42)	2 (1/47)
Sachs et al. (1988)[19]	16	AA, LE, C	Planar	CD, UA	REV	21 (3/14)	0 (0/32)
Hendel et al. (1992)[20]	327	AA, LE, C	Planar	CD, MI	REV	14 (24/167)	—
Lane et al. (1989)[21]	101	AA, LE, C	Planar	CD, MI, UA, IPE	REV	14 (10/71)	3 (1/30)
Mangano et al. (1991)[22]	60	AA, LE	Planar	CD, MI, UA, CHF	NS	27 (6/22)	18 (7/38)
Marwick et al. (1990)[23]	86	AA, LE, C	SPECT	CD, MI, UA	NS	—	—
Baron et al. (1994)[24]	457	AA	SPECT	CD, MI, UA, CHF, VT	NS	19 (31/160)	—
Brewster et al. (1985)[25]	47	AA, LE	Planar	CD, MI, UA	REV	47 (7/15)	0 (0/32)
Cutler et al. (1987)[26]	116	AA	Planar	CD, MI	REV	—	—
McPhail et al. (1989)[27]	60	AA, LE	Planar	CD, MI, CHF	REV	61 (19/31)	10 (3/29)
Younis et al. (1990)[28]	111	AA, LE, C	Planar	CD, MI	REV, ABN	20 (6/46)	2 (2/85)
Makaroun et al. (1990)[29]	46	AA, LE	Planar	CD, MI	REV	25 (5/20)	4 (1/26)
Total numbers	2014					23 (180/782)	5 (27/593)

Abbreviations: AA, abdominal aortic surgery; LE, lower extremity vascular surgery; C, carotid surgery; CD, cardiac death; MI, myocardial infarction; UA, unstable angina; IPE, ischemic pulmonary edema; ISCH, electrocardiographic evidence of myocardial ischemia; CHF, congestive heart failure; VT, ventricular tachyarrhythmia; SPECT, single-photon emission computed tomography; REV, reversible perfusion defect; FIXED, fixed perfusion defect; ABN, abnormal study; NS, no significant scintigraphic predictors found; —, data not published.

mole–thallium-201 imaging prior to having vascular surgery. Eight (17%) of these patients had a perioperative cardiac event—unstable angina in five, nonfatal myocardial infarction in two, and death following an acute myocardial infarction in one. An abnormal planar thallium-201 scan was found to be associated with significantly increased incidence of these postoperative cardiac events ($p < 0.05$). However, the strongest predictor of a perioperative cardiac event was the presence of a reversible myocardial perfusion defect. This finding was present in all 8 of the patients who had a perioperative event, and in 8 of the 40 patients without an event ($p < 0.0001$). Conversely, an isolated fixed defect was not seen in any of the 8 patients with events, and was not associated with increased risk.

Subsequent reports have generally confirmed these findings (Table 30-1). In some of these later series, the patient population studied was limited to those having repair of abdominal aortic aneurysms, but most have also included those having other types of peripheral vascular procedures. Some investigators restricted their definition of a perioperative cardiac event to only nonfatal myocardial infarction or cardiac death, while others included "softer" events such as unstable angina or (presumably ischemic) pulmonary edema. Despite these differences, however, the results reported in these later studies have been reasonably consistent. A normal dipyridamole–thallium-201 study is associated with a high negative predictive value—being associated with a low incidence of perioperative cardiac events. Although several studies have found that a fixed perfusion defect, consistent with either myocardial scarring or severe ischemia, can be associated with increased perioperative risk,[13,30] most have not found this to be the case. Conversely, the presence of a reversible perfusion defect with planar thallium-201 imaging has generally been associated with increased perioperative risk.

Relation to Clinical Evaluation

In accordance with Bayes theorem, the benefit of testing is greatest among patients who have an intermediate probability of disease (or in this case, an event). Several studies have attempted to better define the prognostic value of dipyridamole-thallium-201 testing by correlating its results with clinical risk factors. Eagle et al.,[15] in a study of 200 patients having either aortic or peripheral vascular procedures, correlated a number of clinical risk factors with the results of a qualitative interpretation of planar thallium-201 images obtained with dipyridamole testing. They identified five such risk factors as having independent predictive value for increased perioperative cardiac risk: a Q-wave on the baseline echocardiogram, history of angina pectoris, age greater than 70 years, history of ventricular ectopic activity requiring treatment, and a history of diabetes mellitus requiring treatment. Perioperative cardiac events were defined in this study as unstable angina, pulmonary edema, acute myocardial infarction, or cardiac death. *In the 64 patients who did not have any of these clinical variables* ("low clinical risk"), only two (3.1%) had a perioperative cardiac event (nonfatal in both cases). In these patients, the results of dipyridamole–thallium-201 testing, including the presence of a reversible perfusion defect, did not add significantly to the risk stratification provided by these clinical variables. Conversely, cardiac events occurred in 10 (50%) of the 20 patients with *three or more of these clinical variables* ("high risk"). The event rate was 64% in these patients when a reversible perfusion defect was seen but, although less, remained high (33%) when this finding was absent. *Dipyridamole–thallium-201 testing was most useful for risk stratification in the remaining 116 patients at "intermediate" clinical risk* (one or two of these clinical variables). In these patients, the cardiac event rate was only 3.2% when a reversible perfusion defect was not seen, but was 29.6% when it was. The authors concluded that in patients at low or high clinical risk by this method, dipyridamole–thallium-201 would probably not contribute to clinical decision making regarding preoperative and perioperative management. However, for those in the intermediate risk group, the test can identify patients at higher risk who might benefit from more aggressive management, such as preoperative coronary angiography.

Influence of Extent of Ischemia

The intermediate prognostic significance of a positive test may be increased by considering the extent of ischemia. A report by Levinson et al.[18] analyzed 62 of the 200 patients described by Eagle, in relation to the extent of redistribution seen. Using a semiquantitative technique, they found that none of the 15 patients who had a reversible defect seen *in only one of the three standard planar views* (anterior, left anterior oblique, and lateral) had a perioperative cardiac event. Conversely, the presence of *reversible defects in greater than two views* or vascular distributions was associated with a perioperative ischemic event in 17 (36%) of the 47 patients with thallium-201 redistribution in greater than two views ($p < 0.005$).

Hendel et al.,[20] in a study of 327 patients having vascular surgery, found that a reversible thallium-201 perfusion defect was the most predictive of the clinical and imaging variables analyzed for the occurrence of a nonfatal myocardial infarction, conferring a nearly ninefold increase in relative risk. Thallium-201 redistribution was also associated with an over fourfold increase in relative risk for the occurrence of any kind of perioperative cardiac event, occurring in 14.4% of these patients but only 1% of those with a normal scan. Using a semiquantitative method for assessment of the extent of myocardium involved, patients *with reversible defects of "moderate size or larger"* were found to be at particularly higher risk. This finding increased the predicted incidence of a perioperative event from 8% to 20%.

Lette et al.[14] used both multivariable clinical models and quantitative dipyridamole–thallium-201 scintigraphy to examine their predictive value for perioperative myocardial infarction or cardiac death in 125 patients having vascular surgery. Although the clinical parameters studied were not useful in predicting postoperative outcome, none of the 63 patients who had normal thallium-201 images of fixed perfusion defects had a perioperative cardiac event. However, such events occurred in 13 (21%) of 62 patients with a reversible defect (sensitivity 100%, specificity 21%). Thallium-201 images were further analyzed using scoring systems based on the severity and extent of perfusion defects, including their degree of reversibility. Patients who had cardiac events were found to have significantly *more severe and extensive reversible perfusion defects* as determined by these scores than those without such events ($p < 0.0001$). *Transient left ventricular dilation* was also found to be a marker of increased risk, occurring in four (32%)

patients with cardiac events and four (4%) of those who did not ($p < 0.0001$).

Studies Presenting Negative Findings

Despite the identification of a reversible perfusion defect with dipyridamole–thallium-201 as a marker of increased perioperative risk in most reports, not all investigators have found this to be the case. Mangano et al.[22] studied 60 patients having vascular surgery in whom, unlike most other studies using dipyridamole–thallium-201, treating physicians were blinded to these test results. Perioperative cardiac events (defined in this study as cardiac death, nonfatal myocardial infarction, unstable angina, or congestive heart failure) occurred in 13 patients (22%). Only 6 of these 13 patients had reversible defects, and this finding was not found to be associated with significantly increased risk.

Other studies using tomographic thallium-201 imaging also failed to demonstrate increased cardiac risk in patients with a reversible perfusion defect.[23,24] Both studies limited image interpretation to qualitative, rather than quantitative techniques. In one series of 86 patients,[23] 10 had perioperative cardiac events. Seven of these events occurred, however, in 64 patients with normal scans, while only 3 patients with an abnormal study (fixed or reversible perfusion defect) had an event. Baron et al.[24] studied 457 patients undergoing elective abdominal aortic surgery, and reported postoperative complications in 86 (19%). In this study, several clinical variables, particularly age greater than 65 years, were found to be predictive of increased risk of a perioperative cardiac event. However, neither a reversible nor a fixed thallium-201 perfusion defect (present in 160 and 94 patients, respectively) were found to be predictors of increased risk.

Possible reasons for the lower association of a reversible thallium-201 perfusion defect with perioperative cardiac events in these studies (compared to earlier reports) might include differences in the techniques used in performing and interpreting the studies (i.e., planar vs. tomographic imaging, or qualitative vs. semiquantitative analysis), in patient selection—especially with respect to correlating results of myocardial imaging with clinical risk factors,[14,15] and changes in patient management made due to these findings. For example, tomographic imaging might detect smaller, more subtle reversible perfusion defects than planar studies, leading to a decrease in specificity for predicting perioperative cardiac events if quantitative methods for evaluating the extent and severity of the defect are not employed. The lack of association of a reversible perfusion defect with increased risk in patients at "low" risk by a clinical profile has already been cited.[15] As these studies involved risk stratification in unselected populations, it is probable that patient selection issues contributed to these negative findings. Finally, since physicians treating these patients were aware of the test results in all but two of these studies,[22,27] it is possible that changes in management based on these results (performance of coronary angiography and revascularization, changes in anti-ischemic medical therapy, increased use of intraoperative hemodynamic monitoring, and cancellation of surgery in patients deemed at "high" risk partly on the basis of scintigraphic findings) may also have decreased the "observed" value of dipyridamole–thallium-201 testing (Table 30-1).

Clinical Application for Prediction of Early Events

Despite these potential limitations, however, dipyridamole–thallium-201 imaging can be recommended as an appropriate means for performing cardiac risk-stratification in selected patients prior to vascular surgery. As previously described, criteria for determining which patients are most likely to benefit from this test have been suggested by Eagle et al.[15] based on the presence of specific clinical and electrocardiographic risk factors. Brown[32] suggested that in addition to those patients, the test should also be performed in patients without a cardiac history being considered for vascular procedures (abdominal aortic aneurysm repair and aortobifemoral bypass surgery), which, overall, have a higher risk of cardiac events. Wong et al.[1] also incorporated the criteria developed by Eagle et al.[15] and those based on the Goldman risk indices into a suggested method for risk stratification. All of these methods can be considered reasonable although, pending further study, not absolute guidelines for assessing cardiac risk.

Clinical Application for Prediction of Late Events

Besides their increased cardiac risk during the perioperative period, cardiovascular events are also the major cause of long-term morbidity and mortality in patients who survive vascular surgery. Several studies have evaluated the long-term prognostic value of dipyridamole–thallium-201 testing in such patients.[20,28,30] In one series, Younis et al.[28] reported on 131 patients with peripheral vascular disease who were evaluated using intravenous dipyridamole–thallium-201 testing. Peripheral vascular surgery was performed on 111. All patients were followed for an average duration of 18 ± 10 months. An abnormal thallium scan predicted an increased risk of cardiac death or myocardial infarction not only postoperatively (0% vs. 7%) but also during late follow up (0% vs. 6%). The presence of reversible or combined reversible and fixed thallium defect predicted twofold increases in the risk of cardiac events (Fig. 30-2).

In several other series,[28,30] the scintigraphic finding most strongly associated with increased risk for late cardiac events in patients who survived vascular surgery was the presence of a fixed perfusion defect. Hendel et al.[20] reported on 345 surgical survivors ($n = 312$) and nonsurgically treated patients ($n = 33$) who were followed for a mean period of 30.2 ± 18.3 months. Late cardiac events (myocardial infarction or death from a cardiac etiology) occurred in 53 patients (15.4%), with most of these events being fatal. The event rate was 18.5% for a reversible perfusion defect, 24% for a fixed defect, and 4.9% for a normal study. In a multivariable model, a fixed defect, particularly one of moderate size or greater, was the best predictor of a late cardiac event and increased its relative risk nearly fivefold. This finding was also associated with significantly decreased event-free survival compared to patients without a fixed defect ($p < 0.0001$). The authors concluded that while a reversible defect may better predict occurrence of perioperative cardiac events, occurrence of late events is better predicted by fixed perfusion defects.

Use of New Techniques for Risk Stratification

New Tracers

Other myocardial perfusion agents besides thallium-201, particularly technetium-99m-sestamibi and teboroxime, have been used with exercise or dipyridamole testing to diagnose the presence of CAD and predict risk of later cardiac events.[10,11,31a] However, to date, only limited experience has been reported with these newer agents for assessing perioperative cardiac risk with vascular surgery.[31] In 197 patients having elective vascular surgery after dipyridamole–technetium-99m sestambi tomography, a perioperative cardiac event (nonfatal myocardial infarction, cardiac death, or acute ischemic pulmonary edema) occurred in only 9. These perioperative events were not predicted by either clinical criteria or the results of myocardial perfusion imaging. Conversely, technetium-99m sestamibi tomography did provide prognostic information regarding late cardiac events. Over a mean follow-up period of 21 ± 14 months after testing, cardiac death or nonfatal myocardial infarction occurred in 26 of 172 (15%) medically treated patients who survived vascular surgery without a cardiac or fatal noncardiac event. These cardiac events occurred in 3 of 82 patients with normal technetium-99m-sestamibi studies (4%), compared to 23 of 90 (26%) with abnormal scans ($p < 0.0001$) and 13 of 39 (33%) with reversible defects ($p < 0.001$). Survival without a cardiac event was significantly decreased in patients who had any type of perfusion abnormality compared to those with normal studies (Fig. 30-3). Thus, although the prognostic value of this test for perioperative cardiac events was limited, dipyridamole–technetium-99m-sestam-

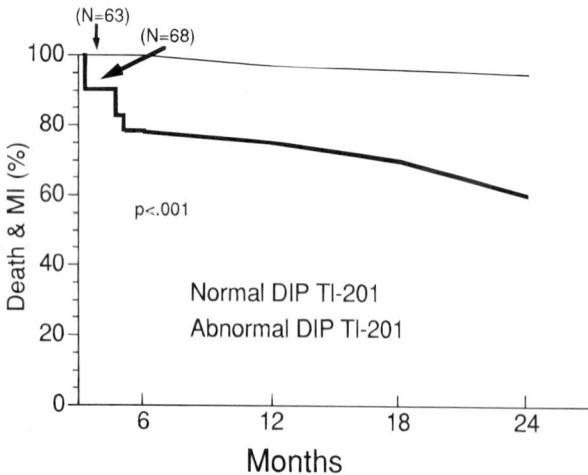

Fig. 30-2. Postoperative long-term cardiac events in patients with peripheral vascular disease stratified by dipyridamole–thallium-201 myocardial perfusion scintigraphy. (From Younis et al.,[28] with permission.)

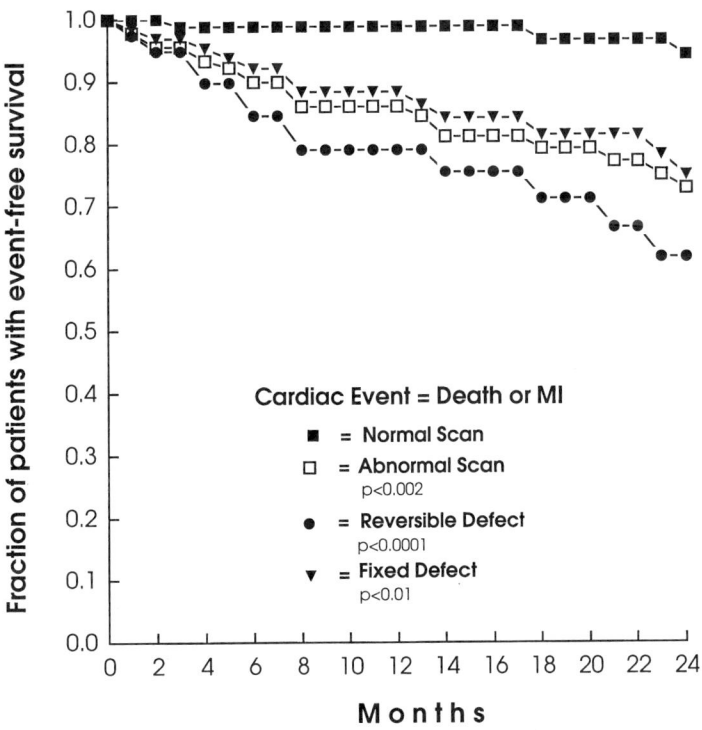

Fig. 30-3. Postoperative late cardiac events in patients with peripheral vascular disease stratified by dipyridamole–technetium-99m-sestamibi scintigraphy. (From Stratmann et al.,[31] with permission.)

ibi imaging was able to identify patients at increased risk of late cardiac events.

New Stressors

As discussed in a previous chapter, adenosine is a potent coronary vasodilator, which can be combined with thallium-201 for diagnosing the presence of CAD. One report[33] evaluated its value for cardiac risk stratification in 60 patients having noncardiac surgery (including 25 vascular procedures), 7 of whom subsequently had perioperative cardiac events. A thallium-201 study with both reversible and fixed perfusion defects was found to be an independent predictor of increased risk. Because most patients in this study underwent nonvascular surgery, however, the applicability of these findings to patients specifically having vascular procedures is uncertain.

Dobutamine induces ischemia by increasing myocardial oxygen demand, and the diagnosis of coronary disease may be made by recognition of a reversible thallium-201 perfusion defect, or a new or worsened segmental wall motion abnormality with two-dimensional echocardiography. A number of studies have evaluated the use of dobutamine testing prior to elective vascular surgery in combination with two-dimensional echocardiography. If myocardial perfusion imaging is desired, and a coronary vasodilator cannot be used (e.g., due to asthma), dobutamine may be combined with thallium-201, although there is limited experience with this combination. Elliott et al.[34] studied 126 patients being prepared for vascular surgery, and reviewed both planar and tomographic thallium-201 images. Of the 109 patients who subsequently underwent vascular reconstruction, 54 (43%) had a *normal thallium-201 study*, and only 1 (2%) had a postoperative cardiac event (nonfatal myocardial infarction). A *fixed perfusion defect*, present in 28 of these patients, was also not associated with significantly increased cardiac risk (event rate 11%). Of the 42 patients of the original group of 126 who had *reversible perfusion defects*, 15 were denied vascular surgery due to a perception of increased cardiac risk, and 9 had subsequent preoperative coronary revascularization, and later underwent vascular reconstruction without a perioperative cardiac event. In the remaining 18 patients with a reversible defect, a postoperative cardiac event occurred in 9 (50%, $p < 0.0001$), including death or nonfatal myocardial infarction in 5. Thus, as with dipyridamole testing, the presence of a reversible perfusion defect with dobutamine thallium-201 testing may identify patients at increased perioperative risk. However, more studies using this method are needed to confirm this finding.

Atrial Pacing Stress

Limited experience has been reported using atrial pacing to induce ischemia, detected using thallium-201 myocardial perfusion imaging for preoperative risk assessment. In a report on 61 patients considered to be at "low" clinical risk studied prior to proposed vascular surgery,[35] atrial pacing produced ischemic (> 1 mm) ST depression in 18 (38%), a fixed thallium-201 perfusion defect was seen in 11 (23%), and a reversible defect in 6 (13%) of the 47 patients who subsequently had an elective vascular procedure. None of these 47 patients had a perioperative cardiac event. In the 14 patients in whom vascular surgery was not done, 6 (43%) had a reversible perfusion defect, and one of these latter patients died suddenly shortly after testing. Six of the total of 12 patients who had reversible perfusion defects underwent subsequent coronary angiography, and all had significant CAD. It was concluded that in patients considered to be at low cardiac risk by clinical criteria, a normal thallium-201 study with atrial pacing or one associated with a fixed perfusion defect confirms this assessment. However, because neither pacing-induced ischemic ST depression nor a reversible perfusion defect was definitely associated with increased perioperative risk, the value of this test for risk stratification in such patients was limited.

ALTERNATIVES AND ADJUNCTS TO MYOCARDIAL PERFUSION IMAGING FOR PERIOPERATIVE RISK STRATIFICATION

Clinical Risk Assessment

As discussed in the previous chapter, initial cardiac risk stratification of patients can be achieved using standard clinical risk indices.[36] The value of the Goldman risk index has been validated by Zelden and Math.[37] The lack of certain cardiac risk factors such as history of angina pectoris or congestive heart failure and the relative complexity of the scoring system led Detsky et al.[38] to develop a modified version of this index. However, while these indices have been found to be useful in the general population of patients having noncardiac surgery, their value is more limited in patients being considered specifically for vascular procedures, which were not well represented in original studies of these scores.[36,37] When the applicability of the original and modified Goldman multifactorial indices was assessed specifically in vascular surgery patients (Table 30-2), they were found to apply fairly well for patients identified as being at moderate to high risk (Classes III and IV). However, in those assessed as being at lower risk (Classes I and III), these indeces underestimated the risk of perioperative cardiac events.1,2,13–15 In one report,[13] a serious cardiac complication (nonfatal myocardial infarction or cardiac-related death) occurred in 7 out of 90 (8%) patients in Goldman Class I and 4 of 26 (15%) in Class II, whereas the "expected" risks for each class were only 1% and 7%, respectively. Likewise, the modified multifactorial index, which includes a history of limiting angina pectoris as one of its risk factors (unlike the original Goldman index), may also underestimate risk in patients without angina due to exercise limitations related to their peripheral vascular disease (e.g., lower extremity amputations, or development of claudication at low levels of exercise).[1]

In summary, clinical risk indices are very useful tools to assess the postoperative cardiac risk in the

Table 30-2. Estimate or Probability of Cardiac Complications Based on Goldman Multifactorial Cardiac Risk Index (%) in Patients Undergoing General versus Aortic Abdominal Surgery

Procedure Points	Class I (<5)	Class II (6–12)	Class III (12–25)	Class IV (>26)	Overall
Major noncardiac	1	4	12	48	4
Abdominal aortic aneurysm	3	10	30	75	10

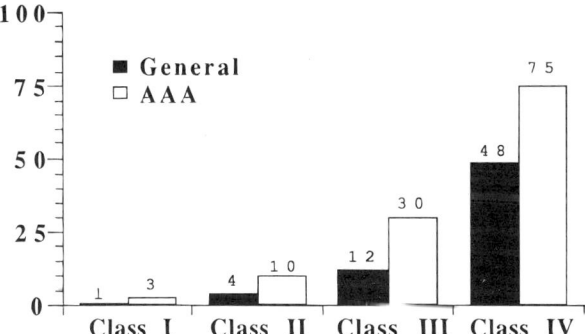

Fig. 30-4. Incidence of postoperative cardiac death in vascular and non vascular surgery patients stratified by Goldman cardiac risk index. (From Goldman,[59] with permission.)

general population. As discussed in more detail in Chapter 29, the predictive accuracy of these indices is limited in vascular patients (Fig. 30-4). The most useful index for this purpose appears to be the Eagle score, the role of which in combination with myocardial perfusion imaging has been discussed.

Coronary Angiography

Because of the high prevalence of significant CAD and attendant risk of preoperative cardiac complications in this population, it has been suggested that coronary angiography should be performed routinely in all patients being considered for vascular surgery.[8,39] Such an approach, however, has serious disadvantages. The procedure is associated with a small but significant risk of serious morbidity and mortality, is costly, and very resource intensive, and does not provide direct information concerning the physiological significance of any coronary lesions identified. Indeed, most patients will not require the procedure, either due to the absence of significant coronary disease or, as reflected in the previously cited event rates, the absence of serious perioperative complications even in those who do have disease.

Exercise Testing

The use of exercise electrocardiogram (ECG) testing for the diagnosis and prognostic evaluation of coronary disease has been discussed in Chapters 1 and 25. In patients with significant lower extremity limitations, arm ergometry may be more feasible than treadmill or bicycle stress. Although it has the advantage of being relatively simple to perform, and the equipment for performing testing is widely available, the workloads obtainable with arm exercise are less than those for those for conventional approaches. Carliner et al.[40] prospectively studied a series of 200 patients scheduled for major noncardiac surgery, 34% of whom were undergoing vascular surgery, and 22% of whom performed arm exercise. Results associated with increased risk were development of ischemic ST depression greater than 1 mm and inability to achieve at least 5 METs. However, the increased risk associated with these factors was not found to be statistically significant, and in a multivariable analysis the only independent predictor of increased risk was an abnormal preoperative 12-lead ECG.

Other studies have examined the potential role of exercise testing specifically in patients being considered for vascular surgery.[7,41–44] Cutler et al.[41] studied 130 patients using either treadmill or arm ergometry exercise, and classified them into four groups based on development of ischemic ST depression and ability to achieve at least 75% of age-predicted maximal heart rate (PMHR) (Table 30-3). A total of 21 patients had a perioperative cardiac event (congestive heart failure, transient ischemia, nonfatal, or fatal myocardial infarction). Of the 45 patients in the *"nondiagnostic"* category (no ischemic electrocardiographic response, but unable to reach 75% PMHR), one had a fatal myocardial infarction and five had perioperative "ischemia." Conversely, the 25 patients at *"high risk"* (ischemic ST depression

Table 30-3. Predictive Value of Preoperative Exercise Test Variables in Vascular Surgery Patients

Predictor	Cardiac Event Rate
≥75% MHR	0
≥75% MHR + ischemia	25
<75% MHR + ischemia	35 + 10 Cardiac Death
≥5 METs	≤1
≤5 METs	8
Exercise duration <2 min	30

Abbreviations: MHR, maximal heart rate.

during exercise testing and unable to reach 75% PMHR) had 10 cardiac complications, including 7 myocardial infarctions, 2 of which were fatal. None of the 35 patients at *"low"* risk (no ischemic ST response and able to achieve 75% PMHR) had a cardiac event, while 6 of the 23 at *"moderate"* risk (ischemic ST response but able to achieve 75% PMHR) had cardiac complications, although none was fatal and only one patient had a myocardial infarction. Based on these data, the authors concluded that exercise stress testing might be useful for risk stratification.

McPhail et al.[42] studied 100 patients using similar exercise testing methods. Perioperative complications (myocardial infarction, congestive heart failure, malignant ventricular arrhythmias, and cardiac death) occurred in 19 patients. The complication rate was 24% in patients who were unable to achieve 85% of PMHR, but only 6% in those able to do so ($p < 0.04$). While the presence and degree of ischemic ST depression were not, in itself, found to be predictors of increased risk, patients with this finding who were *unable to achieve 85% of PMHR* had a cardiac complication rate of 33%, while those who did reach that heart rate had no complications ($p < 0.05$).

In another series of 105 patients,[43] a perioperative cardiac event (arrhythmias, transient ischemic electrocardiographic changes, nonfatal cardiac arrest, and myocardial infarction) was reported to occur in 18 of 26 patients (69%) with exercise-induced *ischemic ST depression*, compared to 13 of 79 (16%) without such changes. However, only 4 of these patients had serious complications (nonfatal cardiac arrest or myocardial infarction), and no information was provided relating these particular events to the results of stress testing (Table 30-4). In a smaller ($n = 39$) series of patients,[45] only 2 of 23 patients (9%) without ischemic ST depression during exercise testing had perioperative cardiac complications, compared to 13 of 16 patients (81%) with ischemic ST depression. However, only 1 of these 13 patients had a fatal cardiac event, while the remainder had relatively minor complications (transient intraoperative ischemia or "severe" ventricular ectopy). In neither of these reports was information given relating overall cardiac events to the heart rate or level of exercise achieved.

Table 30-4. Comparison between Clinical Cardiac Risk Indices Used in Preoperative Assessment of Vascular Patients

	Goldman	Detsky	Eagle
Age >70	Yes	Yes	Yes
Congestive heart failure	Yes	Yes	Yes
Angina	No	Yes	Yes
Old myocardial infarction	Yes	Yes	Yes
Emergent surgery	Yes	Yes	No
Ventricular arrhythmia	Yes	Yes	Yes
Noninvasive test	No	No	Yes

In summary, the value of exercise testing for preoperative cardiac risk stratification in patients being considered for vascular surgery is uncertain, due to the limited number of patients reported, inconsistent results regarding the independent predictive value of ischemic ST depression as a marker of increased risk, variations in the testing methods used, and the inclusion in some studies of relatively minor perioperative cardiac events (such as ventricular arrhythmias) as a "complication." Achievement of 85% of PMHR, particularly in the absence of ischemic ST depression, may identify patients at lower risk[41,42] (Table 30-4). However, most patients studied were unable to reach this level of exercise, perhaps at least partly because of noncardiac limitations (e.g., development of intermittent claudication or limited ability to perform arm exercise). Thus, based on current information, exercise stress testing appears to be of limited value for preoperative evaluation of patients requiring vascular surgery.

Stress Echocardiography

Resting two-dimensional echocardiography is commonly used to assess left ventricular function prior to vascular surgery in patients with known or suspected coronary disease. The prognostic usefulness of this approach was evaluated by Takase et al.[46] who studied 53 consecutive patients that had major surgery and underwent clinical, intravenous dipyridamole–thallium-201 myocardial perfusion study, and echocardiographic left ventricular function assessment. Four patients died or had postoperative myocardial infarction while nine patients developed unstable angina or pulmonary edema. Myocardial perfusion imaging was predictive of ischemic events (cardiac death or myocardial infarction), while left ventricular dysfunction was predictive of perioperative pulmonary edema.

The inability of the majority of vascular patients to perform adequate levels of exercise has lead to the widespread use of pharmacological stress echocardiographic as well as nuclear imaging. Just as the diagnostic accuracy of both techniques appears to be comparable,[47,48] the techniques appear to be similar for prognostic purposes, as discussed in Chapter 31.[49-54] The choice of the noninvasive test used to assess the postoperative risk should probably be based on the clinical expertise, availability, and cost of each of these procedures.

PREOPERATIVE INTERVENTION AND POSTOPERATIVE OUTCOME
Myocardial Revascularization

In patients who are found to have CAD by angiography, performance of coronary revascularization primarily to reduce perioperative risk during subsequent vascular surgery may not confer a net decrease in risk. Overall, patients with prior coronary artery bypass surgery have a lower mortality rate during vascular surgery (1.5%) than those with only suspected (and therefore not revascularized) CAD (6.8%).[2,3] However, in those with significant coronary disease who have not yet had the procedure, the protective effects of coronary artery bypass surgery must be balanced with its risks. The average operative mortality for the procedure in patients with peripheral vascular disease has been reported to be approximately 5%, and increases with advancing age to as high as 16.7% in octogenarians.[2,3] Based on these data, the combined cardiac risk of preoperative coronary bypass surgery and the vascular surgery itself may be greater in some patients than performing the latter without preoperative coronary revascularization.

Preoperative coronary revascularization to reduce cardiac risk during subsequent vascular reconstructive procedures would be most beneficial in patients who have other major indications for the procedure, such as left main CAD, angina pectoris refractory to medical therapy, or triple-vessel CAD with left ventricular dysfunction. In patients without such indications, the protective effect of preoperative coronary revascularization remains controversial. Only limited experience has been reported regarding the use of preoperative coronary angioplasty to reduce cardiac risk during vascular surgery, and its role for the purpose is also uncertain.[2]

Based on all of these factors, patients not already identified as being at "high" risk of perioperative cardiac events by an initial clinical assessment may benefit most by using various noninvasive tests as the next level of evaluation. These tests include exercise, atrial pacing, and pharmacologic "stress" testing, with or without myocardial perfusion imaging or two-dimensional echocardiography, radionuclide ventriculography, and continuous ambulatory ECG monitoring. Patients considered to be at increased risk of perioperative cardiac events based on the results of these studies can then be referred for coronary angiography for further risk stratification.

The identification of high-risk patients is the first step in preoperative assessment, as most of these patients will eventually require intervention to improve their quality of life, prolong survival, or both. No randomized data are available to evaluate the impact of intervention on the outcome of vascular surgery, most likely due to ethical reasons that render the randomization process unacceptable. Few studies have addressed the intervention issue (medical or coronary revascularization) and its effect on reducing the postoperative cardiac events. Foster et al.[55] reported from the CASS registry that the risk of perioperative myocardial infarction and death associated with noncardiac surgery is essentially similar in patients without significant CAD as in patients who had undergone successful coronary revascularization. The risk is estimated to be (1%), which is lower than 2% to 3% risk in patients with CAD who did not undergo revascularization. The influence of preoperative coronary angioplasty was assessed in a recent study from the Mayo Clinic. Huber and colleagues[56] reported 50 patients referred for noncardiac surgery with severe CAD. All patients underwent preoperative coronary angioplasty. Postoperatively, the incidences of death and nonfatal myocardial infarction were 5.6% and 1.9%, respec-

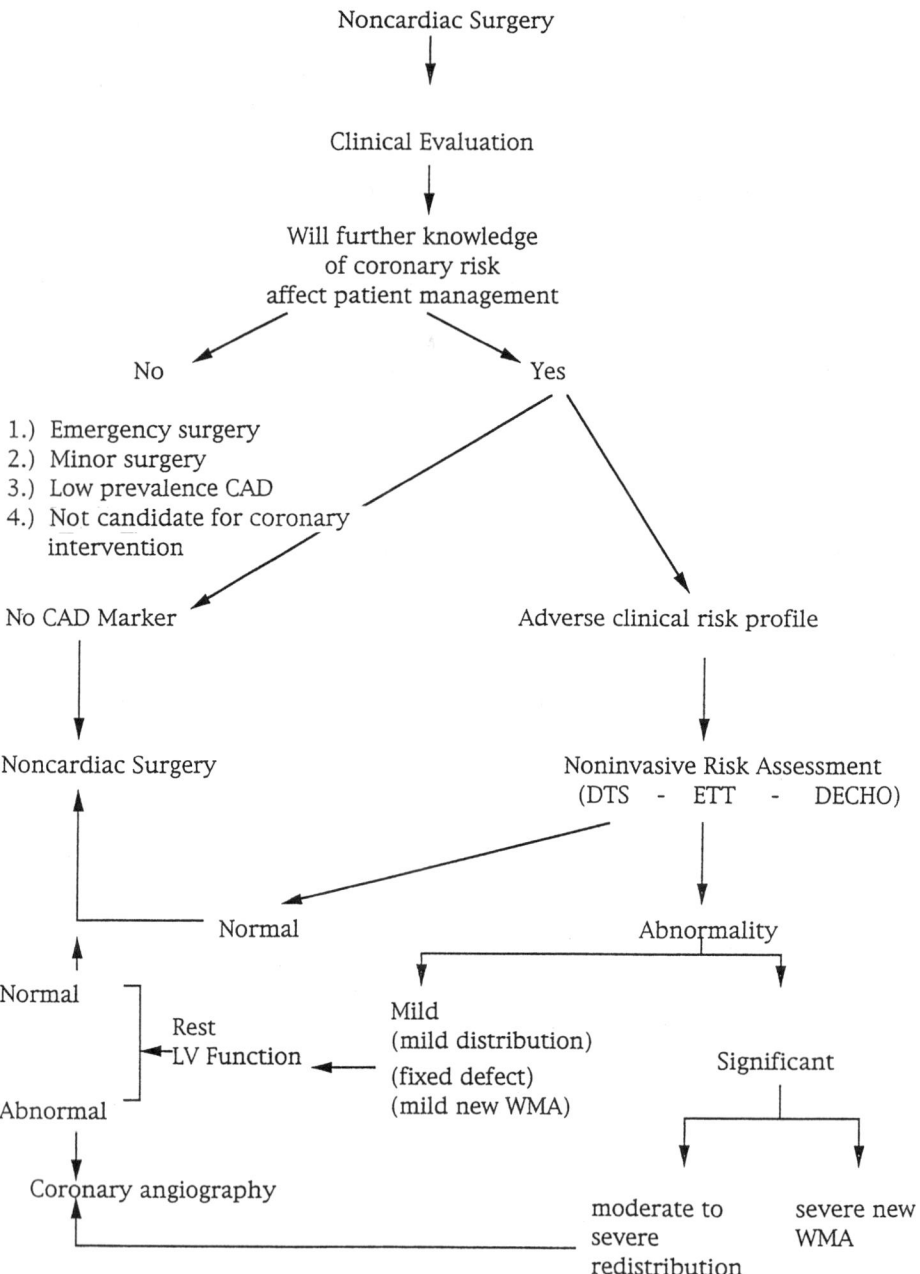

Fig. 30-5. Strategies for preoperative cardiac risk assessment. CAD, coronary artery disease; ETT, exercise test; DST, dipyridamole[201] T1 scintigraphy; DECO, dobutamine stress echocardiography. (From Younis et al.,[60] with permission.)

tively, suggesting a favorable outcome in these relatively high-risk patients.

Medical Therapy

Adjusting medical therapy in patients with coronary disease referred for vascular surgery is common, especially in patients with abnormal stress test results suggesting significant CAD or ischemia. Younis et al.[57] reported the impact of preoperative intervention based on clinical and scintigraphic evaluation in 72 patients who underwent noncardiac surgery and had an abnormal dipyridamole–thallium 201 myocardial perfusion study. Among 36 patients who had a cardiac intervention, 30 patients had adjustments in their antianginal medications, 6 patients had coronary angioplasty, and 14 patients had intraoperative hemodynamics monitoring. The risk modifications using this approach resulted in a significantly lower incidence of postoperative cardiac events (8% vs. 47% for any cardiac events, and 6% vs. 31% for death or myocardial infarction).[57] The use of medical therapy adjustment or indicated coronary revascularization appears to positively influence the postoperative outcome in vascular patients, although randomized trials are still needed to confirm the utility of these approaches.

Cost Effectiveness of Preoperative Cardiac Risk Assessment

The expanding use of vascular reconstructive surgery to include older and higher risk patients has led to an increase in the number evaluated for these interventions, and a subsequent increase in the number of cardiac procedures performed to screen and optimize the perioperative cardiac risk in these patients at an estimated cost of 3 to 4 billion dollars annually. Due to the lack of randomized trials to define the optimal preoperative risk assessment strategy, the cost-effectiveness of any of the procedures performed remains controversial at best. Eagle et al.[58] reported an analysis detailing five different strategies used in preoperative evaluations, and analyzed the cost of each strategy. The use of clinical risk markers followed by dipyridamole stress myocardial perfusion imaging in selected patients and coronary angiography in patients who have high-risk scan (multisegmental defect, moderate reversible defect, or large fixed defect in symptomatic patients) appeared to be the most cost-effective approach at a cost per year of life saved of less than $20,000. Despite the fact that this type of analysis based on retrospective data collection and hypothetical survival could be criticized, it clearly demonstrates the need for a large-scale study to prove its effectiveness in containing cost as well as improving postoperative outcome.

CONCLUSIONS

We demonstrated in this review the usefulness of clinical as well noninvasive cardiac evaluations in the risk stratification of patients evaluated for vascular surgery who have intermediate to high prevalence of significant CAD a priori. The judicious use of cardiac testing after comprehensive clinical evaluation can significantly reduce the postoperative cardiac events and enhance long-term survival (Fig. 30-5). The reduction in the incidence of postoperative cardiac events can substantially reduce the cost of postoperative care and probably justify the cost of this preoperative evaluation.

REFERENCES

1. Wong T, Detsky AS: Preoperative cardiac risk assessment for patients having peripheral vascular surgery. Ann Intern Med 116:743, 1992
2. Gersh BJ, Rihal CS, Rooke TW, Ballard DJ: Evaluation and management of patients with both peripheral vascular and coronary artery disease. J Am Coll Cardiol 18:203, 1991
3. Hertzer NR: Basic data concerning associated coronary disease in peripheral vascular patients. Ann Vasc Surg 1:616, 1987
4. Taylor LM, Jr., Yeager RA, Moneta GL et al: The incidence of perioperative myocardial infarction in general vascular surgery. J Vasc Surg 15:52, 1991
5. Pasternack PF, Grossi EA, Baumann FG et al: The value of silent myocardial ischemia monitoring in the prediction of perioperative myocardial infarction in patients undergoing peripheral vascular surgery. J Vasc Surg 10:617, 1989
6. McPhail NV, Ruddy TD, Calvin JE et al: Comparison of left ventricular function and myocardial perfusion

for evaluating perioperative cardiac risk of abdominal aortic surgery. Can J Surg 33:224, 1990
7. McFalls EO, Doliszny KM, Grund F et al: Angina and persistent exercise thallium defects: Independent risk factors in elective vascular surgery. J Am Coll Cardiol 21:1347, 1993
8. Hertzer NR, Beven EG, Young JR et al: Coronary artery disease in peripheral vascular patients. A classification of 1000 coronary angiograms and results of surgical management. Ann Surg 199:223, 1984
9. Kotler TS, Diamond GA: Exercise thallium-201 scintigraphy in the diagnosis and prognosis of coronary artery disease. Ann Intern Med 113:684, 1990
10. Berman DS, Kiat H, Maddahi J: The new 99mTc myocardial perfusion imaging agents: 99mTc-sestamibi and 99mTc-teboroxime. Circulation 84:17, 1991
11. Taillefer R: Technetium-99m sestamibi myocardial imaging: same-day rest-stress studies and dipyridamole. Am J Cardiol 66:80E, 1990
12. Stratmann HG, Kennedy HL: Evaluation of coronary artery disease in the patient unable to exercise: Alternatives to exercise stress testing. Am Heart J 117:1344, 1989
13. McEnroe CS, O'Donnell TF Jr, Yeager A et al: Comparison of ejection fraction and Goldman risk factor analysis to dipyridamole-thallium 201 studies in the evaluation of cardiac morbidity after aortic aneurysm surgery. J Vasc Surg 11:497, 1990
14. Lette J, Watters D, Lassonde J et al: Multivariate clinical models and quantitative dipyridamole-thallium imaging to predict cardiac morbidity and death after vascular reconstruction. J Vasc Surg 14:160, 1991
15. Eagle KA, Coley CM, Newell JB et al: Combining clinical and thallium data optimizes preoperative assessment of cardiac risk before major vascular surgery. Ann Intern Med 110:859, 1989
16. Boucher CA, Brewster DC, Darling RC et al: Determination of cardiac risk by dipyridamole-thallium imaging before peripheral vascular surgery. N Engl J Med 312:389, 1985
17. Leppo J, Plaja J, Gionet M et al: Noninvasive evaluation of cardiac risk before elective vascular surgery. J Am Coll Cardiol 9:269, 1987
18. Levinson JR, Boucher CA, Coley CM et al: Usefulness of semiquantitative analysis of dipyridamole-thallium-201 redistribution for improving risk stratification before vascular surgery. Am J Cardiol 66:406, 1990
19. Sachs RN, Tellier P, Larmignat P et al: Assessment by dipyridamole-thallium-201 myocardial scintigraphy of coronary risk before peripheral vascular surgery. Surgery 103:584, 1988
20. Hendel RC, Whitfield SS, Villegas BJ et al: Prediction of late cardiac events by dipyridamole thallium imaging in patients undergoing elective vascular surgery. Am J Cardiol 70:1243, 1992
21. Lane SE, Lewis SM, Pippin JJ et al: Predictive value of quantitative dipyridamole-thallium scintigraphy in assessing cardiovascular risk after vascular surgery in diabetes mellitus. Am J Cardiol 64:1275, 1989
22. Mangano DT, London MJ, Tubau JF et al: Dipyridamole thallium-201 scintigraphy as a preoperative screening test. A reexamination of its predictive potential. Study of Perioperative Ischemia Research Group. Circulation 84:493, 1991
23. Marwick TH, Underwood DA: Dipyridamole thallium imaging may not be a reliable screening test for coronary artery disease in patients undergoing vascular surgery. Clin Cardiol 13:14, 1990
24. Baron JF, Mundler O, Bertrand M et al: Dipyridamole-thallium scintigraphy and gated radionuclide angiography to assess cardiac risk before abdominal aortic surgery. N Engl J Med 330:663, 1994
25. Brewster DC, Okada RD, Strauss HW et al: Selection of patients for preoperative coronary angiography: use of dipyridamole-stress-thallium myocardial imaging. J Vasc Surg 2:504, 1985
26. Cutler BS, Leppo JA: Dipyridamole thallium 201 scintigraphy to detect coronary artery disease before abdominal aortic surgery. J Vasc Surg 5:91, 1987
27. McPhail NV, Ruddy TD, Calvin JE et al: A comparison of dipyridamole-thallium imaging and exercise testing in the prediction of postoperative cardiac complications in patients requiring arterial reconstruction. J Vasc Surg 10:51, 1989
28. Younis LT, Aguirre F, Byers S et al: Perioperative and long-term prognostic value of intravenous dipyridamole thallium scintigraphy in patients with peripheral vascular disease. Am Heart J 119:1287, 1990
29. Makaroun MS, Shuman-Jackson N, Rippey A et al: Cardiac risk in vascular surgery. The oral dipyridamole-thallium stress test. Arch Surg 125:1610, 1990
30. L'Italien GJ, Cambria RP, Cutler BS et al: Comparative early and late cardiac morbidity among patients requiring different vascular surgery procedures. J Vasc Surg 21:935, 1995
31. Stratmann HG, Younis LT, Wittry MD et al: Dipyridamole technetium-99m sestamibi myocardial tomography in patients evaluated for elective vascular surgery: prognostic value for perioperative and late cardiac events. Am Heart J 131:923, 1996
31a. Stratmann HG, Williams GA, Wittry MD et al: Exercise technetium-99m sestamibi tomography for car-

diac risk stratification of patients with stable chest pain. Circulation 89:615, 1994
32. Brown KA: Prognostic value of thallium-201 myocardial perfusion imaging. A diagnostic tool comes of age. Circulation 83:363, 1991
33. Shaw L, Miller DD, Kong BA et al: Determination of perioperative cardiac risk by adenosine thallium-201 myocardial imaging. Am Heart J 124:861, 1992
34. Elliott BM, Robison JG, Zellner JL, Hendrix GH: Dobutamine-201Tl imaging. Assessing cardiac risks associated with vascular surgery. Circulation 84:III54, 1991
35. Stratmann HG, Mark AL, Walter KE, Williams GA: Preoperative evaluation of cardiac risk using atrial pacing and thallium-201 scintigraphy. J Vasc Surg 10:385, 1989
36. Goldman L, Caldera DL, Nussbaum SR et al: Multifactorial index of cardiac risk in noncardiac surgical procedures. N Engl J Med 297:845, 1977
37. Zeldin RA, Math B: Assessing cardiac risk in patients who undergo noncardiac surgical procedures. Can J Surg 27:402, 1984
38. Detsky AS, Abrams HB, McLaughlin JR et al: Predicting cardiac complications in patients undergoing noncardiac surgery. J Gen Intern Med 1:211, 1986
39. Hertzer NR, Young JR, Kramer JR et al: Routine coronary angiography prior to elective aortic reconstruction: results of selective myocardial revascularization in patients with peripheral vascular disease. Arch Surg 114:1336, 1979
40. Carliner NH, Fisher ML, Plotnick GD et al: Routine properative exercise testing in patients undergoing major noncardiac surgery. Am J Cardiol 56:51, 1985
41. Cutler BS, Wheeler HB, Paraskos JA, Cardullo PA: Applicability and interpretation of electrocardiographic stress testing in patients with peripheral vascular disease. Am J Surg 141:501, 1981
42. McPhail N, Calvin JE, Shariatmadar A et al: The use of preoperative exercise testing to predict cardiac complications after arterial reconstruction. J Vasc Surg 7:60, 1988
43. Von Knorring J, Lepantalo M: Prediction of perioperative cardiac complications by electrocardiographic monitoring during treadmill exercise testing before peripheral vascular surgery. Surgery 99:610, 1986
44. Arous EJ, Baum P, Cutler BS: The ischemic exercise test in patients with peripheral vascular disease: implications for management. Arch Surg 119:780, 1984
45. McCabe CJ, Reidy NC, Abbott WM et al: The value of electrocardiogram monitoring during treadmill testing for peripheral vascular disease. Surgery 89:183, 1981

46. Takase B, Younis LT, Byers SL et al: Comparative prognostic value of clinical risk indexes, resting two-dimensional echocardiography, and dipyridamole stress thallium-201 myocardial imaging for perioperative cardiac events in major nonvascular surgery patients. Am Heart J 126:1099, 1993
47. Marwick T, Willemart B, D'Hondt AM et al: Selection of the optimal nonexercise stress for the evaluation of ischemic regional myocardial dysfunction and malperfusion. Comparison of dobutamine and adenosine using echocardiography and 99mTc-MIBI single photon emission computed tomography. Circulation 87:345, 1993
48. Quinones MA, Verani MS, Haichin RM et al: Exercise echocardiography versus 201 Tl single-photon emission computed tomography in evaluation of coronary artery disease: Analysis of 292 patients. Circulation 85:1026, 1992
49. Poldermans D, Fioretti PM, Forster T et al: Dobutamine stress echocardiography for assessment of perioperative cardiac risk in patients undergoing major vascular surgery. Circulation 87:1506, 1993
50. Langan EM, Youkey JR, Franklin DP et al: Dobutamine stress echocardiography for cardiac risk assessment before aortic surgery. J Vasc Surg 18:905, 1993
51. Davila-Roman VG, Waggoner AD, Sicard GA et al: Dobutamine stress echocardiography predicts surgical outcome in patients with an aortic aneurysm and peripheral vascular disease. J Am Coll Cardiol 21:957, 1993
52. Eichelberger JP, Schwarz KQ, Black ER et al: Predictive value of dobutamine echocardiography just before noncardiac vascular surgery. Am J Cardiol 72:602, 1993
53. Lane RT, Sawada SG, Segar DS et al: Dobutamine stress echocardiography for assessment of cardiac risk before noncardiac surgery. Am J Cardiol 68:976, 1991
54. Afridi I, Quinones MA, Zoghbi WA, Cheirif J: Dobutamine stress echocardiography: sensitivity, specificity, and predictive value for future cardiac events. Am Heart J 127:1510, 1994
55. Foster ED, Davis KB, Carpenter JA et al: Risk of noncardiac operation in patients with defined coronary disease: the Coronary Artery Surgery Study (CASS) Registry experience. Ann Thorac Surg 41:42, 1986
56. Huber KC, Evans MA, Bresnahan JF et al: Outcome of noncardiac operations in patients with severe coronary artery disease successfully treated preoperatively with coronary angioplasty. Mayo Clin Proc 67:15, 1992
57. Younis L, Stratmann H, Takase B et al: Preoperative clinical assessment and dipyridamole thallium-201 scintigraphy for prediction and prevention of cardiac

events in patients having major noncardiovascular surgery and known or suspected coronary artery disease. Am J Cardiol 74:311, 1994
58. Eagle KA, Coley CM: Cost-effective use of dipyridamole-thallium imaging for cardiac risk stratification. Semin Vasc Surg 4:100, 1991
59. Goldman L: Assessment of the patient with known or suspected ischaemic heart disease for non-cardiac surgery. Br J Anaesth 61:38, 1988
60. Younis LT, Miller DD, Cuattman BR. Preoperative strategies to assess cardiac risk before noncardiac surgery. Clin Cardiol 18:447, 1995

Chapter 31

Pharmacologic Stress Echocardiography for Risk Stratification Prior to Vascular Surgery

Don Poldermans, Paolo M. Fioretti, and Ian R. Thomson

CLINICAL CONTEXT OF THE USE OF STRESS ECHOCARDIOGRAPHY FOR RISK STRATIFICATION

Magnitude of the Problem

The number of patients admitted to the hospital for noncardiac vascular disease is increasing in both Europe and North America. In the Netherlands in 1980, approximately 8,400 such patients were admitted, increasing to 18,000 in 1992. This increment is due largely to the aging of the population, with the number of Europeans over 60 years of age expected to increase by over 60% to 224 million by 2025.[1]

Many of these patients require surgery, with an associated 5% to 10% incidence of cardiac complications and a 1% to 2% mortality. Ideally, patients undergoing major surgery should emerge from the perioperative period intact and survive long enough to enjoy the benefits of successful surgery. However, the occurrence of serious perioperative and late cardiac complications frequently mars an otherwise excellent surgical result. Preoperative cardiac risk stratification defines the probability that individual patients will suffer a major cardiac event. By facilitating decision-making, precise risk assessment has the potential to improve outcome and reduce the cost of surgery.

As discussed in Chapter 29, patients scheduled for elective major noncardiac vascular surgery have a high incidence of underlying coronary artery disease (CAD) and are at especially high risk of both perioperative and late cardiac events.[2-6] Late cardiac events, among which myocardial infarction is the major cause of perioperative and late death, occur in 9% to 12% of survivors within 2 years of surgery.[7-10] Despite increases in the number of elderly patients and in the frequency of extensive comorbidity, the frequency of cardiac complications decreased from 13.6% to 5.6% during the 1980s.[6] One reason for improved perioperative outcome may be a greater recognition by attending physicians of the importance of underlying cardiac disease.

The increasing number of elderly patients with major noncardiac vascular disease and extensive comorbidity will impose an increasing financial burden on health care resources. In view of increasing cost restraints, efficient cardiac risk stratification is potentially very important.

Pathophysiology of Perioperative Cardiac Morbidity

Perioperative cardiac events are principally caused by myocardial ischemia due to CAD.[2] The mechanism of ischemia may derive from perioperative factors that either increase oxygen demand or reduce supply. Myocardial oxygen demand may be increased by tachycardia, hypertension, sympathomimetic drugs, interruption of β-blocker medication, and stress. Oxygen supply may be decreased by plaque rupture with thrombosis, hypotension, vasospasm, anemia, and hypoxemia.

The awareness of perioperative ischemic risk has, somewhat paradoxically, made the intraoperative period relatively low risk compared to the postoperative period. As the patient returns to the routine floor (and, therefore, a setting of decreased monitoring capacity), perhaps after a period in intensive care, the chance of a cardiac event increases. Extravascular fluid is mobilized, and pain increases as adrenergic activity and a hypercoagulable state develop. These factors contribute to the development of peak morbidity and mortality at between 1 and 7 days *after* surgery.[11]

Clinical Approach to Risk Stratification

The current challenge in patients undergoing vascular surgery is to further reduce the frequency of early and late cardiac events in a cost-efficient manner. Risk stratification should define three groups; low-risk patients who can proceed to surgery without intervention, patients in whom perioperative cardiac risk outweighs the potential benefits of surgery, and patients whose risk may be reduced by perioperative therapeutic intervention. In this context, routine coronary angiography, while showing some disease in 90% of patients,[12] could not be justified because not all patients with coronary stenoses warrant intervention.

Various approaches to clinical risk stratification have been discussed. The Goldman index[13] uses nine differentially weighted predictors of cardiac risk that emphasize the importance of underlying CAD, ventricular dysfunction, and surgical stress in the pathogenesis of perioperative cardiac events. Detsky's modification of Goldman's index[14] included additional variables (angina and alveolar pulmonary edema) and introduced a Bayesian approach whereby the cardiac event rates for various surgical procedures defined the pretest probability of complications. The risk index for an individual patient was then used to calculate a likelihood ratio and post-test probability of a cardiac event with the aid of a nomogram.

Despite the sophisticated statistical approach of these clinical risk indices, they lack sensitivity[15] and approximately 40% of perioperative cardiac events occur in patients predicted to be "low risk." This insensitivity may reflect their inability to detect significant, but silent, underlying CAD, especially when exercise capacity is severely limited by noncardiac systemic disease (e.g., chronic pulmonary disease or peripheral vascular disease). This explains an increasing reliance by clinicians on noninvasive tests which detect underlying CAD without requiring physical exercise.

LEFT VENTRICULAR FUNCTION AS A PROGNOSTIC GUIDE

Resting Global Left Ventricular Function

Noninvasive determination of resting global left ventricular ejection fraction (LVEF) has been proposed for perioperative cardiac risk assessment. In 1984, Pasternack et al.[16] used this technique in patients undergoing abdominal aortic aneurysm resection. Among those whose preoperative ejection fraction was greater than 56%, no perioperative myocardial infarctions (MI) occurred, whereas patients whose ejection fraction was less than 35% had a 75% infarction rate. However, other studies have not confirmed these results. Kazmers et al.[17] identified no additional perioperative risk in patients with a low ejection fraction (< 35%), compared to those with better left ventricular function (LVF), but found that the former group had a greatly reduced long-term survival after surgery. Similarly, Rose et al.[46] found that impaired LVF predicted late cardiac events after surgery, but not perioperative events. While equivalent data have not been obtained using resting echocardiography, for other prognostic purposes (such as risk stratification after MI), resting echocardiography has been shown to provide similar data to nuclear ventriculography.

The failure of preoperative resting ventriculography to predict perioperative events suggests that not only ventricular dysfunction but also ischemia is the major determinant of these events. Severe CAD may be present in patients with a normal ejection fraction. Conversely, patients with impaired ejection fraction may have normal coronary arteries. Therefore, preoperative resting analysis of LVF is not recommended for perioperative risk stratification, although it may be a useful predictor of long-term survival.

Response of Left Ventricular Function to Stress

The LVF response to stress is a reliable indicator of myocardial ischemia. The detection of ischemia at nuclear ventriculography is dependent upon the development of alterations in global LVF in response to stress, which usually correlates with more severe coronary disease. In contrast, the detection of ischemia at echocardiography is more dependent on regional changes, which occur with milder disease. As discussed in Chapter 3, stress echocardiography is more sensitive than nuclear ventriculography for the identification of CAD.

Stress echocardiography is a promising tool for preoperative and late cardiac risk stratification. It provides information about resting LVF and inducible myocardial ischemia,[18] the respective hallmarks of perioperative ischemic complications and long-term survival. Additionally, it can detect unsuspected or underappreciated valvular disease. As these patients are unable to exercise maximally, pharmacological stressors are usually required. The following section will discuss the different stressors currently used and compare their prognostic value for perioperative and late cardiac events.

Selection of Echocardiographic Stress Technique

Stress echocardiography relies on exercise or drugs to increase myocardial oxygen demand and/or reduce oxygen supply. In patients with hemodynamically significant CAD, this stress induces transient myocardial ischemia. The onset of ischemia is associated with transient segmental myocardial wall motion abnormalities that are detectable with standard two-dimensional echocardiographic techniques.[19,20] Thus, stress echocardiography detects the functional consequences of physiologically important CAD.

Exercise Stress

Physical exercise was the first stressor to be combined with echocardiography, but it is not usually selected in these patients. In addition to the usual disadvantages of this technique, including technical difficulties, many patients with vascular disease have a limited exercise capacity. For example, using exercise electrocardiography (ECG), McPhail et al.[21] found that 70% of patients were unable to achieve 85% of their predicted maximal heart rate and therefore had a nondiagnostic test. Submaximal stress compromises the sensitivity of exercise echocardiography.

Pharmacological stress echocardiography has been shown to be a satisfactory alternative to exercise in patients who are unable to exercise maximally. The agents used for stress testing include the vasodilators adenosine and dipyridamole and the inotropic agents dobutamine and arbutamine.

Vasodilator Stress

The mechanism of action of the coronary vasodilators is discussed in Chapter 13. Adenosine and dipyridamole exert their effects by increasing local adenosine concentrations either directly or indirectly (reducing the reuptake of endogenously produced adenosine). Adenosine-induced vasodilatation provokes ischemia by causing systemic hypotension and coronary steal, which may be vertical (subepicardial from subendocardial vessels) or horizontal (normal from stenotic arteries). These effects are accentuated by a mild, reflex tachycardia that increases oxygen demand while reducing diastolic time for myocardial perfusion. In susceptible patients the result is ischemia and new wall motion abnormalities. The main difference between adenosine administration and dipyridamole is in their duration of action, with the half-life of adenosine being in seconds, compared to 6 hours for dipyridamole.

Sympathomimetic Stress

Dobutamine is a sympathomimetic amine that directly increases myocardial oxygen demand through positive chronotropic and inotropic effects,[22] and also impairs myocardial oxygen supply by reducing the duration of diastole. The blood pressure usually remains unaffected during dobutamine infusion because of an increase in cardiac output and a decrease in systemic vascular resistance.[23] Dobutamine infusion can be regarded as an exercise simulator. In regions supplied by critically stenotic coronary arteries, dobutamine induces myocardial ischemia and regional dysfunction. The addition of atropine further increases heart rate and improves sensitivity without increasing side effects.[24] Supplemental atropine is especially useful when target heart rates are not achieved during dobutamine infusion in patients who are taking β-adrenergic blocking agents.

The safety of dobutamine stress echocardiography (DSE) for preoperative cardiac risk assessment has been studied in several series.[11,25–29] Only one major adverse event has been recorded using DSE for this purpose. This patient, a 55-year-old male with a history of symptomatic ventricular tachyarrhythmias, developed ventricular fibrillation during the peak dose of dobutamine. He was successfully resuscitated with a single countershock and experienced no sequelae. Minor side effects consisting primarily of minor cardiac arrhythmias and hypotension occur more frequently.[24,30] In a group of 451 patients,[24] significant cardiac arrhythmias occurred in about 4% of patients. These consisted of sustained and nonsustained ventricular tachycardia, paroxysmal atrial fibrillation, and supraventricular tachycardia. There was a strong association between a history of previous ventricular arrhythmias and the risk of dobutamine induced arrhythmias (odds ratio 9.9, 95% CI 2–45). Hypotension, defined as a decrease in systolic blood pressure of greater than 20 mmHg, occurred in about 3% of patients. This mild degree of hypotension was well tolerated, and most patients successfully completed the test. Hypotension occurred significantly less frequently in patients receiving concomitant β-adrenergic blocking agents (odds ratio 4.1, 95% CI 2.1–8.7). Hypertension, defined as a systolic blood pressure greater than 220 mmHg, is a potentially serious complication in patients with abdominal aortic aneurysm, but occurred in only 1% of the patients and no complications of this have been reported. These results are similar to those reported by Picano et al.,[30] in which serious complications occurred in 9 of 2799 patients (0.3%), and cardiac arrhythmias and hypotension were the most frequent side effects. In summary, the complication rate of DSE appears comparable to that of dipyridamole stress testing,[31] and exercise ECG.[32] An alternative stress test, for instance dipyridamole thallium scintigraphy, might be considered in patients with uncontrolled cardiac arrhythmias or severe hypertension.

Arbutamine is a newly developed catecholamine with β-agonist activity. Arbutamine increases heart rate, systolic blood pressure, and myocardial contractility. No studies are yet available using arbutamine stress echocardiography for cardiac risk stratification.

Prediction of Perioperative Events using Stress Echocardiography

Perioperative cardiovascular complications such as cardiac death, MI, unstable angina, and pulmonary edema are potentially avoidable causes of mortality and morbidity in surgical patients. Preoperative cardiac evaluation has the potential to reduce costs and improve outcome by tailoring perioperative and long-term management in accordance with quantified risk. Cardiac risk stratification in this setting is one of the most promising clinical applications of pharmacological stress echocardiography.

Dipyridamole Stress Echocardiography

As discussed, dipyridamole is less effective in inducing new wall motion abnormalities than dobutamine, especially for milder CAD.[33,34] From the standpoint of risk stratification, this lower sensitivity for milder forms of coronary disease may not be a problem. This is because perioperative cardiac complications tend to occur more often in patients with extensive CAD. The evidence for this is the following: (1) during exercise electrocardiography patients who develop ischemia at "low" heart rates have a relatively high perioperative risk,[21] (2) during dipyridamole thallium scintigraphy, extensive and severe redistribution defects are associated with more perioperative complications,[15] and (3) patients with three or more of Eagle's clinical criteria for cardiac disease have an increased perioperative risk compared to patients with fewer risk factors.[11] If patients undergoing vascular surgery are stratified by an overly sensitive test that detects relatively mild CAD, inappropriate interventions may result. For example, patients may be subjected to unnecessary invasive testing or have needed surgery delayed.

These considerations may explain the paradox that dipyridamole stress echocardiography has been shown to effectively stratify cardiac risk, despite its lower sensitivity for moderate CAD.[35] In this study, Tischler reported a positive predictive value of 78%, and a negative predictive value of 99%. Further studies are needed to confirm this favorable positive predictive value, and to ensure that this is not obtained at the cost of a lower negative predictive value.

Dobutamine Stress Echocardiography

A number of studies have employed DSE for preoperative risk stratification,[11,25–28,35a] as summarized in Table 31-1. Unfortunately, the study groups and design are heterogeneous and they are therefore difficult to compare. In some studies, referral bias might have been introduced by lack of consecutive recruitment. Other reports included patients scheduled for either vascular surgery or general surgical procedures; inclusion of less stressful surgical procedures may have reduced the pretest probability of perioperative cardiac events. In most studies the attending physicians were aware of the results of DSE—this knowledge may have altered preoperative patient management, including referral for coronary angiography with or without subsequent myocardial revascularization, or cancellation of surgery. These shortcomings were avoided by Poldermans et al.[11]; all patients referred for vascular surgery were studied consecutively, attending physicians were blinded to the results of DSE, and patient management was not altered—in particular, preoperative coronary angiography and myocardial revascularization were not performed.

The initial study, performed in 136 vascular surgery patients demonstrated that new regional wall motion abnormalities induced by DSE were associated with a greatly increased risk of perioperative cardiac events (Fig. 31-1) including cardiac death, nonfatal MI, and unstable angina (odds ratio 95, 95% CI 11–822). Wall motion abnormalities at rest and clinical and ECG indicators of ischemia during stress were not independently predictive of perioperative events. In order to confirm these preliminary results the study was extended, using the same protocol, to 300 patients,[29] with essentially no change in the findings. Clinical data, even combined into a risk index such as the Detsky score, provided little useful information about risk (Fig. 31-2), and DSE was superior to clinical data for the prediction of perioperative cardiac events (Table 31-2). The absence of diabetes as a risk marker in the Detsky score compromised its predictive value compared to Eagle's clinical risk factors, whose role will be discussed. However, as a screening test DSE had some limitations. These included the cost of routinely screening all vascular surgery patients, and the relatively low positive predictive value (38%) of a positive test.[11]

The cost of using DSE for risk stratification may be reduced by defining a low-risk patient group who do not require this study preoperatively. Patients with none of the clinical risk factors defined by Eagle (age > 70 years, angina, diabetes mellitus, Q-wave infarction by ECG, and symptomatic ventricular tachyarrhythmias) have a low perioperative cardiac risk (1%). In the study of Poldermans et al.,[29] 100 of 300 patients were stratified to this low-risk status and did not require additional stress testing. Patients with three or more clinical risk factors comprised a high-risk group, with a 29% perioperative complication rate. In contrast to the experience of Eagle, using thallium imaging,[36] we found that DSE pro-

Table 31-1. Predictive Value of New Wall Motion Abnormalities Detected by Stress Echocardiographic for Perioperative Cardiac Events in Patients Scheduled for Elective Vascular Surgery

	Stress	Patients	Sensitivity	Specificity	+PV	−PV	Events
Tischler et al. (1991)[35]	Dipyridamole	109	88	98	78	99	CD, MI, UAP, CHF
Williams et al. (1995)[41]	Dipyridamole	130	67	92	38	97	MI, UAP
Lane et al. (1991)[28]	Dobutamine	57	100	56	21	100	CD, MI, UAP
Poldermans et al. (1995)[29]	Dobutamine	300	100	84	38	100	CD, MI, UAP, CHF
Lalka et al. (1992)[27]	Dobutamine	60	85	44	29	95	CD, MI, UAP
Davila-Roman et al. (1993)[25]	Dobutamine	93	100	95	83	100	CD, MI, UAP, CHF
Eichelberger et al. (1992)[26]	Dobutamine	70	100	65	19	100	MI, UAP
Langan et al. (1993)[35a]	Dobutamine	74	100	79	17	100	MI

Abbreviations: +PV, positive predictive value (%); −PV, negative predictive value (%); CD, cardiac death; MI, myocardial infarction; UAP, unstable angina pectoris; CHF, congestive heart failure.

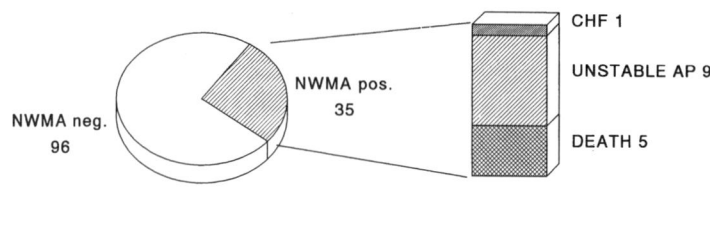

Fig. 31-1. Perioperative cardiac events (cardiac death, nonfatal myocardial infarction, or unstable angina) in 136 patients with subsequent dobutamine–atropine stress test results. AP, angina pectoris; CHF, congestive heart failure; Neg., negative, NWMA, new wall of motion abnormalities; pos., positive.

vided further useful risk stratification in this high risk group. Patients with 3 or more risk factors, and a positive DSE had a perioperative event rate of 55% compared to 0% in patients with a negative test (Fig. 31-3).

The positive predictive value of DSE was improved by adopting a semiquantitative analysis of the results. By considering the heart rate threshold at which ischemia occurred, patients with a positive test were divided into groups, those with the development of ischemia at a low heart rate (< 70% of the age predicted maximum heart rate), or a high heart rate (70% of predicted maximum heart rate). The 38 patients who developed ischemia at a low heart rate were at greatest risk for perioperative cardiac events (positive predictive value of 67%). All fatal complications occurred in this group (Table 31-3). In the 34 patients who developed ischemia at a high heart rate, patients had a lower risk of perioperative cardiac events (16%).

Predictive Value of Different Stressors for Late Events

CAD is a major cause of late morbidity and mortality in survivors of major vascular surgery. For example, Krupski et al.[37] found that late cardiac events occurred in 19% of 129 patients followed-up for 2 years after vascular surgery. This high incidence reflects the severity of underlying CAD. Severe correctable CAD is present in 36% of patients with aortic aneurysm and in 28% of those with lower extremity ischemia.[12] Vascular surgery thereby constitutes an "index event" at which patients with unidentified

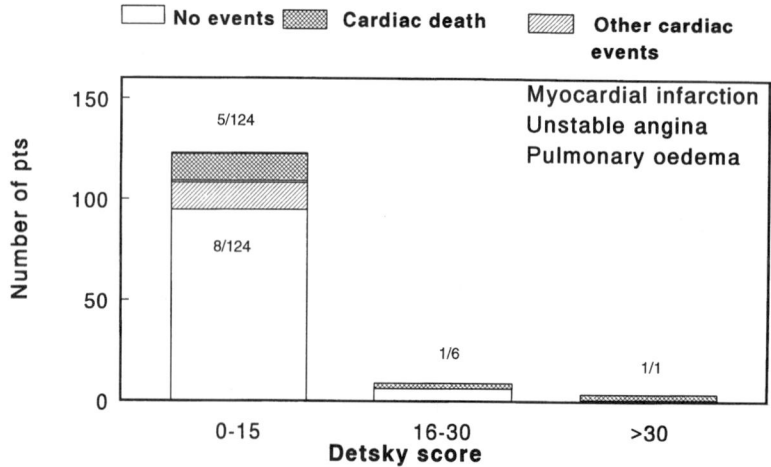

Fig. 31-2. Detsky score and perioperative cardiac events in patients (pts) undergoing major vascular surgery.

Table 31-2. Univariate Analysis of Clinical Data and Stress Test Results

	Cardiac Events (n = 15 patients)	No Cardiac Events (n = 116 patients)	Odds Ratio	Confidence Interval
Age >70 years (No.)	9	46	2.3	0.7–7.8
Sex (M/F)	11/4	100/16	0.44	0.1–1.9
History of angina	7	17	5.1	1.4–18
History of infarction	10	39	4.0	1.1–14.4
Hypertension	4	49	0.5	0.1–1.8
Smoking	8	57	1.2	0.4–3.9
Diabetes	4	11	3.5	0.8–14.8
Aortic/infrainguinal surgery	10/5	84/32	0.8	0.2–2.8
Angina during test	3	10	2.7	0.5–12.7
ST changes during test	7	31	2.4	0.7–8.1
WMA at rest	10	47	2.9	0.9–10.6
Severe LV dysfunction at rest	3	14	1.8	0.4–8.3
NWMA during test	15	20	72	9.0–577

Abbreviations: WMA, any wall motion abnormality; severe LV dysfunction at rest, 10 ot 14 abnormal left ventricular segments; NWMA, new wall motion abnormalities.

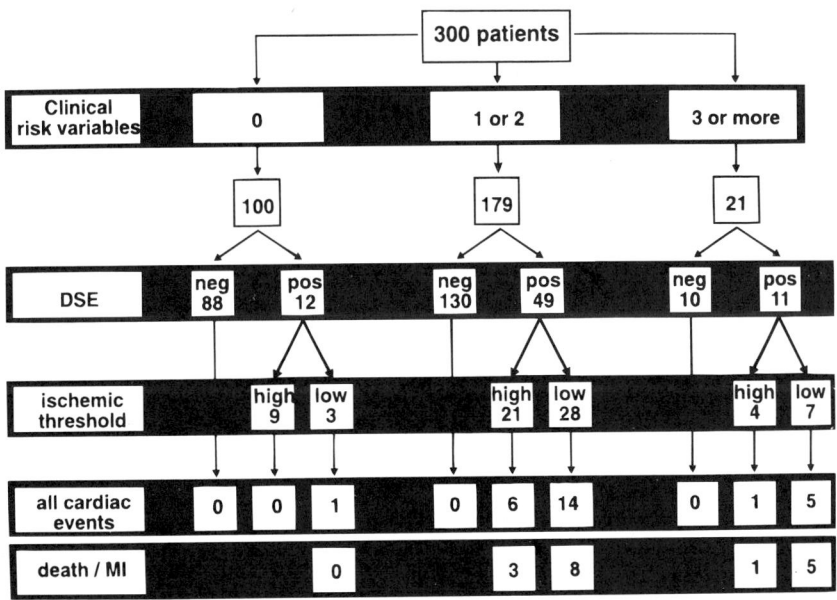

Fig. 31-3. Breakdown of clinical variables and dobutamine–atropine stress test results for perioperative outcomes as applied to a group of 300 patients. Clinical variables are age greater than 70 years, angina, diabetes, Q-wave on electrocardiogram and a history of ventricular ectopic activity. Events refer to cardiac death, nonfatal myocardial infarction (MI), and unstable angina pectoris. Ischemic threshold is the heart rate at which new echocardiographic wall motion abnormalities occurred, divided by the maximal age-corrected heart rate (220 − age). High-threshold is new echocardiographic wall motion abnormalities at greater than 70% of the maximal age-corrected heart rate. Low-threshold is new echocardiographic wall motion abnormalities at less than 70% of the maximal age-corrected heart rate. DSE, dobutamine stress echocardiography; neg, negative, pos, positive.

Table 31-3. Clinical Data and Dobutamine Stress Test Results on Patients with Perioperative Cardiac Death

Patient	Age (years)	AP	MI	Days	WMSI-R	NWMA	Threshold	Extent	Severity
1	70	No	Yes	3	1.48	Yes	68	4	0.24
2	76	No	Yes	5	1.96	Yes	63	5	0.42
3	76	Yes	Yes	5	1.24	Yes	64	6	0.36
4	62	No	No	3	1.00	Yes	62	4	0.24
5	85	No	Yes	7	1.54	Yes	66	4	0.18

Abbreviations: AP, angina pectoris; MI, history of previous myocardial infarction; WMSI-R, wall motion score index at rest; NWMA, new wall motion abnormalities; threshold, heart rate increment at which echocardiographic detected myocardial ischemia occurs ([heart rate at ischemia: age-predicted maximal heart rate] %); extent, number of ischemic segments; severity, difference between wall motion score at peak stress and rest.

CAD may be detected. The preoperative evaluation of candidates should assess the risk of late postoperative cardiac events, since these will determine the likelihood that individual patients will survive to enjoy the benefits of successful surgery.

Several clinical and laboratory variables have been associated with an increased risk of late cardiac events after major surgery. Clinical predictors include a history of CAD or congestive heart failure. Of particular interest is the finding by Mangano et al.[9] that patients who survived a perioperative MI or episode of unstable angina had a 20-fold increase in the odds of a late cardiac event. Noninvasive laboratory indicators of late cardiac risk include LV dilatation and extent of fixed defects and thallium redistribution on dipyridamole thallium scintigraphy,[10] impaired LVF on resting radionuclide ventriculography,[38] and ischemic ST-segment changes during perioperative ambulatory ECG monitoring.[7]

In addition to these conventional risk factors, we have recently shown that inducible ischemia during DSE is also an independent predictor of the risk of late cardiac events in patients with suspected or proven CAD.[39] In a study of 318 survivors of major vascular surgery who had undergone preoperative DSE and clinical evaluation for the presence of cardiac risk factors (smoking, hypertension, angina, diabetes, previous infarction, and age > 70 years), patients were followed for 19 ± 11 months (range 6 to 36) postoperatively and the occurrence of cardiac events was noted. Thirty-two cardiac events occurred (11 cardiac deaths, 11 nonfatal MI, and 10 patients with unstable angina).

Univariate and multivariate regression analysis of clinical history and stress test results was performed for the prediction of late cardiac events. The univariate predictors of late cardiac events, including sensitivity, specificity, and likelihood ratios, are presented in Table 31-4. Baseline clinical parameters, LV dysfunction at rest (> 3 segments), new wall motion abnormalities during stress, and stress-induced angina or ST-segment changes and the occurrence of a nonfatal perioperative cardiac events were significant predictors of late cardiac events. The severity of ischemia during stress and the heart rate threshold for ischemia were not predictive. Multivariate regression analysis was performed on all clinical risk factors and stress test results (Table 31-5). Like Mangano et al.,[9] we found that the occurrence of a nonfatal perioperative cardiac event at the time of major vascular surgery was the most powerful predictor of late cardiac events. New wall motion abnormalities during stress, a history of myocardial infarction, and diabetes mellitus were also independent predictors of late cardiac events. Event-free survival curves for patients with a normal stress test, and those with stress-induced new wall motion abnormalities, are presented in Figure 31-4. There was a significant decrease in event-free survival in patients with new wall motion abnormalities. In the absence of a history of MI and diabetes mellitus (n = 204) the late event rate was 4% with neither risk factor (Table 31-6). Thus, stress testing did not significantly enhance risk stratification in this low-risk group. On the other hand, the late cardiac event rate was 21% in patients with either clinical risk factor. The occurrence of new wall motion abnormalities during stress significantly increased the likelihood of a late cardiac event from 21% to 40% in this group, but a negative test result was not helpful.

Interestingly, a relationship was noted between the extent of ischemia observed during DSE and the

Table 31-4. Use of Preoperative Clinical Data and Stress Test Results to Predict Cardiac Death or MI or Coronary Revascularization after Successful Major Vascular Surgery (n = 318, follow-up period 19 ± 11 Months)

	Pretest (%)	Sensitivity (%)	Specificity (%)	Likelihood Ratio Positive (%)	Likelihood Ratio Negative (%)	Odds Ratio (95% CI)
Perioperative events	10.6					7.8 (3.3–18)
Previous MI		64	75	2.56	0.48	5.3 (2.5–11)
Angina		40	84	2.40	0.71	3.4 (1.6–7.5)
Diabetes mellitus		24	91	2.72	0.82	3.3 (1.4–8.1)
Smoking		52	55	1.18	0.87	1.3 (0.6–2.7)
Hypertension		46	58	1.09	0.94	1.2 (0.5–2.4)
Age >70 years		33	61	0.86	1.08	0.8 (0.4–1.7)
Stress Test Results	10.6					
NWMA		67	78	2.90	0.49	5.7 (2.7–11)
RWMA >3 segments		46	89	4.09	0.61	4.9 (2.3–10)
Angina during test		21	93	3.18	0.84	3.8 (1.5–9.8)
ST segment changes during test		49	78	2.24	0.66	3.4 (1.6–7.1)

Abbreviations: Pretest, pretest probability (%); NWMA, new wall motion abnormalities; RWA, rest wall motion abnormalities; CI, confidence interval.

risk of late cardiac events after vascular surgery. These results are in accordance with previous studies using quantitative dipyridamole thallium scintigraphy,[40] which showed the extent of thallium redistribution to be a significant predictor of late cardiac events.

On the basis of these data, we recommend that dobutamine–atropine stress echocardiography be performed preoperatively in all patients with diabetes mellitus and/or a previous MI. This will provide perioperative risk stratification and predict late cardiac events after successful surgery. Patients with clinical risk factors and a stress-induced ischemia, and survivors of perioperative cardiac events should be followed intensively. Aggressive "anti-ischemic"

Table 31-5. Multivariable Regression Analysis of All Clinical Risk Factors and Stress Test Results

Risk Factors	Odds Ratio (95% CI)
Perioperative cardiac events	5.9 (2.3–15)
NWMA	4.5 (1.9–11)
Previous myocardial infarction	3.8 (2.1–12)
Diabetes mellitus	3.6 (1.3–9.7)

Abbreviations: NWMA, new wall motion abnormalities; CI, confidence interval.

therapy might prolong the period of event-free survival after surgery.

Comparative Utility of Dobutamine and Dipyridamole

The relative accuracy of stress echocardiography using dobutamine and dipyridamole stress has been compared in several studies. As discussed, the use of dipyridamole is associated with significantly lower sensitivity, especially for single-vessel disease. From the prognostic standpoint, the only study comparing both stress modalities is that of Williams et al.[41] In a group of 204 patients, 130 patients' preoperative cardiac risk was assessed by dipyridamole stress echocardiography and in 74 patients by dobutamine stress echocardiography. Perioperative cardiac events, MI, and unstable angina occurred in 13/191 patients (6%). Both studies showed an excellent negative predictive value for perioperative cardiac events (97% and 98%) and a comparable positive predictive value (38% and 27%). Thus, in contrast to the use of these tests for diagnostic purposes, dipyridamole and dobutamine stress echocardiography appear to be interchangeable from the standpoint of prognostic evaluation, and at present there are insufficient data to conclude which is the best "stressor."

When the two agents were compared with respect to side effects during stress testing in a group of 40

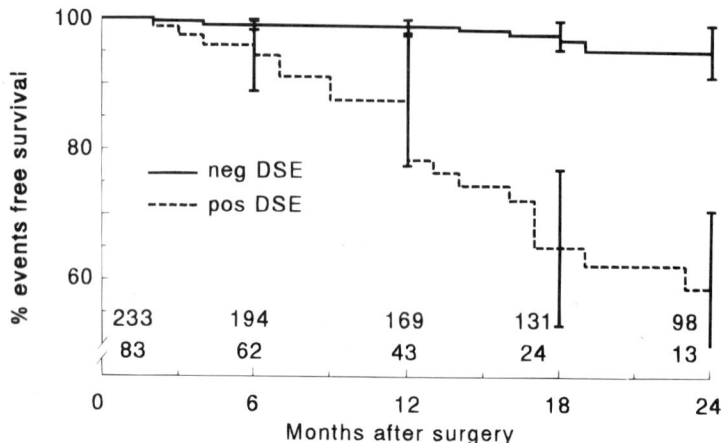

Fig. 31-4. Kaplan-Meier curves for cardiac events (cardiac death, myocardial infarction, or coronary revascularization procedures) during follow-up by results of new wall motion abnormalities (NWMA) during dobutamine-atropine stress tests. Each plot represents the cumulative percentage of patients remaining event free. Vertical lines represent 95% confidence interval point. DSE, dobutamine stress echocardiography; neg, negative; pos, positive.

patients who underwent both tests,[34] some symptom occurred in 88% of patients with dipyridamole compared to 80% during dobutamine infusion. More severe symptoms occurred in 12% of patients with both drugs.

COMPARISON OF STRESS ECHOCARDIOGRAPHY WITH OTHER TESTS FOR RISK STRATIFICATION

Ambulatory ECG Monitoring

In 1989 Raby et al.[42] described the use of 24 to 48 hours of preoperative ambulatory ECG monitoring to assess the perioperative cardiac risk in patients undergoing major vascular surgery. Of 176 patients, 18% had transient episodes of ischemic ST-segment change, the majority of which were asymptomatic. Ischemia on ambulatory monitoring had a sensitivity of 92% and a negative predictive value of 99% for prediction of perioperative cardiac events. By extending monitoring to the perioperative period additional prognostic information of late cardiac events after surgery was provided.[8] Studies by Fleisher et al.[43] and Ouyang et al.[44] have supported these findings, albeit with less favorable sensitivity. Mangano et al.[45] reported cardiac events occurred in 10% to 15% of patients without preoperative ischemia, suggesting that the test does not precisely define a low-risk group. Differences between studies might be related to the relatively small number of end-points, different surgical procedures, and the time at which events occurred after surgery; in the study of Mangano et al.[45] one-third of the events occurred 2 or more weeks after surgery.

Table 31-6. The Likelihood Ratio and Probability of Late Cardiac Events as a Function of the Number of Clinical Risk Factors and Stress Test Results

Number of risk Factors[a]	Events/Number of Patients	Likelihood Ratio	Probability of Cardiac Events	Probability of Cardiac Events with Negative Test	Probability of Cardiac Events with Positive Test
0	8/204	0.38	4%	4% (NS)	5% (NS)
1	24/114	2.40	21%	7% (NS)	40% ($p < 0.01$)

Abbreviations: p value, comparison poststress test results to risk factors; NS, not significant.
[a] Risk factors, previous myocardial infarction and diabetes mellitus.

While ambulatory ECG monitoring has the advantages of being inexpensive and widely available, the presence of resting ECG changes (digitalis use, LV hypertrophy, and bundle branch block) precludes reliable ST-segment analysis in 40% of the recordings.[46] Together with its limited sensitivity, the consideration of feasibility may compromise the application of the technique. While no comparison has been recorded to date with stress echocardiography, it is unlikely that ambulatory monitoring will be as feasible or as sensitive as a stress-imaging approach.

Dipyridamole-Thallium Scintigraphy

Dipyridamole-thallium myocardial perfusion scintigraphy (DTS), often combined with clinical risk assessment, is the most established tool for cardiac risk stratification, and is discussed in Chapter 30. Initial reports indicated that patients who exhibited scintigraphic myocardial perfusion defects during dipyridamole infusion that normalized within 3 to 4 hours or upon reinjection of thallium were at increased risk.[37,47–51] Later studies showed that (1) the extent of redistribution, (2) fixed perfusion defects (no viable myocardium present), and (3) increased lung thallium uptake or transient left ventricular cavity dilatation also had prognostic value.[50] A review from the literature of 1,114 vascular surgery patients studied prior to 1991 showed that preoperative DTS had a sensitivity of 98% and a specificity of 69% for perioperative cardiac events. The predictive value could be increased by using a semiquantitative approach which measured the severity and extent of dipyridamole-induced perfusion defects.[50]

These promising initial results of dipyridamole-thallium scintigraphy were initially questioned by Mangano et al.,[52] who found a sensitivity of 46% and a negative predictive value of only 82%. Although this study has been criticized for its small number of patients and few cardiac events, the results have been confirmed by Baron et al.[53] and Marwick and Underwood.[54] Possible explanations for these disappointing and disparate results with dipyridamole-thallium scintigraphy include the following: (1) the test is now being used widely in a the general population instead of in selected patients with clinical risk factors; (2) clinicians responsible for perioperative care were blinded to the results of dipyridamole-thallium scintigraphy; (3) repeat imaging 3 to 4 hours after thallium infusion may not allow sufficient time for thallium redistribution to regions perfused by severely stenotic coronary arteries. These regions may thus be falsely classified as "fixed defects" when, in fact, they contain viable myocardium; and (4) in patients with severe and diffuse coronary artery disease, thallium uptake may be uniformly reduced, so that discrete perfusion defects are not detectable.

The discrepancy between the reported accuracy of dipyridamole-thallium scintigraphy makes a comparative study between this and stress echocardiographic techniques of critical importance. Unfortunately, no such study has been published to date, although preliminary data in a group of 43 patients suggest that both dipyridamole-thallium scintigraphy and dipyridamole echocardiography have a high negative predictive value (88% vs. 94%), but dipyridamole echocardiography has a superior positive predictive value (37% vs. 67%).[55]

Late cardiac events after successful vascular surgery have also been related to reversible and fixed defects on dipyridamole-thallium scintigraphy.[15,56] In a multivariate analysis, Lette et al.[15] reported the predictors of late cardiac events to be age greater than 70 years, congestive heart failure, reversible defects on dipyridamole-thallium scintigraphy, and LV cavity dilatation during dipyridamole infusion. Markers of chronically or transiently impaired LVF were the best predictors of late cardiac events (congestive heart failure, odds ratio [OR] 5.5, 95% confidence interval [CI] 1.9–16 and left ventricular cavity dilatation, OR 2.9, 95% CI 1.3–6.8). These results agree with those of Kazmers et al.,[38] using resting radionuclide ventriculography, and are also comparable to the late follow-up data for dobutamine echocardiography. The relative prognostic ability of these tests for late events also warrants direct comparison.

GUIDELINES FOR PREOPERATIVE ASSESSMENT USING STRESS ECHOCARDIOGRAPHY

We suggest the following approach for preoperative cardiac risk stratification in patients scheduled for major vascular surgery.

1. *Clinical assessment.* In patients without any risk fac-

tor (age > 70 years, diabetes requiring treatment, angina, Q-waves on ECG, and history of symptomatic ventricular arrhythmias) and adequate exercise capacity, the chance of perioperative cardiac events will be low (1% in our study and 3% in the study of Eagle et al.[36]). Patients in this group can undergo surgery expeditiously and without additional preoperative cardiac investigations or extensive postoperative monitoring.
2. *Dobutamine stress echocardiography.* This test should be performed in all patients with one or more risk factors. Patients with a negative test have an event rate of 1% and can be sent for surgery without extra investigations.
3. *Positive dobutamine stress echocardiography.* Patients who develop ischemia at a high heart rate (70% of the maximum age-related heart rate) are at relatively low risk, with a perioperative event rate of 16%. It is important to realize that no intervention has been demonstrated to reduce perioperative cardiac risk. With this in mind we recommend that medical treatment for ischemia, especially β-adrenergic blocking agents, be initiated preoperatively and maintained throughout the perioperative period. Intraoperative and postoperative ECG monitoring for ischemia is also indicated. Patients who develop ischemia during or after surgery should remain in intensive care and receive additional treatment.

Patients who develop ischemia at a low heart rates represent an extremely high-risk group with a predicted perioperative event rate of 67%, and a mortality rate of 16.7%. The optimal approach in this group has not been established. Available options include cancellation of surgery or substitution of a less invasive procedure like percutaneous transluminal angioplasty (PTA) or stent implantation. A second possibility is evaluation of CAD by angiography and performance of a myocardial revascularization procedure with a view to reducing perioperative and late cardiac event rates. This aggressive approach requires careful prospective evaluation before it can be recommended. The cumulative mortality rate associated with angiography, myocardial revascularization, and subsequent vascular surgery might prove to be substantial in this elderly, high-risk population. We would recommend coronary angiography and myocardial revascularization only in patients with disabling angina despite maximal medical therapy or DSE results that suggest left main or triple vessel disease. The final treatment alternative would be to proceed with essential surgery while utilizing some combination of anti-ischemic and/or antithrombotic therapy, invasive hemodynamic monitoring including perhaps transesophageal echocardiography, perioperative monitoring for ischemia, and a prolonged postoperative intensive care unit admission.

FUTURE DIRECTIONS FOR STRESS TESTING AND PERIOPERATIVE MANAGEMENT

The risk assessment algorithm developed in conjunction with our DSE program is of more than academic interest. First, we have demonstrated that clinical assessment alone followed by DSE in patients with risk factors can define a very large population of patients who can proceed to surgery without extensive investigation or intensive perioperative management. This information has the potential to substantially reduce costs and avoid potentially hazardous tests and interventions. Second, by providing more precise information about risk, we can help patients and their physicians make genuinely informed decisions about the advisability of surgery. This is bound to prevent morbidity and reduce costs. Finally, our ability to quantify cardiac risk in vascular surgery sets the stage for future risk-reduction studies that will define the efficacy of various interventions designed to reduce risk in high-risk subsets of patients.

Design of Subsequent Studies

Future risk-reduction studies will face several problems and must be carefully designed. Potential problems include the following: (1) the number of perioperative cardiac events in noncardiac surgery is decreasing over time due to improved surgical and anaesthetic care, (2) surgeons are likely to refer high-risk candidates for less invasive procedures such as PTA or stents, without extensive cardiac screening, and (3) perioperative cardiac events are heterogeneous and need to be classified uniformly. For example, a "chemical MI," diagnosed solely on a finding of elevated cardiac enzymes, must be clearly differentiated from transmural Q-wave infarction. "Soft" cardiac events such as prolonged ischemia without infarction or congestive heart failure have questionable clinical relevance. Ideally one would study only "hard" cardiac events such as cardiac death and definite MI, but this approach would necessitate studying larger numbers of patients, as the number of "end-points" will be less.

Risk Reduction Strategies

Some risk-reduction strategies that deserve prospective investigation include (1) perioperative β-adrenergic blockade, (2) continuous ECG monitoring with aggressive anti-ischemic management, (3) coronary angiography with prophylactic myocardial revascularization, and (4) antithrombotic therapy.

Perioperative cardiac protection with β-adrenergic blockers in high-risk patients is an attractive approach. β-Blockers have an established role in the treatment of CAD. Treatment with β-blockers during surgery is safe: extensive experience has been acquired in patients undergoing coronary artery bypass grafting (CABG), and no major side effects have been observed during aortic surgery. β-Adrenergic blockers have been demonstrated to reduce the incidence and severity of perioperative myocardial ischemia.[57,58] Although Raby et al.[42] did not detect a relation between short-term heart rate changes and perioperative ischemia, patients who experienced cardiac events had higher peak heart rates, suggesting a potential beneficial effect of β-blockers.

The use of intensive perioperative monitoring seems attractive. Prolonged ischemia during surgery and in the early postoperative period (24 to 48 hours) is highly related with adverse outcome,[59] and a perioperative MI increases the risk of late events 20-fold. This explained the initial enthusiasm of sophisticated techniques like transesophageal echocardiography (TEE) and 12-lead electrocardiography. However, the study of Eisenberg[60] showed that the *intraoperative* use of these new techniques added no additional information about perioperative events compared to clinical data and continuous two-lead ambulatory ECG monitoring. A limitation of this study was the low number of perioperative cardiac complications and the echo technique using only monoplane images. One benefit of intensive intraoperative monitoring may be the selection of patients who would benefit from continued postoperative monitoring in the intensive care unit. Patients with minimal ischemia may be referred to the ward within 24 hours as they have a low risk for cardiac events, in contrast to patients with more marked ischemia.

REFERENCES

1. Smith T: European health challenges. BMJ 303:1395, 1991
2. Mangano DT: Perioperative cardiac morbidity. Anesthesiology 72:153, 1990
3. Sonecha TN, Nicolaides AN: The relationship between intermittent claudication and coronary artery disease- is it more than we think? Vasc Med Rev 2:137, 1991
4. Goldman L: Assessment of perioperative cardiac risk. N Engl J Med 330:707, 1994
5. Massie BM, Mangano DT: Assessment of perioperative risk: have we put the cart before the horse? J Am Coll Cardiol 21:1353, 1993
6. Katz DJ, Stanley JC, Zelenock GB: Operative mortality rates for intact and ruptured abdominal aneurysms in Michigan: An eleven-year statewide experience. J Vasc Surg 19:804, 1994
7. Yeager RA, Moneta GL, Edwards JM et al.: Late survival after perioperative myocardial infarction complicating vascular surgery. J Vasc Surg 20:598, 1994
8. Raby KE, Goldman L, Cook EF et al.: Long-term prognosis of myocardial ischemia detected by Holter monitoring in peripheral vascular disease. Am J Cardiol 66:1309, 1990
9. Mangano DT, Browner WS, Hollenberg M et al.: Long-term cardiac prognosis following noncardiac surgery. JAMA 268:233, 1992
10. Younis LT, Aguirre F, Byers S et al.: Perioperative and long-term prognostic value of intravenous dipyridamole thallium scintigraphy in patients with peripheral vascular disease. Am Heart J 119:1287, 1990
11. Poldermans D, Fioretti PM, Foster T et al.: Dobutamine stress echocardiography for the assessment of perioperative cardiac risk in patients undergoing major non cardiac vascular surgery. Circulation 87:1506, 1993
12. Hertzer NR, Beven EG, Young JR et al.: Coronary artery disease in peripheral vascular patients: a classification of 1000 coronary angiograms and results of surgical management. Ann Surg 199:223, 1984
13. Goldman L, Caldera DL, Nussbaum SR et al.: Multifactorial index of cardiac risk in noncardiac surgical procedures. N Engl J Med 297:845, 1977
14. Detsky AS, Abrams HB, Forbath N et al.: Cardiac as-

sessment for patients undergoing noncardiac surgery. Arch Intern Med 146:2131, 1986
15. Lette J, Waters D, Lassone J et al.: Multivariate clinical models and quantitative dipyridamole-thallium imaging to predict cardiac morbidity and death after vascular reconstruction. J Vasc Surg 14:160, 1991
16. Pasternack PF, Imparato AM, Bear G et al.: The value of radionuclide angiography as a predictor of perioperative myocardial infarction in patients undergoing abdominal aortic aneurysm resection. J Vasc Surg 1:320, 1984
17. Kazmers A, Cerqeira MD, Zierler RE: The role of preoperative radionuclide ejection fraction in direct abdominal aortic aneurysm repair. J Vasc Surg 8:128, 1988
18. Picano E: Stress echocardiography: from pathophysiological toy to diagnostic tool. Circulation 85:1604, 1992
19. Bourdillon PDV, Broderick TM, Sawada SG et al.: Regional wall motion index for infarct and noninfarct regions after reperfusion in acute myocardial infarction: comparison with global wall motion index. J Am Soc Echocardiogr 2:398, 1989
20. Salustri A, Fioretti PM, Pozzoli MMA et al.: Dobutamine stress echocardiography: Its role in the diagnosis of coronary artery disease. Eur Heart J 13:70, 1992
21. McPhail N, Calvin JE, Shariatmadar A et al.: The use of preoperative exercise testing to predict cardiac complications after arterial reconstruction. J Vasc Surg 7:60, 1988
22. Fung AY, Gallagher KP, Buda AJ: The physiologic basis of dobutamine as compared with dipyridamole stress interventions in the assessment of critical coronary stenosis. Circulation 76:943, 1987
23. Poldermans D, Boersma E, Fioretti PM et al.: Cardiac chronotropic responsiveness to β-adrenoceptor stimulation is not reduced in the elderly. J Am Coll Cardiol 25:995, 1995
24. Poldermans D, Fioretti PM, Boersma E et al.: Safety of dobutamine-atropine stress echocardiography in patients with suspected coronary artery disease. Am J Cardiol 73:456, 1994
25. Davila-Roman VG, Waggoner AD, Sicard GA et al.: Dobutamine stress echocardiography predicts surgical outcome in patients with an aortic aneurysm and peripheral vascular disease. J Am Coll Cardiol 21:957, 1993
26. Eichelberger J, Schnarz K, Black E et al.: Medical value of dobutamine echocardiography before vascular surgery. Circulation Suppl. I, 86:I-789, 1992
27. Lalka SG, Sawada SG, Dalsing MC et al.: Dobutamine stress echocardiography as a predictor of cardiac events associated with aortic surgery. J Vasc Surg 15:831, 1992
28. Lane RT, Sawada SG, Segar DS et al.: Dobutamine stress echocardiography as a predictor of perioperative cardiac events. Am J Cardiol 68:976, 1991
29. Poldermans D, Arnese M, Fioretti PM et al.: Improved cardiac risk stratification in major vascular surgery with dobutamine-atropine stress echocardiography. J Am Coll Cardiol 26:648, 1995.
30. Picano E, Mathias W, Pingitori A et al.: Safety and tolerability of dobutamine-atropine stress-echocardiography: a prospective, multicentre study. Lancet 344:1190, 1994
31. Picano E, Marini C, Pirelli S et al.: Safety of intravenous high-dose dipyridamole echocardiography. Am J Cardiol 70:252, 1992
32. Rochmis P, Blackburn H: Exercise test: a survey of procedures, safety and litigation experience in approximately 170000 tests. JAMA 217:1061, 1971
33. Previtali M, Lanzarini L, Tortorici M et al.: Dobutamine versus dipyridamole echocardiography in coronary artery disease. Circulation, Suppl. III, 83:III-27, 1991
34. Martin TW, Seaworth JF, Johns JP et al.: Comparison of adenosine, dipyridamole, and dobutamine in stress echocardiography. Ann Intern Med 116:190, 1992
35. Tischler MD, Lee TH, Hirsch AT et al.: Prediction of major cardiac events after peripheral vascular surgery using dipyridamole echocardiography. Am J Cardiol 68:593, 1991
35a. Langan EM, Youky JR, Franklin DP et al.: Dobutamine stress echocardiography for cardiac risk assessment before aortic surgery. J Vasc Surg 18:905, 1993
36. Eagle KA, Coley CM, Newell JB et al.: Combining clinical and thallium data optimizes preoperative assessment of cardiac risk before major vascular surgery. Ann Intern Med 110:859, 1989
37. Krupski WC, Layug EL, Reilly LM et al.: Comparison of cardiac morbidity rates between aortic and infrainguinal operations. J Vasc Surg 18:609, 1993
38. Kazmers A, Moneta GL, Cerqueira MD et al.: The role of perioperative radionuclide ventriculography in defining outcome after revascularization of the extremity. Surg Gynecol Obstet 171:481, 1990
39. Poldermans D, Fioretti PM, Boersma E et al.: Dobutamine-atropine stress echocardiography and clinical data for predicting late cardiac events in patients with suspected coronary artery disease. Am J Med 97:119, 1994
40. Brown KA: Prognostic value of thallium-201 myocardial perfusion imaging: a diagnostic tool comes of age. Circulation 83:363, 1991
41. Williams MJ, O'Gorman D, Shan K et al.: Dobutamine

vs dipyridamole echo for risk stratification before vascular surgery (Abstr.). J Am Soc Echocardiogr 1995 (in press).
42. Raby KE, Goldman L, Creager MA et al.: Correlation between preoperative ischemia and major cardiac events after peripheral vascular surgery. N Engl J Med 321:1296, 1989
43. Fleisher LA, Hawes AD, Rosenbaum SH: The limited predictive value of dipyridamole thallium imaging in noncardiac surgery patients, abstracted. Anesthesiology 73:A75, 1990
44. Ouyang P, Gerstenbliyh G, Furman WR et al.: Frequency and significance of early postoperative silent myocardial ischemia in patients having peripheral vascular surgery. Am J Cardiol 64:1113, 1989
45. Mangano DT, Browner WS, Hollenberg M et al.: Association of perioperative myocardial ischemia with morbidity and mortality in men undergoing noncardiac surgery. N Engl J Med 323:1781, 1990
46. Rose EL, Liu XJ, Henley M et al.: Prognostic value of noninvasive cardiac tests in the assessment of patients with peripheral vascular disease. Am J Cardiol 71:40, 1993
47. Lette JL, Waters D, Cerino M et al.: Preoperative coronary artery disease risk stratification based on dipyridamole imaging and a simple three-step, three segment model for patients undergoing noncardiac vascular surgery or major general surgery. Am J Cardiol 69:1553, 1992
48. McPhail NV, Ruddy TD, Calvin JE et al.: Comparison of left ventricular function and myocardial perfusion for evaluating perioperative cardiac risk of abdominal aortic surgery. Can J Surg 33:224, 1990
49. Coley CM, Field TS, Abraham SA et al.: Usefulness of dipyridamole-thallium scanning for preoperative evaluation of cardiac risk for nonvascular surgery. Am J Cardiol 69:1280, 1992
50. Levinson JR, Boucher CA, Coley CM et al.: Usefulness of semiquantitative analysis of dipyridamole-thallium-201 redistribution for improving risk stratification before vascular surgery. Am J Cardiol 66:406, 1990
51. Boucher CA, Brewster DC, Darling RC et al.: Determination of cardiac risk by dipyridamole thallium imaging before peripheral vascular surgery. N Engl J Med 312:389, 1985
52. Mangano DT, London MJ, Tubau JF et al.: Dipyridamole thallium-201 scintigraphy as a preoperative screening test: a reexamination of its predictive potential. Circulation 84:493, 1991
53. Baron JF, Mundler O, Bertrand M et al.: Dipyridamole-thallium scintigraphy and gated radionuclide angiography to assess cardiac risk before abdominal aortic surgery. N Engl J Med 330:663, 1994
54. Marwick T, Underwood D: Dipyridamole thallium imaging may not be a reliable screening test for coronary artery disease in patients undergoing vascular surgery. Clin Cardiol 13:14, 1990
55. Vincent M, Marwick T, D'Hondt AM et al.: Prediction of perioperative events at vascular surgery: selection of thallium scintigraphy or echocardiography with dipyridamole stress. Circulation, Suppl. I, 86:3142, 1992
56. Hendel RC, Whitfield SS, Villegas BJ et al.: Prediction of late cardiac events by dipyridamole thallium imaging in patients undergoing elective vascular surgery. Am J Cardiol 70:1243, 1992
57. Slogoff S, Keats AS, Ott E: Preoperative propanolol therapy and aortocoronary bypass operation. JAMA 240:1478, 1978
58. Kataja JHK, Kaukinen S, Viinamaki OVK et al.: Esmolol for treatment of hypertension and tachycardia in patients during and after abdominal aortic surgery. J Cardiothorac Anesth 4:37, 1990
59. Landesberg G, Luria MH, Cotev S et al.: Importance of long-duration postoperative ST-segment depression in cardiac morbidity after vascular surgery. Lancet 341:715, 1993
60. Eisenberg MJ, London MJ, Leung MJ et al. Monitoring for myocardial ischemia during non cardiac surgery. A technology assessment of transesophageal echocardiography. JAMA 268:210, 1992

Chapter 32

Flow Maldistribution Versus Malfunction in Clinical Decision Making

Mario S. Verani

The functional evaluation of coronary artery disease (CAD) often depends on the demonstration of ischemic electrocardiographic (ECG) abnormalities, myocardial perfusion heterogeneity, or stress-induced changes in wall motion (sometimes combined with changes in left ventricular ejection fraction (LVEF) or end-systolic volume). The methods used to elicit and document these changes—exercise ECG, radionuclide techniques, and two-dimensional (2D) echocardiography—have all been well studied and are definitely useful in the noninvasive identification of CAD, but they really assess different pathophysiologic phenomena that can be brought about in patients with coronary stenoses. Hence, because the above techniques fundamentally probe different manifestations of CAD, it should not be anticipated that they would correlate very precisely with one another—and they don't!

The application of the existing techniques to the assessment of patients with CAD, their limitations, and interrelationships, are all based on our current understanding of the pathophysiology of myocardial ischemia, which will be briefly reviewed.

PATHOPHYSIOLOGY OF MYOCARDIAL ISCHEMIA: THE ISCHEMIC CASCADE

Experimental Considerations

Ischemia due to Reduced Coronary Supply

More than 60 years ago, Tennant and Wiggers[1] observed that ligation of a coronary artery in the dog led to nearly immediate cessation of the contraction of the cardiac muscle supplied by this artery; they also observed that the involved muscle became cyanotic and bulged outwardly. Nearly half a century later, the seminal work of John Ross and associates[2,3] and others[4,5] demonstrated that within 30 to 60 seconds after acute coronary occlusion in dogs, elevation of the ECG ST segment promptly developed in leads overlying the ischemic myocardium, associated with paradoxical systolic movement of the involved myocardium, lack of systolic shortening (in fact, systolic thinning occurred), and impaired ventricular relaxation.[6-8]

Ischemia due to Increased Oxygen Demand

Directionally similar changes, albeit less intense, were observed in paced-induced[9] and exercise-induced ischemia.[10] It also became clear that the residual tissue perfusion of the occluded vascular bed is species dependent. In dogs, a species with a rich collateral network, the perfusion in the center of the ischemic area falls to 5% to 15% of normal,[11,12] whereas in goats, pigs, and primates—species with intrinsically poor collateral vessels—the flow often decreases to below 5% of control values.[13] In dogs, and probably in humans too, the reduction in flow is more severe in the subendocardium than in the subepicardium.[12,13]

Changes in Myocardial Perfusion and Function during Acute Ischemia in Humans

Reduced Coronary Supply

With the advent of coronary angioplasty, it became feasible to study the temporal effects of acute, low flow, myocardial ischemia in humans. Inflation of the angioplasty balloon in the coronary artery lumen leads to a sudden, temporary interruption of the coronary blood flow and acute ischemia of the subtended myocardium. The ischemic manifestations commence within a few seconds of the occlusion, reach a maximum within 30 to 50 seconds,[14,15] and evolve in a predictable pattern, beginning with diastolic dysfunction, followed by systolic dysfunction, ischemic ECG changes, and lastly chest pain. The latter occurs in 33% to 70% of patients.[14,16–18]

In a recent study from our group[19] ischemic ST-segment changes occurred in only 17 of 35 patients during balloon inflation of a coronary artery. These changes consisted of ST-segment elevation in 7 and ST-segment depression in 10 patients. Angina during balloon inflation occurred in only 19 of 35 patients. These data confirmed the astute clinician's observation that chest pain and ECG changes are not very sensitive indicators of myocardial ischemia. In contrast, myocardial perfusion defects on technetium-99m (^{99m}Tc)-sestamibi single-photon emission computed tomography (SPECT) occurred in 34 of 35 (97%) patients during balloon inflation of a coronary artery. The only exception was a patient with no detectable perfusion deficit during occlusion of a small posterolateral branch of the circumflex artery. In the same investigation, wall motion abnormalities during balloon inflation, assessed by first-pass radionuclide angiography (RNA), occurred in only 17 (59%) of the patients. Even after excluding patients who had inflation of a circumflex artery, which would cause posterolateral wall motion abnormality, and which could be missed during first-pass RNA performed in the anterior projection, only 12 of 18 patients with transient occlusion of the left anterior descending or right coronary artery developed transient wall motion abnormalities. A decrease in LVEF also occurred often during transient coronary occlusion; the severity of the fall in LVEF, however, was highly dependent on the site of coronary occlusion and was greater during left anterior descending occlusion, intermediate during circumflex occlusion, and smaller during right coronary artery occlusion. Patients with occlusion of the left anterior descending artery had a fall in LVEF from 54 ± 6% at baseline to 40 ± 11% during occlusion; however, when the balloon was inflated in the proximal left anterior descending artery a 50% or greater fall in LVEF occurred, with proportionately smaller decreases during mid and distal left anterior descending occlusion.

In a previous study, using a portable multiwire gamma camera and the generator-produced, short lived ($t\frac{1}{2}$ = 9 minutes) element tantalum-178, we had already demonstrated that the fall in LVEF during transient coronary occlusion is also dependent on the presence of angiographically identified coronary collateral circulation; patients with collateral vessels had a smaller fall in LVEF (mean fall 9%) than those without angiographic collaterals (mean fall 27%).[20] In addition to the changes in regional systolic function and a fall in LVEF, our group has also demonstrated a transient and significant increase in left ventricular end-systolic volume and a significant decrease in stroke volume index (which was compensated by an increase in heart rate sufficient to preserve the cardiac index within normal limits).[19]

Changes in diastolic ventricular function, assessed by the peak diastolic filling rate during first-pass RNA, using the multiwire gamma camera and tantalum-178,[20] also occurred often during transient coronary occlusion, and were significantly correlated with the changes in LVEF ($r = 0.75$). These studies during coronary angioplasty have also led us to conclude that the extent of perfusion abnormality during coronary occlusion is highly dependent on the site of coronary occlusion: occlusion of the left anterior descending artery resulted in a hypoperfused area involving 39% of the left ventricle, compared to 15% for occlusion of the right coronary artery and 15% for left circumflex artery occlusions. Directionally similar results were reported by Haronian et al.[18] Our data during coronary angioplasty also suggest that wall motion changes are less consistent and, at least by first-pass RNA, more difficult to detect than changes in myocardial perfusion during acute ischemia.[19]

Ischemia due to Increased Oxygen Demand

The changes in myocardial perfusion and ventricular function that occur during exercise testing are less severe than the changes produced during transient coronary occlusion.[21] Mahmarian et al.[22] from our institution demonstrated that significantly larger perfusion defects occur in patients with proximal left anterior descending stenoses (30% average defect size) than in those with left circumflex (14% defect size) or right coronary artery stenoses (18% defect size) by exercise thallium tomography. Defects present during exercise were larger when the stenosis involved the proximal rather than the middle or distal left anterior descending artery.[23] The overall extent of left ventricular hypoperfusion is also dependent on the extent of CAD—patients with three-vessel disease generally have a larger perfusion defect size than those with one-vessel disease.[22] Likewise, both the extent of exercise-induced wall motion abnormalities and the fall in LVEF are greater in patients with multivessel disease than in those with single-vessel disease.[24,25]

These clinical data suggest that in ischemia due either to alterations of supply or demand, perfusion changes are more marked than functional changes, examined using nuclear techniques. The extent to which these differences are related to underlying physiology or the modalities involved remains unclear, however.

MYOCARDIAL PERFUSION SCINTIGRAPHY IN THE MANAGEMENT OF CAD

Diagnosis and Assessment of Disease Significance

The extensive experience that now exists with SPECT, which has become the preferred technique for myocardial perfusion scintigraphy, has been reviewed in Chapter 2. Using thallium-201 SPECT during exercise stress, an average sensitivity of 90% and specificity of 70% can be expected, with a normalcy rate approaching 90%.[26-28] The published experience with ^{99m}Tc-sestamibi is not as extensive as that with thallium-201, but nonetheless, similar sensitivity and specificity can be expected with this agent as with thallium-201. ^{99m}Tc-teboroxime is more problematic, because it clears rapidly from the myocardium after its administration, although it has also yielded good diagnostic accuracy.[29] ^{99m}Tc-tetrofosmin is yet another promising myocardial perfusion tracer that will soon compete with sestamibi.

Although SPECT has several advantages over planar myocardial scintigraphy, it cannot be overemphasized that it is often more demanding and requires meticulous quality control to achieve results that approach those of the published reports. Apart from technical factors and interpreter's experience, several elements impact importantly on the test accuracy: exercise intensity, severity of coronary stenosis, presence of anti-ischemic medication, extent of CAD, frequency of prior myocardial infarction, and location of coronary stenosis (see preceding discussion). Computer quantification of SPECT images further enhances the identification of moderate stenoses (involving between 50% and 70% of the luminal diameter stenosis), and stenosis confined to the left circumflex artery.[22,26,27] Quantification also enhances our ability to recognize the presence of multivessel disease and may increase the specificity for right coronary artery stenosis, by decreasing the number of false-positive defects due to tracer attenuation in the inferior left ventricular wall.[22]

The high sensitivity of these techniques makes them attractive for the functional evaluation of known coronary stenoses; such functional evidence of disease significance should be obtained prior to the performance of interventions. Lower values for specificity may, however, be viewed as a problem when the test is used for diagnostic purposes, especially in patients with lower probabilities of coronary disease.

Prognostic Value of Myocardial Perfusion Scintigraphy

The extensive literature documenting the prognostic value of myocardial perfusion scintigraphy in patients with chronic CAD has been reviewed in Chapter 27.[30–33] In addition to the presence of perfusion defects, several variables are important predictors of increased propensity for future cardiac events, including the nature of perfusion defects (whether fixed or transient), the number and extent of perfusion defects, and, in particular, increased lung uptake and transient left ventricular cavity dilatation during stress. These variables are equally important during exercise and pharmacologic stress using dipyridamole or adenosine.

In patients with a recent myocardial infarction, predischarge exercise myocardial perfusion scintigraphy affords a powerful means to stratify patients with respect to subsequent risk for cardiovascular events.[30,34] In patients who are unable to undergo an exercise test, pharmacologic stress scintigraphy with dipyridamole or adenosine is an accurate predictor of future cardiovascular risk.[30,33,35–37] The ability to quantify the extent of perfusion defects and the extent of defect reversibility are recent developments that have refined our ability to stratify risk in patients after an acute myocardial infarction.[36,37] Similarly, in patients with unstable angina who are stabilized after intensive medical therapy, a predischarge myocardial perfusion scintigraphy study done during exercise or pharmacologic stress is an excellent option in the risk stratification of these patients.[30,31,38]

The available data briefly reviewed above, and data reviewed in other chapters of this book, indicate that a wealth of experience surrounds the use of perfusion scintigraphy for prognostic purposes. However, the high predictive values for negative studies are balanced by lower positive predictive values.

RADIONUCLIDE ANGIOGRAPHY IN THE EVALUATION OF CAD

Diagnosis and Assessment of Disease Significance

Before the advent of SPECT, RNA was often used to ascertain the diagnosis of CAD noninvasively. Detection of CAD by this technique is based on the principle that during exercise, deterioration of wall motion occurs in patients with coronary stenosis, who have limited coronary flow reserve. In these patients, the augmentation of myocardial blood flow is not commensurate with the increase in myocardial oxygen demand brought on by exercise. When systolic function deteriorates in a large area of myocardium, the LVEF may also fall, and the end-systolic volume may increase. These changes are in marked contrast with the response of normal subjects during exercise stress, where more vigorous myocardial contraction leads to an increase in LVEF and a decrease in end-systolic volume.

Accuracy

The accuracy of exercise RNA has been discussed in Chapter 3. Using a combined criteria of wall motion abnormality and/or less than 5 ejection fraction units increase during exercise, many investigators achieved sensitivities ranging from 82% to 100% (average 88%) and specificities from 55% to 100% (average 81%).[24] Nonetheless, it was recognized that not uncommonly patients with CAD *who failed to achieve an ischemic end-point during exercise* testing could have a completely normal exercise RNA study. More disturbing was the realization that the ejection fraction response to exercise is in fact a complex phenomenon and may be influenced by factors such as the intensity of exercise, the baseline LVEF value, the presence of valvular heart disease, hypertension, cardiomyopathy, or negative inotropic drugs, and even by gender and age.[24,25,39]

Reasons for the Obsolescence of Radionuclide Angiography in the Diagnosis of CAD

Despite its widespread use for several years, RNA is no longer much used in the diagnosis of CAD in the United States. Several reasons contributed to this development. First, there was a projection problem. Gated RNA is ordinarily performed in the "best septal" left anterior oblique projection, to allow for a clear separation between the left ventricle, the right ventricle, and the left atrium. In this view, only the interventricular septum, the posterolateral wall, and the superimposed inferior wall and left ventricular apex can be delineated. Thus, stenosis of the left anterior descending artery causing exclusive deterioration of the anterolateral wall, or stenosis of the right coronary artery causing exclusive deterioration of the inferobasal region of the left ventricle, could be entirely missed. First-pass RNA would circumvent this problem, because it is usually performed in the anterior view, which displays well the anterolateral and inferior walls, in addition to the left ventricular apex. First-pass RNA, however, fails to show the interventricular septum or the left ventricular posterolateral wall. Hence, lesions of the left anterior descending artery that created a wall motion abnormality solely in the septum, or lesions of the circumflex artery with its resulting posterolateral wall motion abnormality, could also be missed.

Second, there was an exercise problem; during gated RNA patients ordinarily exercise in the supine or semisupine position on a bicycle ergometer to facilitate camera positioning and minimize chest movement during exercise. In this unnatural, awkward position, it is difficult to attain a high level of stress, as evidenced by the lower heart rates achieved by patients. During first-pass RNA, exercise is often performed on a bicycle ergometer in the upright (sitting) position. Even in this position many patients fail to attain the target heart rate because of early leg fatigue.

Third, the detection of the changes in wall motion was highly subjective and variably influenced by the interpreter's skills (and sometimes biases)—which is also a potential problem with 2D echocardiography. Fourth, and perhaps most important, was the advent and rapid acceptance of SPECT, with its enhanced potential to provide a three-dimensional (3D) image of left ventricular perfusion, which was very amenable to computer quantification techniques. This has led to a gradual replacement of both planar perfusion imaging and exercise RNA for the diagnosis of CAD.

The above reasons may also explain the limited use and suboptimal diagnostic accuracy of RNA in combination with other stresses, such as the cold pressor test, dipyridamole, and dobutamine.[25] The failure of these types of stress RNA may reflect the inability of these various stresses to elicit a predictable ischemic response as well as the limited technical resolution of the images.

Prognostic Value of Radionuclide Angiography in CAD

Prognostic Value in Chronic CAD and after Myocardial Infarction

Despite the obsolescence of exercise RNA for diagnostic purposes, exercise RNA remains a powerful predictor of long-term prognosis in patients with or without CAD.[24,39] This important topic has been reviewed in Chapter 26.

In ambulatory patients with chronic CAD, the exercise ejection fraction (determined by first-pass RNA) has been shown to be the single most important prognostic predictor among several clinical, scintigraphic, and angiographic variables.[24,25,39] Moreover, the exercise ejection fraction allows stratification of patients with three-vessel disease and mild anginal symptoms into a high- and a low-risk group for future cardiac events.[21,25]

Several studies have demonstrated that the rest LVEF assessed by RNA is an important predictor of short- and long-term prognosis in patients who had an acute myocardial infarction. The exercise LVEF may be of additional prognostic value in these patients, although it is likely that rest ejection fraction contains most of the prognostic information. In the thrombolytic therapy era, recent evidence ensures a continued, pivotal role for the RNA-determined LVEF in ascertaining the likelihood of patients suffering a subsequent cardiac event.[40] The risk of subsequent cardiac death is also closely related to the LVEF.[37,41,42]

Patients Undergoing Revascularization

Exercise RNA can be used to assess the results of coronary artery bypass grafting (CABG) and coronary angioplasty; successful revascularization leads to improved exercise LVEF, which is often accompanied by a reversion of exercise-induced wall motion abnormalities.[43-45] However, RNA has limited ability to predict CABG patency, just as it is a suboptimal test for localizing the site of coronary stenoses.

In summary, while exercise RNA offers useful prognostic data, its value for diagnostic purposes is limited. The latter is undesirable, as it is infrequent for a study to be performed *purely* for prognostic purposes.

USE OF TWO-DIMENSIONAL ECHOCARDIOGRAPHY FOR THE EVALUATION OF CAD

The rationale for using 2D echocardiography to assess the left ventricular function during different stresses is the same as for RNA. However, in contrast

Table 32-1. Strengths of Echocardiography

Cost and availability
"Versatility" (at a cost!)
Comprehensive assessment of systolic and diastolic function, valves, pericardium
Feasibility to measure chamber volumes, wall thickness, pressure, and systolic thickening
Indirect assessment of hemodynamics: PA pressure, PA wedge, and diastolic function
Stress-induced wall motion abnormalities equal myocardial ischemia (detection of true ischemia)
Technique well standardized
Controlled by cardiologists (income, access, exposure of trainees, etc.)
No radiation exposure

(From Verani,[46] with permission.)

with RNA, where the LVEF can be accurately and reproducibly calculated by a computer, 2D echocardiography relies predominantly on the demonstration of stress-induced regional wall motion deterioration as the hallmark of CAD. However, 2D echocardiography permits the assessment of more left ventricular segments during stress. This provides some benefit over RNA, because of the limited number of left ventricular segments that can be assessed during stress RNA. Moreover, 2D echocardiography is feasible during exercise (treadmill or bicycle) or pharmacologic stress following dipyridamole, adenosine, or dobutamine administration. Stress echocardiography has a number of strengths that render it a very attractive technique to assess patients with suspected CAD (Table 32-1).[46]

Diagnosis and Assessment of Disease Significance

Exercise 2D echocardiography was first reported in 1979 by Feigenbaum's group[47] and its use was for a long time restricted to academic centers, with only more recent achievement of broad usage in clinical practice. As with RNA, 2D echocardiography may be done using a treadmill, or an upright or supine bicycle exercise. When a treadmill is used, the 2D images are obtained before exercise and *immediately after*, rather than *during* peak exercise, because imaging cannot be done while the patient walks on the treadmill. This imposes a delay of several seconds between the termination of exercise and the commencement of imaging; in experienced hands, imaging is initiated within the first 20 to 30 seconds after exercise and completed within 60 seconds. If the delay between the end of exercise and completion of the images is substantially longer, this may pose a significant problem, because the changes in wall motion evoked by exercise may resolve rapidly,[48-51] especially in patients with single-vessel CAD.

The use of upright bicycle exercise may limit the views that can be obtained by 2D echocardiography; subcostal or apical views are more reliably obtained than parasternal views. However, all views may be obtained with the patient lying supine, immediately after exercise. Stress echocardiography can also be done during supine bicycle exercise. However, although this approach is probably more feasible than that with upright exercise, it suffers from the same constraint as exercise RNA, namely leg fatigue requires terminating the test before the target heart rate is achieved and hence results in many submaximal (and suboptimal) exercises.

Studies of exercise 2D echocardiography have reported a range of sensitivities and specificities,[50-63] and are discussed in Chapter 3. This variation reflects patient selection and variable preponderance of prior infarction, coronary stenosis severity and extent, influence of anti-ischemic drugs, and the interpreter's threshold to call an abnormality—more aggressive reading often resulting in high sensitivity with lower specificity and less aggressive reading to the opposite. Limitations or "weaknesses" of 2D echocardiography are summarized in Table 32-2. The inability to define the endocardial edge of certain regions of the left ventricle—especially the lat-

Table 32-2. Weaknesses of Echocardiography

Suboptimal studies in some patients
Poor endocardial border definition
Observer dependency: subjective interpretation ("loose" criteria of abnormality)
Variable "echogenicity" ("the lung factor")
Difficulties diagnosing ischemia superimposed on scar tissue
Cannot be done during treadmill exercise
Less likely to predict multivessel disease correctly
Inability to assess myocardial perfusion noninvasively

(From Verani,[46] with permission.)

eral wall—because of poor lateral resolution of the echocardiography technique may be an important problem. The need for adequate training is critical.

Prognostic Value of Exercise Two-Dimensional Echocardiography

Prognostic Value in CAD and after Myocardial Infarction

The prognostic applications of stress echocardiography have been discussed in Chapters 26 and 30. Fewer studies have assessed the prognostic value of exercise 2D echocardiography than perfusion scintigraphy, reflecting the more recent development of the former as a clinical tool.

Patients with chronic stable coronary disease have an event rate of 34% in those with a positive test and 9% in those with a negative test at a mean follow-up of 12 months.[64] A total event rate of 4.1% over a 2-year follow-up was reported by Sawada et al.[68] in patients with a normal stress 2D echocardiogram. While this rate is twofold or threefold higher than that reported for patients with a normal thallium or sestamibi perfusion scan, these events occurred in patients who exercised submaximally. Thus, the performance of maximal stress with stress echocardiography is mandatory for obtaining reliable results, either for diagnostic or prognostic purposes.

In patients recovering from an acute myocardial infarction, a positive test is associated with cardiac events in more than two-thirds of patients, and a negative test was associated with events in less than one-fourth of patients with a negative test.[65-67] The prognostic value of rest or exercise 2D echocardiography after thrombolytic therapy has not been well documented as yet.

Patients Undergoing Revascularization

The efficacy of exercise 2D echocardiography after intervention has been summarized in Chapter 18.[69-74] Residual ischemia in these circumstances may reflect incomplete revascularization, as well as restenosis or bypass graft occlusion.

Pharmacologic Two-Dimensional Echocardiography

The combination of dipyridamole and adenosine stress in combination with 2D echocardiography is rarely used in the United States. Although these combinations have been found by some investigators to be relatively accurate for the diagnosis of CAD, the overall sensitivity of these modalities is suboptimal for detection of CAD—on average of 63% in a recent review.[46] Recent comparative studies have shown exercise and dobutamine to be more sensitive than dipyridamole 2D echocardiography in patients with suspected CAD.[75]

The rationale of using dobutamine to provoke changes in wall motion in the presence of coronary stenoses depends on the induction of myocardial ischemia by high-dose dobutamine.[76] A recent review of the literature showed a sensitivity and a specificity of 83% and 83%, respectively, although the range of sensitivities was quite wide (59% to 95%).[77-87] Dobutamine 2D echocardiography, however, suffers some of the same limitations as exercise 2D echocardiography, especially with respect to the merely qualitative evaluation of changes in wall motion. When interpreters were asked to grade the confidence level of their own interpretations, only 17% of dobutamine echocardiography studies were read with a high degree of confidence, whereas in 28% of the interpretations the confidence level was low.[88]

WALL MOTION OR PERFUSION PARADIGMS FOR ASSESSING CAD?

Considerations Regarding Accuracy

The previous discussion summarized the reported accuracy of techniques designed to detect flow abnormalities (perfusion scintigraphy) or wall motion abnormalities (RNA or 2D echocardiography). As useful as these reported figures may be, they do not allow a comparison among these diverse techniques, unless *the same* patients are concomitantly studied by these methods. Comparisons between exercise RNA and 2D echocardiography have shown similar accuracies for these techniques for CAD detection,[54] but do not reflect the use of current stress echocardiography techniques, including image digitization.

Studies comparing exercise perfusion scintigraphy and exercise 2D echocardiography are summarized in Table 32-3. There is a slightly higher sensitivity with myocardial perfusion scintigraphy (87% vs. 80%), which is counterbalanced by a slightly higher specificity by 2D echocardiography (89% vs. 86%). Although these studies did not evaluate the

Table 32-3. Exercise 2D Echocardiography versus Myocardial Perfusion Imaging

Reference	Number of patients	Sensitivity (%)		Specificity (%)	
		Echo	MPI	Echo	MPI
Maurer and Nanda (1981)[53]	23	70	74	92	92
Pozzoli et al. (1991)[60]	75	71	84	96	88
Quiñones et al. (1992)[63]	112	74	74	88	81
Amanullah et al. (1992)[89]	27	82	95	80	100
Hecht et al. (1993)[90]	71	90	92	80	65
Galanti et al. (1991)[91b]	53	93	100	96	92
Mean ± SD		80 ± 10	87 ± 11	89 ± 7	86 ± 12

Abbreviations: Echo, echocardiography; MPI, myocardial perfusion imaging; SD, standard deviation.
[a] Sensitivity for individual arteries: 85% (myocardial perfusion imaging) versus 63% (echocardiography) ($p < 0.01$).
(From Verani,[46] with permission.)

detection and localization of individual coronary stenoses, the nonsimultaneous studies that assessed this issue have generally found a higher accuracy of myocardial perfusion scintigraphy for detection of stenosis in individual territories, particularly for left circumflex artery stenosis. Correct prediction of multivessel disease is also higher by myocardial perfusion scintigraphy in most studies. A higher detection of reversible ischemia was achieved by myocardial perfusion scintigraphy, especially in patients with a prior myocardial infarction and ischemia superimposed on or adjacent to an area of infarction.[63]

With respect to dobutamine stress testing, a slightly higher sensitivity was found by myocardial perfusion scintigraphy (83% vs. 79%), whereas 2D echocardiography had a slightly higher specificity (84% vs. 80%). With dobutamine echocardiography, however, it may be more critical to achieve an adequate heart rate response (≥ 85% of the predicted maximum) to enhance the test sensitivity. In patients with an inadequate heart rate response, the sensitivity may be superior by perfusion scintigraphy than by 2D echocardiography.[86] A recent study by Senior et al.[94] reported abnormal myocardial perfusion SPECT in 45 of 54 patients, but ischemia at 2D echocardiography in only 25 (56%) patients during high-dose dobutamine infusion. However, a biphasic response (i.e., an initial improvement at low dose followed by worsening at peak dose) occurred in 44 patients.

A fundamental difference exists between techniques that rely on the demonstration of wall motion abnormality (RNA and 2D echocardiography), as opposed to those that uncover a perfusion abnormality. Although both wall motion deterioration and perfusion defects are good markers of significant coronary stenosis, they are evoked by fundamentally different mechanisms. Wall motion deterioration, on the one hand, is due to myocardial ischemia and depends on its duration, extension, and severity, in addition to its distribution across the left ventricular wall thickness. A perfusion defect, on the other hand, is caused by coronary blood flow heterogeneity. Very brief episodes of ischemia, involving a small area of the left ventricle and compromising less than one-third of the left ventricular wall thickness (as may be the case, for example, of subendocardial ischemia localized to the inner subendocardium) may not be enough to produce a wall motion abnormality sufficiently obvious to be detected by noninvasive means. The tethering effect of the normally hypercontractile myocardium during exercise or dobutamine infusion, upon the abnormally contracting myocardium, may further hamper the detection of a small area of wall motion abnormality. Thus, wall motion deterioration is dependent on the presence of ischemia, which in turn depends on an increase in myocardial oxygen demands in excess of the capacity of the stenosed coronary artery to augment myocardial blood flow and oxygen supply. Moreover, when the target of the test is the development of wall motion abnormality, and the stress is discontinued when the first abnormality is detected, it may lead to an inability to assess the total extent of CAD, since only the territories that *first* manifested ischemia would be identified.

Conversely, a perfusion defect does not require the presence of active ischemia, but rather depends on the existence of myocardial blood flow heterogeneity, which in turn depends on the coronary flow reserve.[95] While this heterogeneity may coexist with ischemia, it may also occur when the blood flow is actually increased in the myocardium perfused by either a normal or a stenosed artery, albeit the increase would be of less magnitude in the latter than in the former (during pharmacologic vasodilation the flow is often increased above baseline in *both* normal and stenosed arteries).

Hence, in a hypothetical scenario, heterogeneous myocardial perfusion may be present during submaximal exercise or pharmacologic stress *before* the onset of myocardial ischemia. If the test is terminated at this point, because of patient fatigue or other reasons, it may not be possible to demonstrate any wall motion change, whereas the perfusion heterogeneity conceivably would be uncovered by myocardial perfusion scintigraphy. How often this hypothetical scenario actually occurs is not known. Recent studies, however, using first-pass RNA concurrently with sestamibi perfusion tomography have confirmed a higher frequency of perfusion abnormalities than of ventricular dysfunction during exercise treadmill testing.[21,96] The addition of regional myocardial function data to the perfusion data provides significantly incremental information with respect to the extent of CAD.[96]

Cost–Benefit Ratio with Myocardial Scintigraphy and Two-Dimensional Echocardiography

At the present time, a stress 2D echocardiography study is considerably less expensive than cardiac scintigraphy, both in terms of hardware and the cost of radionuclide agent, which obviously is not needed for 2D echocardiography. However, the current costs do not take into consideration the physician's time to perform and interpret the test, which may be less with cardiac scintigraphy, which can be acquired in standard fashion by nuclear technologists.

The cost–benefit ratio, however, may not be the appropriate paradigm to determine the ultimate clinical value of these tests. For example, the benefit may be higher with one technique, in terms of more correct identification of the extent of CAD and prediction of future cardiac events, but since the cost of this test is also higher, a cost–benefit ratio will be achieved similar to that of a test that may afford less benefit (more patients with CAD and future cardiac events are missed) but also costs less. Thus, ultimately society as a whole—and hopefully, not only the medical administrators determined to cut costs at any price—must decide whether a more accurate diagnosis and prognosis are worth a higher price tag.

Finally, it is pivotal that physicians and patients know the competency and accuracy level of different laboratories performing these competing modalities in their hospitals or communities. The ultimate decision on which tests the physician will choose among an ever increasing number of choices will be dictated by how much the test results contribute in the management of their patients.

REFERENCES

1. Tennant R, Wiggers CJ: The effect of coronary occlusion on myocardial contraction. Am J Physiol 112:351, 1935
2. Batler A, Froelicher VF, Gallagher KP et al.: Dissociation between regional myocardial dysfunction and ECG changes during ischemia in the conscious dog. Circulation 62:735, 1980
3. Osakada G, Hess OM, Gallagher KP et al.: End-systolic dimension-wall thickness relations during myocardial ischemia in conscious dogs. Am J Cardiol 51:1750, 1983
4. Sunagawa K, Maughan WL, Sagawa K: Effect of regional ischemia on the left ventricular end-systolic pressure-volume relationship of isolated canine hearts. Circ Res 52:170, 1983
5. Lew WYW, Chen Z, Guth B et al.: Mechanisms of augmented segment shortening in nonischemic areas during acute ischemia of the canine left ventricle. Circ Res 56:351, 1985
6. Visner MS, Arentzen CE, Parrish GD et al.: Effects of global ischemia on the diastolic properties of the left ventricle in the conscious dog. Circulation 71:610, 1985
7. Wexler LF, Weinberg EO, Ingwall JS et al.: Acute alterations in diastolic left ventricular chamber distensibility: mechanistic differences between hypoxia and is-

chemia in isolated perfused rabbit and rat hearts. Circ Res 59:515, 1986
8. Takahashi T, Levine MJ, Grossman W: Regional diastolic mechanics of ischemic and nonischemic myocardium in the pig heart. J Am Coll Cardiol 17:1203, 1991
9. Momomura SI, Ferguson JJ, Miller MJ et al.: Regional myocardial blood flow and left ventricular diastolic properties in pacing-induced ischemia. J Am Coll Cardiol 17:781, 1991
10. Miyazaki S, Guth BD, Miura T et al.: Changes of left ventricular diastolic function in exercising dogs without and with ischemia. Circulation 81:1058, 1990
11. Jugdutt BJ, Hutchins GM, Bulkley BH et al.: Myocardial infarction in the conscious dog: three dimensional mapping of infarct, collateral flow and region at risk. Circulation 60:1141, 1979
12. Koyanagi S, Eastham CL, Harrison DG et al.: Transmural variations in the relationship between myocardial infarct size and risk area. Am J Physiol 242:H867, 1982
13. Marcus ML: The Coronary Circulation in Health and Disease. McGraw-Hill, New York, 1983
14. Wohlgerlernter D, Jaffee CC, Cabin HS et al.: Silent ischemia during coronary occlusion produced by balloon inflation: relation to regional myocardial dysfunction. J Am Coll Cardiol 10:491, 1987
15. Jaffee CC, Wohlgerlernter D, Cabin H et al.: Preservation of left ventricular ejection during percutaneous transluminal coronary angioplasty by distal transcatheter coronary perfusion of oxygenated Fluosol DA 20%. Am Heart J 115:1156, 1988
16. Braat SH, deSwart H, Janssen JH et al.: Use of technetium-99m sestamibi to determine the size of the myocardial area perfused by a coronary artery. Am J Cardiol 66:85E, 1990
17. Serruys PW, Wigns W, Van den Brand M et al.: Left ventricular performance, regional blood flow, wall motion and lactate metabolism during transluminal angioplasty. Circulation 70:25, 1984
18. Haronian HL, Remetz MS, Sinusas AJ et al.: Myocardial area at risk defined by technetium-99m sestamibi imaging during coronary angioplasty: comparison with coronary angiography. J Am Coll Cardiol 22:1033, 1993
19. Gallik DM, Obermueller SD, Swarna US et al.: Simultaneous assessment of myocardial perfusion and left ventricular function during transient coronary occlusion. J Am Coll Cardiol 25:1529, 1995
20. Verani MS, Lacy JL, Guidry GW et al.: Quantification of left ventricular performance during transient coronary occlusion at various anatomical sites in humans: a study using tantalum-178 and a multiwire gamma camera. J Am Coll Cardiol 19:297, 1992
21. Borges-Neto S, Puma J, Jones RH et al.: Myocardial perfusion and ventricular function measurements during total coronary artery occlusion in human: a comparison with rest and exercise radionuclide studies. Circulation 89:278, 1994
22. Mahmarian JJ, Boyce TM, Goldberg RK et al.: Quantitative exercise thallium-201 single photon emission computed tomography for the enhanced diagnosis of ischemic heart disease. J Am Coll Cardiol 15:318, 1990
23. Mahmarian JJ, Pratt CM, Boyce TM et al.: The variable extent of jeopardized myocardium in patients with single vessel coronary artery disease: quantification by thallium-201 SPECT. J Am Coll Cardiol 17:355, 1991
24. Borer JS, Supino P, Wencker D et al.: Assessment of coronary artery disease by radionuclide cineangiography. History, current applications, and new directions. Cardiol Clin 12:333, 1994
25. Iskandrian AS, Verani MS: Radionuclide angiography. In Iskandrian AS, Verani MS (eds): Nuclear Cardiac Imaging. FA Davis, 1995 (in press)
26. Mahmarian JJ, Verani MS: Exercise thallium-201 perfusion scintigraphy in the assessment of coronary artery disease. Am J Cardiol 67:2D, 1991
27. Maddahi J, Rodrigues E, Berman DS et al.: State-of-the-art myocardial perfusion imaging. Cardiology Clinics 12:199, 1994
28. O'Keefe JH, Barnhart CS, Bateman TM: Comparison of stress echocardiography and stress myocardial perfusion scintigraphy for diagnosing coronary artery disease and assessing its severity. Am J Cardiol 75:25D, 1995
29. Hendel RC, McSherry B, Karimeddini M et al.: Diagnostic value of a new myocardial perfusion agent, teboroxime (SQ30217), utilizing a rapid planar imaging protocol: preliminary results. J Am Coll Cardiol 16:855, 1990
30. Brown KA: Prognostic value of thallium-201 myocardial perfusion imaging. A diagnostic tool comes of age. Circulation 83:363, 1991
31. Heller GV, Brown KA: Prognosis of acute and chronic coronary artery disease by myocardial perfusion imaging. Cardiol Clin 12:271, 1994
32. Iskandrian AS, Chae SC, Heo J et al.: Independent and incremental prognostic value of exercise single-photon emission computed tomographic (SPECT) thallium imaging in coronary artery disease. J Am Coll Cardiol 22:665, 1993
33. Brown KA: Prognostic value of cardiac imaging in patients with known or suspected coronary artery disease: comparison of myocardial perfusion imaging, stress

echocardiography, and positron emission tomography. Am J Cardiol 75:35D, 1995
34. Gibson RS, Watson DD, Craddock GB et al.: Prediction of cardiac events after uncomplicated myocardial infarction: a prospective study comparing predischarge exercise thallium-201 scintigraphy and coronary angiography. Circulation 68:321, 1983
35. Leppo JA, O'Brien J, Rothendler JA et al.: Dipyridamole-thallium-201 scintigraphy in the prediction of future cardiac events after acute myocardial infarction. N Engl J Med 310:1014, 1984
36. Mahmarian JJ, Pratt CM, Nishimura S et al.: Quantitative adenosine T1-201 single-photon emission computed tomography for the early assessment of patients surviving acute myocardial infarction. Circulation 87:1197, 1993
37. Mahmarian JJ, Mahmarian AC, Marks GF et al.: Role of adenosine thallium-201 tomography for defining long-term risk in patients after acute myocardial infarction. J Am Coll Cardiol 25:1333, 1995
38. Brown KA: Prognostic value of thallium-201 myocardial perfusion imaging in patients with unstable angina who respond to medical treatment. J Am Coll Cardiol 17:1053, 1991
39. Port SC: Recent advances in first-pass radionuclide angiography. Cardiol Clin 12:359, 1994
40. Simoons MV, Vos J, Tijssen JG et al.: Long-term benefit of early thrombolytic therapy in patients with acute myocardial infarction: 5 year follow-up of a trial conducted by the Interuniversity Cardiology Institute of the Netherlands. J Am Coll Cardiol 14:1609, 1989
41. Cerqueira MD, Maynard C, Ritchie JL et al.: Long-term survival in 618 patients from the Western Washington Streptokinase in Myocardial Infarction Trials. J Am Coll Cardiol 20:1452, 1992
42. Zaret BL, Wackers FJTh, Terrin ML et al.: Value of radionuclide rest and exercise left ventricular ejection fraction in assessing survival of patients after thrombolytic therapy for acute myocardial infarction: results of thrombolysis in myocardial infarction (TIMI) phase II study. J Am Coll Cardiol 26:73, 1995
43. Kent KM, Bonow RO, Rosing DR et al.: Improved myocardial function during exercise after successful percutaneous transluminal coronary angioplasty. N Engl J Med 306:441, 1982
44. DePuey EG, Leatherman LL, Leachman RD et al.: Restenosis after transluminal coronary angioplasty detected with exercise-gated radionuclide ventriculography. J Am Coll Cardiol 4:1103, 1984
45. Lewis JF, Verani MS, Poliner LR et al.: Effects of transluminal coronary angioplasty on left ventricular systolic and diastolic function at rest and during exercise. Am Heart J 109:792, 1985
46. Verani MS: Myocardial perfusion imaging versus two-dimensional echocardiography: comparative value in the diagnosis of coronary artery disease. J Nucl Cardiol 1:399, 1994
47. Wann LS, Faris JV, Childress RH et al.: Exercise cross-sectional echocardiography in ischemic heart disease. Circulation 60:1300, 1979
48. Dymond DS, Foster C, Grenier RP et al.: Peak exercise and immediate postexercise imaging for detection of left ventricular functional imaging for detection of left ventricular functional abnormalities in coronary artery disease. Am J Cardiol 53:1532, 1984
49. Presti CF, Armstrong WF, Feigenbaum H: Comparison of echocardiography at peak exercise and after bicycle exercise in evaluation of patients with known or suspected coronary artery disease. J Am Soc Echocardiogr 1:119, 1988
50. Hecht HS, De Bord L, Shaw R et al.: Digital supine bicycle stress echocardiography: a new technique for evaluating coronary artery disease. J Am Coll Cardiol 21:950, 1993
51. Ryan T, Segar DS, Sawada SG et al.: Detection of coronary artery disease with upright bicycle exercise echocardiography. J Am Soc Echocardiogr 6:186, 1993
52. Morganroth J, Chen CC, David D et al.: Exercise cross-sectional echocardiographic diagnosis of coronary artery disease. Am J Cardiol 47:20, 1981
53. Maurer G, Nanda NC: Two dimensional echocardiographic evaluation of exercise induced left and right ventricular asynergy: correlation with thallium scanning. Am J Cardiol 48:720, 1981
54. Limacher MC, Quiñones MA, Poliner R et al.: Detection of coronary artery disease with exercise two-dimensional echocardiography. Circulation 67:1211, 1983
55. Visser CA, van der Wieken RL, Kan G et al.: Comparison of two-dimensional echocardiography with radionuclide angiography during dynamic exercise for the detection of coronary artery disease. Am Heart J 106:528, 1983
56. Armstrong WF, O'Donnell J, Ryan T et al.: Effect of prior myocardial infarction and extent and location of coronary artery disease on accuracy of exercise echocardiography. J Am Coll Cardiol 10:531, 1987
57. Ryan T, Vasey CG, Presti CF et al.: Exercise echocardiography: detection of coronary artery disease in patients with normal left ventricular wall motion at rest. J Am Coll Cardiol 11:993, 1988
58. Sawada SG, Ryan T, Fineberg NS et al.: Exercise echo-

cardiographic detection of coronary artery disease in women. J Am Coll Cardiol 14:1140, 1989
59. Sheikh KH, Bengston JR, Helmy S et al.: Relation of quantitative coronary lesion measurements to the development of exercise-induced ischemia assessed by exercise echocardiography. J Am Coll Cardiol 15:1043, 1990
60. Pozzoli MMA, Fioretti PM, Salustri A et al.: Exercise echocardiography and technetium-99m MIBI single photon emission computed tomography in the detection of coronary artery disease. Am J Cardiol 67:350, 1991
61. Crouse LH, Harbrecht JJ, Vacek JL et al.: Exercise echocardiography as a screening test for coronary artery disease and correlation with coronary arteriography. Am J Cardiol 67:1213, 1991
62. Marwick TH, Nemec JJ, Pashkow FJ et al.: Accuracy and limitations of exercise echocardiography in a routine clinical practice. J Am Coll Cardiol 19:74, 1992
63. Quiñones MA, Verani MS, Haichin RM et al.: Exercise echocardiography versus thallium-201 single-photon emission computed tomography in evaluation of coronary artery disease: analysis of 292 patients. Circulation 85:1026, 1992
64. Krivokapich J, Child JS, Gerber RS et al.: Prognostic usefulness of positive or negative exercise stress echocardiography for predicting coronary events in ensuing twelve months. Am J Cardiol 71:646, 1993
65. Jaarsma W, Visser CA, Kupper AJF et al.: Usefulness of two-dimensional exercise echocardiography shortly after myocardial infarction. Am J Cardiol 57:86, 1986
66. Ryan T, Armstrong WF, O'Donnell JA et al.: Risk stratification after acute myocardial infarction by means of exercise two-dimensional echocardiography. Am Heart J 114:1305, 1987
67. Applegate RJ, Dell'Italia LJ, Crawford MH: Usefulness of two-dimensional echocardiography during low-level exercise testing early after uncomplicated acute myocardial infarction. Am J Cardiol 60:10, 1987
68. Sawada SG, Ryan T, Conley JNJ et al.: Prognostic value of a normal exercise echocardiogram. Am Heart J 120:49, 1990
69. Broderick T, Sawada S, Armstrong WF et al.: Improvement in rest and exercise-induced wall motion abnormalities after coronary angioplasty: an exercise echocardiographic study. J Am Coll Cardiol 15:591, 1990
70. Gentile R, Dillon J, Ryan T et al.: Risk stratification for restenosis after coronary angioplasty by means of exercise echocardiography. Cardiologia 39:651, 1994
71. Abdul-Enein H, Bengtson JR, Adams DB et al.: Effect of the degree of effort on exercise echocardiography for the detection of restenosis after coronary artery angioplasty. Am Heart J 122:430, 1991
72. Mertes H, Erbel R, Nixdorff U et al.: Exercise echocardiography for the evaluation of patients after nonsurgical coronary artery revascularization. J Am Coll Cardiol 21:1087, 1993
73. Sawada SG, Judson WE, Ryan T et al.: Upright bicycle exercise echocardiography after coronary artery bypass grafting. Am J Cardiol 64:1123, 1989
74. Crouse LJ, Vacek JL, Beauchamp GD et al.: Exercise echocardiography after coronary artery bypass grafting. Am J Cardiol 70:572, 1992
75. Dagianti A, Penco M, Agati L et al.: Stress echocardiography: comparison of exercise, dipyridamole and dobutamine in detecting and predicting the extent of coronary artery disease. J Am Coll Cardiol 26:18, 1995
76. Fung AY, Gallagher KP, Buda AJ: The physiologic basis of dobutamine as compared with dipyridamole stress interventions in the assessment of critical coronary stenosis. Circulation 76:943, 1987
77. Martin TW, Seaworth JF, Johns JP et al.: Comparison of adenosine, dipyridamole and dobutamine in stress echocardiography. Ann Intern Med 116:190, 1992
78. Mazeika P, Nihoyannopoulos P, Joshi J et al.: Uses and limitations of high dose dipyridamole stress echocardiography for evaluation of coronary artery disease. Br Heart J 67:144, 1992
79. Sawada SG, Segar DS, Ryan T et al.: Echocardiographic detection of coronary artery disease during dobutamine infusion. Circulation 83:1601, 1991
80. Previtali M, Lanzarini L, Ferrario M et al.: Dobutamine versus dipyridamole echocardiography in coronary artery disease. Circulation, Suppl. 83:III-27, 1991
81. Segar DS, Brown SE, Sawada SG et al.: Dobutamine stress echocardiography: correlation with coronary lesion severity as determined by quantitative angiography. J Am Coll Cardiol 19:1197, 1992
82. Cohen JL, Greene TO, Ottenweller J et al.: Dobutamine digital echocardiography for detecting coronary artery disease. Am J Cardiol 67:1311, 1991
83. Marcovitz PA, Armstrong WF: Accuracy of dobutamine stress echocardiography in detecting coronary artery disease. Am J Cardiol 69:1269, 1992
84. McNeil AJ, Fioretti PM, El-said EM et al.: Enhanced sensitivity for detection of coronary artery disease by addition of atropine to dobutamine stress echocardiography. Am J Cardiol 70:41, 1992
85. Marwick T, Willemart B, D'Hondt AM et al.: Selection of the optimal nonexercise stress for the evaluation of ischemic regional myocardial dysfunction and malperfusion. Circulation 87:345, 1993
86. Marwick T, D'Hondt AM, Baudhvin T et al.: Optimal

use of dobutamine stress for the detection and evaluation of coronary artery disease: combination with echocardiography or scintigraphy, or both? J Am Coll Cardiol 22:159, 1993
87. Simek CL, Watson DD, Smith WH et al.: Dipyridamole thallium-201 imaging versus dobutamine echocardiography for the evaluation of coronary artery disease in patients unable to exercise. Am J Cardiol 72:1257, 1993
88. Marwick TH, D'Hondt AM, Mairesse GH et al.: Comparative ability of dobutamine and exercise stress in induced myocardial ischemia in active patients. Br Heart J 72:31, 1994
89. Amanullah AM, Lindvall K, Bevegard S: Exercise echocardiography after stabilization of unstable angina: correlation with exercise thallium-201 single photon emission computed tomography. Clin Cardiol 15:585, 1992
90. Hecht HS, DeBord L, Shaw R et al.: Supine bicycle echocardiography versus tomographic thallium-201 exercise imaging for the detection of coronary artery disease. J Am Soc Echocardiogr 6:177, 1993
91. Galanti G, Sciagrà R, Comeglio M et al.: Diagnostic accuracy of peak exercise echocardiography in coronary artery disease: comparison with thallium-201 myocardial scintigraphy. Am Heart J 122:1609, 1991
92. Foster T, McNeill AJ, Salustri A et al.: Simultaneous dobutamine stress echocardiography and technetium-99m isonitrile single-photon emission computed tomography in patients with suspected coronary artery disease. J Am Coll Cardiol 21:1591, 1993
93. Gunalp B, Dokumaci B, Uyan C et al.: Value of dobutamine technetium-99m sestamibi SPECT and echocardiography in the detection of coronary artery disease compared with coronary angiography. J Nucl Med 34:889, 1993
94. Senior R, Lahiri A: Enhanced detection of myocardial ischemia by stress dobutamine echocardiography utilizing the "biphasic" response of wall thickening during low and high dose dobutamine infusion. J Am Coll Cardiol 26:26, 1995
95. Gould LK: Noninvasive assessment of coronary stenoses by myocardial perfusion imaging during pharmacologic coronary vasodilatation. I. Physiologic basis and experimental validation. Am J Cardiol 41:267, 1978
96. Palmas W, Friedman JD, Diamond GA et al.: Incremental value of simultaneous assessment of myocardial function and perfusion with technetium-99m sestamibi for prediction of extent of coronary artery disease. J Am Coll Cardiol 25:1024, 1995

Index

Page numbers followed by *f* denote figures; those followed by *t* denote tables.

A

Acetate labeled with carbon-11, in myocardial metabolism assessment, 427–429
Adenosine stress, 238
  in echocardiography, 71, 599
    accuracy of, 248t, 249
    compared to other echocardiographic techniques, 85t
    compared to perfusion imaging, 101–104, 103t
    dipyridamole with, 619
  in electrocardiography, 246–247
  hemodynamic responses to, 242–243
  in perfusion imaging, 235–236
    accuracy of, 247t, 247–249
    compared to dobutamine stress echocardiography, 104–105
    in left bundle branch block with coronary artery disease, 229, 230t
    in preoperative assessment of vascular disease, 587
    prognostic evaluation with, 551f, 552
    in women and in men, 180–181, 181f
  side effects of, 245, 245t
Albumin microspheres, radiolabeled, in myocardial perfusion studies, 424
Ambulatory ECG
  compared to stress echocardiography, 606–607
  left ventricular hypertrophy affecting, 197, 197f
Ammonia labeled with nitrogen-13, in myocardial perfusion studies, 422–423
Angina pectoris
  coronary flow in, 34
  stable
    exercise ECG in, 500t, 500–501, 501t
    perfusion imaging in, 545–547, 546f
  unstable
    exercise ECG in, 501
    perfusion imaging in, 547
    prognostic evaluation in, 494
    and restenosis after angioplasty, 335
    stress echocardiography in, 514

Angiography
  compared to exercise echocardiography, 80t, 83f
  compared to perfusion imaging, 539–540, 540f, 541f–542f
  compared to transtenotic pressure gradient measurements, 296f
  conventional, 266–267
  digital subtraction, 35
  in end-stage renal failure with coronary artery disease, 203–204
  limitations of, 126, 299, 300f
    in restenosis after angioplasty, 328–333, 330f–332f
  in preoperative assessment of vascular disease, 589
  prognostic value of, 495–496, 496f
  quantitative, 267
  radionuclide
    accuracy of, 616
    compared to exercise echocardiography, 619
    in diagnosis and assessment of disease, 616
    exercise with, 69–70, 87, 88t, 517
    in left ventricular function evaluation, 74, 77–79, 79f, 87, 517–521. *See also* Ventriculography, radionuclide
    obsolescence of, 616–617
    prognostic value of, 617
  reference segments in, 301–302, 302f
  repeat studies after angioplasty, 346
  in restenosis after angioplasty, 325–328, 327f, 327t
    limitations of, 328–333, 330f–332f
Angioplasty. *See also* Interventional therapy
  and assessment with stress echocardiography, 355–365
  remodeling after, 325, 326f
  restenosis after, 324f, 324–333. *See also* Restenosis after angioplasty
Antimyosin with flow tracers, in myocardial viability assessment, 410
Aortic stenosis, and risk of noncardiac surgery, 573–574

Arbutamine stress, 236, 239–242, 241f
  accuracy of, 250t, 250–253
  in echocardiography, 241–242, 600
    accuracy of, 250
  hemodynamic responses to, 244
  in perfusion imaging, accuracy of, 250, 250t
  side effects of, 245t, 246
Artifacts
  in intravascular ultrasonography, 304, 304f
  in perfusion imaging, 528
  in women, 179
Asymptomatic patients
  exercise ECG in, 127–128, 130t–131t
    and hemodynamic changes in silent ischemia, 560
    positive tests in, 133, 137–138
  as high-risk subjects, 128
  and prognostic evaluation in silent ischemia, 333–334, 337, 540–544, 544f, 545f
Atherosclerosis. *See also* Coronary artery disease
  in cardiac transplant recipients, 316f, 317f, 317–318
  clinical features of, 34
  coronary flow reserve in, 34, 263, 265f
  fatty streaks in, 34, 126
  intravascular ultrasound in, 267, 269–273, 304–306, 305f–308f
  lesion morphology and ischemia in, 525–527, 526f, 527f
  occult lesions in, 126
  plaques in, 34, 126
    rupture of, 34, 126
  prevalence of, 125–126
  reference segment disease in, 301–302, 302f
  vascular remodeling in, 300–301, 301f
Atrial pacing. *See* Pacing stress
Atropine in stress tests, 236
  with dipyridamole, 236, 237
  with dobutamine, 236, 238, 238f
  with pacing, 242

627

B

Backscatter variations, in stunned myocardium, 488
Bayesian analysis
 in assessment of disease probability in women, 167–168
 in exercise ECG, 3, 158–162
 gender affecting, 147
 in perfusion imaging compared to stress echocardiography, 107–108, 108f
Bicycle exercise
 in echocardiography, 69, 81
  compared to other techniques, 85t
 in electrocardiography, 5–6
 in radionuclide angiography, 70
Blood flow. See Coronary blood flow
Blood pressure
 exercise affecting, 5
 in exercise ECG, 12
  monitoring of, 9
 and risk of noncardiac surgery in hypertension, 574, 578t
BMIPP. See β-Methyliodophenylpentadecanoic acid
Borg Scale in exercise ECG, 8t
Bridging, myocardial, intracoronary studies in, 314
Bruce protocol in exercise ECG, 8
Bundle branch block, left, 223–230. See also Left bundle branch block
Bypass surgery, and assessment with stress echocardiography, 355–365. See also Interventional therapy

C

Calcification
 of atheroma, intravascular ultrasound of, 305–306, 306f, 307f
 coronary, screening for, 135–137, 136f
Carbon-11 acetate, in myocardial metabolism assessment, 427–429
Carbon-11 palmitate, in myocardial metabolism assessment, 426–427
Chest pain syndromes, acute, prognostic evaluation in, 493–494
Chronotropic incompetence, 13
Computerized ECG interpretation, 6, 21–26
Contrast echocardiography, 234, 235f
 in myocardial viability assessment, 486–488
Copper-62-PTSM, in positron emission tomography, 48t, 51
Coronary artery disease
 coronary flow reserve in, 34, 263, 265f

decision tree in suspected disease, 544f, 544–545, 545f
diagnosis in women, 177–178
 multivariate approaches in, 147–164
 perfusion imaging in, 177–187
 stress echocardiography in, 167–174
echocardiography in. See Echocardiography
economic costs of, 126
electrocardiography in. See Electrocardiography
and hypothesis of "stenosis at risk," 525–528
left ventricular dysfunction in, 559–560
localization of lesions using stress echocardiography, 82t, 82–83
 compared to perfusion imaging, 105, 106f
natural history of, 499–500
perfusion imaging in. See Perfusion imaging
prognostic evaluation of, 492–493, 493t
 perfusion imaging in, 525–553
 radionuclide angiography in, 518t, 518–519
 stress echocardiography in, 510, 510t
risk of noncardiac surgery in, 572–573, 577–579, 578t
screening for, 125–141
stenosis measurements. See also Pressure measurements in coronary stenosis
 intravascular ultrasound in, 267, 269–273
 relationship to flow, 268–269, 273–274
vascular disease with, 581, 582f
Coronary blood flow
 in acute ischemia, 34–35
 in angina, 34
 in atherosclerosis, 34
 basal and maximal, relationship of, 261, 263f
 and coronary arterial pressure, 261, 262f
 insufficiency at rest, 35
 measurements of, 35–36, 266–268
  angiography in. See Angiography
  comparison of methods in, 274–275
  Doppler catheter in, 273, 307
  Doppler flow-wire in, 273–274, 307
  invasive, 35–36
  noninvasive, 36
  perfusion imaging in. See Perfusion imaging
  PET scans in, 267–269

transtenotic pressure gradient in, 274, 282–285. See also Pressure measurements in coronary stenosis
 velocity in, 273, 302, 308–309
microcirculation in, 282, 369–370
 pathophysiology of, 282
normal physiology of, 33
reserve, 33, 261–264
 absolute, 264–266, 285, 286t, 288f, 372
 in coronary artery disease, 34, 263, 265f
 and flow velocity, 309–312, 310f, 311f
 fractional, pressure-derived, 274, 285–291
 in left ventricular hypertrophy, 194t, 194–195, 207, 262, 264f, 312
 relation to stenosis, 370–373
 relative, 264–266, 285, 286t, 288f, 372
 schematic models of, 287f, 288f
 stenosis affecting, 268–269, 273–274
 variability of, 266
 velocity measurements, 273, 302, 308–309
  diastolic to systolic ratio in, 309
  and flow reserve, 309–312, 310f, 311f
  proximal to distal ratio in, 309, 310f–311f
Coronary ostia disease, intracoronary studies in, 313
Cost analysis
 of coronary artery disease effects, 126
 of exercise ECG as screening tool, 139–141
 in noninvasive testing, 113–122
  calculation of costs in, 114
  data used in, 116, 116t
  and effectiveness of cardiac care, 113–114
  with intermediate probability of disease, 118–119, 121f
  with low to intermediate probability of disease, 116–118, 117f, 118f, 119f, 120f
  Medicare reimbursements in, 122, 122t
 in preoperative evaluation, 577t
 pretest probability of disease affecting, 115–116
 sensitivity analysis of model in, 114–115, 115t, 119–120
 in preoperative cardiac risk assessment, 577t, 593
 of stress echocardiography compared to perfusion imaging, 621

in women, 172–173, 173t
Culprit lesion identification
    perfusion imaging in, 375, 377, 380
    stress echocardiography in, 356
Cycle ergometers. *See* Bicycle exercise

D

Decision-making
    and exercise ECG in screening for disease, 137f, 137–141, 140f
    and perfusion imaging after revascularization, 380–382
    postinfarction, 552f, 553
    in preoperative risk assessment, 695f
    prognostic evaluation in, 491
    in suspected coronary artery disease, 544f, 544–545, 545f
Detsky score in cardiac risk assessment, 575, 575f, 590t, 598
Diabetes mellitus
    and end-stage renal failure with coronary artery disease, 203–220
    and restenosis after angioplasty, 335
Dialysis patients with end-stage renal failure and coronary artery disease, 204–205
    coronary revascularization in, 204–205, 205f
Digital echocardiography, 73f, 73–74
Digital subtraction angiography, 35
Dipyridamole stress
    atropine with, 236, 237
    dobutamine with, 236, 237, 242, 242f
    in echocardiography, 71, 237–238, 599
        accuracy of, 248t, 249
        adenosine with, 619
        after infarction, 516
        in assessment of angioplasty effects, 358
        compared to dobutamine, 252, 253t, 605–606
        compared to other echocardiographic techniques, 84, 85t
        compared to perfusion imaging, 101–104, 103t
        early after bypass surgery, 363
        in myocardial viability assessment, 357
        in preoperative evaluation of vascular disease, 600–601, 601t
        prognostic value of, 513–514
        in restenosis detection after angioplasty, 360, 360t
        in women, 173–174
    in electrocardiography, 246
    exercise with, 236
    hemodynamic responses to, 242
    oral administration of, 247
    in perfusion imaging, 235, 236, 237f, 237–238
        accuracy of, 247t, 247–249
        compared to dobutamine stress echocardiography, 104–105
        in rubidium-82 PET imaging, left ventricular hypertrophy affecting, 199
        side effects of, 244, 245t
        with technetium-99m-sestamibi, in preoperative assessment of vascular disease, 586–587, 587f
    in thallium scintigraphy
        compared to exercise stress, 534
        compared to stress echocardiography, 607
        in end-stage renal failure with coronary artery disease, 207, 211, 212f
        in left bundle branch block with coronary artery disease, 229, 230t
        in left ventricular hypertrophy, 197f, 197–198
        in preoperative assessment, 576, 582, 583t
        prognostic value of, 530t
        in restenosis prediction, 376
        and transient left ventricular dilatation, 532, 533f, 552
        uptake in low-flow areas, 387
        in vascular disease, 574
Discriminant analysis, diagnostic value of, 155
Dobutamine stress, 236
    accuracy of, 250t, 250–253, 251f, 252f, 252t
    atropine with, 236, 238, 238f
    dipyridamole with, 236, 237, 242, 242f
    in echocardiography, 70–71, 75f, 238f, 238–239, 239f, 240f–241f, 599–600, 619
        accuracy of, 250–253, 251f, 252f, 252t
        after infarction, 515
        in assessment of angioplasty effects, 358
        in bypass graft patency assessment, 364t, 364–365
        in chronic left ventricular ischemic dysfunction, 479–481, 480t, 481f
        combined with scintigraphy, 484–485
        compared to dipyridamole, 252, 253t, 605–606
        compared to exercise ECG, 252–253
        compared to nuclear medicine techniques, 481–484
        compared to other echocardiographic techniques, 84, 85t
        compared to perfusion imaging, 100–101, 103t, 104–105, 620
        compared to vasodilator stress, 252, 253t
        early after infarction, 477–479, 478t, 479f
        in end-stage renal failure with coronary artery disease, 207, 214–220, 215t, 216t, 217f, 218f
        in left bundle branch block with coronary artery disease, 228–229, 229t, 230
        left ventricular hypertrophy affecting, 198
        limitations of, 494
        in myocardial viability assessment, 357, 476–486, 478f
        perfusion imaging with, 253
        in preoperative evaluation of cardiac risk, 576–577
        prognostic value of, 485, 485f, 512–513
        in restenosis detection after angioplasty, 360, 360t
        in vascular disease assessment, 574, 587, 601–602, 602f, 603f, 603t, 604t
    in electrocardiography, 247
        in detection of restenosis, 343
    hemodynamic responses to, 243f, 243–244
    in magnetic resonance imaging, 88–89, 89f, 238
    in perfusion imaging, 238
        accuracy of, 250, 250t
        echocardiography with, 253
    side effects of, 245t, 245–246
    with thallium-201
        in left bundle branch block with coronary artery disease, 230
        in preoperative assessment of vascular disease, 587–588
Doppler echocardiography, 72–73
    in assessment of angioplasty effects, 358–359
Doppler studies, intracoronary, 36, 306–312
    catheter in, 273, 307
    equipment in, 307–308
    flow guidance after interventional therapy, 348
    flow reserve in, 309–312, 310f, 311f
    flow velocity measurements, 273, 302, 308–309
    guidewires in, 273–274, 307–308
    physiology in, 306–307

Doppler studies, intracoronary
(Continued)
  technique in, 312
  turbulence in lesions, 312
Drug therapy
  affecting perfusion imaging, 529
  affecting stress echocardiography, 100
  after positive exercise ECG test, 138–139
  before vascular surgery, 593

E

Eagle score in cardiac risk assessment, 575, 590t
Echocardiography
  contrast, 234, 235f
    in myocardial viability assessment, 486–488
  digital, 73f, 73–74
  Doppler, 72–73
    in assessment of angioplasty effects, 358–359
    in left ventricular hypertrophy, 189–190, 190f
    stress methods in, 198
  in myocardial viability assessment, 475–488
    contrast agents in, 486–488
    dobutamine stress in, 476–486, 478f
  stress methods in, 69t, 69–71. *See also* Stress echocardiography
  transesophageal, 72
    and atrial pacing, 71. *See also* Pacing stress
    in bypass graft patency assessment, 365
    dobutamine stress in, 238, 240f–241f
    transgastric views of left ventricle in, 360f, 362f
  transthoracic, 71, 72f
    in bypass graft patency assessment, 364–365
Electrocardiography
  ambulatory
    compared to stress echocardiography, 606–607
    in left ventricular hypertrophy, 197, 197f
  exercise in. *See* Exercise ECG
  in left bundle branch block, 223
  in left ventricular hypertrophy, 189, 190–191, 197
  pharmacologic stress testing in, 246–247
  in detection of restenosis, 343
Enoximone stress, in echocardiography, 357

Ergometers, cycle. *See* Bicycle exercise
Exercise
  blood pressure in, 5
  capacity for, affecting stress tests, 233, 234f
  cardiovascular responses to, 3t
  in echocardiography. *See* Exercise echocardiography
  in electrocardiography. *See* Exercise ECG
  gender difference in performance of, 168
  heart rate in, 4–5, 12–13, 130
    relationship to ST segment, 24–25, 149–152
    in women, 152–153, 154f
  ischemia from, related to myocardial fractional flow reserve, 292–295, 293f, 294f, 295f
  isometric or static, 3
  isotonic or dynamic, 3
  left bundle branch block in, 223–224
  left ventricular response to
    clinical application of, 68–69
    in ischemia, 68
    in normal subjects, 67–68
  oxygen uptake in, 3–4, 12
  in perfusion imaging. *See* Exercise scintigraphy
  peripheral response to, 4
  with radionuclide angiography, 69–70, 87, 88t, 517
  simulating agents, 236
    in electrocardiography, 247
    hemodynamic responses to, 243f, 243–244
    side effects of, 245t, 245–246
  supine, exertion in, 69
  upright, exertion in, 69
Exercise ECG
  abnormal responses in, 13–19, 16f–18f
  criteria for, 129–132
  accuracy affected by gender, 148, 150t
  after bypass surgery, 363
  after infarction, prognostic value of, 548–549
  in asymptomatic population, 127–128, 130t–131t
    positive tests in, 133, 137–138
  blood pressure in, 12
    monitoring of, 9
  Borg Scale in, 8t
  clinical responses in, 11
  compared to perfusion imaging, 379, 538f, 538–539, 539f, 549
  compared to stress echocardiography, 83, 83f, 252–253
  computerized interpretation of, 6, 21–26

  controversial issues in, 24
  criteria for diagnosis in, 21t
  digital processing of data in, 21, 24
  ST segment and heart rate in, 24–26
  summary of studies with, 22t–23t
  conversion to positive tests in, 130–131
  cycle ergometers in, 5–6. *See also* Bicycle exercise
  development of, 2–3
  diagnostic value of, 1–26, 148
  duration of exercise in, 129
  and results in women, 153
  electrodes and cables in, 7
  endpoints in, 9, 129
  exercise capacity in, 12
  false-positive results in, 132
  in fitness assessment, 133
  heart rate adjustment in, 130
  hemodynamic responses in, 12–13
  in high risk patients, 131–132
  in high-risk professions, 133–135
  increased speed and grade in, 9
  indications for, 1, 504t
  interpretation of
    computerized, 6, 21–26
    newer principles in, 20t
  lead systems in, 7
    sensitivity of, 7–8
  in left bundle branch block with coronary artery disease, 225, 225t
  left ventricular hypertrophy affecting, 196–197, 197f
  limitations of, 67
  and multivariate analysis, 3, 128–129
  maximal exercise scores in, 153–162
  in men, 155–156, 156t, 157t
  in prognostic evaluation, 505t, 505–506
  in women, 156t, 156–158, 157t
  normal ECG responses in, 13
  patient preparation for, 6
  perceived exertion in, 12
  positive tests in
    in asymptomatic subjects, 133, 137–138
    conversion to, 130–131
    false-positive, 132
    and management of patients, 138–139
  and postexercise recovery, 11
  in preoperative evaluation of cardiac risk, 575–576
  pretest examination in, 6–7
  prognostic evaluation with, 499–506
    accuracy of, 128, 130t–131t
    compared to perfusion imaging, 538f, 538–539, 539f, 549
    multivariate analysis in, 505t, 505–506

in non-Q wave infarction, 502
in Q-wave infarction, 502–505
in stable angina, 500t, 500–501, 501t
in unstable angina, 501
in women, 503f, 505
protocols in, 8–9
Bruce, 8
and criteria for abnormalities, 129–131, 132f
optimal, 9
oxygen costs of, 10f
Q waves in, 15
R waves in, 15
in restenosis detection, 340–341, 341t
as screening tool
accuracy of, 127
and clinical decision-making, 137–141
cost effectiveness of, 139–141
indications for, 133–135
for women, 132–133
sensitivity and specificity of, 15, 18–19
ST segment in, 2, 13–15, 14f, 148
analysis in women, 148–149, 168–169
computerized interpretation of, 24–26
criteria for abnormality in, 129–130, 132f
depression of, 13–15, 133, 134f
diagnostic value of, 148
elevation of, 15
in left bundle branch block, 225
relationship to heart rate, 24–25
T waves in, 15
termination of, 9–11
treadmills in, 5–6
U waves in, 15
in vascular disease assessment, 589t, 589–590
in women, 19–21, 132–133, 147–164, 168–169, 177–178
compared to stress echocardiography, 170–171, 171f
factors affecting, 20t
multivariate analysis of, 156–158, 157t
prognostic value of, 504f, 505
workloads in, 8
Exercise echocardiography, 69, 599
in bypass graft patency assessment, 363–364, 364t
compared to perfusion imaging, 100–101, 102t, 104f, 619–621, 620t
compared to pharmacologic tests, 84–85
compared to radionuclide angiography, 619

in diagnosis and assessment of disease, 618–619
in end-stage renal failure with coronary artery disease, 216t, 216–218
prognostic value of, 510–512, 511t, 512t, 619
after infarction, 515
in restenosis detection, 342–343, 343t, 359–360, 360t
serial tests after angioplasty, 362
in women, 169–173
Exercise radionuclide angiography, 69–70, 87, 88t
Exercise scintigraphy
sestamibi in, 467, 534
thallium-201 in
compared to pharmacologic agents, 534
in left bundle branch block with coronary artery disease, 226, 226t
planar imaging in end-stage renal failure with coronary artery disease, 211–213, 213f
in preoperative evaluation, 576, 582
prognostic value of, 530t
in restenosis prediction, 375–376
SPECT images affected by left ventricular hypertrophy, 197f, 197–198
in women, 169, 179t, 179–181

F

Fatty acids labeled with iodine-123, 386, 402–409
iodophenylpentadecanoic acid (IPPA), 403–405
β-methyliodophenylpentadecanoic acid (BMIPP), 406–409
Fluorine-18 fluorodeoxyglucose
in myocardial metabolism assessment, 429–431, 430f
in myocardial viability assessment, 409
compared to dobutamine echocardiography, 484
Fluorodeoxyglucose labeled with fluorine-18
in myocardial metabolism assessment, 429–431, 430f
in myocardial viability assessment, 409
compared to dobutamine echocardiography, 484
Functional recovery related to myocardial viability, 385–386. *See also* Myocardial viability assessment
Functional testing
after interventional therapy, 323–348

exercise ECG in, 340–341, 341t
exercise echocardiography in, 342–343, 343t
new developments affecting, 347–348
perfusion imaging in, 380–382
psychological and work-related issues in, 345
radionuclide ventriculography in, 342
routine use of, 333–334
selective use of, 334–340
and symptomatic status at follow-up, 337–339, 338f–339f
test selection in, 340, 343–344
thallium scintigraphy in, 341–342, 342t
timing of, 344–345
benefits of, 495
and indices for pressure measurements in coronary stenosis, 281–282
left ventricular. *See* Left ventricular function evaluation
in prognostic evaluation, 491–496

G

Gas washout techniques in coronary flow measurement, 36
Glycoprotein IIb/IIIa inhibition, and restenosis after angioplasty, 347
Goldman index of cardiac risk assessment, 572t, 574–575, 575t, 588t, 588–589, 589f, 590t, 598

H

Heart block, left bundle branch, 223–230
Heart failure, and risk of noncardiac surgery, 573
Heart rate in exercise, 4–5, 12–13, 130
relationship to ST segment, 24–25, 149–152
in women, 152–153, 154f
Heart transplant recipients, atherosclerosis in, 316f, 317f, 317–318
Hemodialysis in end-stage renal failure with coronary artery disease, 204–205
Hibernating myocardium, 35, 386, 476
chronic, 479–480
identification of
clinical parameters in, 560
hemodynamic parameters in, 560–561
PET imaging in, 561

Hibernating myocardium *(Continued)*
  prognostic significance of, 562t, 562–565, 563f
  and severe left ventricular dysfunction, 378
High-risk professions, 133–135
High-risk subjects, 131–132
  asymptomatic, 128
Hypertension, and risk of noncardiac surgery, 574, 578t
Hypertrophy of left ventricle. *See* Left ventricular hypertrophy

I

Infarction, myocardial
  non-Q wave, exercise ECG in, 502
  prognostic evaluation of, 494–495
    exercise ECG in, 502–505, 548–549
    with fixed defects, 550
    myocardial viability and residual ischemia in, 550–551
    perfusion imaging in, 547–553, 551f, 552f
    radionuclide angiography in, 519–521, 520t
    with "reverse-redistribution" defect, 550
    with reversible defect, 549–550
    stress echocardiography in, 514–517, 515t
  Q-wave, exercise ECG in, 502–505
  and risk of noncardiac surgery, 573
  risk stratification after, 547–548
Interventional therapy
  in dialysis patients, 204–205, 205f
  functional testing after, 323–348
  intracoronary studies in, 316–317
  perfusion imaging in, 369–382
    indications for, 374–379
    postoperative, 373–374
    preoperative, 373, 373f
    timing of, 374, 374f
  PET metabolic imaging in, 439–451
  prediction of results in. *See* Prognostic evaluation
  and restenosis after angioplasty, 324f, 324–333
  stress echocardiography in, 355–365
    after therapy, 357–365
    indications for, 355, 356t
    limitations of, 365
    prior to therapy, 355–357
  before vascular surgery, 591–593
Intracoronary studies
  in ambiguous lesions, 314
  in cardiac transplant recipients, 316f, 317f, 317–318
  clinical applications of, 312–318
  in coronary ostia disease, 313
  Doppler measurements, 36, 306–312
  indications for, 312–318
  intravascular ultrasound, 267, 269–273, 299–306. *See also* Ultrasound, intravascular
  in ischemia with "normal arteries," 314–315
  in left main lesions, 313, 314f
  in lesions of uncertain severity, 315f, 315–316
  in myocardial bridging, 314
  in percutaneous interventions, 316–317
Iodine-123, fatty acids labeled with, 386, 402–409
  iodophenylpentadecanoic acid (IPPA), 403–405
  β-methyliodophenylpentadecanoic acid (BMIPP), 406–409
Iodophenylpentadecanoic acid (IPPA), 403–405
  myocardial uptake and metabolism of, 403–404, 404f
  in myocardial viability assessment, 404–405, 406f
  structure of, 403f
IPPA. *See* Iodophenylpentadecanoic acid
Ischemia
  coronary flow in, 34–35
  exercise-induced, relation to myocardial fractional flow reserve, 292–295, 293f, 294f, 295f
  from increased oxygen demand, 613–614, 615
  and left ventricular response to exercise, 68
  and "normal coronary arteries," 314–315
  pathophysiology of, 613–615
  perioperative risk of, 597–598
  from reduced coronary supply, 613, 614–615
  silent. *See* Asymptomatic patients

L

Left bundle branch block, 223–230
  coronary artery disease detection in, 225–230
    apical perfusion defects in, 227–228, 228t
    exercise ECG in, 225, 225t
    false-positive perfusion defects in, 226–227
    perfusion scintigraphy in, 225–228, 226t, 227t, 228t
    radionuclide ventriculography in, 228
    reversible septal perfusion defects in, 227, 227t
    stress echocardiography in, 228–229, 229t
  exercise-induced, 223–224
  resting, 223
  wall motion abnormalities in, 224f, 224–225
Left ventricular function evaluation, 67–90
  clinical applications of, 79–89
  detection of reversible dysfunction in, 561–562
  digital echocardiography in, 73f, 73–74
  Doppler echocardiography in, 72–73
  hibernation in. *See* Hibernating myocardium
  imaging techniques in, 71–76
  interpretation of, 76–79
  magnetic resonance imaging in, 74–76
  stress tests with, 87–89
  as prognostic guide, 598–606
  prognostic value of PET in, 559–567
  radionuclide angiography in, 74, 517–521
    interpretation of, 77–79, 79f
    stress tests with, 87
  and response to exercise
    clinical application of, 68–69
    in ischemia, 68
    in normal subjects, 67–68
  and size of left ventricle in women, 182, 183f
  stress methodologies in, 69t, 69–71
    echocardiography, 79–87, 509–517
    interpretation of, 76–77, 77t, 78f
    magnetic resonance imaging, 87–89
    radionuclide angiography, 87
  stunning in. *See* Stunned myocardium
  transesophageal echocardiography in, 72
  and transient dilatation in perfusion imaging, 532, 533f, 552
  transthoracic two-dimensional echocardiography in, 71, 72
Left ventricular hypertrophy, 189–200
  affecting diagnostic tests for coronary artery disease, 195–196, 196t
    in exercise ECG, 196–197, 197f
    in positron emission tomography, 199
    in stress echocardiography, 198
    in stress thallium scintigraphy, 197f, 197–198
  coronary flow reserve in, 194t, 194–195, 207, 262, 264f
  echocardiography in, 189–190, 190f, 198
  electrocardiography in, 189, 190–191, 196–197, 197f

in end-stage renal failure with coronary artery disease, 218–220
and myocardial ischemia, 195
prognosis of, 191–193, 193f
and risk of coronary artery disease, 191, 192f, 192t
in women, 192f, 192t
Lung thallium uptake, 532, 533f
in women, 179

M

Magnetic resonance imaging
dobutamine stress with, 88–89, 89f, 238
in left ventricular function test, 74–76
Medications. See Drug therapy
2-Methoxy-2-isobutyl-isonitrile (MIBI). See Sestamibi labeled with technetium-99m
β-Methyliodophenylpentadecanoic acid (BMIPP), 406–409
distribution compared to flow tracers, 406–407
myocardial uptake and metabolism of, 406, 407f
in myocardial viability assessment, 407–408
structure of, 403f
MIBI. See Sestamibi labeled with technetium-99m
Microcirculation, coronary, 282, 369–370
Microspheres, radiolabeled, in myocardial perfusion studies, 424, 425
Multivariate analysis in exercise ECG tests, 3, 128–129
maximal exercise scores in, 153–162
in men, 155–156, 156t, 157t
variables in, 505t, 505–506
in women, 156t, 156–158, 157t
Myocardial viability assessment
choice of technique in, 463–470
in sequential and combined approaches, 469
clinical role of, 463–464
definitions in, 475–476
echocardiography in, 475–488
contrast agents in, 486–488
dobutamine stress in, 357, 476–486, 478f
perfusion imaging in, prognostic value of, 550–551
PET imaging in, 357, 398–399, 400f, 402, 402t, 431–452, 467–469, 561. See also PET (positron emission tomography)
relation to functional recovery, 385–386
SPECT tracers in, 385–411

N

Nitrates
with sestamibi labeled with technetium-99m, 397t, 401, 467
with thallium-201, 396
Nitrogen-13 ammonia
in myocardial perfusion studies, 422–423
in positron emission tomography, 48t, 49
kinetic models for, 49t, 50f
Nuclear cardiology. See Angiography, radionuclide; Perfusion imaging; Ventriculography, radionuclide

O

Oxygen
costs in exercise protocols, 10f
increased demand causing ischemia, 613–614, 615
myocardial consumption in exercise, 4
uptake in exercise, 3–4, 12
Oxygen-15 water
in myocardial perfusion studies, 423
in positron emission tomography, 48t, 49–50

P

Pacing stress, 242
accuracy of, 253–254
echocardiography with, 242
hemodynamic responses to, 244
in perfusion imaging, 242, 254
side effects of, 246
with thallium-201
in preoperative assessment of vascular disease, 588
prognostic value of, 530t
transesophageal atrial, and echocardiography, 71, 84, 85t, 253–254
after infarction, 516–517
in restenosis detection after angioplasty, 360t, 360–362, 361f
Palmitate labeled with carbon-11, in myocardial metabolism assessment, 426–427
Perfusion imaging, 1–25
adenosine in, 235–236. See also Adenosine stress, in perfusion imaging
advantages and disadvantages of, 98t, 99–100
analysis of data in, 46–48
normal maps in, 48
polar maps in, 47–48
quantitative approaches in, 14–15
semiquantitative approaches in, 46–48
arbutamine stress in, accuracy of, 250, 250t
artifacts in, 528
compared to coronary angiography, 539–540, 540f, 541f–542f
compared to exercise ECG, 379, 538f, 538–539, 539f, 549
compared to nuclear ventriculography, 534–536, 536t
compared to other studies, clinical status in, 536–538, 537f
compared to stress echocardiography, 85–87, 86t, 97–110, 380, 536, 607
in assessment of disease extent, 105–107
Bayesian analysis of, 107–108, 108f
in detection of coronary artery disease, 101, 104f
with dobutamine stress, 100–101, 103t, 104–105, 620
with exercise stress, 619–621, 620t
in localization of coronary artery lesions, 105, 106f
sensitivity and specificity in, 104f, 106f
coronary reserve in, 371–373
cost and availability of, 528
cost-benefit ratio in, 621
in culprit lesion identification in multivessel disease, 375, 377, 380
in diagnosis and assessment of disease, 615–616
diagnostic performance of, 54–57
dipyridamole in, 235, 236, 237f, 237–238. See also Dipyridamole stress
dobutamine stress in, 238
accuracy of, 250, 250t
echocardiography with, 253
dual isotope approach in, 45
in end-stage renal failure with coronary artery disease, 206–214, 208t–210t
exercise stress in. See Exercise scintigraphy
flow tracers in, 36–41, 387–391
indications for, 529
interpretation of, 528–529
in interventional therapy, 369–382
after angioplasty, 375–376, 380, 381
after bypass surgery, 363, 376–378, 381–382
in bypass graft disease identification, 376–378, 377t
and clinical decisions after revascularization, 380–382

Perfusion imaging *(Continued)*
    compared to other techniques, 379–380
    dysfunctioning myocardium in, 381–382
    in early postoperative period, 374–375
    follow-up studies in, 375, 378
    in incomplete revascularization, 379
    indications for, 374–379
    normal left ventricular function in, 380–381
    postoperative, 373–374
    preoperative, 373, 373f
    restenosis prediction in, 375–376
    timing of, 374, 374f
  in left bundle branch block with coronary artery disease, 225–228, 226t, 227t, 228t
  limitations of, 528–529
  medical therapy affecting, 529
  new stressors in, 587–588
  new tracers in, 586–587, 587f
  pacing stress in, 242, 254
  PET images in, 36, 48–54. *See also* PET (positron emission tomography)
  planar imaging in, 45, 54, 55t–56t. *See also* Thallium-201, planar imaging
  in preoperative evaluation of cardiac risk, 576
  in vascular disease, 581–593
  prognostic value of, 525–553, 615–616
    after infarction, 547–553, 551f, 552f
    compared to other techniques, 534–540
    in coronary artery disease, 545–547, 546f
    decision tree in, 552f, 553
    defect extent in, 531, 531f
    normal scintigraphy in, 529–530
    reversible versus fixed defects in, 531–532
    selection of technique in, 551f, 552f, 552–553
    in silent ischemia, 540–544, 544f, 545f
  protocols for, 41–45, 43f
    reinjection protocols in, 38, 42–44, 43f
  SPECT images in, 45–48. *See also* SPECT (single photon emission tomography)
    gated, 46
  technetium-99m-labeled radiopharmaceuticals in, 38–41, 387–388. *See also* Sestamibi labeled with technetium-99m
    protocols for, 43f, 44–45
  techniques in, 45–46
  postinfarction selection of, 551f, 552f, 552–553
  thallium-201 in, 36–38, 387. *See also* Thallium-201
    protocols for, 41–44, 43f
  vasodilator stress in, 234–236
    accuracy of, 247t, 247–249
  in women, 177–187
    accuracy of exercise SPECT in, 179t, 179–180, 180f
    breast attenuation artifacts in, 179
    in diagnosis of coronary artery disease, 179–182
    lung thallium uptake in, 179
    prognostic assessment with, 182–187, 183t–184t, 184f, 185t, 185f–186f
    results with adenosine SPECT thallium imaging, 180–181, 181f
Peripheral vascular disease. *See* Vascular disease
PET (positron emission tomography), 36, 48–54
  combined with dobutamine echocardiography, 484–485
  in coronary flow measurements, 52t, 52–54, 267–268, 424–426
    and coronary stenosis severity, 268–269, 270f–272f
    limitations of, 53–54
  diagnostic performance of, 55t–56t, 57
  in follow-up after revascularization, 378–379
  left ventricular hypertrophy affecting, 199
  methodology in cardiac imaging, 417–420, 418f, 420f
  in myocardial metabolism assessment, 426–431
    carbon-11 acetate in, 427–429
    carbon-11 palmitate in, 426–427
    fluorine-18 fluorodeoxyglucose in, 429–431, 430f
  in myocardial viability assessment, 357, 398–399, 400f, 402, 402t, 431–452, 467–469, 561
    absolute perfusion measurements in, 434–435, 436f
    compared to dobutamine echocardiography, 484
    correlation with histopathologic findings, 445–451, 448f–450f
    fluorine-18 fluorodeoxyglucose in, 439–441, 440t
    metabolic imaging in, 439–451
    oxidative metabolism assessment in, 441–443
    and prediction of functional recovery after revascularization, 440t, 444–445, 467–469, 468t
    quantitative techniques in, 443–444
    relative perfusion measurements in, 432–434, 433f
    rubidium-82 tissue kinetics in, 438–439
    water perfusable index in, 435–438
  nitrogen-13 ammonia in, 422–423, 425
  oxygen-15 water in, 423, 425
  prognostic value of, 559–567
    and management decisions, 564f–565f, 565–566, 567f
  quantitation of tracer concentrations in, 420–422, 421f
  rubidium-82 in, 48t, 50–51, 423, 425
    in left ventricular hypertrophy, 199
    and tissue kinetics in myocardial viability assessment, 438–439
  techniques in, 51–52
  tracers used in, 48t, 48–51
    comparison of, 50f, 51
    metabolic, 426–431, 467–469
    perfusion, 422–426, 467
Pharmacologic stress testing, 69t, 70–71, 233–254. *See also specific pharmacologic agents*
  accuracy of, 247–254
  adenosine in, 238
  arbutamine in, 239–242
  dipyridamole in, 237–238
  dobutamine in, 238f, 238–239, 239f
  in echocardiography, 70–71
    compared to perfusion imaging, 101–104, 103t
    in women, 173–174
  in electrocardiography, 246–247
  exercise simulation in, 236
  hemodynamic responses to, 242–244
  indications for, 122–234
  in perfusion imaging, compared to dobutamine stress echocardiography, 104–105
  side effects of, 244–246, 245t
  vasodilators in, 234–236
Positron emission tomography (PET), 36, 48–54. *See also* PET (positron emission tomography)
Preoperative evaluation in noncardiac surgery, 571–579, 572t
  in aortic stenosis, 573–574
  in coronary artery disease, 572–573, 577–579, 578t
  cost of stress tests in, 577t
  Detsky score in, 575, 575t, 590t, 598
  dobutamine stress echocardiography in, 576–577

Eagle score in, 575, 590t
exercise ECG in, 575–576
Goldman index in, 572t, 574–575, 575t, 588t, 588–589, 589f, 590t, 598
in heart failure, 573
in hypertension, 574, 578t
noninvasive testing in, 575–577
perfusion imaging in, 576
in vascular disease, 576, 581–593
in recent infarction, 573
in vascular disease, 574, 578t
perfusion imaging in, 576, 581–593
Pressure measurements in coronary stenosis, 281–296
anatomic and functional indices in, 281–282
balloon catheters affecting, 282, 283f
fractional flow reserve in, pressure-derived, 274, 285–291
advantages and limitations of, 288–289
collateral, 288
coronary, 287–288
myocardial, 287
relation to exercise-induced ischemia, 292–295, 293f, 294f, 295f
reproducibility of calculations, 202f, 289–291
validation of calculations, 289, 290f, 291f
translesional pressure gradient in, 274, 282–285
compared to coronary angiography, 296f
effects of guidewires in, 284–285, 285f, 286f
fluid-filled guidewires in, 283–284, 284f
high-fidelity guidewires in, 282–283
Prognostic evaluation
in acute coronary syndromes, 493–495
in chronic ischemic left ventricular dysfunction, 493
coronary angiography in, 495–496, 496f
dobutamine echocardiography in, 485, 485f
exercise ECG in, 499–506
accuracy of, 128, 130t–131t
after infarction, 502–505, 548–549
in angina, 500t, 500–501, 501t
multivariate analysis of, 505t, 505–506
in women, 503f, 505
functional testing in, 491–496
in known coronary artery disease, 492–493, 493t
in left ventricular hypertrophy, 191–193, 193f

perfusion imaging in, 525–553, 615–616
in women, 182–187, 183t–184t, 184f, 185t, 185f–186f
positron emission tomography in, 559–567
in preoperative patients, 571–579, 572t, 578t
radionuclide angiography in, 517–521
in silent ischemia, 333–334, 337, 540–544, 544f, 545f
stress echocardiograhpy in, 509–517
Psychological issues in functional tests after interventional therapy, 345

Q

Q waves in exercise ECG, 15
in infarction, 502–505
QRS interval in left bundle branch block, 223

R

R wave in exercise ECG, 15
Radionuclide studies. See Angiography, radionuclide; Perfusion imaging; Ventriculography, radionuclide
Redistribution of thallium-201, 37–38, 38f, 387, 464
Referral bias, and disease diagnosis in women, 147, 171–172, 172f
Remodeling, vascular
after angioplasty, 325, 326f
in atherosclerosis, 300–301, 301f
Renal failure, end-stage, with coronary artery disease, 203–220
angiography in, 203–204
in dialysis patients, 204–205
identification of low-risk patients in, 214
noninvasive diagnostic strategies in, 205–220
perfusion imaging in, 206–214, 208t–210t
stress echocardiography in, 214–220, 215t, 216t, 217f, 218f
in transplantation candidates, 204, 217f, 218f, 219f
Reserve
flow, 33, 261–264
resistance, 282
Resistance in coronary microcirculation, 282
Restenosis after angioplasty, 324f, 324–333

anatomic factors in, 335–336
angiography in, 325–328, 327f, 327t
correlation with functional tests, 328–333
dissociation from clinical symptoms, 328, 329f
clinical implications of, 339–340
clinical symptoms in, 325–328, 327t
dissociation from angiographic findings, 328, 329f
detection with stress echocardiography, 359–362
in incomplete revascularization, 337
prediction with perfusion imaging, 375–376
probability of, 334–336
procedures affecting, 336
residual stenosis in, 336–337
variables affecting, 333t, 335
Revascularization procedures. See Interventional therapy
Ribose infusions, with thallium-201, 387, 396
Risk reduction strategies
after positive exercise ECG test, 138
future studies of, 608–609
Risk stratification
after infarction, perfusion imaging in, 547–548
clinical approach to, 598
before noncardiac surgery, 571–579, 572t
perfusion imaging in, 583–593
stress echocardiography in, 597–609
Rubidium-82 PET imaging, 48t, 50–51
left ventricular hypertrophy affecting, 199
in myocardial perfusion studies, 423, 425
tissue kinetics in myocardial viability assessment, 438–439

S

Scintigraphy for perfusion imaging. See Perfusion imaging
Screening for coronary artery disease, 125–141
calcifications identified in, 135–137, 136f
exercise testing in, 126–135
accuracy of, 127–128
in asymptomatic population, 127–128
and clinical decision-making, 137f, 137–141, 140f
conversion to positive test in, 130–131

Screening for coronary artery disease *(Continued)*
  cost effectiveness of, 139–141
    criteria for abnormality in, 129–130, 132f
    false-positive results in, 132
    hard versus soft endpoints in, 129
    heart rate adjustment in, 130
    in high-risk patients, 131–132
    indications for, 133–135
    multivariate adjustment in, 128–129
    prevalence of positive tests in, 133
    prognostic significance of, 128, 130t–131t
    in women, 132–133
Screening for suitability for exercise testing, 502
Sestamibi labeled with technetium-99m, 38–39, 39f, 43f, 387–388, 615
  in bypass graft disease detection, 377f
  compared to stress echocardiography, 86t
  compared to thallium-201, 388–389, 389f, 390f, 397–398, 398f–400f, 467, 534, 535f, 552–553
  dipyridamole with, in preoperative assessment of vascular disease, 586–587, 587f
  distribution compared to BMIPP, 407
  exercise with, 467, 534
  left ventricular hypertrophy affecting, 198
  in myocardial viability assessment, 396–401, 466–467
    compared to thallium-201, 397–398, 398f–400f
    exercise studies in, 467
    predictive accuracy of, 397t, 397–398
    resting studies in, 466, 467t
    results compared to PET imaging, 398–399, 400f, 402, 402t
  net uptake related to cellular metabolism, 387–388
  nitrates with, 397t, 401, 467
  redistribution images, 401
  in restenosis detection, 342t
  in simultaneous evaluation of flow and function, 467
  in SPECT imaging
    compared to stress echocardiography, 86t
    gated data acquisition in, 46
    in left bundle branch block with coronary artery disease, 226t, 226–228
    in myocardial viability assessment, 396–402

  prognostic value of, 530t
  uptake in low-flow areas, 388
Silent ischemia. *See* Asymptomatic patients
SPECT (single photon emission tomography), 36, 45–48
  compared to stress echocardiography, 86t
  in coronary flow measurements, 45–48
  diagnostic performance of, 54–57, 55t–56t
  gated, 46
  gender differences in accuracy of, 181–183, 183t
  in left bundle branch block with coronary artery disease, 226t, 226–228
    compared to stress echocardiography, 228–229
  in myocardial viability assessment, 385–411
    antimyosin in, 410
    flow tracers in, 387–402
    fluorine-18 fluorodeoxyglucose in, 409
    iodine-123 free fatty acids in, 386, 402–409
    metabolic tracers in, 402–409
    technetium-99m-sestamibi in, 396–402
    thallium-201 in, 389–396
  technetium-99m-sestamibi in
    compared to stress echocardiography, 86t
    gated data acquisition in, 46
    in left bundle branch block with coronary artery disease, 226t, 227t, 228t
    in myocardial viability assessment, 396–402
    prognostic value of, 530t
  thallium in. *See* Thallium-201, in SPECT
ST segment
  analysis in women, 168–169
  in exercise ECG, 2, 13–15, 14f
    criteria for abnormality in, 129–130, 132f
    relationship to heart rate, 24–25
Stents, intracoronary, affecting restenosis, 347–348
Stress ECG
  exercise in, 1–26. *See also* Exercise ECG
  pharmacologic stress in, 246–247
Stress echocardiography
  accuracy of vasodilator stress in, 248t, 249
  adenosine in, 71, 238, 599. *See also* Adenosine stress, in echocardiography
  advantages and disadvantages of, 98t, 98–99
  arbutamine in, 241–242, 600

  accuracy of, 250
  in assessment of angioplasty effects, 357–359, 358t
  in assessment of stenosis significance, 355–356
  in bypass graft patency assessment, 363–365, 364f, 364t
  compared to ambulatory ECG, 606–607
  compared to coronary angiography, 80t, 83f
  compared to exercise ECG, 83, 83f, 252–253
  compared to perfusion imaging, 85–87, 86t, 97–110, 380, 536, 607
    in assessment of disease extent, 105–107
    Bayesian analysis of, 107–108, 108f
    in detection of coronary artery disease, 101, 104f
    in localization of coronary artery lesions, 105, 106f
    sensitivity and specificity in, 104f, 106f
  cost-benefit ratio in, 621
  in culprit lesion identification in multivessel disease, 356
  in detection of coronary artery disease, 79–82
  dipyridamole in, 71, 237–238, 599. *See also* Dipyridamole stress, in echocardiography
  dobutamine in, 238f, 238–239, 239f, 240f–241f. *See also* Dobutamine stress, in echocardiography
  drug therapy affecting, 100
  early after bypass surgery, 363
  in end-stage renal failure with coronary artery disease, 206–214
  exercise in. *See* Exercise echocardiography
  factors affecting sensitivity of, 80t
  imaging techniques with, 71–76, 76f
  interpretation of, 76–77, 77t, 78f, 100
  in interventional therapy, 355–365
    after therapy, 357–365
    indications for, 355, 356t
    limitations of, 365
    prior to therapy, 355–357
  in left bundle branch block with coronary artery disease, 228–229, 229t
  in left ventricular function evaluation, 79–87, 509–517
  left ventricular hypertrophy affecting, 198
  in localization of coronary artery lesions, 82t, 82–83
  in myocardial viability assessment, 356–357, 475–488
  pacing in, 242

transesophageal. *See* Pacing stress, transesophageal atrial
pharmacologic tests in, 70–71
  compared to exercise tests, 84–85
  compared to perfusion imaging, 100–101, 103
  in women, 173–174
in preoperative assessment of vascular disease, 590–591, 597–609
prognostic value of, 509–517, 510t
  after infarction, 514–517, 515t
  compared to perfusion imaging, 536
  in unstable angina, 514
rapid recovery of wall motion in, 81f, 81–82
in restenosis detection after angioplasty, 359–362, 360t
strengths of, 618t
techniques in, 69t
  comparison of, 83–85, 85t
weaknesses of, 618t
in women, 167–174
  compared to exercise ECG, 170–171, 171f
  cost effectiveness of, 172–173, 173t
  pharmacologic stress in, 173–174
Stunned myocardium, 386, 476, 559–560
  backscatter signal in, 488
Surgery
  after positive exercise ECG test, 139
  noncardiac, evaluation of cardiac risk in, 571–579, 572t, 578t. *See also* Preoperative evaluation in noncardiac surgery
  physiologic stresses of, 571–572
  revascularization procedures in. *See* Interventional therapy
Sympathomimetic amines. *See* Arbutamine; Dobutamine

T

T wave in exercise ECG, 15
Teboroxime labeled with technetium-99m, 40–41, 42f, 43f, 586, 615
Technetium-99m-labeled radiopharmaceuticals, 38–41
  protocols for perfusion imaging, 43f, 44–45
    one-day, 44–45
    pre- and postintervention tracer injection, 45
    separate-day, 44
    with significant washout, 45
    without significant washout, 44–45
  sestamibi, 38–39, 39f, 43f, 387–388, 615. *See also* Sestamibi labeled with technetium-99m

teboroxime, 40–41, 42f, 43f, 586, 615
tetrofosmin, 39–40, 40f, 41f, 43f, 615
thallium-201 with, 45
Tetrofosmin labeled with technetium-99m, 39–40, 40f, 41f, 43f, 615
Thallium-201, 36–38
  adenosine with. *See* Adenosine stress, in perfusion imaging
  after angioplasty, 357
  biokinetics of, 36–37, 37f
  compared to stress echocardiography, 85–87, 86t, 97–110, 380, 536, 607
  compared to technetium-99m-sestamibi, 388–389.390f, 397–398, 398f–400f, 467, 534, 535f, 552–553
  dipyridamole with. *See* Dipyridamole stress
  distribution compared to BMIPP, 406–407
  dobutamine with
    in left bundle branch block with coronary artery disease, 230
    in preoperative assessment of vascular disease, 587–588
  exercise with. *See* Exercise scintigraphy
  lung uptake of, 532, 533f
    in women, 179
  in myocardial viability assessment, 389–396, 464–466
    compared to sestamibi, 397–398, 398f, 399f, 400f
    reinjection imaging in, 391–393, 392f, 393t, 394f
    rest-redistribution in, 393t, 393–396, 395f, 464–465, 465t
    results compared to PET imaging, 402, 402t
    stress-early redistribution in, 389–390, 391f
    stress-late redistribution in, 390–391, 393t
  net uptake related to cellular metabolism, 387
  nitrates with, 396
  pacing stress with
    in preoperative assessment of vascular disease, 588
    prognostic value of, 530t
  physical characteristics of, 36
  planar imaging
    compared to SPECT, 532–534
    compared to stress echocardiography, 86t
    diagnostic performance of, 54, 55t–56t
    in end-stage renal failure with coronary artery disease, 206, 211, 212f
    in left bundle branch block with coronary artery disease, 226, 226t

in myocardial viability assessment, 393t, 393–396, 395f
prognostic value of, 45, 530t
prognostic value of, 45, 529–553, 530t
protocols for perfusion imaging, 42–44, 43f
  rest redistribution, 44, 393t, 393–396, 395f, 464–465, 465t
  stress 4-hour and late redistribution, 42
  stress redistribution, 42, 389–391, 391f, 393t
  stress redistribution-reinjection, 42, 391–393, 392f, 393t, 394f, 465–466, 466t
  stress reinjection, 44
redistribution of, 37–38, 38f, 387, 464
in restenosis detection, 341–342, 342t, 360
ribose with, 387, 396
in SPECT
  adenosine with, prognostic value of, 551f, 552
  compared to dobutamine echocardiography, 481–484, 483f
  compared to planar imaging, 532–534
  in diagnosis and assessment of disease, 615
  dipyridamole with, for restenosis prediction, 376
  in end-stage renal failure with coronary artery disease, 207
  and ischemia with left ventricular hypertrophy, 195
  in left bundle branch block with coronary artery disease, 226t, 226–228, 229, 230t
  left ventricular hypertrophy affecting, 197f, 197–198
  in myocardial viability assessment, 389–396
  prognostic value of, 530t, 551f, 552
  in restenosis prediction, 376
technetium-99m-labeled radiopharmaceuticals with, 45
Thermodilution in coronary flow measurements, 36
Thrombolytic therapy, perfusion imaging after, 551
Tomography
  positron emission. *See* PET
  single photon emission. *See* SPECT
Transplantation
  of heart, and atherosclerosis in recipients, 316f, 317f, 317–318
  of kidneys, in end-stage renal failure with coronary artery disease, 204

Treadmills for exercise testing
  in exercise ECG, 5–6
  in exercise echocardiography, 69, 81
    compared to other techniques, 85t
  in radionuclide angiography, 70

U

U wave in exercise ECG, 15
Ultrasound, intravascular, 267, 269–273, 299–306
  abnormal morphology in, 304–306
  after interventional therapy, 348
  artifacts in, 304, 304f
  calcified atheroma in, 305–306, 306f, 307f
  delivery systems in, 303
  equipment for, 302–303
  extent and location of plaque in, 306, 308f
  normal coronary anatomy in, 303f, 304
  plaque content in, 304–305, 305f
  remodeling detection in, 300, 301f
  tomographic orientation of, 300

V

Vascular disease
  coronary angiography in, 589
  coronary artery disease with, 581, 582f
  and effects of myocardial revascularization, 591–593
  exercise testing in, 589t, 589–590
  Goldman risk assessment in, 588t, 588–589, 589f, 590t
  medical therapy adjustments in, 593
  preoperative interventions in, 591–593
    cost effectiveness of, 593
  preoperative perfusion imaging in, 576, 581–593
    accuracy of, 583–584
    dipyridamole-thallium-201 in, 582, 583t
    exercise tests in, 582
    extent of ischemia affecting, 584–585
    negative findings in, 585
    new stressors in, 587–588
    new tracers in, 586–587, 587f
    prediction of early events in, 585–586
    prediction of late events in, 586, 586f
    relation to clinical status, 584
  preoperative stress echocardiography in, 590–591, 597–609
    comparative utility of pharmacologic agents in, 605–606
    compared to other tests, 606–607
    dipyridamole stress in, 600–601, 601t
    dobutamine stress in, 601t, 601–602, 602f, 603f, 603t, 604t
    guidelines for, 607–608
    and pathophysiology of cardiac morbidity, 597–598
    predictive value of different stressors in, 602–605, 605t, 606f, 606t
    and response of left ventricle to stress, 599
    selection of technique in, 599–600
    and risk of noncardiac surgery, 574, 578t
    clinical indices in, 598
Vasodilator stress testing, 234–236. See also Adenosine stress; Dipyridamole stress
  accuracy of, 247t, 247–249, 248t, 249f
  in echocardiography, 71
    compared to dobutamine stress, 252, 253t
    compared to other echocardiographic techniques, 83–84
    compared to perfusion imaging, 101–104, 103t
  in electrocardiography, 246–247
  hemodynamic responses to, 242–243
  in perfusion imaging, compared to dobutamine stress echocardiography, 104–105
  side effects of, 244–245, 245t
Ventricular function tests. See Left ventricular function evaluation
Ventriculography, radionuclide, 77–79, 79f
  in ischemia detection, 599
  in left bundle branch block with coronary artery disease, 228
  prognostic value of, 517–521
    after infarction, 519–521, 520t
    compared to perfusion imaging, 534–536, 536f
    in coronary artery disease, 518t, 518–519
    in restenosis detection, 342
Viability of myocardium. See Myocardial viability assessment

W

Wall motion studies. See Echocardiography
Water
  labeled with oxygen-15, in myocardial perfusion studies, 423
  perfusable index in myocardial viability assessment, 435–438
Women
  diagnosis of coronary artery disease in, multivariate approaches in, 147–164
  exercise ECG in, 19–21, 132–133, 147–164, 168–169, 177–178
    compared to stress echocardiography, 170–171, 171f
    factors affecting, 20t
    multivariate analysis of, 156t, 156–158, 157t
    prognostic value of, 503f, 505
  heart rate in
    in exercise, 152–153
    relation to ST segment, 149–152
  left ventricular hypertrophy in, 192f, 192t
  perfusion imaging in, 177–187
    accuracy of exercise SPECT in, 179t, 179–180, 180f
    breast attenuation artifacts in, 179
    in diagnosis of coronary artery disease, 179–182
    exercise thallium in, 169
    lung thallium uptake in, 179
    prognostic assessment with, 182–187, 183t–184t, 184f, 185t, 185f–186f
    results with adenosine SPECT thallium, 180–181, 181f
    referral bias considerations, 147, 171–172, 172f
  results of noninvasive testing in, 167
  stress echocardiography in, 167–174
    compared to exercise ECG, 170–171, 171f
Work-related issues in functional tests after interventional therapy, 345